ORTHOPAEDIC PHYSICAL THERAPY

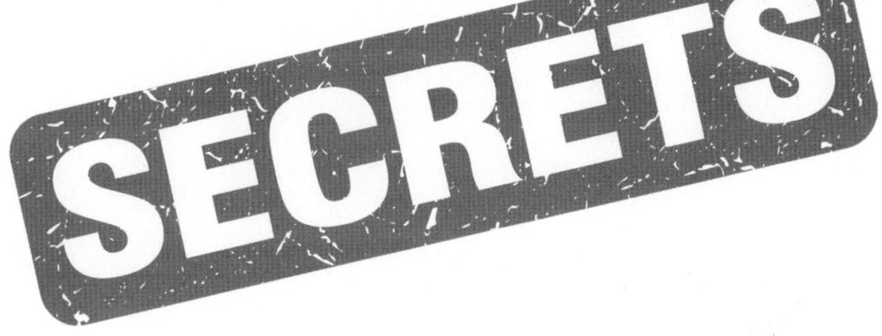

FOURTH EDITION

ORTHOPAEDIC PHYSICAL THERAPY

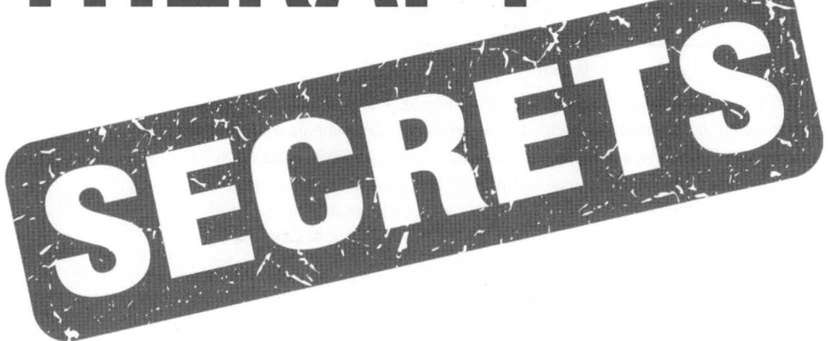

JEFFREY D. PLACZEK, MD, PT
Hand and Upper Extremity Surgeon
Michigan Orthopaedic Surgeons
Medical Director
Bone and Joint Surgery Center of Novi
Ascension Providence Hospital
Novi, Michigan

DAVID A. BOYCE, PT, EDD, OCS, ECS
Clinical Professor
Doctorate of Physical Therapy Program,
Hanover College, CEO/Owner, EMG Stat
Tower, Minnesota

Associate Editors

MARGARET ELAINE LONNEMANN, PT, DPT, OCS, FAAOMPT
Associate Dean, PT Program,
University of St. Augustine for Health Sciences,
St. Augustine, Florida
Program Director, Fellow AAOMPT

PAUL B. LONNEMANN, PT, DPT, OCS, FAAOMPT
Assistant Professor
Physical Therapy, Bellarmine University, Louisville, Kentucky
Physical Therapist
KORT, New Albany, Indiana

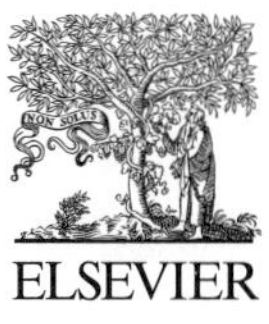
ELSEVIER

Elsevier
3251 Riverport Lane
St. Louis, Missouri 63043

ORTHOPAEDIC PHYSICAL THERAPY SECRETS, FOURTH EDITION ISBN: 978-0-323-84657-8

Senior Content Strategist: Lauren Willis
Senior Content Development Specialist: Shilpa Kumar
Publishing Services Manager: Deepthi Unni
Project Manager: Thoufiq Mohammed
Design Direction: Bridget Hoette

Printed in India

Last digit is the print number: 9 8 7 6 5 4 3 2 1

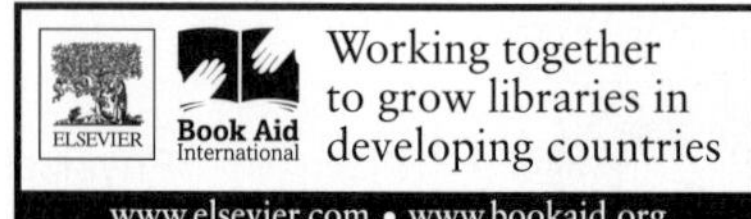

To my father and mother, Edward and Lillian, for their love, support, and discipline. To my wife Laura, my best friend, a true blessing from heaven. To my four angels, Alexis, Baily, Lily, and Addison, my life's true joy and deepest love. To my new little men, Lincoln and Hudson, may they put on the full armor and grow to be great men.

J. Placzek

To my family (Marcia, Elizabeth, Emily, and Cole), colleagues, and patients for constantly challenging me to be my best and press forward. In addition, I dedicate this book to my students, who should read it!

D.A. Boyce

To my family, whose love and unwavering support have been the foundation for my professional journey. To my mentors, patients, and students, your stories, challenges, and triumphs have taught me the true essence of empathy, resilience, and courage.

"The best teacher is not the one who knows most but the one who is most capable of reducing knowledge to that simple compound of the obvious and wonderful." H. L. Mencken

M.E. Lonnemann

To my teachers and students who challenged me to continue to learn. To my parents, who helped me grow to embrace science and wonder. To my wife Elaine for her love, support, and encouragement, and to my boys, Patrick, Peter, Elliott, and Martin, for showing me patience, kindness, and grit.

P.B. Lonnemann

In loving memory of the authors of this text who have passed away since the publication of our first edition.

Jack Echternach (February 23, 1932–July 11, 2013). In memory of Dr. John "Jack" Echternach, Sr, PT, DPT, Ed. D, ECS, FAPTA. A leader, advocate, and mentor who inspired us to love what we do, and do what we love.

Dick Erhard (March 21, 1942–October 4, 2009). A master clinician who mentored numerous physical therapy students and graduate manual therapy residents. A humble and skilled instructor who possessed a wonderful, warm, healing touch and demeanor. Those who were fortunate enough to spend time with him have been blessed and are better people because of it.

Harry Herkowitz (January 13, 1948–June 7, 2013). As the Chairman of Orthopaedic Surgery at William Beaumont Hospital from 1991 to 2013, Dr. Harry Herkowitz was deeply committed to the education of residents and fellows in orthopedics and spine surgery. Dr. Herkowitz provided countless contributions to the realm of orthopedic surgery in research, education, and patient care. He brought out excellence in those around him and expected perfection as a loving father would for his children. He will be remembered warmly by all those he mentored and cared for.

Edward Gerald Tracy (November 2, 1941–March 3, 2004). Professor of Anatomy at the University of Detroit Mercy, Oakland University, Wayne State University, and several hospital appointments teaching residents and interns. Dr. Ed Tracy spent over three decades teaching anatomy to students, inspiring them with his anatomy knowledge and his kind-hearted, calm, and warm personality.

CONTRIBUTORS

H. Agustsson, PhD, DPT
Contributing Faculty
Doctor of Physical Therapy
University of St. Augustine
St. Augustine, Florida

E. Armantrout, PT (retired), DSc
Electrophysiologic Clinical Specialist Emeritus
American Board of Physical Therapy Specialties
Seattle, Washington

N.W. Ayotte, III, PT, MPT, DSc, FAAOMPT
Assistant Professor
School of Movement and Rehabilitation Sciences
Bellarmine University
Louisville, Kentucky

J.A. Bailey, PT, DPT, OCS, CSCS, CPed
President and CEO
Business Center
Rehabilitation Associates of Central Virginia
Lynchburg, Virginia
President
Advisory Board
Lynchburg College Doctor of Physical Therapy Program
Lynchburg, Virginia
Medical Educator
North American Seminars
Franklin, Tennessee

J. Bateman, MD
Oakland Arthritis Center
Bingham Farms, Michigan

C.G. Bise, PT, DPT, PhD, OCS
Assistant Professor
Physical Therapy
University of Pittsburgh
Pittsburgh, Pennsylvania

T.A. 'TAB' Blackburn Jr., MEd, PT (Life)
AT-Retried
AOSSM-Retired

M.L. Bowman, PT, DPT, WCS
Assistant Professor
Physical Therapy
Tennessee State University
Nashville, Tennessee

D.A. Boyce, PT, EdD, OCS, ECS
Clinical Professor
Doctorate of Physical Therapy Program
Hanover College
CEO/Owner
EMG Stat
Tower, Minnesota

D. Boyce, MD, RPh
Physician
Gastroenterology
Charles George VA Medical Center
Ashville, North Carolina

K.A. Brindle, MS, MDs
Associate Professor
Department of Radiology
George Washington University School of Medicine and Health Sciences
Washington, DC

T.J. Brindle, PT, PhD, AT-R
Scientific Program Manager
Office of Research and Development
Department of Veterans Affairs
Washington, DC

M.E. Brooks, DSc, PT, ECS, OCS
Owner and Director
Clinical Electrophysiology
Integrity Diagnostics
Richmond, Kentucky

T.A. Brosky, Jr. PT, DHSc, SCS
Professor
Doctor of Physical Therapy Program
Bellarmine University
Louisville, Kentucky
Dean
School of Movement and Rehabilitation Sciences
Bellarmine University
Louisville, Kentucky

D. Burd, MEd, RD
Instructor in Nursing
Bellarmine University
Louisville, Kentucky

A. Burke-Doe, PT, MPT, PhD
Professor/Program Director
Doctor Physical Therapy
Hawaii Pacific University
Las Vegas, Nevada

J.M. Burnfield, PhD, PT
Director
Institute for Rehabilitation Science and Engineering
Madonna Rehabilitation Hospital
Lincoln, Nebraska

M. Cacko, MPT, OCS
Director
Physical Therapy
Orthopedic Edge Physical Therapy

M. Caid, DO
Adult Reconstructive Surgery
Advanced Orthopaedic Specialists
Brighton, Michigan

C.-n. (Joyce) Chen, PhD
Professor
Department of Physical Therapy and Assistive Technology
National Yang Ming Chiao Tung University
Taipei, Taiwan

C.D. Ciccone, PT, PhD, FAPTA
Professor (Retired)
Physical Therapy
Ithaca College
Ithaca, New York

J. Cronin, OTR/L, CHT
Certified Hand Therapist
Michigan Orthopaedic Surgeons
Novi, Michigan

M.M. Danzl, PT, DPT, PhD, NCS
Chair and Associate Professor
Department of Physical Therapy
Bellarmine University
Louisville, Kentucky

D.J. Denton, PT, DPT, EdD, CIDN, CVT
Director of Clinical Education and Assistant Clinical Professor of Physical Therapy
Doctor of Physical Therapy Program
Hanover College
Hanover, Indiana

L.L. Devaney, PT, ATC, PhD, OCS, FAAOMPT
Associate Professor in Residence
Kinesiology
University of Connecticut
Storrs, Connecticut
Co-Director
UConn Institute for Sports Medicine
Storrs, Connecticut

R.E. DuVall, PT, DHSc, MMSc, OCS, SCS, ATC, FAAOMPT
President
Clinic Operations
Sports Medicine of Atlanta, Inc
Snellville, Georgia
President
NxtGen Institute of Physical Therapy, LLC
Snellville, Georgia
Clinical Director
The Arm Care Academy
Snellville, Georgia

J.L. Echternach, PT, DPT, EDD, ECS, FAPTA
Deceased, Professor
School of Community Health Professions and Physical Therapy
Old Dominion University
Norfolk, Virginia

E. Ennis, PT, EDD, PCS
Senior Program Director
Doctor of Physical Therapy
University of St. Augustine for Health Sciences
St. Augustine, Florida
Co-Owner
All About Families, PLLC
Louisville, Kentucky

R.E. Erhard, PT, DC
Deceased, Assistant Professor
Department of Physical Therapy
University of Pittsburgh
Pittsburgh, Pennsylvania

S.P. Flanagan, PhD, ATC, CSCS
Professor
Department of Kinesiology
California State University
Northridge, California

T.W. Flynn, PT, PhD, OCS, FAAOMPT, FAPTA
Professor
School of Physical Therapy
South College
Knoxville, Tennessee
Owner
Colorado in Motion
Fort Collins, Colorado
Principal
Evidence in Motion
Louisville, Kentucky

J.M. Fritz, PHD, PT, ATC
Distinguished Professor
School of Health, Department of Physical Therapy & Athletic Training
University of Utah
Salt Lake City, Utah

Job A. Gallaher
Nursing Student
University of Michigan
Flint, Michigan

K. Galloway, PT, DSc, ECS
Professor
Physical Therapy
Belmont University
Nashville, Tennessee

G. Gennaoui, DO
Rheumatologist
Rheumatology
The Toledo Clinic
Toledo, Ohio

T. Gibbons, MPT
Physical Therapist
Rehabilitation Services
Henry Ford Health System
Bloomfield Twp, Michigan

J. Girard, DPT, DSc, OCS, FAAOMPT
Clinical Associate Professor
Physical Therapy
Hanover College
Hanover, Indiana

A. Grant, PT, DPT, MTC, CLT
Director, Residency and Fellowship Programs
College of Rehabilitative Sciences
University of St. Augustine for Health Sciences
St. Augustine, Florida

D.G. Greathouse, PT, PhD, ECS, FAPTA
Director
Clinical Electrophysiology Services
Texas Physical Therapy Specialists
Live Oak, Texas
Professor
U.S. Army-Baylor Univ Doctoral Program in Physical Therapy
AMEDD Center of Excellence
Fort Sam Houston, Texas

E.T. Greenberg, PT, DPT, SCS
Associate Professor
Department of Physical Therapy
New York Institute of Technology
Old Westbury, New York

D. Gustitus, OTR/L, CHT
Certified Hand Therapist
Michigan Orthopaedic Surgeons
Novi, Michigan

R.C. Hall, DPT, ATC
Lt Colonel (Ret)
Biomedical Sciences Corps
USAF
Tyler, Texas

J.S. Halle, PT, PhD, ECS (Emeritus)
Emeritus Professor
School of Physical Therapy
Belmont University
Nashville, Tennessee
Adjunct Professor
Medical Education and Administration
Vanderbilt University
Nashville, Tennessee

J. Hanks, PT, PhD, DPT, CLT, Certified DN
Associate Professor
Department of Physical Therapy
University of Tennessee at Chattanooga
Chattanooga, Tennessee

H.N. Herkowitz, MD
Deceased, Chairman
Department of Orthopaedic Surgery
William Beaumont Hospital
Royal Oak, Michigan

S. Ho, PT, DPT, MS, OCS
Adjunct Associate Professor
Biokinesiology and Physical Therapy
University of Southern California
Los Angeles, California
Owner/Director
Ho Physical Therapy
Beverly Hills, California

R.T. Hockenbury, MD
Assistant Clinical Professor
Orthopedic Surgery
University of Louisville
Louisville, Kentucky

J.A. Hyland, PA-C
Physician Assistant
Michigan Orthopaedic Surgeons
Novi, Michigan

D.E. Jacks, PhD
Professor
Physical Therapy
Hanover College
Hanover, Indiana

J.D. Keener, MD, PT
Professor and Chief
Orthopaedic Surgery, Shoulder and Elbow Division
Washington University
St. Louis, Missouri

P.M. King, PT, PhD, FAAOMPT
Professor and Chair
Department of Physical Therapy
Tennessee State University
Nashville, Tennessee
Physical Therapist
Knoxville Physical Therapy
Knoxville, Tennessee

J.R. Krauss, PhD, PT, OCS, FAAOMPT
Professor
School of Health Sciences
Oakland University
Rochester, Michigan
Clinical Director
OMPT Specialists
Auburn Hills, Michigan

K. Kulig, PhD, PT
Professor
Biokinesiology and Physical Therapy
University of Southern California
Los Angeles, California

B.J. Lee, PT, DPT, LAT, FAAOMPT, SCS, OCS, CSCS, USAW
Physical Therapy Clinical Specialist
Texas Health Sports Medicine & Texas Christian University
Texas Health Resources
Fort Worth, Texas
Co-Owner and Educator
Evolution Ed Presented by Clinic to Field Physical Therapy, LLC
Contract Physical Therapist
Texas Christian University
Fort Worth, Texas

M.E. Lonnemann, PT, DPT OCS, FAAOMPT
Associate Dean, PT Program,
University of St. Augustine for Health Sciences
St. Augustine
Florida
Program Director
Fellow AAOMPT

P.B. Lonnemann, PT, DPT, OCS, FAAOMPT
Assistant Professor
Physical Therapy
Bellarmine University
Louisville, Kentucky
Physical Therapist
KORT
New Albany, Indiana

P.D. Loprinzi, PhD
Assistant Professor
Department of Health, Exercise Science and Recreation Management
University of Mississippi
University, Mississippi

J. Magel, PT, PhD, DSc
Research Associate Professor
Department of Physical Therapy and Athletic Training
University of Utah
Salt Lake City, Utah

N. Maiers, PT
Assistant Professor
Physical Therapy
Des Moines University
Des Moines, Iowa

S. Mais, BS, BA, MS, DPT
Associate Professor
Physical Therapy
Chapman University
Irvine, California
Physical Therapist
PT@theBeach
California State University
Long Beach, California

T.R. Malone, EdD, MS, BS
Professor
Physical Therapy
University of Kentucky
Lexington, Kentucky

T.J. Manal, PT, DPT,OCS, SCS, FAPTA
Senior Vice President
Scientific Affairs
American Physical Therapy Association
Alexandria, Virginia
Affiliate Associate Professor
Physical Therapy
University of Delaware
Newark, Delaware

S. Maskalick
Trainer
Bellarmine University
Louisville, Kentucky

K.R. Maywhort, PT, DPT
Certification Program Director and Lead Instructor
Division of Functional Dry Needling
Evidence in Motion
San Antonio, Texas
Faculty Experience Team
Department of Post Professional Education
Evidence in Motion
San Antonio, Texas
Affiliate Faculty
Department of Physical Therapy
Regis University
Denver, Colorado

R.J. McKibben, PT, DSc, ECS
Integrity Rehab Management, LLC
Integrity Diagnostics
Jackson, Georgia

N. Nevin, PT, DPT, OCS, MTC, FAAOMPT
Assistant Professor
Doctor of Physical Therapy
Bellarmine University
Louisville, Kentucky
Physical Therapist
MVMT Institute
Floyds Knobs, Indiana

A.J. Nitz, PT, PhD
Emeritus Professor
Department of Physical Therapy, College of Health Sciences,
University of Kentucky
Lexington, Kentucky

O. Oshikoya, MD, PharmD
Orthopaedic Surgeon
Orthopaedics
Rothman Orthopaedics of Florida
Orlando, Florida
Fellow
Orthopaedics
William Beaumont Hospital
Royal Oak, Michigan

J.P. Owens, BAppSci (Sport Science)
Lecturer
School of Physiotherapy & Exercise Science
Curtin University, Perth
Western Australia

J.G. Owens, MPT
CEO
Clinical Education and Research
Owens Recovery Science, Inc.
San Antonio, Texas

J.J. Palazzo, PT, DSc, ECS
EDX Consultant
Private Practice
NeuroLAB
Novi, Michigan

S. Paris, PhD, PT, FAPTA, Hon LLD (Otago)
President
University of St. Augustine
St. Augustine, Florida

S.D. Patterson, PhD
Doctor
School of Sport, Health & Applied Science
St Mary's University
Twickenham, United Kingdom

L.R. Perazza, PhD
Postdoctoral Fellow
Department of Physical Therapy & Athletic Training
Boston University
Boston, Massachusetts

A.L. Pfeifle, EdD, PT
Professor
Family and Community Medicine
The Ohio State University
Columbus, Ohio
Associate Vice President for Interprofessional Practice and Education
The Ohio State University
Columbus, Ohio

S.R. Piva, PT, PhD, FAPTA
Professor
Physical Therapy
University of Pittsburgh
Pittsburgh, Pennsylvania
Vice Chair for Research
Physical Therapy
University of Pittsburgh
Pittsburgh, Pennsylvania

A. Placzek
Student
Brighton High School
Brighton, Michigan

J. Placzek, MD, PT
Hand and Upper Extremity Surgeon
Michigan Orthopaedic Surgeons
Medical Director
Bone and Joint Surgery Center of Novi
Ascension Providence Hospital
Novi, Michigan

L. Placzek
Nursing Student
University of Michigan
Flint, Michigan

F.D. Pociask, PT, PhD, OCS, FAAOMPT
Associate Professor
Physical Therapy Program
Wayne State University
Detroit, Michigan

C.M. Powers, PT, PhD
Professor
Biokinesiology & Physical Therapy
University of Southern California
Marina del Rey, California

M. Quinn, MD
Medical Director
Orthopaedics
Bloomfield Hand Specialists, P.C./Orthopaedic Surgical Institute
Rochester Hills, Michigan

D. Rico, PT, DPT
Associate Professor
Physical Therapy
Rockhurst University
Kansas City, Missouri

B. Ring, RN
Department of Nursing
University of Michigan
Ann Arbor, Michigan

M.W. Reynolds, PT, DPT, EdD
Associate Professor
Physical Therapy
University of St. Augustine for Health Sciences
St. Augustine, Florida

T.K. Robinson, PT, DSc, OCS
Professor
School of Physical Therapy
Belmont University
Nashville, Tennessee

M.G. Roman, PT, MHA, MMCi
Chief Digital Strategy Officer
Duke Health Technology Solutions
Duke University Health System
Durham, North Carolina

P.J. Roubal, PhD, DPT, OCS
President
Physiomefit
Stuart, Florida

H.D. Saunders
Chief Executive Officer
The Saunders Group, Inc.
Chaska, Michigan

M. Schmidt, PT, DPT, MHA
Director of Rehabilitation Services
Rehabilitation Services
Duke Health
Durham, North Carolina

E. Schrank, DSc, MPT
Electromyographer
Electrophysiology
EMG Testing Services
Parker, Colorado

R.A. Sellin, PT, DSc, ECS
President
EMG/NCV Department
Electrophysiologic Testing, PLC
Lexington, Kentucky

W.G. Seymour, PT, DPT, OCS, FAAOMPT
University of Delaware Physical Therapy
Physical Therapy
University of Delaware
Newark, Delaware

R. Shah, MD
Orthopedic Surgeon
Orthopedic Surgery
University of Texas
Austin, Texas

K. Shaughnessy, PT, DPT, OCS, CSCS
Head Physical Therapist
San Diego Wave
University of Texas
San Diego, California

E. Sigman, PT, DPT, OCS
Assistant Professor of Clinical Physical Therapy
Biokinesiology and Physical Therapy
University of Southern California
Los Angeles, California

M. Skurja, Jr. DPT, ECS (Emeritus)
Chair
Board of Trustees
Rocky Mountain University of Health Professions
Provo, Utah

C.B. Smith, DPT, OMPT
Lecturer
Department of Physical Therapy
Oakland University
Rochester, Michigan

L.A.M. Snow, MD, PhD
Assistant Professor
Department of Rehabilitation Medicine, Division of Physical Therapy
University of Minnesota
Minneapolis, Minnesota

B.A. Stamford, PhD
Professor and Chair
Kinesiology & Integrative Physiology
Hanover College
Hanover, Indiana

B.T. Swanson, PT, DSc, OCS, FAAOMPT
Associate Professor
Department of Rehabilitation Sciences
University of Hartford
West Hartford, Connecticut

C.A. Thigpen, PhD, PT, ATC
Vice President of Care Delivery
Commercial Services
ATI Physical Therapy
Greenville, South Carolina
Adjunct Professor
Physical Therapy
Duke University
Durham, North Carolina

L.D.V. Thompson, PT, PhD
Professor
Department of Physical Therapy
Boston University
Boston, Massachusetts

M.T. Bee, PhD
Professor
Department of Biology
University of Detroit Mercy
Detroit, Michigan

E. Truumees, MD
Professor
Orthopaedic Surgery and Neurosurgery
University of Texas, Dell Medical School
Austin, Texas
Attending Spine Surgeon
Ascension Texas Spine Program
Seton Medical Center
Austin, Texas

J. Tuori, PT, DPT
Physical Therapist
Fitness Science
University of Rochester Medical Center
Rochester, New York

E. Ulanowski, DPT
Associate Professor
Doctor of Physical Therapy Program
Bellarmine University
Louisville, Kentucky

F.B. Underwood, PT, PhD, ECS
Professor Emeritus
Physical Therapy
University of Evansville
Evansville, Indiana

B. Vibert, MD
Spine Surgeon
Orthopaedic Surgery
William Beaumont-Troy
Troy, Michigan

J.A. Viti, PT, MSc, DPT, OCS, FAAOMPT
Assistant Professor
Doctor of Physical Therapy Department
University of St. Augustine for Health Sciences
Ponte Vedra Beach, Florida
Vice President/Partner/PT
First Coast Rehabilitation
St. Augustine, Florida

M.L. Voight, PT, DHSc, OCS, SCS, ATC, FAPTA
Professor
School of Physical Therapy
Belmont University
Nashville, Tennessee
Director of Sports Medicine
Nashville Hip Institute
Nashville, Tennessee

J.M. Whitman, PT, DScPT, OCS, FAAOMPT
Physical Therapy Specialist
Rocklin, California

J.M. Wiater, MD
Chief of Shoulder Surgery
Orthopaedic Surgery
Corewell Health William Beaumont University Hospital
Royal Oak, Michigan
Program Director, Shoulder and Elbow Fellowship
Orthopaedic Surgery
Corewell Health William Beaumont University Hospital
Royal Oak, Michigan
Professor
Orthopaedic Surgery
Oakland University William Beaumont School of Medicine
Rochester, Michigan

M.R. Wiegand, PT, PhD
Interim Vice President for Academic Affairs and Provost
Academic Affairs
Bellarmine University
Louisville, Kentucky
Professor
Physical Therapy Program
Bellarmine University
Louisville, Kentucky

S.K. Young, MD
Anesthesiology & Pain Medicine
Commonwealth Pain and Spine
Louisville, Kentucky

E.D. Zylstra, PT, DPT
Partner
Education
Evidence in Motion
Hudsonville, Michigan

PREFACE

We are pleased to announce the fourth edition of *Orthopaedic Physical Therapy Secrets*. The popularity of this text as a study guide for the orthopedic and sports certification specialty examinations as well as a home and office reference guide has led us into a new updated edition. This year, the electronic edition will be offered in conjunction with the paperback copy. This will allow access via a smart device or simple "old-fashioned" access via your lab coat pocket.

New chapters on the neuroscience of pain, diagnostic ultrasound, cervical spine pathology and treatment, blood flow restriction, and running have been added. Significant updates have been made to the remaining chapters in order to reflect contemporary practice standards, and over 200 new sample test questions similar to those encountered on the specialty exams have been added.

The success of *Orthopaedic Physical Therapy Secrets* is due to the contributions of its authors, who contributed their time and expertise to make this text a popular and sought-after study and reference guide.

J. Placzek, MD, PT
D.A. Boyce, PT, EdD, OCS, ECS

CONTENTS

I Basic Science

II Disease Processes

III Electrotherapy and Modalities

IV Special Topics

V THE SHOULDER

VI THE ELBOW AND FOREARM

VII THE WRIST AND HAND

VIII The Spine

IX The Sacroiliac Joint

X The Hip and Pelvis

XI The Knee

XII The Foot and Ankle

SKELETAL MUSCLE

C.-n. (Joyce) Chen, PhD, L.D.V. Thompson, PT, PhD, L.R. Perazza, PhD, and L.A.M. Snow, MD, PhD

MUSCLE FUNCTION

1. **What are the functions of muscle?**
   - Movement
   - Support and protection
   - Heat generation
   - Energy storage

MUSCLE STRUCTURE

2. **What is the organizational hierarchy of skeletal muscle, and how is it achieved?**
   The hierarchy:
   - Muscle fascicles
   - Muscle fibers or cells
   - Myofibrils (arranged in parallel)
   - Sarcomeres (arranged in series)

   Achieved as follows: The connective tissue that surrounds an entire muscle is called the epimysium; the membrane that binds fibers into fascicles is called the perimysium. Two separate membranes surround individual muscle fibers. The outer membrane of fibers has three names that are interchangeable: basement membrane, endomysium, or basal lamina. An additional thin elastic membrane is found just beneath the basement membrane and is termed the plasma membrane or sarcolemma.

3. **What is the range of muscle fiber lengths?**
   Muscle fiber lengths range from a few millimeters in the intraocular muscles of the eye to greater than 45 cm in the sartorius muscle.

4. **Describe the characteristics of individual muscle fibers.**
   The cross-sectional area of an individual muscle fiber ranges from approximately 2000 to 7500 μm^2, with the mean in the 3000 to 4000 μm^2 range. Whole muscle and muscle fiber lengths vary considerably. For example, the length of the medial gastrocnemius muscle is approximately 25 cm, with fiber lengths of 35 mm, whereas the sartorius muscle length is approximately 50 cm, with fiber lengths of 450 mm. The number of fibers ranges from several hundred in small muscles to more than 1 million in large muscles, such as those involved in hip flexion and knee extension.

5. **What are the characteristics of myofibrils?**
   Individual myofibrils are approximately 1 μm in diameter and comprise approximately 80% of the volume of a whole muscle. The variable number of myofibrils is regulated during the growth-related hypertrophy of muscle fibers. For example, the number of myofibrils ranges from 50 per muscle fiber in the muscles of a fetus to approximately 2000 per fiber in the muscles of an untrained adult. The hypertrophy and atrophy of adult skeletal muscle are associated with resistance training and disuse, respectively, and result from the regulation of the number of myofibrils per fiber. Hypertrophy is associated with an increase in the number of myofibrils, and atrophy is associated with myofibril loss.

6. **Describe the characteristics of the sarcomere (Figure 1-1).**
   - The sarcomere is composed of thick filaments and thin filaments. The thick filaments are composed mainly of myosin. The thin filaments are composed mainly of actin.
   - In the middle of the sarcomere, the areas that appear dark are termed anisotropic. This portion of the sarcomere is known as the A band.
   - Areas at the outer ends of each sarcomere appear light and are known as I bands because they are isotropic with respect to their birefringent properties.
   - The H zone is in the central region of the A band, where there is no overlap of thick filaments and thin filaments.
   - The H zone is bisected by the M line, which consists of proteins that keep the sarcomere in proper spatial orientation as it lengthens and shortens.

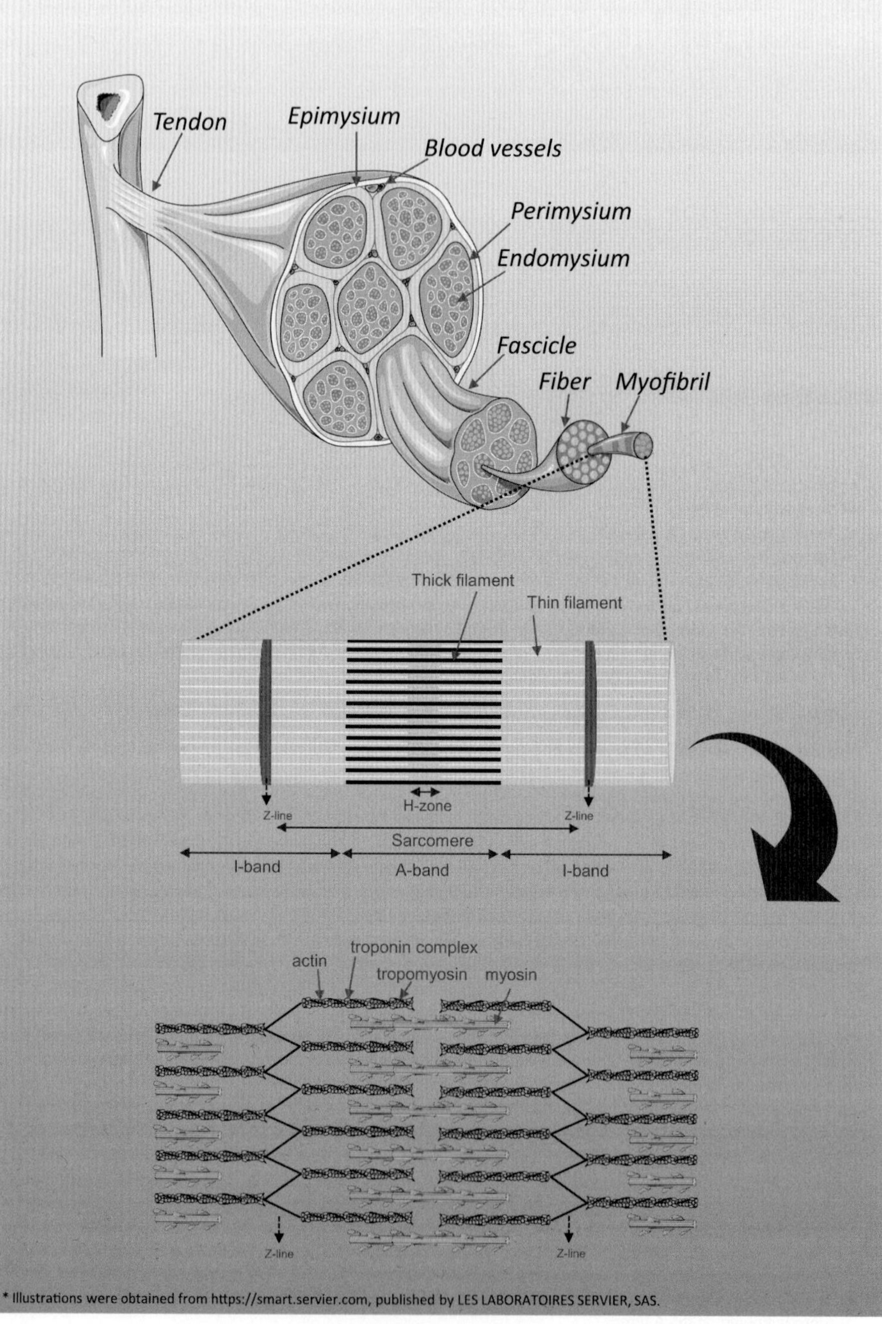
Tendon
Epimysium
Blood vessels
Perimysium
Endomysium
Fascicle
Fiber
Myofibril
Thick filament
Thin filament
H-zone
Z-line
Z-line
Sarcomere
I-band
A-band
I-band
troponin complex
actin
tropomyosin
myosin
Z-line
Z-line
* Illustrations were obtained from https://smart.servier.com, published by LES LABORATOIRES SERVIER, SAS.

Figure 1-1

- At the ends of each sarcomere are the Z discs. The sarcomere length is the distance from one Z disc to the next.

  Optimal sarcomere length in mammalian muscle is 2.4 to 2.5 μm. The length of a sarcomere relative to its optimal length is of fundamental importance to the capacity for force generation.

7. **Identify key proteins within the sarcomere.**
   - The most prominent proteins making up the sarcomere are myosin, actin, tropomyosin, and the troponin complex.
   - The C protein—part of the thick filament is involved in holding the tails of myosin in their correct spatial arrangement.
   - The M line protein—also known as myomesin functions to keep the thick and thin filaments in their correct spatial arrangement.
   - Titin links the end of the thick filament to the Z disc. α-Actinin attaches actin filaments together at the Z disc and desmin links Z discs of adjacent myofibrils together.
   - Spectrin and dystrophin have structural and perhaps functional roles as sarcolemma membrane proteins.

8. **Describe the characteristics of myosin.**
   - Myosin is of key importance for the development of muscular force and velocity of contraction.
   - A myosin molecule is a relatively large protein (approximately 470–500 kD) composed of two identical myosin heavy chains (MHCs) (approximately 200 kD each) and four myosin light chains (MLCs) (16–20 kD each).
   - Light-meromyosin (LMM) is the tail or backbone portion of the myosin molecule, which intertwines with the tails of other myosin molecules to form a thick filament. Heavy-meromyosin (HMM) consists of two subfragments: S-1 and S-2. The S-2 portion of HMM projects out at an angle from LMM, and the S-1 portion is the globular head that can bind to actin. S-1 and S-2 together are also termed a myosin cross-bridge. There are approximately 300 molecules of myosin in one myofilament or thick filament. Approximately one half of the MHCs combine with their HMM at one end of the thick filament; the other half have their HMM toward the opposite end of the thick filament—a tail-to-tail arrangement. When molecules combine, they are rotated 60 degrees relative to the adjacent molecules and are offset slightly in the longitudinal plane. As a consequence of these three-dimensional structural factors, myosin has a characteristic bottlebrush appearance, with HMM projecting out along most of the filament.
   - The MHCs and MLCs are found in slightly different forms called isoforms. The isoforms have small differences in some aspects of their structure that markedly influence the velocity of muscle contraction.

9. **What are the characteristics of actin?**

   Actin consists of approximately 350 monomers and 50 molecules of each of the regulatory proteins—tropomyosin and troponin. The actin monomers are termed G-actin because they are globular and have molecular weights of approximately 42 kD. G-actin normally is polymerized to F-actin (ie, filamentous actin), which is arranged in a double helix. The polymerization from G-actin to F-actin involves the hydrolysis of ATP and the binding of adenosine diphosphate (ADP) to actin; 90% of ADP in skeletal muscle is bound to actin. The actin protein has a binding site that, when exposed, attaches to the myosin cross-bridge. The subsequent cycling of cross-bridges causes the development of muscular force. The actin filaments also join together to form the boundary between two sarcomeres in the area of the A band. α-Actinin is the protein that holds the actin filaments in the appropriate three-dimensional array.

10. **What are the characteristics of the different skeletal muscle fiber types?**

    Fiber type characteristics are detailed in the table.

11. **What is type IIb myosin heavy chain?**

    Myosin heavy chain type IIb is found in animals but not in humans. It has greater maximal shortening velocity and maximal isometric tension than myosin heavy chain type IIx, which is found in both humans and animals.

MUSCLE PHYSIOLOGY

12. **Define a motor unit and the all-or-none principle of muscle contraction.**

    A motor unit is defined as a single motor neuron and all the muscle fibers innervated by that neuron. The all-or-none principle of muscle contraction means that when a motor neuron is activated, all the muscle fibers innervated by that motor neuron contract maximally.

13. **What is the process of motor unit recruitment?**

    When skeletal muscles contract voluntarily against a load, motor units are recruited from lowest threshold to highest threshold.

Table 1.1 Muscle fiber types and motor unit types in humans

PROPERTY	CHARACTERISTICS: TYPE I (S, SO)	CHARACTERISTICS: TYPE IIA (FFR, FOG)	CHARACTERISTICS: TYPE IIX (FF, FG)
Anatomy			
Myosin heavy chain isoform	Type I	Type IIa	Type IIx
Fiber diameter	Small	Intermediate	Large
Z line thickness	Wide	Wide	Narrow
Color	Red	Red	White
Myoglobin	High	High	Low
Capillary supply	Rich	Rich	Poor
Mitochondria	Many	Intermediate	Few
Glycogen content	Low	Intermediate	High
Physiology			
Respiratory type	Aerobic	Aerobic and anaerobic	Anaerobic
Oxidative capacity	High	Intermediate	Low
Glycolytic ability	Low	Intermediate	High
Contraction speed	Slow	Fast	Fast
Force production	Small	Intermediate	Large
Fatigue resistance	High	Intermediate	Low

FF, Fast fatigable; *FFR*, fast fatigue resistant; *FG*, fast glycolytic; *FOG*, fast oxidative glycolytic; *S*, slow; *SO*, slow oxidative.

14. Define excitation-contraction coupling.

Excitation-contraction coupling is the physiologic mechanism whereby an electric discharge at the muscle initiates the chemical events that lead to contraction.

15. Summarize how excitation-contraction coupling occurs in skeletal muscle (Figure 1-2).

1. Action potentials in the alpha motor neuron propagate down the axon to the axon terminals.
2. Acetylcholine, the neurotransmitter at the neuromuscular junction, is released from the axon terminals.
3. Acetylcholine diffuses across the neuromuscular junction and binds with acetylcholine receptors on the sarcolemma of the muscle.
4. A muscle action potential is generated at the motor end plate.
5. The muscle action potential travels along the sarcolemma and into the depths of the transverse tubules, which are continuous with the sarcolemma.
6. The action potential (voltage change) is sensed by the dihydropyridine receptors in the transverse tubules.
7. The dihydropyridine receptors communicate with the ryanodine receptors of the sarcoplasmic reticulum.
8. Calcium is released from the sarcoplasmic reticulum through the ryanodine receptors.
9. Calcium binds to the regulatory protein, troponin C, and the interaction between actin and myosin can occur.
10. Myosin cross-bridges, previously activated by the hydrolysis of ATP, attach to actin.
11. The myosin cross-bridges move into a strong binding state, and force production occurs.

16. Explain the sliding filament theory of muscle contraction.

A muscle shortens or lengthens because the myosin and actin myofilaments slide past each other without the filaments themselves changing length. The myosin cross-bridge projects out from the myosin tail and attaches to an

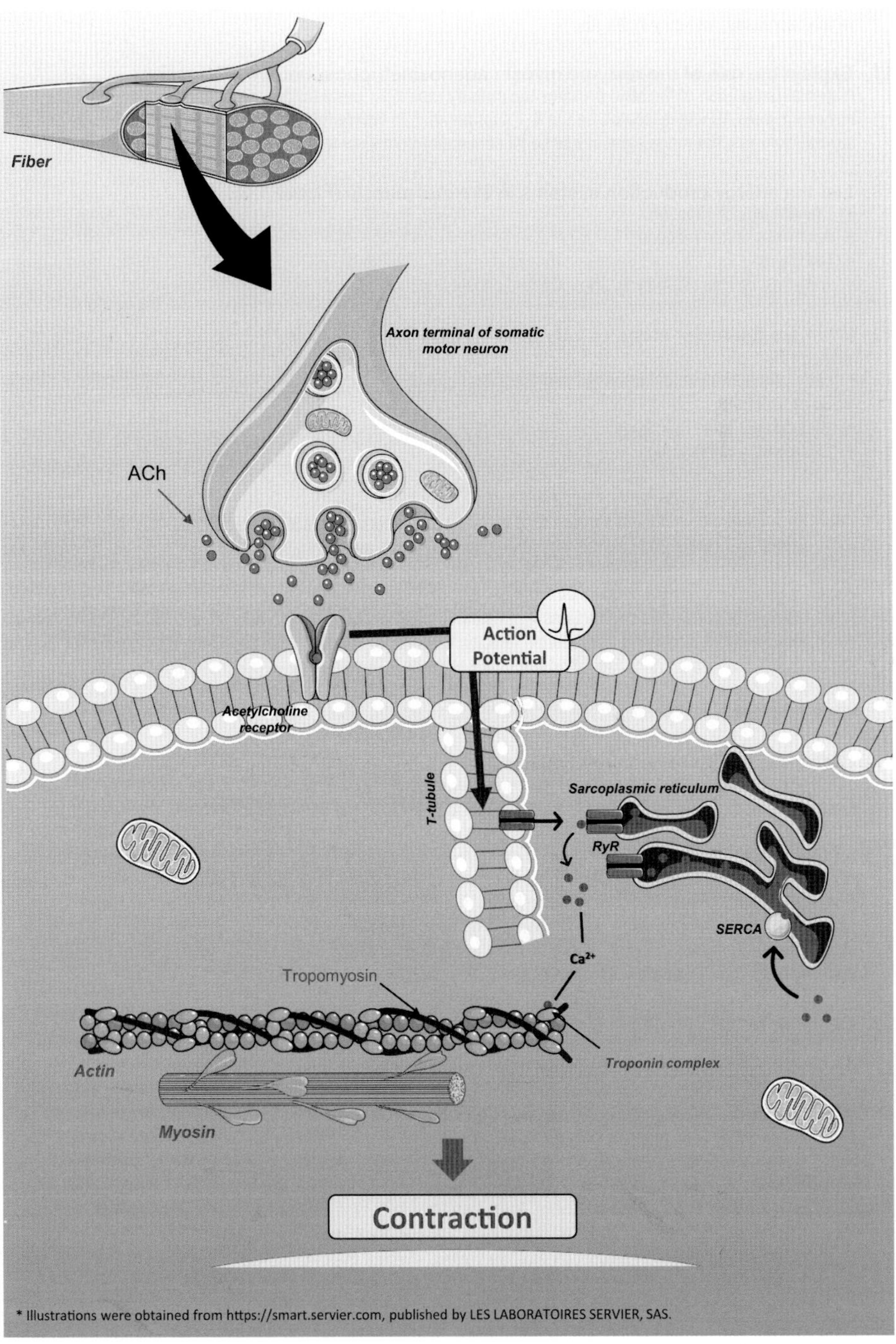
Fiber
Axon terminal of somatic motor neuron
ACh
Action Potential
Acetylcholine receptor
T-tubule
Sarcoplasmic reticulum
RyR
SERCA
Ca2+
Tropomyosin
Troponin complex
Actin
Myosin
Contraction
* Illustrations were obtained from https://smart.servier.com, published by LES LABORATOIRES SERVIER, SAS.

Figure 1-2

actin monomer in the thin filament. The cross-bridges then force the thin filaments to move toward the M line and the sarcomere shortens. The major structural rearrangement during contraction occurs in the region of the I band, which decreases markedly in length.

17. Explain the role of the enzyme myosin adenosinetriphosphatase (ATPase).

A specialized portion of the MHC provides the primary molecular basis for the speed of muscular contraction. The enzyme myosin ATPase is located on the S-1 subfragment. In different fibers, the myosin ATPase can be one of several isoforms that range along a functional continuum from slow to fast.

18. List the energy production systems in skeletal muscle (Figure 1-3).

- Creatine kinase reaction
- Adenylate kinase reaction
- Glycolysis
- Tricarboxylic acid (TCA) cycle and oxidative phosphorylation

19. What are the major steps of fatty acid metabolism in muscle that result in the release of energy?

- Fatty acid activation and transport into the mitochondria
- Beta-oxidation
- Tricarboxylic acid (TCA) cycle
- Oxidative phosphorylation

20. Define the force-velocity relationship.

The muscle contracts at different velocities depending on the force it needs to exert. As the load increases, the force exerted in a concentric (shortening) contraction increases and contraction velocity decreases. When the load exceeds the maximal force capable of being developed in concentric (shortening) or isometric contraction, an eccentric (lengthening) contraction ensues.

The velocity of concentric contractions is considered positive, whereas the velocity of eccentric contractions is considered negative. According to the force-velocity relationship, the force developed during a concentric/shortening contraction is less than the isometric force. The force developed during an eccentric/lengthening contraction exceeds the isometric force by 50% to 100%. An application of the force-velocity relationship is observed in resistance training with heavier weights used during eccentric contractions.

21. Define the length-tension relationship.

The length-tension relationship describes characteristics of sarcomere contraction in maximally stimulated isometric conditions. A contracting sarcomere exerts differing tensions depending on its length prior to contraction. Maximal tension is created at resting length, which corresponds to a sarcomere length of ~2.2 microns. At this length, there is maximal overlap between actin and myosin filaments, so that maximal number of cross-bridges can be formed during contraction. As the length of the sarcomere increases or decreases from resting length, contraction force decreases due to less optimal configurations for actin-myosin cross-bridge formation. Whole muscle application of the length-tension relationship is complex due to effects of stretch-related passive tensions, complex muscle architecture, and submaximal dynamic contractions, as opposed to maximal isometric contractions.

22. Describe factors influencing muscle strength at the muscle fiber level.

The myosin structural state, the ratio of strong binding and weak binding cross-bridges to actin, muscle innervation, motor unit recruitment, and synchronization are all factors influencing muscle strength.

23. What is active insufficiency at the muscle level?

Active insufficiency is a condition that arises when a dual-joint muscle contracts concentrically and shortens while concurrently moving both joints. In such a condition, the muscle is not able to generate great enough tension, nor to shorten enough to achieve full range of motion in both joints simultaneously.

24. Describe the anatomy of muscle spindles, and define their function.

Muscle spindles are stretch receptors located throughout skeletal muscle. They are comprised of three intrafusal fibers, located within the fusiform connective tissue capsule. These fibers are: two nuclear bag fibers and one nuclear chain fiber. Spindles are innervated by two types of sensory afferent neurons (Ia and II) and one gamma motor neuron. The spindles detect changes in muscle length and the rate of the length changes. This sensory information is then transmitted to higher centers in the brain, from which efferent signals are transmitted to the gamma motor neurons in the spinal cord. The gamma motor neuron controls contraction/relaxation of the spindle so that it continually adjusts to the length changes in the muscle. Muscle spindles are primary sensory receptors for proprioception.

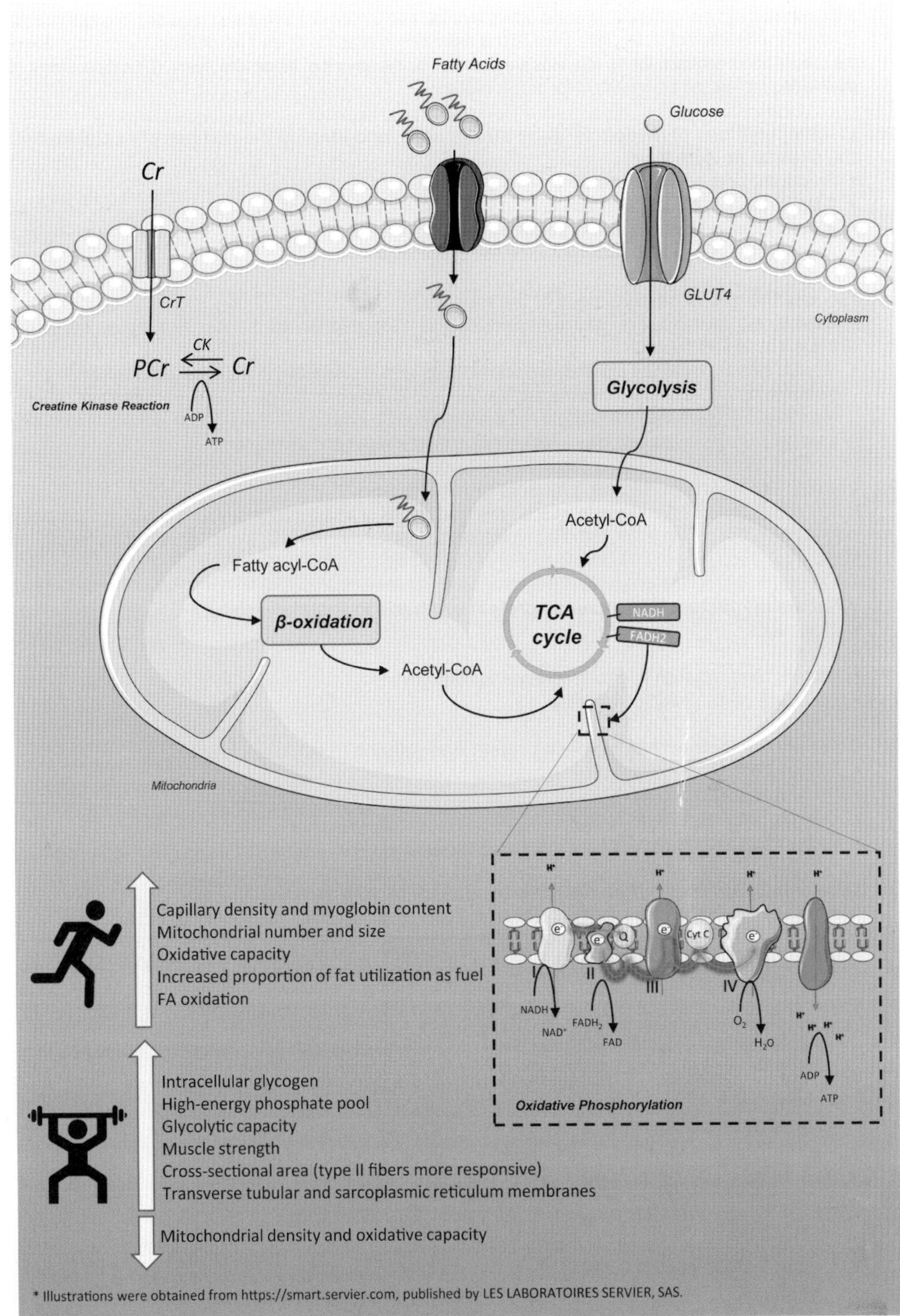
Fatty Acids
Glucose
Cr
CrT
GLUT4
Cytoplasm
CK
PCr
Cr
Creatine Kinase Reaction
ADP
ATP
Glycolysis
Acetyl-CoA
Fatty acyl-CoA
β-oxidation
TCA cycle
NADH
FADH2
Acetyl-CoA
Mitochondria
Capillary density and myoglobin content
Mitochondrial number and size
Oxidative capacity
Increased proportion of fat utilization as fuel
FA oxidation
Intracellular glycogen
High-energy phosphate pool
Glycolytic capacity
Muscle strength
Cross-sectional area (type II fibers more responsive)
Transverse tubular and sarcoplasmic reticulum membranes
Mitochondrial density and oxidative capacity
Cyt C
NADH
NAD+
FADH2
FAD
O2
H2O
ADP
ATP
Oxidative Phosphorylation
* Illustrations were obtained from https://smart.servier.com, published by LES LABORATOIRES SERVIER, SAS.

Figure 1-3

25. **Describe the anatomy of Golgi tendon organs, and define their function.**
Golgi tendon organs (GTO) are stretch receptors located in the tendons near musculotendinous junctions. They are innervated by type Ib afferent neurons, which terminate on tendon fibers that are connected to single muscle fibers of several different motor units. Each GTO is estimated to attach to at least ten different motor units. When the muscle fibers contract, the 1b afferents are activated by the stretch of the tendon fibers. GTOs detect force of muscle contraction and are important for proprioception.

26. **List the functions of myonuclei and satellite cells, and identify the number of nuclei found in the skeletal muscle fiber.**
    - Growth and development of muscle
    - Adaptive capacity of skeletal muscle to various forms of training or disuse
    - Recovery from exercise-induced or traumatic injury
    - Approximately 200 to 3000 nuclei per millimeter of fiber length

27. **Discuss the role of satellite cells in the muscle.**
    - Satellite cells are muscle fiber stem cells. Satellite cells are located beneath the fiber basal lamina, but outside of the muscle fiber membrane.
    - Satellite cells are quiescent until they are activated (eg, start to proliferate) in response to physiological stimuli or muscle trauma. Proliferating satellite cells and their progeny are called myogenic precursor cells or myoblasts. Myoblasts then differentiate and eventually fuse to existing myofibers or fuse together to form new myofibers. Thus, satellite cells play a central role in muscle repair and development.

28. **Identify and define or describe muscle growth factors.**
Muscle growth factors either promote muscle growth and repair or inhibit muscle protein breakdown. Examples include insulin-like growth factor, fibroblast growth factor, hepatocyte growth factor, and transforming growth factor.

29. **What are the factors that increase protein synthesis in skeletal muscle?**
    - Amino acids
    - Insulin
    - Anabolic hormones such as growth hormone and testosterone
    - Resistance training/muscle contraction

30. **What are the factors that increase protein degradation in skeletal muscle?**
    - Inflammation
    - Oxidative stress
    - Catabolic hormones such as cortisol
    - Energy stress such as starvation

31. **Differentiate apoptosis from necrosis as applied to skeletal muscle.**
Apoptosis, or programmed cell death, is a regulated physiologic process critical to cellular homeostasis, which can become dysregulated, leading to disease states including muscle disease or dysfunction. Apoptosis results in cell shrinkage, DNA fragmentation, membrane blebbing, and disassembly into apoptotic bodies (membrane-bound cell fragments). Necrosis is a pathologic process caused by the progressive degradative action of enzymes that is generally associated with severe cellular trauma in muscles, leading to cell death.

32. **What are the hallmarks of muscles undergoing degeneration-regeneration?**
    - Central nuclei
    - Increased variation of fiber sizes

APPLIED MUSCLE ANATOMY AND PHYSIOLOGY

33. **What is a strap or fusiform muscle? List examples of fusiform muscles.**
Muscles that have fibers arranged parallel to their force generation axis are termed strap, fusiform, or longitudinal muscles. In these muscles, the fibers are arranged essentially parallel to the longitudinal axis of the muscle itself. Longitudinal muscles often have longer fiber lengths, with many sarcomeres positioned in series. This fiber and sarcomere arrangement generally allows these muscles to produce a greater range of motion (ROM) and greater contraction velocity than muscles with the same cross-sectional area but with a different fiber arrangement.
Examples:
    - Sartorius (strap)

- Biceps brachii (fusiform)
- Sternohyoid (strap)

34. **Explain the role of pennation in force production.**
Pennation is the angle of muscle fiber orientation relative to the muscle's force generation axis. Pennation angles allow for more fibers to be packed together in an in-parallel arrangement within a given muscle volume. This packing arrangement increases a muscle's physiological cross-sectional area, which is proportional to its maximal force generating capacity. Pennated muscles generally produce greater force than muscles with the same cross-sectional area but with a different fiber arrangement.

35. **Describe the differences among unipennate, bipennate, and multipennate muscles (anatomic characteristics).**
    - In unipennate muscles, all muscle fibers are oriented at the same angle to the axis of muscle force generation. Example: flexor pollicis longus.
    - In bipennate muscles, two populations of muscle fibers are oriented at different angles to the axis of muscle force generation. Example: rectus femoris.
    - In multipennate muscles, many populations of muscle fibers are oriented at many different angles to the axis of muscle force generation. Example: deltoid.

36. **Describe the adaptations in muscle structure and function that occur with progressive resistance exercises.**
Progressive resistance exercise (PRE) is a type of exercise where individuals contract their muscles against resistance that is progressively increased. Progressive resistance training results in the increase of muscle strength and muscle size (hypertrophy), and the number of muscle fibers is minimally affected. The increase of muscle strength occurs earlier than the increase of muscle size because of neural adaptations. Strength may increase by 20% to 30% over 3 months. Both type I and type II fibers hypertrophy with the type II fibers more responsive than type I fibers. The amounts of transverse tubular and sarcoplasmic reticulum membranes increase as well. Intramuscular high-energy phosphate pool increases and phosphagen metabolism improves. Intracellular glycogen and glycolytic capacity increase, too. Oppositely, mitochondrial density per fiber and oxidative capacity of muscle fibers decreases.
A sample of PRE program for a healthy adult is starting from 60% 1 repetition maximum (RM) and gradually increasing to 80% of 1 RM, 8 to 12 repetition, 2 to 3 SET; progress every ~2 weeks over ~3 months. The beginning intensity and the progression are adjusted according to the age, exercise habit, and health of individuals.

37. **Describe the adaptations in muscle structure and function that occur with endurance exercises.**
Endurance exercise is a type of exercise that involves big muscle groups and increases heart rate and ventilation. Capillary density and myoglobin content increase, which improves efficiency in extracting oxygen from blood. Increased capillary density also improves the removal of metabolic byproducts. Mitochondrial number and size increase, especially in the type I fibers. Endurance training improves ability of muscle cells to obtain ATP from oxidative phosphorylation, which decreases the lactic acid production. It increases proportion of energy derived from fat and lowers the proportion of energy derived from carbohydrate. The greater capillary density and oxidative metabolism and the lower rate of glycogen depletion result in the delayed onset of muscle fatigue during sustained exercise.

38. **What are the consequences of muscle disuse?**
    - The most striking consequence is atrophy—a reduction in muscle and muscle fiber cross-sectional area.
    - The muscles develop lower tensions, beyond those expected on the basis of fiber atrophy.
    - There is an increase in fatigability.
    - In the sarcolemma, there is a spread of acetylcholine receptors beyond the neuromuscular junction.
    - The motor nerve terminals are abnormal in showing signs of degeneration in some places and evidence of sprouting in others.
    - There is a loss of motor drive, such that the motor units cannot be recruited fully.
    - A few fibers undergo necrosis, and there is an increase in the endomysial and perimysial connective tissue.

39. **What occurs as a result of lengthening the muscles?**
Sarcomeres are added.

40. **What adaptations occur if muscles are immobilized in a shortened position?**
    - Decreased number of sarcomeres
    - Increased amount of perimysium

- Thickening of endomysium
- Increased ratio of collagen concentration
- Increased ratio of connective tissue to muscle fiber tissue
- Atrophy
- Decreased strength
- Increased stiffness to passive stretch
- Increased fatigability

41. **What are the changes in skeletal muscles that occur with aging?**
    - Decreased size of muscle cells
    - Decreased number of muscle cells
    - Preferential loss of type 2 muscle fibers

42. **Define the term sarcopenia and its operational definition.**
    Sarcopenia is the term used to describe age-related loss of skeletal muscle mass and strength. The operational definition of sarcopenia is low muscle strength and low muscle mass. Muscle strength is determined by grip strength or chair stand test. Skeletal muscle mass is measured by dual-energy x-ray absorptiometry or bioelectrical impedance analysis. The cutoff points for low muscle strength are grip strength less than 27 kg for men and less than 16 kg for women, or more than 15 seconds taken for five chair-stand rises. The cutoff points for low muscle mass is appendicular skeletal muscle mass/height^2 less than 7 kg/m^2 for men and less than 6 kg/m^2 for women.

43. **Define disease-associated muscle atrophy, such as cachexia.**
    Disease-associated muscle atrophy occurs as a result of accelerated proteolysis. This form of skeletal muscle atrophy is systemic and associated with metabolic and/or inflammatory factors.
    Cachexia may be associated with chronic conditions such as congestive heart failure, chronic obstructive pulmonary disease, end stage renal disease, or cancer.

BIBLIOGRAPHY

Cruz-Jentoft, A. J., Bahat, G., Bauer, J., et al. (2019). Sarcopenia: revised European consensus on definition and diagnosis. *Age Ageing, 48*(1), 16–31.

Derrickson, B. (2017). *Human physiology.* Hoboken, NJ: Wiley.

Enoka, R. M. (2015). *Neuromechanics of human movement* (5th ed.). Champaign, IL: Human Kinetics Publishers.

Lieber, R. L. (2011). *Skeletal muscle structure, function, & plasticity: the physiological basis of rehabilitation* (3rd ed.). Philadelphia, PA: Lippincott Williams & Wilkins.

Liguori, G., Feito, Y., Fountaine, C. J., & Roy, B. (Eds.), (2022). *ACSM's Guidelines for Exercise Testing and Prescription* (11th ed.). Philadelphia, PA: Wolters Kluwer.

McArdle, W. D., Katch, F. I., & Katch, V. L. (2015). *Exercise physiology: nutrition, energy, and human performance* (8th ed.). Philadelphia, PA: Wolters Kluwer Health/Lippincott Williams & Wilkins.

Neumann, D. (2016). *Kinesiology of the musculoskeletal system: foundations for rehabilitation* (3rd ed.). St. Louis, MO: Elsevier.

Proske, U., & Gandevia, S. C. (2012). The proprioceptive senses: their roles in signaling body shape, body position and movement, and muscle force. *Physiological Reviews, 92*, 1651–1697.

Rodriguez-Outeirino, L., Hernandez-Torres, F., Ramirez-de Acuna, F., et al. (2021). Muscle satellite cell heterogeneity: does embryonic origin matter? Frontiers in Cell and Developmental Biology, 9, 750534.

Widmaier, E. P., Raff, H., & Strang, K. (2019). *Vander's human physiology: the mechanisms of body function* (15th ed.). New York, NY: McGraw-Hill Education.

Yin, H., Price, F., & Rudnicki, M. A. (2013). Satellite cells and the muscle stem cell niche. *Physiological Reviews, 93*(1), 23–67.

CHAPTER 1 QUESTIONS

1. **Which of the following is significantly shorter in length when muscle contracts concentrically?**
   a. Sarcomere
   b. Myosin
   c. Actin
   d. Sarcoplasmic reticulum

2. **You were doing bench press training in a gym to strengthen your triceps. Your trainer said that you can tolerate use of a greater weight when lowering the weight to your chest than you can when pressing a weight above your chest (extending the arms). The statement of your trainer is the application of which principle of muscle physiology?**
   a. Sliding filament theory of muscle contraction
   b. Force-velocity relationship

c. Length-tension relationship
d. All-or-none principle

3. A 30-year-old person visits a physical therapist to get advice about training for a marathon. This person is hoping to run the marathon after training for 12 months and to remain injury free during the training. This person has had a sedentary activity level for the prior 3 years. What type of muscle function will the physical therapist need to emphasize for this person's training, which muscle fiber type will be most involved, and what is the primary metabolic pathway being trained?
   a. Muscle strength, type 2x, glycolysis
   b. Muscle endurance, type 2x, tricarboxylic acid cycle, and oxidative phosphorylation
   c. Muscle strength, type 1, glycolysis
   d. Muscle endurance, type 1, tricarboxylic acid cycle, and oxidative phosphorylation

CHAPTER 2

BIOMECHANICS

S.P. Flanagan, PhD, ATC, CSCS and K. Kulig, PhD, PT

1. **Does kinematic similarity ensure kinetic similarity?**
No. Kinematics is the description of motion without reference to the cause of motion. Kinetics refers to the causes of motion (forces). Although two movements may appear similar (kinematics), the underlying forces causing those movements (kinetics) may be very different. This fact should be appreciated when using readily available motion analysis tools (such as recording movements on smartphones or tablets). For example, some patients who have undergone ACL reconstructive surgery and subsequent rehabilitation have gait patterns that look typical compared with noninjured controls but are produced by altered joint kinetics (larger contributions from the hip and decreased contributions from the knee). These differences have been found to persist even a year after surgery.

2. **Explain how impulse can be manipulated to prevent injury.**
Impulse is the area under the force-time curve and accounts not only for the magnitude of the force but also for the duration over which the force is applied. Impulse determines the change in a body's momentum, which is the product of mass and velocity. Applying a smaller force over a longer period of time will have the same impulse (and effect on a body's momentum) as applying a larger force over a shorter period of time. Increasing the time of the impact, which can be accomplished by cushioned shoes and/or flexing the knees when making contact with the ground, can attenuate the magnitude of an impact force and may decrease the risk of injury.

3. **What are some considerations to keep in mind when using elastic resistance?**
Elastic materials, such as bands and tubes, are often used as a form of resistance and follow Hooke's law (the force is proportional to the stiffness and elongation). The stiffness is determined by the manufacturer (which uses different colors for different levels of stiffness) and will decrease with time as the material fatigues. It is also important to keep in mind that the elongation is related to the resting length of the band or tube and not just the elongation during the exercise. For example, consider two scenarios. In the first, an exercise starts with the band at its resting length and is elongated by a certain amount, "x." In the second scenario, the exercise starts slightly elongated by a certain amount "a" but is still elongated by the amount "x." In the first case, the amount of elongation is "x," and in the second case the elongation is "a + x." The band is providing greater resistance in the second scenario, even though the elongation during exercise is the same. This highlights the need to ensure patients are using the same starting length each time they perform an exercise.

4. **Define commonly used biomechanical terms and equations.**

Common Biomechanical Terms and Equations

		EQUATION		UNITS	
TERM (LINEAR; ANGULAR)	PHYSICAL MEANING	LINEAR	ANGULAR	LINEAR (METRIC, US CUSTOMARY)	ANGULAR (METRIC, US CUSTOMARY)
Displacement (Δx; $\Delta\theta$)	A change in position	$x_2 - x_1$	$\theta_2 - \theta_1$	m ft	deg rad
Velocity (υ; ω)	A change in displacement with respect to a change in time	$\Delta x/\Delta t$	$\Delta\theta/\Delta t$	m/sec ft/sec	deg/sec rad/sec
Acceleration (a; α)	A change in velocity with respect to a change in time	$\Delta v/\Delta t$	$\Delta\omega/\Delta t$	m/sec^2 ft/sec^2	deg/sec^2 rad/sec^2
Force; Moment (F; M)	A push or pull by one object on another object; turning effect of a force	$\Sigma F = ma$	$\Sigma M = I\alpha$	N lb	N-m lb-ft

Common Biomechanical Terms and Equations

TERM (LINEAR; ANGULAR)	PHYSICAL MEANING	EQUATION: LINEAR	EQUATION: ANGULAR	UNITS: LINEAR (METRIC, US CUSTOMARY)	UNITS: ANGULAR (METRIC, US CUSTOMARY)
Momentum (H; L)	Resistance to change in velocity	$L = m\upsilon$	$H = I\omega$	kg•m/sec	kg•m²/sec
Impulse (I)	Effect of a force/torque during the time the force/torque acts	$\int F\,dt$	$\int M\,dt$	N-s lb-sec	N-m-sec lb-ft-sec
Work (W)	A change in energy	$\int F\,dx$	$\int M\,d\theta$	J ft-lb	
Gravitational potential energy	Energy caused by position	mgh		J	
Elastic potential	Energy caused by deformation	$\frac{1}{2}ks^2$		J	
Kinetic energy	Energy caused by motion	$\frac{1}{2}m\upsilon^2$	$\frac{1}{2}I\omega^2$	J	
Power (P)	Time rate of doing work	$W/\Delta t$		W hp	
Stress (Pressure) σ	Magnitude of force dispersed over an area	F/A		N/m^2 lb/in^2	
Strain	Amount of deformation	$\Delta L/L_0$		Unitless measure	

5. **What is the relation between the linear motion at the joint surface and the angular motion of a bone around the joint axis?**
A theoretical construct, developed to describe this relation and advocated by Kaltenborn, is known as the convex-concave rule. In brief, if the convex surface of one bone is moving on the fixed concave surface of another bone, rotation and translation will occur in opposite directions. Additionally, if the concave surface of one bone is moving on the fixed convex surface of another bone, rotation and translation occur in the same direction. This rule should be appreciated when joint mobilizations are performed. It is proposed that in order to restore rotational motion at a joint, a linear mobilization is performed in relation to the treatment plane, which is parallel to the concave joint surface. Mobilization can be performed on either segment in accordance with the convex-concave rule.

6. **Has the convex-concave rule been experimentally verified?**
No, at least not for all joints. For example, it has been demonstrated that the glenohumeral joint contradicts the convex-concave rule during external rotation when the humerus is abducted to 90 degrees, and there is no clear consensus that the femur translates anteriorly when the knee is flexing in a weight-bearing position. However, these findings may not violate the convex-concave rule if the amount of translation in the direction of rolling is less than what the curvature of the convex segment would predict. The amount of rolling in one direction may be greater than the sliding in the opposite direction. This "rule" pertains to the shape of the articular surfaces but does not account for the regional characteristics of the para-articular tissues, which may present as directional restrictions. Therefore, the application of the convex-concave rule to treatment may need to be further informed by directly assessing a restriction of gliding at a joint.

7. **What is the difference between a segment angle and a joint angle?**
A segment angle is the angle that the distal point of a segment (eg, foot, shank, thigh) makes with respect to some reference line (such as the horizontal for sagittal plane movements). A joint angle is the angle made by two segments (eg, the knee angle is the angle between the shank and thigh). Joint angles can be stated as either internal (included) or external (anatomic) angles. An internal angle is the angle between the longitudinal axes of

the two segments comprising a joint, while the external angle is the angular displacement from the anatomic position. For example, in the anatomic position, the internal knee angle is 180 degrees, while the external angle is 0 degrees. If this angle were decreased by 30 degrees, the internal angle would be 150 degrees and the external angle would be 30 degrees.

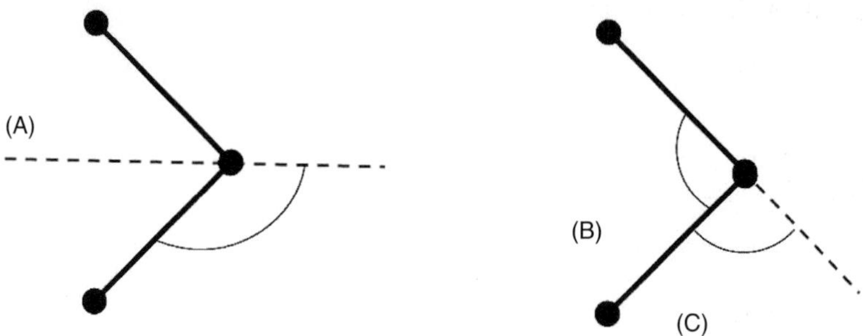

A graphic depiction of the three types of angles: (A) absolute angle from the horizontal; (B) relative, internal angle; and (C) relative, external angle.

It is important to understand the distinction between these three measures and to be consistent in their use. In observational gait analysis, for example, ankle and knee measures are usually external relative angles, while the thigh is usually an absolute angle with respect to the vertical; many motion capture systems, on the other hand, report internal angles for all joints.

8. **Provide examples of the concept of moment.**
   The moment of a force ("moment" for short), or torque, is the turning effect of a force. A force will have a tendency to rotate a body according to its magnitude, its direction, and the perpendicular distance between its line of application and the axis of rotation (this perpendicular distance is known as the moment arm). Knowing that the moment is the product of the force and the moment arm, the length of the moment arm can be manipulated to increase or decrease the force required to complete a task. For example, low back injury prevention strategies are based on the premise of decreasing the moment about the low back during lifting by keeping the load as close to the spine as possible, thus reducing the moment arm of the external resistance. Similarly, flexing the elbows during abduction will decrease the moment arm about the shoulder, thus making the movement easier to perform. On the other hand, during manual muscle testing, the therapist can increase the demand on a muscle by applying the resistance as far from the joint's axis of rotation as possible.

9. **What is the effect of a muscle's force on a joint system?**
   Just as forces can be combined together to determine a resultant, forces can also be broken into components. The components are useful in identifying the different effects of a force on a joint. For example, a muscle force can be divided into the component that is perpendicular to the bone (causing it to rotate and create a shear force across a joint) and the component that is parallel to the bone (usually increasing the compressive force across a joint). Therefore, in addition to causing movement at a joint, all muscle forces will affect the amount of compression at a joint. During rehabilitation of certain joint pathologies, it may be necessary to identify which therapeutic exercises will increase the force of a muscle (to strengthen it) without applying excessive compressive forces across the joint. For example, performing unilateral (as opposed to bilateral) exercises for the lumbar extensors will decrease compressive forces on the spine while increasing the demand on those muscles.

10. **Explain how torque-producing capabilities of a muscle vary over a joint's range of motion.**
    Over the range of motion of a joint, the magnitudes of moment arms and forces may vary. The amount of force a muscle can produce is influenced by several properties, including the length-tension relationship, which states that a muscle that is too stretched or too shortened cannot actively produce as high amounts of force as it can when the muscle is at its optimal length. For example, when using the deltoid to abduct the shoulder from 0 to 180 degrees, the moment arm of the deltoid increases and the force-producing capabilities also increase to a position of optimal length and then decrease. These variations result in an initial increase of torque production, until the optimal position is reached, and then a relatively constant amount of torque production from the deltoids ensues for the remainder of the range of motion. Based on this, it is important to keep the same manual muscle testing position, especially if the therapist wants to compare among patients or examine the effect of training over a period of time.

11. Can a muscle's action at a joint change?

Yes. A muscle's action at a joint is determined by the magnitude of the force and the direction of the force vector (a line roughly extending from the effective origin to the effective insertion). Tendon-transfer surgeries will often make use of this fact when a certain muscle group is paralyzed. Additionally, with flat feet (pes planus) the tibialis anterior's role can change from that of a subtalar invertor to an evertor. Even in the absence of pathology, this can occur most notably at the hip. For example, the piriformis is an external rotator when the hip is in a neutral position but becomes an internal rotator when the hip is flexed beyond 90 degrees.

12. When a study refers to a net joint moment, what does that mean, and what are the assumptions behind it?

One of the greatest limitations in biomechanics is that we cannot, with current technology, directly measure muscle forces in a noninvasive way. However, we can measure the acceleration of the limbs and forces between the body and the ground to calculate the net joint moment (NJM), which is the moment required to accelerate a limb in accordance with Newton's second law. Despite the fact that muscles and other soft tissue structures contribute to the NJM, and cocontractions of the antagonists can make the actual moment much greater than the NJM, we usually equate high NJMs with high muscle forces needed to produce that moment. So when a research study suggests that exercise A has a greater extensor NJM at the knee than exercise B, it assumes that there is no cocontraction of the hamstrings during both exercises, and exercise A has a higher demand on the quadriceps. Studies will typically report internal moments (as described previously) or external moments (which are a result of external forces and inertia). Internal moments are equal in magnitude and opposite in direction to the external moment.

13. What is joint instability, and how does it differ from hypermobility?

Joint stability is the ability of a joint to maintain a posture or trajectory similar to an undisturbed behavior in the presence of a perturbation. Although joint instability would represent the lack of this ability, the definition used by investigators and clinicians within studies is inconsistent, with three main definitions: (1) excessive and occasionally uncontrolled range of motion resulting in frank joint dislocation; (2) small, abnormal movement in an otherwise normal range of motion that may result in pain because of "impingement" at the joint; and (3) a small amount of force necessary to move a joint through its range of motion (or low stiffness). Joint hypermobility describes a laxity of the joint, where there is increased extensibility and range of motion, and is often used interchangeably with instability by clinicians. However, a hypermobile joint may still be stable because of muscular influence and motor coordination.

14. How are force and strength related?

Force is a push or pull of one object on another. Force is a vector quantity, having both a magnitude and a direction. Strength may be thought of as the ability to produce or absorb force. Measures of strength typically determine the maximum force a muscle or muscle group can produce.

15. Does the amplitude of the electromyography (EMG) signal quantify a muscle's force-producing (absorbing) capability?

No. A muscle's force-producing (absorbing) capability is primarily determined by the:

- Type of muscle action (concentric, eccentric, isometric)
- Velocity of lengthening or shortening (force-velocity relation)
- Length of a muscle (length-tension relation)
- Physiologic cross-sectional area of the muscle
- Number of motor units within a muscle that are activated (intramuscular coordination)
- Rate of motor unit activation (rate-coding)
- Intrinsic force-generating capability of the muscle (specific tension)
- Contractile history of the muscle (eg, prestretch)

The EMG signal quantifies the number of motor units and their rate of activation within the electrode field. In addition, because electrode placement can affect the number of motor units within the field, it is important to compare relative values (usually normalized to a maximum voluntary isometric contraction) rather than absolute values when comparing differences in EMG signals.

16. What are the benefits of having three different types of muscle actions?

Skeletal muscles are required to produce force, reduce (or absorb) force, or stabilize against a force. There is a different type of muscle action to fulfill each of these roles. A concentric muscle action produces force—the muscle moment is greater than the moment of an external force, and movement occurs in the direction of the muscle moment. An eccentric muscle action reduces force—the muscle moment is less than the moment of an external force, and movement occurs in the direction opposite of the muscle moment. The eccentric muscle action reduces the external force and consequently decreases the acceleration caused by it. An isometric muscle action stabilizes against a force—the muscle moment is equal and opposite to the moment created by an external force, and no movement occurs.

17. **What information can be obtained from studying the force-velocity curve?**
Examining this relationship reveals that greater force can be produced isometrically (when the velocity is zero) than can be produced concentrically, and greater force can be produced eccentrically than can be produced isometrically.

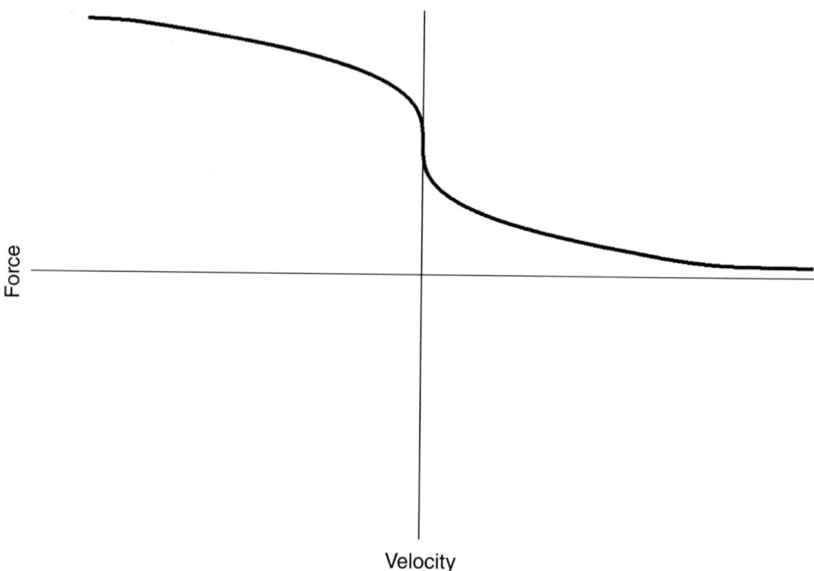

The force-velocity relation.

Peak eccentric force is estimated to be between 120% and 140% of peak isometric force. Additionally, there is a negative relationship between force and velocity in the concentric range and a positive one between force and velocity in the eccentric range.

18. **Is there a mechanical variable that can identify the types of muscle actions?**
Yes, mechanical power is the product of the net joint moment (NJM) and the angular velocity. If the NJM and the angular velocity are in the same direction, the power is positive and a concentric muscle action is controlling the velocity. If the NJM and angular velocity are in opposite directions, the work is negative and an eccentric muscle action is controlling the velocity. If there is an NJM but no angular velocity, the power is zero because there is no angular velocity, but the presence of an NJM indicates an isometric muscle action is preventing a velocity.

19. **Why is eccentric strength important in the prevention of injury?**
Although energy can be absorbed by all of the tissues of the body (eg, bone, ligament, muscle-tendon), the muscle-tendon complex has the greatest potential to safely absorb or distribute energy within the body. Eccentric muscle actions are the primary means by which energy is safely absorbed by the body. If the muscles cannot produce enough force and/or undergo the appropriate length changes, then other tissues must absorb this energy. Because the other tissues are not as capable of absorbing or distributing energy, energy levels can quickly exceed the tissues' limits, resulting in injury.

20. **Explain the length-tension relationship of muscle.**
The amount of force or tension that a muscle can produce varies with the length of the muscle at the time of contraction. Maximum force is produced when the muscle is approximately at its resting length. When the fibers shorten beyond resting length, the force production decreases slowly at first and then rapidly. There is a progressive decline as the fibers are lengthened beyond resting length. This relationship can be used to help explain why surgically lengthened muscles are weak postoperatively (see figure). Although muscles typically do not operate over the entire length, this relationship helps explain the positions used for manual muscle tests, particularly for biarticular muscles. Biarticular muscles are typically tested with one end of the muscle lengthened and the other end shortened to place the muscle in the middle of its operating range. For example, when testing the hamstrings' action at the hip, the hip is usually extending (muscle shortening) while the knee is extended (muscle in a lengthened position).

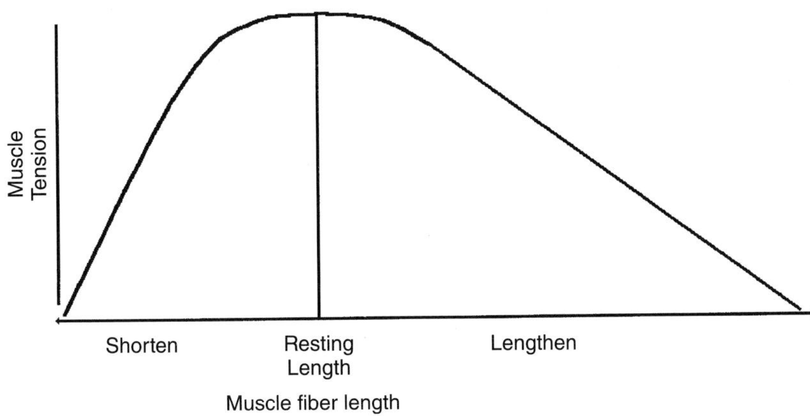

Length-tension curve.

21. **What is the stretch-shortening cycle?**
The stretch-shortening cycle (SSC) involves 1) a well-timed preactivation of the muscle before an eccentric muscle action; 2) a short, rapid eccentric action; and 3) an immediate transition from an eccentric muscle action to a concentric muscle action. The subsequent concentric action is more forceful than it typically is because it was proceeded by the rapid eccentric action. The SSC is involved in many movements, from gait to jumping and throwing. Plyometric exercises are usually used to improve utilization of the stretch-shortening cycle.

22. **Is excessive force the cause of pain and injury?**
Not directly. A better measure would be stress (force per unit area), which gives an indication of how that force is distributed. Although the term stress is used in reference to internal forces and pressure is used for external forces, clinically they can be used synonymously without much difficulty. Although a certain amount of stress is desirable, too much is believed to be the cause of injury and pain. Patellofemoral pain syndrome is believed to be the result of too much force (from the quadriceps) over too little area (patellofemoral contact area). The smaller contact area seems to have a stronger relationship to symptoms than does the increased amount of force. The insensate and poorly vascularized foot, in association with connective tissue changes, is vulnerable to increases in pressure and consequently the development of pressure sores. If the body weight transmitted to the foot can be dispersed over a larger surface area of the foot, the magnitude of pressure is decreased as is the chance for ulceration. The same factors apply to a person confined to prolonged bed rest; pressure sores may develop on areas where bony prominences contact the bed.

23. **What is the tissue response to a force (stress), and how is it measured?**
The tissue response to a force (or load) is deformation, which is a change in the size or shape of the tissue. Deformation is usually expressed as the quotient of the change in tissue dimension (eg, length) divided by the tissue's original dimension (eg, length), or strain. Laboratory experiments usually apply a given force (N) to a tissue of known cross-sectional area (mm^2) and specified length (mm), in which the resulting deformation (mm) is measured. Simple calculations will produce the applied stress and resulting strain. In vivo, force, either exerted by subject (active) or caused by an apparatus (passive), is measured using a dynamometer and the deformation (here displacement) is measured using an imaging technique (ie, ultrasound). Not all tissues can be measured in this way; some musculotendinous units are accessible to testing in vivo, but cartilage is not.

24. **What information can be ascertained from studying force-deformation curves?**
Typically, plotting force on the vertical axis and the corresponding deformation on the horizontal axis produces a force-deformation curve, which graphically represents the relationship between the two (see figure).
Several important tissue qualities can be determined from this curve, including:

- Ultimate strength—the point on the curve where the tissue fails
- Yield point—the point at which a permanent deformation occurs
- Elastic region—the portion of the curve preceding the yield point

- Plastic region—the portion of the curve following the yield point
- Stiffness—the slope of the curve in the elastic range
- Energy—the area under the curve

When force is normalized to the area over which it is distributed and deformation is normalized to the resting dimension, we will have a stress on the vertical axis and strain on the horizontal axis. This curve provides insight into the material properties of the studied tissue, and its slope is the Young's modulus.

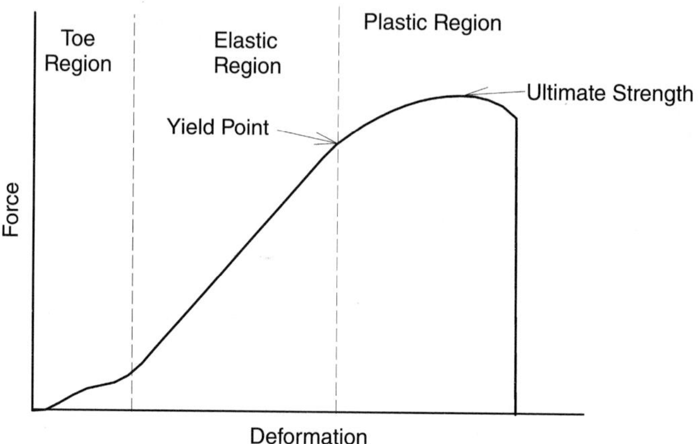

Force-deformation curve.

25. **Do human tissues respond to all stresses in the same way?**

No. Depending on the tissue and its role, tissues respond quite differently, and this difference in response is called anisotropism. For example, a tendon responds well to tension, but not as well to shear, and not at all to compression. Cartilage, on the other hand, responds well to compression. Human bone can handle compressive force best (such as pushing both ends of the bone toward each other), followed by tension (such as pulling both ends of the bone away from each other), and then shear force (such as pushing the top of the bone to the right and the bottom of the bone to the left). A bending force basically subjects one side of the bone to compression, while the other side experiences tension; therefore, the side subjected to tension usually fails first (immature bone may fail in compression first). For torsional loading (such as twisting the top part of the bone, while holding the bottom of the bone in a fixed position), fracture patterns typically show that the bone fails as a result of shear forces and then tension.

26. **When the force is applied to the tissue externally, does the tissue return to its original state after the force is removed?**

It depends on the amount of force applied. At lower levels of force the tissue returns to its original form, and therefore this stage is called the elastic region. It is in the elastic region that the characteristics of the tissue are stable and therefore are used to describe the tissue's stiffness. If the force continues to increase, it reaches a transitional point—the yield point. The yield point is where the material changes from the elastic range to the plastic range. Beyond this yield point, permanent deformation will occur even after the load is removed.

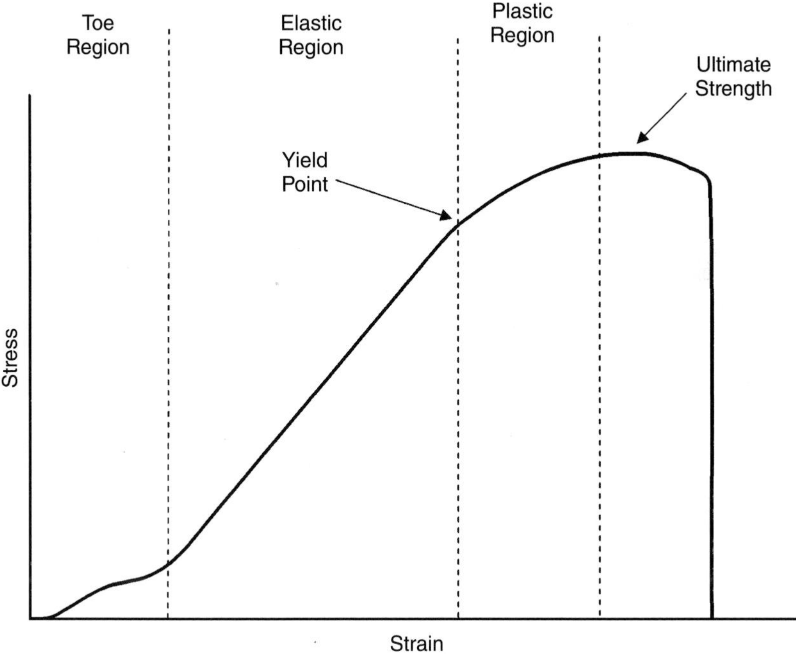

The stress-strain relation.

27. **Give an example of the clinical implications of the force-deformation curve.**
The force-deformation curve can be appreciated clinically most easily during ligamentous testing. If a pain-inducing force did not exceed the yield point, the ligament would return to its original length with no detectable changes in joint laxity. This injury would be classified as a first-degree sprain. If the injurious force exceeded the yield point but did not reach the ultimate strength of the ligament, the ligament would experience a permanent deformation that would be manifested as an increase in joint laxity. This injury would be classified as a second-degree sprain. If the injurious force exceeded the ultimate strength of the ligament, the ligament would catastrophically fail, and the subsequent force applied during ligamentous testing would be met with no resistance. This injury would be classified as a third-degree sprain.

28. **Discuss some factors that affect the biomechanical properties of tendons and ligaments.**

The Most Commonly Cited Factors Affecting the Biomechanical Properties of Tendons and Ligaments

FACTOR	PHYSIOLOGIC EFFECT ON COLLAGEN	MECHANICAL EFFECT
Physical activity	↑Glycosaminoglycan content ↑Cross-linking ↑Alignment of fibers	Strengthens
Disuse/immobilization	↑Turnover ↑Reducible cross-linking ↑Nonuniform orientation ↓Glycosaminoglycan and water content	Weakens
Aging	↓In number and quality of cross-links ↓In fibril diameter	Weakens

The Most Commonly Cited Factors Affecting the Biomechanical Properties of Tendons and Ligaments		
FACTOR	**PHYSIOLOGIC EFFECT ON COLLAGEN**	**MECHANICAL EFFECT**
Corticosteroid use	↓Collagen synthesis ↓Stiffness ↓Ultimate stress ↓Energy to failure	Weakens
Pregnancy-induced hormones NSAIDs	↑Collagen degradation Variable, depending on specific drug	Increases laxity Inconclusive

29. **Is cartilage the same in all joints?**

No. There are morphologic, biomechanical, metabolic, and histologic differences between types of cartilage in the joints of the lower extremities. Those differences, in part, are the reason why osteoarthritis is more prominent in the knee and hip joints than in the ankle joint.

30. **Do all tissues adapt at the same rate?**

No. An obvious example would be the difference in change in volume response to resistive exercise by a muscle and a tendon. A tendon adapts to change more slowly than muscle because it has fewer cells (in this case, tenocytes) that are capable of facilitating adaptation. Bone adapts more slowly than muscle. Evidence on the rate of adaptation of ligaments, cartilage, and intervertebral discs is scarce, but it is believed that they develop more slowly than muscle. It is important to realize, during rehabilitation, that a muscle will regain its strength before the other tissues of the musculoskeletal system, and therefore muscle strength alone is not a good indicator of the rehabilitation process.

31. **What does it mean that a tendon is more compliant?**

A more compliant tendon, typically accompanying degeneration, is a tendon where more displacement (m) occurs as a result of the same amount of force (N) produced by the muscle, on the contralateral extremity. Compliance is the inverse of stiffness, which is the change in force over displacement (N/m). Mechanical stiffness and patient-reported perceived sensation of stiffness are not related.

32. **Are tissue responses to a submaximal stress time dependent?**

Yes, tissue responses do change with time of application (or loading rate). Even if the amount of load is in the elastic range, but applied for a longer time, it will continue to cause a deformation. This type of deformation is reversible and is called creep. Creep is caused by the exudation of interstitial fluid. The fluid exits most rapidly at first and diminishes gradually over time. Human cartilage takes 4 to 16 hours to reach creep equilibrium, and this is why humans become slightly shorter as the day passes. Creep can also be associated with injury. Prolonged flexion of the lumbar spine results in a creep of the posterior ligaments, which decreases joint stiffness and may predispose the low back to injury. It is prudent to advise patients to allow this flexion-creep to reverse itself before performing activities that require lumbar stability.

33. **What is hysteresis?**

When viscoelastic tissue is loaded and then subsequently unloaded, the amount of stress is lower for a given amount of strain. This phenomenon is a consequence of the tissue's viscosity and is called hysteresis. The area between the loading and unloading curves (shaded area, see figure) is a measure of hysteresis and represents the difference between the energy absorbed and released by the tissue, which is usually lost in the form of heat (although it could cause tissue damage).

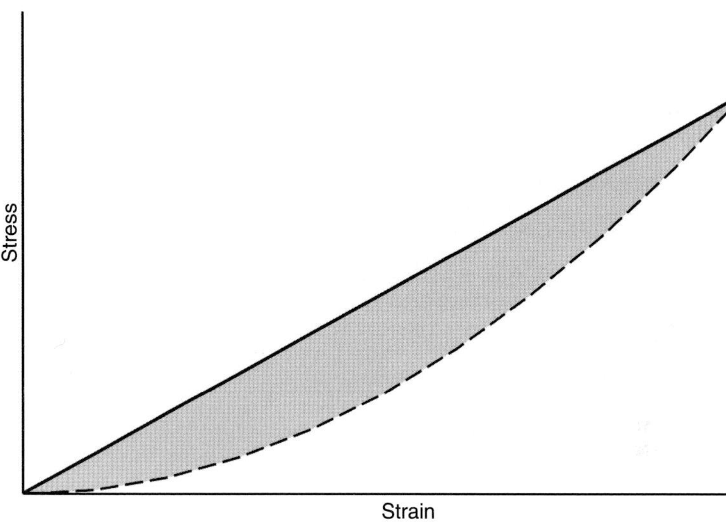

The hysteresis loop.

Repeated loadings, as well as acute and chronic stretching, increase a tendon's compliance and decrease the amount of hysteresis. These changes increase the energy returned during the stretch-shortening cycle (improving performance) and can decrease the risk of injury.

34. **What is friction, and is it good or bad?**
Friction is a force, parallel to the contact surface, that opposes motion between two objects' surfaces. The interlocking of irregularities in the contact surfaces causes friction. The magnitude of the friction force will depend on the material characteristics of the two contacting surfaces and will be lower if there is relative motion between the two surfaces.

Friction may be good or bad, depending on the situation. A certain amount of friction between the ground and our shoes is necessary for efficient movement and to prevent slipping, but it also wears the soles of our shoes. High friction forces between the ground and the shoe increase the risk of ankle and knee injuries in sports where there is a lot of sudden turning or stopping, and repetitive friction forces to the skin can cause blisters. High friction forces at the joint surfaces cause wear, which leads to articular degeneration.

35. **Do movement screens have diagnostic value?**
It is doubtful. Although a movement screen may alert you that something could be wrong with the way a person is moving, it cannot tell you the cause of a dysfunction. Additionally, some dysfunctions may not even be picked up by visual inspection as a result of compensations. The concept of a support moment highlights the need to be cautious when evaluating multijoint movement. Collapse of the lower extremity requires flexion at all three joints (ankle, knee, and hip). A sufficiently large NJM at the ankle or hip can prevent flexion at the knee, and vice versa. Summing all three NJMs is called a support moment, and the support moment has been shown to be less variable during repeated gait trials than any of the individual NJMs. The support moment demonstrates how a decrease in one NJM can be compensated for by an increase in another and helps explain why kinematic specificity does not ensure kinetic specificity.

36. **What is motor abundancy?**
Motor abundancy (also called motor redundancy) refers to the fact that we have more degrees of freedom (both kinematic and kinetic) than necessary to accomplish most tasks. This means that we can accomplish most tasks in several different ways. For example, several combinations of glenohumeral, elbow, and wrist rotations can place the hand at the same point in space, and several combinations of hip, knee, and ankle flexion angles can lead to the same squat depth.

37. **How might compensatory motion lead to injury?**
Compensatory motion stems from motor abundancy: we have several different ways of accomplishing the same task, but they are not all equivalent. Compensatory motions can be either good or bad. They allow us to complete a task in the presence of musculoskeletal impairments or errors in motor control. However, if the stresses on the compensating structure(s) exceed their capacity, an injury at the site(s) of compensation may result. Thus, the source(s) of the injury (impairment) and site(s) of the injury (compensation) can be different. While it is important to treat the site(s), it is also necessary to treat the source(s) so that the injury does not reoccur. For example, someone with limited mobility in the hips may compensate with increased mobility in the spine. This may cause excessive stresses on the spinal tissues and create pain. In such instances, one must address hip mobility to relieve stress on the spinal tissues.

38. **What is the difference between mechanical versus material properties?**
Mechanical properties are the result of material properties and the amount of material. Material property of a tissue indicates what the material is made of, and how it is organized and distributed. For example, let's take two lower extremity tendons that for the sake of argument have the same stiffness (mechanical property). However, the second tendon has a larger cross-sectional area and the same length. That may suggest a different material property exhibited by that tendon. To quantify the material property, we would need to determine both tendons' strain (change in length normalized to the resting length). Finally, the linear region of the stress-strain curve will estimate the material property (Young's modulus) of both tendons. Here, the tendon with the large cross-sectional area will have a lesser material property value.

39. **What is coupled motion?**
Biomechanically speaking, coupled motion is the occurrence of consistent association of motion that can be described around two axes. An example of coupled motion can be at the same joint (ie, tibia external rotation with terminal knee extension) or at neighboring joints (tibia internal rotation with calcaneal eversion). The primary causes of kinematic coupling are articular and para-articular morphology.

40. **Why is it important that we can produce more force eccentrically than concentrically?**
Producing more force eccentrically than concentrically is a built-in safety mechanism. It means that we can lower more weight than we can raise, and we can absorb more energy than we can generate. As an example, we have the potential to safely land from any height that we can jump up to. If we could produce more force concentrically than eccentrically, then this would not be the case.

41. **What do people mean by an "energy leak" and how does it relate to injury?**
The conservation of energy states that energy cannot be created nor destroyed; it can move from one place to another or change from one form to another—but the energy must go somewhere. Injury occurs when either the magnitude or the rate of energy entering a tissue exceeds its capacity to absorb it. Soft tissues absorb energy as they elongate during a joint rotation. Generally speaking, the muscle-tendon complex (MTC) can absorb the greatest amount of energy with rotations that occur in the sagittal plane. An "energy leak" usually occurs with an out-of-plane movement that causes osteoligamentous structures (or smaller muscles) to elongate and absorb too much energy. An example of an energy leak would be when valgus collapse occurs during the landing from a jump. The energy going into the body from impact is usually absorbed by the lower extremity MTCs as they rotate into flexion. Excessive frontal or transverse plane movement at the hip and/or subtalar joint can cause ligaments at the knee, such as the ACL or MCL, to absorb energy they are ill equipped to handle and result in a noncontact injury.

42. **What is mechanical jerk and why is it important?**
Mechanical jerk is the time rate of change of acceleration, or how quickly acceleration is changing. Thus, jerk tells us something about how quickly forces (and ultimately, stresses) are changing during a movement. Smooth movements are thought to minimize jerk. Abrupt starts and stops are associated with large jerk. In a point-to-point task such as reaching, jerk is minimized at the beginning and end of the movement. In contrast, a boxing punch would have a large jerk at the beginning and end of the movement. The boxer may anticipate a target (such as a heavy bag or an opponent) will create large jerk at the moment of impact of the punch. If the boxer misses the target, large accelerations at end range may create injury at the elbow or shoulder.

43. **What is the difference between an anatomical and functional antagonist?**
An anatomical antagonist is a muscle whose uniarticular torque counteracts the uniarticular torque of another muscle. However, during multijoint movements this relationship may not be antagonistic. For example, during isolated knee motion or isolated hip motion, torque created by the rectus femoris and the hamstrings oppose each other. In contrast, during the concentric portion of a squat (due to differences in moment arms at both the knee and hip) both the rectus femoris and the hamstrings are acting concentrically. In this case, they would be

functional agonists. Therefore, it is important to realize that you cannot interpret relationships during multijoint movement from anatomical classifications.

44. **What is limb stiffness, and can it be altered?**
Limb stiffness can be expressed as a ratio of ground reaction force to change in limb length. For example, when landing from a jump the ground reflects the acceleration of the center of mass while the lower extremity joints flex. Hip, knee, and ankle dorsiflexion make the limb length shorter by a certain linear amount. The easiest way to alter limb stiffness is to manipulate limb length. By increasing the flexion in the lower limb joints, the jumper produces a less stiff limb and by limiting the joint flexion, the jumper's limb behaves stiffer.

45. **List biomechanical factors that affect a joint implant.**
   - Initial stability—based mainly on the surgery technique used and the implant design
   - Late stability—determined by bone growth and remodeling of the bone around the implant (biologic fixation); if cement is used, late stability is determined by the bone-cement and cement-implant interfaces
   - Stress shielding—affects the bone around the implant as the load typically goes through the stronger implant and not the bone surrounding it
   - Wear of the implant—cobalt-chrome implants are typically used for the femoral head to decrease frictional wear on the acetabular component; ceramic acetabular cups and femoral heads are used because of their low coefficient of friction, but their implant strength has been questioned in some studies (they break and you never get all the fine ceramic debris out of the joint); highly cross-linked plastic has been used for acetabular components, but microscopic wear over time has proven to create an environment of aseptic loosening at the bone/cement/implant interfaces
   - Wear debris—polyethylene wear can cause osteolysis and potential aseptic loosening
   - Changing the anatomic alignments—by the manner in which the implant is installed or the correction of any preoperative deformity (hip dysplasia, knee varum, or valgum)

46. **List factors that affect the stability of an external fixator.**
   - Pin diameter—bending stiffness increasing by an order of the fourth power as the diameter increases
   - Number of pins used
   - Distance from the surface to the bone
   - Stiffness of the frame
   - Number of fixation planes
   - Bone integrity into which the pins are placed (infection, avascular necrosis/poor vascularity)

47. **What happens to the strength of an intramedullary rod when its diameter is increased?**
Strength increases as the rod size increases by an order of the third power.

48. **What happens biomechanically with improper fixation size?**
In the case of total knee arthroplasty (TKA), if the plastic tibial insert is too big, then the space is "over-stuffed" and the knee will not have full flexion or extension capability. If the insert is too small, then the joint is unstable and the ligamentous and capsular structures are too lax; the muscular length tension characteristics are also compromised and both scenarios are often accompanied by pain.
In the case of total hip arthroplasty (THA), if the acetabular component is too big, then the femoral implant "fulcrums" against the lip of the cup with flexion and can cause dislocation. If the stem is too long, then leg length discrepancy may occur. If the femoral head is too big, then range of motion is decreased in all planes. If any of the components is too small, then risk of joint dislocation increases. Furthermore, the muscular length tension characteristics are disrupted, and the supporting capsule and ligaments are lax. The patients often feel weak and walk with a limp.

49. **How do holes in the bone (ie, missing screw or following removal of plate) affect its strength?**
   - Decreases the cross-sectional area of the bone; less bone at the hole and strength is decreased
   - Decreases strength by causing a stress concentration point, determined by the geometry of the hole and bone
   - A hole of 20% of the bone diameter decreases strength by 50%

50. **How long does it take for strength to return to normal levels after the removal of a screw?**
It takes between 4 months and 1 year for strength to return to normal (provided typical bone physiology).

51. **List the types of metals that are closest biomechanically to bone.**

WITH REGARD TO MODULUS:	WITH REGARD TO BIOCOMPATIBILITY:
• Aluminum	• Titanium (and titanium alloys)
• Titanium (and titanium alloys)	• Cobalt-chromium
• Stainless steel	• Stainless steel
• Cobalt-chromium	• Aluminum

52. **How much strength does a well-placed lag screw add to fracture fixation?**
One should be able to assume that the strength of the fixation is determined by the pull-out strength of the lag screw, or approximately a 40% increase in strength over plating alone.

BIBLIOGRAPHY

Adams, M. A., Bogduk, N., Burton, K., & Dolan, P. (2002). *The biomechanics of back pain.* Edinburgh: Churchill Livingstone.
Baeyens, J. P., van Roy, P., & Clarys, J. P. (2000). Intra-articular kinematics of the normal glenohumeral joint in the late preparatory phase of throwing: Kaltenborn's rule revisited. *Ergonomics, 43*, 1726–1737.
Cerny, K. (1984). Kinesiology versus biomechanics: a perspective. *Physical Therapy, 64*, 1809.
Flanagan, S. P. (2014). *Biomechanics: A case-based approach.* Burlington: Jones and Bartlett Learning.
Hatze, H. (1974). The meaning of the term "biomechanics". *Journal of Biomechanics, 7*, 189–190.
Kubo, K., Kanehisa, H., & Fukunaga, T. (2002). Effects of resistance and stretching training programmes on the viscoelastic properties of human tendon structures in vivo. *Journal of Physiology, 538*, 219–226.
Latash, M. L. (2012). The bliss (not problem) of motor abundance (nor redundancy). *Experimental Brain Research, 217*, 1–5.
McGill, S. M. (2007). *Low back disorders: evidence-based prevention and rehabilitation* (2nd ed.). Champaign: Human Kinetics.
McGill, S. M., & Brown, S. (1992). Creep response of the lumbar spine to prolonged full flexion. *Clinical Biomechanics, 7*, 43–46.
Meriam, J. L., & Kraige, L. G. (1997). *Engineering mechanics: dynamics.* New York, NY: John Wiley and Sons.
Neumann, D. A. (2002). *Kinesiology of the musculoskeletal system: foundations for physical rehabilitation.* St. Louis, MO: Mosby.
Neumann, D. A. (2012). The Convex-Concave Rules of arthrokinematics: flawed or perhaps just misinterpreted? *Journal of Orthopaedic & Sports Physical Therapy, 42*, 53–55.
Rasch, P. J., & Burke, R. K. (1971). *Kinesiology and applied anatomy: the science of human movement* (4th ed.). Philadelphia: Lea & Febiger.
Simoneau, G. G., Bereda, S. M., Sobush, D. C., & Starsky, A. J. (2001). Biomechanics of elastic resistance in therapeutic exercise programs. *Journal of Orthopaedic & Sports Physical Therapy, 31*, 16–24.
Smidt, G. L. (1984). Biomechanics and physical therapy: a perspective. *Physical Therapy, 64*, 1807–1808.
Song, Y., Ito, H., Kourtis, L., et al. (2012). Articular cartilage friction increases in hip joints after the removal of acetabular labrum. *Journal of Biomechanics, 45*(3), 524–530.
Venes, D. (2009). *Taber's cyclopedic medical dictionary* (21st ed.). Philadelphia, PA: FA Davis.
Whiting, W. C., & Zernicke, R. F. (2008). *Biomechanics of musculoskeletal injury* (2nd ed.). Champaign: Human Kinetics.
Winter, D. A. (1980). Overall principle of lower-limb support during stance phase of gait. *Journal of Biomechanics, 13*, 923–927.
Zajac, F. E., Neptune, R. R., & Kautz, S. A. (2002). Biomechanics and muscle control of human walking—Part 1: introduction to concepts, power transfer, dynamics and simulations. *Gait & Posture, 16*, 215–232.
Zatsiorsky, V. M. (1998). *Kinematics of human motion.* Champaign: Human Kinetics.
Zatsiorsky, V. M. (2002). *Kinetics of human motion.* Champaign: Human Kinetics.

CHAPTER 2 QUESTIONS

1. **You wish to perform joint mobilizations on a patient who is unable to achieve full knee extension by 5 degrees. Which of the following is the correct direction of the tibial mobilization?**
   a. An anterior-posterior mobilization parallel to the tibial plateau
   b. An anterior-posterior mobilization perpendicular to the femoral shaft
   c. A posterior-anterior mobilization parallel to the tibial plateau
   d. A posterior-anterior mobilization perpendicular to the femoral shaft

2. **You wish to perform a manual muscle test for glenohumeral abduction. Where should you place your hand to produce the greatest moment about the joint?**
   a. At the patient's humeral head
   b. At the patient's humeral epicondyle
   c. At the patient's ulnar styloid process

3. **You wish to perform a manual muscle test for the gluteus maximus. What is the correct position of the knee while the hip is extending?**
   a. Extended
   b. Flexed

4. **A volleyball player landed on the opponent's foot after blocking a shot. Her subtalar joint excessively inverted and her anterior talofibular ligament sustained a second-degree sprain. What type of deformation did the tissue undergo?**
   a. Elastic
   b. Plastic
   c. Sustained

CHAPTER 3

SOFT TISSUE INJURY AND REPAIR

A.J. Nitz, PT, PhD

1. **What is the body's initial response to soft tissue injury? How is it identified?**
   The inflammatory response is characterized by a chemically mediated amplification cascade that represents the body's initial reaction to injury, whether caused by trauma, surgery, or metabolic or infectious disease. The principal signs of the inflammatory response are erythema (rubor), swelling (tumor), elevated tissue temperature (calor), and pain (dolor). Local vasodilation, fluid leakage into the extracellular and extravascular spaces, and impaired lymphatic drainage are responsible for the erythema, swelling, and increased tissue temperature. The fourth cardinal sign of inflammation—pain—is the result of mechanical distention and pressure of the soft tissues and chemical irritation of pain-sensitive nerve receptors.

2. **Describe the phases of soft tissue healing.**
   The acute inflammatory phase begins immediately after injury and lasts 24 to 48 hours, although some aspects may continue for up to 3 weeks. The proliferative phase may begin early in the inflammatory phase but is thought to be most extensive approximately 21 days after injury. The matrix formation/remodeling phase begins 3 weeks after injury and may last for up to 2 years, although in many cases the majority of remodeling has occurred by 2 months. Because the time frames for these three phases overlap considerably, the accepted delineations should be used as general guidelines only.

3. **Describe the basic vascular and cellular activities associated with the inflammatory reaction and the primary function of each activity.**
   Blood vessels at the site of injury initially undergo vasoconstriction, which is mediated by norepinephrine and usually lasts from a few seconds to a few minutes. If serotonin is released by mast cells in the area of injury, a secondary prolonged vasoconstriction occurs to slow blood loss in the affected region. Additional cellular activities after soft tissue injury include margination of leukocytes, which adhere to the vessel wall, and chemotaxis (movement of white blood cells through the extravascular space toward the site of injury), which begins the process of phagocytosis and removes the cellular debris caused by the injury.

4. **Identify the key chemical mediators of the inflammatory response.**
   Both histamine and serotonin (5-HT) are released from granules of mast cells in the area of the injury. Histamine results in elevated vascular permeability, whereas serotonin is a potent vasoconstrictor. Kinins, notably bradykinin, also cause a marked increase in vascular permeability, much as histamine does. It is now recognized that numerous cytokines and growth factors are involved in the cellular response to inflammation and injury. Proinflammatory prostaglandins are believed to sensitize pain receptors, attract leukocytes to the inflamed area, and increase vascular permeability by antagonizing vasoconstriction. Though slightly different in their specific point of biochemical interaction, the primary mode of action of aspirin, nonsteroidal antiinflammatory drugs (NSAIDs), and steroids is to inhibit prostaglandin synthesis by deactivation of a key enzyme (cyclooxygenase).

5. **Which cell type is especially prominent in the proliferative and matrix formation phases of connective tissue healing?**
   The fibroblast is the most common connective tissue cell. It is responsible for synthesizing and secreting most of the fibers and ground substance of connective tissue. Soft tissue injury signals the fibroblast to multiply rapidly and mobilizes free connective tissue cells to the injured area. Tissue bleeding, in the case of trauma-induced inflammation, will result in deposition of fibrin and fibronectin in the tissues. These substances form a substratum that enhances the adhesion of various cells during later stages of repair.

6. **Describe the elements that comprise the connective tissue matrix.**
   The connective tissue matrix is comprised of fibrous elements (such as collagen, elastin, and reticulin) and ground substance, which consists principally of water, salts, and glycosaminoglycans (GAGs). The matrix provides the strength and support of the soft tissue and also serves as the means for diffusion of tissue fluid and nutrients between capillaries and cells.

7. **What general factors affect connective tissue repair after tissue injury?**
   Healing after soft tissue injury is affected by the availability of a number of factors, including blood supply, proteins, minerals, and amino acids. Enzymes and hormones also play a role in tissue healing, as do mechanical stress and infection. Steroids suppress the mitotic activity of fibroblasts, which results in diminished deposition of

collagen fibers and reduction in tensile strength. Antibiotic medicines inhibit protein synthesis and may adversely affect wound healing and scar formation. Disease processes such as diabetes mellitus significantly retard wound healing because small-vessel disease inhibits normal collagen synthesis.

8. **What is the association of antibiotic medicines and acute tendinopathy and tendon ruptures?**

Fluoroquinolones (FQs) (Cipro) are a popular class of antibiotics with broad-spectrum coverage for a number of gram-negative pathogens. Beginning first in 1983 there have been many anecdotal and case-controlled studies reporting the incidence of tendon ruptures associated with FQs, with 90% occurring in the Achilles tendon. Tendon rupture is nearly always preceded by spontaneous onset of pain within 2 to 3 cm of the insertion point, thought to be closely correlated with reduced vascularization at this site. Other tendons reported to be affected include the biceps brachii, supraspinatus, and extensor pollicis longus.

9. **What risk factors are associated with FQ antibiotic-induced tendon rupture?**

Identified risk factors associated with FQ (eg, Cipro)-induced tendon rupture or tendinopathy include age over 60, previous corticosteroid use, renal failure, diabetes mellitus, and a history of musculoskeletal disorders such as other tendon ruptures. The latency period between the administration of FQ antibiotic treatment and occurrence of tendinopathy has a median onset of 6 days with half of tendon ruptures occurring within 1 week of taking the medicine. FQs are known to cause direct toxicity to type 1 collagen synthesis and promote collagen degradation.

10. **What influence does nutrition play in the soft tissue repair process?**

Collagen biosynthesis is especially sensitive to the availability of proper nutrients. Lack of vitamins C and A impedes the process of collagen synthesis. Glucosamine, found within collagen type II, is the critical compound in connective tissue repair and production. Glucosamine is the precursor for compounds important to connective tissue health, such as chondroitin sulfate and hyaluronic acid, and increases proteoglycan production. Whether dietary supplements such as glucosamine have a significant and lasting effect on joint disease has not been well established in controlled clinical trials, though mounting evidence suggests that such supplements are beneficial. Recent studies indicate that glucosamine may limit the advancement of joint space narrowing associated with osteoarthritis, resulting in improved functional scores. Minerals such as zinc contribute to the normal rate of cell proliferation and ultimate wound strength.

11. **What role does aging play in altering the soft tissue injury healing process?**

Age-related effects on wound healing include attenuated metabolic activity, decreased vascular supply, diminished cellular biosynthesis, delayed collagen remodeling, and decreased wound strength. Despite these differences, many of which have been confirmed in animal studies, clinical experience indicates that older patients often undergo surgical treatment with no adverse healing responses related to aging.

12. **How does tendinitis differ from tendinosis?**

Historically, painful tendon conditions were referred to as “tendinitis” and were assumed to be an inflammatory condition. Over time, however, further analysis revealed that the condition was not attended by inflammatory cells but was a degenerative change in the tendon—more accurately referred to as “overuse tendinosis.” Tendinitis (paratendinitis) is a rather rare condition that may occur occasionally in the Achilles tendon but almost always in conjunction with a primary tendinosis. The paratenon, a double-layered sheath of loose areolar tissue, is attached to the outer connective tissue surface of tendons that do not have a synovial lining. Paratendinitis refers to inflammation and thickening of the paratenon sheath. The pathology of tendinosis is characterized by a loss of collagen continuity and an increase in ground substance, vascularity, and cellularity. Research indicates that substance P, a neuropeptide known to contribute to tendon pain, is upregulated with tendon overuse. The cellularity increase associated with tendinosis results from fibroblasts and myofibroblasts, but inflammatory cells are absent. Because of this new understanding, it has been recommended that the term *tendinopathy* replace the term *tendinitis* for describing tendon pathology.

13. **What is the appropriate treatment for tendinosis?**

Treatment efforts to reduce pain and tenderness include ice application, oral NSAID administration, iontophoresis, rest, and cortisone injection. However, because tendinosis is by definition a chronic condition, treatment usually focuses on a controlled eccentric training program, often lengthy (10–12 weeks or more in some cases) in duration.

For Achilles tendinopathy, the most widely adopted approach is the Alfredson protocol of eccentric heel-drop exercises. This high-volume regimen (slow resistance loading) has been shown to be particularly effective in athletic patients, though less so in nonathletic and older patients. Evidence clearly points toward exercise and mechanical loading as the best documented strategy for treating patients with tendinosis. Progressive, plyometric-based loading represents an integral element in tendinosis rehabilitation, though specific dosing of exercise for various conditions remains an area in need of additional research.

14. **What is the role of the nervous system in contributing to the pain of tendinopathies?**
There is growing recognition of the important role that the central nervous system plays in the persistence of pain associated with tendinopathies. Sensitization of the peripheral and central nervous system has been documented for patients with persistent tendon pain. Decreased mechanical pain thresholds, suggesting widespread hyperalgesia, have been reported in human subjects with both upper and lower extremity tendinopathies.

15. **What interventions might be useful for central sensitization pain associated with persistent tendinopathies?**
Therapeutic neuroscience education has been shown to be useful for helping patients with longstanding musculoskeletal pain, though this intervention has been primarily directed at patients with pain of spinal origin. Trigger point dry needling has also been a tool used to address chronic pain associated with tendinopathies. The specific underlying physiologic effects of dry needling remain elusive, but many researchers indicate it is most likely to have a positive effect on the local and central sensitization effects of persistent pain. This remains an area of considerable research at present.

16. **What tissue changes occur in response to a period of immobilization after soft tissue injury?**
Immobility after soft tissue injury alters the rate of the biological process of remodeling. Changes that result in this alteration include an increased density of cells (usually fibroblasts), the presence of myofibroblasts, a reduction in hyaluronic acid and chondroitin sulfate levels in the periarticular connective tissue, and a 4% to 6% reduction in water content of the same tissues after only 9 weeks of immobilization. Further changes include a shift in the balance between collagen synthesis and degradation, which results in a reduction in total collagen.

17. **What is the effect of immobilization on stiffness and strength of injured soft tissue?**
Experimental evidence in rabbits indicates that 9 weeks of immobilization results in a 50% reduction in the normal breaking strength of the medial collateral ligament. At the same time a significant increase in the intermolecular cross-links of collagen leads to contracture formation. Therefore, the remodeled connective tissue after immobilization is both thicker (tendency toward contracture) and weaker, possibly because of the random alignment of collagen fibers.

18. **How do stress and motion affect connective tissue repair after injury?**
Stress and motion have a profound effect on the quality of soft tissue repair after injury or surgery. Many studies have documented that scar tissue forms earlier in mobilized tendons, is well oriented, and is not attended by adhesions, in contrast to scar tissue that develops without physiologic stresses. Exposure of scar tissue to physiologic tensile forces during the healing process results in a more mature and stronger union of tendon and ligament. Healing of articular cartilage involves a greater amount of collagen and glycosaminoglycans, less cellularity, and fewer scar tissue adhesions when accompanied by modest joint movements. Some experimental evidence indicates that ultrasound application to tenotomized Achilles tendons improves tensile strength of the tissue if administered during postoperative days 2 to 4. This response appears to be time dependent and may be related to limiting the inflammatory response and encouraging fibroplasia and fibrillogenesis. In a similar manner, high-voltage electrical stimulation appears to augment protein synthesis and the ultimate strength of the tendon if applied during the early stages of healing.

19. **After ligament and tendon repair or reconstruction, when is the soft tissue the strongest and when is it the weakest?**
Much of the information related to this question has been derived from studies using animal models (primates and others) and should be interpreted with caution. General data indicate that the strength of the patellar tendon autograft used in anterior cruciate ligament reconstruction cases is strongest on the day that it is surgically implanted. As the tissue heals in its new location, its strength diminishes to significantly <50% during the first 4 to 8 weeks postoperatively. In the ensuing 3 to 6 months, there is a slow transformation of collagen type and revascularization of the graft tissue. Stiffness and load to failure continue to increase for many months, and at 1 year the tissue is reported to have achieved 82% of its original strength. The clinical implications are fairly straightforward: protect the graft in the early stages of rehabilitation, encourage closed-chain axial loading activity to minimize shear forces (joint translation), and emphasize maximal motor unit activation throughout the rehabilitation process.

20. **What is the response of articular cartilage to chondroplasty (microfracture technique, abrasion, and drilling) of the undersurface of the patella?**
The microfracture technique is used to stimulate tissue repair of full-thickness articular cartilage defects. A drill is used to make multiple perforations in the subchondral bone in the area of the cartilage defect in an effort to produce a "super clot." Over a period of 8 weeks or more the super clot heals with a hybrid mixture of fibrocartilage and type II (hyaline-like) collagen. This hybrid repair tissue may be functionally better than fibrocartilage alone; early animal and human studies suggest that it is durable enough to function like articular cartilage.

21. **Describe the scientific evidence supporting articular cartilage repair.**
Reproduced chondrocyte cells harvested from the patient are injected under a periosteal flap covering the articular defect. Two-year follow-up studies of patients with femoral condyle transplants indicate excellent results; most patients developed hyaline-like cartilage in the defect site. Patellar lesions have not done as well, possibly because of shear forces or noncorrection of underlying malalignment abnormalities. Research is encouraging for focal chondral defects but not for generalized osteoarthritis of the joint. In addition, there is evidence that articular cartilage exposed to electric and electromagnetic fields can lead to a sustained upregulation of growth factors, enhancing its viability. The degradative enzymes in the synovial fluid of osteoarthritic joints are not conducive to cell transfer with cartilage transplant experimental procedures.

22. **What growth factors are involved with soft tissue healing?**
- Chemotactic factors—prostaglandins, complement, platelet-derived growth factor (PDGF), and angiokines
- Competence factors—activate quiescent cells, PDGF, and prostaglandins
- Progression factors—stimulate cell growth, such as IL-1 and somatomedins
- Enhancing factors—fibronectin and osteonectin

23. **What is the effect of NSAIDs on muscle recovery?**
Short-term use (<1 week) of NSAIDs after muscular strain may improve recovery. However, long-term use (>1 month) may result in decreased recovery.

24. **What factors affect allograft strength?**
Freeze-drying reduces the immunogenic response but also decreases strength. Greater than 3-megarad irradiation will also decrease strength. Less radiation (2 megarads) in combination with ethylene oxide will decrease graft strength. Allografts have a slower, less predictable recovery than autografts.

25. **What growth factors may aid in soft tissue repair?**
Platelet-rich plasma (PRP) (Orthobiologics) has been shown to improve soft tissue healing in horses with improved collagen abundance and organization. Recent clinical studies of patients with a variety of musculoskeletal conditions (lateral epicondylitis, rotator cuff disease, Achilles tendon ruptures, knee osteoarthritis) show inconsistent evidence of improvement following PRP injections. Macrophage-secreted myogenic factors may someday play a role in inducing muscle repair. Specific chondrocyte growth factors and bone morphogenetic protein (BMP) have shown promise in improving cartilage repair.

Bibliography

Akeson, W. H., Woo, S. L., Amiel, D., Coutts, R. D., & Daniel, D. (1973). The connective tissue response to immobility: biochemical changes in periarticular connective tissue of the immobilized rabbit knee. *Clinical Orthopaedics, 93*, 356–361.

Alford, J. W., & Cole, B. J. (2005). Cartilage restoration, Part 1: basic science, historical perspective, patient education, and treatment options. *The American Journal of Sports Medicine, 33*, 295–306.

Alfredson, H., Pietila, T., Jonsson, P., & Lorentzon, R. (1998). Heavy-load eccentric calf muscle training for the treatment of chronic Achilles tendinosis. *The American Journal of Sports Medicine, 26*, 360–366.

Boesen, A. P., Boesen, M. I., Hansen, R., et al. (2020). Effect of platelet-rich plasma on nonsurgically treated acute Achilles tendon ruptures: a randomized, double-blinded prospective study. *American Journal of Sports Medicine, 48*, 2268–2276.

Cagnie, B., Dewitte, V., Barbe, T., et al. (2013). Physiologic effects of dry needling. *Current Pain and Headache Reports, 17*, 348.

Carter, C. A., Jolly, D. G., Worden, C. E., Sr., Hendren, D. G., & Kane, C. J. M. (2003). Platelet rich plasma promotes differentiation and regeneration during equine wound healing. *Experimental and Molecular Pathology, 74*, 244–255.

Chen, F. S., Frenkel, S. R., & DiCesare, P. E. (1997). Chondrocyte transplantation and experimental treatment options for articular cartilage defects. *The American Journal of Orthopedics, 6*, 396–406.

Ciccone, C. D., & Wolf, S. L. (1990). Non-steroidal anti-inflammatory drugs. In C. D. Ciccone (Ed.), *Pharmacology in rehabilitation* (pp. 160–172). Philadelphia, PA: FA Davis.

Coronado, R. A., Simon, C. B., Valencia, C., & George, S. Z. (2014). Experimental pain responses support peripheral and central sensitization in patients with unilateral shoulder pain. *Clinical Journal of Pain, 30*, 143–151.

Curwin, S. L. (1998). The etiology and treatment of tendinitis. In M. Harris (Ed.), *Oxford textbook of sports medicine* (2nd ed., pp. 610–627). Oxford: Oxford University Press.

Devereux, D. F., Thibault, L., Boretos, J., & Brennan, M. F. (1979). The quantitative and qualitative impairment of wound healing by adriamycin. *Cancer, 43*, 932.

English, T., Wheeler, M. E., & Hettinga, D. L. (1997). Inflammatory response of synovial joint structure. In T. R. Malone, T. McPoil, & A. J. Nitz (Eds.), *Orthopedic and sports physical therapy* (3rd ed., pp. 81–113). St. Louis, MO: Mosby.

Enwemeka, C. S. (1989). Inflammation, cellularity and fibrillogenesis in regenerating tendon: Implications for tendon rehabilitation. *Physical Therapy, 69*, 816–825.

Frank, C., Amiel, D., & Woo, S. L. -Y. (1985). Normal ligament properties and ligament healing. *Clinical Orthopaedics, 196*, 15–25.

Goodson, W. H., & Hung, T. K. (1977). Studies of wound healing in experimental diabetes mellitus. *The Journal of Surgical Research, 22*, 211.

Goodson, W. H., & Hunt, T. K. (1979). Wound healing and aging. *The Journal of Investigative Dermatology, 73*, 88.

Gross, M. T. (1992). Chronic tendinitis: pathomechanics of injury, factors affecting the healing response and treatment. *The Journal of Orthopaedic and Sports Physical Therapy, 16*, 248–261.

Huang, K., Giddins, G., & Wu, L. D. (2020). Platelet-rich plasma versus corticosteroid injections in the management of elbow epicondylitis and plantar fasciitis: an updated systematic review and meta-analysis. *American Journal of Sports Medicine, 48*, 2572–2585.
Jo, C. H., Lee, S. Y., Yoon, K. S., Oh, S., & Shin, S. (2020). Allogeneic platelet-rich plasma versus corticosteroid injection for the treatment of rotator cuff disease: a randomized controlled trial. *Journal of Bone and Joint Surgery, 102*, 2129–2137.
Khan, K. M., Cook, J. L., Taunton, J. E., & Bonar, F. (2000). Overuse tendinosis, not tendinitis. Part 1: A new paradigm for a difficult clinical problem. *The Physician and Sports Medicine, 28*, 38–48.
Kingma, J. J., de Knikker, R., Wittink, H. M., & Takken, T. (2007). Eccentric overload training in patients with chronic Achilles tendinopathy: a systematic review. *British Journal of Sports Medicine, 41*, e3.
Kloth, L. C., & McCulloch, J. M. (1995). The inflammatory response to wounding. In J. M. McCulloch, L. C. Kloth, & J. A. Feedar (Eds.), *Wound healing alternatives in management* (2nd ed., pp. 3–15). Philadelphia, PA: FA Davis.
Lieber, R. L., Bjorn-Ove, L., & Friden, J. (1997). Sarcomere length in wrist extensor muscles. *Acta Orthopaedica Scandinavica, 68*, 249–254.
Lineaweaver, W., Howard, R., Soucy, D., et al. (1985). Topical antimicrobial toxicity. *Archives of Surgery, 120*, 267.
Magnussen, R. A., Dunn, W. R., & Thomson, A. B. (2009). Non-operative treatment of midportion Achilles tendinopathy: a systematic review. *Clinical Journal of Sport Medicine, 19*, 54–64.
Medzhitov, R. (2008). Origin and physiologic roles of inflammation. *Nature, 454*, 428–435.
Modolin, M., Bevilacqua, R. G., Margarido, N. F., & Lima-Goncalves, E. (1985). Effects of protein depletion and repletion on experimental wound contraction. *Annals of Plastic Surgery, 15*, 123.
Reginster, J. Y., Deroisy, R., Rovati, L. C., et al. (2001). Long-term effects of glucosamine sulphate on osteoarthritis progression: a randomized, placebo-control clinical trial. *Lancet, 357*, 251–256.
Rio, E., Moseley, L., Purdam, C., et al. (2014). The pain of tendinopathy: physiological or pathophysiological? *Sports Medicine, 44*, 9–23.
Tang, S., Wang, X., Wu, P., et al. (2020). Platelet-rich plasma vs autologous blood vs corticosteroid injections in the treatment of lateral epicondylitis: a systematic review, pairwise and network meta-analysis of randomized controlled trials. *Physical Medicine & Rehabilitation, 12*, 397–409.
Uygur, E., Aktas, B., & Yilmazoglu, E. G. (2021). The use of dry needling vs. corticosteroid injection to treat lateral epicondylitis: a prospective, randomized, controlled study. *Journal of Shoulder and Elbow Surgery, 30*, 134–139.
van Ark, M., Rio, E., Cook, J., et al. (2018). Clinical improvements are not explained by changes in tendon structure or ultrasound tissue characterization after an exercise program for patellar tendinopathy. *American Journal of Physical Medicine & Rehabilitation, 97*, 708–714.
Van Story-Lewis, P. E., & Tennenbaum, H. C. (1986). Glucocorticoid inhibition of fibroblast contraction of collagen gels. *Biochemical Pharmacology, 35*, 1283.
Videman, T. (1987). Connective tissue and immobilization. *Clinical Orthopaedics, 221*, 26–32.
Wagner, S., Coerper, S., Fricke, J., et al. (2003). Comparison of inflammatory and systemic sources of growth factors in acute and chronic human wounds. *Wound Repair and Regeneration, 11*, 253–260.
Weiss, E. L. (1995). Connective tissue in wound healing. In J. M. McCulloch, L. C. Kloth, & J. A. Feedar (Eds.), *Wound healing alternatives in management* (2nd ed., pp. 16–31). Philadelphia, PA: FA Davis.
Williams, R. J., Attia, E., & Wickiewicz, T. L. (2000). The effect of ciprofloxacin on tendon, paratenon, and capsular fibroblast metabolism. *American Journal of Sports Medicine, 28*, 364–369.
Woo, S. L., Horibe, S., & Ohland, K. (1990). The response of ligaments to stress deprivation and stress enhancement. In D. Daniel, W. Akeson, & J. O'Connor (Eds.), *Knee ligaments: structure, function, injury and repair* (pp. 337–350). New York, NY: Raven Press.
Woo, S. L. -Y., Gelberman, R. H., Cobb, N. G., et al. (1981). The importance of controlled passive mobilization on flexor tendon healing. *Acta Orthopaedica Scandinavica, 52*, 615–622.
Yu, C., & Guiffre, B. M. (2005). Achilles tendinopathy after treatment with fluoroquinolone. *Australasian Radiology, 49*, 407–410.

CHAPTER 3 QUESTIONS

1. **Which is a risk factor associated with Achilles tendon rupture related to FQ antibiotic administration?**
   a. Age range of 20 to 40
   b. No prior history of corticosteroid use
   c. History of diabetes mellitus
   d. History of liver failure

2. **The most widely adopted and evidence-based approach for the treatment of tendinosis/tendinopathy is:**
   a. Steroid injection at the lesion site
   b. Eccentric exercises (eg, Alfredson protocol)
   c. Progressive concentric strength training of the musculo tendinous unit
   d. Iontophoresis of 4% acetic acid solution to the tendon lesion

3. **Which of the following growth factors for soft tissue healing is correctly matched with the appropriate agent?**
   a. Regression factors—interleukin 4
   b. Enhancing factors—prostaglandins
   c. Chemotactic factors—platelet-derived growth factor (PDGF)
   d. Immunoglobulin M (IgM)

BONE INJURY AND REPAIR

A.J. Nitz, PT, PhD

1. **What are the components that make up bone?**
   - Cells
   - Ground substance
   - Fibrous tissue network

   The cellular component consists of osteoblasts, which produce and initiate mineralization of new bone and cartilage, and osteoclasts, which are essential for the removal of the callus for lamellar bone to be laid down. A third cell type found in mature adult bone is the osteocyte.

   The ground substance component of bone contains mostly calcium phosphate, glycosaminoglycans, and hyaluronic acid. Calcium phosphate helps to add rigidity and hardness to the bone.

   The fibrous component consists of collagen fibers, which help resist tensile stress, and elastin fibers, which add a resilient aspect to the bone.

2. **Describe the effects of aging on bone structure.**
   The most commonly known age-related change is a calcium-related loss of mass and density. This loss ultimately causes the pathologic condition of osteoporosis. Osteoporosis is a major bone mineral disorder in older adults that decreases the bone mineral content; as a result, bone mass and strength decline with age. In geriatric patients, the hormonal system regulating calcium metabolism is less efficient and responds poorly to the challenge of a calcium-incorporating process, such as callous formation. Aging influences tissues (ie, the kidneys, gastrointestinal tract, and endocrine system) of the body that affect calcium metabolism and bone physiology. Thus the process of fracture healing in the geriatric patient is altered to some extent. Calcitonin, a hormone associated with decreasing serum calcium levels and possibly the remodeling of bone, has a decreased responsiveness to a calcium challenge with age. This decrease in calcitonin response may account, in part, for the slow bone healing in geriatric patients. Bones of older adults can withstand about half the strain of the bones of younger adults. Bones of older adults are less pliable and less able to store energy. Although there are physiologic changes that occur during the aging process that can affect bone health, the more sedentary lifestyle of many older individuals also may account for many of the age-associated changes in bone health.

3. **How does Wolff's law apply to bone healing?**
   The ability of bone to adapt by changing size, shape, and structure depends on the mechanical stress on the bone. When optimal stress is placed on bone, there is greater bone deposition than bone reabsorption. This results in hypertrophy of periosteal bone and increased bone density. When bone is subjected to less than optimal stress, reabsorption of periosteal bone can occur, resulting in a decrease in strength and stiffness. Optimal stress within an appropriate range is essential for bone strength.

4. **List the different types of bone fractures.**
   - Compound (open)—occurs when sharp ends of the broken bone protrude through the victim's skin or when some projectile penetrates the skin into the fracture site
   - Closed—skin remains intact
   - Perforating (eg, gunshot-bullet penetration)—may involve loss of bone from the effect of high-level energy at the fracture site
   - Depressed or fissured—occurs when a sharply localized blow depresses a segment of cortical bone below the level of the surrounding bone (eg, a skull fracture)
   - Greenstick—occurs on one side of the bone but does not tear the periosteum of the opposite side (seen in children)
   - Spiral—caused by opposite rotatory forces pulling on the bone (twisting)
   - Oblique—oriented at an angle of $\geq$30 degrees to the axis of the bone
   - Transverse—oriented at a right angle to the axis of the bone
   - Avulsion—may be produced by a sudden muscle contraction, with the muscle pulling off the portion of the bone to which it is attached; also may result from traction on a ligamentous or capsular attachment
   - Comminuted—involves multiple fracture fragments
   - Stress—results from stresses repeated with excessive frequency to a bone
   - Pathologic—arises in abnormal or diseased bones; pathologic conditions that can lead to fractures include carcinomas, infection, and osteoporosis

5. **What is a bone bruise and how does it relate to bone fractures?**
Bone bruise (bone marrow contusion) is now considered to be one of four types of bone injuries that fall under the general heading of *fracture*—the others being stress fractures, osteochondral fractures, and frank fractures (described in the list earlier in #4). The distribution of bone marrow edema has been likened to a footprint left behind by the musculoskeletal injury and is produced by compression and traction forces impacting adjacent bones. Availability of definitive imaging by MRI has provided evidence that bone edema (bone bruising) may persist for many months following musculoskeletal injury and is thought to account for some of the post-injury pain experienced by patients. Further analysis indicates that there are actually three types of bone bruises:
   a. Subperiosteal hematoma—a concentrated accumulation of blood underneath the periosteum after high-force trauma and most often seen in the lower extremities
   b. Interosseous bone bruise—occurs most often with repetitive, high-compression forces that damage the blood supply in the bone marrow; usually occurs in the knee and ankle of professional athletes (eg, football and basketball players and elite runners)
   c. Subchondral lesion—occurs beneath the cartilage layer of a joint and is usually caused by extreme compression or shear forces. Often there is microscopic separation of the cartilage and the underlying bone and is, again, most often seen in football and basketball players

6. **How are bone bruises identified?**
Bone bruises are not visible with plain film radiographs, though this imaging modality may confirm that a frank fracture has not occurred. Most often bone bruises are visualized by means of T1- or T2-weighted fat-suppressed MRI. Patients with bone bruises tend to have a prolonged clinical recovery time with antalgic gait, slower recovery of motion, and persistent effusion compared with those with similar joint injuries who do not also have this complication.

7. **Discuss the stages of bone healing.**
The first stage is referred to as the inflammatory phase, or the granulation stage, fracture stage, or clot stage. During this phase surviving cells are sensitized to chemical messengers that are involved in the healing process. Macrophages, neutrophils, and platelets release cytokines including PDGF and TNF-alpha and may be detected as early as 24 hours following the bone injury. The lack of TNF-alpha, in particular, results in delay of endochondral and intramembranous ossification. This initial aspect of the first stage is probably completed within 7 days. A second feature of the initial stage is the development of a clot around the fracture site (not seen in stress fracture healing). After the formation of the clot, granulation tissue forms in the space between the fracture fragments. This granulation tissue activates macrophages, whose function is to remove the clot. This second aspect of the initial stage lasts about 2 weeks.

The second stage is known as the reparative phase or callous stage and can be divided further into soft callous and hard callous stages. Osteoblasts and chondrocytes within the granulation tissue begin to synthesize cartilage and weave bone matrices (soft callus). Approximately 1 week later, the newly formed soft callus begins to mineralize. This mineralization concludes several weeks later with the formation of a fracture (hard) callus. The hard callus is detectable on radiographs because of the calcium it contains. The creation and mineralization of the callus can require 4 to 16 weeks to complete.

The third stage is called the remodeling or consolidation phase and involves several processes. First the callus is replaced by woven bone, which in turn is replaced with packets of new lamellar bone. The callus plugging the marrow cavity is removed, restoring the cavity. It has been estimated that the complete replacement of the callus with functionally competent lamellar bone can take 1 to 4 years.

8. **Name some conditions that have a negative effect on the bone healing process.**

TECHNICAL FACTORS*	BIOLOGICAL FAILURES†	MISCELLANEOUS CONDITIONS
Infection	Vascular injury	Poor nutrition
Poor reduction	Failure to make or mineralize callus (because of metabolic abnormalities)	Alcohol abuse
Distraction	Formation of scar and fat tissue instead of callus	Smoking
Repeated gross motion of fracture fragments	Inability to replace woven bone with lamellar bone (eg, children with osteogenesis imperfecta)	—

TECHNICAL FACTORS*	BIOLOGICAL FAILURES†	MISCELLANEOUS CONDITIONS
Loss of local blood supply because of injury and/or surgical procedure	—	—

*In these situations, the potential for normal healing is present, but problems during the treatment have prevented the healing process from proceeding, resulting in delayed union or nonunion.
†Biological failures refer to abnormalities in the biology of the healing process that delay or prevent union even with proper treatment. Smoking, in particular, has been singled out as a factor associated with delayed healing and rates of infection. It is believed that the reduced peripheral blood supply results in delayed healing of bone and accounts for the higher infection risk that patients who smoke experience following bone fracture.

9. **Discuss the effect that smoking has on the bone healing process.**

In studies in which animals were administered nicotine, a significant decrease in callous formation and an increase in the prevalence of nonunions were documented. Nicotine-exposed bones have been shown to be significantly weaker in a three-point bending test compared with controls. Smoking and nicotine have been shown to delay the revascularization and incorporation of bone grafts and to increase the pseudarthrosis rate in spinal fusion patients. One study found that patients with fractured tibias who smoked took 62% longer to heal than nonsmokers. Nicotine has been shown to have a direct inhibitory effect on bone cellular proliferation and function. These changes, taken together with the vascular effects, result in a decrease in the quantity and maturity of the fracture callus. It has been estimated that the risk of fractures is two to six times higher in patients who smoke because of reduced bone density in these patients. Somewhat unexpectedly, current and previous smokers have been shown to be significantly more likely to develop infections (including osteomyelitis) after fractures. Damaged soft tissue and impaired nerve function (neurogenic inflammation) can impede fracture healing by increasing the metabolic demand of the tissue repair system and limiting the benefit of supportive muscle function around the fracture site. Such failures usually require downward revision of the rehabilitation timetable and ultimate recovery potential for the patient.

10. **What steps may be taken by a patient to promote accelerated fracture healing?**

a. Traumatic fractures of the long bones and patients with multiple fractures require as much as three times the caloric intake compared with normal nutritional demands.
b. Specifically, increasing protein intake enhances growth factors, such as insulin-like growth factor-1, which exerts a beneficial effect on skeletal integrity and bone renewal in particular.
c. Vitamins C, D, and K, along with mineral intake and antiinflammatory nutrients, should be increased. Antiinflammatory nutrients (antioxidants) repair oxidative damage that would otherwise suppress fracture healing. Such antioxidants include vitamins E and C, lycopene, and alpha-lipoic acid.

11. **Discuss the effect calcium nutrition has on bone healing.**

Nutritional deficiencies have a significant impact on the rate of fracture healing. Vitamin D and calcium are particularly crucial for bone healing; one recent study showed 84% of patients with nonunion were found to have metabolic issues with 66% of these demonstrating vitamin D deficiencies. Calcium plays an important role in helping attain peak bone mass during bone development and in preventing fractures later in life. The daily recommended allowance of calcium for nonpregnant, nonlactating women is 800 mg/day. This level increases to 1500 mg/day in postmenopausal, estrogen-depleted women. It is estimated that 75% of all women ingest less than the recommended daily allowance. Men tend to meet their calcium needs more successfully by consuming twice as much calcium at the same age. Multiple factors can affect the bioactivity of calcium. High-fat or high-fiber diets can interfere with or decrease the activity of calcium. Large doses of zinc supplementation or megadoses of vitamin A can lower calcium bioactivity. High-protein diets can decrease calcium reserves by increasing urinary excretion of calcium.

12. **What other factors affect calcium absorption?**

Alcohol consumption can decrease the absorption of calcium by a direct cytotoxic effect on the intestinal mucosa. Various medications, such as glucocorticoids, heparin, and anticonvulsants, can affect calcium activity.

Vitamin D increases serum calcium levels by enhancing intestinal absorption of calcium and enhancing parathyroid hormone–stimulating reabsorption of bone. A low level of vitamin D impairs the ability of the body to adapt to low levels of calcium intake and may contribute to the pathogenesis of osteoporosis. Intake of vitamin D alone has never been shown to improve fracture healing.

13. **Define closed reduction, open reduction, and rigid external fixation in fracture treatment.**
 - Closed reduction—use of casting or traction
 - Open reduction—surgical intervention using plates, screws, or other internal fixation devices
 - Rigid external fixation—combination of closed and open reduction using percutaneous pins and external stabilizing bars

14. **What are the advantages of closed reduction?**
 Avoidance of surgery, reduction of the fracture, and usually (except in the case of traction) a shorter hospital stay are all advantages of closed reduction. Usually the patient can safely begin gentle range of motion exercises several weeks before the fractured limb is strong enough to return to normal weight-bearing function or to withstand resistance at the fracture site. In later stages of fracture healing, splints can be worn to protect the fractured limb, which is to be removed at intervals to permit joint mobilization or bathing.

15. **List advantages and disadvantages of open reduction.**
 Advantages:
 - Precise bone reduction
 - Early mobilization of joints
 - Immediate stability, allowing earlier return to full function

 Disadvantages:
 - Increased possibility of infection
 - Increased hospital stay
 - Metal devices may require subsequent removal

16. **How does rigid fixation affect bone healing?**
 When rigid fixation is used, there is no stimulus for the production of the external callus from the periosteum or the internal callus from the endosteum (secondary bone healing). Instead the fracture healing occurs directly between the cortex of one fracture fragment and the cortex of the other fracture fragment (primary bone healing). Primary bone healing involves a direct repair of the bone lesion by new bridging osteons that become oriented through haversian remodeling to the long axis of the bone.

17. **What effects can internal fixation have on bone healing?**
 - Improper placement or tightening of plates, screws, nuts, or bolts in bone surgery may cause bone reabsorption because of local stress concentration or decreased vascular perfusion.
 - Plates that are too rigid may cause bone atrophy secondary to preventing the bone from perceiving intermittent compressive stress.
 - If the hardware needs to be removed, a secondary inflammatory response occurs that leads to weakening of the bone; the bone needs to be protected until it regains strength.
 - If the plates are left in place, problems with stress along the plate-bone interface can occur.

18. **List some advantages of weight-bearing activities after sustaining a fracture.**
 - Enhanced rehabilitation (eg, improved range of motion)
 - Shorter hospital stay
 - Less overall postfracture morbidity

19. **Describe a radiologic sign of a fracture of the radial head/neck.**
 Fat-pad signs constitute radiologic evidence of an effusion in the elbow joint and appear as areas of translucency on the lateral radiograph of the elbow flexed to a right angle. The fat-pad sign has an overall high negative predictive value (87%). The absence of the fat-pad sign can exclude a fracture and is a reliable indicator of the absence of a fracture. The presence of a fat-pad sign should only raise the suspicion of a fracture being present, however, because there may be a positive fat-pad sign with no fracture.

20. **What is the most commonly overlooked fracture in adults at the time of injury?**
 Carpal scaphoid fractures are easily overlooked. Because fractures of the scaphoid may result in loss of blood supply to the bone and consequent avascular necrosis, most physicians elect to treat wrist injuries as a fracture (immobilization) until properly interpreted radiographs indicate otherwise.

21. **Discuss the role of ultrasound in the treatment of acute fractures.**
 Low-intensity pulsed ultrasound (LIPUS) stimulation can accelerate the normal repair process in a fresh fracture and may help stimulate the healing process of nonunions. In animal models low-intensity pulsed ultrasound at 0.1 to 0.5 W/cm^2 accelerated fracture healing. Pulsed ultrasound at higher doses (1.0–2.0 W/cm^2) significantly inhibited the synthesis of collagen and noncollagenous protein, however. In clinical double-blind

studies, ultrasound has been shown to decrease significantly the time for overall healing of grade I open tibial fractures and distal radial fractures. Ultrasound has been shown to reduce significantly the prevalence of delayed union in nonsmokers and smokers. In animal studies ultrasound increased bone mineral content and density, increased peak torque, and accelerated the overall endochondral ossification process. Ultrasound stimulation may increase the mechanical properties of the healing fracture callus by stimulating earlier synthesis of extracellular matrix proteins in cartilage. The exact mechanism for enhancement of fracture healing with LIPUS stimulation is not clear but is thought to include alteration of protein expression, elevation of vascularity, and the development of mechanical strain gradient. Recent systematic reviews of the literature regarding LIPUS clinical studies have questioned the quality of the supporting research to date. However, the current evidence indicates that LIPUS may be useful for comminuted and/or open fractures that involve patients with associated risk comorbidities such as older age, smoking history, those with diabetes, and malnourished individuals. Simple fractures in otherwise healthy people should not be the target of LIPUS therapy according to the most recent evidence.

22. **What effect does bioelectric stimulation have on fracture healing?**
Implantable electric stimulation and pulsed electromagnetic field (surface application) have been used for healing nonunion tibial fractures with some success. Electric stimulation generally is thought to convert fibrous connective tissue to bone, possibly by simulating mechanical stress in the bone. The best results with implantable electrodes in animal studies have been associated with the cathode located in the fracture gap and the anode in adjacent bone or in the soft tissue. Ionic migration in response to external direct current is believed to be one probable explanation for the apparent efficacy of electric stimulation on bone healing.

23. **What is the effect of medications on bone healing?**
Bisphosphonates are recognized as a cause of osteoporotic fractures with long-term usage with recent studies demonstrating longer healing times for surgically treated wrist fractures in patients on bisphosphonates; long-term usage has also been reported to be associated with atypical subtrochanteric/femoral shaft fractures.
Systemic corticosteroids have a potentially deleterious effect on bone healing with studies showing a 6.5% higher rate of intertrochanteric fracture nonunions.
Long-term NSAIDs have been shown to prolong healing time because of COX enzyme inhibition. Quinolones are known to be toxic to chondrocytes and diminish fracture repair. Although there is still no well-defined answer, prostaglandins are known to participate in the inflammatory response and to stimulate osteoclasts as well as increase osteoblastic activity and subsequent new bone formation. It has become clear with recent studies that long-term excessive use of these medications may reduce normal bone healing.

24. **What are stress fractures, and how do they occur?**
Fatigue or stress fractures occur in otherwise healthy individuals usually in response to a sudden increase in physical activity of several weeks' duration. First described in military training as "march fractures," they are now fairly common in young individuals engaged in athletic activities and almost always represent a form of training error. In weight-bearing bones the overactivity causes microscopic fractures (debonding of osteons) that do not totally heal from day to day, eventually resulting in macroscopic bone failure and severe pain during ambulation or running. Though more common in the lower extremities, they can also occur in the medial epicondyle of the elbow with excessive throwing. Standard treatment involves early identification and rest of the involved extremity with avoidance of high-impact activities until healing has occurred. Signs of healing include resolution of bone tenderness with palpation and radiographic indication of healing—bone sclerosis.

25. **What is the best imaging method for detecting stress fractures?**
In spite of severe pain experienced by the patient, initial plain film radiographs of individuals suspected of a stress fracture are usually normal (up to 3–4 weeks after the initial onset of symptoms). Consequently, MRI and technetium bone scans are considered the best imaging studies for identifying stress fractures. Bone scans, in particular, may show signs of bone uptake as early as 72 hours after the onset of symptoms. However, radionucleotide (bone) scans have a disadvantage, compared with MRI, of exposing the patient to ionizing radiation. The American College of Radiology also recommends computerized tomography without contrast for early detection of a stress fracture, if MRI is contraindicated.

26. **What is bone transplantation (replacement), and why is it used?**
Bone transplantation (replacement) is an aggressive surgical technique whereby an entire diseased bone is excised and a cadaveric allograft replacement is transplanted in its place. This is usually necessitated by malignant bone tumors—primary or metastatic—and most of the descriptions in the current literature are of cases of femur transplantation. The alternative is typically an above-knee amputation or a hip disarticulation. Allograft replacement of the femur is prone to a number of complications, such as refracture, infection, nonunion, and resorption of the graft.

27. **What treatments are available for nonunions?**
    - Autogenous bone grafting and appropriate stable fixation
    - Vascularized bone grafting
    - Use of allografts or autografts with the addition of platelet-rich plasma (contains high levels of PDGF and TGF-β1)
    - Use of bone morphogenic proteins such as BMP-2
    - Mesenchymal stem cells
    - Muscle-derived stem cells

28. **How do Salter-Harris fractures influence the pediatric population?**
    The growth plate appears on a radiograph as a lucent line near the joint, and a fracture through that line can be missed easily unless there is some disturbance in the alignment of the bone. When there is an injury to the growth plate, growth disturbances may occur in that bone. The younger the patient, the greater the growth potential remaining; however, there is also the danger of significant growth disturbance.

29. **What are the roles of various growth factors on bone healing?**
    - BMP—Bone morphogenic protein induces metaplasia of undifferentiated perivascular mesenchymal cells into osteoblasts.
    - PDGF—Platelet-derived growth factor is chemotactic for inflammatory cells at the fracture site.
    - TGF-β—Transforming growth factor-β stimulates the production of type II collagen and proteoglycans at the fracture callus.
    - IGF-II—Insulin-like growth factor II stimulates type I collagen production and cellular proliferation.

BIBLIOGRAPHY

Ahl, T., Dalen, N., & Selvik, G. (1988). Mobilization after operation of ankle fractures: good results of early motion and weight bearing. *Acta Orthopaedica Scandinavica, 59*, 302–306.

Cimino, W., Ichtertz, D., & Slabaugh, P. (1991). Early mobilization of ankle fractures after open reduction and internal fixation. *Clinical Orthopaedics, 267*, 152–156.

Colson, D. J., Browett, J. P., Fiddian, N. J., & Watson, B. (1988). Treatment of delayed and nonunion of fractures using pulsed electromagnetic fields. *Journal of Biomedical Engineering, 10*, 301–304.

Cook, S. D., Ryaby, J. P., McCabe, J., et al. (1997). Acceleration of tibia and distal radius fracture healing in patients who smoke. *Clinical Orthopaedics, 337*, 198–207.

Eckardt, H., Christensen, K. S., Lind, M., et al. (2005). Recombinant human bone morphogenetic protein 2 enhances bone healing in an experimental model of fractures at risk of nonunion. *Injury, 36*, 489–494.

Einhorn, T. A., Levine, B., & Michel, P. (1990). Nutrition and bone. *The Orthopedic Clinics of North America, 21*, 43–50.

Frost, H. M. (1989a). The biology of fracture healing: an overview for clinicians: Part I. *Clinical Orthopaedics, 248*, 283–293.

Frost, H. M. (1989b). The biology of fracture healing: an overview for clinicians: Part II. *Clinical Orthopaedics, 248*, 294–309.

Hadjiargyrou, M., McLeod, K., Ryaby, J. P., & Rubin, C. (1998). Enhancement of fracture healing by low intensity ultrasound. *Clinical Orthopaedics, 355*(Suppl), S216–S229.

Harder, A. T., & An, Y. H. (2003). The mechanism of the inhibitory effects of nonsteroidal anti-inflammatory drugs on bone healing: A concise review. *The Journal of Clinical Pharmacology, 43*, 807–815.

Hayes, C. W., Brigido, M. K., Jamadar, D. A., & Propeck, T. (2000). Mechanism-based pattern approach to classification of complex injuries of the knee depicted at MR imaging. *Radiographics, 20*, S121–S134.

Hulth, A. (1989). Current concepts of fracture healing. *Clinical Orthopaedics, 249*, 265–284.

Khasigian, H. A. (1980). The results of treatment of nonunions with electrical stimulation. *Orthopedics, 31*, 32.

Kristiansen, T. K., Ryaby, J. P., McCabe, J., Frey, J. J., & Roe, L. R. (1997). Accelerated healing of distal radial fractures with the use of specific, low intensity ultrasound. *Journal of Bone and Joint Surgery, 75A*, 961–973.

Levangie, P. K., & Norkin, C. C. (2005). *Joint structure and function: a comprehensive analysis* (4th ed.). Philadelphia, PA: FA Davis.

Levine, J. D., Dardick, S. J., Basbaum, A. I., & Scipio, E. (1985). Reflex neurogenic inflammation: I. Contribution of the peripheral nervous system to spatially remote inflammatory responses that follow injury. *Journal of Neuroscience, 5*, 1380–1386.

Orthopedic and sports physical therapy Malone, T. R., McPoil, T., & Nitz, A. J. (Eds.), (1997). (3rd ed.). St. Louis: Mosby.

McRae, R. (Ed.), (1994). *Practical fracture treatment* (3rd ed.). New York, NY: Churchill Livingstone.

Meller, Y., Kestenbaum, R. S., & Shany, S. (1985). Parathormone, calcitonin, and vitamin D metabolites during normal fracture healing in geriatric patients. *Clinical Orthopaedics, 199*, 272–279.

Mooney, V. (1990). A randomized double-blind prospective study of efficacy of pulsed electromagnetic fields for interbody lumbar fusion. *Spine, 15*, 708–712.

Raikin, S. M., Landsman, J. C., Alexander, V. A., Froimson, M. I., & Plaxton, N. A. (1998). Effect of nicotine on the rate and strength of long bone fracture healing. *Clinical Orthopaedics, 353*, 231–237.

Sanders, T. G., Medynski, M. A., Feller, J. F., & Lawhorn, K. W. (2000). Bone contusion patterns of the knee at MR imaging: footprint of the mechanism of injury. *Radiographics, 20*, S135–S151.

Skaggs, D. L., & Vmirzayan, R. (1999). The posterior fat pad sign in association with occult fracture of the elbow in children. *Journal of Bone and Joint Surgery, 81A*, 1429–1433.

Thayer, L. S., Tiffany, E. M., & Carreira, D. S. (2021). Current concepts review: addressing smoking in musculoskeletal specialty care. *Journal of Bone and Joint Surgery, 103*, 2145–2152.

CHAPTER 4 QUESTIONS

1. **Bone bruises (bone marrow contusions) are most often visualized with which of the following imaging modalities:**
   a. Plain film radiographs
   b. Dexa-scan bone density imaging
   c. T1- or T2-weighted fat-suppressed MRI
   d. Bone scan—scintigraphy

2. **A variety of factors affect the bone healing process. Which of the following factors is NOT thought to impact bone healing?**
   a. Vascular injury
   b. Poor reduction
   c. Smoking
   d. Gender

3. **Which of the below promotes *accelerated* fracture healing?**
   a. Decreasing caloric intake
   b. Increasing protein intake
   c. Decreasing vitamin and antioxidant
   d. Increasing fat intake

CHAPTER 5

EXERCISE PHYSIOLOGY

B.A. Stamford, PhD, P.D. Loprinzi, PhD, and S. Maskalick

1. **What factor is considered to be the best indicator of an individual's level of aerobic capacity?**
   Maximum oxygen uptake (VO_{2max}) is the best indicator of aerobic capacity.

2. **How is VO_{2max} determined?**
   VO_{2max} is the product of cardiac output (heart rate × stroke volume) and arteriovenous oxygen difference (A – VO_2 diff). This is an example of the application of the Fick equation (VO_2 = cardiac output × arterial O_2/venous O_2 difference).

3. **How is VO_{2max} measured?**
   VO_{2max} is measured via various methodologies, including, for example:
   a. Laboratory assessment entails the use of sophisticated equipment that accurately measures percentages of expired O_2 and CO_2 plus the amount of air expired per minute (ventilatory volume). The amount of O_2 inspired per minute minus the amount expired is the VO_2, and when the VO_2 is pushed to ultimate capacity it is the VO_{2max}.
   b. Laboratory prediction tests can be used. Because VO_2 and heart rate are closely related, the heart rate response during various forms of exercise (ie, cycle ergometer) can be inserted into a prediction equation for the determination of VO_{2max}. The lower the heart rate during exercise the greater the predicted VO_{2max}.
   c. Field-based tests also can predict VO_{2max}. For example, the distance covered in the Cooper 12-minute walk/run test can be inserted into a prediction equation for the determination of VO_{2max}. The greater the distance covered the greater the predicted VO_{2max}.
   d. If the above tests are not available, it's possible to grossly approximate VO_{2max} from nonexercise algorithms taking into consideration the patient's self-reported physical activity, age, gender, and body mass index.

4. **Why is VO_{2max} considered the best indicator of aerobic fitness?**
   It is dependent on several factors:
   Aerobic fitness is the product of "central" and "peripheral" factors working together. Central factors determine the ability to "deliver" O_2 to the working muscles. Delivery depends upon the heart (cardiac output = heart rate × stroke volume), the lungs (ventilatory volume), the blood (hemoglobin), and the vessels (capillarization). The ability to "take up and utilize" the oxygen that has been delivered is determined by peripheral factors located in the working muscles. Specifically, the size and density of mitochondria present in the working muscles determine the ability to use oxygen to produce the energy required for muscular contractions.

5. **What are limiting factors in determining VO_{2max}?**
   - In individuals with asthma, chronic bronchitis, or emphysema, ventilatory compromise
   - In individuals with peripheral vascular disease, decreased tissue perfusion
   - In healthy individuals, the "central" component (maximal cardiac output) typically is the limiting factor. However, the "peripheral" component (size and density of mitochondria in the working muscle) also can be a limiting factor. In other words, it's possible that a huge amount of oxygen can be "delivered" to working muscles, but they may not be able to "use" it effectively to produce energy.

6. **Are the VO_{2max} values the same in an individual performing various exercises (eg, treadmill, cycling, arm ergometry)?**
   No. In general, the greater the amount of muscle mass used in the exercise, the greater the oxygen requirement. Since there can be only "one" *maximal* VO_2 level, the highest levels that are below the max level should be considered the VO_2 peak. Thus, if the highest level of VO_2 achieved on a cycle ergometer or arm crank ergometer is less than on a treadmill test, the cycle ergometer and arm crank values would represent a VO_2 peak for each mode of exercise.
   NOTE: If one is trained on the cycle ergometer, this could result in a higher VO_2 when compared to the treadmill. Thus, the cycle ergometer test could yield a VO_{2max}. This is an example of the concept of "task specificity."

7. **Why is the "central" factor (delivery of O_2) and the "peripheral" factor (utilization of O_2) greater in individuals who engage in regular physical activity?**

Chronic, sustained physical activity improves both the "central" (delivery) and "peripheral" (utilization) components. Greater delivery results primarily from training adaptations that include a greater cardiac output caused by an increase in stroke volume. Increased capillarization also helps delivery. The ability to take up and use more oxygen that has been delivered is dependent upon an increase in mitochondrial size and density in the working muscles.

8. **How does the VO_{2max} of a well-trained man compare with the VO_{2max} of a well-trained woman?**

When VO_{2max} is expressed per kilogram of body weight, the VO_{2max} of a well-trained man is approximately 20% higher than that of a well-trained woman. If VO_{2max} is expressed relative to lean body mass, it is only about 9% higher in men. The cause of the difference is not known, but it may be a result of a greater oxygen-carrying capacity in men caused by a higher hemoglobin content, larger blood volume, and higher cardiac output.

9. **Define other common indicators of physical fitness (a high VO_{2max}).**

- Blood lactate threshold—the intensity of exercise when there is a sudden increase in the amount of anaerobic metabolic activity reflected in a sudden increase (the threshold) in blood lactate concentration. The greater the intensity of exercise *before* the blood lactate threshold occurs, the greater the ability to work aerobically (with oxygen).
- Ventilatory threshold—a noninvasive indication of the blood lactate threshold. When blood lactate concentration suddenly increases, the accompanying metabolic acidosis triggers greater CO_2 production during the buffering process. CO_2 strongly stimulates ventilatory volume to suddenly increase (the threshold), which is easily detectable. As indicated above, the greater the intensity of exercise *before* the ventilatory threshold occurs, the greater the ability to work aerobically (with oxygen).

10. **Differentiate between physical activity, exercise, and physical fitness.**

- Physical activity is defined as any movement produced by a person's skeletal muscles that result in the expenditure of energy. NEAT (nonexercise activity thermogenesis) is any extraneous and unintentional muscular contractions that expend energy (ie, toe-tapping, fidgeting, etc.)
- Exercise is defined as a subset of physical activity that is planned, structured, and repetitive with the goal of the improvement or maintenance of a person's physical fitness
- Physical fitness is a set of attributes that can be either health- or skill-related and the degree of which can be measured with specific performance tests

11. **What are the five components of physical fitness?**

    1. Cardiovascular fitness—also known as cardiorespiratory fitness, is the ability of the heart, lungs, and vascular system to deliver oxygen-rich blood to working muscles during sustained physical activity. It also entails the ability of working muscles to utilize delivered oxygen.
    2. Muscular strength—the amount of force a muscle or muscle group can exert against a resistance, assessed with a 1-repetition maximal lift for isotonic exercise, or a maximal isometric contraction against an immovable object.
    3. Muscular endurance—the ability of a muscle or muscle group to repeat a physically challenging movement many times or to hold a particular position for an extended time.
    4. Flexibility—the ability of a joint to move through its full range of motion, from a flexed to an extended position.
    5. Body composition—the amount of fat in the body compared with the amount of lean mass. Body density is determined (eg, hydrostatic weighing) and results are inserted into a prediction equation that yields body fat reported as a percentage of whole-body mass (% fat).

12. **What is the effect of regular exercise on cardiometabolic parameters?**

Exercise has the potential to reduce levels of C-reactive protein (CRP), homocysteine, triglycerides, fasting glucose and insulin, hemoglobin A1c, and blood pressure. The effect of exercise to lower total cholesterol and low-density lipoprotein (LDL) cholesterol is modest (a reduced intake of saturated fat is more effective). Higher-intensity, high-volume exercise can increase high-density lipoprotein (HDL) cholesterol.

13. **What is the effect of regular exercise on neurologic parameters?**

Exercise is associated with a reduced risk of Parkinson's disease, Alzheimer's disease, and cognitive function, with possible mechanisms occurring from exercise-induced changes in the cerebral blood flow and metabolism, decreases in cortical accumulation of amyloid-β peptides, and increases in brain-derived neurotrophic factors.

14. What is oxygen deficit?

Oxygen deficit occurs when exercise begins and before achieving a steady-state (plateau) in VO_2. It is the difference between the amount of oxygen that is consumed at the onset of exercise and the amount of oxygen that is required. The energy deficit is covered anaerobically.

15. What effect does warming up have on the oxygen deficit?

It decreases it. Warming up increases blood flow, muscle temperature, and mitochondrial respiration, and these factors enable oxygen to be delivered to and used by working muscles more rapidly at the onset of exercise. There is less time for a deficit to develop, and this results in a smaller deficit.

16. How do the resting stroke volume, heart rate, and cardiac output of a well-trained athlete compare with those of a sedentary individual?

The resting stroke volume of an athlete is greater than that of a sedentary individual. Two major factors are involved. Early in training, there is an increase in plasma volume that contributes to greater end-diastolic volume. After considerable training, an athlete's cardiac muscle (ventricles) will hypertrophy, resulting in increased contractility.

The resting heart rate of sedentary males on average is 70 to 72 beats/minute, while in sedentary females it is 78 to 82 beats/min, the difference attributable to a larger male heart.

Well-trained male and female endurance athletes have a considerably lower resting heart rate. Here's why. Cardiac output (heart rate × stroke volume) at rest is similar in endurance athletes and sedentary individuals. The greater stroke volume in athletes allows for fewer heartbeats to achieve the same resting cardiac output.

17. How does the stroke volume response to exercise in the upright position differ between individuals who are physically fit and those who are not?

In a trained individual, stroke volume continues to increase until VO_{2max} is reached; in an untrained individual, stroke volume increases as exercise intensity increases up to about 50% of VO_{2max} and then remains steady. Maximal stroke volume is higher in fit individuals, and the stroke volume for any submaximal exercise intensity is higher in a fit individual.

18. How do heart rate, stroke volume, mean total peripheral resistance, mean arterial blood pressure, and respiratory rate change when exercise is performed using the upper extremities compared with a similar amount of exercise using the lower extremities?

These changes occur because vasodilation occurs in exercising muscles, and vasoconstriction occurs in nonexercising muscles (helping to reroute blood where it is needed most).

Upper extremity (arm) exercise involves smaller muscles than lower extremity (leg) exercise. This means with arm exercise (a smaller muscle mass), there is more overall vasoconstriction throughout the body (because vasoconstriction occurs in the larger nonexercising legs).

Conversely, with leg exercise (a larger muscle mass) there is less overall vasoconstriction throughout the body (because vasoconstriction occurs in the smaller nonexercising arms).

Greater overall vasoconstriction throughout the body during upper extremity exercise causes an increase in total peripheral resistance, resulting in higher heart rate, lower stroke volume, higher mean arterial pressure, and higher respiratory rate.

19. What is the acute response of systolic and diastolic blood pressure to aerobic exercise?

During acute incremental exercise, systolic blood pressure increases while diastolic blood pressure remains steady or slightly decreases. Post acute exercise systolic and diastolic pressure can lower in both hypertensive and normotensive individuals, often referred to as postexercise hypotension.

20. Describe the normal interaction of inotropes and chronotropes during exercise.

During exercise, the initial chronotropes and inotropes are the sympathetic nerves that directly innervate and stimulate the heart. Inotropes influence contractility, whereas chronotropes influence heart rate.

These terms, inotropic and chronotropic agents, also are used for classifying cardiac medications according to the impact imposed.

A slightly delayed chronotrope and inotrope effect comes from the adrenal medulla. When sympathetic nerves innervating the adrenal medulla are stimulated, epinephrine and norepinephrine are released into the blood. These hormones travel to the heart and perpetuate the response that was initiated by the sympathetic nerves.

(NOTE: In general, nerves impart an immediate and transient impact, whereas the impact of hormones is slower acting but longer lasting.)

21. **What effect does a low partial pressure of oxygen (Po_2) have on blood vessel diameter in the lung and in the systemic circulation?**
Vessels in the lung constrict when exposed to a low Po_2, whereas vessels in the systemic circulation dilate. The constriction of vessels in the lung shunts blood to the areas of the lung that are better ventilated. This results in better ventilation-perfusion matching, which causes more effective oxygenation of blood.
Dilation of systemic vessels enables more blood to be delivered to the area. This results in better oxygenation of the localized tissues.

22. **Discuss the effect long-term endurance training has on the heart and on blood volume.**
Increases in plasma volume occur shortly after the initiation of intense endurance training. This appears to be caused by an increase in plasma albumin levels, which osmotically draws fluid into the vasculature. Higher plasma volumes cause an increase in venous return, left ventricular end-diastolic volume, and stroke volume. These changes can occur within 1 week of the initiation of endurance training. Hypertrophy of myocardial muscle also occurs with endurance training, but this is a slower process.

23. **Describe the contributions of stored adenosine triphosphate (ATP), creatine phosphate, glycolysis, and aerobic metabolism toward providing ATP during intense exercise over time.**
- Stored ATP is used primarily for maximal intensity exercise, causing fatigue after about 4 seconds.
- If the intensity of exercise is such that fatigue occurs within 10 seconds, creatine phosphate is used to supply the energy to replenish the ATP stores during the last 6 seconds of exercise.
- Intense exercise lasting between 10 seconds and 2 minutes depends on anaerobic glycolysis (lactate production) to produce ATP. The maximal intensity of exercise is not as great as it was when creatine phosphate was being used.
- For intense exercise lasting longer than 2 minutes, aerobic metabolism provides most of the ATP and is supplemented by anaerobic glycolysis as intensity increases. The anaerobic contribution is progressively greater beyond the lactate threshold.

24. **What can be done to improve the systems for providing ATP during intense exercise?**
To improve the ability of creatine phosphate to provide energy, several bouts of intense exercise should be performed for 5 to 10 seconds with a 30- to 60-second rest between bouts. This is an example of high-intensity interval training (HIIT).
To improve anaerobic capacity, several bouts of intense exercise should be performed for at most 1 minute in duration (for example, maximal effort quarter-mile runs) with 3 to 5 minutes of recovery between bouts. This is called repetition training.
To improve aerobic capacity (VO_{2max}), perform longer duration interval training. An example is a maximal effort interval of half-mile runs for, say, 3 minutes each. After each run, brisk walk for an equal amount of time (3 minutes), then repeat for several bouts.

25. **What are the main muscle fiber types and their characteristics?**
Type I—slow oxidative (also called slow-twitch)
Type IIa—fast oxidative, glycolytic (also called intermediate)
Type IIx—fast glycolytic (also called fast-twitch) – also known as type IIb
NOTE: There are other "fine-tuned" classifications, but the above three classifications are accepted, in general.

PROPERTIES	TYPE I	TYPE IIA	TYPE IIX
Motor unit type	Slow oxidative	Fast oxidative glycolytic	Fast glycolytic
Motor unit type	Slow	Fast	Fast
Diameter	Small	Medium	Large
Twitch velocity	Low	Intermediate	High
Twitch force	Small	Medium	Large
Resistance to fatigue	High	Intermediate	Low
Glycogen content	Low	High	High
Capillary density	Rich	Rich	Poor
Myoglobin content	High	High	Low

PROPERTIES	TYPE I	TYPE IIA	TYPE IIX
Color	Dark red	Dark red	Pale
Mitochondrial density	High	High	Low
Oxidative capacity	High	Moderate-high	Low

26. **Which type of muscle fiber is activated during moderate-intensity, long-duration exercise, such as jogging?**
Slow-twitch (type I) fibers are primarily activated.

27. **Which type of muscle fiber is activated during high-intensity, short-term exercise, such as sprinting?**
Slow-twitch type I fibers are always activated first regardless of the type of activity (according to the "size principle" – size meaning the size of the motor nerves that innervate muscle fibers. Smaller motor nerves have a lower threshold of stimulation). Soon, the main muscle fibers involved in sprinting are activated, as larger motor nerves that innervate type IIa and type IIx fibers are stimulated.

28. **Why are specific muscle fiber types activated during different kinds of exercise?**
The activation of a particular motor unit depends on the size of the α-motor neuron that innervates it (the "size principle"). Type I fibers are always activated first because they are the most easily activated. Type II fibers are stimulated only if the intensity of the exercise requires it. In other words, the body hopes type I fibers will get the job done, but if not, reluctantly, the body will resort to recruiting type IIa and ultimately type IIx fibers.

29. **Explain why movements become less precise and refined as low-intensity exercise is continued for a prolonged period.**
Initially, low-intensity exercise uses motor units consisting of slow-twitch muscle fibers. These motor units have fewer muscle fibers per unit than motor units with fast-twitch fibers. Fewer fibers per motor unit means better control. If it becomes necessary (for a variety of reasons) to recruit fast-twitch fibers, precision is compromised because fast-twitch motor units have more muscle fibers per unit, which results in less precise control of movements.

30. **Can the three muscle fiber types be changed as a result of exercise?**
This has been a highly controversial topic for many years. On one extreme, some believe fiber types are genetically determined and shall always remain the same, regardless of the nature of training. On the other extreme, some believe that with the "proper training" it's possible to convert type I fibers into type II and vice versa. Who is correct?

Current knowledge suggests that changes are possible but are modest. Thus a major change from type 1 to type IIX, or vice versa, seems unlikely. Rather, it's more likely that changes occur from each extreme (type I or type IIx) toward the intermediate fibers (type IIa). It's possible, in other words, to make type IIa fibers somewhat more like type I, or somewhat more like type IIx, depending on the type of training involved.

31. **What changes occur in muscle with endurance training?**
Endurance training results in improvements in oxygen delivery and use. This is caused by an increased capillarization, plus increases in myoglobin and mitochondria size and number. Type IIx muscle fibers may be altered to be more like type IIa. The cross-sectional area of the muscle decreases, resulting in shorter diffusion distances for oxygen and carbon dioxide.

32. **What changes occur in muscle with resistance training, and how long does it take for those changes to occur?**
Resistance training causes the synthesis of proteins in thick and thin filaments, increasing the cross-sectional area. The ratio of mitochondrial volume to contractile protein volume decreases, thus reducing aerobic capacity of the muscle, hindering performance in endurance activities. Type IIx muscle fibers become more like type IIa, and this change can occur quickly, within the first few weeks of training. Increases in contractile filaments resulting from protein synthesis take much longer.

33. **What causes improvements in strength with resistance training?**
In the first 2 weeks, 90% of the improvements are attributed to neural changes, including improvements in the recruitment pattern of motor units, increases in CNS activation, more synchronization of motor units, and less neural inhibition. Once these neuronal changes have been maximized, further increases in strength must come about as a result of muscle hypertrophy (an increase in contractile proteins).

34. **What is the cause of athletic amenorrhea?**
Athletic amenorrhea (loss of the menstrual cycle, resulting from heavy physical training) may be Mother Nature's way of preventing conception at times that threaten a developing fetus. A greatly reduced storage of body fat may be a factor.

More specifically, women who train heavily have higher levels of catecholamines, cortisol, and β-endorphins. These hormones inhibit the release of luteinizing hormone and follicle-stimulating hormone, which results in decreased levels of estradiol. Studies have shown that physical and emotional stress, diet, and the presence of menstrual irregularity before training also contribute. However, the exact mechanism is not known.

35. **Is it true that pregnant women who are physically fit deliver more easily?**
There is some evidence to suggest this, but there is also evidence stating otherwise. However, the perception of pain may be less in physically fit women.

36. **Summarize some physiologic changes that occur during pregnancy that affect exercise.**
The American College of Obstetrics and Gynecology (ACOG) recognizes the following:
   a. After the first trimester, the supine position results in relative obstruction of venous return by the enlarging uterus and a significant decrease in cardiac output.
   b. Stroke volume and cardiac output during steady-state exercise are increased significantly.
   c. Exercise during pregnancy induces a greater degree of hemoconcentration than an exercise in the nonpregnant state.
   d. There is a 10% to 20% increase in baseline oxygen consumption during pregnancy.
   e. Because of the increased resting oxygen requirements and the increased work of breathing brought about by physical effects of the enlarged uterus on the diaphragm, decreased oxygen is available for the performance of aerobic exercise during pregnancy.
   f. There is a shift in the physical center of gravity that may affect balance.
   g. Basal metabolic rate and heat production increase during pregnancy.
   h. Approximately 300 extra kilocalories per day are required to meet the metabolic needs of pregnancy; this caloric requirement is increased further in pregnant women who exercise regularly.
   i. Pregnant women use carbohydrates during exercise at a greater rate than do nonpregnant women; adequate carbohydrate intake for exercising pregnant patients is essential.

37. **What are the American College of Sports Medicine (ACSM) guidelines for physical activity?**
ACSM's physical activity guidelines for healthy adults recommend participating in at least 30 minutes of moderate-intensity physical activity 5 days per week or 150 minutes total of moderate-intensity exercise. For vigorous intensity physical activity, 20 minutes for 3 days per week is recommended.

38. **What are the ACSM guidelines for muscular fitness?**
ACSM recommends that a strength training program should be performed a minimum of two nonconsecutive days each week, with one set of 8 to 12 repetitions for healthy adults or 10 to 15 repetitions for older and frail individuals. In total, 8 to 10 exercises should be performed that target the major muscle groups.

39. **List the ACSM guidelines for an exercise program to decrease body weight.**
   a. The most successful program to decrease body weight is one that combines exercise with dieting. Such a program decreases weight, decreases fat mass, and maintains or increases fat-free mass. If one diets without exercising (especially if there is an extreme reduction in caloric intake as occurs on semi-starvation "crash" diets), one may lose more weight than by combining diet and exercise, but the fat-free mass is lost in addition to fat mass.
   b. An aerobic exercise program is very effective. However, resistance training also can be beneficial, even though the caloric expenditure is substantially less. This is because any addition of muscle mass increases resting metabolic rate, resulting in expending additional calories even when not exercising.
   c. Exercise should be performed at least 3 days per week at an intensity and duration to expend 250 to 300 kilocalories per exercise session for a 75-kg person. This usually requires a duration of at least 30 to 45 minutes for a person in average physical condition.

40. **What are the ACSM guidelines for sustaining weight loss?**
For sustaining weight loss, the ACSM recommendation is to engage in >250 minutes/week of moderate-intensity physical activity.

41. **Describe the "fit-but-fat" paradigm.**
   - An individual could have adequate cardiorespiratory capacity but still be of an undesirable bodyweight.
   - Evidence suggests that overweight (and possibly obese) adults who are physically active may be just as healthy, or even healthier, than inactive normal weight adults.

42. What are the ACSM guidelines for an exercise program to preserve bone health?

a. Types of exercise should be weight-bearing that apply compressional stress to bones. Endurance exercises include tennis, stair climbing, and jogging intermittently during walking and jumping activities such as volleyball and basketball. Resistance exercises (weight lifting) should involve all major muscle groups.
b. Intensity should be moderate to high, in terms of bone-loading forces.
c. The frequency of weight-bearing endurance activities should be 3 to 5 times per week, and resistance exercise 2 to 3 times per week.
d. Duration should be 30 to 60 minutes per day.
e. The older adult should also perform activities to improve balance for the prevention of falls.

43. How do exercise and training affect the endocrine system and the resting levels of hormones?

Most hormone levels increase during submaximal, short-term exercise except for insulin, which decreases, and thyroid hormones, which do not change. Resting levels of ACTH, cortisol, catecholamines, insulin, and glucagons decrease with training. This may be related to greater energy stores or a decreased perception of stress.

44. Discuss prolonged, moderate-intensity exercise training and blood glucose levels in individuals with type 1 and type 2 diabetes.

Blood glucose levels do not seem to change with a prolonged exercise program in individuals with type 1 diabetes, but they decrease in individuals with prediabetes (metabolic syndrome) and type 2 diabetes. Exercise causes the cells of prediabetic and type 2 diabetic patients to be less resistant to insulin, but the effect is acute and must be renewed daily. Moderate endurance exercise performed at an intensity of 60% to 75% of VO_{2max} reduces insulin resistance; however, higher intensity exercise has recently been shown to be more effective. Resistance training also is effective.

Most type 2 diabetic patients are overweight. Chronic exercise may help reduce body fat percentage, which results in an increase in the number of insulin receptors, an increase in their sensitivity, or both, which in turn helps to reduce insulin resistance.

Exercise may help to reduce cholesterol level in type 2 diabetic patients. This is an indirect effect as cholesterol is not a fuel. Rather, exercise stimulates enzymes that move LDL from the blood into the liver where it can be converted to bile or excreted. Thus, the more you exercise the more LDL is removed, lowering the total serum cholesterol.

This effect, along with the effect of exercise to cause weight loss, decreases cardiovascular risk, the most significant benefit of performing exercise. Although exercise has not been shown to improve blood glucose levels in individuals with type 1 diabetes, it is still recommended for the same reasons that exercise is recommended for individuals without diabetes.

45. Does exercise affect the prevalence of upper respiratory tract infections (URTI)?

Few studies have addressed the effect of moderate-intensity exercise on URTI. Preliminary results indicate a decrease in URTI with moderate exercise. More evidence indicates an increased prevalence of URTI during heavy endurance training and 1 to 2 weeks after a marathon-type event. This reflects the stimulatory effects of moderate exercise on the immune system, plus the transient suppressed effects of heavy endurance training. However, upon full recovery from heavy training, the immune system may be improved (graphically a "J" shaped relationship).

46. Should patients with chronic obstructive pulmonary disease (COPD) be encouraged to exercise?

Ambulation distance and feeling of well-being can increase significantly with an exercise program in individuals with mild or moderate COPD. There is controversy regarding the benefits of exercise for individuals with severe COPD. Some studies have shown improvements in endurance, whereas others have found no change. Only patients with stable COPD are encouraged to participate in an exercise program in a nonmedical setting.

47. How does the heart rate response to exercise differ between normal individuals and individuals who have had heart transplants?

In normal individuals, heart rate increases rapidly with moderate exercise as a result of a decrease in parasympathetic nerve activity and an increase in sympathetic nerve activity. Transplanted hearts are denervated. Any change in heart rate must be caused by changes in circulating levels of catecholamines, which takes more time than altering nerve activity. It takes longer for the heart rate to increase when exercise is initiated, and it takes longer for it to return to resting levels after exercise.

48. **How does resting heart rate differ between normal individuals and individuals who have had heart transplants?**
Resting heart rate is higher in individuals who have had a heart transplant because they no longer have the normal parasympathetic tone to slow the intrinsic rate of depolarization of the sinoatrial node.

49. **Why are individuals with thoracic-level spinal cord injuries at risk for fainting after exercising in the upright position with the upper extremities?**
There is no sympathetic innervation to the lower limb vasculature, and there may not be any innervation to the adrenal glands (depending on how high the injury is). This results in a lack of vasoconstriction of the vessels of the lower extremities, venous pooling occurs, and syncope follows.

50. **What is the most common problem associated with exercising in cold environments?**
When people know they are going to be exercising in cold environments, they usually overdress, resulting in hyperthermia.

51. **List strategies to avoid hypothermia and hyperthermia when exercising in a cold environment.**
- Dress in layers that can be removed as the exercise progresses.
- Stay dry; heat is lost much more rapidly when you are wet than when you are dry.

52. **Describe the physiologic changes that occur with exercising in the cold.**
Compared with a thermoneutral environment, exercising in the cold results in less lipid metabolism and free fatty acid use but greater lactate production and higher ventilation, oxygen consumption, respiratory heat loss, and peripheral heat loss.

53. **List possible causes for decreased maximal muscle strength and power with hypothermia.**
- Increased viscosity of skeletal muscle
- Increased resistance to blood flow
- Decreased maximal nerve conduction velocity

54. **What are the two most common problems associated with exercising in hot environments?**
Dehydration and hyperthermia are the two most common problems in this situation.

55. **How can dehydration and hyperthermia be avoided?**
These problems cannot be avoided completely, but they can be limited by ingesting fluid while exercising. There appears to be a similar benefit between ingestion of pure water compared with carbohydrate and electrolyte drinks as far as controlling core temperature and cardiovascular changes.

56. **Describe the physiologic changes that occur with exercising in the heat.**
The principal physiologic responses of exercise in the heat include skin and muscle vasodilation, nonactive tissue vasoconstriction, maintenance of blood pressure, and sweating. The hypothalamus plays a crucial role in thermoregulatory integration.

57. **Does living at high altitude improve exercise tolerance at high altitude?**
Yes. The exercise response of subjects at a high altitude who live at moderate altitudes compared with subjects who live at sea level shows that individuals who live at a moderate altitude have less of a decrease in VO_{2max} and blood lactate accumulation. They also have larger maximal ventilation during maximal exercise. Hematocrit levels increase after about 25 days of exposure to high altitude, which should increase performance. Some studies indicate that pulmonary function, cardiac output, muscle enzyme capacity, and lean body mass decrease at high altitudes. World-class athletes performing endurance exercises consistently seem to perform better if they train at a moderate altitude.

BIBLIOGRAPHY

American College of Obstetricians and Gynecologists, (1994). *Exercise during pregnancy.* Washington, DC: ACOG (technical bulletin 189).

American College of Sports Medicine, (1998). Position stand: The recommended quantity and quality of exercise for developing and maintaining cardiorespiratory and muscular fitness, and flexibility in healthy adults. *Medicine and Science in Sports and Exercise, 30,* 975–991.

American College of Sports Medicine, (2002). Position stand: Progression models in resistance training for healthy adults. *Medicine and Science in Sports and Exercise, 34,* 364–375.

American College of Sports Medicine, (2004a). Position stand: Exercise and hypertension. *Medicine and Science in Sports and Exercise, 36,* 533–546.

American College of Sports Medicine, (2004b). Position stand: Physical activity and bone health. *Medicine and Science in Sports and Exercise, 36,* 1985–1993.

American College of Sports Medicine., (2009). *ACSM's guidelines for exercise testing and prescription* (8th ed.). Philadelphia, PA: Lippincott Williams and Wilkins.
Artal Mittelmark, R., et al. (1991). Exercise guide for pregnancy. In R. A. Mittelmark, R. A. Wiswell, & B. L. Drinkwater (Eds.), *Exercise in pregnancy* (2nd ed., pp. 299–319). Baltimore, MD: Williams & Wilkins.
Bacon, S. L., Sherwood, A., Hinderliter, A., & Blumenthal, J. A. (2004). Effects of exercise, diet and weight loss on high blood pressure. *Sports Medicine, 34,* 307–314.
Cardoso, C. G., Jr., et al., Gomides, R. S., Queiroz, A. C. C., et al. (2010). Acute and chronic effects of aerobic and resistance exercise on ambulatory blood pressure. *Clinics (Sao Paulo), 65*(3), 317–325.
Casa, D. J. (1999). Exercise in the heat. I. Fundamentals of thermal physiology, performance implications, and dehydration. *Journal of Athletic Training, 34*(3), 246–252.
Doub, T. J. (1991). Physiology of exercise in the cold. *Sports Medicine, 11*(6), 367–381.
Fahay, T. D. (1994). Endurance training. In M. Shangold & G. Mirkin (Eds.), *Women and exercise: Physiology and sports medicine* (2nd ed., pp. 73–86). Philadelphia, PA: FA Davis.
Hasson, S. M. (ed.), (1994). *Clinical exercise physiology.* St. Louis, MO: Mosby.
Katch, F. I., & McArdle, W. D. (1993). *Introduction to nutrition, exercise, and health* (4th ed.). Philadelphia, PA: Lea & Febiger.
Loprinzi, P. D., Lee, H., & Cardinal, B. (2013). Dose response association between physical activity and biological, demographic, and perceptions of health variables. *Obesity Facts, 6*(4), 380–392.
Loprinzi, P. D., Herod, S. M., Cardinal, B. J., & Noakes, T. D. (2013). Physical activity and the brain: A review of this dynamic, bi-directional relationship. *Brain Research, 1539,* 95–104.
Loprinzi, P., Smit, E., & Lee, H., et al. (2014). The "Fit but Fat" paradigm addressed using accelerometer- determined physical activity data. *North American Journal of Medical Sciences, 6*(7), 295–301.
MacIntosh, B. R., Gardiner, P. F., & McComas, A. J. (2006). *Skeletal muscle: Form and function* (2nd ed.). Champaign, IL: Human Kinetics.
McArdle, W. D., Katch, F. I., & Katch, V. L. (2001). *Exercise physiology* (5th ed.). Philadelphia, PA: Lippincott Williams & Wilkins.
McMurray, R. G., & Hackney, A. C. (2000). Endocrine responses to exercise and training. In W. E. Garrett & D. T. Kirkendall (Eds.), *Exercise and sport science* (pp. 135–161). Philadelphia, PA: Lippincott Williams & Wilkins.
Moffatt, R. J., & Stamford, B. A. (Eds.). (2006). *Lipid metabolism and health.* Boca Raton, FL: CRC Press, Taylor & Francis Group.
Nieman, D. C. (2000). Exercise, the immune system, and infectious disease. In W. E. Garrett & D. T. Kirkendall (Eds.), *Exercise and sport science* (pp. 177–190). Philadelphia, PA: Lippincott Williams & Wilkins.
Powers, S. K., Howley, E. T., & Quindry, J. (2021). *Exercise physiology: Theory and application to fitness and performance* (11th ed.). New York, NY: McGraw-Hill.
Robergs, R. A., & Roberts, S. O. (1997). *Exercise physiology: Exercise, performance, and clinical applications.* St. Louis, MO: Mosby.
Roberts, S. O. (1997). Principles of prescribing exercise. In S. O. Roberts, R. A. Robergs, & P. Hanson (Eds.), *Clinical exercise testing and prescription theory and application* (pp. 235–259). Boca Raton, FL: CRC Press.
Shephard, R. J., & Astrand, P. O. (Eds.). (1992). *The encyclopedia of sports medicine endurance in sport.* London: Blackwell Scientific.
Stamford, B. A. (2001). *Weight loss reader: Sane strategies for losing body fat and keeping it off.* Louisville, KY: Biosynergic Health Press.
Staron, S. S., & Hikida, R. S. (2000). Muscular responses to exercise and training. In W. E. Garrett & D. T. Kirkendall (Eds.), *Exercise and sport science* (pp. 163–176). Philadelphia, PA: Lippincott Williams & Wilkins.
Tipton, C. M. (1999). Exercise and hypertension. In R. J. Shephard & H. S. Miller (Eds.), *Exercise and the heart in health and disease* (2nd ed., pp. 463–484). New York, NY: Marcel Dekker.
Viru, A., & Viru, M. (2000). Nature of training effects. In W. E. Garrett & D. T. Kirkendall (Eds.), *Exercise and sport science* (pp. 67–95). Philadelphia, PA: Lippincott Williams & Wilkins.
Wendt, D., van Loon, L. J. C., & van Marken Lichtenbelt, W. D. (2007). Thermoregulation during exercise in the heat strategies for maintaining health and performance. *Sports Medicine, 37*(8), 669–682.
Zernicke, R. F., Salem, G. F., & Alejo, R. K. (1996). Endurance training. In B. Reider (Ed.), *Sports medicine: the school age athlete* (pp. 3–16). Philadelphia, PA: WB Saunders.

CHAPTER 5 QUESTIONS

1. **Which of the following factors is considered the best indicator of an individual's level of aerobic capacity?**
   a. Maximum oxygen uptake (VO_{2max})
   b. Resting heart rate
   c. Ventilatory threshold
   d. Blood lactate threshold

2. **Which of the following muscle fiber types is activated primarily during prolonged, low-intensity exercise?**
   a. Type I
   b. Type IIa
   c. Type IIb
   d. Type IIx

3. **Which of the following is a method to assess cardiorespiratory fitness?**
   a. Indirect calorimetry
   b. Field-based tests
   c. Nonexercise prediction equation
   d. All of the above

4. **Greater utilization of oxygen by working muscles is dependent upon:**
   a. Cardiac output increased by an increase in maximal heart rate
   b. Cardiac output increased by an increase in stroke volume
   c. An increase in size and density of mitochondria in working muscles
   d. An increase in % oxygen saturation

5. **Oxygen deficit occurs when:**
   a. Exercise begins and prior to achieving a steady state
   b. Exercise is over and there is the need to replenish CP and ATP stores
   c. There is an excess supply of O_2 that is greater than the demand
   d. There is no anaerobic metabolism

6. **Resting VO_2 in highly trained endurance athletes compared to the untrained is:**
   a. Much greater due to a higher stroke volume
   b. Much lower due to a greater efficiency of the cardiovascular system
   c. Much greater due to a higher stroke volume and higher plasma volume
   d. About the same despite a greater stroke volume

7. **Thermoregulatory integration is triggered and largely controlled by the:**
   a. Cerebral cortex
   b. Hypothalamus
   c. Cerebellum
   d. Thermoregulatory control center in the brain stem

CHAPTER 6

ARTHRITIS

J. Bateman, MD and G. Gennaoui, DO

1. **List the common causes and types of arthritis.**
   - Osteoarthritis
   - Autoimmune-related arthritis like rheumatoid arthritis, seronegative arthritis, and systemic lupus erythematous
   - Crystaline-induced arthritis—gout and pseudogout
   - Infectious-related arthritis like septic arthritis from bacterial infection, a viral illness, or Lyme disease

2. **List tools used to help differentiate between the different types of arthritis.**
   - A good complete medical history with a focus on the distribution and pattern of the pain and whether it is inflammatory or noninflammatory in nature
   - Synovial fluid cell counts, crystal analysis, and cultures
   - Imaging including x-rays, ultrasound, and MRI
   - Lab work looking for specific antibodies or other disease markers

3. **What are the differences between inflammatory and noninflammatory joint pain, and why is it important?**
   It is critical to distinguish between the two types of pain as they have different causes.

Table 6.1 Differences between inflammatory and non-inflammatory joint pain

	INFLAMMATORY	NONINFLAMMATORY
General cause	Autoimmune disease	Mechanical, osteoarthritis
Morning stiffness	>60 minutes	<30 minutes
Timing of pain	Worse in the morning	Worse at night
Pain with activity	Better with activity	Worse with activity
Physical exam	Erythema, swelling	No swelling, bony enlargement
Synovial fluid cell count	>2000 WBCs	200–2000 WBCs
ESR, CRP lab values	Elevated	Normal

4. **What is osteoarthritis (OA) and who gets it?**
   Osteoarthritis is the most common degenerative joint disease commonly referred to as wear and tear of the joints. It is characterized by the breakdown of cartilage in the joints leading to bony changes, deterioration of tendons and ligaments, and muscle atrophy. It is generally seen in the elderly and commonly involves joints of the hands, spine, hips, knees, and great toes.

5. **How common is OA and what are the risk factors?**
   OA is the most common type of arthritis. Prevalence increases with age, and it has been estimated to be noted radiographically in >80% of individuals >75 years of age. Lifetime risk of developing OA has been estimated at 46% in the knee and 25% in the hip in one study. Risk factors include trauma, obesity, heavy physical workload, genetic factors, and anatomic factors.

6. **What are Heberden and Bouchard nodes?**
   These hard bumps are a form of exostosis and osteophyte formation seen in osteoarthritis located at the DIP (Heberden) and PIP (Bouchard) joints of the hand. The nodes are usually painless but can become inflamed and be painful, especially when they are first developing.

7. **What is erosive osteoarthritis?**
   Erosive osteoarthritis is a severe and aggressive subset of OA that has inflammatory-like features seen at the DIP and PIP joints of the hand.

8. **How is OA treated?**
Currently, there is no treatment to reverse or even slow the joint damage from OA. Treatment is geared towards pain management and functional improvement. Options include NSAIDs (both topical and oral), duloxetine, physical modalities (heart/cold therapy, ultrasound), orthoses, exercise, weight loss, physical therapy, injections, and sometimes surgery. Chronic narcotic use is strongly discouraged.

9. **What are proven beneficial therapy modalities to treat OA?**
Studies have shown that strength training increases strength, reduces pain, and improves function in patients with OA. Aquatic therapy and balance perturbation therapy has been shown to reduce pain and improve function as well. Other treatments like electrical stimulation or manual therapy can be used to supplement current treatment; however, the evidence for their impact on these variables is equivocal.

10. **What is rheumatoid arthritis (RA) and who gets it?**
RA is a chronic autoimmune disease characterized by inflammatory joint pain in the hands and feet. It is the most common autoimmune arthritis, affecting approximately 1% of the population worldwide and 1.3 million Americans, 75% of whom are female. RA can start at any age; however, most people are diagnosed between ages 30 and 50. Genetic influences are important. More severe disease is associated with HLA-DR 4 subtypes.

11. **What labs help in the diagnosis of RA? Are they needed to make a diagnosis?**
Rheumatoid factor (RF) and anti-cyclic citrullinated peptide (anti-CCP) antibodies are both labs that can be ordered that, when in high titer, can help with the diagnosis of rheumatoid arthritis; however, they are not diagnostic and are negative in 30% of patients with RA. Having inflammatory joint pain in a typical distribution of the hands and feet for >6 weeks alone can be diagnostic. RF is an antibody that precipitates immune complex formation. It is associated with nodule formation, extraarticular disease, and more severe joint disease. The RF sensitivity and specificity for RA is 60% to 70% and 78%, respectively. Anti-CCP antibody is a test that is more specific (98%) and similar sensitivity (70%) at detecting RA.

12. **Why is it important to diagnose RA?**
RA causes inflammation in synovial joints leading to pain, swelling, and destruction of cartilage, bone, and ligamentous structures. This can lead to severe deformities and impaired function. The challenge in RA now is to make the diagnosis and start treatment early, as this has been proven to prevent joint damage. Untreated RA is also associated with systemic inflammation that has been proven to increase cardiovascular morbidity and mortality. This can be mitigated by controlling the systemic inflammatory process with DMARD therapy.

13. **What are the x-ray findings of RA versus OA?**
In RA, changes in hand x-rays may occur in order of appearance: soft tissue swelling, periarticular osteopenia, marginal erosions, uniform joint space narrowing, and malalignment. These changes are typically seen in the MCPs, wrists, and PIPs. DIPs are not involved in RA. For osteoarthritis, subchondral sclerosis, asymmetric joint space narrowing, and osteophyte and bone cyst formation are generally found. These changes are seen at first carpometacarpal joint, DIPs, and PIPs in OA.

14. **What are common hand and wrist deformities associated with RA?**
- Subluxation and ulnar deviation at metacarpophalangeals (MCPs)
- Swan neck deformity (flexion at DIP, extension at proximal interphalangeal [PIP])
- Boutonnière deformity (extension at DIP, flexion at PIP)
- Flexion, radial deviation, and subluxation at wrist
- Extensor tendon rupture at wrist

15. **How does RA affect the spine?**
Rheumatoid arthritis is a disease of the synovial tissue, which in the spine, is seen at the atlanto-axial joint of C1-C2. Inflammation here can cause erosion of the dens or loosening of the transverse ligament that holds the dens in place. Subluxation here can cause compression of the cervical spinal cord. The discs and the rest of the spine are otherwise not clinically involved in RA.

16. **What are possible medical emergencies with RA?**
- Cervical myelopathy from subluxation at C1-C2 can occur, usually in a patient with long-standing, polyarticular, and deforming RA. Even minor trauma may precipitate symptoms. Patients may have paresthesias, weakness, and hyperreflexia.
- Infection is a significant risk, especially with immunosuppressive drugs. Consider especially with monoarticular joint flares.
- Rarely, in the age of aggressive medical therapy, rheumatoid vasculitis can be seen with mononeuritis multiplex (multiple unrelated peripheral nerve deficits), skin lesions, and internal organ involvement.

- Painful red eye may relate to inflammation in a variety of structures of the eye, some of which are vision-threatening. Urgent ophthalmologic evaluation is indicated.
- Cardiovascular disease is increased in RA. Relative inactivity may minimize any warning signs.

17. **Is physical and exercise therapy an effective treatment of rheumatoid arthritis?**
The effect of therapy is still unclear; however, there are studies that show statistical significance on the benefits of supervised exercise therapy on quality of life, physical function, and pain management. Based on the desirable effects with reasonable quality of evidence, the American Physical Therapy Association updated their guidelines in 2021 and presented a strong recommendation to offer exercise therapy and education to patients aligned with their needs.

18. **How do children present with juvenile inflammatory arthritis?**
Different patterns of involvement have been identified and are listed here. By definition, onset is before the age of 16.
- Systemic onset with fevers, serositis, rash, arthritis, and other organ involvement
- Oligoarticular (most common presentation) with four or fewer joints involved at onset
- Polyarticular onset, behaves like adult RA
- Psoriatic arthritis
- Enthesitis-related

Synovitis in children is typically not severely painful. Limping, activity modification, or noted swelling in joint(s) are more likely to bring a child to medical attention. A very painful swollen joint or joints should raise the concern of leukemia in a child.

19. **Name the four seronegative arthropathies.**
- Ankylosing spondylitis
- Reactive arthritis (previously called Reiter's syndrome)
- Psoriatic arthritis
- Enteropathic arthritis associated with inflammatory bowel disease

20. **What clinical features do seronegative arthropathies share?**
- Enthesitis (inflammation at sites of insertion of tendons or ligaments into bone)
- Sacroiliitis and other axial skeletal involvement
- Asymmetric, peripheral pauciarticular inflammatory arthritis
- Extraarticular disease involving the gastrointestinal or genitourinary systems, skin, and eye
- Association with HLA-B27 (in patients with spondylitis)

21. **List clinical features of psoriatic arthritis.**
- Psoriatic skin lesions (nail changes are common)
- Asymmetric peripheral arthritis with DIP involvement
- Sausage digits and other tendinitis
- Occasional spondylitis and sacroiliitis
- Occasional arthritis deformans with telescoping of digits

22. **What is reactive arthritis?**
Reactive arthritis is a seronegative arthritis that is triggered by infection, typically by *Chlamydia, Campylobacter, Salmonella, Shigella*, or *Yersinia*. The classic triad of arthritis, conjunctivitis, and urethritis is seen in a minority of cases.

23. **How does the back pain of ankylosing spondylitis differ from mechanical back pain?**

Table 6.2 Differences between ankylosing spondylitis and mechanical back pain

	ANKYLOSING SPONDYLITIS	MECHANICAL BACK PAIN
Age of onset	Late teens to 20 s	Any age (more common in older age)
Timing of onset	Insidious, nontraumatic	Often sudden, traumatic
Pain with rest	Increased	Decreased
Pain with activity	Decreased	Increased
Stiffness	+++	±, usually <15 min

24. **How is AS treated?**
    - Education and exercise are still very important.
    - Extension exercises three times daily (swimming recommended), attention to erect posture, and sleeping without a pillow to prevent kyphosis are recommended.
    - Nonsteroidal antiinflammatory drugs (NSAIDs) can help relieve pain and stiffness.
    - Tumor necrosis factor (TNF) inhibitors have been shown to cause clinical improvement in the axial skeleton. There are not enough data to prove that bony fusion is changed by therapy.
    - Methotrexate and sulfasalazine improve inflammation in peripheral joints but are not helpful for spinal disease.

25. **Describe x-ray findings in AS.**
    - Erosion, pseudowidening, sclerosis, and ultimately fusion of sacroiliac joints
    - Squaring of vertebrae with shiny corners
    - Syndesmophyte formation (ossification of the outer layer of the intervertebral disc), leading to bamboo spine
    - Fusion of apophyseal joints

26. **Can exercise be used as a treatment for AS and improve disease activity?**
    The Assessment of Spondylo Arthritis international Society (ASAS)/European League Against Rheumatism recommend regular exercise as a nonpharmacologic treatment of AS. Many studies show exercise programs improved physical function and disease activity including for patients on medical treatment. A combination of biologic therapy and physical activity has a synergistic effect and improves pain, function, respiratory capacity, and quality of life and decreases cardiovascular risk.

27. **What are red flags PTs should know about AS?**
    Persistent localized back pain after a fall should raise a concern of fracture with pseudoarthrosis. Bone density is typically low because of a lack of normal biomechanical forces across the vertebrae. If much of the spine is fused, there can be a great deal of movement at the fracture site, preventing normal healing.

28. **What is systemic lupus erythematosus (SLE) and how is it diagnosed?**
    SLE is a multisystem inflammatory disease that may cause fever, fatigue, rash, blood count abnormalities, renal disease, serositis, lung disease, nervous system changes, joint pain, and other problems. It is a clinical diagnosis and at this time, there are only classification criteria used for research purposes to help diagnose the disease.

29. **What are antinuclear antibodies (ANA) and how are they used in SLE?**
    ANA are antibodies that target small proteins in the nucleus. When present in large amounts, they could suggest an underlying autoimmune disease. It is present in 99% of patients with SLE and often used as a screening test. However, false positive results are common (up to 30%–40%) and also very nonspecific as many other diseases have positive ANAs including scleroderma, Sjogren's syndrome, autoimmune hepatitis, and autoimmune thyroid diseases. Additionally, certain medications can cause a positive ANA as well.

30. **Describe typical lupus arthritis.**
    - Arthralgias are most common, without visible joint swelling.
    - When inflammation is present, it often involves the small joints of the hands in a similar pattern to RA.
    - The arthritis is not erosive, although joint deformities may be seen (eg, Jaccoud's arthropathy—chronic deforming nonerosive rheumatoid like arthritis with possible MP deviation and/or swan neck deformities).

31. **What are musculoskeletal problems SLE patients can develop?**
    - Arthralgia and arthritis
    - Osteonecrosis
    - Tendonitis and tendon rupture
    - Fibromyalgia
    - Steroid myopathy
    - Polymyositis

32. **What causes gout?**
    Gout is caused by the accumulation of uric acid crystals in synovial joints. When polymorphonuclear leukocytes are attracted to the joint and try to engulf the crystals, they release digestive enzymes and proinflammatory mediators, causing an acute gout flare presenting with severe pain, swelling, and warmth of the affected joints. This can lead to joint damage and large collections of uric acid crystals called tophi.

33. **Describe a typical episode of acute gout.**
    Acute gout episodes typically begin with the sudden onset of severe burning pain, often in the middle of the night, usually involving the first metatarsophalangeal (MTP) joint. The pain may be so severe that even the weight of

the bed sheets may be unbearable. The joint appears red, swollen, and hot to the touch. Episodes usually resolve within 7 to 10 days. They may be precipitated by alcohol consumption, trauma, surgery, or immobilization. As the disease progresses, other joints can be involved as well including the midfoot, ankles, knees, shoulders, hands, and wrists.

34. **How is an acute gout flare treated?**
If one joint is affected, an intraarticular corticosteroid injection is usually effective in controlling symptoms. Colchicine can be used; however, it is much less effective if started >24 hours from symptom onset. If multiple joints are involved, systemic treatment with NSAIDs and even oral/IV steroids are needed. Allopurinol or febuxostat are medications that lower the uric acid level. The dosing of these medications should not be changed in the setting of an acute flare, as changes in the uric acid level can precipitate flaring.

35. **How is gout diagnosed?**
Gout is diagnosed with certainty by identifying intracellular uric acid crystals in the synovial fluid of an affected joint. A classic presentation of an acute gout flare with first MTP involvement is very suggestive. Serum uric acid levels are not diagnostic as <20% of patients with elevated serum uric acid levels develop gout and 30% of patients with gout do not have elevated uric acid levels at the time of a joint flare-up.

36. **What causes pseudogout?**
Calcium pyrophosphate crystals initiate inflammation.

37. **How are gout and pseudogout differentiated?**
Examination of synovial fluid under a polarizing microscope helps differentiate gout from pseudogout: uric acid crystals are needle-like and negatively birefringent, whereas pseudogout crystals are rod-shaped and positively birefringent.

38. **How does pseudogout differ from gout?**
Calcium pyrophosphate deposition disease can present similarly to gout (pseudogout), to RA (pseudo-RA), or as aggressive osteoarthritis (OA). Calcium pyrophosphate deposits (chondrocalcinosis) often can be seen on radiographs as opacities in the knee joint space or in the triangular fibrocartilage of the wrist. Definitive diagnosis requires examination of joint fluid. Aspiration of fluid often is adequate to relieve symptoms with pseudogout. Local steroid injection, colchicine, or NSAIDs are used for flaring.

39. **What is the differential diagnosis of a single red hot joint?**
Infection is the most dangerous condition associated with this diagnosis and must immediately be ruled out by testing a sample of synovial fluid. Other diagnoses include acute gout, hemarthrosis with or without trauma, pseudogout, RA, seronegative arthropathy, and other less common etiologies (eg, tumor or pigmented villonodular synovitis).

40. **What are common types of inflammatory muscle disease?**
   - Polymyositis is an autoimmune disease manifested by symmetric weakness in the proximal muscles of the upper and lower extremities.
   - Dermatomyositis also causes proximal weakness and inflammation of the skin.
   - Inclusion body myositis causes asymmetric weakness, especially in the quadriceps, wrists, and finger flexors.

41. **Is exercise safe and beneficial in patients with myositis?**
Exercise has proven to be safe in patients with stable active and inactive muscle disease. Aerobic exercise and strength training were studied individually and in combination showing an improvement of functional capacity, walking distance, and quality of life in patients studied. Additionally, both aerobic exercise and isometric strength training did not alter CPK levels.

42. **List uses and potential side effects of medications commonly used to treat types of arthritis.**

Table 6.3 Medications used in the treatment of athritis

MEDICATION	MECHANISM OF ACTION	COMMON USAGE	SIDE EFFECTS
NSAIDs and COX-2 inhibitors	Inhibits cyclooxygenase and formation of thromboxanes, prostaglandins, and prostacyclins	OA, soft tissue injuries, inflammatory arthritis	GI upset and ulceration, renal dysfunction, heart disease, bleeding

Table 6.3 Medications used in the treatment of athritis

MEDICATION	MECHANISM OF ACTION	COMMON USAGE	SIDE EFFECTS
Glucocorticoids	Inhibits expression of proinflammatory cytokines by immune cells and adhesion molecules	RA, SLE, other inflammatory disorders	Infection (including TB), weight gain, diabetes, muscle weakness, bone loss, poor healing
Antimalarials (hydroxychloroquine)	Reduces toll-like receptor signaling and cytokine production	RA, SLE	Vision change, rarely myopathy
Colchicine	Inhibits microtubule assembly disrupting inflammasome activation, inflammatory cell chemotaxis, and generation of leukotrienes and cytokines	Gout, pseudogout	Diarrhea, rarely bone marrow suppression
Sulfasalazine	Inhibits prostaglandins resulting in an anti-inflammatory effect	RA, psoriatic arthritis	Rash, hepatitis, bone marrow suppression
Methotrexate	Inhibits dihydrofolate reductase that leads to increased T cell apoptosis and a diminished immune response	RA, psoriatic arthritis, other inflammatory conditions	Infection (including TB), skin cancers, lymphomas, heart failure
Leflunomide	Inhibits pyrimidine synthesis and activated T cells	RA, psoriatic arthritis	Diarrhea, weight loss, neuropathy, hypertension, infection
TNF alpha inhibitors	Inhibits TNF alpha that modulates biologic responses responsible for leukocyte migration	RA, psoriatic arthritis, other inflammatory conditions	Infection (including TB), skin cancers, lymphomas, heart failure
Rituximab	Depletes B cells by binding to CD20 and causing their cell death	RA, myositis, other inflammatory disorders	Infection (including TB), low WBC
IL12/23 inhibitors	Inhibit interleukin 12 and 23 inhibiting naïve T-cells to differentiate and produce IFN-γ and IL-17	Psoriasis, psoriatic arthritis	Infection (including TB)
IL-17 inhibitors	Inhibit interleukin 17 that recruits immune cells like monocytes and neutrophils to sites of inflammation	Psoriasis, psoriatic arthritis, ankylosing spondylitis	Infection, inflammatory bowel disease
JAK inhibitors	Inhibit the JAK/SAT signaling pathway inhibiting several cytokine interactions	Rheumatoid arthritis	Infection (including TB), skin cancers, lymphomas, blood clots
IL-6 inhibitors	Inhibit interleukin 6 that is a proinflammatory cytokine produced by many cell types	Rheumatoid arthritis, giant cell arteritis	Infection (including TB), low WBC, liver toxicity

Bibliography

Aletaha, D., Neogi, T., Silman, A. J., et al. (2010). Rheumatoid arthritis classification criteria. *Arthritis and Rheumatism, 62*(9), 2269–2581.

Brakke, R., Singh, J., & Sullivan, W. (2012). Physical therapy in persons with osteoarthritis. *PMR, 4*(5 Suppl), S53–S58.

Chen, D., Shen, J., Zhao, W., et al. (2017). Osteoarthritis: toward a comprehensive understanding of pathological mechanism. *Bone Research, 5*, 16044.

Cronstein, B. N., & Aune, T. M. (2020). Methotrexate and its mechanisms of action in inflammatory arthritis. *Nature Reviews Rheumatology, 16*, 145–154.

Dalbeth, N., Lauterio, T. J., & Wolfe, H. R. (2014). Mechanism of action of colchicine in the treatment of gout. *Clinical Therapeutics, 36*(10), 1465–1479.

Fink, C. W. (1995). Proposal for the development of classification criteria for idiopathic arthritides of childhood. *Journal of Rheumatology, 22*, 1566.

Habers, G., & Takken, T. (2011). Safety and efficacy of exercise training in patients with an idiopathic inflammatory myopathy— A systematic review. *Rheumatology, 50*(11), 2113–2124.

Jacobsson, L., Turesson, C., Nilsson, J. -A., et al. (2007). Treatment with TNF blockers and mortality risk in patients with rheumatoid arthritis. *Annals of the Rheumatic Diseases, 66*, 670–675.

Pécourneau, V., Degboé, Y., Barnetche, T., et al. (2018). Effectiveness of exercise programs in ankylosing spondylitis: a meta-analysis of randomized controlled trials. *Archives of Physical Medicine and Rehabilitation, 99*(2), 383–389. e1.

Peter, W. F., Swart, N. M., Meerhoff, G. A., & Vliet Vlieland, T. P. M. (2021). Clinical practice guideline for physical therapist management of people with rheumatoid arthritis. *Physical Therapy, 101*, pzab127.

Santos, A., Misse, R. G., Borges, I. B. P., Perandini, L. A. B., & Shinjo, S. K. (2021). Physical exercise for the management of systemic autoimmune myopathies: recent findings, and future perspectives. *Current Opinion, 33*, 563–569.

Schurich, A., Raine, C., Morris, V., & Ciurtin, C. (2018). The role of IL-12/23 in T cell–related chronic inflammation: implications of immunodeficiency and therapeutic blockade. *Rheumatology, 57*(2), 246–254.

Sieper, J., Rudwaleit, M., Baraliakos, X., et al. (2009). The Assessment of SpondyloArthritis international Society (ASAS) handbook: a guide to assess spondyloarthritis. *Annals of the Rheumatic Diseases, 68*(Suppl 2), ii1–ii44.

Silman, A. J., MacGregor, A. J., Thomson, W., et al. (1993). Twin concordance rates for rheumatoid arthritis: Results from a nationwide study. *British Journal of Rheumatology, 32*(10), 903.

Solomon, D., Kavanaugh, A. J., Schur, P. H., & American College of Rheumatology Ad Hoc Committee on Immunologic Testing Guidelines, (2002). Evidence-based guidelines for the use of immunologic tests: Antinuclear antibody testing. *Arthritis and Rheumatism, 47*, 434–444.

Vallbracht, I., Rieber, J., Oppermann, M., et al. (2004). Diagnostic and clinical value of anti-cyclic citrullinated peptide antibodies compared with rheumatoid factor isotypes in rheumatoid arthritis. *Annals of the Rheumatic Diseases, 63*, 1079–1084.

Wen, Z., & Chai, Y. (2021). Effectiveness of resistance exercises in the treatment of rheumatoid arthritis: a meta-analysis. *Medicine (Baltimore), 100*(13), e25019.

Wolfe, F., Mitchell, D. M., Sibley, J. T., et al. (1994). The mortality of rheumatoid arthritis. *Arthritis and Rheumatism, 37*(4), 481–494.

CHAPTER 6 QUESTIONS

1. **A 68-year-old female with rheumatoid arthritis on TNF inhibitor and methotrexate comes for physical therapy after carpal tunnel release. She mentions that her right knee is painful. You notice a warm large effusion with limited range of motion. The best approach is to:**
   a. Increase immunosuppressive medication
   b. Start antibiotic therapy immediately
   c. Obtain synovial fluid for analysis and wait for culture
   d. Obtain synovial fluid and then start antibiotics

2. **A patient with longstanding ankylosing spondylitis comes for treatment of back pain that began after a minor fall. The pain is constant, worse with bending forward. He has been compliant with his treatment with TNF inhibitor. On exam he has very limited movement of his neck in any direction, limited distraction at the lower spine (abnormal Schober's test), and point tenderness in the mid thoracic spine to palpation. What is the next step?**
   a. Change DMARD because the TNF inhibitor appears to be losing effectiveness.
   b. Evaluate radiologically for a nonhealing fracture in the thoracic spine.
   c. Check blood cultures for possible infection.
   d. Heat, massage, and stretches for muscle spasm.

3. **A patient with crystal-proven gout comes in with a swollen knee. He has had three episodes of gout over the past 5 years. The knee has been swollen, warm, and painful for 4 days. Which is the preferred treatment?**
   a. Colchicine
   b. Allopurinol
   c. Oral steroid therapy
   d. Intra-articular corticosteroid injection

4. A 35-year-old Caucasian woman comes in with complaints of severe pain "from head to toe," rated 12/10, worst in the lower back and worse the day after she has any increase in activity. She is very sore in the mornings and feels exhausted. She is not able to take nonsteroidals because of a history of peptic ulcer disease. On exam she has full range of small and large joints and has muscular tenderness. Strength testing is difficult because of her complaints of pain. Therapies might include:
   a. Corticosteroids
   b. Tricyclic antidepressants
   c. Mild narcotic analgesia
   d. TNF inhibitor

5. A 44-year-old African-American female is being seen for joint pains in her hands. On exam, the patient has ulnar deviation and swan neck deformities with some synovitis noted at the MCPs that is worse on the right compared to the left hand. The deformities, however, are reducible and not identified on x-ray. What is the cause of this patient's deformity?
   a. Rheumatoid arthritis
   b. Jaccoud's arthropathy
   c. Psoriatic arthritis
   d. Gout

6. State whether each of the following is true or false.
   a. A patient can have arthritis caused by both gout and infection.
   b. Rheumatoid arthritis only involves joints in the hands and feet.
   c. Nail involvement in psoriasis is related to enthesopathy at the DIP joints in the hand.
   d. ANA antibodies are only positive in systemic lupus erythematosus.

CHAPTER 7

DEEP VENOUS THROMBOSIS

M. Quinn, MD

1. **Define Virchow's triad.**
   Virchow's triad represents the risk factors for the development of a deep venous thrombosis (DVT).

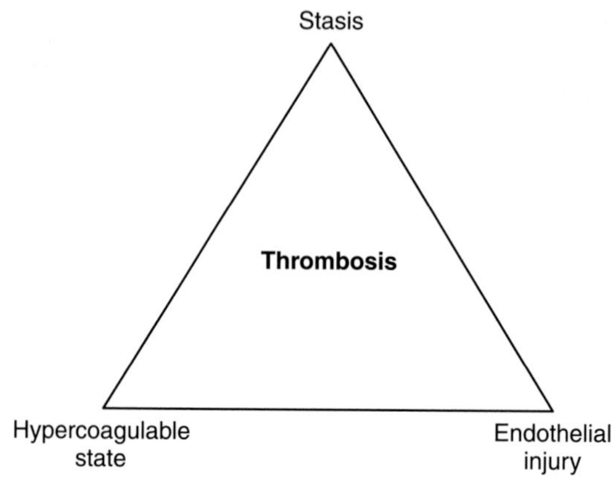

Virchow's triad.

1. Endothelial injury—change to the vascular wall that serves as a potent thrombogenic influence. It may be caused directly by trauma (including surgical) or indirectly by hematoma formation or thermal injury.
2. Alteration in blood flow—arterial turbulence or venous stasis contributes to the development of thrombi. Stasis occurs during the time spent on the operating table and postoperatively because of immobilization or impaired ambulation.
3. Hypercoagulability—alteration in the blood coagulation mechanism that predisposes one to thrombosis. A transient hypercoagulable state may exist as a part of the normal host response to surgery.

2. **List states that are associated with hypercoagulability.**

GENETIC
- Antithrombin C deficiency
- Protein C deficiency
- Protein S deficiency
- Factor V Leiden deficiency
- Prothrombin G20210A mutation

ACQUIRED
- Postoperative
- Malignancy
- Postpartum
- Congestive heart failure
- Prolonged bed rest or immobilization
- Advanced age
- Severe trauma
- Nephrotic syndrome
- Cancer
- Obesity
- Oral contraceptives
- Prior thromboembolism

3. **What is the most common inherited thrombophilia?**
Factor V Leiden is the most prevalent inherited thrombophilia, accounting for approximately 20% of patients with DVT. It is present in 3% to 5% of people of northern European descent. The risk of thromboembolism is increased by a factor of 7 in persons who are heterozygous for the Leiden mutation and 80 times for persons who are homozygous for the mutation.

4. **In the general population, how frequently does DVT occur?**
In the general population, DVT occurs at a rate of approximately 1 in 1000 people.

5. **How common are genetic factors in association with hypercoagulability?**
Approximately 20% to 30% of patients with DVT have a predisposing genetic factor.

6. **When do venous thrombi develop?**
   - DVT may begin during the surgical procedure.
   - Patients may present with signs and symptoms of DVT 24 to 48 hours postoperatively.
   - The risk of late postoperative DVT is recognized to continue for 3 months.

7. **Describe the incidence of DVT after total joint arthroplasty.**
Patients who undergo total hip arthroplasty or total knee arthroplasty are at high risk for DVT. If no prophylaxis is used, DVT occurs in 40% to 80% of these patients. Thromboembolic prophylaxis, early mobilization, and modern surgical techniques have reduced the incidence of fatal pulmonary embolism to 0.18%. Despite prophylaxis, venous thromboembolism remains the most common reason for emergency department readmission and death after a total joint arthroplasty.

8. **Does the type of anesthetic used during surgery affect the incidence of DVT?**
Regional epidural anesthesia has been associated with a reduction in overall, proximal, and distal DVT. Epidural anesthesia may reduce the overall incidence of DVT by 40% to 50%. Hypotensive anesthesia may also be beneficial.

9. **List the clinical signs and symptoms of DVT.**
   - Calf pain
   - Engorged veins
   - Swelling
   - Edema
   - Calf cramping
   - Low-grade fever
   - Warmth
   - Palpable cord along the course of the involved vein
   - Erythema
   - Pain along the course of the involved vein

10. **Is DVT easily clinically diagnosed?**
No. DVT may be difficult to diagnose on the basis of physical examination. In one study, the diagnosis was confirmed with diagnostic studies in less than half of those suspected of having a DVT. Most venous thrombi are clinically silent. A clinician may not rely on physical examination findings alone to diagnose a DVT.

11. **What is Homans' sign?**
Homans' sign is calf pain with forced passive foot dorsiflexion; it is a physical examination finding suggestive of DVT.

12. **List differential diagnoses of DVT.**
   - Muscle strain
   - Nerve compression syndromes
   - Cellulitis
   - Lymphedema
   - Superficial thrombophlebitis
   - Arterial occlusion
   - Chronic venous insufficiency
   - Baker's cyst

13. **Name the most dreaded complication from DVT.**
Pulmonary embolism (PE) is the most feared complication.

14. **Describe the signs and symptoms of PE.**
PE may be the first clinical sign of a DVT. The most common signs of PE are tachycardia, low oxygen saturation, and shortness of breath. However, the clinical presentation of PE is notoriously unreliable. The clinical signs of PE are nonspecific, and, as with DVT, diagnostic studies are needed to confirm the diagnosis.
A classic presentation of pulmonary embolism consists of pleuritic chest pain and dyspnea (40%). Patients also may present with cough, diaphoresis, apprehension, altered mental status, hemoptysis, tachypnea, tachycardia (most common finding, 85%), rales, fever, bulging neck veins (30%), and a pleural friction rub. In one study, nearly 40% of patients who had a DVT, but no symptoms of pulmonary embolism, had evidence of pulmonary embolism on diagnostic studies. Massive pulmonary embolism may present as syncope or sudden death. Two-thirds of patients who suffer a fatal pulmonary embolus do so within 30 minutes of becoming symptomatic.

15. **What are the electrocardiogram (ECG) findings of pulmonary embolism?**
Typical ECG findings include ST segment depression or T wave inversion, right axis deviation, or right bundle branch block. The classic ECG pattern S1Q3T3 is rare.

16. **What long-term complications are associated with DVT?**
Chronic venous insufficiency secondary to venous dilation and valvular incompetence is a typical long-term DVT complication. At 5 years post DVT, symptoms may include:
- Night pain (45%)
- Pigmentation changes (50%)
- Pain with prolonged standing (39%)
- Venous ulceration (7%)
- Edema (52%)

17. **Discuss the modalities that are available to prevent the formation of a DVT.**
- Aspirin—the benefit for patients after joint arthroplasty is not conclusively proven. Aspirin has been proven to be a safe drug, but more studies are needed to prove its efficacy for prevention of thromboembolism. Aspirin has been found to be effective in decreasing DVT when combined with exercise and graded stockings or leg pumps.
- Heparin—may be given subcutaneously in the perioperative period. It may be given as a fixed dosage (5000 units every 8 to 12 hours) or as an adjusted low dosage (3500 units every 8 hours; then adjust the dose to desired anticoagulation). The therapeutic effect is most commonly measured using the activated partial thromboplastin time (aPTT).
- Low-molecular-weight heparin (LMWH)—typically given at a fixed dosage without the need for outpatient monitoring. However, it may be associated with a slightly increased incidence of postoperative bleeding and wound problems. Many consider LMWH to be the "gold standard" for VTE prophylaxis in orthopaedic surgery patients. An uncommon but potentially serious complication of LMWH is heparin-induced thrombocytopenia (HIT syndrome).
- Warfarin (Coumadin)—a vitamin K antagonist and the anti-coagulation effect may take several days to reach therapeutic levels. Patients often are placed on heparin or LMWH until the warfarin is therapeutic. The use of vitamin K antagonists requires monitoring, and the most common way to measure therapeutic effect is the prothrombin (PT) test.
- Fondaparinux—a selective factor Xa inhibitor. An advantage of fondaparinux over other injectable agents such as LMWH is that it does not inactivate thrombin (factor IIa), does not affect platelets, and does not cross-react with the serum of patients diagnosed with HIT.
- Direct oral anticoagulants (DOAC)—newer oral anticoagulants have the advantage of the ability to be administered at fixed doses without the need for laboratory monitoring.
  - *Rivaroxaban*—A direct inhibitor of activated factor X(Xa). Sold under the brand name Xarelto.
  - *Dabigatran*—A selective, reversible, direct thrombin inhibitor. Sold under brand name Pradaxa.
  - *Apixaban*—Also a direct activated factor X(Xa) inhibitor. Sold under brand name Eliquis.
- Dextran—should be used cautiously. The additional fluid volume may result in heart failure in patients with low cardiac reserve. A decrease in renal function also may occur from excessive diuresis after administration of dextran.
- Mechanical—a variety of mechanical modalities exist including early mobilization. External pneumatic compression devices decrease the risk of DVT without bleeding risk by decreasing venous stasis and stimulating fibrinolytic activity. Calf and thigh sleeves exist, as well as pneumatic foot pumps. The devices should not be used on patients who have an acute DVT or lower extremity fracture. Compression stockings also may help prevent venous thrombosis.

18. **What actions should a therapist take if a DVT is suspected?**
The therapist should hold therapeutic intervention and immediately inform the physician. The patient should be non–weight-bearing on the affected lower extremity until he or she is evaluated by the physician. Diagnostic tests

may be ordered by the physician to confirm the suspicion. Historically, patients with DVT were admitted to the hospital and placed on bed rest. Today, mobilization may begin as early as 24 hours after anticoagulation therapy has been initiated. Early mobilization may help prevent long-term complications.

19. **Discuss diagnostic tests for identifying DVT.**
    - D-dimer—a substance in the blood that is often elevated in patients with DVT or PE. D-dimer assays are fast, accurate, and readily available. The negative predictive value of the high-sensitivity d-dimer assay is about 94%. However, d-dimer is useful only for ruling out DVT. Positive results are not diagnostic for DVT.
    - Duplex ultrasound—the screening test of choice for initial evaluation of patients with suspected DVT. Color flow Doppler imaging improves the ability to detect a clot. In patients with asymptomatic DVT, the sensitivity and specificity have been found to be 89% and 100%, respectively. When used as a screening tool in asymptomatic patients, the sensitivity and specificity are 62% and 97%, respectively. Duplex ultrasound imaging is highly operator dependent, and these values vary widely among institutions. It is less sensitive for detecting calf vein thrombi than those located more proximally.
    - Venography—the gold standard for the diagnosis of DVT in the calf and thigh, with sensitivity and specificity almost 100%. The procedure is not an ideal screening test because of cost and potential morbidity related to the test. It is not recommended in the initial evaluation given the invasive nature, technical difficulty, and risks.
    - Impedance plethysmography—measures the change in blood volume in the calf while a thigh cuff is inflated. It is not readily available in the United States. May give false positive results.
    - ^{125}I-Fibrinogen scanning—90% accurate in detecting calf vein DVT. It may be falsely positive in the thigh after total hip arthroplasty in which there is fibrin present at the surgical site.
    - Magnetic resonance imaging—also may be used to image DVT, particularly in the pelvis (100% sensitivity, 95% specificity), where it is more sensitive than venography. Magnetic resonance imaging is equally sensitive for detection of DVT in the thigh but inferior in the calf (87% sensitivity and 97% specificity).

20. **If the presence of a DVT is confirmed, what treatments are available?**
    Anticoagulation is the treatment of choice for venous thromboembolism.
    - Heparin or LMWH is initiated to prevent propagation and promote stabilization of the clot.
    - Anticoagulation therapy is often continued for at least 3 months for DVT caused by surgery or other transient risk factors.

21. **What are the mechanisms of action of heparin, LMWH, warfarin, aspirin, fondaparinux, and the newer oral anticoagulants?**
    - Heparin—produces its major anticoagulant effect by inactivating thrombin and activated factor X (factor Xa)
    - LMWH—derived from heparin by chemical or enzymatic depolymerization to yield fragments approximately one-third the size of heparin. LMWH acts similarly to heparin, but compared with the unfractionated form, LMWH has a greater ratio of antifactor Xa/antifactor IIa activity, greater bioavailability, and longer duration of action.
    - Warfarin—acts by inhibiting the synthesis of vitamin K-dependent clotting factors, which include factors II, VII, IX, and X, and the anticoagulant proteins C and S
    - Aspirin—inhibits platelet cyclooxygenase, a key enzyme in thromboxane A2 (TXA2) generation. TXA2 triggers reactions that lead to platelet activation and aggregation.
    - Fondaparinux—antithrombotic effect is as a result of antithrombin III (ATIII)-mediated selective inhibition of factor Xa. By selectively binding to ATIII, fondaparinux sodium potentiates (about 300 times) the innate neutralization of factor Xa by ATIII. Neutralization of factor Xa interrupts the blood coagulation cascade.
    - Rivaroxaban—inhibits both free and bound factor Xa in the prothrombinase complex. It is a selective direct factor Xa inhibitor.
    - Dabigatran—reversibly binds to the active site on the thrombin molecule, preventing thrombin-mediated activation of coagulation factors. It also can inactivate thrombin even when thrombin is fibrin bound. It reduces thrombin-mediated inhibition of fibrinolysis.
    - Apixaban—a highly selective and reversible direct inhibitor of free and clot-bound factor Xa. It has no direct effect on platelet aggregation.

22. **Define PTT, PT, and INR.**
    - PTT (partial thromboplastin time)—used to monitor anticoagulation if patient is taking heparin
    - PT (prothrombin time)—used to monitor anticoagulation if the patient is taking warfarin
    - INR (international normalized ratio)—represents measured PT adjusted by reference thromboplastin so that all laboratories have a universal result of patient PT; usually kept between 2 and 3 for treatment or prevention of DVT

BIBLIOGRAPHY

Buller, H. R., Davidson, B. L., Decousus, H., et al. (2004). Fondaparinux or enoxaparin for the initial treatment of symptomatic deep venous thrombosis: a randomized trial. *Annals of Internal Medicine, 140*, 867–873.

Della Valle, C. J., Steiger, D. J., & Di Cesare, P. E. (1998). Thromboembolism after hip and knee arthroplasty: diagnosis and treatment. *Journal of the American Academy of Orthopaedic Surgeons, 6*, 327–336.

Diamond, S., Goldbweber, R., & Katz, S. (2005). Use of D-dimer to aid in excluding deep venous thrombosis in ambulatory patients. *American Journal of Surgery, 189*, 23–26.

Flevas, D. A., Megaloikonomos, P. D., Dimopoulos, L., et al. (2018). Thromboembolism prophylaxis in orthopaedics: an update. *EFORT Open Reviews, 3*(4), 136–148.

Grabowski, G., Whiteside, W., & Kanwisher, M. (2013). Venous thrombosis in athletes. *Journal of the American Academy of Orthopaedic Surgeons, 21*, 108–117.

Haas, S. (2000). Deep vein thrombosis: beyond the operating table. *Orthopedics, 6*, 629–632.

May, B. (2022, Jan 21). Updated CHEST Guidelines on Antithrombotic Therapy in Venous Thromboembolism. Pulmonary Advisor.

Simon, S. R. (1994). *Orthopaedic basic science.* Rosemont, IL: American Academy of Orthopaedic Surgeons.

Tornetta, P., & Bogdan, Y. (2012). Pulmonary embolism in orthopaedic patients: diagnosis and management. *Journal of the American Academy of Orthopaedic Surgeons, 20*, 586–595.

Wilbur, J., & Shian, B. (2012). Diagnosis of deep venous thrombosis and pulmonary embolism. *American Family Physician, 86*, 913–919.

CHAPTER 7 QUESTIONS

1. **A patient presents to the outpatient PT clinic for therapy following a left total knee arthroplasty. The patient notes some calf tenderness and the therapist appreciates increased swelling in the lower extremity. The patient has no cough or shortness of breath. The next best step would be:**
   a. Send the patient home and advise rest and pain medications. Resume therapy when the pain is better.
   b. Massage the calf to relieve the discomfort in addition to the prescribed PT.
   c. Hold therapy and contact the physician's office while the patient is in the clinic.
   d. Call 911 for transport to the nearest emergency center.

2. **What drug is not used for the treatment of confirmed DVT, but may be used as prophylaxis?**
   a. Heparin
   b. Coumadin
   c. Aspirin
   d. Arixtra

3. **What is the most common genetic risk factor for increased risk of DVT?**
   a. Factor V Leiden
   b. Protein C deficiency
   c. Protein S deficiency
   d. Osteogenesis imperfecta

4. **What is the initial test of choice for diagnosis of DVT?**
   a. MRI
   b. Venography
   c. Duplex ultrasound
   d. d-dimer

5. **Which drug does not match its mechanism of action?**
   a. Heparin—inactivating thrombin and activated factor X (factor Xa)
   b. Warfarin—inhibiting the synthesis of vitamin K–dependent clotting factors
   c. Aspirin—inhibits platelet cyclooxygenase
   d. Fondaparinux—inhibits bound and free thrombin

ELECTROTHERAPY

F.D. Pociask, PT, PhD, OCS, FAAOMPT and J.R. Krauss, PhD, PT, OCS, FAAOMPT

MUSCLE AND NERVE ANATOMY AND PHYSIOLOGY

1. **Define cellular membrane potentials.**
   Human cells are electrically charged or polarized, the inside of the cell being relatively negative in charge compared with the outside of the cell. The polarization is a result of the unequal distribution of ions on either side of the cell membrane. This polarity can be measured as a difference in electrical potential between the inside and the outside of the cell and is referred to as the membrane resting potential. Nerve cells are specialized in detecting changes in their surroundings. A rapid change in the membrane resting potential resulting in nerve depolarization and repolarization in response to stimulus is referred to as an action potential and is the basis for the transmission of a nerve impulse. Clinical applications of electrotherapy commonly generate action potentials in sensory and motor nerves.

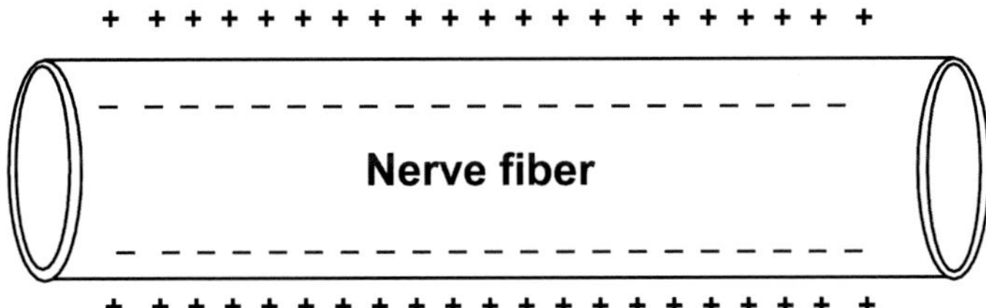

2. **Define refractory period.**
   Immediately after a nerve impulse is triggered, an ordinary stimulus is not able to generate another impulse. This brief period is termed the refractory period. The refractory period consists of two phases, the absolute refractory period and the relative refractory period. A subsequent action potential cannot be generated during the absolute refractory period. During the relative refractory period, a higher intensity stimulus can trigger an impulse.

3. **What is saltatory, or jumping conduction?**
   Saltatory (ie, jumping) conduction of a nerve impulse occurs in myelinated nerve axons because myelin is an excellent insulator with a high resistance to current flow. Because myelin does not cover the nodes of Ranvier, current flows from one node of Ranvier to the next. The action potentials do not travel along the entire length of the axon; consequently, the nerve impulses can travel much faster in myelinated axons compared with unmyelinated axons. This jumping of nerve impulses is much more efficient from a metabolic and physiologic standpoint. Fewer sodium and potassium ions are necessary to cross the cell membrane during the nerve impulse, and as a result, resting potentials are reestablished at a much faster rate, while conserving metabolic energy.

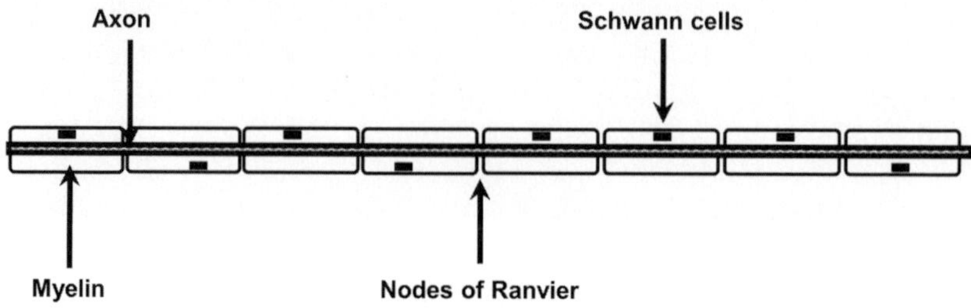

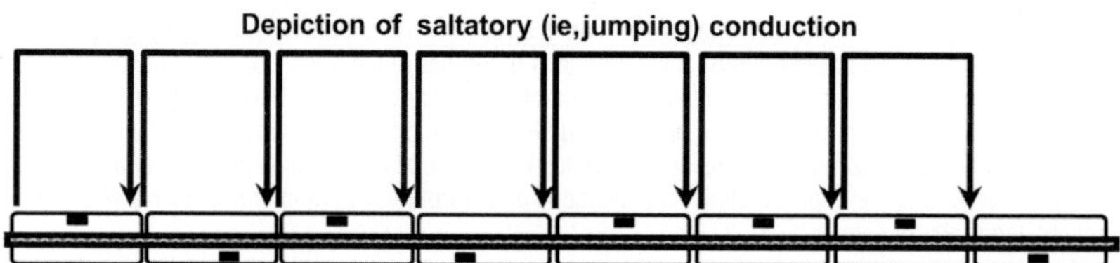

4. What are the approximate conduction velocities for myelinated and unmyelinated nerve fibers?
   - Larger myelinated ≈ 80–120 m/sec.
   - Small myelinated ≈ 10–30 m/sec.
   - Unmyelinated ≈ 0.5–2.0 m/sec.

PHYSICS OF ELECTRICAL FORCES

5. What is an electrical current?
   Current describes the rate of electron flow. The Ampere or amp (A) is the unit of measurement for electron flow. Clinically, intensity (I) is frequently used to denote current.

6. Clinically, therapeutic intensities should not exceed what amperage?
   Typical therapeutic intensities do not exceed 80 to 100 mA.

7. What is voltage?
   The rate of current flow depends on a source of free electrons, positive ions, materials that allow the electrons to flow, and the electromotive force that concentrates electrons in one place. The volt (V) is the International System of Units measure of electrical potential or electromotive force (ie, electric pressure), whereas voltage is the driving force of the electrons. One volt is the electromotive force required to move 1 amp of current through a resistance of 1 ohm.

8. What is resistance?
   Resistance describes the opposition to the flow of alternating and direct currents (ie, electron flow inhibitor). The ohm (Ω) is unit of measurement for electrical resistance.

9. How does Ohm's law express the relationship between current (I), voltage (V), and resistance (R)?
   $V = IR$
   $I = V/R$
   $R = V/I$
   Therefore:
   - When resistance decreases, current increases.
   - When resistance increases, current decreases.
   - When voltage decreases, current decreases.
   - When voltage increases, current increases.
   - When voltage is zero, current is zero.

10. **What factors may increase skin resistance to electrical currents over a treatment region and how can these factors be minimized?**

FACTORS INCREASING SKIN RESISTANCE	RECOMMENDATIONS TO DECREASE SKIN RESISTANCE
Cold skin temperature	Warm the skin
Excessive body hair	Remove excess hair
Oily skin or poor hygiene	Clean the skin or provide hygiene recommendations
Electrode type, interface, and surface dimensions	Select electrodes and an electrolytic interface best suited for the intended application and increase the cross-sectional area of the electrode if permissible

WAVEFORM CHARACTERISTICS

11. **What is the waveform of a current?**

The waveform is a graphic representation of the current flow over time. Waveforms are typically classified as direct (monophasic), alternating (biphasic), or pulsed current and are further defined by waveform units of measurement and output characteristics of electrical simulators. For example, electrical simulators may produce symmetric or asymmetrical biphasic, or sinusoidal or rectangular waveforms, as well as a wide variety of modulated waveforms. Many modern electrical simulators can produce a variety of waveforms; however, claims by manufacturers describing superiority of one waveform over anther typically lack scientific validation.

12. **Define frequency of an electrical current.**

The frequency is the number of pulses of electrical current that occur in a second, expressed as cycles per second (cps), Hertz (Hz), or pulses per second (pps). Clinically, "rate" and "pulse rate" are frequently used to describe frequency.

13. **Define pulse duration and phase duration.**

Pulse duration is the length of time the current is flowing per cycle and phase duration is the length of time the current is flowing for one phase of a pulse; both are typically expressed in microseconds (μs).

14. **Draw and label the following waveform characteristics: (1) pulse duration, (2) phase duration, and (3) amplitude.**

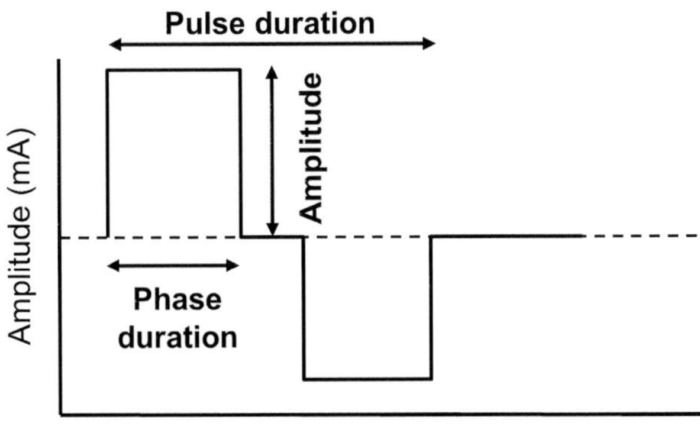

15. **Describe the clinical relevance of frequency, phase duration, and amplitude.**

Frequency contributes to the type of contraction (eg, twitch or tetanic), as well as theorized endogenous opiate pain effects. Phase duration contributes to the comfort of the stimulation, the amount of chemical change that occurs in the treated tissues, and nerve discrimination. A duration of 50 to 100 μs typically is used for sensory stimulation, and 200 to 300 μs is typically used for motor stimulation. Amplitude is less discriminatory than phase duration and pulse rate; low intensities (ie, amplitudes) are customarily used for sensory stimulation and higher intensities are customarily used for motor stimulation.

16. **Define rise time, fall time, and duty cycle.**
    - Rise time—the time that it takes the wave to travel from zero to its peak amplitude.
    - Fall time—the time that it takes the wave to travel from its peak amplitude to zero.
    - Duty cycle—the relative proportion of time between the stimulation period and the rest period expressed as a percentage.

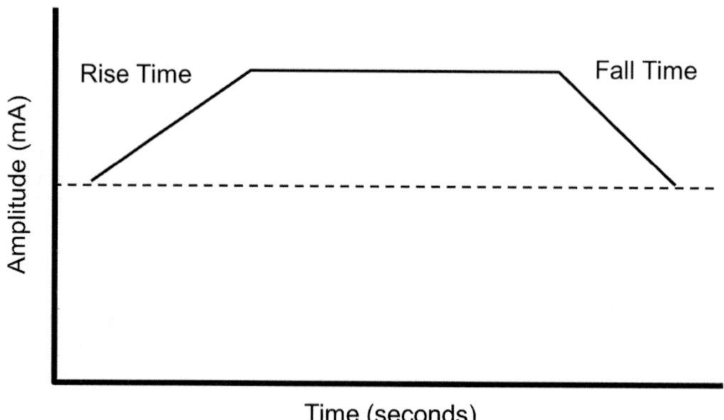

PRINCIPALS OF ALTERNATING, DIRECT, AND PULSED CURRENTS

17. **What are the criteria used to describe direct current?**
    Direct current (DC) is the flow of electrons in one direction for >1 second. A current is considered DC if it meets the following criteria:
    - Flow of electrons is unidirectional.
    - Polarity is constant.
    - Current produces a twitch response only at the time of make (ie, when the circuit is closed).
    - Cell membrane is hyperpolarized when the current is on.
    - Duration of current flow is >1 second.
    - Polar effects may occur under or around the electrode with extended treatment durations (eg, iontophoresis).

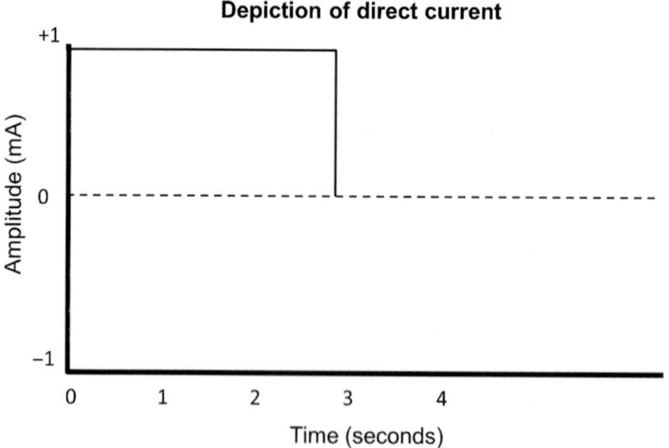

18. What are the criteria used to describe alternating current (AC)?

AC is characterized by sine wave modulation and has a constantly fluctuating voltage and a symmetric pattern. A current is termed AC if it meets the following criteria:

- Magnitude of flow of electrons changes.
- Direction of flow reverses.
- No polar effects should occur under or around the electrode.

Depiction of alternating current

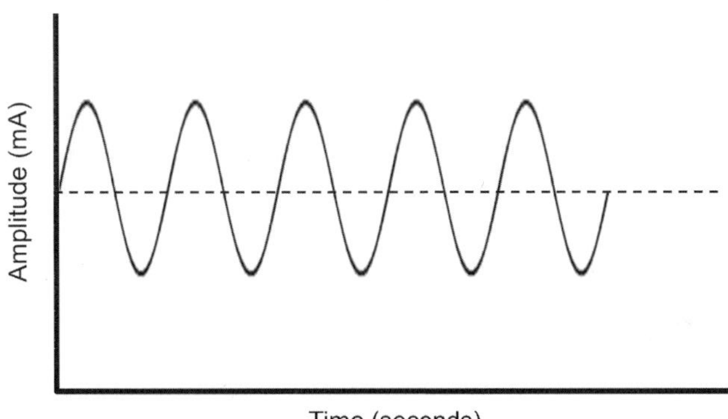

19. Does medium-frequency stimulation (MFS) differ from low-frequency stimulation in terms of skin resistance (capacitive impedance)?

Yes. When electrical current passes through cutaneous tissues, by surface electrodes, an opposition to the flow of current is encountered. When electrical currents are introduced into the body, ions accumulate at tissue interfaces, and cell membranes create a charge that opposes the applied voltage. This opposing voltage is referred to as reactance or capacitive impedance. The capacitive impedance can be calculated using the following formula:

$$\mathbf{Z} = \frac{\mathbf{1}}{\mathbf{C(F)} \times \mathbf{2} \times \mathbf{f(H \cdot z)}}$$

where Z=capacitive impedance, C=polarization capacitance of tissues in farads (constant), and F=frequency of current. This formula shows that capacitance impedance decreases as the frequency increases. Accordingly, medium frequency currents are capable and effective at stimulating deep and superficial tissues. For example, a 4100 Hz frequency and a 4000 Hz frequency will produce a constant beat frequency of 100 Hz. This will give the effect of deep painless treatment secondary to the medium frequency, and the low 100 Hz effect will be delivered deep in the tissues.

20. Describe the key attributes of interferential currents.

With true interferential current (IFC), two separate AC current generators produce electrical currents that vary in relation to one another in amplitude or frequency, or both. Where these two distinct currents meet in the tissue, an electrical interference pattern is created based on the summation or the subtraction of the respective amplitudes or frequencies. With a sinusoidal wave pattern, when oscillations from two unlike frequencies or amplitudes are out of phase and blend (heterodyne), they produce the interference effect for which this modality was given its name. The typical depiction of the interference pattern is that which may be produced in homogeneous tissues, which would differ in human tissues. With IFC, the patient perceives the resulting signal or beat signal produced by the heterodyned alternating current as amplitude-modulated electrical pulses.

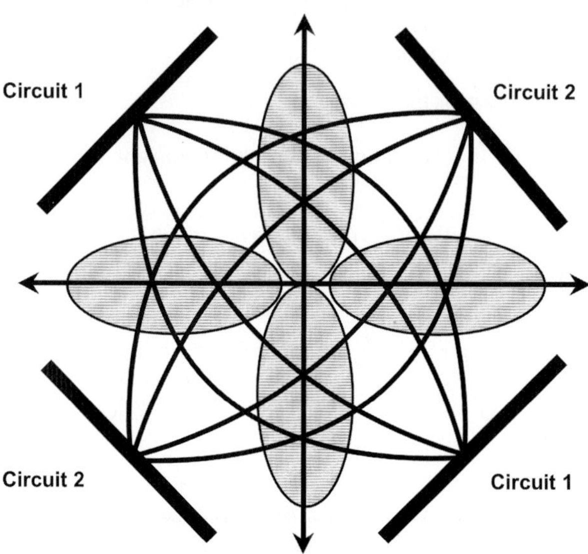

The beat signal is comparable to low-frequency pulse rates and is operationally the stimulation frequency of the waveform, which may be set to mimic frequencies comparable to low frequency protocols. For example, a 4100-Hz frequency and a 4200-Hz frequency could produce a constant beat frequency of 100 Hz. The phase duration of the delivered current can be easily calculated as follows:

$$\textbf{Frequency} = \frac{\textbf{1}}{\textbf{2} \times \textbf{Phase Duration}}$$

21. **What is premodulated IFC?**
Premodulated IFC is a medium-frequency sinusoidal waveform with increasing and decreasing current amplitude produced by a single current generator and delivered using two electrodes.

22. **Is premodulated or true IFC superior to the other?**
No. True IFC may be more comfortable and reach deeper and larger tissue areas as compared to premodulated IFC. Premodulated IFC may provide more simplified setups and may limit potential misapplications of true IFC. However, there is no conclusive evidence supporting the superiority of one form of IFC over the other for the management of common pain conditions, or to pain relief that may be provided by low frequency current generators. Additional studies are warranted.

23. **What is Russian protocol and how did it originate?**
Russian current or the 10/50/10 protocol (ie, 10 seconds on, 50 seconds off, repeat 10 times) is customarily defined as a medium-frequency sinusoidal waveform modulated (ie, burst) at 50 Hz, with a burst duration and interburst interval of 10 ms, using 10 ms on and 10 ms off periods at a maximum tolerable level, repeated 10 times with rest periods of 50 seconds or 10 stimulation/rest cycles. The Russian neuromuscular electrical stimulation (NMES) protocol was introduced by Yakov Kots in the late 1970s. Kots and his colleagues claimed the Russian current could produce a pain-free contraction with greater force than a maximal voluntary contraction and lasting strength gains in athletes. The studies conducted by Kots and corresponding data were never made available for scientific scrutiny and North American scientists have not been able to reproduce the proclaimed findings. Manufacturers of electrostimulation devices introduced Russian protocol stimulation devices in the 1980s based on Kots' unsubstantiated claims.

24. **Is the Russian protocol superior to voluntary exercise or other forms of NMES?**
No. While the Russian protocol has been shown to increase muscle strength as a form of NMES, there is no evidence showing that the Russian protocol is more effective to voluntary exercise training alone or more effective or comfortable than other forms of NMES.

25. **Does electrode construction and pressure influence stimulation performance during NMES?**
Euler et al. examined the effectiveness of dry and wet textile electrodes in combination with pressure. They concluded that wet textile electrodes (0.9 % saline solution) perform better than dry electrodes. However, the performance of dry textile electrodes improved when combined with an intermediate to high-pressure application of >20 mmHg (eg, the use of a compression stocking). They also concluded that 16 cm electrode areas were better than 32 cm in terms of stimulation comfort and efficiency.

26. **Does NMES therapy improve muscle performance in critically ill patients?**
There is evidence within the literature that NMES preserves muscle mass, joint range of motion, improves outcomes of ventilation, and reduces activity limitations in critically ill patients. However, due to inconsistencies with the reported literature, further research is warranted with longer follow-up periods and standardized outcome measures.

27. **What are the optimal parameters and application timeframe for the use of NMES for postoperative quadriceps strength in patients recovering from knee surgery?**
There is limited quality patient-oriented evidence supporting the use of NMES to aid in the recovery of quadriceps strength after knee surgery. It is recommended that NMES be implemented during the first 2 postoperative weeks at a frequency of ≥50 Hz, at maximal tolerable intensity, using a biphasic current, large electrode, and a duty cycle ratio of 1:2 (eg, 10 seconds on and 20 seconds off) to 1:3 and a 2- to 3-second ramp. Further research is warranted.

28. **Describe high-voltage pulsed current and the unique characteristics of this waveform.**
High-voltage twin-peaked pulsed current is unique because it cannot be readily classified as alternating or direct current. The typical high-volt current stimulator produces a twin-peak monophasic waveform. Because the waveform is fixed and small in duration, two peaks are required to depolarize nerve cells.

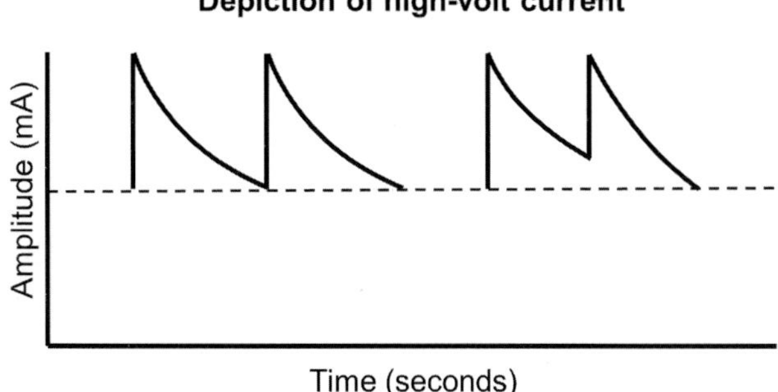

High-volt current stimulators are constant voltage units capable of delivering amplitudes >100 volts. They also have a high peak current; however, the average current is only 50% of the peak current. High-volt units typically have two electrode leads, one active and one dispersive, with the active electrodes being much smaller than the dispersive electrode. A variety of hand applicators and probes are available for the high-volt unit. A polarity switch is present and can be used to set the polarity of the active electrode.

29. **Describe how high voltage pulsed current differs from direct current.**

HIGH VOLTAGE	DIRECT CURRENT
• Used to excite peripheral nerves	• Useless in exciting peripheral nerves
• Useless in exciting denervated tissues	• Used to excite denervated tissues
• Creates minimal to no thermal reaction under electrodes	• Creates thermal and chemical reactions under electrodes
• Ineffective current for iontophoresis	• Effective current for iontophoresis
• Affects superficial and deep tissues	• Affects superficial tissues
• Allows discriminating between sensory, motor, and painful stimulation	• Discrimination is almost impossible, and stimulation is usually uncomfortable
• Used in a variety of sensory, edema control and wound healing applications	• Restricted benefit to a limited number of clinical presentations and pathologies
• Polarity under active electrode can be selected as positive or negative	• Polarity under active electrode is always negative

30. **Is high-voltage monophasic pulsed current (HVMPC) more effective than standard wound care (SWC) for treating stage II-IV pressure ulcers?**
Studies consistently demonstrate that HVMPC plus SWC were more effective than SWC alone, or SWC plus sham HVMPC, in treating stage II-IV pressure ulcers. Level 1 evidence studies indicate that HVMPC improves healing of pressure ulcers, reducing wound surface area, and when combined with SWC increased the probability of complete healing. Proposed applications for HVMPC include wound management, pain modulation, muscle reeducation, and reduction of spasm reduction. However, all applications, with the exception of wound management (eg, pressure ulcers), are best accomplished with other forms of electrotherapy. Electrically induced activity of inflammatory cells and cellular actions in the initial phases of tissue repair comprise the multitude of proposed mechanisms for the use of HVMPC in wound management.

31. **What is H-Wave® device stimulation?**
H-Wave® device stimulation (HWDS) is a form of transcutaneous electrotherapy that utilizes a proprietary waveform intended to stimulate contractions of the lymphatic smooth muscles and is intended for the treatment of edema, inflammation, and pain. H-wave parameters are described as a bipolar waveform with a pulse amplitude less than 10 mA, a fixed 16 ms pulse duration, and a frequency between 2 Hz and 60 Hz.

32. **Is H-Wave® device stimulation effective?**
Predominately low quality to limited moderate quality HWDS studies have reported positive and mixed findings for the use of H-Wave® for pain reduction, increased function, and lower medication use across numerous conditions. Additional studies are warranted.

33. **What is patterned electrical neuromuscular stimulation?**
Patterned electrical neuromuscular stimulation (PENS) is a form of NMES that claims to mimic normal muscle-firing patterns of healthy individuals as derived from electromyographic data of muscle agonist-antagonist pairs. PENS utilizes a low volt pulsed current at a frequency of 50 Hz and a short-phase duration of 70 microseconds. PENS protocols describe triphasic (agonist–antagonist–agonist), biphasic (agonist–antagonist), and functional rehabilitation stimulation patterns.

34. **Is PENS effective?**
Overall limited empirical evidence, which predominately includes low quality to limited moderate quality PENS literature, has reported positive, mixed, and no statistical or clinically meaningful effects. Positive effects have been reported for disuse atrophy, pain, muscle activation, and functional tasks across several orthopaedic conditions, as well as muscle activation and kinematics in healthy subjects. Additional studies are warranted.

ELECTRODES AND ELECTRODE PLACEMENT

35. **What is the relationship between interelectrode distance and depth of penetration?**
Current travels through areas of least resistance; electrodes placed at greater distances from each other should be expected to provide deeper penetration, provided that other factors remain constant.

36. **Name three common electrode placement strategies for NMES.**
    1. Unipolar method: the active electrode is placed on the motor point, and the dispersive electrode is placed on some other point such as the nerve trunk.
    2. Bipolar method: two electrodes of equal size are placed along the length of the muscle belly. The active electrode is usually placed over the motor point.
    3. Quadripolar method: four electrodes of equal size are used. This application is typically reserved for interferential currents in which two electrodes from each channel crisscross the treatment region.

37. **Compare and contrast electrode size in terms of current density and spread, selectivity and discrimination.**

SMALL ELECTRODES	LARGE ELECTRODES
Greater current density	Less current density
Decreased current spread	Increased current spread
More selective	Less selective
Greater discrimination	Less discrimination

STIMULATION OF HEALTHY AND DENERVATED TISSUES

38. **Discuss Pflüger's law and its implications in the stimulation of human tissues.**
    According to Pflüger's law, healthy muscle contracts with less current if stimulated by the cathode compared with stimulation by the anode. When stimulating a muscle with a direct current, the cathode should be the active electrode because the amount of current required to acquire a muscle contraction is less with the active cathode than with the anode:

$$\text{CCC} > \text{ACC} > \text{AOC} > \text{COC}$$

where CCC=cathode closing current, ACC=anode closing current, AOC=anode opening current, COC=cathode opening current, closing=starting the current, and opening=stopping the current.

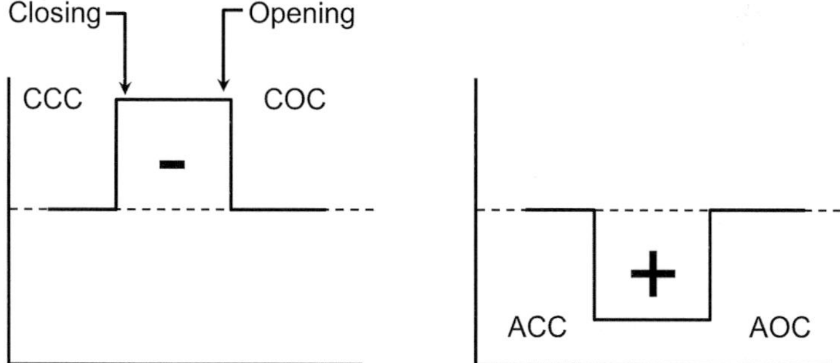

39. **What is accommodation?**
    Accommodation is the increased threshold of excitable tissue when a slowly rising stimulus is used. Both nerve and muscle tissues are capable of accommodating an electrical stimulus; nerve tissue accommodates more rapidly than muscle tissue. Understanding the process of accommodation is important when stimulating healthy muscle by the motor axon because the electrical stimulus must be applied somewhat rapidly to avoid accommodation.

40. **What is the strength-duration curve?**
    The strength-duration curve describes the relationship between the strength of the stimulus (intensity) and the duration of the stimulus (on time) required to reach a specified level of activation. By varying the intensity and duration of an electrical stimulus, it is possible to plot a strength-duration curve. The strength-duration curve gives

a graphic representation of the excitability of nerve and muscle tissues. Although the strength-duration curves are comparable for healthy nerve and muscle tissues, they are different from denervated nerve and muscle tissues. As a result, we are clinically able to stimulate healthy, innervated muscles with a stimulus of adequate amplitude and of short duration. It also is shown by this curve that greater amplitudes of stimulus and longer durations are necessary to stimulate denervated muscles effectively.

TEST	NORMAL	DENERVATING	DENERVATED	REINNERVATING	REINNERVATED
Chronaxie	< 1 msec	begins to rise	30 to 50 msec	begins to decrease	approaches normal
Strength Duration Curve	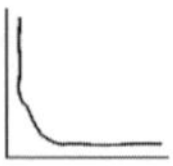	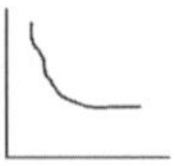	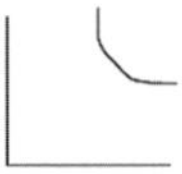	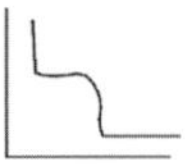	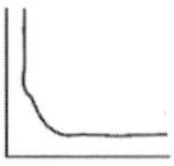
Reaction of degeneration	AC = DC	DC > AC	DC only	AC begins	AC = DC
Nerve Conduction	40 to 60 m/sec	No conduction after 3 days	No conduction	Conduction increases	WNL

CLINICAL APPLICATION

41. List common indications for electrical stimulation.

- Pain management.
- Edema management.
- Maintaining and improving range of motion.
- Neuromuscular facilitation and reeducation.
- Muscle strengthening.
- Reduction of muscle spasm.

42. What are common contraindications and precautions for electrotherapy application?

Contraindications (Absolute and Relative):

- Patients with synchronous or demand type pacemakers, cardiac defibrillators, or unstable arrhythmias.
- Placement of electrodes across or around the heart.
- Placement of electrodes over an area suspected of arterial or venous thrombosis or thrombophlebitis.
- Patients prone to seizures.
- Placement of electrodes over the uterus during pregnancy, especially during the first trimester (delivery itself may present with relative precautions).
- Placement of electrodes over pharyngeal, carotid sinus orbital, and transcranial areas.
- Placement of electrodes over protruding metal.
- Patients that experience adverse reactions to electrotherapy application.

Precautions:

- Allergies to tapes, gels, electrodes, etc., used during treatment.
- Areas of absent or decreased sensation.
- Electrically sensitive patients.
- Patients with a history of cardiac disease.
- Patients with severe hypotension or hypertension.
- Placement of the electrode over an area with significant adipose tissue.
- Placement of the electrode over damaged skin, except for certain tissue healing protocols.
- Placement of the electrode over or near the stellate ganglion.
- Patients who are unable to communicate clearly.

43. Outline a suitable protocol for neuromuscular facilitation and reeducation including purpose, rationale, indications, parameters, and special considerations.

- Purpose—to barrage the central nervous system (CNS) with appropriate sensory information.
- Rationale—by supplying the proper sensory input of what a muscle contraction or limb movement feels like, and visual information about the appearance of the action, electrical stimulation can enhance a motor response.
- Indications—any patient for whom a motor- and sensory-augmented muscle response would assist in better performance of his or her own voluntary actions.

- Parameters—pulse duration, 100 to 200 μs for small muscles and 200 to 250 μs for large muscles; pulse rate, 35 to 50 Hz or desired tetanic contraction; intensity, to a tolerable motor level or sufficient level for functional activity goals; ramp 1 to 3 seconds up/down as tolerated or activity specific; on/off, 1:1 ratio set or hand-held switch; treatment time, 5 to 30 minutes, 1 to 3 times/day, 3 to 7 days/week, 1 to 2 weeks. Adjust parameters as indicated and as tolerated by the patient.
- Special considerations—facilitation and reeducation require active participation by the patient and may be limited by patient tolerance, cooperation, and attention span.

44. **Outline a suitable protocol for muscle strengthening in terms of purpose, rationale, indications, parameters, and special considerations.**
    - Purpose—to increase muscle strength, encourage muscle hypertrophy, and facilitate normal motor response.
    - Rationale—electrical stimulation can be used to help patients achieve a volitional contraction sufficient to increase strength and prevent disuse atrophy if they are unable to do so on their own.
    - Indications—any patient in need of increasing girth and strength of an atrophied muscle.
    - Parameters—pulse duration, 125 to 200 μs for small muscles and 250 to 350 μs for large muscles; pulse rate, 35 to 80 Hz or desired tetanic contraction; intensity, motor at 10% to 20% maximal voluntary contraction (MVC) in injured muscle and 50% to 60% MVC in uninjured muscle; ramp 1 to 5 seconds up/down as tolerated or activity specific; on/off, 1:5 ratio; treatment time, 10 to 20 minutes, or activity specific, 10 to 20 reps every 2 to 3 hours while awake, 3 to 5 days/week, 2 to 3 weeks. Adjust parameters as indicated and as tolerated by the patient.
    - Special considerations—this program should be used with patients with sufficient innervation to make muscle strengthening practical. It is important to avoid muscle fatigue with this type of stimulation.

45. **Should the presence or absence of a knee extensor lag be a criterion for using or not using NMES after ACL reconstruction?**
    No. No strong relationship has been found between knee extensor lag and treatment outcomes after use of NMES.

46. **Discuss important considerations and treatment parameters for maintaining joint range of motion.**
    Protocols should typically begin with simple one-plane joint movements, use antigravity starting positions with a rest period between movements, and progress to antigravity positions without a rest period between movements (ie, flexion-rest-extension-rest) and repeat as tolerated. Reasonable treatment parameters are as follows: intensity, to a tolerable motor level; frequency, 35 to 50 Hz or desired tetanic contraction; phase duration, 125 to 200 μs; ramp, 4 to 5 seconds progressing to 3 seconds; on/off, as required to achieve desired range of motion; treatment time, 30 min/day, 50 repetitions. Adjust parameters as indicated and as tolerated by the patient.

47. **Discuss key considerations and treatment parameters for edema control.**
    Muscular activity is an important aspect of lymphatic and venous flow. The contraction of skeletal muscles by electrical stimulation can produce a muscle contraction capable of aiding lymphatic and venous flow. The intervention can be enhanced further by combining it with other forms of management, such as elevation, rest, and compression. Muscle pumping protocols are also valuable for pain modulation. Reasonable stimulation parameters should focus on producing a nonfatiguing muscle contraction: pulse rate, 35 to 50 Hz or desired tetanic contraction; phase duration, 100 to 200 μs; intensity, visible muscle contraction, time of treatment, 20 to 30 minutes, two to three times per day as part of a home program, 1 to 2 weeks; electrode placement, muscle bulk of an involved region. Adjust parameters as indicated and as tolerated by the patient.

48. **What are the suitable parameters and rationale for conventional, low-rate, and brief intense transcutaneous electrical nerve stimulation (TENS)?**

	CONVENTIONAL	LOW RATE	BRIEF INTENSE
Indications	Acute, superficial pain, and/or first-time application	Sub-acute to chronic pain	Prior to or in conjunction with other interventions
Phase duration	50 to 80 μs	150 to 300 μs	>250 μs
Pulse rate	100 to 150 Hz	2 to 10 Hz	125 Hz (can be varied)
Intensity	Sensory just below motor	Extremely high sensory to a visible contraction	Extremely high sensory to a visible contraction
Treatment duration	15 to 30 minutes up to 24 hours if needed	30 to 45 minutes	10 to 15 minutes

Continued

	CONVENTIONAL	LOW RATE	BRIEF INTENSE
Onset of relief	10 to 20 minutes	20 to 40 minutes	1 to 10 minutes
Possible carryover	30 minutes to 2 hours	Several hours to a day	Short (<30 minutes)
Proposed rationales for pain reduction	Gate control theory of pain, endogenous opiate pain control theory, and descending pain control theory, as well as potential counterirritant and placebo effects.		

Electrotherapy protocols may vary greatly in literature. Electrotherapeutic interventions must be selected based of factors such as the condition being treated, the stage of injury, the electrical stimulation device being utilized, available evidence and clinical practice guidelines, indications, and contraindications. All electrotherapeutic intervention should be carefully scrutinized before they are applied to patient care.

49. Is TENS effective in the management of chronic pain in adults?

Evidence is inconclusive. A review by Gibson et al. (2019) of evidence from Cochrane Reviews on the effectiveness of TENS in the management of chronic pain in adults was "unable to conclude with any confidence that, in people with chronic pain, TENS is harmful, or beneficial for pain control, disability, health-related quality of life, use of pain-relieving medicines, or global impression of change" (p. 2). Very low quality of the evidence was identified as one principal factor for this conclusion. Two additional systematic reviews from the Cochrane Database reported insufficient evidence for the use of TENS in patients with chronic neck pain and the use of TENS for neuropathic pain in adults.

50. Is TENS effective in the management of acute pain in adults?

TENS may be effective in reducing the intensity of acute pain in some patients. A second update of a Cochrane Review by Johnson et al. (2015) on the transcutaneous electrical nerve stimulation for acute pain reported "tentative evidence that TENS reduces pain intensity over and above that seen with placebo (no current) TENS when administered as a stand-alone treatment for acute pain in adults" (p. 2). The authors reported that quality of evidence was moderate to low, making definitive conclusions impossible.

51. Is biofeedback recommended following knee arthroscopic surgery?

In addition to cryotherapy and NMES, surface electromyographic (sEMG) biofeedback is recommended following arthroscopic surgery to assist in pain relief, recovery of muscle strength, and knee function. In contrast, a continuous passive motion (CPM) device is not recommended due to its limited effectiveness in restoring knee range of motion.

Bibliography

Beatti, A., Rayner, A., Chipchase, L., & Souvlis, T. (2011). Penetration and spread of interferential current in cutaneous, subcutaneous and muscle tissues. *Physiotherapy, 97*(4), 319–326.

Bellew, J. W. (2016). Clinical electrical stimulation: application and techniques. In J. W. Bellew, S. L. Michlovitz, & T. P. Nolan (Eds.), *Michlovitz's modalities for therapeutic intervention* (pp. 287–327). Philadelphia, PA: F.A. Davis Company.

Bickel, S. C., Gregory, C. M., & Bellew, J. W. (2016). Electrotherapy for musculoskeletal disorders. In J. W. Bellew, S. L. Michlovitz, & T. P. Nolan (Eds.), *Michlovitz's modalities for therapeutic intervention* (pp. 373–397). Philadelphia, PA: F.A. Davis Company.

Burch, F. X., Tarro, J. N., Greenberg, J. J., & Carroll, W. J. (2008). Evaluating the benefits of patterned stimulation in the treatment of osteoarthritis of the knee: a multi-center, randomized, single-blind, controlled study with an independent masked evaluator. *Osteoarthritis Cartilage, 16*(8), 865–872.

Cameron, M. H., Shapiro, S., & Ocelnik, M. (2018a). Electrical currents for muscle contraction. In M. H. Cameron (Ed.), *Physical agents in rehabilitation: an evidence-based approach to practice* (pp. 238–257). St. Louis, MO: Elsevier/Saunders.

Cameron, M. H., Shapiro, S., & Ocelnik, M. (2018b). Introduction to electrotherapy. In M. H. Cameron (Ed.), *Physical agents in rehabilitation: an evidence-based approach to practice.* St. Louis, MO: Elsevier/Saunders.

Cobo-Vicente, F., San Juan, A. F., Larumbe-Zabala, E., et al. (2021). Neuromuscular electrical stimulation improves muscle strength, biomechanics of movement, and functional mobility in children with chronic neurological disorders: a systematic review and meta-analysis. *Physical Therapy, 101*(10), pzab170.

Conley, C. E. W., Mattacola, C. G., Jochimsen, K. N., et al. (2021). A comparison of neuromuscular electrical stimulation parameters for postoperative quadriceps strength in patients after knee surgery: a systematic review. *Sports Health, 13*(2), 116–127.

de Freitas, G. R., Szpoganicz, C., & Ilha, J. (2018). Does neuromuscular electrical stimulation therapy increase voluntary muscle strength after spinal cord injury? A systematic review. *Topics in Spinal Cord Injury Rehabilitation, 24*(1), 6–17.

DeJong, G., Hsieh, C. J., Vita, M. T., et al. (2020). Innovative devices did not provide superior total knee arthroplasty outcomes in post-operative rehabilitation: results from a four-arm randomized clinical trial. *The Journal of Arthroplasty, 35*(8), 2054–2065.

Draper, D. O., Jutte, L. S., & Knight, K. L. (2021a). Application procedures: Electrotherapy. In D. O. Draper, L. S. Jutte, & K. L. Knight (Eds.), *Therapeutic modalities: the art and science* (pp. 321–361). Philadelphia, PA: Wolters Kluwer.

Draper, D. O., Jutte, L. S., & Knight, K. L. (2021b). Principles of electricity for electrotherapy. In D. O. Draper, L. S. Jutte, & K. L. Knight (Eds.), *Therapeutic modalities: the art and science* (pp. 299–320). Philadelphia, PA: Wolters Kluwer.

Euler, L., Juthberg, R., Flodin, J., et al. (2021). Textile electrodes: influence of electrode construction and pressure on stimulation performance in neuromuscular electrical stimulation (NMES). *Annual International Conference IEEE Engineering in Medicine and Biology Society, 2021*, 1305–1308.

Facci, L. M., Nowotny, J. P., Tormem, F., & Trevisani, V. F. (2011). Effects of transcutaneous electrical nerve stimulation (TENS) and interferential currents (IFC) in patients with nonspecific chronic low back pain: randomized clinical trial. *Sao Paulo Medical Journal, 129*(4), 206–216.

Gatewood, C. T., Tran, A. A., & Dragoo, J. L. (2017). The efficacy of post-operative devices following knee arthroscopic surgery: a systematic review. *Knee Surgery, Sports Traumatology, Arthroscopy, 25*(2), 501–516.

Gibson, W., Wand, B. M., & O'Connell, N. E. (2017). Transcutaneous electrical nerve stimulation (TENS) for neuropathic pain in adults. *The Cochrane Database of Systematic Reviews, 9*, CD011976.

Gibson, W., Wand, B. M., Meads, C., Catley, M. J., & O'Connell, N. E. (2019). Transcutaneous electrical nerve stimulation (TENS) for chronic pain—an overview of Cochrane Reviews. *The Cochrane Database of Systematic Reviews, 4*(4). CD011890-CD011890.

Girgis, B., & Duarte, J. A. (2018). High voltage monophasic pulsed current (HVMPC) for stage II-IV pressure ulcer healing. A systematic review and meta-analysis. *Journal of Tissue Viability, 27*(4), 274–284.

Glaviano, N. R., Marshall, A. N., Mangum, L. C., et al. (2019). Impairment-based rehabilitation with patterned electrical neuromuscular stimulation and lower extremity function in individuals with patellofemoral pain: a preliminary study. *Journal of Athletic Training, 54*(3), 255–269.

Glaviano, N. R., & Saliba, S. A. (2016). Immediate effect of patterned electrical neuromuscular stimulation on pain and muscle activation in individuals with patellofemoral pain. *Journal of Athletic Training, 51*(2), 118–128.

Glaviano, N. R., Huntsman, S., Dembeck, A., Hart, J. M., & Saliba, S. (2016). Improvements in kinematics, muscle activity and pain during functional tasks in females with patellofemoral pain following a single patterned electrical stimulation treatment. *Clinical Biomechanics, 32*, 20–27.

Gorgey, A. S., & Dudley, G. A. (2008). The role of pulse duration and stimulation duration in maximizing the normalized torque during neuromuscular electrical stimulation. *The Journal of Orthopaedic and Sports Physical Therapy, 38*(8), 508–516.

Hooker, D. N., & Prentice, W. E. (2021). Basic principles of electricity and electrical stimulating currents. In W. E. Prentice (Ed.), *Therapeutic modalities in rehabilitation* (pp. 105–186). New York, NY: McGraw Hill.

Johnson, M. I., Paley, C. A., Howe, T. E., & Sluka, K. A. (2015). Transcutaneous electrical nerve stimulation for acute pain. *The Cochrane Database of Systematic Reviews, 2015*(6). CD006142.

Martimbianco, A. L. C., Porfirio, G. J., Pacheco, R. L., Torloni, M. R., & Riera, R. (2019). Transcutaneous electrical nerve stimulation (TENS) for chronic neck pain. *The Cochrane Database of Systematic Reviews, 12*, CD011927.

Ozcan, J., Ward, A. R., & Robertson, V. J. (2004). A comparison of true and premodulated interferential currents. *Archives of Physical Medicine and Rehabilitation, 85*(3), 409–415.

Samuel, S. R., & Maiya, G. A. (2015). Application of low frequency and medium frequency currents in the management of acute and chronic pain-a narrative review. *Indian Journal of Palliative Care, 21*(1), 116–120.

Tanaka, M., Hirayama, Y., Fujita, N., & Fujino, H. (2013). Comparison of premodulated interferential and pulsed current electrical stimulation in prevention of deep muscle atrophy in rats. *Journal of Molecular Histology, 44*(2), 203–211.

Wang, T. J., Sung, K., Wilburn, M., & Allbright, J. (2019). Russian stimulation/functional electrical stimulation in the treatment of foot drop resulting from lumbar radiculopathy: a case series. *Innovations in Clinical Neuroscience, 16*(5-6), 46–49.

Ward, A. R., & Shkuratova, N. (2002). Russian electrical stimulation: The early experiments. *Physical Therapy, 82*(10), 1019–1030.

Ward, A. R., Lucas-Toumbourou, S., & McCarthy, B. (2009). A comparison of the analgesic efficacy of medium-frequency alternating current and TENS. *Physiotherapy, 95*(4), 280–288.

Williamson, T. K., Rodriguez, H. C., Gonzaba, A., et al. (2021). H-Wave® device stimulation: a critical review. *Journal of Personalized Medicine, 11*(11), 1134.

CHAPTER 8 QUESTIONS

1. **Select the waveform characteristic that BEST contributes to the comfort of stimulation, the amount of chemical change that occurs in the treated tissues, and nerve discrimination.**
   a. Amplitude
   b. Frequency
   c. Phase duration
   d. Current

2. **Select the form of electrotherapy that is BEST suited for the treatment of pressure ulcers.**
   a. H-Wave® device stimulation
   b. High-voltage monophasic pulsed current
   c. Premodulated interferential current
   d. Patterned electrical stimulation

3. **Select the form of electrotherapy that is BEST suited to help patients in recovering muscle strength following surgery.**
   a. Conventional TENS
   b. High-voltage monophasic pulsed current
   c. sEMG biofeedback
   d. Patterned electrical neuromuscular stimulation

CHAPTER 9

IONTOPHORESIS, ULTRASOUND, PHONOPHORESIS, AND PHOTOBIOMODULATION THERAPY

F.D. Pociask, PT, PhD, OCS, FAAOMPT and J.R. Krauss, PhD, PT, OCS, FAAOMPT

IONTOPHORESIS

1. **Define iontophoresis.**
   Iontophoresis is a noninvasive and targeted method of transdermal drug delivery that drives negatively or positively charged ion solutions through the skin and into underlying tissues by means of a low-amplitude direct electrical current.

2. **Describe how Leduc's classic strychnine experiment established ionized molecules can penetrate intact skin.**
   In 1908 Leduc showed that ionic medication could penetrate intact skin and produce local and systemic effects in animals. Two rabbits were placed in series in the same direct current circuit so that the current had to pass through both rabbits to complete the circuit. The electrical current entered the first rabbit by a positive electrode soaked in strychnine sulfate and exited the rabbit by a negative electrode soaked in water. The current then entered the second rabbit by an anode soaked in water and exited by a cathode soaked in potassium cyanide. When a current of 40 to 50 mA was used, the first rabbit exhibited tetanic convulsions secondary to the introduction of the strychnine ion, and the second rabbit died quickly, secondary to cyanide poisoning. When the animals were replaced and the flow of current was reversed, they were not harmed because the strychnine ion was not repelled by the positive pole and the cyanide was not repelled by the negative pole.

3. **What are potential advantages of iontophoresis?**
   - Able to deliver antiinflammatory medication locally without gastrointestinal or systemic effects noted with injection or oral medication
   - No carrier fluids are required
   - Noninvasive application
   - Portable wired and self-contained wireless patches provide greater treatment options
   - Relatively painless for most patients

4. **What are the potential disadvantages of iontophoresis?**
   - Depth of penetration and treatment area are limited
   - Electrodes are costly
   - Numerous treatments may be required to obtain results
   - Setup and application are time consuming
   - Skin irritation may occur
   - Unknown concentrations of drugs delivered to tissues

5. **What type of current is used for iontophoresis?**
   A continuous direct current is characteristically used for iontophoresis. The current is on for the duration of the treatment, the flow of electrons is unidirectional, and polarity is constant.

6. **Why is continuous direct current effective for performing iontophoresis?**
   The positively charged electrode (ie, anode) repels or delivers positively charged ionic drugs and the negatively charged electrode (ie, cathode) repels or delivers negatively charged ions into the skin and tissues under the active or dispersive electrode.

7. **Can modulated pulsed currents be used for iontophoresis?**
   Research on the use of modulated pulsed currents is limited and includes in vivo and in vitro animal studies, as well as human epidermal membranes in vitro. Evidence supporting the efficacy of modulated pulsed currents is predominately absent and these currents have not shown to enhance iontophoretic transport compared to direct

currents. Further investigations are necessary to identify the potential benefits of modulated pulsed currents, which may include a decreased risk of local electrochemical skin irritation.

8. **What are the typical dosages and methods of delivery for iontophoretic drug delivery?**
Iontophoresis treatment dosage is expressed in milliamperes-minutes (mA-min), which reflects the direct current amplitude measured in milliamps and the duration of treatment time measured in minutes. For example, a 4.0 mA current delivered for 10 minutes results in a 40 mA-min treatment dose. In contrast, self-contained wireless patches provide comparable iontophoresis dosages at much smaller current intensities, usually 80 mA/min, for a longer treatment time (eg, 3–24 hours). However, there is little agreement of optimal dosage, particularly for different orthopaedic conditions, and the specific parameters required to achieve it.

9. **How many serial iontophoresis treatments are safe?**
While there is no clear consensus, the total number of ionophoretic treatments, as well as the time between individual applications, will vary based on the ion or medication being used. One to six treatments of dexamethasone have been shown to be safe and effective in the management of specific orthopaedic conditions when administered alone and delivered 1 to 3 days apart within 15 days.

10. **What is the depth of iontophoretic drug delivery?**
The depth of iontophoretic drug delivery below the surface of the skin is uncertain; however, authors have reported depths ranging from 3 to 20 mm. It has been shown that lidocaine iontophoresis can reach a depth of 3 mm in the gastrocnemius muscle when delivered at a 40 mA-min dose and 2% lidocaine can be delivered up to 5 mm below the surface of the skin when combined with epinephrine and passive delivery occurs for at least 50 minutes after active delivery is concluded. It has also been suggested that longer periods of passive drug delivery following active delivery, greater interelectrode distance, and longer durations of active treatment at lower amplitudes may facilitate greater depths of drug delivery in human tissues. Additional studies are warranted.

11. **List commonly used ions, their polarity, proposed indications, and concentrations.**

ION	POLARITY	INDICATIONS	CONCENTRATION
Dexamethasone	Negative	Inflammation	0.4 (4 mg/mL)
Lidocaine	Positive	Local anesthetic effects	4%–5%
Salicylates	Negative	Inflammation	2%–3%
Tap water	Alternate	Hyperhidrosis	100%
Zinc oxide	Positive	Dermal ulcers and wounds	20%
Acetic acid	Negative	Calcium deposits	2%–5%
Iodine	Negative	Scar tissue adhesions	5%–10%

Proposed indications and concentrations of ions vary in literature and with factors such as the condition being treated, the stage of injury, treatment parameters and the transdermal delivery system. Ions, ionic concentrations and treatment parameters should be carefully scrutinized before they are applied to patient care.

12. **Should ionophoretic patches be removed immediately following active treatment?**
Maybe. While typical treatment durations for wired delivery system range from 10 to 40 minutes, limited evidence suggests that the active (ie, medicated) electrode may be worn for up to 3 to 24 hours after the electrical current is stopped to allow for passive diffusion of medication. Equally, newer wireless patches typically require a longer treatment duration (eg, up to 24 hours), which may include time for passive diffusion of medication. Following manufacturer recommendations and carefully monitoring for adverse skin reactions are important considerations for determining when the patch should be removed.

13. **What factors influence the efficacy of iontophoresis?**
- The time of application of the current
- The intensity of the current
- The cross-sectional area of the skin in contact with the electrodes
- The integrity of the skin surface and skin thickness under the electrodes
- The electrical impedance of the tissues being treated
- The selected ion has a therapeutic effect on the patient's condition
- The concentration of ions in solution

- The pH of the iontophoretic solution
- The quality of the iontophoretic patch and phoresor system
- The difference in current density between the active and dispersive electrodes

14. **List contraindications for iontophoresis.**
Contraindications for iontophoresis include damaged skin in the area of application, drug allergies or sensitivity to the ion used for treatment, potential drug interactions, and general contraindication to electrotherapy.

15. **Summarize the efficacy of iontophoresis in the management of common orthopaedic conditions.**
Although iontophoresis is commonly used in clinical practice for the management of numerous orthopedic conditions, efficacy data are conflicting. Well-controlled and larger-scale clinical trials of sufficient duration are needed to better understand the effectiveness of iontophoresis in the management of musculoskeletal disorders. At present, orthopaedic conditions that appear to benefit from dexamethasone iontophoresis include epicondylitis, TMJ dysfunction, midportion Achilles tendinopathy, and short-term (ie, 2–4 weeks) relief of plantar heel pain resulting from plantar fasciitis. Additionally, lidocaine iontophoresis appears to be effective in pain relief and the study of ketoprofen iontophoresis is promising in terms of a greater potential for direct penetration into local tissues underneath the skin. The efficacy of acetic acid iontophoresis used in the treatment of other orthopaedic conditions, such as calcific tendinitis of the shoulder, remains unclear. Equally, iontophoresis is not currently recommended for the management of patellofemoral pain, mild to moderate carpal tunnel syndrome, adhesive capsulitis, and intermediate and long-term (ie, 1–6 months) relief of plantar heel pain resulting from plantar fasciitis.

16. **What is the difference between phonophoresis and iontophoresis?**
Phonophoresis utilizes ultrasound to facilitate transdermal drug delivery of topical medications and iontophoresis utilizes low-amplitude direct electric current to facilitate the delivery of ionic drugs.

ULTRASOUND

17. **How is ultrasound generated, and what is a piezoelectric effect?**
The natural quartz or synthetic crystal housed within the sound head, classified as a piezoelectric material, will mechanically respond or deform when subjected to alternating current (AC) by expanding and contracting at the same frequency at which the current changes polarity. This process is described as a piezoelectric effect.

18. **What is the beam nonuniformity ratio (BNR)?**
BNR is the measure of the variability of the ultrasound wave intensity produced by the machine. If the machine is set at 1.5 W, BNR is the range of possible intensities actually delivered by the machine. The lower the ratio, the more uniform the machine output, resulting in a more uniform treatment. A higher ratio, 8 W, for example, means that when the machine is set at 1 W, it could deliver in the range of 1 to 8 W.

19. **What is the effective radiating area (ERA) of a transducer?**
ERA is the effective radiating area that corresponds to the part of the sound head that produces the sound wave. The ERA should be close to the size of the sound head or transducer. If it is smaller than the sound head, it may be misleading when treating the patient. The recommended treatment area is only two to three times the ERA.

20. **What are nonthermal and thermal ranges of therapeutic ultrasound?**
Intensities between 0.1 and 0.3 W/cm^2 are considered nonthermal, and intensities above approximately 0.3 W/cm^2 are considered thermal.

21. **What are the reported and theorized nonthermal effects of ultrasound?**
    - Increased cell membrane permeability
    - Increased vascular permeability
    - Increased blood flow in chronically ischemic tissue
    - Collagen synthesis
    - Phagocytosis
    - Promotes tissue regeneration
    - Breaks down scar tissue in acute injuries
    - Kills bacteria and viruses in chronic situations

22. **What are the reported and theorized thermal effects of ultrasound?**
    - Preferentially heats collagen-rich tissues
    - Increased tissue elasticity of collagen-rich tissue

- Increased blood flow
- Increased pain threshold
- Decreased muscle spasm
- Decreased pain and joint stiffness
- Mild inflammatory response

23. **How does ultrasound frequency relate to depth of penetration?**
Increasing the frequency of ultrasound causes a decrease in its depth of penetration and concentration of the ultrasound energy in the superficial tissues. For example, the approximate depth of penetration at 1 MHz is 2 to 5 cm, and the approximate depth of penetration at 3 MHz is 1 to 2 cm.

24. **Does the ultrasound transducer speed affect the intramuscular tissue temperature?**
It has been reported that the speed of the ultrasound transducer over the treatment area does not affect the underlying tissue temperature if the ultrasound treatment is applied within a set treatment area of two times the size of the transducer. Speeds of 2 to 3, 4 to 5, and 7 to 8 cm/sec were studied.

25. **Will tissue temperature increases in human muscle vary between pulsed and continuous ultrasound application when administered at equivalent temporal average intensities?**
The literature suggests that equivalent temporal average intensities will produce similar increases in intramuscular tissue temperature. For example, 3 MHz at a 50% duty cycle and an intensity of 1.0 W/cm^2 over a 10-minute period produced similar heating compared with 3 MHz at a 100% duty cycle and an intensity of 0.5 W/cm^2 over a 10-minute treatment.

26. **List contraindications for ultrasound.**
Application of ultrasound is contraindicated over or adjacent to cancerous lesions, infections, growth plates, pacemakers, healing fractures, and plastic implants.

27. **Is a metal implant an absolute contraindication for the use of ultrasound?**
No. However, caution should be exercised because ultrasound is contraindicated over plastic implants and joint cement, which are often components of a total joint replacement.

28. **Is ultrasound effective in treating calcific tendinitis of the shoulder?**
Yes. It has been suggested that ultrasound treatment helps resolve calcifications and is associated with short-term improvements in pain and quality of life. In a study by Ebenbichler and colleagues, patients received 24 15-minute sessions of 25% pulsed ultrasound (0.89 MHz at 2.5 W/cm^2) over a 6-week period. After 6 weeks of treatment, calcifications resolved in 19% of patients and decreased by at least 50% in 28% of patients (compared with 0 and 10% in those receiving sham ultrasound). At the 9-month follow-up, calcifications resolved in 42% of patients and improved in 23% of patients receiving ultrasound (compared with 8% and 12% in those receiving sham ultrasound).

29. **Is there evidence supporting the use of static ultrasound application over conventional ultrasound application?**
Studies have shown that the use of high-power pain threshold ultrasound over myofascial trigger points is effective at improving pain level, pressure pain threshold, and neck pain disability scores. A study by Majlesi and Unalan in 2004 specifically showed improvements in pain and active cervical spine ROM with this static technique applied to patients with acute upper trapezius trigger points. Alfredo et al. compared the effects of continuous and pulsed ultrasound combined with strengthening exercises on 100 participants with Grade 2–4 knee osteoarthritis. They determined that prolonged applications of continuous ultrasound combined with exercises are effective in providing pain, mobility, functionality, and activity in participants with knee osteoarthritis. The application parameters for the continuous ultrasound were 1 MHz frequency, 1.5 w/cm^2 intensity, duty cycle 100%, and an application of 5 minutes on the medial side and 5 minutes on the lateral side of the knee.

30. **Is there evidence supporting the use of low-intensity pulsed ultrasound?**
Research suggests that low-intensity pulsed ultrasound is effective in promoting tendon healing and reducing inflammation (ie, acute tendinitis). Animal models have also shown that this technique may attenuate the progression of cartilage degeneration and increase articular cartilage formation in arthritic conditions. More research is needed to support these effects in humans.

31. **Is ultrasound effective in treating carpal tunnel syndrome?**
Maybe. A study by Ebenbichler and colleagues suggests that ultrasound may be effective in reducing pain and improving electroneurographic variables (eg, motor distal latency and nerve conduction velocity) in patients with carpal tunnel syndrome. In this study, 20 sessions of ultrasound treatment were performed over a 6 week

period (1 MHz, 1.0 W/cm^2, pulsed mode 1:4, 15 minutes per session). A more recent study by Boonhong and Thienkul compared phonophoresis and standard ultrasound in the treatment of carpal tunnel. Both were applied at a frequency of 1 MHZ and 1.0 W/cm^2. They concluded that there was no significant difference between either treatment.

32. **Is ultrasound effective in treating plantar fasciitis?**
Katzap and colleagues examined the effect of adding ultrasound to a stretching program for patient's experiencing plantar fasciitis. They concluded that ultrasound did not have any additive benefit to calf and plantar fascia stretching.

33. **Is there sufficient support for the use of ultrasound in a physical therapy treatment program?**
Based on a review of randomized controlled trials (RCTs) published between 1975 and 1999 in which ultrasound was used for patient treatment, it was suggested that there is little evidence to support the use of active therapeutic ultrasound versus placebo ultrasound. It was also noted that 25 out of the 35 studies reviewed were methodologically inaccurate, and the 10 remaining studies had significant variability in dosages used and patient problems treated; further research is required to answer this question. Noori et al. reviewed the benefits of ultrasound on the management of chronic low back and neck pain. They concluded that there was insufficient evidence that therapeutic ultrasound improved pain or quality of life in patients with nonspecific chronic low back pain. In addition, they concluded there was insufficient evidence to recommend the routine use of ultrasound therapy in the treatment of chronic neck pain.

PHONOPHORESIS

34. **How does phonophoresis work?**
It was once thought that ultrasound exerted pressure on the drug, driving it through the skin. However, ultrasound exerts only minimal pressure. Another explanation is that ultrasound changes the permeability of the stratum corneum (ie, the most superficial skin layer) through thermal and nonthermal effects. Ultrasound performed before the application of a drug to the skin has been found to increase drug penetration, supporting this theory.

35. **When performing phonophoresis, what dosage is preferred?**
In several animal studies Griffin and colleagues demonstrated that ultrasound allowed cortisone to penetrate paravertebral muscles and nerves under a variety of treatment dosages (eg, 1.0 W/cm^2 for 5 minutes, 3.0 W/cm^2 for 5 minutes, 0.3 W/cm^2 for 17 minutes, and 0.1 W/cm^2 for 51 minutes, with frequencies that ranged from 0.09 to 3.6 MHz). Griffin's work demonstrated the greatest penetration with higher intensities at shorter durations and with lower intensities at longer durations. Results favored lower intensities at longer durations in terms of greatest delivery of cortisone to muscles and nerves. Clinically, modest intensities at longer durations using a nonstationary sound mode of application within carefully constrained areas of treatment are recommended for patient comfort and to prevent tissue damage. Further investigations are necessary

36. **When performing phonophoresis, what concentrations of hydrocortisone are most effective?**
A study by Kleinkort and Wood suggests that treatments using 10% hydrocortisone are more effective than those using 1% hydrocortisone for relieving pain associated with tendinitis or bursitis. Further investigations are necessary

37. **How many serial phonophoresis treatments are safe?**
While there is no clear consensus, the total number of ionophoretic treatments, as well as the time between induvial applications, will vary based on the ion or medication being used. One to six treatments of dexamethasone have been shown to be safe and effective in the management of specific orthopaedic conditions when administered alone and delivered 1 to 3 days apart within 15 days.

38. **What are examples of drugs that can be administered by phonophoresis?**
The following drugs have been identified as phonophoretic agents: dexamethasone (0.4% ointment), hydrocortisone (0.5%–1.0% ointment), iodine (10% ointment), lidocaine (5% ointment), magnesium sulfate (2% ointment), salicylates (10% trolamine salicylate or 3% sodium salicylate ointment), and zinc oxide (20% ointment).

39. **Provide an example of a topical nonsteroidal antiinflammatory drug (NSAID) that may be administered by phonophoresis.**
Fastum gel (ketoprofen 2.5%) has been shown to be an effective phonophoretic agent. Phonophoretic application of this drug appears to be superior to topical application. In a study by Cagnie and colleagues, the concentration of

ketoprofen in synovial tissue was significantly greater in the groups receiving phonophoresis with either continuous (ie, 1 MHz at 1.5 W/cm^2) or pulsed (20%) ultrasound than in the group receiving only topical application.

40. **What is the most efficiently transmitted topical antiinflammatory media used in phonophoresis?**
    Fluocinonide 0.05% (Lidex) gel and methyl salicylate 15% (Thera-Gesic) cream transmit ultrasound the best—97% relative to water.

41. **Is phonophoresis effective in treating lateral epicondylitis?**
    Maybe. A study by Baskurt and colleagues suggests that phonophoresis of 10% naproxen (pulsed 1:1, 1 MHz and 1 watt/cm^2) may be equally as effective as 10% naproxen iontophoresis in reducing pain and improving grip strength in patients with lateral epicondylitis. Thakur et al. also concluded that 10% naproxen delivered through iontophoresis and phonophoresis (1 MHz and 1 watt/cm^2) were equally effective in reducing pain, improving grip strength, and functional status for patients with lateral epicondylitis.

42. **Is phonophoresis effective in improving pain and function in knee osteoarthritis?**
    Maybe. A study by Said Ahmed and colleagues concluded the use of dexamethasone phonophoresis resulted in greater improvement in pain and function in patients with knee OA than therapeutic ultrasound combined with exercise and TENS. The effect size of phonophoresis was clinically significant and higher than that reported for intraarticular steroid injection from pooled data in the literature.

PHOTOBIOMODULATION THERAPY

43. **What is photobiomodulation therapy?**
    The North American Association for Photobiomodulation Therapy (Anders, 2015) defines Photobiomodulation Therapy (PBMT) as "a form of light therapy that utilizes non-ionizing forms of light sources, including LASERS, LEDs, and broad-band light, in the visible and infrared spectrum."

44. **What are other terms used to describe PBMT?**
    Other terms used to describe PBMT and photobiomodulation (PBM) devices include phototherapy, laser therapy, light therapy, therapeutic laser, soft laser, cold laser, low-energy laser, low-level laser therapy (LLLT), high-intensity laser therapy (HILT), biostimulation, and monochromatic infrared energy.

45. **List examples of light sources and photobiomodulation technologies used in PBMT.**
    - Coherent light sources
        - LLLT
        - HILT
    - Noncoherent light sources
        - Light-emitting diodes (LEDs)
        - Super luminescent diodes (SLDs)

46. **What are the differences between light waves omitted from LASERs, LEDs, and SLDs?**
    Light amplification by stimulated emission of radiation (laser) produces light in which all photons are the same wavelength (ie, monochromatic), in phase (ie, coherent), and directional. The properties of laser light produce high energy in a narrow beam. LEDs produces light in which all photons are the same wavelength (ie, monochromatic), out of phase (ie, noncoherent), and with limited directionality. The properties of LEDs produce light that is nondirectional and spreads out widely. SLDs produce near monochromatic and noncoherent light that is more directional and spreads out less than light produced by LEDs.

47. **Describe how LASER, LEDs, and SLDs may be best matched to clinical applications of PBMT.**
    Laser diodes produce directional light composed of a single wavelength that is most suitable for treating small areas at various depths of penetration as determined by the wavelength of the applicator. LEDs produce diffuse light most suitable for treating larger areas and superficial tissues, and SLDs produce light that is most suitable for treating intermediate sized areas and superficial to moderately deep tissues as determined by the wavelength of the applicator.

48. **List key PBMT parameters.**
    Important parameters include wavelength (nm), frequency (Hz) and duty cycle (%), power density or irradiance (mW/cm^2), treatment time (sec), energy density or fluence (J/cm^2), beam size (cm), and total energy (J).

49. **What is the relationship between wavelength and depth of penetration?**
Light with longer wavelengths will typically penetrate deeper than light with shorter wavelengths. However, factors such as the tissues being treated (eg, fat and water content), blood concentration, PMD device parameters (eg, peak power), and light sources (eg, pulsed and continuous) will affect depth of penetration.

50. **Should photobiomodulation devices be identified by the color of the light they produce?**
No. Photobiomodulation devices should be identified by wavelength (eg, 650 nm) and not the color of the light they produce because tissues respond differently to light within the same wavelength and according to their wavelength within the light spectrum (eg, visible and near-infrared).

51. **What is the power density (irradiance) of a PMD device?**
The power density or irradiance is the average power produced by the PMD device measured in milliwatts watts (mW), divided by the beam size (cm^2) and reported in mW/cm^2. Power density differs between PMD devices.

52. **How is PMDT dose typically reported?**
PMDT dose may be reported as energy density or fluence (J/cm^2) or as total energy (J).

53. **How is energy density calculated and how is it modified?**
Energy density, fluence, or PMDT dose is the amount of power per unit area and is calculated by the formula: Energy density (J/cm^2) = Irradiance (W/cm^2) × Time (s). Energy density may be modified by altering the time of application and/or the energy density.

54. **How is total energy calculated?**
Total energy is calculated by the formula: Total energy (J) = Energy density (J/cm^2) × Beam Size (cm^2).

55. **Are PBMT dosage recommendations available for musculoskeletal disorders?**
Yes. The World Association for Laser Therapy (WALT) provides detailed low level laser therapy/photobiomodulation therapy dosage recommendations for common musculoskeletal disorders. The recommendations are freely available on the WALT website. Additional dosage recommendations are available in scientific journals, from various PMDT organizations, and from PMD device manufacturers. Dosage recommendations, as well as PBM devices and PBMT parameters, should be closely scrutinized before they are applied to patient care.

56. **List contraindications for PBMT.**
History of malignant carcinoma and irradiation of the abdomen or lower back during pregnancy, the neck region in individuals with hyperthyroidism, the retina, and reproductive organs are routinely described in literature as contraindications for PBMT. Other potential contraindication should be considered as warranted.

57. **Summarize the efficacy of PBMT in the management of common orthopaedic conditions.**
Although PBMT is used in the healing of soft tissue injuries and the management of acute or chronic inflammation, edema, and pain with few to no reported side effects, efficacy data are conflicting. Efficacy data are further complicated by the wide variety of available devices and applicators (eg, cluster and mixed, arrays combining laser, LED, and SLD photodiodes) and the lack of rationale and agreement for selecting treatment parameters and dosage (eg, light source, wavelength, power density, duty cycle, application technique, treatment time, and the number of required sessions). Additionally, the mechanisms underlying PBMT effects on human tissues are not fully understood. Commutatively, extremely low quality to limited moderate quality PBMT literature have reported positive, mixed, and negative effects and the benefits of PBMT in mainstream physical therapy practice are not entirely clear.

There is contradictory evidence suggesting PBMT may provide shorter term improvements in pain and aspects of disability for numerous orthopedic conditionings, including nonspecific low back pain (ie, pain education and improved disability measures) temporomandibular arthralgia pain (ie, reduced arthralgia pain and improved jaw movement), heal pain from plantar fasciitis (ie, pain reduction and improved disability measures), osteoarthritis, and tendinopathies, to name a few. There is conflicting evidence supporting the use of PBMT in the management of acute ankle sprains and moderate evidence against the use of PBMT in the management of carpal tunnel syndrome and patellofemoral pain. Well-controlled and larger-scale clinical trials of sufficient duration are needed to better understand the effectiveness of PBMT in the management of musculoskeletal disorders and to establish reliable and reproducible treatment parameters.

BIBLIOGRAPHY

Aisaiti, A., Zhou, Y., Wen, Y., et al. (2021). Effect of photobiomodulation therapy on painful temporomandibular disorders. *Scientific Reports*, *11*(1), 9049.

Alfredo, P. P., Junior, W. S., & Casarotto, R. A. (2020). Efficacy of continuous and pulsed therapeutic ultrasound combined with exercises for knee osteoarthritis: A randomized controlled trial. *Clinical Rehabilitation*, *34*(4), 480–490.

Alkilani, A.Z., McCrudden, M.T., & Donnelly, R.F. (2015). Transdermal drug delivery: Innovative pharmaceutical developments based on disruption of the barrier properties of the stratum corneum. Pharmaceutics, 7(4), 438–470.

Amirjani, N., Ashworth, N. L., Watt, M. J., Gordon, T., & Chan, K. M. (2009). Corticosteroid iontophoresis to treat carpal tunnel syndrome: A double-blind randomized controlled trial. *Muscle & Nerve, 39*(5), 627–633.

Anders, J.J. (2015). Nomenclature consensus meeting. Retrieved November 20, 2021, from https://www.naalt.org/whitepapers/2014-naalt-walt-meeting-nomenclature-breakout/.

Anderson, C. R., Morris, R. L., Boeh, S. D., Panus, P. C., & Sembrowich, W. L. (2003). Effects of iontophoresis current magnitude and duration on dexamethasone deposition and localized drug retention. *Physical Therapy, 83*(2), 161–170.

Bagniefski, T., & Burnette, R. R. (1990). A comparison of pulsed and continuous current iontophoresis. *Journal of Controlled Release, 11*(1), 113–122.

Baskurt, F., Ozcan, A., & Algun, C. (2003). Comparison of effects of phonophoresis and iontophoresis of naproxen in the treatment of lateral epicondylitis. *Clinical Rehabilitation, 17*(1), 96–100.

Bellew, J. W., Michlovitz, S. L., & Nolan, T. P. (2016). *Michlovitz's modalities for therapeutic intervention* (6th ed.). Philadelphia, PA: F.A. Davis Company.

Berliner, M. N. (1997). Skin microcirculation during tapwater iontophoresis in humans: Cathode stimulates more than anode. *Microvascular Research, 54*(1), 74–80.

Boonhong, J., & Thienkul, W. (2020). Effectiveness of phonophoresis treatment in carpal tunnel syndrome: A randomized double-blind, controlled trial. *PM & R, 12*(1), 8–15.

Cagnie, B., Vinck, E., Rimbaut, S., & Vanderstraeten, G. (2003). Phonophoresis versus topical application of ketoprofen: Comparison between tissue and plasma levels. *Physical Therapy, 83*(8), 707–712.

Calin, M. A., Badila, A., Hristea, A., Manea, D., Savastru, R., & Nica, A. S. (2019). Fractionated irradiation in photobiomodulation therapy of ankle sprain. *American Journal of Physical Medicine & Rehabilitation, 98*(8), 692–698.

Cameron, M. H. (2018a). *Physical agents in rehabilitation: An evidence-based approach to practice* (5th ed.). St. Louis, MO: Elsevier/Saunders.

Cameron, M. H. (2018b). Lasers and light. In M. H. Cameron (Ed.), *Physical agents in rehabilitation: An evidence-based approach to practice* (pp. 305–326). St. Louis, MO: Elsevier/Saunders.

Cameron, M. H., Shapiro, S., & Ocelnik, M. (2018). Electrical currents for soft tissue healing. In M. H. Cameron (Ed.), *Physical agents in rehabilitation: An evidence-based approach to practice* (pp. 271–288). St. Louis, MO: Elsevier/Saunders.

Chow, R., Liebert, A., Tilley, S., Bennett, G., Gabel, C. P., & Laakso, L. (2021). Guidelines versus evidence: What we can learn from the Australian guideline for low-level laser therapy in knee osteoarthritis? A narrative review. *Lasers in Medical Science, 36*(2), 249–258.

Chung, H., Dai, T., Sharma, S. K., Huang, Y. -Y., Carroll, J. D., & Hamblin, M. R. (2012). The nuts and bolts of low-level laser (light) therapy. *Annals of Biomedical Engineering, 40*(2), 516–533.

Ciccone, C. D. (2003). Does acetic acid iontophoresis accelerate the resorption of calcium deposits in calcific tendinitis of the shoulder? *Physical Therapy, 83*(1), 68–74.

Clijsen, R., Brunner, A., Barbero, M., Clarys, P., & Taeymans, J. (2017). Effects of low-level laser therapy on pain in patients with musculoskeletal disorders: A systematic review and meta-analysis. *European Journal of Physical and Rehabilitation Medicine, 53*(4), 603–610.

Coglianese, M., Draper, D. O., Shurtz, J., & Mark, G. (2011). Microdialysis and delivery of iontophoresis-driven lidocaine into the human gastrocnemius muscle. *Journal of Athletic Training, 46*(3), 270–276.

Costello, C. T., & Jeske, A. H. (1995). Iontophoresis: applications in transdermal medication delivery. *Physical Therapy, 75*(6), 554–563.

da Luz, D. C., de Borba, Y., Ravanello, E. M., Daitx, R. B., & Döhnert, M. B. (2019). Iontophoresis in lateral epicondylitis: A randomized, double-blind clinical trial. *Journal of Shoulder and Elbow Surgery, 28*(9), 1743–1749.

Draper, D. O., Coglianese, M., & Castel, C. (2011). Absorption of iontophoresis-driven 2% lidocaine with epinephrine in the tissues at 5 mm below the surface of the skin. *Journal of Athletic Training, 46*(3), 277–281.

Draper, D. O., & Jutte, L. S. (2021). Application procedures: Electrotherapy. In D. O. Draper, L. S. Jutte, & K. L. Knight (Eds.), *Therapeutic modalities: The art and science* (pp. 231–362). Philadelphia, PA: Wolters Kluwe.

Ebenbichler, G. R., Resch, K. L., Nicolakis, P., et al. (1998). Ultrasound treatment for treating the carpal tunnel syndrome: Randomised "sham" controlled trial. *BMJ, 316*(7133), 731–735.

Ebenbichler, G. R., Erdogmus, C. B., Resch, K. L., et al. (1999). Ultrasound therapy for calcific tendinitis of the shoulder. *New England Journal of Medicine, 340*(20), 1533–1538.

Erickson, M., Lawrence, M., Jansen, C. W. S., Coker, D., Amadio, P., & Cleary, C. (2019). Hand pain and sensory deficits: Carpal tunnel syndrome. *Journal of Orthopaedic & Sports Physical Therapy, 49*(5), CPG1–CPG85.

Gallo, J. A., Draper, D. O., Brody, L. T., & Fellingham, G. W. (2004). A comparison of human muscle temperature increases during 3-MHz continuous and pulsed ultrasound with equivalent temporal average intensities. *Journal of Orthopaedic and Sports Physical Therapy, 34*(7), 395–401.

Glass, J. M., Stephen, R. L., & Jacobson, S. C. (1980). The quantity and distribution of radiolabeled dexamethasone delivered to tissue by iontophoresis. *International Journal of Dermatology, 19*(9), 519–525.

Gökoğlu, F., Fındıkoğlu, G., Yorgancoğlu, Z. R., Okumuş, M., Ceceli, E., & Kocaoğlu, S. (2005). Evaluation of iontophoresis and local corticosteroid injection in the treatment of carpal tunnel syndrome. *American Journal of Physical Medicine & Rehabilitation, 84*(2), 92–96.

Griffin, J.E., & Touchstone, J.C. (1963). Ultrasonic movement of cortisol into pig tissues. I. Movement into skeletal muscle. American Journal of Physical Medicine, 42, 77–85.

Griffin, J.E., Touchstone, J.C., & Liu, A.C. (1965). Ultrasonic movement of cortisol into pig tissue. II. Movement into paravertebral nerve. American Journal of Physical Medicine, 44, 20–25.

Gudeman, S. D., Eisele, S. A., Heidt, R. S., Jr., Colosimo, A. J., & Stroupe, A. L. (1997). Treatment of plantar fasciitis by iontophoresis of 0.4% dexamethasone. A randomized, double-blind, placebo-controlled study. *American Journal of Sports Medicine, 25*(3), 312–316.

Heiskanen, V., & Hamblin, M. R. (2018). Photobiomodulation: Lasers vs. light emitting diodes? *Photochemical & Photobiological Sciences, 17*(8), 1003–1017.

Helmstädter, A. (2001). The history of electrically-assisted transdermal drug delivery ("iontophoresis"). Pharmazie, 56(7), 583–587.

Helmy, A. M. (2021). Overview of recent advancements in the iontophoretic drug delivery to various tissues and organs. *Journal of Drug Delivery Science and Technology, 61*, 102332.

Huang, Z., Ma, J., Chen, J., Shen, B., Pei, F., & Kraus, V. B. (2015). The effectiveness of low-level laser therapy for nonspecific chronic low back pain: A systematic review and meta-analysis. *Arthritis Research & Therapy, 17*, 360.

Jewell, D. V., Riddle, D. L., & Thacker, L. R. (2009). Interventions associated with an increased or decreased likelihood of pain reduction and improved function in patients with adhesive capsulitis: A retrospective cohort study. *Physical Therapy, 89*(5), 419–429.

Jing, G., Zhao, Y., Dong, F., et al. (2021). Effects of different energy density low-level laser therapies for temporomandibular joint disorders patients: A systematic review and network meta-analysis of parallel randomized controlled trials. *Lasers in Medical Science, 36*(5), 1101–1108.

Kassan, D. G., Lynch, A. M., & Stiller, M. J. (1996). Physical enhancement of dermatologic drug delivery: Iontophoresis and phonophoresis. *Journal of the American Academy of Dermatology, 34*(4), 657–666.

Katzap, Y., Haidukov, M., Berland, O. M., Itzhak, R. B., & Kalichman, L. (2018). Additive effect of therapeutic ultrasound in the treatment of plantar fasciitis: A randomized controlled trial. *The Journal of Orthopaedic and Sports Physical Therapy, 48*(11), 847–855.

Kedzierski, T., Stanczak, K., Gworys, K., Gasztych, J., Sibinski, M., & Kujawa, J. (2012). Comparative evaluation of the direct analgesic efficacy of selected physiotherapeutic methods in subjects with knee joint degenerative disease—preliminary report. *Ortopedia, Traumatologia, Rehabilitacja, 14*(6), 537–544.

Kleinkort, J. A., & Wood, F. (1975). Phonophoresis with 1 percent versus 10 percent hydrocortisone. *Physical Therapy, 55*(12), 1320–1324.

Knight, K. L., & Draper, D. O. (2013). Therapeutic modalities: The art and science: (2nd ed.). Philadelphia, PA: Lippincott Williams & Wilkins.

Kuryliszyn-Moskal, A., Kita, J., Dakowicz, A., Chwiesko-Minarowska, S., Moskal, D., & Lewis, C. (2004). Ultrasound efficacy. *Physical Therapy, 84*(10), 984. author reply 984–985; discussion 985–987.

Li, L. C., & Scudds, R. A. (1995). Iontophoresis: An overview of the mechanisms and clinical application. *Arthritis Care & Research, 8*(1), 51–61.

Lobo, S., & Yan, G. (2018). Improving the direct penetration into tissues underneath the skin with iontophoresis delivery of a ketoprofen cationic prodrug. *International Journal of Pharmaceutics, 535*(1–2), 228–236.

Lopes-Martins, R. A. B., Marcos, R. L., Leal-Junior, E. C. P., & Bjordal, J. M. (2018). Low-level laser therapy and World Association for Laser Therapy dosage recommendations in musculoskeletal disorders and injuries. *Photomedicine and Laser Surgery, 36*(9), 457–459.

Majlesi, J., & Unalan, H. (2004). High-power pain threshold ultrasound technique in the treatment of active myofascial trigger points: A randomized, double-blind, case-control study. *Archives of Physical Medicine and Rehabilitation, 85*(5), 833–836.

Martin, R. L., Chimenti, R., Cuddeford, T., et al. (2018). Achilles pain, stiffness, and muscle power deficits: Midportion Achilles tendinopathy revision 2018. *Journal of Orthopaedic & Sports Physical Therapy, 48*(5), A1–A38.

Martin, R. L., Davenport, T. E., Reischl, S. F., et al. (2014). Heel pain-plantar fasciitis: Revision 2014. *Journal of Orthopaedic & Sports Physical Therapy, 44*(11), A1–33.

Morrisette, D. C., Brown, D., & Saladin, M. E. (2004). Temperature change in lumbar periarticular tissue with continuous ultrasound. *Journal of Orthopaedic and Sports Physical Therapy, 34*(12), 754–760.

Nambi, G., Kamal, W., Es, S., Joshi, S., & Trivedi, P. (2018). Spinal manipulation plus laser therapy versus laser therapy alone in the treatment of chronic non-specific low back pain: A randomized controlled study. *European Journal of Physical and Rehabilitation Medicine, 54*(6), 880–889.

Navratil, L., & Kymplova, J. (2002). Contraindications in noninvasive laser therapy: Truth and fiction. *Journal of Clinical Laser Medicine & Surgery, 20*(6), 341–343.

Newman, N., & Homan, K. (2021). Photobiomodulation therapy. In W. E. Prentice (Ed.), *Therapeutic modalities in rehabilitation* (pp. 505–551). New York, NY: McGraw Hill.

Nirschl, R. P., Rodin, D. M., Ochiai, D. H., Maartmann-Moe, C., & Group, D.-A.-S. (2003). Iontophoretic administration of dexamethasone sodium phosphate for acute epicondylitis. A randomized, double-blinded, placebo-controlled study. *American Journal of Sports Medicine, 31*(2), 189–195.

Noori, S. A., Rasheed, A., Aiyer, R., et al. (2020). Therapeutic ultrasound for pain management in chronic low back pain and chronic neck pain: A systematic review. *Pain Medicine, 21*(7), 1482–1493.

Post, R., & Nolan, T. P. (2016). Electromagnetic waves-laser, diathermy, and pulsed electromagnetic fields. In J. W. Bellew, S. L. Michlovitz, & T. P. Nolan (Eds.), *Michlovitz's modalities for therapeutic intervention* (pp. 167–210). Philadelphia, PA: F.A. Davis Company.

Prentice, W. E. (2021). *Therapeutic modalities in rehabilitation* (6th ed.). New York, NY: McGraw Hill.

Rigby, J., & Castel, C. (2021). Photobiomodulation (light and laser) therapy. In D. O. Draper, L. S. Jutte, & K. L. Knight (Eds.), *Therapeutic modalities: The art and science* (pp. 417–432). Philadelphia, PA: Wolters Kluwer.

Rigby, J. H., Draper, D. O., Johnson, A. W., Myrer, J. W., Eggett, D. L., & Mack, G. W. (2015). The time course of dexamethasone delivery using iontophoresis through human skin, measured via microdialysis. *Journal of Orthopaedic & Sports Physical Therapy, 45*(3), 190–197.

Rigby, J. H., Hagan, A. M., Kelcher, A. R., & Ji, C. (2020). Dexamethasone sodium phosphate penetration during phonophoresis at 2 ultrasound frequencies. *Journal of Athletic Training, 55*(6), 628–635.

Rigby, J. H., Mortensen, B. B., & Draper, D. O. (2015). Wireless versus wired iontophoresis for treating patellar tendinopathy: A randomized clinical trial. *Journal of Athletic Training, 50*(11), 1165–1173.

Robertson, V. J., & Baker, K. G. (2001). A review of therapeutic ultrasound: Effectiveness studies. *Physical Therapy, 81*(7), 1339–1350.

Romani, W. A., Perrin, D. H., Dussault, R. G., Ball, D. W., & Kahler, D. M. (2000). Identification of tibial stress fractures using therapeutic continuous ultrasound. *Journal of Orthopaedic and Sports Physical Therapy, 30*(8), 444–452.

Roustit, M., Blaise, S., & Cracowski, J. L. (2014). Trials and tribulations of skin iontophoresis in therapeutics. *British Journal of Clinical Pharmacology, 77*(1), 63–71.

Saepang, K., Li, S. K., & Chantasart, D. (2021). Effect of pulsed direct current on Iontophoretic delivery of pramipexole across human epidermal membrane in vitro. *Pharmaceutical Research, 38*(7), 1187–1198.

Said Ahmed, M., Boles Saweeres, E., Abdelkader, N., Abdelmajeed, S., & Fares, A, (2019). Improved pain and function in knee osteoarthritis with dexamethasone phonophoresis: A randomized controlled trial. *Indian Journal of Orthopaedics, 53*(6), 700–707.

Schiffman, E. L., Braun, B. L., & Lindgren, B. R. (1996). Temporomandibular joint iontophoresis: A double-blind randomized clinical trial. *Journal of Orofacial Pain, 10*(2), 157–165.

Scifers, J., & Prentice, W. (2021). Iontophoresis. In W. Prentice (Ed.), *Therapeutic modalities in rehabilitation* (6th ed.). New York, NY: McGraw Hill. (p. cm).

Stefanou, A., Marshall, N., Holdan, W., & Siddiqui, A. (2012). A randomized study comparing corticosteroid injection to corticosteroid iontophoresis for lateral epicondylitis. *Journal of Hand Surgery American, 37*(1), 104–109.

Taylor, D. N., Winfield, T., & Wynd, S. (2020). Low-level laser light therapy dosage variables vs treatment efficacy of neuromusculoskeletal conditions: A scoping review. *Journal of Chiropractic Medicine, 19*(2), 119–127.

Thakur, R., Patole, K., & Mitra, M. (2017). To compare the effect of naproxen applied by topical iontophoresis and phonophoresis in treatment of lateral epicondylitis. *Indian Journal of Physiotherapy & Occupational Therapy, 11*(3), 96–100.

Tomazoni, S. S., Almeida, M. O., Bjordal, J. M., et al. (2020). Photobiomodulation therapy does not decrease pain and disability in people with non-specific low back pain: A systematic review. *Journal of Physiotherapy, 66*(3), 155–165.

Tripodi, N., Feehan, J., Husaric, M., Sidiroglou, F., & Apostolopoulos, V. (2021). The effect of low-level red and near-infrared photobiomodulation on pain and function in tendinopathy: A systematic review and meta-analysis of randomized control trials. *BMC Sports Science, Medicine and Rehabilitation, 13*(1), 91.

Weaver, S. L., Demchak, T. J., Stone, M. B., Brucker, J. B., & Burr, P. O. (2006). Effect of transducer velocity on intramuscular temperature during a 1-MHz ultrasound treatment. *Journal of Orthopaedic and Sports Physical Therapy, 36*(5), 320–325.

Willy, R. W., Hoglund, L. T., Barton, C. J., et al. (2019). Patellofemoral pain. *Journal of Orthopaedic & Sports Physical Therapy, 49*(9), CPG1–CPG95.

World Association for Laser Therapy. (2010). Guidelines for treatment with laser therapy. Retrieved November 30, 2021, from https://energy-laser.com/guide-lines-for-treatment-with-laser-therapy/.

Yarrobino, T. E., Kalbfleisch, J. H., Ferslew, K. E., & Panus, P. C. (2006). Lidocaine iontophoresis mediates analgesia in lateral epicondylalgia treatment. *Physiotherapy Research International, 11*(3), 152–160.

CHAPTER 9 QUESTIONS

1. **A 32-year-old recreational tennis player with increasing complaints of lateral elbow pain over the past 4 weeks is examined by a physical therapist. Clinical findings include point tenderness over the extensor carpi radialis brevis muscle and common extensor tendon insertion up to 2 cm distal to the lateral epicondyle, pain with resisted wrist extension, and pain and weakness with grip strength testing. Which of the following is the most appropriate application of an electrophysical agent?**
   a. Iontophoresis with dexamethasone utilizing the cathode as the active electrode with a dosage of 4.0 mA x 10 minutes for a total of six treatments 1 to 3 days apart
   b. Iontophoresis with dexamethasone utilizing the anode as the active electrode for a dosage of 4.0 mA x 10 minutes for a total of six treatments 1 to 3 days apart
   c. Iontophoresis with dexamethasone utilizing the cathode as the active electrode with a dosage of 80 mA x 20 minutes for a total of six to eight treatments 1 to 2 days apart
   d. Iontophoresis with dexamethasone alternating between the anode and cathode as the active electrode for a dosage of 4.0 mA x 10 min for a total of six treatments 2 days apart

2. **Which of the following ultrasound parameters should be administered to achieve thermal effects in superficial tissues?**
   a. Frequency = 1.0 MHz, Intensity = 0.3 w/cm^2, Treatment area = two times the ERA
   b. Frequency = 1.0 MHz, Intensity = 1.0 w/cm^2, Treatment area = three times the ERA
   c. Frequency = 3.0 MHz, Intensity = 0.5 w/cm^2, Treatment area = four times the ERA
   d. Frequency = 3.0 MHz, Intensity = 1.5 w/cm^2, Treatment area = two times the ERA

3. **A patient presents with osteoarthritis of the left medial compart of the knee. Which of the following biophysical agent is MOST appropriate for this patient?**
   a. Ultrasound at 3 MHz and .5 W/cm^2
   b. Phonophoresis with 10% naproxen at 1 MHz and 1 watt/cm^2
   c. Iontophoresis with 8% acetic acid at a dose of 80 mA-min
   d. Photobiomodulation therapy using a high-intensity laser at a dose of 40 Joules

CHAPTER 10

STRETCHING

D.A. Boyce, PT, EdD, OCS, ECS

1. **What is stress relaxation?**

   Stress relaxation is a physical property of viscoelastic structures, such as a muscle-tendon unit (MTU). If an MTU is elongated to a specific length and held in that position, the internal tension within the MTU decreases with the passage of time. Clinically, this is what occurs during a static stretch of an MTU.

2. **Define creep.**

   Creep occurs when an MTU is elongated to a specific length and then allowed to continue to elongate as stress relaxation occurs. Clinically, this is what occurs when a therapist performs a stretch in which joint range is increased during the stretch repetition. Creep is partially responsible for the immediate increase in joint range of motion (ROM) during a stretch repetition.

3. **When stretching a muscle joint complex, what structures are influenced?**
   - Joint capsule
   - Ligaments
   - Nerves
   - Vessels
   - Skin
   - MTU

4. **What is ballistic stretching?**

   Ballistic stretching places the muscle joint complex at or near its limit of available motion and then cyclically loads the muscle joint complex (bouncing motion at the end ROM). The rate and amplitude of the stretch are variable. Ballistic muscle stretching is indicated for preconditioning a muscle joint complex for activities such as sprinting, high jump, or other events that depend on the elastic energy in an MTU to enhance the performance of a particular movement pattern.

5. **Define dynamic stretching, or dynamic warm-up.**

   Dynamic stretching is activities or movements that involve muscles and joints moving through partial or full range of motion at a submaximal level of intensity. Movements that simulate or are a part of the functional activity to be performed should be incorporated into the dynamic warm-up. Dynamic stretching is not associated with strength or performance deficits and has been found to improve jumping and running performance.

6. **Define static stretching.**

   Static stretching is a technique that places a muscle joint complex in a specific ROM until a stretch is perceived. The position is held for a specific period of time and repeated as necessary to increase joint ROM.

7. **Describe some commonly used proprioceptive neuromuscular facilitation (or active inhibition) stretching techniques.**
   - Hold-relax—the muscle to be stretched is placed in a lengthened but comfortable starting position. The patient is instructed to contract the target muscle for approximately 5 to 10 seconds. After the 10-second contraction, the patient is instructed to relax the target muscle completely as the therapist passively increases joint ROM. This is repeated for a specific number of repetitions. Intensity of the stretch is limited by the patient.
   - Hold-relax-antagonist contraction—the muscle to be stretched is placed in a lengthened but comfortable starting position. The patient is instructed to contract the target muscle for approximately 5 to 10 seconds. After the 10-second contraction, the patient is instructed to relax and then contract the muscle opposite (reciprocally inhibiting the target muscle) the target muscle, actively increasing joint ROM. Intensity of the stretch is limited by the patient.
   - Antagonist contraction—the muscle to be stretched is placed in a lengthened but comfortable starting position. The patient is instructed to contract the muscle opposite (reciprocally inhibiting the target muscle) the target muscle, actively increasing joint ROM. Intensity of the stretch is limited by the patient.

8. **Summarize the benefits of static, dynamic, and PNF stretching techniques.**

   When attempting to increase ROM, all types of stretching are effective. PNF stretching produces the greatest immediate gains in range of motion. Static stretching has been found to improve range of motion; however, it can decrease in strength prior to an activity. On the other hand, dynamic stretching can improve performance and is recommended prior to an activity.

9. **What is the optimal number of static stretch repetitions?**
The optimal number of static stretch repetitions is four. Boyce and Brosky in 2008 found that passive stretching beyond five repetitions results in insignificant gains in hamstring length and that the greatest increase in range of motion occurs during the first stretch repetition.

10. **What is the optimal amount of time that a static stretch should be held?**
The literature reports stretching durations from 6 seconds to 60 minutes. When looking at immediate increases in range of motion, the literature recommends (on average) stretch times between 15 and 60 seconds. Overwhelmingly the literature reports that prolonged stretching times impair performance. Additionally, it has been found that shorter stretch times <30 seconds result in the least performance impairments, and stretch times of 6 seconds (repeated six times) can improve ROM while significantly lessening the negative impairment effects of static stretching. Thus stretch durations between 6 to 30 seconds are advocated.

11. **What is the optimal intensity of a static stretch?**
Stretching to the point of discomfort (POD) is a common practice and is often believed to yield the greatest results. The vast majority of the literature has found that stretching to the POD results in decreased performance measures (decreased force production, jump height, and balance). Literature examining stretch intensities under a person's POD reports results of improved ROM and has been found to have less negative effects on performance.

12. **What are common stretching practices of athletes?**
A recent study that collected over 3000 surveys concluded the following:
- 89% of athletes use stretching for recovery
- 72% of athletes stretch after training
- 50% of athletes use stretching as a pre-exercise routine
- Static stretching is the most commonly used form of stretching in athletes (88%)

13. **How often must static stretching be performed to maintain gains experienced during a static stretch session?**
Bohannon found that stretch gains lasted 24 hours after a stretching session of the hamstrings. Zito reported no lasting effect of two 15-second passive stretches of the ankle plantar flexors after a 24-hour period. Clinically, this suggests that stretching should be performed at least every 24 hours.

14. **If an individual statically stretches on a regular basis, how long will the gains be retained?**
According to Zebas, after a 6-week regimen of stretching, gains realized during that period were retained for a minimum of 2 weeks and in some subjects a maximum of 4 weeks.

15. **Does static muscle stretching alter performance?**
According to a recent review, the majority of the literature surrounding performance measures such as force production, isokinetic power, and vertical jump are impaired with static stretching. Impairments caused by static stretching can last upward of 2 hours in some instances. It should be noted that in some instances static stretching can improve performance of activities that require slower submaximal force production such as jogging and submaximal running or in jumping and hopping activities with longer contact times. Additionally, shorter stretch durations (<30 seconds) have less negative effects on dynamic activities. Finally, it is recommended that static stretching should be avoided in activities that require high-speed rapid movements or when explosive/reactive forces are required.

16. **Does dynamic stretching alter performance?**
Yes. Dynamic stretching is preferred to static stretching when preparing for physical activity. According to the literature surrounding dynamic stretching, it has been shown that dynamic stretching enhances athletic performance and in some cases improves ROM similar to static stretching. Dynamic stretching activities should be carried out at a frequency of 50 to 100 beats per minute. Dynamic stretching of at least three stretch repetitions of 30 seconds' duration per muscle group is advocated. A 10-minute dynamic warm-up consisting of dynamic stretching, light aerobic activity, skipping, and hopping is best to prepare for physical activity.

17. **Does static stretching decrease the chance of injury?**
Several studies have found that static stretching alone does not reduce injury. However, a dynamic warm-up that consists of stretching, strengthening, balance training, sport-specific drills, and landing drills carried out for at least 3 months reduces injury.

18. **Does static stretching decrease muscle soreness?**
Stretching focused on the reduction of delayed-onset muscle soreness (DOMS) after exercise has not been found effective at reducing pain. Some reports in the literature say that stretching can reduce DOMS; however, it is not statistically significant.

19. **Is static stretching effective at reducing the effects of spasticity?**
A systematic review by Bovend'Erdt et al. in 2008 found the effects of stretching on spasticity to be inconclusive because of a lack of quality research in this area.

20. **Does static stretching reduce joint contracture?**
The exact cause of joint contracture is unknown; however, it is generally agreed upon that neurologic and non-neurologic factors contribute to the formation of joint contractures. A 2010 Cochrane Review concluded that for persons suffering with neurologic or nonneurologic joint contracture, stretching did not have clinically important immediate, short-term, or long-term effects on joint mobility. Additionally, it was found that pain, spasticity, activity limitation, participation restriction, or quality of life did not improve when stretching was employed for joint contracture.

21. **Should a muscle joint complex be warmed up to optimize the effects of a stretch?**
Not necessarily. Logically, it seems that increasing the tissue temperature before stretching would increase viscoelastic properties of the soft tissue surrounding a muscle joint complex; however, research has shown that stretching with or without a warm-up yields similar results.

22. **Does age influence the extensibility of muscle and tendon?**
It does appear that with increasing age the extensibility of the muscle tendon unit decreases (related directly to the calf muscle tendon unit). This is important with regard to normal ambulation, balance, and fall prevention in the older adult. A flexibility program directed toward the calf musculature appears to be a logical prevention program for the older adult.

23. **Is foam rolling more effective than static stretching at improving flexibility?**
There is evidence to support that foam rolling with static stretching or foam rolling alone does improve flexibility over static or dynamic stretching alone.

24. **Does stretching the gastrocnemius muscle in subtalar supination result in greater ankle dorsiflexion range of motion?**
It is often theorized that stretching the gastrocnemius muscle in a subtalar neutral position will result in increased gastrocnemius muscle length because the totality of the stretch will be directed more specifically toward the target muscle (gastrocnemius) rather than the stretch force being dissipated across the midtarsal and subtalar joints. The literature suggests that there is no significant difference in the dorsiflexion ROM gains between individuals who stretched while maintaining the subtalar joint in supination versus pronation.

25. **Does stretching alter joint position sense?**
A brief stretching regimen of three stretches held for 30 seconds had no effect on knee joint position sense.

26. **Is stretching effective at reducing neck pain?**
According to the neck pain clinical practice guidelines published by the Orthopedic Section of the American Physical Therapy Association in 2008, only limited literature is available regarding the use of stretching and neck pain. Compared with manual therapy of the cervical spine, stretching of the cervical spine has been found to be equally effective. Stretching of the suboccipitals, scalenes, levator scapulae, upper trapezius, and pectoralis major and minor muscle groups should be considered in patients with neck pain.

27. **Is stretching effective at reducing hamstring injuries?**
According to a 2012 Cochrane Review, there is conflicting evidence to suggest that stretching the hamstrings will reduce hamstring injury. There is evidence to suggest that stretching after hamstring injury and exercise can reduce time to return to full activity.

28. **Is stretching effective at reducing patellofemoral pain syndrome (anterior knee pain)?**
According to a recent review, the most effective manner to treat patients with patellofemoral pain syndrome is a combined physical therapy program, including strength training of the quadriceps and hip abductors and stretching of the quadriceps muscle group.

29. **Is stretching effective at reducing heel pain?**
Stretching has been found to be no more effective than taping and bracing. The main pain-relieving benefits of stretching occur in the first 2 weeks to 4 months after the onset of stretching. Specific plantar fascia stretches may provide better short-term results versus Achilles stretching. Recommendations for frequency and number of repetitions are two to three times per day with a sustained hold of 15 to 30 seconds to as long as 3 minutes.

30. **Can stretching of the jaw muscles influence performance in athletes?**
Evidence suggests that stretching performed twice daily for 10 minutes in mandibular submaximal jaw opening position resulted improved performance in cross-fit athletes. Proposed mechanisms are a decrease in the trigeminal reflex (which results in decreased heart rate and blood pressure), improved blood lactate recovery, and improving oxygen conserving mechanisms.

31. **Should stretching be required as a major component of physical fitness?**
Recent literature examining the effects of flexibility found that flexibility and mortality did not correlate, meaning that flexible people don't live longer, and those that are not flexible don't die earlier. Flexibility does not predict falls in the elderly, is not a predictor of low back pain, and is not associated with quality of life. Alternatives to stretching are the performance of a less strenuous version of the activity as a warm-up to the activity. It should be noted that the American College of Sports Medicine still recommends daily stretching.

BIBLIOGRAPHY

Babault, N., Rodot, G., Champelovier, M., & Cometti, C. (2021). A survey on stretching practices in women and men from various sports or physical activity programs. *International Journal of Environmental Research and Public Health, 18*(8), 3928.

Bohannon, R. (1984). Effect of repeated eight-minute muscle loading on the angle of straight leg raising. *Physical Therapy, 64*, 491–497.

Bovend'Eerdt, T. J., Newman, M., Barker, K., Dawes, H., Minelli, C., & Wade, D. T. (2008). The effects of stretching in spasticity: a systematic review. *Archives of Physical Medicine and Rehabilitation, 89*(7), 1395–1406.

Boyce, D. (2008). Determining the minimal number of cyclic passive stretch repetitions recommended for an acute increase in an indirect measure of hamstring length. *Physiotherapy Theory and Practice, 24*(2), 113–120.

Childs, J. D., Cleland, J. A., Elliott, J. M., et al. (2008). Neck pain: clinical practice guidelines linked to the International Classification of Functioning, Disability, and Health from the Orthopaedic Section of the American Physical Therapy Association. *Journal of Orthopaedic and Sports Physical Therapy, 38*(9), A1–A34.

Gajdosik, R., Vander Linden, D., & Williams, A. (1999). Influence of age on length and passive elastic stiffness characteristics of the calf muscle-tendon unit of women. *Physical Therapy, 79*, 827–838.

Herman, K., Barton, C., Malliaras, P., & Morrissey, D. (2012). The effectiveness of neuromuscular warm-up strategies, that require no additional equipment, for preventing lower limb injuries during sports participation: a systematic review. *BMC Medicine, 10*, 75.

Katalinic, O. M., Harvey, L. A., Herbert, R. D., Moseley, A. M., Lannin, N. A., & Schurr, K. (2010). Stretch for the treatment and prevention of contractures. *Cochrane Database of Systematic Reviews, 9*, CD007455.

Larsen, R., Lund, H., Christensen, R., Røgind, H., Danneskiold-Samsøe, B., & Bliddal, H. (2005). Effect of static stretching of quadriceps and hamstring muscles on knee joint position sense. *British Journal of Sports Medicine, 39*, 43–46.

Mason, D. L., Dickens, V. A., & Vail, A. (2012). Rehabilitation for hamstring injuries. *Cochrane Database of Systematic Reviews, 12*, CD004575.

McPoil, T. G., Martin, R. L., Cornwall, M. W., Wukich, D. K., Irrgang, J. J., & Godges, J. J. (2014). Heel pain: clinical practice guidelines linked to the International Classification of Functioning, Disability, and Health from the Orthopaedic Section of the American Physical Therapy Association. *Journal of Orthopaedic and Sports Physical Therapy, 38*(4), A1–A18.

Nuzzo, J. L. (2020). The case for retiring flexibility as a major component of physical fitness. *Sports Medicine, 50*, 853–870.

Page, P. (2012). Current concepts in muscle stretching for exercise and rehabilitation. *International Journal of Sports Physical Therapy, 7*(1), 109–119.

Rixe, J. A., Glick, J. E., Brady, J., & Olympia, R. P. (2013). A review of the management of patellofemoral pain syndrome. *The Physician and Sportsmedicine, 41*(3), 19–28.

Smith, C. A. (1994). The warm up procedure: to stretch or not to stretch. *Journal of Orthopaedic and Sports Physical Therapy, 19*, 12–16.

Su, H., Chang, N. J., Wu, W. L., Guo, L. Y., & Chu, I. H. (2017). Acute effects of foam rolling, static stretching, and dynamic stretching during warm-ups on muscular flexibility and strength in young adults. *Journal of Sport Rehabilitation, 26*(6), 469–477.

Sweeting, D., Parish, B., Hooper, L., & Chester, R. (2011). The effectiveness of manual stretching in the treatment of plantar heel pain: a systematic review. *Journal of Foot and Ankle Research, 4*, 19.

Taylor, D. C. (1990). Viscoelastic properties of muscle tendon units: the biomechanical effects of stretching. *The American Journal of Sports Medicine, 18*, 24–32.

Tonlorenzi, D., Conti, M., & Traina, G. (2022). The influence of mandibular stretching on athletes subjected to high intensity workout. *Archives Italiennes de Biologie, 159*(3–4), 178–186.

Yeung, S. S., Yeung, E. W., & Gillespie, L. D. (2011). Interventions for preventing lower limb soft-tissue running injuries. *Cochrane Database of Systematic Reviews, 7*, CD001256.

Zito, M. (1997). Lasting effects of one bout of two 15-second passive stretches on ankle dorsiflexion range of motion. *Journal of Orthopaedic and Sports Physical Therapy, 26*, 214–220.

CHAPTER 10 QUESTIONS

1. **When looking at acute increases in range of motion when performing static stretching, what is the optimal number of stretch repetitions?**
   a. 1
   b. 2
   c. 3
   d. 4

2. **Which of the following is *true* regarding static or dynamic stretching?**
   a. Stretching to the point of discomfort results in the greatest increases in range of motion.
   b. Stretching to the point of discomfort has no effect on performance impairment.
   c. Stretching has no effect on delayed onset muscle soreness.
   d. Stretching is effective at reducing spasticity.

3. **Which of the following is *not true* regarding stretching?**
   a. Static stretches held for <30 seconds do not impair performance.
   b. Dynamic stretching reduces and impairs performance.
   c. Static stretching is effective at reducing joint contracture.
   d. Specific plantar fascia stretches are advocated for in the treatment of plantar/heel pain.

MANUAL THERAPY

*C.G. Bise, PT, DPT, PhD, OCS, S.R. Piva, PT, PhD, FAPTA, and R.E. Erhard, PT, DC**

1. **What is manual therapy?**

   When the term manual therapy is used alone, it has been described internationally as the use of skilled hand movements performed by physical therapists, chiropractors, or other health professionals to improve tissue extensibility, increase range of motion, induce relaxation, mobilize or manipulate soft tissue and joints, modulate pain, and reduce soft tissue swelling, inflammation, or restriction. Hands-on procedures such as mobilization, manipulation, massage, stretching, and deep pressure are all components of manual therapy. General orthopaedic manual therapy (OMT) techniques are used by a number of professions and may include thrust and nonthrust manipulation, passive and active-assist forms of stretching, and other novel hands-on interventions.

2. **What is orthopaedic manual physical therapy?**

   In the United States, orthopaedic manual physical therapy is a subspecialty of orthopaedic physical therapy. It has been described by the International Federation of Orthopaedic Manipulative Physical Therapists as a specialized area of physiotherapy/physical therapy for the "management of neuro-musculoskeletal conditions, based on clinical reasoning, using highly specific treatment approaches including manual therapy techniques and therapeutic exercises. Orthopaedic Manual Physical Therapy also encompasses, and is driven by, the available scientific and clinical evidence and the biopsychosocial framework of each individual patient."

3. **When is manual therapy treatment indicated?**

   The Guide to Physical Therapist Practice states: Physical therapists select, prescribe, and implement manual therapy techniques when the examination findings, diagnosis, and prognosis indicate use of these techniques to decrease edema, pain, spasm, or swelling; enhance health, wellness, and fitness; enhance or maintain physical performance; increase the ability to move; or prevent or remediate impairment in body functions and structures, activity limitations, or participation restrictions to improve physical function. Joint-specific techniques are indicated when the motion impairment is caused by loss of the normal joint motion as a result of a reversible joint hypomobility. Manual therapy is typically contraindicated when the motion impairment is caused by excessive joint mobility. Motion impairment caused by weakened or shortened muscles is often an indication to use soft tissue techniques. Once pain has been reduced and joint mobility improved with the application of manual therapy, it is easier for a patient to regain normal movement patterns and restore maximal function. Current research has shown that manual therapy, when combined with therapeutic exercise, provides a superior outcome to manual therapy alone. Therefore, current evidence recommends manual therapy to be used in combination with exercise during the episode of care.

4. **What is joint play?**

   Mennell defined joint play as "a movement that cannot be produced by the action of voluntary muscles." Joint play movements include distraction, compression, roll, glide, and spin. Loss of joint play frequently impairs range of motion. Manual therapy techniques use joint play movements for treating joint impairments.

5. **Is manual therapy always passive?**

   Some manual therapy techniques are passive. However, many manual therapy techniques use the patient's muscle contraction to assist or augment the treatment applied by the therapist. In these cases, the patient's participation is an expected, extra force that enhances the technique. Manual therapy occurs in response to existing extrinsic forces (the therapist or gravity force) or intrinsic forces (patient's muscle contraction or breathing) acting on the patient's body. Physical therapists who specialize in orthopaedic manual physical therapy use manual treatment with controlled mechanical loading to facilitate efficient hands-on treatment whether passive movement, passive-assisted movement, active movement, or touch-facilitated exercise.

6. **Describe the basic types of manipulations.**

   Manipulation consists of techniques utilizing skilled passive movements to joints and/or soft tissues that are applied at varying speeds and amplitudes. Thrust manipulation employs high-velocity, low-amplitude therapeutic movement within or at the end range of motion of a joint, whereas nonthrust manipulation uses all of the same principles for soft tissue and joint impairments without the thrust component. Following are more specific definitions of various types of manipulations.

---

*Deceased.

- Joint manipulation (thrust)—a localized, single passive movement using a high-velocity, low-amplitude thrust to bring the joint beyond its physiologic barrier. The result is distraction or translation of the joint surfaces. It does not exceed the anatomic barrier.
- Joint mobilization (nonthrust)—uses repetitive passive movements to return full range of motion and decrease pain. It moves joints within the physiologic ROM and uses three types of motion application: graded oscillation, progressive loading, and sustained loading.
- Muscle energy/osteopathic approach (nonthrust)—uses patient's active muscle contraction after joint is passively taken to restrictive barrier. It is indicated when the limiting factor to motion is the neuromuscular system. The osteopathic approach uses postisometric relaxation principles and also employs thrust manipulation when deemed necessary.
- Soft tissue mobilization—aims at enhancing the status of muscle activity and/or extensibility in tissues. It may produce effects on muscular, nervous, lymph, and circulatory systems. It can utilize instruments to assist in the treatment of soft tissues when deemed necessary.

7. **What is a physiologic and anatomic barrier?**
   - The physiologic barrier is the point at which voluntary range of motion in a joint is limited by soft tissue tension. This is sometimes referred to as the end-feel of the joint. When the joint reaches the physiologic barrier, further motion toward the anatomic barrier can be induced.
   - The anatomic barrier is the point at which passive range of motion of a joint is limited by bone contour, soft tissues (especially ligaments), or both. The anatomic barrier serves as the final limit to motion in an articulation. Movement beyond the anatomic barrier can cause tissue damage.

8. **Define direct and indirect manual therapy techniques.**
   - Direct technique—movement and force are in the direction of the motion restriction. Direct technique allows maximal restoration of movement; however, it may be painful when pain and muscle guarding are present.
   - Indirect technique—movement and force are not both in the direction of the motion restriction. This technique is indicated in acute stages and helps to facilitate blood flow and fluid movement.

9. **What is the difference between general and specific manual therapy techniques?**
   - General technique—the force is transmitted to a number of joints that have been determined to be hypomobile. A disadvantage of the general technique is that it can increase motion in an unstable joint not previously detected.
   - Specific technique—the force is localized to one joint; therefore, force transmission is minimized through the uninvolved joints.

10. **Is there evidence that specific thrust manipulation techniques are delivered accurately to the targeted segment?**

    No. Studies have compared the target location of the technique with the location of the joints that actually produced an audible pop (cavitation) in response to manipulation therapy. It has been reported that spinal manipulation is accurate about half of the time. However, part of this accuracy was because of most procedures being associated with multiple audible joint cavitations, and in most cases, at least one audible cavitation emanated from the target joints. Therefore, it seems that the clinical success of spinal manipulation is not dependent on the accurate delivery of that therapy to a specific targeted spinal joint.

11. **What is the pop?**

    Popping of the joint frequently accompanies a manipulative thrust. The crack noise or joint cavitation is the result of generation or collapse of a gaseous bubble in the synovial fluid. Cineradiographic studies reported increased joint space and carbon dioxide gas production/breakdown after thrust manipulation. Because carbon dioxide is a gas with higher miscibility within the synovial fluid, this increase has been suggested to be the mechanism responsible for an increase in range of motion in the joint after manipulation. It has also been hypothesized that the cavitation would initiate certain reflex relaxation of the periarticular musculature. After the manipulation, the joint takes approximately 15 minutes to rearrange the gas particles and allow for another cavitation sound. Some people believe that if there is no noise after a thrust manipulation, nothing has happened; this belief is incorrect. Studies have shown no relationship between the occurrence of an audible pop during joint manipulation and improvement in pain, ROM, and disability in patients with nonradicular low back pain.

12. **Describe the grading systems for joint mobilization.**

    Different grading systems exist for joint mobilization. Two of the most widely used grading systems are proposed by Maitland and Kaltenborn.

    The Maitland system is based on joint oscillation techniques and has five different grades as follows:
    - Grade 1—slow, small-amplitude movements performed at the beginning of the range.
    - Grade 2—slow, large-amplitude movements that do not reach the resistance or limit of the range.

- Grade 3—slow, large-amplitude movements performed through the resistance and up to the limit of the range.
- Grade 4—slow, small-amplitude movements performed through the resistance and at the limit of the range.
- Grade 5—small-amplitude, high-velocity movements (thrust) performed beyond the pathologic limitation of the range.

Grades 1 and 2 are used mainly to reduce pain, grades 3 and 4 are used primarily to increase mobility, and grade 5 is used for the thrust technique and is indicated when resistance limits movement in the absence of pain in that direction.

The Kaltenborn system is based on sustained hold gliding techniques and traction. Kaltenborn has three grades of traction and two grades of gliding as follows:

Traction

- Grade 1—traction force of extremely small amplitude, that nullifies the compression forces acting on a joint (musculature tension, cohesive forces, atmospheric pressure) where the joint is loosened but there is no appreciable separation of the joint surfaces.
- Grade 2—slack is taken up in the tissues surrounding the joint.
- Grade 3—beyond the slack, traction force is applied so that tissues crossing the joint are stretched.

Gliding

- Grade 2—translatoric gliding occurs until slack in joint is taken up and tightened.
- Grade 3—after slack is taken up and more force is applied, the tissues (capsular) crossing the joint are stretched.
- * There is no grade 1 glide according to Kaltenborn.

13. **Is there evidence that orthopaedic manual physical therapy is effective?**
Results vary across systematic reviews but all show that OMPT provides similar or superior outcomes versus a variety of comparable interventions. Many systematic reviews involving disorders of the knee, neck, shoulder, thoracic spine, and hip, as well as conditions such as headaches, cervical and lumbar radiculopathy, lateral elbow pain, acute and chronic low back pain, and ankle sprains have substantiated the outcomes of OMPT.

14. **Is there evidence that manual therapy is effective in treating cervicogenic headache?**
Systematic reviews suggest that thrust and nonthrust manipulation is effective for patients with cervicogenic headache. A more recent trial of patients with cervicogenic headaches compared a control group to groups receiving cervical thrust and nonthrust manipulation, strengthening of the deep neck flexor and scapular muscles, and a combined manual therapy and exercise group. The results showed significant reductions in headache symptoms in all treatment groups versus the control group. At 7- and 12-week follow-up visits, the combined exercise and manual therapy group showed some advantages over the other groups. Another RCT evaluated the effectiveness of manual therapy versus usual care at a general practitioner's office. The authors found that mobilizations to the cervical and thoracic spine, combined with exercise and postural correction, reduced headache frequency and intensity. Eighty-one percent of the participants in the manual therapy group experienced at least a 50% decline compared with only 40% in the usual care group. The evidence suggests that manual therapy is an effective intervention alone; however, when paired with exercise, the treatment effects are superior to the independent interventions.

15. **Is there evidence that manual therapy is effective in treating conditions of the extremities?**

HIP JOINT

- A recent randomized trial compared manual therapy (thrust and nonthrust manipulations of the hip joint) with an exercise therapy program in patients with osteoarthritis of the hip. Success rates after 5 weeks were 81% in the manual therapy group and 50% in the exercise group. Furthermore, patients in the manual therapy group had significantly better outcomes on pain, stiffness, hip function, and range of motion.
- Current clinical practice guidelines recommend the use of manual therapy for patients with mild hip osteoarthritis. Manual therapy should be used to decrease pain and increase mobility of the joint. This recommendation is based on moderate evidence. Current clinical practice guidelines advocate, in the absence of contraindication, the use of manual therapy for patients with nonarthritic hip pain. Manual therapy can include nonthrust manipulation for capsular restriction and soft tissue techniques to treat muscular and fascial impairments. This recommendation is based on expert opinion.

KNEE JOINT

- One study compared a group who received manual therapy combined with exercise to a placebo group. Subjects in the manual therapy group received joint mobilization techniques to the lumbopelvic region, hip, knee, and/or ankle, depending on whether they exhibited pain or reduced mobility. The manual therapy plus exercise group showed improvements in pain, stiffness, and function. The control group did not change. Yet the combination of manual therapy and exercise resulted in positive effects.
- A systematic review in 2011 found evidence for the use of manual therapy in patient with knee osteoarthritis (OA), but the heterogeneity of the studies prohibited meta-analysis and a definitive conclusion when combining manual therapy and exercise.

- An RCT in 2013 showed equivocal results for manual therapy and exercise in terms of outcomes. A follow-up cost-effectiveness analysis showed manual therapy and exercise together were the preferred treatment when compared with exercise and usual care for knee OA.

SHOULDER JOINT

- Manual therapy used alone or combined with exercise has shown to be effective in the treatment of patients with shoulder problems. One trial studied the effectiveness of manipulative therapy for the shoulder girdle in addition to usual medical care. At 12 and 52 weeks after treatment, the manipulation group reported better rates of full recovery. A consistent between-group difference in severity of the shoulder pain, disability, and general health favored manipulative therapy.
- An RCT compared a group of patients with shoulder impingement syndrome who performed supervised flexibility and strengthening exercises with a group who performed that same exercise program plus received manual physical therapy treatment. They reported significantly more improvement in pain and function in the exercise plus manual therapy group.
- Current clinical practice guidelines for adhesive capsulitis report studies showing a beneficial effect from manual therapy, but there is little evidence to establish its efficacy versus other interventions. The recommendation, based on weak evidence, is that joint mobilization be targeted to the glenohumeral and be used to decrease pain and increase range of motion.
- A recent RCT compared manual therapy with corticosteroid injections for shoulder impingement. Both groups demonstrated approximately 50% improvement in outcome scores, but the corticosteroid group required additional visits to their primary care physician, additional injections, and utilized additional physical therapy resources. As with other equivocal outcomes, manual therapy proved to be superior in terms of efficiency and cost.
- Finally, there has been evidence presented that the use of thoracic manipulation may benefit those patients with subacromial impingement. Though follow-up was only 48 hours after, thoracic manipulation provided statistically significant decreases in patients' reported pain and disability.

ELBOW JOINT

- Limited evidence indicates that mobilization with movement may help reduce painful movements and improve grip strength in patients with lateral epicondylalgia.
- A randomized trial of mobilization with movement (MWT) and exercise versus corticosteroid injections versus wait and see showed those treated with MWT and exercise had decreased pain and improved function. MWT was not superior to injections at the 52-week follow-up, but those who received MWT sought significantly less treatment than those who received injections.
- A systematic review showed short- and long-term benefits from mobilization with movement in patients with lateral epicondylalgia. There is, however, limited evidence to support one particular technique over another.

There is clear evidence that manual therapy has an immediate effect on the joints discussed. Alone there appears to be short-term benefit. The current evidence (and previous investigations) calls attention to the interaction effect between manual therapy and exercise. Each by itself is effective but almost all trials show the superiority of the combination of manual therapy and exercise.

16. **What are the expected side effects of spinal manipulation?**

Reactions after spinal manipulation are very common in clinical practice. A recent study reported that approximately 61% of patients complain of at least one postmanipulative reaction. The most common side effects are stiffness (20%), local discomfort (15%), headache (12%), radiating discomfort (12%), fatigue (12%), muscle spasms (6%), dizziness (4%), and nausea (3%). Most reactions begin within 4 hours and generally disappear within 24 hours after treatment. Women are more likely to report side effects than men.

17. **Does manual therapy affect the visceral organs?**

There is some emerging evidence to support a relationship between organ manipulation and mobilization and decreased pain in specific areas of the body. Some patients report improvement in their gastrointestinal discomfort or in constipation after thoracic or lumbar manipulation. Joint dysfunction facilitates the corresponding spinal cord segment, which can excite any of the neural elements arising from that segment, causing adverse visceral symptoms. There is a belief that when joint lesion is addressed, it may suppress or attenuate visceral complaints. To date, however, little evidence exists to validate the direct and indirect effects of manual therapy for visceral problems.

18. **Can manual therapy straighten a spinal deformity?**

When there are structural spinal deformities, such as scoliosis or hyperkyphosis, manipulation and mobilization have not been shown to decrease the progression, reverse, or straighten acquired spinal deformities.

19. **Can manual therapy restore spinal curvatures?**

When there is a temporary loss of spinal curvature, such as in a lateral lumbopelvic list or in a straightened cervical spine because of muscle spasm, nonaggressive manipulative techniques can be used to decrease spasm and increase movement.

20. **How does manual therapy help to increase range of motion and decrease pain and disability?**
The specific in vivo effects of manual therapy are not known, but suggested theories include:
- Manual therapy moves or frees the mechanical impediment (loose body, disc material, synovial fringe, or meniscoid entrapment) to joint movement, permitting movement and halting nociceptive input and associated reflex muscle spasm.
- Improvement in range of motion helps to relieve pain that is the direct result of such hypomobility.
- Manual therapy stretches or ruptures periarticular scar tissues.
- Manual therapy may improve nerve conductivity and circulation by means of increasing the space where nerves and blood vessels exit or cross.
- Manual therapy improves muscle function and decreases stress on bones and ligaments by improving the distribution of joint forces and levers.
- Manual therapy initiates a number of neurophysiologic effects that can be linked to the favorable outcomes seen when treating musculoskeletal issues.
- Manual therapy may initiate a neurochemical response that can be linked to favorable outcomes when treating musculoskeletal impairments.

21. **Should joint hypomobility be treated in the absence of symptoms?**
No. Despite the fact that some clinicians advocate a prophylactic treatment for joint hypomobility, there is no evidence that this approach prevents dysfunction.

22. **What is end-feel and how is it classified?**
End-feel is the resistance felt by an examiner at the end range of joint passive range of motion. Proper assessment can assist and guide diagnosis and treatment. End-feels can be normal or pathologic, depending on the movement they accompany at a particular joint and where in the range of movement they occur. Pathologic end-feels are muscle spasms, sensation of soft end-feel, springy rebound, and severe pain without any motion restriction (empty end-feel).
Typical end-feels:
- Bone to bone—abrupt stop to the movement that is felt when two hard surfaces meet (eg, passive extension of the elbow)
- Capsular—feeling of immediate stop of movement with some give (eg, end range of shoulder flexion)
- Tissue approximation—limb segment cannot be moved farther because the soft tissues surrounding the joint cannot be further compressed (eg, end range of knee flexion)
- Empty—patient complains of severe pain from the movement without the examiner perceiving an increase in resistance to the movement; indicates acute inflammation or extraarticular lesions
- Springy block—rebound is felt at the end of the range; results from displacement of an intraarticular structure
- Spasm—feeling of a muscle coming actively into play during the passive movement; indicates the presence of an acute or subacute condition
- Soft—results from soft tissue approximation or soft tissue stretching (eg, resistance felt at the end range of knee flexion)

23. **What are the general contraindications to manual therapy?**
- Fracture
- Instability of the target joint
- Infectious arthritis
- Tumors
- Joint ankylosis
- Acute inflammatory disorders
- Lack of diagnosed joint lesion
- Presence of pathologic end-feel

24. **List specific contraindications for thrust manipulation.**
- Cranial nerve signs or symptoms and dizziness of unknown origin (specific for cervical spine)
- Sacroperineal numbness or loss of bowel and bladder control (specific for lumbar spine)
- Painful movements in all joint directions or just one degree of movement free of pain and restriction
- Bilateral or multisegmental neurologic signs or symptoms
- Paralysis in nonperipheral nerve distribution
- Hyperreflexia or positive pathologic reflexes
- Presence of emotional disorders
- Patient taking anticoagulant medication or steroidal medication for a long period
- Patient apprehension
- Clinician not proficient in the indicated technique

- Down syndrome
- Long-term steroid usage
- Rheumatoid arthritis

25. **Describe the convex-concave rule, and explain how it influences manual therapy.**
Though this theory is currently debated, the classic definitions are still applied to manual techniques. When a convex joint surface moves on a fixed concave joint surface, joint rolling and gliding occur in opposite directions. Conversely, when a concave joint surface is moved on a fixed convex joint surface, rolling and gliding occur in the same direction. If only one of these motions occurred, the joint surface could become compressed toward the side of movement and the intraarticular structures may be impinged. This theory of physiologic movement informs clinicians when deciding the direction in which to apply manual therapy. When performing a nonthrust joint manipulation (mobilization), the therapist moves a bone with a convex joint surface in the direction opposite to the restriction, whereas nonthrust manipulation of a concave joint surface is performed in the same direction as the restriction.

26. **Describe loose-packed and close-packed positions.**
    - Loose-packed position—resting position in which the joint capsule is most relaxed, the articular surfaces are least congruent, and the greatest amount of joint play is possible. This resting position does not take into account extraarticular structures, such as muscles and fascia. Most joint manipulations are performed in this position and are progressed to the close-packed position.
    - Close-packed position—the joint capsule and ligaments are tight or at maximal tension. In this position, there is maximal contact between the concave and convex articular surfaces, and separation between the articular surfaces by traction forces is difficult.

27. **How do the loose-packed and close-packed positions influence manual therapy treatment?**
Knowledge of these positions allows clinicians to determine which movement compresses and tightens the joint and which movement distracts and loosens the joint. The loose-packed position is the position used for testing joint play and for starting treatment of restricted joint movement. The close-packed position is used to avoid joint movement. As an example, in order to isolate the mobilizing force to a particular level of the spine, the adjacent vertebral joints are locked in the close-packed position.

28. **Define capsular pattern.**
Cyriax described the capsular pattern as a predictable pattern of limitation in joint movement when the entire joint capsule has been shortened. Cyriax goes on to suggest that these patterns are a result of lesions in the joint capsule or the synovial membrane. These patterns indicate loss of mobility of the entire joint capsule from fibrosis, effusion, or inflammation, which may occur in arthrosis, arthritis, prolonged immobilization, or acute trauma. Joints not controlled by muscles, such as the sacroiliac or tibiofibular joints, do not exhibit a capsular pattern.

29. **Compare loose-packed position, close-packed position, and capsular pattern for all joints.**

JOINT	LOOSE-PACKED	CLOSE-PACKED	CAPSULAR PATTERN
Temporomandibular	Mouth slightly open	Teeth clenched	Limited mouth opening
Cervical spine	Midway between flexion and extension	Maximal extension	Limited in all motion, except flexion
Sternoclavicular	Arm resting by side	Maximal shoulder elevation	Limited full elevation; pain at end ranges
Acromioclavicular	Arm resting by side	Arm abducted 90°	Limited full elevation; pain at end ranges
Glenohumeral	55° shoulder abduction, 30° horizontal adduction	Maximal abduction and external rotation	Loss in external rotation > loss in abduction > loss in internal rotation
Humeroulnar	70° flexion, 10° supination	Full extension and supination	Loss of flexion > loss in extension
Humeroradial	Extension and supination	90° flexion, 5° supination	Loss of flexion > loss in extension

JOINT	LOOSE-PACKED	CLOSE-PACKED	CAPSULAR PATTERN
Radioulnar: proximal	70° flexion, 35° supination	5° supination, full extension	Limited pronation = limited supination
Radioulnar: distal	10° supination	5° supination	Limited pronation = limited supination
Radiocarpal	Neutral, slight ulnar deviation	Full extension, radial deviation	Limited flexion = limited extension
Midcarpal	Neutral, slight flexion and ulnar deviation	Full extension	Equal limitation in all directions
Trapeziometacarpal	Neutral	Full opposition	Limited abduction > extension
Carpometacarpal	Neutral	Full opposition	Equal limitation in all directions
Metacarpophalangeal	Slight flexion, ulnar deviation	Full flexion	
Interphalangeal	Slight flexion	Full extension	Limited flexion > extension
Thoracic spine	Midway between flexion and extension	Maximal extension	Side-bending and rotation > extension > flexion
Lumbar spine	Midway between flexion and extension	Maximal extension	Equal limitation of side-bending and rotation; extension > flexion
Hip	30° flexion, 30° abduction, slight external rotation	Full extension, abduction, internal rotation	Flexion and internal rotation > abduction > adduction > external rotation
Tibiofemoral	25° flexion	Full extension and external rotation	Limited flexion > extension
Talocrural	10° plantar flexion, neutral inversion/eversion	Full dorsiflexion	Plantar flexion > dorsiflexion
Subtarsal	10° plantar flexion, neutral inversion/eversion	Full inversion	Limitation in varus
Midtarsal	10° plantar flexion, neutral inversion/eversion	Full supination	Supination > pronation
Tarsometatarsal	Neutral supination and pronation	Full supination	
Metatarsophalangeal	Neutral	Full extension	Extension > flexion
Interphalangeal	Slight flexion	Full extension	Limited extension

BIBLIOGRAPHY

Abbott, J. H., Patla, C. E., & Jensen, R. H. (2001). The initial effects of an elbow mobilization with movement technique on grip strength in subjects with lateral epicondylalgia. *Manual Therapy*, *6*, 163–169.

Anwer, S., Alghadir, A., Zafar, H., & Brismee, J. M. (2018). Effects of orthopaedic manual therapy in knee osteoarthritis: a systematic review and meta-analysis. *Physiotherapy*, *104*(3), 264–276.

Bang, M. D., & Deyle, G. D. (2000). Comparison of supervised exercise with and without manual physical therapy for patients with shoulder impingement syndrome. *Journal of Orthopaedic and Sports Physical Therapy*, *30*, 126–137.

Bennell, K. L., Egerton, T., Martin, J., et al. (2014). Effect of physical therapy on pain and function in patients with hip osteoarthritis: A randomized clinical trial. *JAMA*, *311*(19), 1987–1997.

Bergman, G. J., Winters, J. C., Groenier, K. H., et al. (2004). Manipulative therapy in addition to usual medical care for patients with shoulder dysfunction and pain: A randomized, controlled trial. *Annals of Internal Medicine, 141*, 432–439.

Bialosky, J., Bishop, M., & Price, D. (2009). The mechanisms of manual therapy in the treatment of musculoskeletal pain: A comprehensive model. *Manual Therapy, 14*(5), 531–538.

Bisset, L., Beller, E., Jull, G., Brooks, P., Darnell, R., & Vicenzino, B. (2006). Mobilisation with movement and exercise, corticosteroid injection, or wait and see for tennis elbow: Randomised trial. *BMJ, 333*(7575), 939.

Bizzarri, P., Buzzatti, L., Cattrysse, E., & Scafoglieri, A. (2018). Thoracic manual therapy is not more effective than placebo thoracic manual therapy in patients with shoulder dysfunctions: A systematic review with meta-analysis. *Musculoskeletal Science & Practice, 33*, 1–10.

Bove, A. M., Smith, K. J., Bise, C. G., et al. (2018). Exercise, manual therapy, and booster sessions in knee osteoarthritis: Cost-effectiveness analysis from a multicenter randomized controlled trial. *Physical Therapy, 98*(1), 16–27.

Boyles, R. E., Ritland, B. M., Miracle, B. M., et al. (2009). The short-term effects of thoracic spine thrust manipulation on patients with shoulder impingement syndrome. *Manual Therapy, 14*(4), 375–380.

Brennan, G. P., Fritz, J. M., Hunter, S. J., Thackeray, A., Delitto, A., & Erhard, R. E. (2006). Identifying subgroups of patients with acute/subacute "nonspecific" low back pain: Results of a randomized clinical trial. *Spine (Phila Pa 1976), 31*(6), 623–631.

Bronfort, G., Assendelft, W. J., Evans, R., Haas, M., & Bouter, L. (2001). Efficacy of spinal manipulation for chronic headache: A systematic review. *Journal of Manipulative and Physiological Therapeutics, 24*, 457–466.

Bronfort, G., Haas, M., Evans, R. L., & Bouter, L. M. (2004). Efficacy of spinal manipulation and mobilization for low back pain and neck pain: A systematic review and best evidence synthesis. *Spine, 4*, 335–356.

Browder, D. A., Erhard, R. E., & Piva, S. R. (2004). Intermittent cervical traction and thoracic manipulation for management of mild cervical compressive myelopathy attributed to cervical herniated disc: A case series. *Journal of Orthopaedic and Sports Physical Therapy, 34*, 701–712.

Cagnie, B., Vinck, E., Beernaert, A., & Cambier, D. (2004). How common are side effects of spinal manipulation and can these side effects be predicted? *Manual Therapy, 9*, 151–156.

Campbell, B. D., & Snodgrass, P. T. S. J. (2010). The effects of thoracic manipulation on posteroanterior spinal stiffness. *Journal of Orthopaedic and Sports Physical Therapy, 40*(11), 685–694.

Childs, J. D. (2004). A clinical prediction rule to identify patients with low back pain most likely to benefit from spinal manipulation: A validation study. *Annals of Internal Medicine, 141*, 920–928.

Childs, J. D., Cleland, J. A., Elliott, J. M., et al. (2008). Neck pain: Clinical practice guidelines linked to the International Classification of Functioning, Disability, and Health from the Orthopedic Section of the American Physical Therapy Association. *Journal of Orthopaedic and Sports Physical Therapy, 38*(9), A1–A34.

Cleland, J. A., Childs, J. D., McRae, M., Palmer, J. A., & Stowell, T. (2005). Immediate effects of thoracic manipulation in patients with neck pain: A randomized clinical trial. *Manual Therapy, 10*, 127–135.

Cleland, J. A., Flynn, T. W., Childs, J. D., & Eberhart, S. (2007). The audible pop from thoracic spine thrust manipulation and its relation to short-term outcomes in patients with neck pain. *Journal of Manual & Manipulative Therapy, 15*(3), 143–154.

Cook, C. E., Donaldson, M., & Lonnemann, E. (2021). "Next steps" for researching orthopedic manual therapy. *Journal of Manual & Manipulative Therapy, 29*(6), 333–336.

Coulter, I. D., Crawford, C., Vernon, H., et al. (2019). Manipulation and mobilization for treating chronic nonspecific neck pain: A systematic review and meta-analysis for an appropriateness panel. *Pain Physician, 22*(2), E55–E70.

Desjardins-Charbonneau, A., Roy, J. S., Dionne, C. E., Fremont, P., MacDermid, J. C., & Desmeules, F. (2015). The efficacy of manual therapy for rotator cuff tendinopathy: a systematic review and meta-analysis. *Journal of Orthopaedic & Sports Physical Therapy, 45*(5), 330–350.

Deyle, G. D., Henderson, N. E., Matekel, R. L., Ryder, M. G., Garber, M. B., & Allison, S. C. (2000). Effectiveness of manual physical therapy and exercise in osteoarthritis of the knee: A randomized, controlled trial. *Annals of Internal Medicine, 132*, 173–181.

Enseki, K., Harris-Hayes, M., White, D. M., et al. (2014). Nonarthritic hip joint pain. *Journal of Orthopaedic and Sports Physical Therapy, 44*(6), A1–A32.

Falsiroli Maistrello, L., Rafanelli, M., & Turolla, A. (2019). Manual therapy and quality of life in people with headache: Systematic review and meta-analysis of randomized controlled trials. *Current Pain and Headache Reports, 23*(10), 78.

Flynn, T., Fritz, J., Whitman, J., et al. (2002). A clinical prediction rule for classifying patients with low back pain who demonstrate short-term improvement with spinal manipulation. *Spine, 27*, 2835–2843.

Flynn, T., Fritz, J. M., Wainner, R. S., & Whitman, J. M. (2003). The audible pop is not necessary for successful spinal high-velocity thrust manipulation in individuals with low back pain. *Archives of Physical Medicine and Rehabilitation, 84*, 1057–1060.

French, H. P., Brennan, A., White, B., & Cusack, T. (2011). Manual therapy for osteoarthritis of the hip or knee—a systematic review. *Manual Therapy, 16*(2), 109–117.

Fritz, J. M., Cleland, J. A., & Childs, J. D. (2007). Subgrouping patients with low back pain: Evolution of a classification approach to physical therapy. *Journal of Orthopaedic and Sports Physical Therapy, 37*(6), 290–302.

Herd, C. R., & Meserve, B. B. (2008). A systematic review of the effectiveness of manipulative therapy in treating lateral epicondylalgia. *Journal of Manual & Manipulative Therapy, 16*(4), 225–237.

Hoeksma, H. L., Dekker, J., Ronday, H. K., et al. (2004). Comparison of manual therapy and exercise therapy in osteoarthritis of the hip: A randomized clinical trial. *Arthritis Rheumatology, 51*, 722–729.

IFOMPT Constitution 2012, 2016, 2020 at https://www.ifompt.org/site/ifompt/IFOMPT%20Constitution%202020%20%20Final%20Document%20GM%202020%20and%20Post%20GM%20amendment.pdf

Jull, G., Trott, P., Potter, H., et al. (2002). A randomized controlled trial of exercise and manipulative therapy for cervicogenic headache. *Spine (Phila Pa 1976), 27*, 1835–1843.

Karas, S., & Olson Hunt, M. J. (2014). A randomized clinical trial to compare the immediate effects of seated thoracic manipulation and targeted supine thoracic manipulation on cervical spine flexion range of motion and pain. *Journal of Manual and Manipulative Therapy, 22*(2), 108–114.

Kelley, M. J., Shaffer, M. A., Kuhn, J. E., et al. (2013). Shoulder pain and mobility deficits: Adhesive capsulitis. *Journal of Orthopaedic & Sports Physical Therapy, 43*(5), A1–A31.

Kuligowski, T., Skrzek, A., & Cieslik, B. (2021). Manual therapy in cervical and lumbar radiculopathy: A systematic review of the literature. *International Journal of Environmental Research and Public Health, 18*(11), 6176.

Lucado, A. M., Dale, R. B., Vincent, J., & Day, J. M. (2019). Do joint mobilizations assist in the recovery of lateral elbow tendinopathy? A systematic review and meta-analysis. *Journal of Hand Therapy*, *32*(2), 262–276 e1.

Noten, S., Meeus, M., Stassijns, G., Van Glabbeek, F., Verborgt, O., & Struyf, F. (2016). Efficacy of different types of mobilization techniques in patients with primary adhesive capsulitis of the shoulder: A systematic review. *Archives of Physical Medicine and Rehabilitation*, *97*(5), 815–825.

Olson, K. (2016). *Manual physical therapy of the spine* (2nd ed). Elsevier.

Paige, N. M., Miake-Lye, I. M., Booth, M. S., et al. (2017). Association of spinal manipulative therapy with clinical benefit and harm for acute low back pain: Systematic review and meta-analysis. *JAMA*, *317*(14), 1451–1460.

Pieters, L., Lewis, J., Kuppens, K., et al. (2020). An update of systematic reviews examining the effectiveness of conservative physical therapy interventions for subacromial shoulder pain. *Journal of Orthopaedic & Sports Physical Therapy*, *50*(3), 131–141.

Pinto, D., Robertson, M. C., Abbott, J. H., et al. (2013). Manual therapy, exercise therapy, or both, in addition to usual care, for osteoarthritis of the hip or knee. 2: Economic evaluation alongside a randomized controlled trial. *Osteoarthritis and Cartilage*, *21*(10), 1504–1513.

Reiman, M. P., Bolgla, L. A., & Loudon, J. K. (2012). A literature review of studies evaluating gluteus maximus and gluteus medius activation during rehabilitation exercises. *Physiotherapy Theory and Practice*, *28*(4), 257–268.

Rhon, D. I., Boyles, R. B., & Cleland, J. A. (2014). One-year outcome of subacromial corticosteroid injection compared with manual physical therapy for the management of the unilateral shoulder impingement syndrome: A pragmatic randomized trial. *Annals of Internal Medicine*, *161*(3), 161–169.

Ross, J. K., Bereznick, D. E., & McGill, S. M. (2004). Determining cavitation location during lumbar and thoracic spinal manipulation: Is spinal manipulation accurate and specific? *Spine*, *29*, 1452–1457.

Rubinstein, S. M., de Zoete, A., van Middelkoop, M., Assendelft, W. J. J., de Boer, M. R., & van Tulder, M. W. (2019). Benefits and harms of spinal manipulative therapy for the treatment of chronic low back pain: systematic review and meta-analysis of randomised controlled trials. *BMJ*, *364*, l689.

UK BEAM Trial Team. (2004). United Kingdom back pain exercise and manipulation (UK BEAM) randomised trial: Effectiveness of physical treatments for back pain in primary care. *BMJ*, *329*, 1377.

Salamh, P., Cook, C., Reiman, M. P., & Sheets, C. (2017). Treatment effectiveness and fidelity of manual therapy to the knee: A systematic review and meta-analysis. *Musculoskeletal Care*, *15*(3), 238–248.

Schiller, L. (2001). Effectiveness of spinal manipulative therapy in the treatment of mechanical thoracic spine pain: A pilot randomized clinical trial. *Journal of Manipulative and Physiological Therapeutics*, *24*(6), 394–401.

Stanton, T. R., Fritz, J. M., Hancock, M. J., et al. (2011). Evaluation of a treatment-based classification algorithm for low back pain: A cross-sectional study. *Physical Therapy*, *91*(4), 496–509.

Vernon, H., McDermaid, C. S., & Hagino, C. (1999). Systematic review of randomized clinical trials of complementary/alternative therapies in the treatment of tension-type and cervicogenic headache. *Complementary Therapies in Medicine*, *7*, 142–155.

Weiss, H. R., Dieckmann, J., & Gerner, H. J. (2002). Effect of intensive rehabilitation on pain in patients with Scheuermann's disease. *Studies in Health Technology and Informatics*, *88*, 254–257.

Yazbek, P. M., Ovanessian, V., Martin, R. L., & Fukuda, T. Y. (2011). Nonsurgical treatment of acetabular labrum tears: A case series. *Journal of Orthopaedic and Sports Physical Therapy*, *41*(5), 346–353.

CHAPTER 11 QUESTIONS

1. **Which of the following manual therapy techniques can be considered harmful when used by inexperienced or untrained practitioners?**
   a. Joint manipulation
   b. Joint mobilization
   c. Muscle energy
   d. Soft tissue mobilization

2. **During assessment, your patient complains of severe pain during a movement of the shoulder and volitionally increases his resistance to movement. Which of the following Cyriax-described end-feels best classifies his condition?**
   a. Capsular
   b. Springy
   c. Spasm
   d. Empty

3. **When subgrouping patients with LBP, which of the following is NOT one of the criteria that predicts success with the application of spinal manipulative therapy?**
   a. Hypomobility of the lumbar spine
   b. No symptoms distal to the knee
   c. SLR >90 degrees
   d. An onset of symptoms <16 days

4. **There appears to be an interaction effect when SMT is combined with which of the following interventions?**
   a. Ultrasound
   b. Electrical stimulation
   c. Exercise
   d. Biopsychosocial interventions

CHAPTER 12

MASSAGE AND MYOFASCIAL MOBILIZATION

J.R. Krauss, PhD, PT, OCS, FAAOMPT and C.B. Smith, DPT, OMPT

1. **Briefly discuss the common approaches to massage and myofascial mobilization.**

   Massage techniques differ in origin and the basic premise behind their effectiveness. Classic Western massage was developed in Europe and the United States over the past two centuries. Western massage is based on the Western medical disease model, with mechanical and neurologic rationales supporting its use as therapy. Contemporary massage, bodywork, and Asian bodywork are widely diverse in their rationale, including energy balancing, myofascial softening and lengthening, and traditional Chinese medicine and meridian theories.

2. **How does massage generate pain relief?**

   Several mechanisms have been proposed and researched as possible sources of pain relief after the massage. These include mechanisms within local tissues, the peripheral nervous system, the spinal cord, and the cortex. One of the oldest theories is that light to moderate mechanical stimulation of cutaneous and subcutaneous tissues increases activity in somatosensory neurons, which may inhibit activity in pain-mediating neurons in the spinal cord. This is based on the gate control theory of pain developed by Melzack and Wall in 1965. Another proposed theory is that increased activation of the descending pain inhibitory system, starting in the periaqueductal gray matter (PAG) and continuing to the dorsal horn of the spinal cord, may reduce pain. In conjunction with this theory is the belief that opioid receptors in the PAG are activated due to massage (Bialosky et al. 2009). Last, Lund et al. in 2002 investigated the mechanisms behind the effects of massage on animals. They concluded that long-term pain relief effects of massage might be attributed, at least in part, to the oxytocinergic system and its interaction with the opioid system. Although this mechanism is not well understood, it is theorized that increased endogenous oxytocin may result in a greater synthesis of endogenous opioids.

3. **Does massage decrease depression?**

   Field et al. in 2004 studied massage therapy effects on depressed pregnant women. Participants received two 20-minute massage therapy sessions by their significant others for 16 weeks of pregnancy, starting during the second trimester. By the end of the study, the massage group had higher dopamine and serotonin levels and lower cortisol and norepinephrine levels. Field et al. in 2012 compared the effects of yoga, massage therapy, or standard prenatal care on prenatal depression and neonatal outcomes for 84 prenatally depressed women. Following 12 weeks of twice-weekly yoga or massage therapy sessions (20 minutes each), both therapy groups, versus the control group, had a greater decrease in depression, anxiety, and back and leg pain. In addition, both groups had greater gestational age and birth weight than the control group. Choi and Lee in 2015 examined the effects of foot reflexology massage on fatigue, stress, and depression of postpartum women. They concluded that foot reflexology massage applied once per day for 3 consecutive days lowered fatigue, urine cortisol, and depression levels compared to control. In 2011 Krohn et al. and Poland et al. in 2013 examined the effects of massage on depression in patients with breast cancer or HIV, respectively. Both authors concluded that massage could reduce depression in both of these patient populations. Finally, Reychler et al. in 2017 explored the benefits of massage therapy delivered for 1 hour per week for 4 weeks for HIV patients. While they did not detect a positive impact of massage on depression in their study, they did identify reduced anxiety and hyperventilation compared to controls.

4. **Does massage boost the immune system and reduce inflammation?**

   There is a growing body of evidence supporting the positive effects of massage on boosting the immune system and reducing inflammation. Regarding inflammation specifically, Crane et al. in 2012 studied the effects of massage on 11 young males with exercise-induced muscle damage. They analyzed the biopsies acquired from the vastus lateralis at baseline, after 10 minutes of massage, and after 2.5 hours of recovery. They concluded that massage was clinically beneficial in reducing inflammation and promoting mitochondrial biogenesis. Relating to the immune system, Ang et al. in 2012 compared the effects of massage therapy versus sham therapy on 120 preterm infants. They concluded that infants who received $\geq$5 consecutive days of massage demonstrated higher natural killer cytotoxicity. Mendes and Procianoy compared the effects of adding maternal massage four times a day to the face and limbs of very low-birth-rate infants. They concluded that maternal massage therapy decreased the length of hospital stay and the incidence of late-onset neonatal sepsis. Rapaport et al. in 2010 and 2012 studies compared the effects of Swedish massage therapy versus a light touch control group on oxytocin (OT), arginine-vasopressin (AVP), adrenal corticotropin hormone (ACTH), cortisol (CORT), circulating phenotypic lymphocyte markers, and mitogen-stimulated cytokine function. They concluded that compared with the touch control condition, a single massage session or 5 weeks of Swedish massage stimulated a sustained pattern of increased circulating phenotypic lymphocyte markers and decreased mitogen-stimulated cytokine production and had minimal effect on hypothalamic-pituitary-adrenal function. In contrast, twice-weekly massage produced a different response pattern with increased OT levels, decreased AVP, decreased CORT, minimal effects on circulating lymphocyte phenotypic markers, and a slight increase in mitogen-stimulated interferon-gamma, tumor necrosis factor-alpha, and interleukin (IL)-1b and IL-2 levels, suggesting increased production of proinflammatory cytokines. Sornkayasit et al. in 2021 evaluated the effects of traditional Thai massage (TTM) and the immune response in elderly individuals. They found that six sessions of TTM provided for 1 hour resulted in an elevated percentage of conventional CD4+ T cells and a decreased percentage of senescent C4+ T cells. These senescent CD4+ T cells are considered a pathological T cell subpopulation and a biomarker of immunosenescence associated with low-grade systemic inflammation.

5. **Does massage improve lymphatic drainage?**
Medline Plus defines manual lymphatic drainage (MLD) as a "light massage therapy technique that involves moving the skin in particular directions based on the structure of the lymphatic system," which is used to "encourage drainage of fluid and waste through the appropriate channels." MLD typically involves a slight stretching of the skin without significant downward pressure into the underlying body tissue. Vairo et al. in 2009 and Majewski-Schrage and Snyder in 2016 reviewed a combined total of 12 articles. They concluded that MLD might be effective in treating musculoskeletal injuries by decreasing pain and edema and improving range of motion. In addition, aspartate aminotransferase and lactate dehydrogenase, both byproducts of physical exertion, were also decreased in skeletal muscle following MLD. These mechanisms are hypothesized to assist in expediting regenerative and repair mechanisms following mechanical loads from physical activity. Provencher et al. in 2021 in their systematic review also concluded that MLD was beneficial for reducing edema and pain, enhancing ROM, and improving patient quality of life and satisfaction following musculoskeletal injuries.

6. **Does massage decrease blood pressure?**
Cambron et al. in 2006 examined the effects of six different massage techniques on 150 participants. Techniques included Swedish, deep tissue, myofascial release, sports, trigger point, and craniosacral. The authors concluded that clients receiving Swedish massage (effleurage and pétrissage) experienced the greatest reduction in blood pressure. Those who received trigger point therapy and sports massage experienced an increase in blood pressure. Limits to the generalization of the results of this study include a small sample size and lack of control regarding treatment duration and technique standardization. Arslan et al. in 2021 examined the effects of foot and back massage on blood pressure and sleep quality in females with essential hypertension. A total of six treatment sessions of foot and back massage were applied for 30 minutes, twice a week, for 3 weeks. They identified a significant ($p < 0.001$) reduction in systolic and diastolic blood pressure and improved sleep quality in the massage group compared to controls. Erzincanli and Kasar in 2021 examined the effect of hand massage on pain, anxiety, and vital signs in patients before venipuncture procedure. They noted a significant ($p < .05$) reduction in anxiety and blood pressure compared to controls.

7. **Does massage increase tissue temperature?**
Drust et al. in 2003 examined the effects of massage on intramuscular temperature in the vastus lateralis in humans. They concluded that when comparing massage with ultrasound, changes in muscle temperature were significantly higher for a massage at 1.5 to 2.5 cm below the skin. They also determined that thigh skin temperatures were significantly higher in massage-treated patients. More recently, Sefton et al. in 2010 demonstrated, through thermography, that massage therapy produced significant increases in temperature over time in the anterior upper chest, posterior neck, upper back, right arm, and middle back. Additionally, the temperatures remained above baseline levels after 60 minutes. Portillo-Soto et al. in 2014 compared the effects of the Graston Technique and massage therapy on calf blood flow, using skin temperature measures on the lower leg. They concluded that following 10 minutes of either technique, skin temperatures were elevated, with massage generating a clinically significant higher temperature than Graston. In this study, temperatures increased immediately following treatment, peaked at 25 minutes, and remained elevated at 60 minutes post treatment. Finally, Chatchawan et al. explored the immediate effects of self-Thai foot massage, and therapist-applied Thai foot massage (TFM) on skin blood flow, skin temperature, and range of motion of the foot and ankle in type 2 diabetic patients. They concluded that skin blood flow and range of motion significantly improved for both groups. However, skin temperature only changed for the TFM group.

8. **Does massage improve muscle flexibility?**
Hopper et al. in 2005 examined the effects of classic soft tissue mobilization (STM) and dynamic STM on hamstring length in 45 healthy male subjects. The dynamic STM consisted of classic STM followed by distal to proximal longitudinal strokes performed during passive, active, and eccentric loading of the hamstring. They concluded that dynamic STM significantly increased hamstring flexibility compared with classic STM and controls. In a separate study, Hopper et al. in 2005 examined the effects of dynamic STM and classic STM on hamstring length

in 50 female field hockey players. This study measured passive straight leg raise and passive knee extension before, after, and 24 hours post intervention. They concluded that both massage techniques significantly improved hamstring length immediately after massage and had no carryover 24 hours post intervention. Huang et al. in 2010 examined the effects of no massage, 10 seconds of massage, and 30 seconds of massage on hip flexion angle, passive leg tension, and electromyography (EMG) in 10 women ages 21 to 23 years old. Treatments were randomized over 3 days. Treatment effects were greatest for the 30 seconds of massage, which resulted in a 7.2% increase in hip angle. There was no significant difference in passive tension or EMG for either the control or the treatment. They concluded that this musculotendinous massage might be used in place of, or in adjunct to, static stretching to improve hamstring flexibility. Forman et al. in 2014 examined the effects of deep stripping massage strokes (DSMS) in isolation or combined with eccentric resistance on hamstring length in 89 participants. In this study, DSMS consisted of longitudinally directed deep pressure strokes over the hamstring muscles, applied for 10 seconds, and repeated 15 times with the hamstring relaxed or held in eccentric contraction. They concluded that DSMS + eccentric contraction and DSMS alone improved flexibility by 10.7% and 6.3%, respectively. Kaur and Sinha in 2020 examined the effects of massage on the flexibility of hamstrings and agility in female athletes. He concluded that Swedish massage of the posterior thigh increased flexibility of hamstring muscles, which persisted for 5 days after cessation of massage. Finally, Kim et al. in 2020 examined the effects of electroacupuncture and manual acupuncture on hip and knee flexion ROM and quadriceps function (strength and activation). They concluded that both hip and knee flexion ROM increased but reduced quadriceps muscles strength immediately following treatment.

9. Does massage aid in recovery from exercise and competition?

A systematic review with meta-analysis performed in 2018 evaluated the impact of multiple recovery techniques on delayed onset muscle soreness (DOMS), perceived fatigue, muscle damage, and inflammatory markers after physical exercise. It was found that massage was the most powerful procedure that induced significant benefits in DOMS and perceived fatigue regardless of whether the individual was an athlete or sedentary. Furthermore, they found that massage was also the most effective recovery technique in reducing concentrations of circulating creatine kinase and interleukin-6 in the blood, which are both elevated in response to muscle damage and inflammation associated with exercise. Multiple studies have found that massage does not affect blood lactate concentrations (Hemmings, Hilbert, Ce), regardless of the depth of massage used (superficial or deep) (Ce). However, the use of blood lactate levels has been questioned on whether it is a valid indicator of postexercise recovery due to the naturally short half-life of blood lactate compared to other elevated enzymes and inflammatory markers (Barnett).

Naderi et al. in 2021 more specifically examined the effects of massage on older individuals (>60 years) following exercise-induced muscle damage (EIMD) in the calf muscles. Fifteen minutes of massage to the calf muscles was performed immediately following the exercise protocol and again at 24, 48, and 72 hours post exercise. They found that repeated massage reduced muscle soreness, loss of proprioception, facilitated the recovery of muscle strength, and alleviated the fear of falling and balance impairments caused by EIMD. This study suggests that older individuals that plan to engage in a strength training program may benefit from massage to attenuate EIDM symptoms and related impairments in strength and balance to reduce the risk of falling in the days following exercise.

10. Does massage decrease the frequency of chronic tension headaches?

Quinn et al. in 2002 investigated the effect of massage therapy on chronic nonmigraine headaches. Chronic tension headache sufferers received structured massage therapy treatment to the neck and shoulder muscles. They concluded that headache frequency was significantly reduced within the first week of treatment and continued throughout the study. The duration of headaches also tended to decrease during the massage treatment period. Headache intensity was unaffected by massage. Chatchawan et al. in 2014 investigated the effects of 3 weeks of Thai traditional massage (TTM) on pressure pain threshold and headache intensity in patients with chronic tension-type and migraine headaches. While TTM resulted in significant ($p < .01$) increase in pressure pain threshold immediately following treatment, and at 3 and 9 weeks post treatment, compared to controls, there was no significant difference in headache intensity between groups. Espi-Lopez et al. investigated the effect of manipulation plus massage therapy versus massage therapy alone on tension-type headaches. Following four treatment sessions applied over 4 weeks, they concluded that while massage provided relief for tension-type headaches, the effect was stronger on range of upper cervical motion when combined with cervical manipulation.

11. Does massage increase range of motion in patients with cervicogenic headache?

Hopper et al. in 2013 investigated the short-term effects of soft tissue massage applied to the neck muscles. Range of motion was measured using the flexion-rotation test immediately after preintervention and postintervention after each of the three treatment sessions and 2 weeks following the final treatment. They concluded that the range of motion increased significantly from treatment sessions one to three. Improvement was greatest after the first and second treatments and remained stable after the final treatment to the 2-week follow-up. Limits to the generalization of the results of this study include a small sample size, the limited age range of participants, and a lack of a control group. Rostron in 2021 reported on a patient with migraines and cervical spondylosis who was treated with Swedish massage, myofascial trigger point release, and proprioceptive neuromuscular facilitation (PNF) stretching. They concluded that massage therapy was effective in increasing cervical ROM.

12. **Does massage improve adverse neural tension signs and symptoms?**

De-la-Llave-Rincon et al. in 2012 examined the effects of soft tissue mobilization and nerve slider neurodynamic technique on the numeric pain rating score (NPRS) and pain pressure threshold over the median, radial, and ulnar nerves; the C5-C6 zygapophyseal joint; the carpal tunnel; and the tibialis anterior muscle. Participants consisted of 18 women with a clinical and electromyographic diagnosis of carpal tunnel syndrome. Each participant received both treatments at potential entrapment sites of the median nerve. The authors concluded that the combination of soft tissue mobilization and neurodynamic technique decreased pain intensity for up to 1 week post treatment but did not change pressure pain sensitivity. Saban et al. in 2014 compared the effects of deep massage therapy (DMS) and neural mobilization with a self-stretch program to ultrasound with the same self-stretch program for 69 participants experiencing heel pain. They concluded that both treatment protocols resulted in short-term improvement and that the DMS treatment was significantly more effective than the ultrasound treatment. Krauss et al. in 2012 examined the effects of functional massage, a technique using soft tissue massage and nonpainful joint motion, on the straight leg raise test in 12 asymptomatic young adults. The massage was applied along the course of the sciatic nerve in the posterior thigh and leg. Participants demonstrated an average improvement in ROM of 11.6 degrees immediately following treatment and 5.3 degrees at a 1-week follow-up. Limits to this study include the small sample size, lack of a control group, and a limited age range of participants. Puntumetakul et al. in 2019 examined the short-term effects of thoracic manipulation, used alone or in conjunction with the Thai massage, on pain and neural extensibility in patients with chronic mechanical neck pain. They noted a significant reduction in cervical pain and improved pain threshold during Upper Limb Neurodynamic Test 1: elbow extension for both intervention groups. However, they did not note any improvement in pain tolerance during elbow extension for either.

13. **What is the origin, nature, and purpose of functional massage?**

Co-developed by Krauss and Evjenth, functional massage integrates soft tissue massage (in the form of manual soft tissue compression and decompression) and nonpainful joint motion (both angular and translatoric). The goals of functional massage are to: 1) manage musculotendinous and periarticular soft tissue pain and tension and 2) aid in the management of impaired segmental and/or joint motion, impaired muscle function/performance, and impaired neural dynamics caused by, or associated with, musculotendinous and/or periarticular soft tissue pain, and/or tension, and/or gliding restrictions. During functional massage the joint is repeatedly moved so that musculotendinous and/or periarticular soft tissues are lengthened/tensed and shortened/slackened while massage pressure is applied. Functional massage is used to reduce pain and improve mobility. By integrating joint motion and massage it is theorized that proprioceptors from both the joint and the muscle are stimulated, potentially increasing the treatment's counterirritation effects at the spinal cord level. In addition, muscle activity during the massage may range from passive to fully active, allowing for a passive intervention to be morphed into an active assistive and/or a fully active motion. Finally, functional massage integrates soft tissue broadening, lengthening, and gliding of the muscles, tendons, fascia, and nerves that occur during normal body function. Indications for functional massage include musculoskeletal and periarticular soft tissue pain and/or stiffness and resultant impairment(s) in muscle performance, joint mobility, tendon and neural mobility, and soft tissue edema/swelling. Contraindications for functional massage include severe hypomobility and injuries, medical conditions, and/or medication-related conditions resulting in severe vascular or connective tissue fragility. Sobeck et al. in 2016 examined the effectiveness of functional massage on pain and range of motion in patients with orthopedic impairments of the extremities. Using a test-retest design, they collected data on pain and range of motion (ROM) for patients experiencing shoulder, knee, and ankle orthopedic impairments. They noted a statistically significant and clinically significant increase in ROM and a statistically significant reduction in NPRS post a single treatment of functional massage. Krauss et al. in 2019 examined the effects of functional massage on the straight leg raise and fingertip to floor tests in asymptomatic individuals using a pre-test, post-test experimental study design. Participants received either 20 minutes of functional massage, placebo ultrasound, or no treatment using a double-blind design. They concluded that functional massage resulted in a statistically and clinically significant increase in the straight leg raise by 16 degrees, $p < .000$, maintaining 13 degrees of motion, $p < .000$ compared to control and placebo, both of which demonstrated no significant ROM changes.

14. **What is the purpose of Cyriax transverse friction massage?**

Cyriax transverse friction massage provides movement to the muscle or tendon while inducing traumatic hyperemia in order to stimulate healing.

15. **What are the basic principles of transverse friction massage?**

- The soft tissue lesion must be properly treated.
- Friction is given across the grain of the soft tissue.

- The therapist's fingers must move together with the patient's skin.
- Friction must have sufficient depth and sweep.
- The patient must be comfortable.
- Tendon is put on stretch, whereas muscle is massaged in a relaxed position.

16. **Does transverse friction massage induce healing?**
No well-performed studies have shown histologic support for the promotion of healing of soft tissue with transverse friction massage. Walker examined the use of transverse friction massage on medial collateral ligaments of rabbits and found no difference between massaged and control rabbits. However, the experimentally induced sprain may have been insufficient to promote an inflammatory response. In a recent systematic review, Joseph et al. in 2012 concluded that there is limited evidence supporting the use of deep friction massage (DFM) in combination with Mill's manipulation in the treatment of elbow tendinopathy and in combination with joint mobilization for the treatment of supraspinatus tendinopathy in the presence of outlet syndrome. Olaussen et al. in 2015 also concluded that deep, transverse friction massage, Mills manipulation, stretching, and eccentric exercises showed no clear benefit in treating lateral epicondylitis. Thus, there remains a lack of evidence examining the isolated efficacy of DFM.

Bibliography

Ang, J. Y., Lua, J. L., Mathur, A., et al. (2012). A randomized placebo-controlled trial of massage therapy on the immune system of preterm infants. *Pediatrics, 130*(6), e1549–e1558.

Arslan, G., Ceyhan, O., & Mollaoglu, M. (2021). The influence of foot and back massage on blood pressure and sleep quality in females with essential hypertension: a randomized controlled study. *Journal of Human Hypertension, 35*(7), 627–637.

Barnett, A. (2006). Using recovery modalities between training sessions in elite athletes: does it help? *Sports Medicine, 36*(9), 781–796.

Bell, J. (2008). Massage therapy helps to increase range of motion, decrease pain and assist in healing a client with low back pain and sciatica symptoms. *Journal of Bodywork and Movement Therapies, 12*(3), 281–289.

Bialosky, J. E., Bishop, M. D., Price, D. D., Robinson, M. E., & George, S. Z. (2009). The mechanisms of manual therapy in the treatment of musculoskeletal pain: a comprehensive model. *Manual Therapy, 14*(5), 531–538.

Birk, T. J., McGrady, A., MacArthur, R. D., & Khuder, S. (2000). The effects of massage therapy alone and in combination with other complementary therapies on immune system measures and quality of life in human immunodeficiency virus. *Journal of Alternative and Complementary Medicine, 6*, 405–414.

Cambron, J. A., Dexheimer, J., & Coe, P. (2006). Changes in blood pressure after various forms of therapeutic massage: a preliminary study. *Journal of Alternative and Complementary Medicine, 12*(1), 65–70.

Cè, E., Limonta, E., Maggioni, M. A., Rampichini, S., Veicsteinas, A., & Esposito, F. (2013). Stretching and deep and superficial massage do not influence blood lactate levels after heavy-intensity cycle exercise. *Journal of Sports Sciences, 31*(8), 856–866.

Chatchawan, U., Eungpinichpong, W., Sooktho, S., Tiamkao, S., & Yamauchi, J. (2014). Effects of Thai traditional massage on pressure pain threshold and headache intensity in patients with chronic tension-type and migraine headaches. *Journal of Alternative and Complementary Medicine, 20*(6), 486–492.

Chatchawan, U., Jarasrungsichol, K., & Yamauchi, J. (2020). Immediate effects of self-Thai foot massage on skin blood flow, skin temperature, and range of motion of the foot and ankle in type 2 diabetic patients. *Journal of Alternative and Complementary Medicine, 26*(6), 491–500.

Choi, M. S., & Lee, E. J. (2015). Effects of foot-reflexology massage on fatigue, stress and postpartum depression in postpartum women. *Journal of Korean Academy of Nursing, 45*(4), 587–594.

Crane, J. D., Ogborn, D. I., Cupido, C., et al. (2012). Massage therapy attenuates inflammatory signaling after exercise-induced muscle damage. *Science Translational Medicine, 4*(119), 119ra13.

De-la-Llave-Rincon, A. I., Ortega-Santiago, R., Ambite-Quesada, S., et al. (2012). Response of pain intensity to soft tissue mobilization and neurodynamic technique: a series of 18 patients with chronic carpal tunnel syndrome. *Journal of Manipulative and Physiological Therapeutics, 35*(6), 420–427.

Drust, B., Atkinson, G., Gregson, W., French, D., & Binningsley, D. (2003). The effects of massage on intramuscular temperature in the vastus lateralis in humans. *International Journal of Sports Medicine, 24*, 395–399.

Erzincanli, S., & Kasar, K. S. (2021). Effect of hand massage on pain, anxiety, and vital signs in patients before venipuncture procedure: a randomized controlled trial. *Pain Management Nursing, 22*(3), 356–360.

Espi-Lopez, G. V., Zurriaga-Llorens, R., Monzani, L., & Falla, D. (2016). The effect of manipulation plus massage therapy versus massage therapy alone in people with tension-type headache. A randomized controlled clinical trial. *European Journal of Physical and Rehabilitation Medicine, 52*(5), 606–617.

Field, T., Diego, M., Hernandez-Reif, M., Medina, L., Delgado, J., & Hernandez, A. (2012). Yoga and massage therapy reduce prenatal depression and prematurity. *Journal of Bodywork and Movement Therapies, 16*(2), 204–209.

Field, T., Diego, M. A., Hernandez-Reif, M., Schanberg, S., & Kuhn, C. (2004). Massage therapy effects on depressed pregnant women. *Journal of Psychosomatic Obstetrics and Gynecology, 25*, 115–221.

Fields, H. L., & Basbaum, A. I. (1994). Central nervous system mechanisms of pain modulation. In P. D. Wall & R. Melzack (Eds.), *Textbook of pain* (pp. 243–257). Edinburgh: Churchill Livingstone.

Forman, J., Geertsen, L., & Rogers, M. E. (2014). Effect of deep stripping massage alone or with eccentric resistance on hamstring length and strength. *Journal of Bodywork and Movement Therapies, 18*(1), 139–144.

Hammer, W. I. (1999). *Functional soft tissue examination and treatment by manual methods* (2nd ed.). Gaithersburg, MD: Aspen Publishers.

Harris, J. A. (1996). Descending antinociceptive mechanisms in the brainstem: their role in the animal's defensive system. *Journal of Physiology—Paris, 90*, 15–25.

Hinds, T., McEwan, I., Perkes, J., Dawson, E., Ball, D., & George, K. (2004). Effects of massage on limb and skin blood flow after quadriceps exercise. *Medicine & Science in Sports & Exercise, 36*, 1308–1313.

Holey, E., & Cook, E. (1998). *Therapeutic massage.* Philadelphia, PA: WB Saunders.

Hopper, D., Bajaj, Y., Kei Choi, C., et al. (2013). A pilot study to investigate the short-term effects of specific soft tissue massage on upper cervical movement impairment in patients with cervicogenic headache. *Journal of Manual and Manipulative Therapy, 21*(1), 18–23.

Hopper, D., Conneely, M., Chromiak, F., Canini, E., Berggren, J., & Briffa, K. (2005). Evaluation of the effect of two massage techniques on hamstring muscle length in competitive female hockey players. *Physical Therapy in Sport, 6*(3), 137–145.

Hopper, D., Deacon, S., Das, S., et al. (2005). Dynamic soft tissue mobilisation increases hamstring flexibility in healthy male subjects. *British Journal of Sports Medicine, 39*(9), 594–598. discussion 598.

Huang, S. Y., Di Santo, M., Wadden, K. P., Cappa, D. F., Alkanani, T., & Behm, D. G. (2010). Short-duration massage at the hamstrings musculotendinous junction induces greater range of motion. *Journal of Strength and Conditioning Research, 24*(7), 1917–1924.

Joseph, M. F., Taft, K., Moskwa, M., & Denegar, C. R. (2012). Deep friction massage to treat tendinopathy: a systematic review of a classic treatment in the face of a new paradigm of understanding. *Journal of Sport Rehabilitation, 21*(4), 343–353.

Kaur, K., & Sinha, A. G. K. (2020). Effectiveness of massage on flexibility of hamstring muscle and agility of female players: an experimental randomized controlled trial. *Journal of Bodywork and Movement Therapies, 24*(4), 519–526.

Kim, D., Jang, S., & Park, J. (2020). Electroacupuncture and manual acupuncture increase joint flexibility but reduce muscle strength. *Healthcare (Basel), 8*(4), 414.

Krauss, J., Amato, L., Brettfeld, C., Nobani, B., & Ung, S. (2015). The effects of functional massage on the straight leg raise test in asymptomatic individuals: a pilot case study. Unpublished manuscript.

Krauss, J., Anderson, B., Delmottee, B., et al. (2012). The effects of functional massage on the straight leg raise test in asymptomatic individuals. A pilot case series. In J. Chevan & P. Clapis (Eds.), *Management of low back pain: A comparison of approaches in physical therapy* (pp. 67–93). Burlington, MA: Jones and Bartlett Learning.

Krauss, J., Wilczewski, T., Narayan, A., & Charney, S. (2019). The effects of functional massage on the straight leg raise and fingertip to floor tests in asymptomatic individuals: pre-test, post-test experimental study. Unpublished manuscript.

Krohn, M., Listing, M., Tjahjono, G., et al. (2011). Depression, mood, stress, and Th1/Th2 immune balance in primary breast cancer patients undergoing classical massage therapy. *Support Care Cancer, 19*(9), 1303–1311.

Lederman, E. (1997). *Fundamentals of manual therapy, physiology, neurology, and psychology.* New York, NY: Churchill Livingstone.

Lund, I., Ge, Y., Long-Chuan, Y., et al. (2002). Repeated massage-like stimulation induces long-term effects on nociception: contribution of oxytocinergic mechanism. *European Journal of Neuroscience, 16*, 330–338.

Majewski-Schrage, T., & Snyder, K. (2016). The effectiveness of manual lymphatic drainage in patients with orthopedic injuries. *Journal of Sport Rehabilitation, 25*(1), 91–97.

Mendes, E. W., & Procianoy, R. S. (2008). Massage therapy reduces hospital stay and occurrence of late-onset sepsis in very preterm neonates. *Journal of Perinatology, 28*(12), 815–820.

Naderi, A., Aminian-Far, A., Gholami, F., Mousavi, S. H., Saghari, M., & Howatson, G. (2021). Massage enhances recovery following exercise-induced muscle damage in older adults. *Scandinavian Journal of Medicine & Science in Sports, 31*(3), 623–632.

Olaussen, M., Holmedal, O., Mdala, I., Brage, S., & Lindbaek, M. (2015). Corticosteroid or placebo injection combined with deep transverse friction massage, Mills manipulation, stretching and eccentric exercise for acute lateral epicondylitis: a randomised, controlled trial. *BMC Musculoskeletal Disorders, 16*, 122.

Poland, R. E., Gertsik, L., Favreau, J. T., et al. (2013). Open-label, randomized, parallel-group controlled clinical trial of massage for treatment of depression in HIV-infected subjects. *Journal of Alternative and Complementary Medicine, 19*(4), 334–340.

Portillo-Soto, A., Eberman, L. E., Demchak, T. J., & Peebles, C. (2014). Comparison of blood flow changes with soft tissue mobilization and massage therapy. *Journal of Alternative and Complementary Medicine, 20*(12), 932–936.

Provencher, A. M., Giguere-Lemieux, E., Croteau, E., Ruchat, S. M., & Corbin-Berrigan, L. A. (2021). The use of manual lymphatic drainage on clinical presentation of musculoskeletal injuries: a systematic review. *Complementary Therapies in Clinical Practice, 45*, 101469.

Puntumetakul, R., Pithak, R., Namwongsa, S., Saiklang, P., & Boucaut, R. (2019). The effect of massage technique plus thoracic manipulation versus thoracic manipulation on pain and neural tension in mechanical neck pain: a randomized controlled trial. *Journal of Physical Therapy Science, 31*(2), 195–201.

Quinn, C., Chandler, C., & Moraska, A. (2002). Massage therapy and frequency of chronic tension headaches. *American Journal of Public Health, 92*, 1657–1661.

Rapaport, M. H., Schettler, P., & Bresee, C. (2010). A preliminary study of the effects of a single session of Swedish massage on hypothalamic-pituitary-adrenal and immune function in normal individuals. *Journal of Alternative and Complementary Medicine, 16*(10), 1079–1088.

Rapaport, M. H., Schettler, P., & Bresee, C. (2012). A preliminary study of the effects of repeated massage on hypothalamic-pituitary-adrenal and immune function in healthy individuals: a study of mechanisms of action and dosage. *Journal of Alternative and Complementary Medicine, 18*(8), 789–797.

Reychler, G., Caty, G., Arcq, A., et al. (2017). Effects of massage therapy on anxiety, depression, hyperventilation and quality of life in HIV infected patients: a randomized controlled trial. *Complementary Therapies in Medicine, 32*, 109–114.

Rostron, S. (2021). The effects of massage therapy on a patient with migraines and cervical spondylosis: a case report. *International Journal of Therapeutic Massage & Bodywork, 14*(3), 15–21.

Saban, B., Deutscher, D., & Ziv, T. (2014). Deep massage to posterior calf muscles in combination with neural mobilization exercises as a treatment for heel pain: a pilot randomized clinical trial. *Manual Therapy, 19*(2), 102–108.

Salvo, S. G. (1999). *Massage therapy principles and practice.* Philadelphia, PA: WB Saunders.

Sefton, J. M., Yarar, C., Berry, J. W., & Pascoe, D. D. (2010). Therapeutic massage of the neck and shoulders produces changes in peripheral blood flow when assessed with dynamic infrared thermography. *Journal of Alternative and Complementary Medicine, 16*(7), 723–732.

Sobeck, C., Lenk, L., Knipper, S., Rhoda, A., Stickler, L., & Stephenson, P. (2016). The effectiveness of functional massage on pain and range of motion measurements in patients with orthopedic impairments of the extremities. *International Musculoskeletal Medicine, 38*(1), 21–25.

Sornkayasit, K., Jumnainsong, A., Phoksawat, W., Eungpinichpong, W., & Leelayuwat, C. (2021). Traditional Thai massage promoted immunity in the elderly via attenuation of senescent CD4+ T cell subsets: a randomized crossover study. *International Journal of Environmental Research and Public Health, 18*(6), 3210.

Tappan, F. M., & Benjamin, P. J. (1998). Tappan's handbook of healing massage techniques: classic, holistic, and emerging methods. Norwalk, CT: Appleton & Lange.

Vairo, G. L., Miller, S. J., McBrier, N. M., & Buckley, W. E. (2009). Systematic review of efficacy for manual lymphatic drainage techniques in sports medicine and rehabilitation: an evidence-based practice approach. *Journal of Manual & Manipulative Therapy, 17*(3), e80–89.

Walker, J. M. (1984). Deep transverse frictions in ligament healing. *Journal of Orthopaedic and Sports Physical Therapy, 6*, 89–94.

CHAPTER 12 QUESTIONS

1. **Your patient presents with low back pain and avoids all trunk movements. When asked why they won't flex their low back they respond that they know it will hurt. Upon examination you determine that the patient has tense and painful lumbar paraspinal muscles in a neutral position. You explain your findings to the patient and how the patient's muscle stiffness will benefit from massage and myofascial mobilization. Following treatment with these interventions, you re-examine the patient and note improved forward bending. Which of the following would best account for this post intervention improvement?**
   a. Pain neuromodulation
   b. Increased skin temperatures
   c. Reduced lymphedema
   d. Improved muscle flexibility
   e. All of the above may account for the improvement post intervention

2. **Your patient is participating in physical therapy following a recent right total knee arthroplasty. They are currently experiencing diffuse swelling anteriorly and posteriorly and restricted knee extension and flexion. In addition to providing patient education on edema management, and an appropriate home education program, you are considering whether applying massage would be beneficial. Based on the evidence, which of the following is the best evidence-informed massage approach for this case?**
   a. Applying friction massage will enhance the healing of the surgical incision.
   b. Swedish massage applied to the hamstring muscle will be the best initial treatment to restore knee extension.
   c. Lymphedema massage to the posterior knee will be the best initial treatment to improve knee flexion and extension.
   d. Massage should be used post treatment to reduce exercise-induced muscle damage following the patient's in-clinic exercise.

3. **[illegible] patient is seeking physical therapy assistance in managing a recent lumbar disc herniation. They are currently experiencing symptoms radiating into the right lower extremity, including paresthesia in their lateral leg. Which of the following massage treatments would be the most beneficial treatment for this case?**
   a. Functional massage of the lumbar paraspinals combined with lumbar traction
   b. Self-Tia foot massage applied to the right foot
   c. Swedish massage applied to the right peroneal muscles
   d. Manual lymph drainage applied to the lumbar paraspinals

SPINAL TRACTION

J.A. Viti, PT, MSc, DPT, OCS, FAAOMPT and H.D. Saunders

1. **What are the theoretical effects of spinal traction and evidence to support it?**
Spinal traction is theorized to have several effects. Among these are distraction or separation of the vertebral bodies, a combination of distraction and gliding of the facet joints, tensing of the ligamentous structures of the spinal segment, widening of the intervertebral foramen, straightening of spinal curves, and stretching of the spinal musculature. There is evidence that a disc protrusion can be reduced and spinal nerve root compression symptoms relieved with the application of relatively high-force spinal traction (approximately 50% of the body weight). Epidurography studies demonstrate temporary reduction in disc protrusions, along with clinical improvement. Onel et al. (1989) used computed tomography (CT) to demonstrate lumbar disc reduction in 21 of 30 patients (70%) and theorized that the reduction was a result of a suction effect caused by decreased intradiscal pressure. The change in intradiscal pressure caused by traction has also been theorized to positively affect the disc's nutrition.

Using MRI, Chung et al. (2002) found an increase in the cervical vertebral column length and partial (over 50%) to complete resolution of cervical disc herniation in 21 of 29 patients utilizing an inflatable traction device worn around the neck, traction was applied statically at 13.5 kg (30 lb) for 20 minutes. Sari et al. (2003) studied 13 patients with cervical disc herniation receiving static cervical traction at 20 kg (44 lb) in slight flexion for 20 minutes. These subjects were evaluated using computerized tomography (CT) before traction and during traction at 20 minutes. They found a mean decrease in the herniated disc area of 11.66 mm^2, an increase in spinal canal area of 11.21 mm^2, and spinal column lengthening between C2 and C7 levels of 1.39 mm. Authors concluded that cervical traction increased intervertebral disc space, stretches the posterior longitudinal ligaments, and results in effective regression of herniated disc volume.

Liu et al. (2008) found an increase in cervical foraminal area and height and area in normal subjects with traction forces of 5 kg (11 lb), 10 kg (22 lb), and 15 kg (33 lb). Increases at 5 and 10 kg were statistically significant. While there was an additional increase at 15 kg, it was not statistically significant.

2. **What are the indications for spinal traction?**
Given these theoretical effects, the significant indications are herniated disc or radiculopathy, any condition in which mobilization and stretching of soft tissue are desired, and any condition in which opening the neural foramen is desired. Studies by Jellad et al. (2009), Fritz et al. (2014), Blanpied et al. (2017), and Romeo et al. (2018) recommended traction for patients with cervical radiculopathy and or neck pain with radiating arm pain.

3. **What are the contraindications for spinal traction?**
Traction is contraindicated in patients with structural disease secondary to tumor or infection, rheumatoid arthritis, severe vascular compromise, and any condition for which movement is contraindicated. Relative contraindications include acute strains and sprains and inflammatory conditions that may be aggravated by traction. Strong traction applied to patients with spinal joint instability may cause further strain. Traction should be avoided if the patient has had recent spinal fusion. Because spinal fusion techniques and healing rates vary from patient to patient, the surgeon should be consulted before applying traction if the fusion is less than 1 year old. Other relative contraindications may include pregnancy, osteoporosis, hiatal hernia, and claustrophobia.

4. **How much force is optimal for cervical traction?**
Forces recommended for cervical traction range from 11 pounds to 50 pounds based on a patient's size and body type. Colachis and Strohm (1965) demonstrated that a traction force of 30 lb produced separation of the cervical spine and that a 50-lb force produced more separation than a 30-lb force.

Sari et al. (2003) studied 13 patients with cervical disc herniation, 8 of which had a herniated disc at the C5/6 level. Patients received static cervical traction at 20 kg (44 lb) in slight flexion for 20 minutes. Patients were evaluated using CT before traction and during traction at 20 minutes. Authors found a mean decrease in the herniated disc area of 11.66 mm^2, an increase in spinal canal area of 11.21 mm^2, and spinal column lengthening between C2 and C7 levels of 1.39 mm. Intervertebral discal space widening occurred at C5/6. Authors concluded that cervical traction had a significant biomechanical effect on spinal structures.

Cleland et al. (2005) had good outcomes in patients with cervical radiculopathy with intermittent cervical traction for 15 minutes at 25 degrees of flexion starting at 18 pounds and progressing 1 to 2 pounds per session as per patient tolerance. Hold times were 30 seconds and release times were 10 seconds. The amount of pull during the release time was 12 pounds.

Liu et al. (2008) found that in normal subjects, the average foraminal height increased by 3.75%, 8.67%, and 10.43% at 5 kg (11 lb), 10 kg (22 lb), and 15 kg (33 lb), respectively. The increase at 5 and 10 kg was statistically significant. While there was a further increase at 15 kg, it was not statistically significant.

Jellad et al. (2009) noted a reduction in neck and arm pain as well as perceived disability utilizing manual traction at 6 kg (13 lb) with 20 pulls for 20 seconds with 10-second rest periods. They noted even greater improvement in patients receiving mechanical traction utilizing two static 25-minute pulls with a 10-minute rest period starting at 5 kg (12 lb) increasing to 11 kg (26.5 lb) over 12 sessions.

5. **Is cervical traction effective for the treatment of cervical radiculopathy?**

One MRI study showed either complete or partial reduction of herniated disc in 21 of 29 patients who received 30-lb seated traction with an inflatable traction device. Honet and Puri (1976) provided a progressively more intense cervical traction treatment, depending on severity of symptoms and neurologic findings. Subjects received traction treatment at home, in an outpatient facility, or in the hospital. The percentage of patients with excellent or good outcomes was 92% in the home treatment category, 77% in the outpatient treatment category, and 65% in the hospital treatment category.

Moeti and Marchetti (2001) performed a case series using cervical traction with other physical therapy interventions with 15 subjects with cervical radiculopathy. The majority of patients exhibited significant improvements in NPRS scores and NDI scores. Eight of the patients experienced complete resolution of symptoms, but three exhibited no significant change in pain level or disability.

Cleland et al. (2005) found significant improvements in Patient Specific Functional Scale (PSFS) and Neck Disability Index (NDI) in 10 of 11 patients with cervical radiculopathy who received intermittent cervical traction, manual physical therapy, and strengthening after 6 to 10 treatment sessions and at 6-month follow-up.

Jellad et al. (2009) found that in subjects with cervical radiculopathy, adding manual or mechanical traction to groups receiving conventional rehabilitation significantly reduced cervical pain, radicular pain, and self-perceived disability at the end of 12 sessions of treatment and at 6 months.

Fritz et al. (2014) found that adding cervical traction to a standard exercise program led to improved disability scores and a greater improvement in neck and arm pain in patients with cervical radiculopathy. Supine traction with a motorized traction device was more effective than over the door traction.

Blanpied et al. in the Clinical Practice Guidelines (2017) recommend intermittent cervical traction combined with other interventions such as stretching, strengthening, and manipulation for patients with chronic neck pain with radiating pain.

Yang et al. (2017) found that cervical traction provided short-term relief of neck pain but no significant change in disability. Subjects studied had complaints of neck pain but not radiating arm pain.

Romeo et al. (2018) in a systematic review and meta-analysis of randomized controlled trials found moderate quality evidence that mechanical cervical traction combined with other physical therapy procedures was more effective than physical therapy procedures alone in reducing pain and disability in patients with cervical radiculopathy.

6. **Is cervical traction effective for treatment of cervicogenic headache?**

No clinical trials have been performed using cervical traction to treat cervicogenic headache, but two case studies have suggested that cervicogenic headache can be treated successfully with traction. Using 25- to 30-lb home traction and cervical exercise, Olson reported success with two difficult cases of headache caused by chronic whiplash. The cervical exercise consisted of postural correction and stabilization exercises. Blanpied et al. (2017) in the Clinical Practice Guidelines recommend manual therapy procedures such as manipulation and passive stretching in addition to strengthening and endurance exercise for patients with headaches of musculoskeletal origin but did not include cervical traction in their recommendations.

7. **What are the important treatment variables for cervical traction?**

- Chin halter versus occipital wedges—when traction was provided with a standard head halter with a chin strap, force is transmitted through the chin strap to the teeth, and the temporomandibular joints become weight-bearing structures. A common problem from administering cervical traction is aggravation of the temporomandibular joints because of the force applied at the chin. It is generally advisable to use a cervical traction system that pulls from the occiput, rather than placing pressure on the chin. If the patient has known temporomandibular joint dysfunction, a chin halter should never be used.
- Force and application—to effectively treat cervical radiculopathy, herniated disc, or other conditions requiring a separation of the intervertebral space, the traction force should be great enough to cause movement at the spinal segment. Based on the evidence available in the literature, a force of 11 to 50 lb is recommended, for Moetti et al. (2001) performed intermittent mechanical traction with a pull of 18 to 35 lb for 10 to 30 seconds with a release time of 5 to 10 second at 5 to 10 lbs.
- Clealand et al. (2005) performed intermittent mechanical traction initiated at 18 lb increased 1 to 2 lb per session for 6 to 10 sessions with a 10 second release time at 12 lbs.

- Jellad et al. (2009) performed intermittent manual traction at 6 kg (13 lb) for 20-second pulls with 10-second rests for 20 repetitions. They also performed static traction in supine using a weight bearing pulley system starting at 5 kg (11 lb) and progressing to 12 kg (26.5 lb) over 12 treatment sessions. Traction was applied for 25 minutes with a 10-minute rest followed by an additional 25 minutes.
- Fritz et al. (2014) had the best results with intermittent mechanical traction initiated at 12 pounds and increased as tolerated. Traction was applied with a 60-second pull and release for 20 seconds at 50% of the traction pull amount. Treatment duration was 15 minutes.
- Patient position—we recommend the supine position to facilitate patient relaxation, proper force application, and optimal cervical angle. The supine position is favored in the literature.
- Cervical angle—cervical traction is typically performed with the head and neck in some degree of flexion. Some clinicians believe that the greater the angle of flexion, the greater the intervertebral separation in the lower cervical spine.

Wong et al. (1992) performed cervical traction on 17 normal adults aged 18 to 30 (7 male, 10 female). Intermittent cervical traction at 13.5 kg (30 lb) was applied for 8 seconds followed by a 6-second rest for 20minutes. Measurements were taken utilizing radiographs. In all cases, anterior and posterior intervertebral spaces were increased in the neutral position and at 30 degrees of flexion but not at 15 degrees of extension.

Favorable outcomes were found by Cleland et al. (2005) at 25 degrees of flexion and Fritz et al. (2014) positioning subjects at 15 degrees of flexion. Jellad et al. (2009) had good results performing intermittent manual and mechanical traction either in neutral, slight flexion, or slight extension based on patient comfort level.

- Mode (static or intermittent)—Moetti et al. (2001), Clealand et al. (2005), and Fritz et al. (20014) demonstrated favorable outcomes with mechanical intermittent cervical traction. Jelad et al. (2009) demonstrated favorable outcomes with intermittent manual traction and also demonstrated favorable results with mechanical static traction for 25 minutes with a 10-minute rest period followed by another 25 minutes of static traction.
- Time for the studies cited in this chapter—the duration of traction was performed for 15 to 25 minutes.

8. **How much force is optimal for lumbar traction?**

There is consensus in the literature that a force of 40% to 50% of the patient's body weight is necessary to cause vertebral separation. In one of the earliest lumbar traction studies, Cyriax reported a visible separation between lumbar vertebrae with static traction of 120 lb for 15 minutes. Other studies have reported measurable separation in the lumbar spine at forces ranging from 80 to 200 lb. Judovich advocated a force equal to one half the patient's body weight on a friction-free surface as the minimum force necessary to produce therapeutic effects in the lumbar spine. Fritz et al. (2007) found improvement in patients with peripheralization of pain with extension or positive contralateral SLR with prone static traction at 40% to 60% body weight for 12 minutes, in combination with an extension-oriented intervention.

Bilgilovsky et al. (2018) found short-term improvements in patients with prone and supine 90/90 intermittent traction using 30-second holds and 10 seconds rest for 15 minutes starting at 25% of the body weight and progressing as tolerated to no more than 50% of the patient's body weight. Greater improvements were found with prone traction.

9. **Is lumbar traction effective for lumbar radiculopathy?**

Epidurography and CT investigations have shown that high-force traction can reduce disc protrusions and relieve spinal nerve root compression symptoms. Despite these findings, lumbar traction is currently out of favor in the literature. Four reviews summarizing lumbar traction studies have concluded that there is no significant benefit for patients treated with lumbar traction compared with a control group. However, wide variations of methods and techniques were described in the studies cited. Some of the studies that showed lumbar traction to be ineffective were performed with low forces. In many of the studies, patient selection criteria were poorly defined. Most studies tended to group all patients with low back pain together and did not distinguish between subgroups or by diagnosis. The only two studies that looked specifically at traction for herniated disc did not use forces generally considered sufficient to separate the intervertebral spaces.

Fritz et al. (2007) studied 64 patients with low back and leg pain with signs of nerve root compression. Subjects were randomized to receive a 6-week extension-oriented intervention with or without prone static traction. At 2 weeks the traction group showed greater improvements in disability scores and fear avoidance beliefs, but at 6 weeks there was no significance in the groups. Two variables associated with greater improvements in traction were peripheralization of pain with extension movements and positive contralateral SLR. Authors stated that past studies of more heterogenous groups have not yielded positive results from traction intervention, but the study of subgroups with more specific signs and symptoms may yield more positive results.

Delitto et al. (2012) in The Clinical Practice Guidelines stated there is conflicting evidence for the effectiveness of intermittent lumbar traction for patients with low back pain. There is preliminary evidence that a subgroup of patients with nerve root compression and peripheralization of symptoms or a positive crossed straight leg raise may benefit from intermittent prone lumbar traction.

Bilgilisoy et al. (2018) studied 125 subjects with chronic back pain and lumbosacral nerve root involvement randomly divided into three groups. Groups were divided into physical therapy only, physical therapy combined with prone traction, or physical therapy combined with supine traction. Each group received 15 treatment sessions. At the end of treatment the group receiving prone traction exhibited statistically significant improvements in Oswestry Disability Index scores and the Visual Analog Scale compared to the PT only group. The results of the supine traction group were also better than the PT only group but the differences were not statistically significant. The ODI scores were improved by 74.4% for the prone traction group, 53.8% for the supine traction group, and 40% for the PT only group. No long-term follow-up was performed.

10. **What are the most important treatment variables for lumbar traction?**
    - Force—to effectively treat lumbar radiculopathy, herniated disc, or other conditions requiring a separation of the intervertebral space, the traction force should be great enough to cause movement at the spinal segment.

    Fritz et al. (2007) found improvement in patients with prone static traction at 40% to 60% body weight for 12 minutes. Bilgilovsky et al. (2018) found short-term improvements in patients with prone and supine 90/90 intermittent traction using 30-second holds and 10-second rest for 15 minutes starting at 25% of the body weight and progressing as tolerated to no more than 50% of the patient's body weight.
    - Spinal position—the position of the spine during traction is an important treatment variable. In our experience, disc herniation is most effectively treated with the patient lying prone with a normal lordosis. However, this position is not always possible because a patient with an acute herniated disc may not tolerate any position of normal lordosis. If this is the case, the treatment must be given in flexion initially with the goal of gradually working toward neutral lumbar lordosis. Foraminal (lateral) stenosis is usually more effectively treated with the lumbar spine in a flexed (flattened) position initially, with the goal of achieving a neutral lordosis when possible. Soft tissue stiffness/hypomobility and degenerative disc or joint disease may be treated in a neutral position, or some degree of flexion or extension, depending on the goals of treatment. Patient comfort and the patient's ability to remain relaxed during the treatment are important considerations when choosing the most beneficial position, and no absolute rule applies. Variations of flexion, extension, and lateral bending should be tried to find the most beneficial position for each patient.

    Fritz et al. (2007) found improvement in patients with prone static traction and Bilgilovsky et al. (2018) found short-term improvements in patients with prone and supine 90/90 intermittent traction.
    - Mode (static or intermittent) and time—Fritz et al. (2007) found improvement in patients with prone static traction for 12 minutes. Bilgilovsky et al. (2018) found short-term improvements in patients with prone and supine 90/90 intermittent traction using 30-second holds and 10-seconds rest for 15 minutes.

11. **Does spinal traction change somatosensory evoked potentials (SSEPs)?**
    SSEP latencies were decreased after cervical traction in patients with radiculopathy and cervical sprain. In patients with severe myelopathy, latencies may increase. Traction may improve conduction by improving blood flow to cervical nerve roots.

12. **Does positional distraction help reduce leg pain in patients with lumbosacral radiculopathy?**
    Positional distraction is a technique where the patient lies on the unaffected side over a soft bolster with the affected segment positioned over the bolster. This bends the spine over the bolster, opening the foramen on the affected side. The hips are then flexed until the spinous processes of the affected segment are felt to spread apart, which further opens the affected foramen. Rotation of the trunk toward the ceiling is then performed to move the bottom scapula and shoulder out from under the patient, thus further increasing side bending and further opening the foramen on the top side. Care should be taken not to rotate down to the affected segment as the rotation could place undue stress on the disc.

    Creighton (2001) found an average foraminal opening on 4 mm at L3, L4, and L5 using a lateral radiograph on 10 subjects. Mitchell et al. (2013) found that subjects with true neurological signs had significantly less pain, more centralization of pain, and increased SLR in patients who received positional distraction for 5 minutes compared to control subjects who laid on side for the same amount of time. While useful clinically, very little research has been performed on the effectiveness of positional distraction, making further outcomes research warranted.

Bibliography

Beurskens, A., de Vet, H. C., Köke, A. J., et al. (1997). Efficacy of traction for nonspecific low back pain: 12-week and 6-month results of a randomized clinical trial. *Spine, 22*, 2756–2762.

Bilgilisoy Filiz, M., Kiliç, Z., Uçkun, A., et al. (2018). Mechanical traction for lumbar radicular pain: supine or prone? A randomized controlled trial. *American Journal of Physical Medicine & Rehabilitation, 97*(6), 433–439.

Blanpied, P. B., Gross, A. R., Elliott, J. M., et al. (2017). Neck pain: revision 2017. *Journal of Orthopedic & Sports Physical Therapy, 47*(7), A1–A83.

Cameron, M. (2013). *Traction physical agents in rehabilitation,* (4th ed.). St. Louis, MO: Elsevier; pp. 361–389.

Chung, T. S., Lee, Y. -J., Kang, S. -W., et al. (2002). Reducibility of cervical disk herniation: evaluation at MR imaging during cervical traction with a nonmagnetic traction device. *Radiology, 225*, 895–898.

Cleland, J., Whitman, J. M., Fritz, J. M., & Palmer, J. A. (2005). Manual physical therapy, cervical traction and strengthen in patients with cervical radiculopathy. A case series. *Journal of Orthopedic & Sports Physical Therapy, 35*, 802–811.

Colachis, S., & Strohm, M. (1965a). Cervical traction: relationship of traction time to varied tractive force with constant angle of pull. *Archives of Physical Medicine, 46*, 815–819.

Colachis, S., & Strohm, M. (1965b). A study of tractive forces and angle of pull on vertebral interspaces in cervical spine. *Archives of Physical Medicine, 46*, 820–830.
Constantoyannis, C., Konstantinou, D., Kourtopoulos, H., & Papadakis, N. (2002). Intermittent cervical traction for cervical radiculopathy caused by large-volume herniated disks. *Journal of Manipulative and Physiological Therapeutics, 25*, 188–192.
Creighton, D. S. (2001). Positional distraction, a radiological confirmation. *Journal of Manual & Manipulative Therapy, 1*(3), 83–86.
Cyriax, J. (1950). The treatment of lumbar disk lesions. *BMJ, 2*, 14–34.
Franks, A. (1967). Temporomandibular joint dysfunction associated with cervical traction. *Annals of Physical Medicine, 8*, 38–40.
Delitto, A., George, S. Z., Van Dillen, L., et al. (2012). Low back pain. *Journal of Orthopaedic & Sports Physical Therapy, 42*(4), A1–57.
Fritz, J. M., Lindsay, W., Matheson, J. W., et al. (2007). Is there a subgroup of patients with low back pain likely to benefit from mechanical traction? *Spine, 32*(26), E793–800.
Fritz, J. M., Thackeray, A., Brennan, G. P., & Childs, J. D. (2014). Exercise only, exercise with mechanical traction, or exercise with over-door traction for patients with cervical radiculopathy, with and without consideration of status on a previously described subgrouping rule: a randomized clinical trial. *Journal of Orthopaedic & Sports Physical Therapy, 44*(2), 45–57.
Harris, P. (1977). Cervical traction: Review of literature and treatment guidelines. *Physical Therapy, 57*, 910.
Hattori, M., Shirai, Y., & Aoki, T. (2002). Research on the effectiveness of intermittent cervical traction therapy using short-latency somatosensory evoked potentials. *Journal of Orthopaedic Science, 7*, 208–216.
Honet, J. C., & Puri, K. (1976). Cervical radiculitis: treatment and results in 82 patients. *Archives of Physical Medicine and Rehabilitation, 57*, 12–16.
Jellad, A., Salah, Z. B., Boudokhane, S., et al. (2009). The value of intermittent cervical traction in recent cervical radiculopathy. *Annals of Physical and Rehabilitation Medicine, 52*(9), 638–652.
Judavich, B. D. (1955). Lumbar traction therapy—elimination of physical factors that prevent lumbar stretch. *JAMA, 159*(60), 549–550.
Komori, H., Shinomiya, K., Nakai, O., et al. (1996). The natural history of herniated nucleus pulposus with radiculopathy. *Spine, 21*, 225–229.
Liu, J., Ebraheim, N. A., Sanford, C. G., Jr., et al. (2008). Quantitative changes in cervical neural foramen resulting from axial traction: in vivo imaging study. *The Spine Journal, 8*, 619–623.
Mathews, J. (1972). The effects of spinal traction. *Physiotherapy, 58*, 64–66.
Mitchell, U., Wooden, M. J., & Mckeough, D. M. (2013). The short term effect of positional distraction. *The Journal of Manual & Manipulative Therapy, 9*(4), 213–221.
Moetti, P., & Marchetti, G. (2001). Clinical outcome from mechanical intermittent cervical traction for the treatment of cervical radiculopathy: a case series. *Journal of Orthopaedic and Sports Physical Therapy, 31*, 207–213.
Olivero, W. C., & Dulebohn, S. C. (2002). Results of halter cervical traction for the treatment of cervical radiculopathy: retrospective review of 81 patients. *Neurosurgical Focus, 12*, 1–3.
Olson, V. (1997a). Case report: chronic whiplash associated disorder treated with home cervical traction. *Journal of Back and Musculoskeletal Rehabilitation, 9*, 181–190.
Olson, V. (1997b). Whiplash-associated chronic headache treated with home cervical traction. *Physical Therapy, 77*, 417–423.
Onel, D., Tuzlaci, M., Sari, H., & Demir, K. (1989). Computed tomographic investigation of the effect of traction on lumbar disc herniations. *Spine, 14*, 82–90.
Philadelphia Panel, (2001). Philadelphia panel evidence-based clinical practice guidelines on selected rehabilitation interventions for low back pain. *Physical Therapy, 81*, 1641–1674.
Prentice, W. (2011). *Spinal traction therapeutic modalities in rehabilitation* (pp. 489–522) (4th ed.). New York, NY: McGraw-Hill.
Romeo, A., Vanti, C., & Boldrini, V., et al. (2018). Cervical radiculopathy: effectiveness of adding traction to physical therapy—a systematic review and meta-analysis of randomized controlled trials. *Physical Therapy, 89*(4), 231–242.
Saal, J., Saal, J. A., & Yurth, E. F. (1996). Nonoperative management of herniated cervical intervertebral disc with radiculopathy. *Spine, 21*, 1877–1883.
Sari, H., Akarirmak, Ü., Karacan, I., & Akman, H. (2003). Evaluation of the effects of cervical traction on spinal structures by computerized tomography. *Advances in Physiotherapy, 5*, 114–121.
van der Heijden, G., Beurskens, A. J., Koes, B. W., et al. (1995). The efficacy of traction for back and neck pain: a systematic, blinded review of randomized clinical trial method. *Physical Therapy, 75*, 93–104.
Wong, A., Lee, M., Chang, W., & Tang, F. (1997). Clincal trial of cervical traction with electromyographic biofeedback. *American Journal of Physical Medicine & Rehabilitation, 76*(1), 19–25.
Yang, J. -D., Tam, K. -W., Huang, T. -W., et al. (2017). Intermittent cervical traction for treating neck pain A meta-analysis of random controlled trials. *Spine, 42*(13), 959–965.
Yates, D. (1972). Indications and contraindications for spinal traction. *Physiotherapy, 58*, 55.

CHAPTER 13 QUESTIONS

1. **Cervical traction has been found to be most effective in which of the following?**
   a. Muscle strain
   b. Cervical radiculopathy
   c. Headaches
   d. Postural neck ache

2. **All of the following appear to be indications of patients who respond to lumbar traction, EXCEPT:**
   a. Peripheralization of pain with extension
   b. Positive contralateral SLR
   c. Nerve root compression
   d. Muscle strain

3. **Patients receiving positional distraction should be positioned:**
    a. In Prone
    b. In side lying on the painful side with the painful side touching the bolster
    c. Supine 90/90
    d. Side lying on the unaffected side with the hips flexed to the affected segment

4. **The parameters that have been found to be effective for lumbar traction is:**
    a. Static traction at 40% to 60% of the body weight in supine 90/90 for 1 hour
    b. Intermittent traction at 25% to 50% of the body weight in supine 90/90 for 15 minutes
    c. Intermittent traction at 70% to 100% of the body weight in prone
    d. Static traction at 10% to 20% of the body weight in prone

CHAPTER 14

NORMAL AND PATHOLOGIC GAIT

J.M. Burnfield, PhD, PT and C.M. Powers, PT, PhD

1. **What is the average adult walking velocity?**
    - On level surfaces, approximately 80 m/min
    - In men, 82 m/min
    - In women, 78 m/min

2. **Does walking velocity decline with age?**
Yes. Declines of 3% to 11% in healthy adults >60 years old have been reported.

3. **Name contributors to an individual's walking velocity.**
    - Step (or stride) length
    - Cadence

4. **What is considered normal stride and step length?**
    - Stride length is the distance from ipsilateral heel contact to the next ipsilateral heel contact during gait (ie, right-to-right or left-to-left heel contact). Normal adult stride length averages approximately 1.39 m, with the mean stride length of men (1.48 m) being slightly longer than that of women (1.32 m).
    - Step length is the distance between ipsilateral and contralateral heel contact (eg, right-to-left heel contact) and is on average equal to half of stride length.

5. **What is normal cadence?**
Cadence is the number of steps per minute.
    - In adults without pathology, average 116 steps/min
    - In women, 121 steps/min
    - In men, 111 steps/min

6. **Define gait cycle.**
Gait cycle is a repetitive pattern that extends from heel contact to the next episode of heel contact of the same foot. The gait cycle can be further subdivided into a period of stance, when the limb is in contact with the ground (approximately 60% of the gait cycle), and a period of swing, when the limb is not in contact with the ground (approximately 40% of the gait cycle).

7. **Describe the functional tasks associated with normal gait.**
Functionally, each gait cycle can be divided into three tasks:
    - Weight acceptance
    - Single limb support
    - Swing limb advancement

During weight acceptance, body weight is accepted onto the limb that has just completed swinging forward. The limb must attenuate impact forces arising from the abrupt transfer of body weight, while remaining stable and allowing continued forward progression of the body.

During single limb support, only the stance limb is in contact with the ground, and the limb must remain stable while allowing continued forward progression of the body over the foot.

Swing limb advancement includes the phase when weight is being transferred from the reference limb to the opposite limb as well as the entire reference limb swing period. During swing limb advancement, the limb must elevate to clear the ground, advance forward, and prepare for the next period of stance.

8. **Describe the key motions and muscular activity patterns at the ankle, knee, and hip during weight acceptance.**
At the beginning of weight acceptance, the ankle is positioned in neutral, the knee observationally appears to be fully extended (it is actually in 5 degrees of flexion), and the hip is flexed approximately 20 degrees (relative to vertical) in the sagittal plane. These combined joint positions allow the heel to be the first part of the foot to contact the ground. During weight acceptance, as the foot lowers to the ground, the ankle moves into 5 degrees of plantar flexion, controlled by eccentric activity of the dorsiflexors. The knee moves into 20 degrees of flexion, controlled by eccentric activity of the quadriceps. The hip remains in 20 degrees of flexion, primarily owing to isometric activity of the single joint hip extensors.

9. **Describe the key motions and muscular activity patterns at the ankle, knee, and hip during single limb support.**
Movement of the ankle from 5 degrees of plantar flexion to 10 degrees of dorsiflexion is controlled by eccentric activity of the calf. Energy is stored in the noncontractile components of the Achilles tendon. The knee moves from 20 degrees of flexion to what observationally appears to be full extension (actually 5 degrees of flexion by motion analysis), in part as a result of concentric activity of the quadriceps (early single limb support) in combination with passive stability achieved when the ground reaction force vector moves anterior to the knee joint (late single limb support). The hip moves from 20 degrees of flexion to 20 degrees of apparent hyperextension (a combination of full hip extension, anterior pelvic tilt, and backward pelvic rotation), in part as a result of concentric activity of the single joint hip extensors (early single limb support) in combination with passive stability achieved when the ground reaction force vector moves posterior to the hip joint.

10. **Describe the key motions and muscular activity patterns at the ankle, knee, and hip during swing limb advancement.**
Initially, as the more proximal joints begin to flex, the foot remains in contact with the ground. Elastic recoil energy stored in the noncontractile components of the Achilles tendon is released and the ankle moves passively into a position of 15 degrees of plantar flexion. Once the foot lifts from the ground, the ankle moves to neutral dorsiflexion owing to concentric activity of the pretibial muscles. The knee initially moves into 40 degrees of flexion (while the foot is still on the ground) primarily as a result of passive forces. As the foot lifts from the ground, the knee moves into 60 degrees of flexion, owing to concentric activity of knee flexors (biceps femoris short head, gracilis, and sartorius). During late swing limb advancement, the knee fully extends, in part as a result of momentum and quadriceps activity. The hip moves from 20 degrees of apparent hyperextension to 25 degrees of flexion by the middle of swing because of a combination of hip flexor muscle activity and momentum. In late swing, hip flexion decreases to 20 degrees as the hamstrings decelerate further progression of the leg.

11. **What factors contribute to shock absorption during weight acceptance?**
- Eccentrically controlled knee flexion to 20 degrees allows for dissipation of forces generated by the abrupt transfer of body weight onto the limb.
- Movement of the foot into 5 degrees of eversion functions to unlock the midtarsal joints (talonavicular and calcaneocuboid), creating a more flexible foot that is able to adapt to uneven surfaces. The rate of this motion is controlled by eccentric activity of the tibialis anterior and posterior.

12. **What allows for stance stability during single limb support?**
- Stability arises primarily from the action of the calf muscles that restrain excess forward collapse of the tibia. As a result, the knee and hip are able to achieve a fully extended position with only minimal muscle activation.
- In late single limb support, a reduction in the amount of subtalar joint eversion functions to lock the midtarsal joints and creates a rigid forefoot over which body weight progresses.

13. **What allows for foot clearance during swing limb advancement?**
- Early in swing limb advancement, knee flexion to 60 degrees (owing to passive and active factors) assists in clearing the limb.
- As swing limb advancement progresses, hip flexion to 25 degrees, in combination with ankle dorsiflexion to neutral, becomes critical to achieve foot clearance.

14. **Name the key factors that are essential to ensure forward progression during the gait cycle.**
- Forward progression during weight acceptance results primarily from eccentric activity of the dorsiflexors, which not only lower the foot to the ground but also draw the tibia forward.
- During single limb support, eccentric calf activity allows controlled forward progression without tibial collapse.
- The 20 degrees of apparent hyperextension achieved at the hip contributes to a trailing limb posture that increases step length and forward progression.
- As body weight unloads rapidly from the trailing limb during preswing, elastic recoil energy stored in the Achilles tendon during single limb support is released and the tibia is driven forward.
- During swing limb advancement, knee extension and hip flexion to 20 degrees in late swing contribute to forward progression and step length.

15. **Describe the role of the heel, ankle, forefoot, and toe "rockers" during gait.**
Collectively, the four rockers reflect a combination of joint motions and muscle actions that contribute to the smooth transition of body weight from the heel to the forefoot during stance. The heel rocker occurs during weight acceptance. Eccentric activity of the pretibial muscles lowers the forefoot to the ground and draws the tibia forward, allowing body weight to roll across the heel. Next is the ankle rocker, occurring during the first half of single limb support. The ankle moves from 5 degrees of plantar flexion to slight dorsiflexion. A gradual increase in eccentric calf muscle activity allows the tibia to remain stable as body weight progresses in front of the ankle. The

forefoot rocker occurs during the last half of single limb support. A modulated increase in eccentric calf muscle activity permits the ankle to move into 10 degrees of dorsiflexion (without collapsing) and the heel to rise. Body weight smoothly transitions across the forefoot. The toe rocker occurs during preswing. As body weight shifts to the opposite limb, elastic recoil energy stored in the Achilles tendon during single limb support plantar flexes the ankle. The tibia advances forward over the medial forefoot and great toe.

16. What is the functional significance of normal subtalar joint eversion/inversion during the stance phase of gait?

During weight acceptance, subtalar eversion is important for unlocking the midtarsal joints (calcaneocuboid and talonavicular) and creating a more flexible foot that is able to adapt to uneven surfaces. During single limb support, a reduction in the amount of subtalar eversion (motion toward inversion) functions to lock the midtarsal joints, creating a rigid forefoot lever over which body weight can progress.

17. What effects would a weak tibialis anterior have on gait?

- Either a forefoot/foot flat initial contact or a foot slap immediately after initial contact (lack of eccentric control)
- Footdrop during swing
- Excessive hip and knee flexion (steppage gait) to clear the toes during swing

18. Describe common foot/ankle gait alterations in individuals with posterior tibial tendon dysfunction.

During the stance period of gait, posterior tibial tendon dysfunction can result in excess forefoot abduction and dorsiflexion as well as hindfoot eversion and plantar flexion. Forefoot abduction may contribute to the "too many toes" sign often used clinically to characterize posterior tibial tendon dysfunction. Heel rise may be delayed or absent.

19. Describe gait deviations that likely would be evident in a patient with plantar fasciitis or a heel spur.

Patients typically exhibit a forefoot initial contact, avoiding the pressure associated with heel impact during weight acceptance. As the plantar fascia becomes tight with the combination of heel rise and metatarsal-phalangeal joint dorsiflexion during late stance, patients may avoid this posture by prematurely unweighting the limb.

20. What are the consequences of a triple arthrodesis on gait function?

- Loss of subtalar joint motion results in reduced shock absorption during weight acceptance.
- The inability to supinate in terminal stance diminishes the forefoot rocker effect.
- The ability to progress beyond the supporting foot is compromised.
- Stride length is diminished.

21. Describe the effect of calf weakness on ankle function during gait.

Calf weakness results in the inability to control forward advancement of the tibia, causing excessive dorsiflexion during single limb support and a lack of heel rise during late stance. As a result of the inability to control the tibia through eccentric action, the tibia advances faster than the femur, causing knee flexion during stance. The flexed knee posture necessitates activity of the quadriceps muscles, which normally are quiescent during single limb support.

22. Describe the effect of a plantar flexion contracture on ankle function during gait.

A plantar flexion contracture (>15 degrees) results in either a flat-foot or a forefoot-initial contact. This disrupts normal advancement of the tibia and may limit the knee from flexing to dissipate the forces associated with weight acceptance. During single limb support, the primary limitation is the inability to progress over the foot. Because 10 to 15 degrees of ankle dorsiflexion is necessary for normal stance phase function, compensatory mechanisms are necessary. Progression may be augmented through a premature heel rise, forward trunk lean, knee hyperextension, or a combination thereof. The inability to achieve a neutral ankle position during swing also necessitates compensatory movements to ensure foot clearance.

23. What are the characteristics of quadriceps avoidance?

Quadriceps avoidance manifests as reduced knee flexion during weight acceptance. This compensatory strategy results in decreased quadriceps demand and diminished muscular forces acting across the knee.

24. With what orthopaedic conditions could quadriceps avoidance be associated?

- Patellofemoral pain
- Anterior cruciate ligament deficiency
- Quadriceps weakness
- Quadriceps inhibition (owing to pain or effusion)

25. **Discuss the penalty associated with a knee flexion contracture.**
A knee flexion contracture (>20 degrees) results in excessive knee flexion during weight acceptance, during single limb support, and at the end of swing limb advancement. The penalties include altered shock absorption during weight acceptance and instability during single limb support. Excessive knee flexion during stance requires greater amounts of quadriceps activity to support the flexed knee posture, increasing the energy cost of gait. Excess knee flexion at the end of swing limb advancement shortens step length.

26. **Name typical compensatory strategies associated with reduced knee flexion range of motion.**
Hip hiking or circumduction on the affected side is necessary to clear the foot during swing. Simultaneously, the opposite heel may lift from the ground (vault) to help with foot clearance of the affected limb.

27. **What is the penalty associated with reduced knee flexion range of motion?**
The muscle activity associated with compensatory strategies increases the energy cost of gait.

28. **What is a Trendelenburg gait pattern?**
It is a contralateral pelvic drop during single limb support, usually caused by weakness of the ipsilateral hip abductors.

29. **Describe a typical compensation associated with Trendelenburg gait.**
A lateral trunk lean to the same side as the weakness functionally serves to move the body's center of mass over the involved hip, reducing the demand on the ipsilateral hip abductors.

30. **Discuss the penalty associated with a hip flexion contracture.**
A hip flexion contracture results in inadequate hip extension during late stance. Failure to obtain a trailing limb posture during late stance limits forward progression and stride length. To compensate for the lack of hip extension, an anterior pelvic tilt may be employed.

31. **Explain the effect of hip extensor weakness on gait function.**
Because adequate hip extensor strength is necessary to support the flexed hip posture during weight acceptance, reduced hip flexion is typically observed at initial contact, resulting in a reduced stride length. Also, a posterior trunk lean is commonly seen during weight acceptance as this posture reduces the external hip flexion moment and thus the demand on the hip extensors.

32. **How does decreased proprioception influence gait?**
Individuals with proprioceptive deficits (secondary to peripheral nerve injury, partial spinal cord injury, or brain lesions) require additional sensory input regarding joint position. Typically this can be achieved through a forward trunk lean (to augment visual feedback) or through a more abrupt transfer of weight during the loading response (to augment sensory feedback).

33. **How does an ankle fusion alter gait and energy consumption?**
Persons who have sustained an ankle fusion often substitute for losses in talocrural joint motion (ie, dorsiflexion) by increasing midfoot and forefoot motion. This permits forward progression over the supporting foot in late stance. Stride length is often reduced, resulting in a slower walking velocity. Gait compensations resulting from an ankle fusion cause individuals to expend a slightly greater amount of energy during walking.

34. **What are the energy costs of using various assistive devices (eg, crutches, standard walker, wheeled walker, cane) when compared with using no equipment?**

Energy Cost Associated with Walking Using Assistive Devices

Assistive device	Energy cost
Crutches	Energy demand increased from 30% to 80%, in part because of increased demands placed on arms and shoulder girdle muscles
Standard walker	Oxygen consumption increased >200%
Front-wheeled walker	Less impact compared with standard walker
Cane	No significant contribution

35. **How are energy costs of assistive devices affected by the presence of significant gait pathology?**
When significant gait pathology is present (eg, excess ankle dorsiflexion and knee flexion secondary to a weak calf), use of an assistive device may lessen the energy demands of ambulation by reducing the demands on lower extremity muscles, allowing achievement of a more normal, energy-efficient gait pattern.

36. How does osteoarthritis of the knee influence gait?

- Patients walk with a slower velocity, owing to reductions in stride length and cadence.
- To avoid joint pain/instability, some patients may use a stiffened-knee strategy during gait (eg, not fully extending their knee during stance or not fully flexing their knee during early swing).

37. How does the energy cost of walking with a total hip fusion compare with that of walking with a total hip arthroplasty?

HIP FUSION

The average rate of oxygen consumption increases 32% when compared with normal values at the same walking speed. Increased energy cost likely results from the compensations required for forward progression during gait (eg, excess lumbar lordosis and an anterior pelvic tilt to enable the fused hip to achieve a trailing limb posture in late stance).

TOTAL HIP ARTHROPLASTY

Energy expenditure (1 year postoperatively) is approximately 17% less compared with walking with a fused hip.

38. What influences do various levels of amputation have on walking velocity and energy cost?

- In persons with unilateral amputations, the more proximal the level of amputation (eg, transfemoral vs. transtibial) the slower the customary walking speed and the greater the energy cost of walking (milliliters of oxygen per kilogram of body weight per meter of walking).
- Energy expenditure, heart rate, and oxygen consumption are typically lower during ambulation with a prosthesis as compared with ambulation with crutches.

39. What are common gait deviations in a person with a transtibial amputation?

- Limited dorsiflexion during single limb support
- Diminished plantar flexion in preswing
- Forward trunk lean
- Reduced knee flexion during weight acceptance

40. List the pros and cons of using an ankle-foot orthosis (AFO) for the treatment of footdrop.

Advantages and Disadvantages of Using an Ankle-Foot Orthosis (AFO) to Manage Footdrop

PROS	CONS
• Assists with foot clearance during swing	• If AFO is too rigid, then during weight acceptance:
• Reduces the need for compensatory maneuvers	• normal movement of ankle into plantar flexion is disrupted
	• heel rocker effect is accentuated, resulting in increased knee flexion and greater quadriceps demand

41. Compared to traditional nonmicroprocessor controlled knee units, what impact do microprocessor controlled knees have on ambulation for individuals with a transfemoral amputation?

Individuals with transfemoral amputations walk faster, more efficiently, and with greater stability when using a microprocessor controlled knee unit than when using a traditional nonmicroprocessor controlled prosthetic knee.

42. Describe the effect of hip abductor weakness on pelvis, hip, and knee motion during gait.

Hip abductor weakness results in the inability to control the hip/pelvis in the frontal plane during weight acceptance and single limb support. Common gait deviations associated with hip abductor weakness include a contralateral pelvic drop and/or excessive hip adduction. In addition, the adducted hip may place the knee in a valgus position during stance. A typical compensation for hip abductor weakness is to lean the trunk toward the stance limb to reduce the external frontal plane moment at the hip (compensated Trendelenburg pattern).

Bibliography

Burnfield, J. M., Eberly, V. J., Gronely, J. K., et al. (2012). Impact of stance phase microprocessor-controlled knee prosthesis on ramp negotiation and community walking in K2 level transfemoral amputees. *Prosthetics and Orthotics International*, *36*, 95–104.

Eberly, V. J., Mulroy, S. J., Gronley, J. K., et al. (2013). Impact of a stance phase microprocessor-controlled knee prosthesis on level walking in lower functioning individuals with a transfemoral amputation. *Prosthetics and Orthotics International*, *38*, 199–203.

Foley, M. P., Prax, B., Crowell, R., & Boone, T. (1996). Effects of assistive devices on cardiorespiratory demands in older adults. *Physical Therapy*, *76*, 1313–1319.

Heiden, T. L., Lloyd, D. G., & Ackland, T. R. (2009). Knee joint kinematics, kinetics and muscle co-contraction in knee osteoarthritis patient gait. *Clinical Biomechanics*, *24*, 833–841.

Highsmith, M. J., Kahle, J. T., Bongiorni, D. R., et al. (2010). Safety, energy efficiency, and cost efficacy of the C-Leg for transfemoral amputees: a review of the literature. *Prosthetics and Orthotics International, 34*, 362–377.

Kaufman, K. R., Bernhardt, K. A., & Symms, K. (2018). Functional assessment and satisfaction of transfemoral amputees with low mobility (FASTK2): a clinical trial of microprocessor-controlled vs. non-microprocessor-controlled knees. *Clinical Biomechanics, 58*, 116–122.

Perry, J., & Burnfield, J. M. (2010). *Gait analysis: normal and pathological function* (2nd ed.). Thorofare, NJ: Slack, Inc.

Perry, J., Burnfield, J. M., Newsam, C. J., & Conley, P. (2004). Energy expenditure and gait characteristics of a person with bilateral amputations walking with the "C-Leg" compared to stubby and conventional articulating prostheses. *Archives of Physical Medicine and Rehabilitation, 85*, 1711–1717.

Reischl, S. F., Powers, C. M., Rao, S., & Perry, J. (1999). The relationship between foot pronation and rotation of the tibia and femur during walking. *Foot and Ankle International, 20*, 513–520.

Rose, J., & Gamble, J. G. (2005). *Human walking* (3rd ed.). Baltimore, MD: Lippincott Williams & Wilkins.

Rancho Los Amigos National Rehabilitation Center & The Pathokinesiology Service and the Physical Therapy Department, (2001). *Observational gait analysis.* Downey, CA: Los Amigos Research and Education Institute, Inc.

Wang, J., Mannen, E. M., Siddicky, S. F., et al. (2020). Gait alterations in posterior tibial tendonitis: a systematic review and meta-analysis. *Gait & Posture, 76*, 28–38.

Waters, R. L., & Mulroy, S. (1999). The energy expenditure of normal and pathologic gait. *Gait & Posture, 9*, 207–231.

CHAPTER 14 QUESTIONS

1. **The range of normal walking velocities for young and middle-aged adults is:**
   a. 66 to 70 m/min
   b. 72 to 76 m/min
   c. 78 to 82 m/min
   d. 86 to 90 m/min

2. **You observe excessive knee flexion, too much ankle dorsiflexion, and lack of a heel rise during the terminal stance phase of gait. The most likely cause of this combination of deviations is weakness of the:**
   a. Plantar flexors
   b. Quadriceps
   c. Hamstrings
   d. Gluteals

3. **Common gait deviations associated with weakness of the hip extensors include:**
   a. Increased hip flexion during weight acceptance and a forward (anterior) trunk lean
   b. Decreased hip flexion during weight acceptance and a forward (anterior) trunk lean
   c. Increased hip flexion during weight acceptance and a backward (posterior) trunk lean
   d. Decreased hip flexion during weight acceptance and a backward (posterior) trunk lean

4. **During stance, common gait deviations associated with hip abductor weakness include:**
   a. Ipsilateral trunk lean, contralateral pelvic drop, and ipsilateral knee valgus
   b. Ipsilateral trunk lean, contralateral pelvic drop, and ipsilateral knee varus
   c. Contralateral trunk lean, ipsilateral pelvic drop, and ipsilateral knee valgus
   d. Contralateral trunk lean, contralateral pelvic drop, and ipsilateral knee varus

5. **The primary muscles contributing to stability during single limb support are the:**
   a. Hip extensors
   b. Hip abductors
   c. Knee extensors
   d. Ankle plantar flexors

PHARMACOLOGY IN ORTHOPAEDIC PHYSICAL THERAPY

C.D. Ciccone, PT, PhD, FAPTA

1. **Summarize properties of common opioid analgesics.**

Common Opioid Analgesics

GENERIC NAME	TRADE NAME	ADMINISTRATION ROUTES	ONSET OF ANALGESIC ACTION (MIN)	PEAK ANALGESIC EFFECT (MIN)	DURATION OF ANALGESIC ACTION (HR)
Butorphanol	Stadol	IM	Within 15	30–60	3–4
		IV	2–3	4–5	2–4
		Intranasal	Within 15	60–120	4–5
Codeine	Paveral	Oral	30–45	60–120	4
		IM	10–30	30–60	4
		Sub-Q	10–30	Unknown	4
Hydrocodone	Hycodan	Oral	10–30	30–60	4–6
Hydromorphone	Dilaudid, Hydrostat	Oral	30	30–90	4–5
		IM	15	30–60	4–5
		Sub-Q	15	30–90	4–5
		Rectal	15–30	30–90	4–5
Levorphanol	Levo-Dromoran	Oral	10–60	90–120	4–5
		IV	Unknown	Within 20	4–5
		Sub-Q	Unknown	60–90	4–5
Meperidine	Demerol	Oral	15	60	2–4
		IM	10–15	30–50	2–4
		IV	Immediate	5–7	2–3
		Sub-Q	10–15	40–60	2–4
Methadone	Methadose	Oral	30–60	90–120	4–12
		IM	10–20	60–120	4–6
		Sub-Q	10–20	60–120	4–6
Morphine	Duramorph, MS Contin, many others	Oral	Unknown	60	4–5
		IM	10–30	30–60	4–5
		IV	Rapid	20	4–5
		Sub-Q	20	50–90	4–5
		Epidural	6–30	60	Up to 24
		Intrathecal	Rapid	Unknown	Up to 24
Nalbuphine	Nubain	IM	Within 15	60	3–6
		IV	2–3	30	3–6
		Sub-Q	Within 15	Unknown	3–6

Continued

Common Opioid Analgesics—cont'd					
GENERIC NAME	**TRADE NAME**	**ADMINISTRATION ROUTES**	**ONSET OF ANALGESIC ACTION (MIN)**	**PEAK ANALGESIC EFFECT (MIN)**	**DURATION OF ANALGESIC ACTION (HR)**
Oxycodone	OxyContin, Roxicodone	Oral	10–15	60–90	3–6
Oxymorphone	Opana	Oral	Unknown	Unknown	4–6
		IM	10–15	30–90	3–6
		IV	5–10	15–30	3–6
		Sub-Q	10–20	Unknown	3–4
Pentazocine	Talwin	Oral	15–30	60–90	3
		IM	15–20	30–60	2–3
		IV	2–3	15–30	2–3
		Sub-Q	15–20	30–60	2–3
Propoxyphene	Darvon	Oral	15–60	120–180	4–6

IM, Intramuscular; IV, intravenous; Sub-Q, subcutaneous.
Information adapted with permission from Ciccone C. D. (2013) *Davis's Drug Guide for Rehabilitation Professionals*, Philadelphia, PA: FA Davis.

2. List the common NSAIDs and compare them.

Common Nonsteroidal Antiinflammatory Drugs		
GENERIC NAME	**TRADE NAME**	**SPECIFIC COMMENTS—COMPARISON WITH OTHER NSAIDS**
Aspirin	Many trade names	The original NSAID used for analgesic and antiinflammatory effects; also used frequently for antipyretic and anticoagulant effects
Diclofenac	Voltaren	Substantially more potent than naproxen and several other NSAIDs; may be more selective for the COX-2 isoenzyme than other NSAIDs; adverse side effects occur in 20% of patients
Diflunisal	Dolobid	Has potency 3 to 4 times greater than aspirin in terms of analgesic and antiinflammatory effects but lacks antipyretic activity
Etodolac	Lodine	Effective as analgesic/antiinflammatory agent with fewer side effects than most NSAIDs; may be more selective for the COX-2 isoenzyme than other NSAIDs; may have gastric-sparing properties
Fenoprofen	Nalfon	GI side effects fairly common but usually less intense than those occurring with similar doses of aspirin
Flurbiprofen	Ansaid	Similar to aspirin's benefits and side effects; also available as topical ophthalmic preparation (Ocufen)
Ibuprofen	Motrin, many others	First nonaspirin NSAID also available in nonprescription form; fewer GI side effects than aspirin, but GI effects still occur in 5% to 15% of patients
Indomethacin	Indocin	Relatively high incidence of dose-related side effects; problems occur in 25% to 50% of patients
Ketoprofen	Orudis, Oruvail, others	Similar to aspirin's benefits and side effects but has relatively short half-life (1–2 hr)
Ketorolac	Toradol	Can be administered orally or by intramuscular injection; parenteral doses provide postoperative analgesia equivalent to opioids
Meclofenamate	Meclomen	No apparent advantages or disadvantages compared with aspirin and other NSAIDs

Common Nonsteroidal Antiinflammatory Drugs		
GENERIC NAME	**TRADE NAME**	**SPECIFIC COMMENTS—COMPARISON WITH OTHER NSAIDS**
Meloxicam	Mobic	Relatively fewer gastric side effects than piroxicam; may be more selective for the COX-2 isoenzyme than other NSAIDs
Nabumetone	Relafen	Effective as analgesic/antiinflammatory agent with fewer side effects than most NSAIDs
Naproxen	Anaprox, Naprosyn, others	Similar to ibuprofen in terms of benefits and adverse effects
Oxaprozin	Daypro	Analgesic and antiinflammatory effects similar to aspirin; may produce fewer side effects than other NSAIDs
Piroxicam	Feldene	Long half-life (45 hr) allows once daily dosing; may be somewhat better tolerated than aspirin
Sulindac	Clinoril	Relatively little effect on kidneys (renal-sparing) but may produce more GI side effects than aspirin
Tolmetin	Tolectin	Similar to aspirin's benefits and side effects but must be given frequently (4 times daily) because of short half-life (1 hr)

GI, Gastrointestinal.
From Ciccone C. D. (2015) *Pharmacology in Rehabilitation* (5th ed.). Philadelphia, PA: FA Davis.

3. How do opioid analgesics decrease pain?

Opioids bind to specific neuronal receptors located at synapses in the brain and spinal cord. These synapses are responsible for transmitting painful sensations from the periphery to the brain. Opioid drugs bind to protein receptors on the presynaptic terminal of these synapses and inhibit the release of pain-mediating chemicals, such as substance P. Opioids also bind to receptors on the postsynaptic neuron and cause hyperpolarization, which decreases the excitability of the postsynaptic neuron. These drugs limit the ability of these central nervous system synapses to transmit painful sensations to the brain.

Opioids can also activate descending CNS pathways that suppress pain at the spinal cord level. These pathways originate in the midbrain and travel caudally to the dorsal horn of the spinal cord where they release neurotransmitters such as norepinephrine and serotonin onto synapses that normally mediate painful impulses. By suppressing these synapses, afferent pain impulses that enter the dorsal horn are not transmitted rostrally to the pain centers in the brain. Thus, opioids appear to exert some of their analgesic effects by activating these descending pathways, thereby suppressing afferent pain impulses reaching the spinal cord.

Finally, opioid drugs may affect neurons outside the central nervous system. Opioid receptors have been identified on the distal ends of peripheral sensory neurons that transmit pain. Opioid drugs can bind to these peripheral receptors and decrease pain sensation by decreasing the sensitivity of nociceptive nerve endings.

4. Discuss side effects of opioids that can be especially troublesome in patients receiving physical therapy.

Sedation and mood changes (eg, confusion, euphoria, dysphoria) can be bothersome because patients receiving physical therapy may be less able to understand instructions and participate in therapy sessions. Opioid drugs cause respiratory depression because they decrease the sensitivity of the respiratory control center in the brain stem. Although respiratory depression is not especially troublesome at therapeutic doses, this side effect can be serious or fatal if patients overdose on opioid medications (see question 9). Orthostatic hypotension (a decrease in blood pressure when the patient becomes more upright) may occur during opioid use, and therapists should look for signs of dizziness and syncope, especially during the first 2 to 3 days after a patient begins taking opioid analgesics. Opioids are associated with several gastrointestinal side effects, including nausea, cramps, and vomiting. Constipation may also occur, and this side effect can be a serious problem if these drugs are used for extended periods in people who are susceptible to fecal impaction (eg, people with spinal cord injuries).

5. What is the difference between opioid tolerance, dependence, and addiction?

Tolerance occurs when the dose of the opioid must be increased to achieve a therapeutic analgesic effect. For example, a patient might initially get adequate pain control from 30 mg of oral morphine every 4 hours, but this dose must be increased after 2 to 3 weeks of daily use to achieve the same level of pain control. **Dependence**

is the onset of withdrawal symptoms when the opioid is suddenly discontinued after several weeks of daily use. **Addiction** is typically defined as a *"chronic, relapsing disease characterized by compulsive drug-seeking and use despite negative consequences, and by long-lasting changes in the brain"* (National Institute on Drug Abuse). Addiction is also referred to as opioid use disorder and is characterized by patients craving these drugs and continually seeking sources of opioids to maintain "normal" function and prevent them from going into withdrawal.

6. **Will tolerance, dependence, and addiction occur in every patient on chronic opioid analgesic therapy (COAT)?**
   Virtually all patients receiving COAT (which is typically defined as 90 days or more of daily use) will develop tolerance and dependence as defined above. That is, the dose will usually need to be progressively increased during the period of administration, and the patient will experience withdrawal symptoms such as shivering, sweating, muscle cramps, and GI problems when the drug is suddenly discontinued. Although the exact reasons for tolerance and dependence are unclear, it seems that these responses are cellular adaptations in neurons and other tissues caused by repeated stimulation of these tissues by the opioid drugs. As such, tolerance and dependence are predictable physiological events that should be expected in most if not all patients on COAT. Addiction, however, tends to occur in only a small percent of patients receiving COAT for non-cancer chronic pain, providing that these patients did not have a history of opioid abuse or addiction. Although exact estimates vary from study to study, it appears that the risk of addiction is less than 5 percent in all patients receiving COAT for non-cancer chronic pain and is less than 1 percent if these patients are screened carefully for any current or past history of substance abuse. In other words, the vast majority of patients on COAT will not abuse opioids following therapeutic administration or continue to crave and seek out additional sources of the drug after it is discontinued.

7. **Why do certain people become addicted to opioids?**
   The reasons for opioid addiction are complex and not fully understood. As indicated, addiction occurs in only certain patients, which suggests that there are predisposing genetic factors, or social and environmental factors, that make that patient vulnerable to addiction. Indeed, the risk of addiction increases substantially if these drugs are given to a patient who has had problems with addiction to other substances such as alcohol, or if the patient has used opioids recreationally. It appears that these patients may experience long-lasting structural and functional adaptations of mesolimbic pathways in the brain, which result in the need to repeatedly stimulate these pathways with opioids to activate the "reward" systems in that part of the brain. Continual stimulation from the opioid becomes the new "normal" in the patient's brain and must therefore be maintained on a regular basis for the patient to go about their daily tasks and avoid going into withdrawal.

8. **What are the signs of opioid overdose?**
   High or excessive opioid doses cause somnolence, pinpoint pupils, shallow breathing, bradycardia, vomiting, and pale, blue, or cold/clammy skin. Dangerously high doses and potentially fatal overdoses cause loss of consciousness, limp body, and respiratory failure.

9. **Why is opioid overdose an emergency, and how can it be treated?**
   As indicated in question 4, opioids inhibit the respiratory control center in the brainstem. This effect is dose dependent, and at some point an excessive dose will cause breathing to slow down or stop completely. This effect is usually the cause of death in opioid overdose. Emergency treatment is in the form of opioid antagonists such as naloxone (Narcan). These drugs block opioid receptors, and a high dose of the blocker will displace the opioid from binding sites on brainstem respiratory control neurons, thus restoring respiratory function. Opioid blockers such as naloxone can be administered in many ways including nasal spray, lingual/sublingual routes, and various types of injection (IV, IM, SC). Drugs such as Narcan should be available in clinical settings so that trained personnel can administer them to patients who overdose on opioids.

10. **Are any drugs used to treat opioid addiction or prevent relapse in patients previously addicted to these drugs?**
    Yes, methadone is often used to treat patients who become addicted to opioids. Methadone (Methadose) is a strong opioid agonist, which means that it binds to, and activates, the same receptors as morphine and other opioids. But, methadone can be given orally and provides milder and more sustained opioid effects than other opioids such as heroin. So, methadone is basically substituted for other opioids, with the hope that methadone can be withdrawn slowly while other interventions such as counseling and psychosocial support are instituted. Buprenorphine (Subutex) is also used to treat opioid addiction. This drug is a partial agonist for specific opioid receptors, which means that this drug binds to these receptors but does not fully activate them. The result is that the patient experiences milder opioid effects without experiencing cravings or going into withdrawal. Buprenorphine can be combined with an opioid blocker (naloxone) in a product called Suboxone. The idea is that adding naloxone will reduce the chance that the patient will misuse this product or try to supplement it with other opioids. Likewise, naltrexone (Vivitrol) is a sustained-release form of a different opioid blocker that can be used to prevent relapse in patients who have gone through withdrawal and are fully detoxified from prior opioid use.

Regular use of naltrexone can negate any effects of the opioid and prevent fatal overdose if the patient starts to abuse these drugs again.

11. **Can opioids be combined with non-opioids to provide pain relief?**
Yes, several non-opioid analgesics can be used with opioids, thus reducing the amount of an opioid needed to effectively treat pain. These "opioid-sparing" strategies often combine the opioid with acetaminophen or an NSAID. Opioids can also be used along with drugs such as gabapentin (Neurontin) and pregabalin (Lyrica) that mimic the inhibitory effects of GABA in the CNS (see question 23). Regarding acetaminophen, an opioid can be combined in the same pill with acetaminophen to provide analgesia while keeping the dose of the opioid fairly low. These products are often identified by a "-cet" or "-tab" suffix at the end of the trade name. For example, Percocet is the trade name for a product containing acetaminophen and oxycodone, Lortab is acetaminophen combined with hydrocodone, and so forth. The dose of acetaminophen is usually fixed at 325 mg per dose, while the dose of the opioid can vary depending on the patient's needs. Clinicians, however, should be aware that certain patients might not get adequate pain control from acetaminophen and that acetaminophen is often ineffective in certain conditions such as acute low back pain. Hence, patients taking these opioid/acetaminophen combinations should be monitored carefully because the dose of the opioid may not be adequate if the patient is not getting any benefit from the acetaminophen.

12. **Can opioids increase pain in certain patients?**
Yes. Certain patients who take opioids for an extended period of time may experience increased pain after taking opioids, a phenomenon known as opioid-induced hyperalgesia (OIH). This phenomenon is not fully understood, but seems to occur in specific patients who become tolerant to these drugs. In these patients, opioids activate rather than suppress CNS nociceptive pathways. Several complex neuronal changes seem to underlie this effect, including activation of descending pathways that promote pain, prolonged and sustained activity (potentiation) of specific pain-mediating synapses, changes in post synaptic receptor function, and neuroinflammation. It is not clear why OIH occurs in only certain patients, and susceptibility is probably related to genetic factors that predispose these patients to this effect. Nonetheless, clinicians should be aware that pain may not decrease, and may actually increase, in certain patients when opioids are administered. Pain should therefore be monitored carefully in these patients, especially within the first hour or so after the patient receives a dose of the opioid. An increase in pain may represent OIH, and this response should be reported to the physician.

13. **List advantages and disadvantages of using a patient-activated electronic drug delivery system, known commonly as patient-controlled analgesia (PCA), to administer opioids**
Advantages:
- Increases patient satisfaction because the patient feels more in control of his or her ability to manage pain.
- Administers smaller doses more frequently than conventional dosing, thus decreasing the chance that an excessive dose of the opioid will cause side effects such as sedation.
- Provides more consistent pain control by avoiding the large peaks and troughs typically seen with conventional dosing (eg, a large dose given every 4 hours or so).

Disadvantages:
- Patients with cognitive problems or fear of addiction might not understand how to use the PCA device.
- Possible human error in programming the PCA device (the PCA pump can be programmed incorrectly and overdose or underdose the patient).
- Various technical problems (pump failure, displacement, or blockage of intravenous catheters).

14. **List the primary effects of NSAIDs**
- Decreased pain (analgesia)
- Decreased inflammation (antiinflammatory)
- Decreased fever (antipyresis)
- Decreased blood clotting (anticoagulation)

15. **How do NSAIDs exert their primary beneficial effects?**
NSAIDs work by inhibiting the synthesis of prostaglandins. Prostaglandins are lipid-like compounds that are synthesized by cells throughout the body. These compounds help regulate normal cell activity, and they are synthesized as part of the cellular response to injury. Prostaglandins can increase sensitivity to pain, help promote inflammation, raise body temperature during fever, and increase platelet aggregation and platelet-induced clotting. Prostaglandin biosynthesis is catalyzed within the cell by the cyclooxygenase (COX) enzyme. This enzyme transforms a 20-carbon precursor (arachidonic acid) into the first prostaglandin (PGG2). Cells then use PGG2 to form various other prostaglandins depending on their physiologic status and whether or not they are injured. By acting as a potent inhibitor of the COX enzyme, NSAIDs block the production of all prostaglandins in the cell.

16. **How do prescription NSAIDs differ from nonprescription (over-the-counter) NSAIDs?**
When used to treat pain and inflammation, prescription NSAIDs do not differ appreciably from an equivalent dose of a nonprescription product. The recommended dosage of nonprescription NSAIDs may be relatively lower than prescription NSAIDs. The major difference between prescription and over-the-counter NSAIDs is their cost; prescription products may be substantially more expensive than their nonprescription counterparts.

17. **Discuss potential problems associated with the long-term use of NSAIDs.**
NSAIDs are relatively safe when taken at recommended doses for long periods (eg, several weeks or months). The most common side effect associated with these drugs is gastric irritation. Most NSAIDs inhibit the production of prostaglandins that help protect the gastric mucosa, and loss of these beneficial prostaglandins renders the mucosa vulnerable to damage from gastric acids. This problem can be minimized by taking each dose with food or by administering NSAIDs with other medications (proton pump inhibitors, histamine type-2 receptor blockers) that reduce the effects or secretion of gastric acid. Other potential problems during long-term use include hepatic and renal toxicity. These problems are especially prevalent if other risk factors are present, including preexisting liver and kidney dysfunction, excessive alcohol consumption, and excessive or unnecessary use of other prescription drugs. NSAIDs probably should not be used for extended periods in people who have one or more of these risk factors.

18. **Can NSAIDs inhibit healing of bone and soft tissues?**
As indicated in question 15, NSAIDs inhibit prostaglandin biosynthesis. Certain prostaglandins, however, appear to be important during bone healing because these prostaglandins increase the activity of osteoblasts and osteoclasts that promote new bone formation. It follows that NSAIDs could impair bone healing by depriving bone of these important prostaglandins. Much of the evidence for this detrimental effect has been derived from studies using laboratory animals and in vitro cellular models. Nonetheless, retrospective clinical studies have found a significant relationship between NSAID use and nonunion of the femoral diaphysis; a relationship was also observed in patients who used NSAIDs postoperatively after spinal fusion surgery compared with patients who did not use these drugs. Consequently, many clinicians feel it is prudent to avoid use of NSAIDs immediately following fracture and bone surgery.

The effects of NSAIDs on soft tissue healing (cartilage, tendons, ligaments, skin) remain unclear. Laboratory and in vitro studies suggest that NSAIDs can impair cell growth and regeneration that could lead to impaired tendon and ligament healing. The majority of human studies, however, failed to find any detrimental effect of conventional (nonselective) NSAIDs on soft tissue healing when these drugs were used at therapeutic doses. Conversely, some evidence suggests that COX-2 selective drugs such as celecoxib (Celebrex) (see the next question) may inhibit tendon healing following surgical tendon repairs in humans. Hence, selective COX-2 inhibitors might not be ideal for controlling pain after certain soft tissue injuries or surgeries, and nonselective NSAIDs (ibuprofen, naproxen, and so forth) might be a better choice in these situations.

19. **What are the COX-2 inhibitors?**
These are drugs that inhibit a specific subtype of the COX enzyme. There are two major subtypes of this enzyme known as COX-1 and COX-2. The COX-2 subtype is produced within various cells that are injured or damaged, and the COX-2 enzyme synthesizes prostaglandins associated with pain and inflammation. Drugs such as celecoxib (Celebrex) that are more selective for the COX-2 enzyme can help control production of prostaglandins that cause pain and inflammation, while sparing the production of beneficial prostaglandins, including the prostaglandins that help protect the stomach lining. Hence, these drugs can decrease pain and inflammation similar to the conventional NSAIDs, with less chance of causing gastric irritation in some patients. An additional benefit is that COX-2 inhibitors do not inhibit platelet function, and therefore do not need to be stopped before surgery to prevent bleeding complications. Celecoxib is the only COX-2 inhibitor that is available in the United States at the present time.

20. **Are COX-2 inhibitors safe?**
COX-2 inhibitors can produce side effects such as headache, abdominal pain, and diarrhea. Moreover, there is concern that these drugs may increase the risk of serious cardiovascular problems, including heart attack and stroke. For this reason, two of the original COX-2 drugs, rofecoxib (Vioxx) and valdecoxib (Bextra), were withdrawn from the market. Research continues to determine if COX-2 drugs such as celecoxib have an acceptable risk-benefit ratio in certain patients. It seems reasonable that people who are at risk for cardiovascular disease should use these drugs cautiously, or perhaps avoid them altogether.

21. **How is acetaminophen similar or different from NSAIDs?**
Acetaminophen is similar to NSAIDs because acetaminophen produces analgesic and antipyretic effects. A primary therapeutic difference is that acetaminophen does not cause irritation of the gastric mucosa and is often preferred as an analgesic in patients who are prone to stomach upset from NSAIDs. Acetaminophen also differs from NSAIDs because acetaminophen does not have any appreciable antiinflammatory or anticoagulant effects.

The lack of antiinflammatory effects is important because patients with pain and inflammation will not be getting as much benefit from acetaminophen as they would when taking an NSAID. Finally, acetaminophen is more toxic to the liver than NSAIDs. Patients should be aware of acetaminophen's potential hepatoxicity, especially if high doses are taken, or the patient already has some degree of liver failure.

22. Can analgesics be applied topically or transdermally to decrease pain?

Certain analgesics can be applied to the skin to treat pain in fairly superficial structures. Trolamine salicylate (an aspirin-like drug) is available in several over-the-counter creams; this drug penetrates the skin and decreases pain in underlying tissues, such as muscle and tendon. Penetration of trolamine and certain other NSAIDs (ketoprofen) can be enhanced by ultrasound (phonophoresis) or by electric current (iontophoresis).

Local anesthetics such as lidocaine can be administered transdermally via a medicated patch that is placed directly over the painful area. Again, the intent is to focus the drug into the tissues directly beneath the patch. Certain opioids, including morphine and fentanyl, can also be administered transdermally. The goal of this administration is to achieve systemic levels that ultimately reach the central nervous system rather than to treat a specific subcutaneous structure or tissue. The use of opioid patches or other transdermal techniques (including iontophoresis) may offer a noninvasive way to provide fairly sustained administration and pain relief with opioid medications.

Several other agents can be applied topically and are often available in over-the-counter products. Some products contain capsaicin, a chemical derived from chile peppers that produces a burning sensation when applied to the skin via creams and lotions. This burning sensation may act initially as a counterirritant to override other painful impulses being transmitted along sensory pathways. Repeated use of capsaicin may also deplete sensory neurons of pain-mediating neurotransmitters, thus decreasing the ability of nociceptive neurons to relay painful information toward the CNS. Topical products can also contain other counterirritants such as menthol, camphor, or a combination of these and other chemicals. These products may offer temporary relief of musculoskeletal pain in some patients. Occasional use is not usually harmful, but excessive use should probably be discouraged.

23. Are medications from other drug categories effective in treating chronic pain?

Yes. Conventional antidepressants such as nortriptyline (Aventyl, Pamelor) and amitriptyline (Elavil), and some of the newer antidepressants such as paroxetine (Paxil) and venlafaxine (Effexor), are often incorporated in the analgesic regimen for people with various types of chronic pain such as fibromyalgia and chronic back and neck pain. In some patients depression may be present along with chronic pain, so it seems reasonable that managing the depression will help provide better outcomes when also trying to manage pain. There is evidence, however, that antidepressants can help improve pain even when a patient is not clinically depressed. Antidepressants prolong the activity of neurotransmitters in the brain such as norepinephrine, dopamine, and serotonin. It follows that their analgesic effects are probably related to their ability to affect these same neurotransmitters, but the exact reason they are effective in treating pain remains to be determined.

Certain antiseizure drugs such as gabapentin (Neurontin) and pregabalin (Lyrica) are also helpful in treating chronic pain, especially neuropathic pain. Again, the reason for their analgesic effects is not clear but seems to be related to their ability to mimic the inhibitory effects of GABA in the CNS. Specifically, these drugs inhibit presynaptic activity of neurons in certain pain pathways. These drugs appear to block calcium channels on presynaptic neurons, thus limiting calcium entry and reducing the release of pain-mediating neurotransmitters from these neurons. Hence, gabapentin, pregabalin, and other antiseizure drugs might decrease neurotransmission in specific afferent pain pathways, thereby reducing nociceptive input that is causing certain types of chronic pain.

24. List the common antiinflammtory steroids (glucocorticoids) that are administered orally or by injection to treat musculoskeletal conditions.

Common Glucocorticoids

GENERIC NAME	TRADE NAME	ORAL DOSE (MG)*	INTRAARTICULAR DOSE (MG)†	INTRALESIONAL/ SOFT TISSUE DOSE (MG)‡
Betamethasone	Celestone	0.6–7.2	Small joint: 1.5–3.0; Larger joints: 6–12	3–6
Cortisone	Cortone acetate	25–300	N/A	N/A
Dexamethasone	Decadron, others	0.75–9.0	N/A	N/A
Hydrocortisone	Cortef, others	20–240	N/A	N/A

Continued

Common Glucocorticoids—cont'd				
GENERIC NAME	TRADE NAME	ORAL DOSE (MG)*	INTRAARTICULAR DOSE (MG)†	INTRALESIONAL/ SOFT TISSUE DOSE (MG)‡
Methylprednisolone	Medrol, others	4–48	Small joint: 4–10; Larger joints: 10–80	4–30
Prednisolone	Prelone, others	5–60	N/A	N/A
Prednisone	Rayos, others	5–60	N/A	N/A
Triamcinolone	Kenalog, others	8–16	Small joint: 2.5–5; Larger joints: 5–15	2.5–15

N/A: not applicable; these drugs are not approved for intraarticular or soft tissue injections.
*Typical daily adult and adolescent dose, administered orally in single or divided doses.
†Examples of small joints: metacarpophalangeal, interphalangeal; larger joints include: wrist, elbow; shoulder; ankle; knee; hip.
‡Intralesional/soft tissue sites typically include injection into a bursa, tendon sheath, and so forth.

25. **How do glucocorticoids decrease inflammation?**
Glucocorticoids enter the cell, bind to a specific receptor in the cytoplasm, and form a glucocorticoid-receptor complex that moves to the cell's nucleus. At the nucleus, the drug-receptor complex increases the transcription of genes that code for antiinflammatory proteins (eg, certain interleukins, neutral endopeptidase) while inhibiting genes that code for inflammatory proteins (eg, cytokines, inflammatory enzymes). Glucocorticoids also inhibit directly the function of various cells involved in the inflammatory response, including macrophages, lymphocytes, and eosinophils.

26. **How do glucocorticoids compare with NSAIDs in terms of efficacy and safety?**
Glucocorticoids are generally much more effective than NSAIDs in reducing inflammation, but glucocorticoids are not as safe as NSAIDs, and glucocorticoid use can produce several serious side effects when these drugs are administered systemically for periods of 3 weeks or more. Glucocorticoids, for example, can cause hypertension, muscle wasting, glucose intolerance, gastric ulcers, and glaucoma. Patients may be more prone to infections because these drugs suppress the immune system. Prolonged glucocorticoid administration causes adrenocortical suppression, in which the adrenal gland stops synthesizing endogenous glucocorticoids (cortisol) because of the negative feedback effect of the drugs on the endocrine system. Because it takes the adrenal gland several days to regain normal function and begin synthesizing cortisol, adrenocortical suppression can be life-threatening if the glucocorticoid drug is suddenly discontinued. Consequently, patients who receive systemic doses of glucocorticoids for extended periods should not discontinue these medications suddenly, but should gradually taper off the dosage under medical supervision.

27. **Which side effect of glucocorticoids can be especially troublesome in patients receiving physical therapy, and how can this side effect be managed?**
One of the most troublesome side effects of glucocorticoids is the tendency of these drugs to cause breakdown (catabolism) of muscle, tendon, bone, and other supporting tissues. Catabolic side effects can be managed by subjecting muscle and other tissues to resistance exercise. For example, renal transplant patients receiving glucocorticoids to prevent organ rejection were trained using an isokinetic cycle ergometer, and these patients experienced an increase in thigh girth and thigh muscle area of 9% to 44% compared with healthy control subjects. This relative protection against muscle atrophy is variable and depends on the type and intensity of the exercise, the dosage of the glucocorticoid, and the amount of catabolism that may already be present because of high glucocorticoid dosage and prolonged administration. Nonetheless, judicious use of progressive resistance training and other strengthening techniques (eg, walking, aquatic exercise) can be invaluable in minimizing the catabolic side effects.

28. **Is there a critical dosage or frequency of administration that contraindicates further intraarticular injections of glucocorticoids?**
It is generally believed that a given joint should receive no more than three to four injections within a 12-month period, with a recommended maximum duration of this treatment of no more than 2 years.

29. **What are the fluoroquinolones?**
They are a group of antibacterial drugs that includes ciprofloxacin (Cipro) and ofloxacin (Floxin). These drugs have a fairly broad antibacterial spectrum and are used frequently to treat urinary tract infections, respiratory tract infections, and other infections caused by gram-negative bacteria.

30. **Why are the fluoroquinolones potentially harmful to patients with orthopaedic conditions?**
Some patients experience tendinopathy (pain, tenderness), especially in the Achilles tendon and other large tendons that are subjected to high amounts of stress. The exact reasons for this effect are unclear, but fluoroquinolone-induced tendinopathy can be severe and lead to tendon rupture. Risk factors include advanced age, renal failure, use of glucocorticoids, and a history of tendinopathy caused by these drugs. Therapists should be especially cognizant of tendinitis in patients who are taking these drugs, and any increase in tendon problems should be brought to the attention of the medical staff. Exercise involving the affected tendon should be discontinued until the source of the pain and tenderness can be evaluated.

31. **What medications are available to treat skeletal muscle spasms associated with orthopaedic impairments (eg, nerve root impingement or direct injury to the muscle)?**
Diazepam (Valium) and a diverse group of drugs such as carisoprodol (Soma), cyclobenzaprine (Flexeril), and other centrally acting muscle relaxants are available to treat these conditions. The drugs commonly used to control muscle spasms act on the central nervous system and attempt to reduce excitatory input onto the α-motor neuron. Valium increases the inhibitory effects of γ-aminobutyric acid (GABA) in the spinal cord. GABA, an inhibitory neurotransmitter in the central nervous system, tends to decrease neuronal activity, including the activity of the α-motor neuron that activates skeletal muscle. Valium increases GABA-mediated inhibition of the α-motor neuron, which, in turn, causes decreased muscle activation, with subsequent relaxation of muscles that are in spasm. The actions of other centrally acting muscle relaxants are poorly understood. Carisoprodol, for example, may affect GABA receptors in a manner similar to diazepam, whereas cyclobenzaprine may increase the inhibitory effects of serotonin in the brainstem. On the other hand, all the centrally acting muscle relaxants cause sedation, and it seems likely that any muscle relaxant properties of these drugs are caused by their sedative effects.

32. **Discuss the efficacy of the drugs commonly used to treat skeletal muscle spasm.**
Antispasm drugs typically have been shown to be more effective than placebo in reducing the pain associated with skeletal muscle spasms. These drugs, however, may not be any more effective than simple analgesic medications such as NSAIDs when treating orthopaedic conditions that include spasms. All of the commonly prescribed antispasm drugs cause sedation, and the ability of these drugs to relax skeletal muscle is probably related more to their sedative properties than to a direct effect on muscle spasms. Many practitioners are forgoing use of these muscle relaxants in lieu of pain medications and other nonpharmacologic interventions, including physical therapy.

33. **How do antispasm medications differ from drugs used to treat spasticity?**
Antispasm medications consist primarily of diazepam (Valium) and other drugs that act in the central nervous system and attempt to decrease excitation of the α-motor neuron. Diazepam also can be used to treat spasticity (i.e., increased stretch reflex activity secondary to central nervous system lesions). The other conventional antispasm drugs (eg, carisoprodol, cyclobenzaprine) are typically used only for spasms. Antispasticity drugs, including baclofen (Lioresal), tizanidine (Zanaflex), gabapentin (Neurontin), dantrolene (Dantrium), and botulinum toxin (Botox), act at various sites to decrease the hyperexcitability of skeletal muscle. Baclofen, tizanidine, and gabapentin act within the spinal cord to increase inhibition and decrease excitation of the α-motor neuron. Dantrolene acts directly on the skeletal muscle cell and causes relaxation by inhibiting the release of calcium from the sarcoplasmic reticulum. Botulinum toxin can be injected directly into spastic muscles and causes relaxation by inhibiting the release of acetylcholine at the neuromuscular junction. Botulinum toxin can be used to treat severe, chronic muscle spasms in conditions such as torticollis.

34. **What are the primary medications used to treat osteoarthritis?**
Acetaminophen and NSAIDs are the primary medications used in the treatment of osteoarthritis. NSAIDs can be used as an alternative or as a supplement to acetaminophen, especially in more advanced stages of osteoarthritis where some inflammation (synovitis) may occur secondary to other degenerative changes in the joints. Other drugs can be used to help restore joint function and prevent further degeneration. Viscosupplementation involves injection of hyaluronan directly into the joint in an attempt to restore viscosity of the synovial fluid. Another strategy uses over-the-counter dietary supplements, such as glucosamine and chondroitin sulfate, to provide substrates for the formation of healthy articular cartilage and synovial fluid.

35. **Is there evidence that dietary supplements (eg, glucosamine, chondroitin) can improve joint function in people with osteoarthritis?**
There is limited evidence to support the use of dietary supplements containing glucosamine, chondroitin, or a combination of both products. Although some early studies suggested these supplements might decrease joint pain and increase function in osteoarthritis, many of these studies had design or methodological flaws that limited their interpretation. More recent, high-quality studies and systematic reviews cast doubt on the effects of these supplements in the general population. Nonetheless, it has been suggested that these supplements may help certain patients, such as those who have a high degree of cartilage turnover and might benefit from supplements

that provide substrates needed to sustain this turnover. Given the relative safety of these interventions, these nutritional supplements might therefore be worth a trial in certain people with osteoarthritis.

36. **Discuss the primary pharmacologic strategies available for treating rheumatoid arthritis.**
    - NSAIDs typically are the first drugs used to control pain and inflammation, and these agents often are the cornerstone of treatment throughout the course of the disease.
    - Glucocorticoids are especially effective in controlling inflammation, but these drugs must be used cautiously because of their catabolic properties and other side effects. Glucocorticoids often are used for short periods to help control flare-ups or acute exacerbations of rheumatoid arthritis.
    - Disease-modifying antirheumatic drugs (DMARDs) include methotrexate (Mexate, Rheumatrex), etanercept (Enbrel), adalimumab (Humira), anakinra (Kineret), abatacept (Orencia), azathioprine (Imuran), and several other agents. These drugs are grouped together because they can slow or reverse the joint destruction that typifies rheumatoid arthritis. DMARDs seem to work by suppressing the immune response that causes the degenerative changes associated with rheumatoid arthritis. DMARDs tend to be fairly toxic, and their use is limited to patients who are able to tolerate long-term administration.

37. **Why are local anesthetics used to treat acute and chronic pain?**
    Local anesthetics (eg, lidocaine, bupivacaine) block transmission of action potentials in nerve axons. This effect occurs because these drugs inhibit sodium channels from opening in the nerve membrane, rendering the membrane inexcitable for a short period. By blocking transmission in sensory axons, local anesthetics prevent painful sensations from reaching the brain. These drugs can be administered in conditions such as reflex sympathetic dystrophy (also known as complex regional pain syndrome) to try to interrupt painful afferent sensations and to decrease efferent sympathetic discharge to the affected extremity. By using a PCA pump and delivery system, local anesthetics can be administered epidurally to the area surrounding the spinal cord. This type of anesthesia can be especially helpful in decreasing severe pain and improving quality of life in conditions such as cancer.

38. **How are local anesthetics used to manage pain during and after surgery?**
    Local anesthetics can be applied near a peripheral nerve to provide regional anesthesia and allow surgery to a specific body part supplied by that nerve. For example, injecting a local anesthetic near the median nerve can provide anesthesia to the wrist and hand so that carpal tunnel surgery can be performed. Likewise, a local anesthetic can be injected into the epidural or subarachnoid space near the spinal cord to provide anesthesia below the level of injection, thus allowing more extensive surgeries such as hip or knee arthroplasty. Use of local anesthetics can offer advantages over general anesthesia because the local anesthetic does not suppress activity in the brain and other organs, and recovery from the local anesthetic can be quicker and less problematic in older adults and patients with organ dysfunction.

    Local anesthetics can also be applied for the first few days after surgery to maintain the anesthetic effect and provide postoperative pain control. This procedure is known as a continuous nerve block and is done by inserting a small catheter near the peripheral nerve that supplies the surgical area and steadily administering a small amount of the local anesthetic onto the nerve. For example, a nerve block can be applied to the femoral nerve in the anterior thigh to provide pain control after knee surgeries. Nerve blocks are often very effective in providing postoperative pain control because the patient cannot feel the body part where the surgery was performed. Clinicians must realize, however, that the loss of sensation is often accompanied by a loss of motor function and joint proprioception, thus making it difficult or impossible for the patient to control and stabilize the joint. Extra care must therefore be taken when exercising the joint, and external support (eg, a knee immobilizer) may be needed if the patient needs to bear weight on the joint.

39. **How can medications decrease the risk of thromboembolic disease in patients recovering from hip arthroplasty and other surgeries?**
    Anticoagulant drugs such as heparin and warfarin (Coumadin) are invaluable in maintaining normal hemostasis after surgery. Heparin is a sugarlike molecule that delays blood clotting by decreasing the activity of thrombin (the active form of clotting factor II) and by inhibiting the active form of clotting factor X. Heparin acts rapidly but typically must be administered parenterally by intravenous or subcutaneous routes. Warfarin and similar oral anticoagulants are administered by mouth, and these drugs work by decreasing the production of certain clotting factors in the liver. Oral anticoagulants take several days to affect blood clotting because they have a delayed effect on clotting factor biosynthesis. Heparin and oral anticoagulants often are used sequentially to control excessive clotting; drug therapy begins with parenteral administration of heparin but is switched after a few days or weeks to oral anticoagulants (warfarin), which can be administered for several weeks or months to maintain normal coagulation after surgery.

    Other strategies to reduce blood clotting and decrease the risk of thromboembolism include drugs that directly inhibit thrombin (eg, argatroban [Acova], bivalirudin [Angiomax], dabigatran [Pradaxa], desirudin [Iprivask], lepirudin [Refludan]), or inhibit the active form of clotting factor X (eg, apixaban [Eliquis], fondaparinux [Arixtra], rivaroxaban [Xarelto]). These drugs offer an alternative anticoagulant strategy, especially in patients who may not tolerate more conventional agents such as heparin and warfarin.

Mechanism of action of anticoagulant medications

DRUG(S)	SITE OF ACTION IN COAGULATION CASCADE	ANTICOAGULATION STRATEGY
• Heparin (unfractionated)	• Clotting factor X • Thrombin	• Unfractionated heparin (UFH) is a mixture of heparin molecules that increase the ability of antithrombin III (an endogenous plasma protein) to inhibit the active form of clotting factor X and thrombin • Smaller amounts of UFH primarily affect clotting factor X, while larger amounts primarily affect thrombin • Inhibition of clotting factor X prevents conversion of prothrombin to its active form (thrombin) • Inhibition of thrombin prevents conversion of fibrinogen to its active form (fibrin)
Low-molecular-weight heparins (LMWHs) Dalteparin (Fragmin) Enoxaparin (Lovenox) Tinzaparin (Innohep)	• Clotting factor X • Thrombin	• LMWHs are extracted from UFH (see above) • LMWHs increase the effects of antithrombin III (similar to UFH) • LMWHs primarily inhibit the active form of clotting factor X, with a lower ability to inhibit thrombin
Warfarin (Coumadin)	• Vitamin K-dependent clotting factors: II, VII, IX, X • Anticoagulant proteins C and S	• Inhibit the synthesis of vitamin K-dependent clotting factors and anticoagulant proteins by inhibiting the regeneration of vitamin K in the liver • Lower amounts of these clotting factors result in decreased clotting and reduced risk of venous thrombosis
Direct thrombin inhibitors Argatroban (Acova) Bilvalirudin (Angiomax) Dabigatran (Pradaxa) Desirudin (Iprivask) Lepirudin (Refludan)	• Thrombin	• Bind directly to thrombin • Inhibit the ability of thrombin to convert fibrinogen to its active form (fibrin)
Clotting factor X inhibitors Apixaban (Eliquis) Fondaparinux (Arixtra) Rivaroxaban (Xarelto)	• Clotting factor X	• Inhibit the active form of clotting factor X by either: • binding directly to clotting factor X (apixaban, rivaroxaban) or • increasing the effects of antithrombin III (fondaparinux) • Inhibition of clotting factor X reduces the ability of this factor to convert prothrombin to thrombin
• Aspirin • Clopidogrel (Plavix)	• Platelets	• Aspirin inhibits platelet activity by inhibiting the biosynthesis of prostaglandins, including the thromboxanes • Thromboxanes normally stimulate platelet aggregation and clotting • Reduced thromboxane biosynthesis decreases platelet-induced clots • Clopidogrel metabolites bind $P2Y_{12}$ADP receptors on platelets inhibiting the glycoprotein GPIIb/IIIa complex and thus platelet aggregation

40. **Is aspirin effective in preventing deep venous thrombosis?**
Yes. Aspirin exerts anticoagulant effects by inhibiting the production of prostaglandins that cause platelets to aggregate and participate in clot formation. Aspirin can be administered alone or with other anticoagulants (heparin, warfarin), especially in patients who are at high risk for developing deep venous thrombosis.

41. **Is ambulation safe for a patient newly diagnosed with deep vein thrombosis?**
There is no evidence that ambulation increases the risk of pulmonary embolism after an uncomplicated DVT. That is, immediate ambulation seems to be safe provided that the patient does not have a current or recent pulmonary embolism (symptomatic or asymptomatic) or other risk factors that would increase the likelihood of an embolism (eg, malignant cancer, prolonged immobilization, advanced age). An adequate level of anticoagulant therapy using heparin, warfarin, or alternative agents should also be achieved before starting ambulation. Graduated compression stockings should also be considered because there is evidence that proper use of these garments can prevent complications related to DVT.

42. **What drugs are contraindications to upper cervical manipulation?**
Anticoagulant drugs such as heparin, warfarin, and conventional NSAIDs (ie, aspirin and other antiplatelet drugs) can increase the risk of vertebral artery damage and bleeding in patients receiving upper cervical manipulation. The direct thrombin inhibitors and clotting factor X inhibitors (see question 39) will also reduce blood clotting, and it follows that these drugs may also increase the risk of vertebral artery damage and bleeding during cervical manipulation. Although the exact incidence of vertebral artery damage is unclear, cervical manipulation should be used cautiously in patients taking these drugs. Therapists should at least avoid using upper cervical manipulation until laboratory tests indicate that the patient's clotting time is being maintained within normal limits. If these tests indicate relatively normal hemostasis, upper cervical manipulation should still be used cautiously, and the velocity and force of the manipulation must be reduced to decrease the risk of bleeding caused by vertebral artery damage.

43. **Discuss medications that are currently available to treat osteoporosis.**
- Calcitonin, a hormone normally produced within the body, can be administered to help increase the storage of calcium and phosphate in bone.
- Estrogen is likewise important in the hormonal control of bone mineral content in women, and estrogen replacement (using patches or oral supplements) can be especially valuable in certain women after menopause.
- Bisphosphonates are a group of drugs that help stabilize bone mineral content by binding directly to calcium in the bone and preventing excessive calcium turnover. Common bisphosphonates include alendronate (Fosamax), ibandronate (Boniva), pamidronate (Aredia), risedronate (Actonel), and zoledronic acid (Reclast).
- Denosumab (Prolia) is a monoclonal antibody that binds to a protein called nuclear factor-kappa ligand (RANKL). RANKL is secreted by osteoblasts, and it facilitates bone breakdown and reabsorption by activating osteoclasts. Denosumab binds to RANKL, thus inhibiting its ability to activate osteoclasts. Reduced osteoclast activity results in decreased bone reabsorption and increased bone density.
- Calcium supplements can help provide a dietary source of this essential mineral, and vitamin D supplements can increase absorption of calcium and phosphate from the gastrointestinal tract.

44. **What is heterotopic ossification?**
It is the abnormal formation of bone in muscle and other periarticular tissues. This condition is one of the most common complications that occurs in patients recovering from hip arthroplasty and similar surgical procedures.

45. **Discuss drugs that are effective in treating heterotopic ossification.**
NSAIDs can substantially reduce the prevalence of heterotopic ossification associated with orthopaedic surgeries and other conditions (eg, fracture, rheumatoid arthritis). Treatment with NSAIDs has been successful in reducing the prevalence and severity of heterotopic ossification after total hip arthroplasty. These drugs inhibit prostaglandin biosynthesis, and their ability to limit heterotopic ossification undoubtedly is related to a reduction of proinflammatory prostaglandins in periarticular soft tissues. These drugs seem to work best when used prophylactically, and they often are administered a day or so before surgery and continued for 1 to 6 weeks after surgery.

46. **Discuss how cardiovascular medications affect exercise responses.**
Certain cardiovascular medications blunt the cardiac response to an exercise bout. β-Blockers typically decrease heart rate and myocardial contractility, resulting in a decrease in blood pressure and heart rate at submaximal and maximal workloads. Digitalis increases myocardial contraction force and can increase left ventricular ejection fraction in patients with heart failure. Other cardiovascular drugs, such as diuretics, vasodilators, antiarrhythmics, angiotensin-converting enzyme inhibitors, and calcium channel blockers, can have variable effects on exercise responses, depending on the drug and dosage used, the type of cardiac disease, and the presence of comorbidity.

47. List specific concerns for physical therapists regarding cardiac medications and exercise.

a. Exercise tolerance may improve when the drug is in effect. This is true even for drugs that blunt cardiac function (eg, β-blockers) because the drug may control symptoms of angina and arrhythmias, allowing the patient to exercise longer and at a relatively higher level.

b. Exercise prescriptions must take into account the medication effects. Formulas that estimate exercise intensity based on age, resting heart rate, and other variables may not be accurate because these formulas fail to account for the effect of each medication on these variables. On the other hand, maximal or submaximal exercise testing will only indicate the patient's exercise capacity at the specific point in time when the medication was acting on the patient. That is, the exercise test will reflect the patient's exercise capacity when the drug was at a specific dose and concentration in their blood stream. Hence, rating of perceived exertion might be one of the best ways to prescribe exercise intensity and monitor the patient's responses when the patient is actually engaging in physical activity while taking cardiac medications.

c. Therapists should look carefully for medication-related side effects and adverse effects while the patient is exercising. These effects may be latent when the patient is inactive, but exercise may unmask certain side effects, such as arrhythmias and abnormal blood pressure responses.

48. Can lipid-lowering medications cause skeletal muscle damage?

Lipid-lowering drugs such as the statins (eg, simvastatin [Zocor], atorvastatin [Lipitor]) are generally well tolerated. In susceptible patients, however, they can cause myopathy that is characterized by skeletal muscle pain, weakness, and inflammation (myositis). In severe cases, myopathy can lead to severe muscle damage (rhabdomyolysis) with disintegration of the muscle membrane and release of myoglobin and other muscle proteins into the bloodstream. This situation can lead to renal damage because the kidneys must try to filter and excrete large quantities of muscle protein. Hence, any patient who spontaneously develops muscle pain and weakness while taking lipid-lowering drugs should be referred to his or her physician immediately to rule out the possibility of drug-induced myopathy.

49. Can physical agents affect drug absorption, distribution, and metabolism?

Physical agents (eg, heat, cold, and electricity) can have dramatic effects on drug disposition in the body; this is especially true for drugs that are injected into a specific area. Insulin typically is administered through subcutaneous injection into adipose tissue in the trunk or extremities. Insulin is absorbed into the bloodstream more rapidly if heat and other physical interventions (eg, electric stimulation, massage, exercise) are applied to the injection site. Application of cold agents delays insulin absorption.

Use of physical agents or manual interventions at the site of the injection should be avoided when the rate of absorption must remain constant or the goal is to keep a drug localized in a specific area. Conversely, heat, massage, and exercise could be applied to a certain area of the body with the idea that a systemically administered drug (ie, a drug that is in the bloodstream) might reach the area more easily because of an increase in local blood flow and tissue metabolism. This idea has not been proved conclusively.

50. What is meant by "medical marijuana?"

Medical marijuana is typically used to describe the use of chemicals known as cannabinoids when treating various clinical conditions. Cannabinoids are found in the marijuana plant and can be ingested by smoking dried leaves of the plant, or by oral or topical administration of various products that contain these chemicals. The marijuana plant contains 60 to 100 different cannabinoids, but two cannabinoids known as Δ^9-tetrahydrocannabinol (THC) and cannabidiol (CBD) seem to have the most clinical relevance. THC produces most of psychoactive and hallucinogenic effects associated with recreational marijuana use, whereas CBD may help modulate immune function and provide certain beneficial effects without unwanted psychoactive effects. Hence, many products now contain only CBD, and these products have been advocated as a way to control conditions such as anxiety, pain, spasticity, and seizures.

51. How do cannabinoids work in the human body?

Cannabinoids such as THC and CBD exert their effects by binding to specific cannabinoid receptors that are located on many tissues throughout the human body. This situation is analogous to the endogenous opioid system, where the body produces chemicals such as endorphins, enkephalins, and dynorphins that control pain and affect other tissues by binding to specific opioid receptors on those tissues. The endogenous cannabinoid system is different from the endogenous opioid system in that the cannabinoid system produces chemicals or "endocannabinoids" such as anandamide and 2-arachidonylglycerol (2-AG), and these substances bind to endogenous cannabinoid receptors. So, the endogenous cannabinoid system can be considered as another way the human body produces specific chemicals in certain situations to modulate function in many tissues. It follows that ingesting natural or synthetic cannabinoids can exert specific effects on various tissues that contain cannabinoid receptors, much in the same way that opioid drugs affect tissues with opioid receptors.

52. **Can cannabinoids be used to treat musculoskeletal pain?**
    Cannabinoids have been advocated as a way to reduce pain in many conditions. In particular, CBD has been reported as a way to control pain without impairing cognitive function due to hallucinogenic effects. However, the evidence for CBD's analgesic effects is somewhat anecdotal or observational, and there is a relative lack of large, well-controlled clinical trials on the analgesic effects of CBD products. Nonetheless, patients often obtain these products in nonprescription oils or topical creams. Unfortunately, the actual content and amount of CBD in these products is often questionable. Products containing adequate amounts of CBD could potentially have analgesic effects that are mediated through the body's cannabinoid receptors. But, again, the lack of quality control in most CBD products, combined with a relative lack of well-controlled clinical trials, makes it difficult to say whether these substances can have meaningful analgesic effects in specific musculoskeletal conditions.

Bibliography

Adcock, I. M., & Mumby, S. (2017). Glucocorticoids. *Handbook of Experimental Pharmacology, 237*, 171–196.

Aletaha, D., & Smolen, J. S. (2018). Diagnosis and management of rheumatoid arthritis: A Review. *JAMA, 320*, 1360–1372.

Amin, M. R., & Ali, D. W. (2019). Pharmacology of medical cannabis. *Advances in Experimental Medicine & Biology, 1162*, 151–165.

Arwi, G. A., & Schug, S. A. (2020). Potential for harm associated with discharge opioids after hospital stay: A systematic review. *Drugs, 80*, 573–585.

Ballantyne, J. C. (2015). Opioid therapy in chronic pain. *Physical Medicine and Rehabilitation Clinics of North America, 26*, 201–218.

Bell, J., & Strang, J. (2020). Medication treatment of opioid use disorder. *Biological Psychiatry, 87*, 82–88.

Brat, G. A., Agniel, D., Beam, A., et al. (2018). Postsurgical prescriptions for opioid naive patients and association with overdose and misuse: Retrospective cohort study. *BMJ, 360*, j5790.

Browne, C. J., Godino, A., Salery, M., & Nestler, E. J. (2020). Epigenetic mechanisms of opioid addiction. *Biological Psychiatry, 87*, 22–33.

Chatsis, V., & Visintini, S. (2018). *Early mobilization for patients with venous thromboembolism: A review of clinical effectiveness and guidelines.* Ottawa, ON: Canadian Agency for Drugs and Technologies in Health.

Chotiyarnwong, P., & McCloskey, E. V. (2020). Pathogenesis of glucocorticoid-induced osteoporosis and options for treatment. *Nature Reviews Endocrinology, 16*, 437–447.

Ciccone, C. D. (2017). Medical marijuana: Just the beginning of a long, strange trip? *Physical Therapy, 97*, 239–248.

Ciccone, C. D. (2018). Medications. In: DeTurk W. & Cahalin L (Eds.): *Cardiovascular and pulmonary physical therapy* (3rd ed.). New York, NY: McGraw-Hill.

Coffa, D., & Snyder, H. (2019). Opioid use disorder: Medical treatment options. *American Family Physician, 100*, 416–425.

Coluzzi, F., Bifulco, F., Cuomo, A., et al. (2017). The challenge of perioperative pain management in opioid-tolerant patients. *Therapeutics and Clinical Risk Management, 13*, 1163–1173.

Corder, G., Castro, D. C., Bruchas, M. R., & Scherrer, G. (2018). Endogenous and exogenous opioids in pain. *Annual Review of Neuroscience, 41*, 453–473.

Dunne, R. B. (2018). Prescribing naloxone for opioid overdose intervention. *Pain Management, 8*, 197–208.

Farmer, A. D., Holt, C. B., Downes, T. J., et al. (2018). Pathophysiology, diagnosis, and management of opioid-induced constipation. *Lancet Gastroenterology and Hepatology, 3*, 203–212.

Fishbain, D. A., Cole, B., Lewis, J., et al. (2008). What percentage of chronic nonmalignant pain patients exposed to chronic opioid analgesic therapy develop abuse/addiction and/or aberrant drug-related behaviors? A structured evidence-based review. *Pain Medicine, 9*, 444–459.

Fisher, E. S., & Curry, S. C. (2019). Evaluation and treatment of acetaminophen toxicity. *Advances in Pharmacology, 85*, 263–272.

Ghosh, N., Kolade, O. O., Shontz, E., et al. (2019). Nonsteroidal anti-Inflammatory drugs (NSAIDs) and their effect on musculoskeletal soft-tissue healing: A scoping review. *JBJS Reviews, 7*, e4.

Handin, R. I. (2016). The history of antithrombotic therapy: The discovery of heparin, the vitamin K antagonists, and the utility of aspirin. *Hematology/Oncology Clinics of North America, 30*, 987–993.

Hur, M., Park, S. K., Koo, C. H., et al. (2017). Comparative efficacy and safety of anticoagulants for prevention of venous thromboembolism after hip and knee arthroplasty. *Acta Orthopaedica, 88*, 634–641.

Imam, M. Z., Kuo, A., & Smith, M. T. (2020). Countering opioid-induced respiratory depression by non-opioids that are respiratory stimulants. *F1000Research, 9*, F1000.

Johal, H., Vannabouathong, C., Chang, Y., et al. (2020). Medical cannabis for orthopaedic patients with chronic musculoskeletal pain: Does evidence support its use? *Therapeutic Advances in Musculoskeletal Disease, 12*, 1759720X20937968.

Joshi, G., Gandhi, K., Shah, N., et al. (2016). Peripheral nerve blocks in the management of postoperative pain: Challenges and opportunities. *Journal of Clinical Anesthesia, 35*, 524–529.

Kiyatkin, E. A. (2019). Respiratory depression and brain hypoxia induced by opioid drugs: Morphine, oxycodone, heroin, and fentanyl. *Neuropharmacology, 151*, 219–226.

Krasselt, M., & Baerwald, C. (2019). Celecoxib for the treatment of musculoskeletal arthritis. *Expert Opinion on Pharmacotherapy, 20*, 1689–1702.

Lang, T. R., Cook, J., Rio, E., & Gaida, J. E. (2017). What tendon pathology is seen on imaging in people who have taken fluoroquinolones? A systematic review. *Fundamental & Clinical Pharmacology, 31*, 4–16.

Lisowska, B., Kosson, D., & Domaracka, K. (2018a). Positives and negatives of nonsteroidal anti-inflammatory drugs in bone healing: The effects of these drugs on bone repair. *Drug Design, Development and Therapy, 12*, 1809–1814.

Lisowska, B., Kosson, D., & Domaracka, K. (2018b). Lights and shadows of NSAIDs in bone healing: The role of prostaglandins in bone metabolism. *Drug Design, Development and Therapy, 12*, 1753–1758.

Listos, J., Łupina, M., Talarek, S., et al. (2019). The mechanisms involved in morphine addiction: An overview. *International Journal of Molecular Sciences, 20*, 4302.

Lorentzon, M. (2019). Treating osteoporosis to prevent fractures: Current concepts and future developments. *Journal of Internal Medicine, 285*, 381–394.

Maurer, G. E., Mathews, N. M., Schleich, K. T., et al. (2020). Understanding cannabis-based therapeutics in sports medicine. *Sports Health, 12*, 540–546.

Mercadante, S., Arcuri, E., & Santoni, A. (2019). Opioid-induced tolerance and hyperalgesia. *CNS Drugs, 33*, 943–955.
Meyers, C., Lisiecki, J., Miller, S., et al. (2019). Heterotopic ossification: A comprehensive review. *JBMR Plus, 3*, e10172.
Nardi-Hiebl, S., Eberhart, L. H. J., Gehling, M., et al. (2020). Quo vadis PCA? A review on current concepts, economic considerations, patient-related aspects, and future development with respect to patient-controlled analgesia. *Anesthesiology Research and Practice, 2020*, 9201967.
Nielsen, S. M., Tarp, S., Christensen, R., et al. (2017). The risk associated with spinal manipulation: An overview of reviews. *Systematic Reviews, 6*, 64.
Nikolic, D., Banach, M., Chianetta, R., et al. (2020). An overview of statin-induced myopathy and perspectives for the future. *Expert Opinion on Drug Safety, 19*, 601–615.
Palmer, N., & Kohane, I. (2018). Postsurgical prescriptions for opioid naive patients and association with overdose and misuse: Retrospective cohort study. *BMJ, 360*, j5790.
Pergolizzi, J. V., Jr, Magnusson, P., Raffa, R. B., et al. (2020). Developments in combined analgesic regimens for improved safety in post-operative pain management. *Expert Review of Neurotherapeutics, 20*, 981–990.
Ramachandran, A., & Jaeschke, H. (2018). Acetaminophen toxicity: Novel insights Into mechanisms and future perspectives. *Gene Expression, 18*, 19–30.
Richards, M. M., Maxwell, J. S., Weng, L., et al. (2016). Intra-articular treatment of knee osteoarthritis: From anti-inflammatories to products of regenerative medicine. *The Physician and Sportsmedicine, 44*, 101–108.
Roeckel, L. A., Le Coz, G. M., Gavériaux-Ruff, C., & Simonin, F. (2016). Opioid-induced hyperalgesia: Cellular and molecular mechanisms. *Neuroscience, 338*, 160–182.
See, S., & Ginzburg, R. (2008). Skeletal muscle relaxants. *Pharmacotherapy, 28*, 207–213.
Stein, C. (2018). New concepts in opioid analgesia. *Expert Opinion on Investigational Drugs, 27*, 765–775.
Strang, J., Volkow, N. D., Degenhardt, L., et al. (2020). Opioid use disorder. *Nature Reviews Disease Primers, 6*, 3.
Urits, I., Peck, J., Orhurhu, M. S., et al. (2019). Off-label antidepressant use for treatment and management of chronic pain: Evolving understanding and comprehensive review. *Current Pain and Headache Reports, 23*, 66.
Vandewalle, J., Luypaert, A., De Bosscher, K., & Libert, C. (2018). Therapeutic mechanisms of glucocorticoids. *Trends in Endocrinology and Metabolism, 29*, 42–54.
Vowles, K. E., McEntee, M. L., Julnes, P. S., et al. (2015). Rates of opioid misuse, abuse, and addiction in chronic pain: A systematic review and data synthesis. *Pain, 156*, 569–576.
Wang, A., Leong, D. J., Cardoso, L., & Sun, H. B. (2018). Nutraceuticals and osteoarthritis pain. *Pharmacology & Therapeutics, 187*, 167–179.
Wang, S. (2019). Historical review: Opiate addiction and opioid receptors. *Cell Transplantation, 28*, 233–238.
Wang, S. C., Chen, Y. C., Lee, C. H., & Cheng, C. M. (2019). Opioid addiction, genetic susceptibility, and medical treatments: A review. *International Journal of Molecular Sciences, 20*, 4294.
Xantus, G., Zavori, L., Matheson, C., et al. (2021). Cannabidiol in low back pain: Scientific rationale for clinical trials in low back pain. *Expert Review of Clinical Pharmacology, 14*, 671–675.
Yaftali, N. A., & Weber, K. (2019). Corticosteroids and hyaluronic acid injections. *Clinical Journal of Sports Medicine, 38*, 1–15.
Yoo, J. S., Ahn, J., Buvanendran, A., & Singh, K. (2019). Multimodal analgesia in pain management after spine surgery. *Journal of Spine Surgery, 5*(Suppl 2), S154–S159.

CHAPTER 15 QUESTIONS

1. Which drugs inhibit heterotopic bone formation?
   a. Muscle relaxers
   b. NSAIDs
   c. Acetaminophen
   d. Opioids

2. What class of antibiotics is associated with tendinopathies?
   a. Macrolides
   b. Fluoroquinolones
   c. Cephalosporins
   d. Aminoglycosides

3. Which is not a side effect of opioid analgesics?
   a. Sedation
   b. Respiratory depression
   c. Orthostatic hypotension
   d. Diarrhea

4. What anticoagulant does not affect factor X?
   a. Eliquis
   b. Plavix
   c. Coumadin
   d. Heparin

5. What drug is contraindicated in the case of cervical manipulation?
   a. Xarelto
   b. Bupivacaine
   c. Gabapentin
   d. Hydrocodone

6. What drug can cause muscle damage?
   a. Cipro
   b. Lipitor
   c. Augmentin
   d. Skelaxin

EVALUATION OF MEDICAL LABORATORY TESTS

D. Boyce, MD, RPh

1. **List various nondisease states that can result in an abnormal laboratory test result.**
   - Pregnancy
   - Exercise
   - Posture
   - Food intake and nutritional state
   - Drugs, alcohol, and vitamin and dietary supplements
   - Specimen complications (hemolysis, stasis, sampling error, storage, and exposure)
   - Circadian rhythms, diurnal variation
   - Technician error
   - Reference range variations among different laboratories
   - Normal variations based on patient age, gender, race, and body weight

2. **What two characteristics are important for diagnostic laboratory testing?**
   Sensitivity and specificity. Sensitivity is the percentage of persons with the disease who are correctly identified by the test. Specificity is the percentage of persons without the disease who are correctly excluded by the test. Clinically, these concepts are important for confirming or excluding disease during screening. Ideally, a test should provide a high sensitivity and specificity. Sensitivity = TP/(TP + FN) and Specificity = TN/(TN + FP). Abbreviations: TP, true positive; TN, true negative; FP, false positive; FN, false negative.

3. **Explain the concepts of positive predictive value (PPV) and negative predictive value (NPV).**
   PPV is defined as the percentage of persons with a positive test result who actually have the disease. NPV is the percentage of persons with a negative test result who do not have the disease. Predictive value therefore is the probability that a person's test result (positive or negative) is correct. PPV = TP/(TP + FP) and NPV = TN/(TN + FN).

4. **Where is albumin produced and what are its functions?**
   Albumin is synthesized in the liver. Albumin functions to maintain osmotic pressure in the vasculature and also serves as a transport protein. Hypoalbuminemia leads to abnormal distribution of body water. This occurs because of decreased osmotic pressure within the vasculature and resultant tissue edema. Albumin serves to transport various drugs, ions, pigments, bilirubin, and hormones.

5. **What is the normal range for serum albumin levels?**
   Normal levels are 3.5 to 5.5 g/dL.

6. **What conditions result in decreased albumin levels (hypoalbuminemia)?**
   - Poor absorption of albumin (malabsorption, malnutrition)
   - Decreased synthesis of albumin (chronic liver disease)
   - Catabolic states (infection, burns, malignancy, chronic inflammation)
   - Increased losses of albumin (hemorrhage, renal disease, protein-losing enteropathies)
   - Albumin dilution

7. **Where does alkaline phosphatase originate?**
   Liver (cells of the biliary tract), intestine (mucosal cells of the small intestine), placenta (pregnancy), and bone (osteoblasts) are sources of alkaline phosphatase. Biliary obstruction and Paget's disease (liver and bone) can result in a marked increase in alkaline phosphatase levels compared with intestinal or placental sources.

8. **Explain alkaline phosphatase elevation as it relates to bone.**
   Any bone lesions (such as sarcoma or metastatic lesions) that produce increased osteoblastic activity will result in elevated alkaline phosphatase levels. Normal bone growth in children and adolescents will also result in alkaline phosphatase elevations.

9. **What are the two hepatic conditions that result in elevation of alkaline phosphatase concentration?**
   - Extrahepatic obstruction—obstruction of the large, extrahepatic bile ducts occurs with bile duct stones, strictures, or tumors. This obstructive process of the biliary system can result in significant enzyme elevation.
   - Intrahepatic obstruction—processes within the liver parenchyma can also lead to alkaline phosphatase elevation because of interference with bile flow or transport. Examples include leukemia, sarcoidosis, amyloid, malignancy, primary biliary cirrhosis (PBC), and primary sclerosing cholangitis (PSC).

10. **How can liver- versus bone-related elevations in alkaline phosphatase levels be differentiated?**
    Measure 5′-nucleotidase, gamma-glutamyl transpeptidase (GGTP), or fractionation of alkaline phosphatase. If nucleotidase or GGTP is elevated, alkaline phosphatase elevations are caused by a liver, not bone, source. Nucleotidase is present in the bile canaliculi of the liver. GGTP is not present in bone or placental tissue; therefore, elevations are because of an underlying liver condition.

11. **What is the normal range for alkaline phosphatase?**
    The normal range is 25 to 100 units/L.

12. **What are aminotransferases?**
    Aminotransferases are enzymes involved in liver synthetic function and/or liver injury. Elevations in both aspartate transaminase (AST) and alanine transaminase (ALT) levels occur with liver inflammation, necrosis, or biliary obstruction. These enzymes are found in many other tissues besides the liver. Together with alkaline phosphatase and bilirubin, aminotransferase evaluation can help the clinician determine the pattern or cause of underlying liver disease.

13. **What are nonhepatic sources of AST and causes for its elevation?**
    In addition to liver, AST is found in the heart, kidney, and skeletal muscle. When AST is elevated without elevation of ALT, a nonhepatic source (ie, muscle, heart) should be considered. Examples include 1) skeletal muscle injury from intramuscular injection, muscle trauma with severe/prolonged exercise, polymyositis, and seizure disorder or 2) myocardial damage as seen in acute myocardial infarction. Both of these nonhepatic conditions can result in isolated AST elevation.

14. **List the common pancreatic causes for elevated amylase and lipase levels.**
    - Acute or chronic pancreatitis
    - Pancreatic pseudocyst
    - Pancreatic trauma

    Amylase is the most sensitive test for pancreatitis; lipase is the most specific indicator of pancreatitis. Often the degree of enzyme elevation does not correlate with the severity of disease.

    Alcohol and gallstones are the most common causes of acute pancreatitis. Chronic pancreatitis is a result of chronic alcohol abuse, hypercalcemia, hyperlipidemia, trauma, or hereditary causes. Any of these conditions can result in elevated amylase/lipase values.

15. **List some of the nonpancreatic causes for elevated amylase and lipase levels.**
    - Salivary gland disorders (amylase)
    - Intestinal perforation or ischemia (amylase and lipase)
    - Perforated peptic ulcer (amylase and lipase)

16. **What are antinuclear antibodies (ANAs)?**
    ANAs are used to detect the presence of antinucleoprotein factors associated with certain autoimmune diseases. ANAs are γ-globulins that react with the nuclei of various tissues. The ANA test is reported as a pattern and a titer. The presence of a positive result can 1) occur in normal individuals, 2) may not indicate disease, or 3) may indicate persons destined to develop disease. ANA positivity usually requires confirmatory testing with other disease-specific tests—eg, anti–double-stranded DNA (anti-dsDNA), anti-Smith antibody (anti-Sm antibody), or antiscleroderma antibody, depending on the suspected disease.

17. **List diseases associated with a positive ANA (conditions associated with the disease or specific laboratory abnormality in parentheses).**
    - Systemic lupus erythematosus (SLE) (anti-dsDNA, anti-Sm antibody)
    - Rheumatoid arthritis (rheumatoid factor [RF], erythrocyte sedimentation rate [ESR])
    - Scleroderma/CREST (calcinosis, Raynaud's, esophageal, sclerodactyly, telangiectasia) (Scl-70 [antitopoisomerase antibodies]/anticentromere)
    - Polymyositis

- Drugs (antideoxyribonucleoprotein [anti-DNP])
- Mixed connective tissue disease (antiribonucleoprotein [anti-RNP])
- Sjögren's syndrome (anti-SSA, anti-SSB [antinuclear antibodies detected in patients with Sjögren's syndrome])
- Chronic hepatitis
- Tuberculosis

18. **What is bilirubin and what are its two forms?**
Bilirubin is a byproduct of hemolysis (red blood cell destruction). It is taken up by the liver, conjugated, and secreted into bile. It is eliminated in the stool and urine. Bilirubin exists in a conjugated and an unconjugated form.

19. **Why does jaundice occur with hyperbilirubinemia?**
Jaundice is yellow discoloration of the skin because of bile deposition in the skin and sclerae. Jaundice can result from abnormal processing of bilirubin, excess bilirubin production, biliary obstruction, or liver damage. Jaundice is clinically evident when the total bilirubin level is >2.5 mg/dL.

20. **What conditions are associated with hyperbilirubinemia?**
- Liver disease (hepatitis, cirrhosis, biliary obstruction)
- Hereditary disorders (Gilbert syndrome, Dubin-Johnson syndrome, Crigler-Najjar disease)
- Drugs
- Hemolysis

21. **What is blood urea nitrogen (BUN)?**
BUN is the end product of protein catabolism. BUN is formed in the liver and excreted by the kidneys. Impairment in kidney function, protein intake, and protein catabolism will affect BUN levels. It is used clinically as an estimate of renal function along with serum creatinine levels.

22. **What are the causes of elevated BUN levels?**
- Inadequate excretion because of kidney disease/impairment
- Urinary obstruction
- Dehydration
- Drugs (aminoglycosides, diuretics)
- Gastrointestinal bleeding
- Decreased renal blood flow (shock, congestive heart failure [CHF], myocardial infarction [MI])

23. **What is the normal range for BUN levels?**
Typical BUN levels range from 8 to 18 mg/dl.

24. **Where is the majority of calcium stored in the body?**
Almost 98% to 99% is found in bone; 1% is found in the intracellular/extracellular space.

25. **What factors affect serum calcium levels?**
- Parathyroid hormone
- Calcitonin
- Vitamin D
- Estrogens and androgens
- Carbohydrates and lactose

These factors have a wide range of effects on calcium homeostasis (ie, GI tract absorption, renal excretion and reabsorption, and bone calcium mobilization).

26. **What conditions are associated with hypercalcemia?**
Hyperparathyroidism, malignancy, sarcoidosis, Paget's disease, vitamin D intoxication, and thiazide diuretics are all causes of hypercalcemia. The two most common causes are hyperparathyroidism and malignancy.

27. **What are the signs and symptoms of hypercalcemia?**
The phrase "bones, stones, and psychiatric overtones" is often used to remember signs and symptoms of hypercalcemia. Here, bones refer to bone pain, stones to nephrolithiasis, and psychiatric overtones to confusion and altered concentration. Hypercalcemia is defined as a serum calcium concentration >10.5 mg/dl.

28. **What are the signs and symptoms of hypocalcemia?**
- Neuromuscular irritability: Chvostek's sign (facial twitch after tapping facial nerve), Trousseau's sign (carpopedal spasm after inflation of blood pressure cuff), tetany, and paresthesias
- Psychiatric disturbances
- Cardiovascular abnormalities (arrhythmias, CHF)

29. **What causes the neuromuscular irritability (tetany) seen with hypocalcemia?**
Neuromuscular irritability occurs as a result of the decrease in the excitation threshold of neural tissue, with a resultant increase in excitability, repetitive response to a stimulus, and continued activity of the affected tissue.

30. **What is the prothrombin time (PT), and what does its value signify?**
Prothrombin time is a measurement of the clotting ability of five plasma coagulation factors (prothrombin, fibrinogen, factor V, factor VII, and factor X). The PT is commonly used for monitoring warfarin therapy (an anticoagulant) and evaluating liver function (liver normally produces clotting factors).

31. **How does warfarin function as an anticoagulant?**
It interferes with vitamin K–dependent clotting factors (II, V, VII, X). As a result, the PT will increase (or prolong) and coagulation will be delayed.

32. **What conditions can lead to an increased PT?**
    - Anticoagulant use (warfarin)
    - Vitamin K deficiency
    - Liver disease (with decreased clotting factor production)
    - Factor deficiency (II, V, VII, X)

33. **What medical therapy requires monitoring of the PTT (partial thromboplastin time)?**
Heparin use requires monitoring of the PTT because heparin is involved in the intrinsic clotting pathway. Heparin acts as a cofactor for antithrombin III and downregulates coagulation. Heparin is used for treatment of pulmonary embolism, prophylaxis of deep vein thrombosis, and treatment of various coronary conditions such as acute MI.

34. **What is the INR (international normalized ratio)?**
INR = patient PT divided by the mean PT for the laboratory reference range. INR provides a universal result indicative of what the patient's PT result would have been if measured using the primary World Health Organization International Reference reagent.

35. **What components constitute the CBC (complete blood count)?**
    - Red blood cell (RBC) count
    - White blood cell (WBC) count
    - Differential white cell count (Diff)
    - Platelet (Plt) count
    - Hemoglobin (Hgb) level
    - Hematocrit (Hct) level
    - Red cell indices (MCV, MCH, MCHC)

36. **What are the causes of leukocytosis (elevated WBC count)?**
Acute infections, hemorrhage, trauma, malignant disease, toxins, drugs, tissue necrosis/inflammation, and leukemia can all contribute to elevated WBC count.

37. **Within the differential white cell count (Diff), name the five white blood cell types, their percentages, and what they protect against.**
    - Neutrophils (58%)—bacterial infections
    - Eosinophils (3%)—allergic disorders and parasitic infections
    - Basophils (1%)—parasitic infections
    - Monocytes (5%)—severe infections
    - Lymphocytes (30%)—viral infections

38. **List the causes of neutrophilia.**
Acute bacterial infections, acute MI, stress, malignancy, and leukemias can all cause neutrophilia.

39. **List the causes of neutropenia.**
Neutropenia can be caused by viral infections, aplastic anemias, drugs, radiation, and leukemias.

40. **List the causes of eosinophilia.**
The acronym NAACP is used to remember the causes of eosinophilia, where N = neoplasms, A = allergies, A = Addison's disease, C = collagen vascular disorders, and P = parasitic infections.

41. **What is the ESR (erythrocyte sedimentation rate), and what does its value signify?**
ESR is the rate at which erythrocytes precipitate out of unclotted blood in 1 hour. Inflammation, infections, malignancy, and various collagen vascular diseases increase the ESR because they facilitate erythrocyte aggregation. This affects the rate at which erythrocytes precipitate in a tube (increased aggregation/heaviness = increased rate of descent/sedimentation = increased ESR value).

42. **What are some common conditions that lead to an increased ESR?**
- Infections
- Inflammatory diseases
- Collagen vascular diseases
- Malignancy
- Anemia

43. **What are the clinical applications of the ESR?**
ESR is a nonspecific index of inflammation. It should not be used as a screening tool in asymptomatic patients. It is indicated in the diagnosis and monitoring of temporal arteritis and polymyalgia rheumatica. It may also be helpful in monitoring therapy in rheumatoid arthritis, Hodgkin's disease, and other inflammatory disorders. ESR values can increase with age in the normal population and tend to be slightly higher in **females**. Normal values are 0 to 15 mm/hr (males) and 0 to 20 mm/hr (females).

44. **What are the symptoms of hypoglycemia, and what is the most common cause of this condition?**
Adrenergic and neuroglycopenic derangements occur as a result of hypoglycemia. Symptoms and signs include weakness, sweating, tremors, tachycardia, headache, confusion, seizure, and coma. By definition, blood glucose levels <50 mg/dl are considered hypoglycemic. The most common cause of hypoglycemia is excessive insulin dosage/administration.

45. **What three criteria must be met to diagnose hypoglycemia?**
- Presence of symptoms (adrenergic and/or neuroglycopenic)
- Low plasma glucose level in a symptomatic patient
- Relief of symptoms after ingestion of carbohydrates

46. **What are the symptoms of hyperglycemia?**
The "3 Ps" are used to remember symptoms of hyperglycemia: polydipsia, polyphagia, and polyuria.

47. **What are some of the complications of hyperglycemia and long-standing diabetes?**
Retinopathy, neuropathy (peripheral and autonomic), nephropathy, and infections are some of the complications.

48. **What is the average life span of platelets, and where are they produced?**
The life span of platelets is 7 to 10 days. Platelets are produced in the bone marrow from megakaryocytes. Platelets are necessary for blood clotting and contribute to vascular integrity, adhesion, aggregation, and subsequent platelet plug formation.

49. **What are the symptoms of thrombocytopenia?**
Symptoms include mild to severe hemorrhage, petechiae, purpura, epistaxis, hematuria, bruising, menorrhagia, and gingival bleeding. Platelet counts $>50 \times 10^9$/l are usually adequate to prevent major bleeding. Spontaneous bleeding is not uncommon with counts $<10 \times 10^9$/l.

50. **What are the three major causes of thrombocytopenia?**
- Splenic sequestration of platelets
- Increased platelet destruction
- Decreased platelet production

Splenic sequestration, or hypersplenism, can result in the pooling of platelets in the spleen and a subsequent decrease in the number of circulating platelets available for clotting.

51. **What specific clinical conditions cause thrombocytopenia?**
Thrombocytopenia can be caused by idiopathic thrombocytopenic purpura (ITP), anemias (aplastic and hemolytic), massive blood transfusions, pneumonia, infections, drugs, HIV, splenomegaly, disseminated intravascular coagulation (DIC), and thrombotic thrombocytopenic purpura (TTP). Most of these conditions cause platelet injury, platelet consumption, or platelet loss.

52. **What is thrombocytosis?**
Thrombocytosis is an increased platelet count, defined as $>400 \times 10^9/l$. This can be a primary (essential thrombocythemia), secondary (eg, leukemia, myeloma, polycythemia, splenectomy, hemorrhage, infections, or drugs), or transient process (after exercise, stress, or epinephrine injection). Clinically, thrombocytosis can cause thrombosis or bleeding or can remain asymptomatic.

53. **What are some basic facts about potassium?**
Potassium (K +) plays a major role in nerve conduction and muscle function. Total body potassium stores are roughly 3500 mEq. About 90% to 95% of potassium is intracellular and functions as a buffer. K + is the body's major cation. Approximately 5% to 10% of K + is extracellular. Routine blood testing measures only the small extracellular portion and not total body potassium. The majority of K + (90%) is excreted by the kidneys, with the remainder lost in stool and sweat.

54. **What factors influence K + levels?**
K + levels are influenced by acid-base status, hormone status, renal function, gastrointestinal loss, and nutritional status.

55. **What are the common causes of hypokalemia?**
- Cellular shift (resulting in extracellular to intracellular movement): alkalosis, insulin administration, and β-agonists
- Gastrointestinal loss: diarrhea, vomiting, nasogastric (NG) suction, laxative use, and fistulas
- Renal loss: diuretic use, magnesium deficiency, renal tubular acidosis, and Bartter syndrome
- Sweating, severe burns
- Poor dietary intake, starvation, and licorice

56. **What is a normal K + level?**
Normal K + levels are 3.5 to 5 mEq/L.

57. **What are common causes of hyperkalemia?**
- Cellular shift (resulting in intracellular to extracellular movement): cell damage (muscle injury, hemolysis, internal bleeding, burns, surgery, and acidosis) causes hyperkalemia by releasing/shifting intracellular K + into the extracellular space (blood)
- Decreased urinary excretion: renal excretion is the main elimination pathway for potassium; therefore, renal failure or decreased urinary K + excretion results in hyperkalemia
- Increased potassium intake
- Spurious: spurious causes result from hemolyzed specimen, fist clenching during blood draw, and severe thrombocytosis/leukocytosis

58. **What are the symptoms of hypokalemia and hyperkalemia?**
- Hypokalemia—muscle weakness, paralysis, cardiac arrhythmias, and electrocardiogram (ECG) changes
- Hyperkalemia—weakness, paresthesias, cardiac arrhythmias, and ECG changes

59. **What is rheumatoid factor (RF)?**
RF is an anti-γ-globulin antibody thought to be directed against the Fc portion of the IgG molecule. A large portion of patients with rheumatoid arthritis (RA) are RF positive, but the role RF plays in RA is uncertain. About 25% of patients with rheumatoid arthritis are RF negative but may become positive later in their disease course. RF is not a screening test for RA. In addition to rheumatoid arthritis, RF can be seen in systemic lupus erythematosus (SLE), chronic inflammatory processes, old age, infections, liver disease, multiple myeloma, sarcoid, and Sjögren's syndrome.

60. **How is RF reported?**
RF is reported as a titer. Values greater than 1:80 are significant; values of 1:640 and higher can be seen in rheumatoid arthritis. Higher titers can correlate with disease severity/activity.

61. **What is the human leukocyte antigen (HLA) test?**
HLAs are major histocompatibility antigens that are found on all nucleated cells and detected most easily on lymphocytes. The HLA complex is located on chromosome 6 and affects immune system functions.

62. **What is the purpose of HLA testing?**
HLA testing determines the degree of histocompatibility between a donor and recipient when organ transplantation is contemplated. The degree of HLA "matching" between donor and recipient will impact graft survival and rejection.

63. **What are other functions of HLA testing?**
HLA testing is also used in various rheumatologic disorders. The presence of a certain HLA antigen may be associated with an increased susceptibility to a specific disease, but it does not mandate the development of that disease in the patient.

64. **List the disease and corresponding HLA antigen.**

DISEASE	HLA ANTIGEN
Ankylosing spondylitis	B27
Reiter syndrome	B27
Multiple sclerosis	B27, Dw2, A3, B18
Myasthenia gravis	B8
Psoriasis	A13, B17
Graves' disease	B27
Rheumatoid arthritis	Dw4, DR4

65. **What percentage of patients with ankylosing spondylitis are HLA-B27 positive?**
About 90% of patients with ankylosing spondylitis are HLA-B27 positive.

66. **What is C-reactive protein (CRP)?**
CRP is a protein that is present in the blood during periods of inflammation (infection, tissue damage). Besides blood, it can be found in peritoneal, pleural, synovial, and pericardial fluid. Diseases such as rheumatoid arthritis, SLE, inflammatory bowel disease, bacterial infection, and malignancy result in increased CRP levels.

67. **What is a normal value for CRP?**
A normal value for CRP is <0.8 mg/dl. The presence of CRP can be detected 16 to 24 hours after the inciting inflammatory event.

68. **What is the importance of creatine phosphokinase/creatine kinase (CPK/CK)?**
CK is an enzyme found in high levels in skeletal muscle (MM), cardiac muscle (MM and MB), and brain tissue (BB). Tissue injury results in CPK enzyme elevations, and the specific isoenzyme (MM, MB, BB) reflects the affected organ or source.

69. **List some of the more common causes of CK-MM (skeletal) elevation.**
The MM isoenzyme is found in skeletal muscle. Common causes for elevation include rhabdomyolysis, myositis, crush injury/trauma, polymyositis, dermatomyositis, vigorous exercise, muscular dystrophy, seizures, and IM injection.

70. **What are the causes of CK-MB elevation?**
Myocardial infarction, muscular dystrophy, myocarditis, and cardiac surgery all contribute to CK-MB elevation.

71. **What are the causes of CK-BB elevation?**
CK-BB elevation can be caused by severe brain injury, hyperthermia, Reye's syndrome, and uremia.

72. **What are the general functions of sodium?**
In general, sodium affects acid-base balance, osmotic pressure balance, and nerve transmission. Sodium concentrations are regulated by the renal system, CNS, and endocrine systems acting in concert. Despite wide variations in sodium intake, serum levels are maintained within a narrow therapeutic range. The normal serum sodium level is 135 to 148 mEq/l. Changes in body water and salt balance are determined/monitored by serum sodium levels.

73. **What factors play a role in sodium homeostasis?**
Renal blood flow, carbonic anhydrase activity, aldosterone, pituitary hormones, renin, and antidiuretic hormone are important in sodium homeostasis.

74. **What are the symptoms of hyponatremia?**
Manifestations vary with the degree of hyponatremia and the rapidity of onset. Confusion, muscle cramps, lethargy, anorexia, and nausea are seen with moderate hyponatremia or gradual onset of hyponatremia. Severe hyponatremia or rapid onset can lead to seizures or coma.

75. What are the causes of hyponatremia?
There are many causes: 1) hypotonic (isovolemic, hypovolemic, or hypervolemic); 2) isotonic; or 3) hypertonic. Within these categories are renal losses (diuretic use, urinary obstruction), extrarenal losses (vomiting, diarrhea, burns, third spacing), adrenal insufficiency, syndrome of inappropriate antidiuretic hormone (SIADH), water intoxication, renal failure, NSAID use, ACE inhibitor use, CHF, nephrosis, cirrhosis, pseudohyponatremia, and hyperglycemia.

76. How are hyponatremia and hypernatremia similar?
The clinical manifestations (confusion, lethargy, seizures, and coma) relate to the degree of hyponatremia or hypernatremia and the rapidity of onset of the electrolyte disturbance.

77. A patient with low serum sodium levels, tachycardia, hypotension, vomiting, diarrhea, and diuretic use has what form of hyponatremia?
This patient is volume depleted and is suffering from hypovolemic hyponatremia. Treatment is isotonic fluid replacement.

78. A patient with low serum sodium levels, edema, CHF, cirrhosis, and renal failure has what form of hyponatremia?
This patient is volume overloaded and is suffering from hypervolemic hyponatremia. Both sodium and water are increased, but water is increased proportionally more than sodium. Treatment is sodium and water restriction and diuretic therapy.

79. What are the causes of hypernatremia?

- Isovolemic (decreased total body water + normal total body sodium levels): diabetes insipidus, skin loss
- Hypervolemic (increased total body water + marked increase in body sodium levels): iatrogenic administration of high sodium solutions, salt intake
- Hypovolemic (loss of body water > loss of body sodium): renal losses, GI losses, respiratory losses, and skin losses

80. List some normal laboratory values.

TEST	LOW VALUE	HIGH VALUE
WBC count	<5000/mm^3	>10,000/mm^3
Neutrophils	<55%	>70%
Lymphocytes	>20%	>40%
Monocytes	<2%	>8%
Eosinophils	<1%	>4%
Basophils	<0.5%	>1%
RBC (male)	<4.7 million/mm^3	>6.1 million/mm^3
RBC (female)	<4.2 million/mm^3	>5.4 million/mm^3
MCV	<80 mm^3	>95 mm^3
MCH	<27 pg	>31 pg
MCHC	<32 g/dl	>36 g/dl
Hemoglobin (male)	<14 g/dl	<16 g/dl
Hemoglobin (female)	<12 g/dl	<14 g/dl
Hematocrit (male)	<45%	>52%
Hematocrit (female)	<37%	>47%
Platelets	<150,000 mm^3	>400,000 mm^3
ESR (male)	Up to 15 mm/hr is normal	

TEST	LOW VALUE	HIGH VALUE
ESR (female)	Up to 20 mm/hr is normal	
CPK (male)	<12 units/ml	>70 units/ml
CPK (female)	<10 units/ml	>55 units/ml
ANA	Normal findings are no ANA detected in a titer with a dilution of >1:32	
CRP	—	>1 mg/dl
Rheumatoid factor	Abnormal if present	

81. **What do these figures represent?**

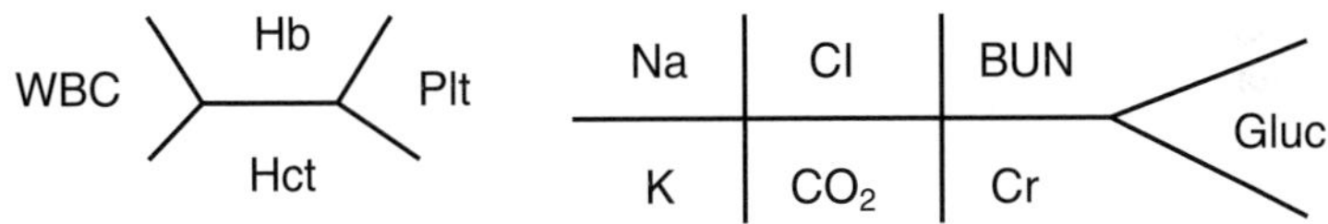

Laboratory values are usually recorded as follows:

- WBC, white blood cell count
- Hb, hemoglobin level
- Hct, hematocrit level
- Plt, platelet count
- Na, sodium concentration
- K, potassium concentration
- Cl, chloride concentration
- CO_2, bicarbonate concentration
- BUN, blood urea nitrogen level
- Cr, creatinine level
- Gluc, glucose level

82. **What is the role of Hemoglobin A1C?**
HA1C is a measure of "chronic glycemia" and correlates with average blood glucose levels over the preceding 2 to 3 months. HA1C is used to both diagnose prediabetes, type 1 and 2 diabetes, and monitor response to diabetic treatments.

83. **Besides Hemoglobin A1C (HA1C), what is the other traditional marker of hyperglycemia?**
Fasting glucose and HA1C are considered the traditional markers of hyperglycemia. Fasting glucose is an acute and direct measurement of blood glucose. HA1C indirectly measures glycated hemoglobin that correlates with various glucose levels.

84. **What is a normal HA1C value?**
Normal HA1C range is 4% to 5.6%. Values between 5.7% and 6.4 % represent prediabetes. Levels greater than 6.5 % represents diabetes.

85. **What is brain natriuretic peptide (BNP)?**
BNP is a natriuretic hormone released from the heart and ventricles. BNP is elevated in setting of heart failure secondary to cardiac wall stretching and subsequent release of hormone from cardiac muscle.

86. **What is the role of measuring BNP in the clinical setting?**
BNP levels help distinguish cardiac versus noncardiac causes of shortness of breath. Normal levels help rule out heart failure as a cause for dyspnea.

87. **What are normal and abnormal BNP values?**
Normal BNP = <100 pg/ml. Elevated BNP = >400 pg/ml. Patients with shortness of breath due to heart failure have BNP values >400 pg/ml.

88. **Are BNP values between 100 pg/ml and 400 pg/ml specific for heart failure?**
No, this range of BNP elevation can be seen in left ventricle dysfunction, pulmonary embolism, renal failure, pulmonary hypertension, etc. and is considered a gray area and therefore inconclusive.

89. **What labs are used to assess thyroid function?**
Serum TSH, Serum total, and free T3 and T4.

90. **What are markers of hypothyroidism and hyperthyroidism?**
Elevated serum TSH equates with hypothyroidism. Decreased TSH correlates with hyperthyroidism.

91. **What are classic symptoms of hyperthyroidism?**
Sweating, heat intolerance, thinning of hair, lid lag, tachycardia, diarrhea, weight loss.

92. **What are classic symptoms of hypothyroidism?**
Fatigue, weakness, cold intolerance, weight gain, constipation, bradycardia, depression.

BIBLIOGRAPHY

Henry, J. B. (1996). *Clinical diagnosis and management by laboratory methods* (19th ed.). Philadelphia, PA: WB Saunders.
McDonagh, T. A. (1998). Biochemical detection of left-ventricular systolic dysfunction. *Lancet, 351*, 9.
McMorrow, M. E., & Malarkey, L. (1998). *Laboratory and diagnostic tests: a pocket guide.* Philadelphia, PA: WB Saunders.
Pagana, K. D., & Pagana, T. J. (1992). *Mosby's diagnostic and laboratory test reference.* St. Louis, MO: Mosby.
Rave, R. (1995). *Clinical laboratory medicine: clinical application of laboratory data* (6th ed.). St. Louis, MO: Mosby.
Vaughn, G. (1999). *Understanding and evaluating common laboratory tests.* Stamford, CT: Appleton & Lange.

CHAPTER 16 QUESTIONS

1. A 70-year-old male taking medication for hypertension and diabetes develops profound muscle weakness after 4 days of vomiting and diarrhea. The patient has a history of chronic, stable constipation. Serum potassium level is 2.3 mEq/l (range 3.5–5.0 mEq/l). Which of the following is not associated with his symptoms of severe hypokalemia?
   a. Vomiting
   b. Diuretic use
   c. Acidosis
   d. Diarrhea
   e. Alkalosis

2. Which of the following are not associated with hypercalcemia?
   a. Malignancy
   b. Sarcoidosis
   c. Hyperparathyroidism
   d. Vitamin D deficiency
   e. Thiazide diuretics

3. Severe hemorrhage, petechiae, purpura, epistaxis, hematuria, and bruising are signs of which condition?
   a. Leukocytosis
   b. Thrombocytosis
   c. Thrombocytopenia
   d. Hypoalbuminemia
   e. Hypocalcemia

4. A 70-year-old male presents to the emergency department with shortness of breath, pitting edema, and lower extremity cellulitis. Patient is diagnosed with congestive heart failure and uncontrolled diabetes. What BNP and HA1C values would you expect in this patient?
   a. BNP <100 pg/ml and HA1C 4%–5.6%
   b. BNP <100 pg/ml and HA1C >6.5%
   c. BNP >400 pg/ml and HA1C 4%–5.6%
   d. BNP >400 pg/ml and HA1C >6.5%

5. **True or False: Fasting blood glucose represents acute blood glucose control whereas HA1C reflects chronic glycemic states.**

   True, HA1C provides a 2 to 3 month "history" or snapshot of patients' blood glucose control. This is helpful as various HA1C values correlate with an average blood glucose value over the past 2 to 3 months.

6. **A 65-year-old female presents with tachycardia, weight loss and diarrhea. You make a clinical diagnosis of hyperthyroidism. What lab values are consistent with this diagnosis?**

   a. TSH elevated
   b. TSH decreased
   c. TSH normal
   d. Free T3 decreased

CHAPTER 17

ELECTRODIAGNOSTIC TESTS: NERVE CONDUCTION STUDIES AND NEEDLE ELECTROMYOGRAPHY

M.E. Brooks, DSc, PT, ECS, OCS, R.J. McKibben, PT, DSc, ECS, and E. Armantrout, PT (retired), DSc

1. **What are the most common electrodiagnostic (EDX) tests performed in clinical practice?**
The most commonly performed tests are nerve conduction studies (NCS) and needle electromyography (EMG).
During NCS, an external electrical stimulus is applied to a mixed peripheral nerve. That stimulus is of an intensity to generate a sensory nerve action potential (SNAP) or a compound motor nerve action potential (CMAP). SNAPs are recorded cutaneously from another portion of the nerve while a CMAP is recorded cutaneously from a muscle that the nerve innervates.
Needle EMG involves recording of subcutaneous bioelectric potentials generated by the motor unit, both at rest and during muscle contraction. Findings generated by both tests are interpreted by the clinician during the EDX examination as decisions on what additional NCS or EMG tests to be performed are based on the findings gathered in real time by the examiner.

2. **What is the clinical usefulness of NCS and Needle EMG?**
Electrodiagnostic tests including both NCS and EMG are an extension of the clinical examination of the neuromuscular system. As such, they are considered to be tests and measurements. While these tests generally give information on the physiologic status of the peripheral nervous system, some information about the status of the central nervous system may also be obtained.
NCS evaluates the status of the myelin sheath of both afferent (sensory) fibers and efferent (motor) fibers of the peripheral nerves. Some information may be obtained about the status of sensory nerve axon damage. EMG assesses the status of the motor axons and to a lesser extent the status of motor myelin.
NCS and EMG studies are used to identify normal or abnormal peripheral neurophysiologic function and can identify the location, chronicity, and severity of the abnormal process. They are useful in assessing presence, location, and prognosis of peripheral neurophysiological dysfunction.
NCS and EMG studies in and of themselves are not diagnostic. The diagnosis of a neuromuscular condition is obtained from the patient's history, symptoms, system review, other laboratory and imaging tests, and a comprehensive neuromusculoskeletal examination that may include an NCS and EMG study.

3. **When is most appropriate to refer for an NCS/EMG examination?**
NCS and EMG studies are helpful in assessing conditions affecting the peripheral nerves, the motor unit (anterior horn cell, motor axon, neuromuscular junction), and muscles. Common symptoms experienced by a patient when the peripheral is affected include abnormal skin sensation/numbness and tingling, muscle weakness and fatigability, muscle atrophy, and pain.
Conditions commonly assessed by NCS and EMG studies include compressive neuropathies such as carpal tunnel syndrome, cervical or lumbosacral radiculopathy, peripheral polyneuropathy, myopathy, neuromuscular junction disorders, and motor neuron disease. NCS and EMG studies are of limited or no use in detection of central nervous system disorders, joint disease, and pain in the absence of neuromuscular abnormalities.

4. **What are examples of compression neuropathies and diseases of nerve and muscle that NCS/EMG studies can assess?**
Focal Neuropathies
   - Carpal tunnel syndrome (median neuropathy at the wrist)
   - Cubital tunnel syndrome (ulnar neuropathy at the elbow)
   - Saturday night palsy (radial neuropathy at spiral groove)
   - Radial tunnel syndrome (radial neuropathy in forearm/elbow)
   - Pronator teres syndrome (median neuropathy at/about elbow)
   - Handlebar palsy (ulnar neuropathy at wrist/palm)
   - Rucksack palsy (long thoracic nerve)
   - Suprascapular nerve palsy
   - Axillary neuropathy following shoulder dislocation
   - Tarsal tunnel syndrome (posterior tibial neuropathy at ankle/foot)
   - Peroneal neuropathy at the fibular head

- Meralgia Paresthetica (lateral femoral cutaneous neuropathy)
- Brachial or lumbosacral plexopathy

Radiculopathy

- Cervical radiculopathy
- Thoracic radiculopathy
- Lumbosacral Radiculopathy

Plexopathy

- Brachial plexopathy
- Parsonage-Turner syndrome
- Diabetic amyotrophy
- Lumbosacral plexopathy

Polyneuropathy

- Diabetic
- Toxic (alcoholic, heavy metal, uremic)
- Inflammatory
- Hereditary
- Idiopathic

Myopathy

- Poly or dermatomyositis, inclusion body, muscular dystrophy, myotonia

Motor Neuronopathy

- ALS, post-polio syndrome, spinal muscular atrophy

Neuromuscular Junction Disorders

- Myasthenia gravis, myasthenic syndrome, botulism

5. **What are the common terms used to describe NCS findings?**

Latency: The time interval measured in milliseconds (ms) from when the electrical stimulus is applied to the nerve and when the SNAP or CMAP is recorded from the surface electrodes. Latency is described as normal or prolonged. A prolonged latency may be indicative of damage to the myelin or a cool temperature, both of which cause slowing of the action potential.

Amplitude: The measured size of the action potential. It reflects the number of axons that are depolarized and contributes to the size of the action potential. SNAP amplitude is measured in microvolts (μV) and CMAP amplitude is measured in millivolts (mV). Amplitude is described as normal or low (diminished). Low amplitude responses may be indicative of axon loss or conduction blocking. Cool limb temperatures may cause an increase in amplitude, especially in sensory nerves.

Nerve Conduction Velocity (NCV): NCV is the speed of conduction of an action potential over a specific measured distance. It is measured in meters/second (m/s). It is calculated by dividing the distance of the segment by the time it takes the action potential to traverse the segment. NCV is described as normal or slowed. As with latency, a slowed NCV may be indicative of myelin damage or cool limb temperature.

Duration: Duration is the time interval from initial deflection of an action potential recording from the baseline and return to the baseline. It also is measured in milliseconds (ms). It reflects the number and synchrony of the depolarized axons. Duration is described as normal or prolonged. Prolonged duration again may be indicative of myelin damage, or in normal nerves due to cool temperature or normal temporal dispersion due to limb length.

6. **What are the common terms used to describe EMG findings?**

Insertional Activity: The electrical activity that occurs with mechanical depolarization of the muscle fibers due to needle insertion and movement through the muscle. It is measured in milliseconds (ms). Insertional activity is described as normal, decreased, or increased. Decreased insertional activity is typically seen in chronic conditions where the muscle fibers have become fibrotic due to denervation or muscle fiber necrosis. Increased insertional activity is indicative of an unstable muscle membrane, due to denervation or in early muscle fiber necrosis. Typically increased insertional activity is seen in acute or ongoing conditions. Normal insertional activity is between 50 and 350 ms.

Resting Activity: Normal resting muscle is electrically silent. However, if the muscle membrane is unstable, due to either denervation or muscle fiber necrosis, the muscle fibers (or groups of muscle fibers) may spontaneously generate muscle fiber action potentials. Typically these include fibrillation potentials and/or positive sharp waves. Other types of spontaneous resting activity may include fasciculations, complex repetitive discharges, or myotonic discharges. Under certain circumstances spontaneous activity may be seen in normal muscle. These include fasciculations and if the needle is near the neuromuscular junction (end plate spikes or end plate potentials).

Voluntary Activity: Involves the contraction of the muscle and assessment of the motor unit action potential (MUAP) configuration (morphology) and ability to generate additional motor units (recruitment). A normal motor unit has four or less phases (number of times the potential crosses the baseline), an amplitude of less than 5 mV, a duration of less than 12 ms, and a firing frequency of 10 to 12 Hz (cycles per second). MUAPs with four or greater phases are called polyphasic and in neurogenic conditions may be associated with a larger than normal amplitude and prolonged duration. Myopathic MUAPs may exhibit shorter than normal duration polyphasic motor units that are low amplitude.

Recruitment: The ability of a muscle to sequentially recruit additional MUAPs as the degree of voluntary contraction increases. Muscles increase force by increasing firing frequency of motor units and recruiting additional motor units to meet resistance demands. In normal muscle contraction, a motor unit will initially fire around 5 Hz and the recruitment of a second MUAP usually occurs when the firing frequency of the first MUAP is around 10 Hz. The first will continue to increase frequency and reach a firing frequency of about 15 Hz when the third unit is recruited and so on. The inability of a muscle to recruit additional MUAPs when firing at a rate of more than 12 to 15 Hz is called reduced recruitment. This is seen in neurogenic conditions and occurs because there are not enough motor units to meet resistance demands. Subsequently, the ability to recruit additional MUAPs is significantly reduced and the functional MUAPs may continue to fire at higher and higher frequencies, often >30 Hz. In myopathic conditions, MUAPs may fire with very minimal contraction. This is called early (or myopathic) recruitment.

Interference Pattern: Interference pattern is the ability to fill the screen with firing MUAPs. While abnormal interference patterns may be seen in pathology, it may also be indicative of decreased effort due to pain, anxiety, or an attempt to simulate weakness.

7. What are examples of pathologic processes assessed with NCS/EMG?

Focal Demyelination and Conduction Block: There are two main types of myelin damage. Paranodal demyelination involves a widening of the distance between nodes of Ranvier. This type of demyelination leads to slowing of neural transmission (prolonged latency and slowed NCV). Internodal demyelination involves the loss of entire nodal segments (nodes of Ranvier). This type of demyelination leads to a blocking of action potential transmission across the site of the nodal segments (partial or complete conduction block). Focal demyelination may typically be seen in compressive neuropathies such as carpal tunnel syndrome.

Diffuse Demyelination: Diffuse demyelination is typically seen in diffuse processes such as polyneuropathy and is seen in multiple sites along the nerve.

Axon Loss: This process involves damage to and/or loss of motor or sensory axons. With NCS, sensory axon pathology may present as a lower than normal amplitude SNAP or an absent response. Motor axon pathology may show a lower than normal amplitude with NCS or abnormal needle EMG findings with insertion, rest, and volitional testing. Axon loss may be seen in focal neuropathies, radiculopathy, polyneuropathy, and motor neuron disease.

Mixed Lesions: Mixed lesions may involve focal NCV slowing, conduction block, or axon loss.

Prognostic Assessment: Generally demyelinating processes have a good prognostic outlook. Sensory axon loss with an intact SNAP generally has a good prognosis. Motor axon loss with retention of greater than 20% to 25% of motor axons has a good prognosis. However, motor axon loss of greater than 75% to 80% of axons has a guarded, less favorable prognosis and is likely to be protracted.

8. What are the normal values for nerve conduction study parameters?

Normative values vary among EDX laboratories due to methodological differences in testing. There are many published normative data sets for a variety of NCS procedures. The table below reflects examples of typically expected: values of latency, amplitude, and NCV for upper and lower extremity nerves. Caution is advised when interpreting data based on a single NCS finding as it is most appropriate to demonstrate corroborative EDX findings to confirm abnormal NCS function.

	DISTAL LATENCY	AMPLITUDE	CONDUCTION VELOCITY
Upper limb motor nerve (8-cm distance)	<4.2 ms	>4 mV	>50 m/sec
Sensory nerve (14-cm distance)	<3.5 ms	>10 μV	>40 m/sec
Lower limb motor nerve (8-cm distance)	<6.0 ms	>2 mV	>39 m/sec
Sensory nerve (14-cm distance)	<4.0 ms	>10 μV	>35 m/sec

9. What are some limitations of NCS/EMG studies?

EDX findings generally are highly specific but less sensitive. Often in subtle neuropathic processes such as early/mild radiculopathy or transient focal neuropathies such as radial tunnel syndrome or pronator syndrome, NCS/EMG studies may be normal when a patient has a clinical presentation of certain neuropathic processes.

Radiculopathies are nerve injuries that are preganglionic (proximal to the dorsal root ganglion) and sensory nerve studies will be normal unless the injury is distal to the dorsal root ganglion. When sensory fibers are primarily involved the EMG will be normal. It takes 14 to 21 days for acute muscle membrane instability findings such as fibrillations and positive sharp waves to develop and be detected by EMG. In a completely transected nerve or in severe conduction block, voluntary motor units are absent in muscles innervated by the nerve distal to the lesion site.

Also, NCS records only the largest diameter motor and sensory fiber function. Small diameter nerve fiber injury or disease is not detectable by NCS and EMG studies.

10. What is the sensitivity and specificity of NCS and EMG?

In general EDX studies are highly specific and moderately sensitive.

CONDITION	DETERMINES	SENSITIVITY	SPECIFICITY
Carpal tunnel syndrome	Slowing, conduction block +/or axonal loss	>85%	95%
Ulnar neuropathy at the elbow	Slowing, conduction block +/or axonal loss	37%–86%	95%
Cervical radiculopathy	Presence & location of axonal injury of the motor nerve root	50%–71%	65%–85%
Lumbosacral radiculopathy	Presence & location of axonal injury of the motor nerve root	29%–92%	37%–100%
Distal symmetric polyneuropathy	Type and severity of neuropathy	80%–83%	72%–89%
Tarsal tunnel syndrome	Conduction delay, conduction block +/or axonal loss	Unknown	Unknown
Peroneal neuropathy at fib head	Conduction delay, conduction block +/or axonal loss	Unknown	Peroneal neuropathy at fib head

11. Can NCS and EMG differentiate between myopathy vs neuropathy?

Yes. In myopathy, NCS studies are generally normal except in severe cases. Extensive muscle fiber necrosis seen in severe myopathies or end stage myopathies may exhibit lower than normal CMAP amplitudes. Slowing of NCS parameters is not a hallmark of myopathy as myelin and axons are not affected.

During needle EMG, myopathies will present with abnormal resting activity, MUAP morphology, and recruitment. Muscles examined at rest will show evidence of membrane instability including fibrillations, positive sharp waves, and complex repetitive or myotonic discharges. During contraction motor units will be short duration, low amplitude, and polyphasic (SLAPP). Additionally, with minimal contraction, the interference pattern will be full (early recruitment). These findings will typically be seen in the most affected (weak or atrophied) muscles and in a proximal > distal distribution.

In a neuropathy NCS abnormalities may include slowing of conduction, low amplitude or absent responses, and prolonged duration and/or abnormal temporal dispersion).

EMG findings may include abnormal insertional activity and spontaneous findings due to muscle membrane instability (denervation), highly polyphasic or larger than normal amplitude MUAPs, and abnormal recruitment including reduced numbers of volitional MUAPs or a fast firing recruitment pattern.

12. Can neuromuscular junction disorders be evaluated by NCS/EMG studies?

Yes. NCS studies are an integral tool in the evaluation of neuromuscular junction disorders.

Typically sensory NCS findings are normal. However, during motor NCS studies, CMAP amplitudes may be variable. In postsynaptic conditions such as myasthenia gravis, the CMAP amplitudes initially will be normal. However, as the muscles fatigue, the CMAP amplitudes will become lower in amplitude. In presynaptic conditions such as myasthenic syndrome (Lambert Eaton myasthenic syndrome) and botulism, the CMAP amplitude will initially be smaller and then increase in amplitude with muscle exertion.

Repetitive nerve stimulation studies (RNS), a specialized NCS study, are also clinically useful. In post synaptic conditions, when a stimulus is applied at 3 to 5 Hz, an amplitude decrease of greater than 10% between the first and fifth CMAPs is considered abnormal and indicative of a postsynaptic condition affecting the neuromuscular junction.

During needle EMG, MUAPs may exhibit a variability in amplitude or may drop out altogether. This is due to blocking of acetylcholine uptake on the postsynaptic membrane.

13. **What is a somatosensory evoked potential (SSEP) study? When is an SSEP study appropriate?**

SSEP is the study of sensory nerve pathways between the extremity and the dorsal column in the spinal cord to the somatosensory cortex. It is performed by stimulating the peripheral nerve and recording through multiple channels at more proximal segments along the nerve, including one or more sites along the spine and at the somatosensory cortex. When a weakness or loss of sensation is significant and there are signs that the location of the lesion could be of central nervous system (spinal cord or brain) origin, the use of SSEP is appropriate. SSEP would be more likely to show a nerve root (preganglionic) sensory nerve lesion than an NCS/EMG study.

14. **Since EMG changes are sporadic in the first 3 weeks of injury, is there any value in requesting an EDX examination before then?**

Yes. An NCS study immediately after the onset of the condition or injury will help to determine if the nerve is still in continuity and establish a baseline for further serial studies.

Typically it takes 5 to 7 days for a motor axon and 9 to 11 days for a sensory axon to undergo complete Wallerian degeneration. When stimulating distal to the site of injury, the SNAP or CMAP initially may be normal since Wallerian degeneration has not yet occurred. Subsequently as Wallerian degeneration occurs, the SNAP or CMAP will decrease in amplitude. If it is a complete lesion, after 7 to 11 days there will be no recordable response. Preservation of a SNAP or CMAP after this time period is generally a good prognostic sign.

Needle EMG findings may be variable. While it may take up to 3 weeks to observe widespread muscle membrane instability with EMG in motor axon loss, abnormalities may be seen, particularly in more proximal muscles, within the first week. Recruitment abnormalities may also be seen immediately, depending on the number of motor axons affected.

15. **Can the severity of a focal neuropathy be graded using NCS and EMG?**

Yes. Most clinicians grade severity of focal neuropathies. There are many scales published for several focal neuropathic conditions (ie, median neuropathy at the wrist, ulnar neuropathy at the elbow, etc.). While they vary to some degree, there are consistent traits that electrodiagnosticians employ that maintain reasonable consistency when determining severity of neuropathy. The following table describes a suggested severity rating scale that can be applicable to any focal neuropathy.

SEVERITY GRADE	ABNORMAL EDX FINDINGS
Normal	All NCS and EMG findings are normal.
Very mild	Abnormal NCS only with most sensitive NCS tests (short-segment or comparison studies).
Mild	Abnormal sensory NCS with preserved SNAP amplitudes and/or abnormal motor latencies/NCVs within 10%–15% above/below the limits of normal.
Moderate	Abnormal sensory NCS with reduced SNAP amplitudes and/or abnormal motor latencies/NCVs exceeding 10%–15% above/below the limits of normal with preserved motor amplitudes. Mild EMG changes.
Severe	Absent sensory NCS and/or reduced motor amplitude above 80% of normal limits. Moderate to Advanced EMG changes.
Very Severe	Motor amplitudes less than 80% of normal. Advanced EMG changes.

16. **What is Wallerian degeneration and how long does it take a peripheral nerve lesion to recover?**

Wallerian degeneration is disruption of the myelin and axons along the entire length of the nerve below the site of an axonal lesion. In compressive lesions, generally the endoneurium remains intact, leaving a conduit for a regenerating axon to reach its target organ in a healthy body. However, it is often slowed when metabolic comorbidities are present. The approximate rate of nerve regeneration is 6 mm per day for a root level lesion, 2 mm per day for a forearm level lesion, and 1 mm per day for a hand or lower leg level lesion. If a target organ (muscle fiber) is not reinnervated within 12 to 18 months, the myofiber will atrophy and become nonviable.

CASE STUDY

A 21-year-old male long jumper had a 4-week history of right foot weakness along with numbness and tingling in the lateral leg and dorsal foot, which reportedly followed daily training room treatments of ice application secured with a tight elastic wrap for a lateral distal hamstring strain over the past month. Manual muscle test demonstrated 2/5 strength of dorsiflexion, eversion, toe extension, and great toe extension. Sensation was decreased to pinprick along the dorsum of the foot. Patellar and Achilles monosynaptic reflexes were 2 + and symmetrical bilaterally.

Electrodiagnostic examination exhibited a common fibular conduction velocity of 20 m/sec across the fibular head segment and 40 m/sec in the distal lower leg segment. The CMAP amplitude was 400 μV with stimulation above the fibular head and 2.0 mV with stimulation below the fibular head. The CMAP amplitude on the unaffected side was 6 mV. The superficial fibular sensory nerve response was not elicited on the affected side and was intact and normal on the unaffected side. Needle EMG demonstrated positive sharp waves and fibrillation potentials in the right anterior tibialis, fibularis longus, and extensor hallucis longus, along with reduced fast firing motor unit recruitment. The remainder of the needle EMG examination, including the short head of the biceps femoris, tibialis posterior, medial gastrocnemius, and lumbosacral paraspinals was unremarkable.

17. From the information given above, describe the location of the nerve injury, the neural structures involved, severity, and prognosis.

The NCS and EMG studies are consistent with a severe focal neuropathy of the common fibular nerve at or about the fibular head (distal to innervation of the short head of the biceps femoris) with evidence of motor and sensory axonopathy and demyelination. Focal demyelination is confirmed by the isolated slowing of the deep fibular nerve across the fibular head segment and drop in amplitude with proximal stimulation consistent with significant partial conduction block. Acute denervation is confirmed by the presence of positive sharp waves and fibrillation potentials along with reduced, fast firing motor unit recruitment in the right common fibular nerve distribution distal to the innervation of the short head biceps femoris as well as a distal motor amplitude below the lower limit of normal. Prognosis is good given the preservation of distal motor amplitude, but the injury will take several months to recover assuming also that the mechanism of the injury is resolved.

BIBLIOGRAPHY

AANEM Practice Guidelines. http://www.aanem.org/Practice/Practice-Guidelines.aspx. Accessed 07/07/14.

APTA, (2014). *Guide to physical therapy practice* (3rd ed.). Alexandria, VA: APTA.

Dolan, C., & Bromberg, M. (2010). Nerve conduction pitfalls and pearls in the diagnosis of peripheral neuropathies. *Seminars in Neurology, 30*(4), 436–442.

Dumitru, D. (2001). *Electrodiagnostic medicine* (2nd ed.). Philadelphia, PA: Hanley & Belfus.

Heise, C. O., Machado, F. C., DeAmorim, S. C., et al. (2012). Combined nerve conduction index in diabetic polyneuropathy. *Arquivos de Neuro-Psiquiatria, 70*(5), 330–334.

Kimura, J. (2013). *Electrodiagnosis in disease of nerve and muscle* (4th ed.). New York, NY: Oxford University Press.

Menorca, R. M., Fussel, T. S., & Elfar, J. C. (2013). Nerve physiology: mechanisms of injury and recovery. *Hand Clinics, 29*(3), 317–330.

O'Sullivan, S. B., McKibben, R. J., & Portney, L. G. (2019). Examination of motor function: motor control and motor learning. In S. B. O'Sullivan, T. J. Schmitz, & G. Fulk (Eds.), *Physical rehabilitation* (7th ed.). McGraw Hill. APTA Guide to Physical Therapist Practice 4.0. American Physical Therapy Association. Published 2023. Accessed [DATE]. https://guide.apta.org.

CHAPTER 17 QUESTIONS

1. Slowed NCV and conduction block implicate involvement of what neural structures?
   a. Axons
   b. Myelin
   c. Neuromuscular junction
   d. Dorsal root ganglion

2. Which EMG findings are suggestive of a myopathic process?
   a. Reduced insertional activity
   b. Requires maximal contraction to recruit motor units
   c. Larger than normal amplitude motor units
   d. Short duration, low amplitude polyphasic motor units

3. A 35-year-old male fell on an outstretched arm 6 weeks ago and developed pain and paresthesias in the medial arm forearm and digits IV-V. He has weakness in intrinsic hand muscles including the thenar muscles and weakness in digital extension. NCS shows low amplitude median/ulnar/radial motor responses with no response in the ulnar and medial cutaneous in the forearm. There are fibrillations and positive sharp waves with reduced and fast firing recruitment in the APB, FDI, EDC, and triceps. There are no findings noted in the lower cervical paraspinals. Based on these findings, which of the following is the most likely involved?
   a. C8 spinal nerve
   b. Lower trunk
   c. Medial cord
   d. Ulnar nerve

ORTHOPAEDIC NEUROLOGY

N. Nevin, PT, DPT, OCS, MTC, FAAOMPT, M.M. Danzl, PT, DPT, PhD, NCS, E. Ulanowski, DPT, and M.R. Wiegand, PT, PhD

1. **What are the common myotomes tested in an upper and a lower quarter screening examination?**

SPINAL SEGMENT LEVEL	MYOTOME (A GROUP OF MUSCLES SUPPLIED BY ONE VENTRAL NERVE ROOT)
C3-4	Shoulder elevators and cervical rotators
C5	Shoulder abductors and external rotators
C6	Elbow flexors and wrist extensors
C7	Elbow extensors and wrist flexors
C8	Thumb and finger extensors
T1	Hand intrinsic muscles
L2-3	Hip flexors
L3-4	Knee extensors
L4-5	Ankle dorsiflexors
L5	Hallux extensors and hip abductors
L5-S1	Knee flexors
S1	Plantar flexors

2. **What are the common dermatomes tested in an upper and a lower quarter screening examination?**

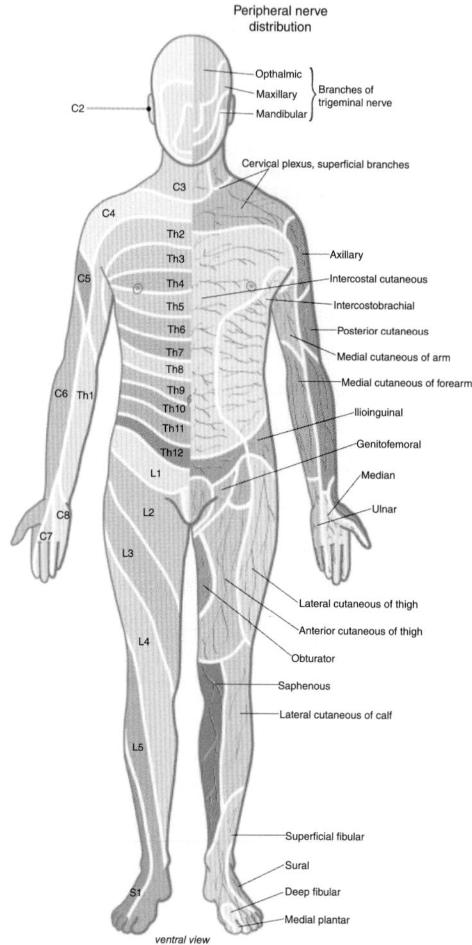

Dermatome and peripheral nerve distributions, anterior view. (Brouwer, B. A., Joosten, B., Kleef, M. (2018). Spinal cord stimulation for peripheral neuropathic pain. In *Neuromodulation* (ed 2). Elsevier.)

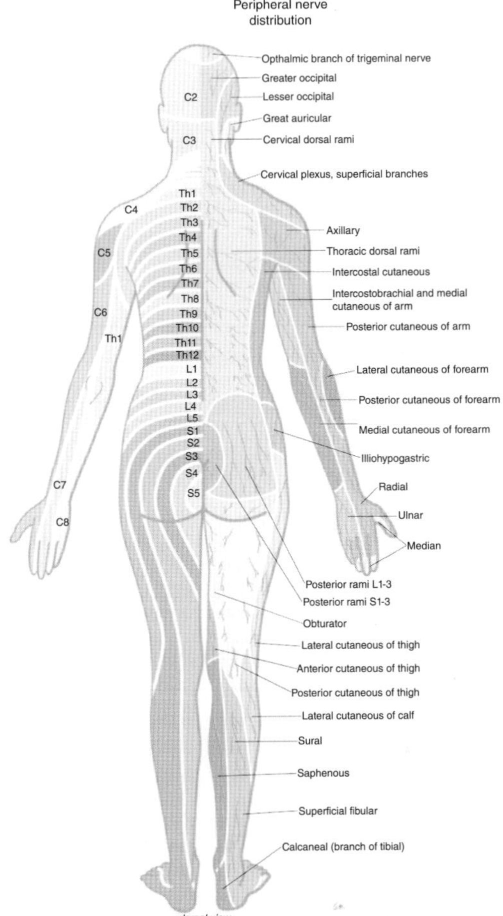

Dermatome and peripheral nerve distributions, posterior view. (Brouwer, B. A., Joosten, B., Kleef, M. (2018). Spinal cord stimulation for peripheral neuropathic pain. In *Neuromodulation* (ed 2). Elsevier.)

SPINAL ROOT	DERMATOME (AREA OF SKIN SUPPLIED BY ONE DORSAL NERVE ROOT)
C1	Top of head
C2	Side of head
C3-4	Lateral neck and top of shoulder
C5	Lateral shoulder and arm
C6	Lateral forearm, thumb, and second digit of the hand
C7	Third and fourth digits of the hand
C8	Fourth and fifth digits of the hand
T1-2	Medial forearm and arm
L1-2	Groin

Continued

SPINAL ROOT	DERMATOME (AREA OF SKIN SUPPLIED BY ONE DORSAL NERVE ROOT)
L2-3	Anterior and medial thigh
L4	Medial lower leg
L5	Lateral lower leg and dorsum of foot
S1	Posterior lateral thigh and lower leg and lateral foot
S2	Plantar surface of foot
S3	Groin and medial thigh to knee
S4	Perineum region, genitals

3. **What are commonly tested deep tendon reflexes?**

STRETCH REFLEX	SPINAL ROOT LEVEL/CRANIAL NERVE
Jaw jerk	Trigeminal nerve (cranial nerve V)
Biceps	C5 - C6
Brachioradialis	C5 - C6
Triceps	C7 - C8
Quadriceps femoris	L3 - L4
Medial hamstrings, extensor digitorum brevis	L5
Achilles tendon	S1 - S2

4. **Classify the cranial nerves, their functions, and how they are tested.**

CRANIAL NERVE (CN)	FUNCTION	TEST	CLINICAL NOTE
I—Olfactory	Olfaction (smell)	Patient eyes closed. Place common strong smells (e.g., coffee, orange, vanilla, cinnamon, cloves, peppermint) under each naris (closing untested side); avoid substances such as ammonia that can stimulate CN V and result in false positive.	Cigarette smoking, cocaine use, inflammation, rhinitis, and sinus issues can interfere with smell ability. Smell may be lost posttrauma because of tearing of olfactory stria from cribriform plate of ethmoid bone (e.g., whiplash, closed head injury). Anosmia or hyposmia posttraumatic brain injury or skull fracture may be indicative of cerebrospinal fluid (CSF) rhinorrhea in which CSF leaks into nasal cavity. Anosmia is a common symptom of COVID-19 with an incident rate of 34%–68%.

CRANIAL NERVE (CN)	FUNCTION	TEST	CLINICAL NOTE
II—Optic	Vision acuity, visual fields, pupil constriction	Test visual acuity using a Snellen chart (patient stands 20 feet from chart, reads lowest line possible). Test visual fields (minimally lateral, upper, lower; can add in quadrant testing and central areas). Pupillary light reflex (sensory component); rapid constriction of pupil with light followed by dilation when light removed.	Accurate assessment of visual fields greatly aids in localization of neurologic dysfunction. For example, bitemporal hemianopsia is a common clinical presentation of tumors within the pituitary gland.
III—Oculomotor	Medial rectus, superior rectus, inferior rectus, and inferior oblique extraocular muscles (elevates eyelid, turns eye up, down, in); pupil constriction; lens accommodation	Assess conjugate eye movements by asking patient to track moving object (finger, pen) in an "H" pattern and for convergence; both eyes move smoothly, symmetrically in same direction at same speed and magnitude; no nystagmus. Pupillary light reflex (parasympathetic motor component).	Ptosis often associated with stroke or head injury. Mydriasis and anisocoria indicative of CN III palsy. Dysfunction of CN III, IV, or VI produces diplopia with head held in neutral position. Patients often present with cervical deviation to correct diplopia. Cervical deviation may be mistaken for a torticollis deformity.
IV—Trochlear	Superior oblique extraocular muscle (moves eye down and in)	Test the patient's ability to move eyes diagonally downward and toward midline.	See CN III
V—Trigeminal	Sensation from face (including cornea and anterior tongue) and motor innervation of muscles of mastication and talking	Perform sensory testing of face in ophthalmic, maxillary, and mandibular branch distributions (sharp/dull discrimination with safety pin or paperclip, light touch with cotton wisp); check ability to clench teeth and open mouth. Gently brush cornea to test afferent limb of corneal blink reflex (patient should blink eye). Test jaw jerk reflex.	An upper motor lesion produces little dysfunction because of bilateral cortical input to the lower motor neuron innervating the muscles of mastication. Lower motor neuron lesion results in unilateral paralysis and atrophy of muscles of mastication. Brief repetitive sharp and excruciating pain in CN V distributions associated with trigeminal neuralgia.
VI—Abducens	Lateral rectus extraocular muscle (abducts eye)	Test the patient's ability to move eyes away from midline.	See CN III.

Continued

CRANIAL NERVE (CN)	FUNCTION	TEST	CLINICAL NOTE
VII—Facial	Muscles of facial expression, taste from anterior tongue, tearing, and salivation	Check symmetry and smoothness of facial expressions at rest and during voluntary movement (e.g., close eyes tightly, close lips tightly). Test corneal blink reflex. Test taste sensation in anterior two-thirds of tongue (sweet, salty, sour).	Swelling within facial canal results in weakness in ipsilateral facial muscles and loss of taste from ipsilateral anterior two-thirds of tongue (Bell's palsy). There will be drooping of the cheek and eye (ptosis) on the involved side.
VIII—Vestibulocochlear	Hearing and vestibular function (balance)	Rub fingers by each ear (patient should hear equally from both ears). Rinne test (patient eyes closed, vibrating tuning fork on one mastoid process until sound no longer heard, then move vibrating tines in front of ipsilateral external ear canal; assess hearing acuity); Weber test (vibrating tuning fork on vertex of skull; sound should be fairly equal bilaterally). Move head slowly side to side to assess vestibulocochlear reflex; eyes should move in opposite direction of head movement. Check for nystagmus.	Common cause of cochlear portion damage to this nerve is an acoustic neuroma—a tumor of the Schwann cells that myelinate this nerve.
IX—Glossopharyngeal	Gag reflex, swallowing, taste from posterior tongue, and salivation	Assess gag reflex. Assess taste sensation in posterior tongue (bitterness).	Lesions of this nerve seldom occur alone. Sudden pain of unknown cause that begins in throat and radiates down side of neck in front of ear to posterior mandible usually precipitated by swallowing or protrusion of jaw is known as glossopharyngeal neuralgia.

CRANIAL NERVE (CN)	FUNCTION	TEST	CLINICAL NOTE
X—Vagus	Phonation, swallowing, and thoracic and abdominal viscera regulation	Ask the patient to say "ah"; observe elevation of soft palate.	CN X lesion causes unilateral soft palate paralysis in which one side rises less than nonaffected side (uvula deviates toward nonaffected side). Lesions result in hoarse voice and difficulty swallowing. Patient often complains of food and fluid regurgitation into nasal cavity.
XI—Accessory (or spinal accessory)	Trapezius and sternocleidomastoid muscle innervation	Test trapezius and sternocleidomastoid muscle strength.	Usually related to radical neck surgery (as in resection of laryngeal carcinomas) that involves dissection of lymph nodes. CN XI lesion results in weakness with rotating neck to opposite side and with elevating the ipsilateral scapula.
XII—Hypoglossal	Tongue musculature innervation (for chewing, swallowing, speech articulation)	Assess for symmetric movement of tongue when patient sticks tongue straight out.	Upper motor neuron lesion results in weakness without atrophy and deviation to side opposite lesion. Lower motor neuron lesion results in paralysis and atrophy of tongue muscles on affected side, and tongue deviates to same side as lesion. Common causes are metastatic tumors or cerebral infarction.

5. **Define terminology describing common sensory impairments.**

The root word *esthesia* means "feeling" or "sensation."

- **Hypoesthesia or hypesthesia**—diminished sensation.
- **Hyperesthesia or hypersensitivity**—heightened sensitivity to sensory stimuli.
- **Anesthesia**—the complete lack of sensation in a particular dermatome, peripheral nerve distribution, or region. The prefix an- means "none."
- **Paresthesia**—abnormal and negatively perceived sensation, often described as burning, pricking (e.g., pins and needles), tickling, tingling, or numbness. The prefix para- means "aside" or "beyond."
- **Dysesthesia**—unpleasant or disagreeable sensations in response to a usually benign stimulus. The prefix dys- generally means "bad." Dysesthesia, or "difficult sensation," is described as "Dante-esque type of pain."
- **Allodynia**—exaggerated or painful response to sensory stimuli that should not be painful.

6. **Define the terms light touch, two-point discrimination, and stereognosis.**
   - **Light touch**—ability to perceive the application of soft brushing to the skin (e.g., camel hair brush, cotton ball wisp, thin facial tissue). The sensation is carried by the anterolateral system (spinothalamic) and dorsal column-medial lemniscal system. Complete absence of light touch sensation is associated with peripheral nerve or spinal cord damage.
   - **Two-point discrimination**—ability to perceive the application of two points of contact applied simultaneously to the skin as two discrete points. The threshold is the smallest distance between points that is still perceived as two points. The determination of this is a function of the density of Merkel receptors in the skin (palm, high density of receptors; back, low density) and the integrity of the dorsal column-medial lemniscal system. Static two-point discrimination sense is transmitted to the spinal cord by slowly adapting large diameter (type I) afferent nerves, while moving two-point discrimination testing evaluates rapidly adapting fibers. The posterior column-medial lemniscus pathway is responsible for carrying information involving fine, discriminative touch. Therefore, two-point discrimination can be impaired by damage to this pathway or to a peripheral nerve.
   - **Stereognosis**—ability to recognize the form and characteristics (e.g., size, shape, weight, consistency, texture) of common objects (e.g., keys, coins, pencil, paper clip, comb, fork) placed in the hand without visual clues. A patient should be able to name familiar objects within 5 seconds of contact. If the patient is unable to name the object, and other touch sensory modalities are intact, it suggests damage in the contralateral parietal cortex.

7. **What is the reliability of various forms of sensory testing?**

   Semmes-Weinstein Monofilament Testing for Light Touch A single 5.07 filament (bends at 10 grams of force) is the best indicator for protective sensation in the feet. Reports of interrater reliability for the assessment of light touch using Semmes-Weinstein monofilaments range from good to only slight or fair, while intrarater reliability is moderate to good. Inconsistency of standardized testing measures and variations in peripheral nerve tested and the presence or absence of pathology in the patient may explain the variation in reports on light touch reliability.

   Vibration Sensibility Testing Vibratory sense is an important neuropathy screen. Vibration testing stimulates Pacinian corpuscles and assesses the function of large diameter rapidly adapting peripheral nerves and the dorsal column-medial lemniscal central pathways. Using mechanical testing devices, the intrarater reliability of the assessment of vibration sense is good. Moderate reliability is reported for interrater reliability. Age and height were associated with minimal threshold values of the feet but not of the hands as determined through multiple regression analysis.

   Two-Point Discrimination Sensibility Testing Reliability ranges considerably from good to poor and is influenced by age, sex, patient cooperation, peripheral nerve tested, symptomatic versus asymptomatic, ability to attend to the stimulus, and testing procedures (e.g., starting position of wide versus narrow distances, amount of pressure applied, instrument used). Results from any sensory testing procedures are not recommended for use as the sole means of developing diagnoses of peripheral or central nervous system origin.

8. **Define the deep sensations of kinesthesia and proprioception.**

   Kinesthesia, or joint movement sense, is the awareness of single joint or body segment movement in terms of degree, velocity, and direction. The tester moves the patient's extremity or joint passively through a small range of motion (~10 degrees) by holding bony prominences with a fingertip grip. The patient is asked to describe the direction (e.g., up, down, in, out) and the range (e.g., initial, mid, terminal) while the extremity/joint is in motion. Impaired kinesthesia indicates dysfunction in the peripheral nerves, spinal cord, brainstem, or cerebrum.

   Proprioception, or joint position sense, is awareness of single joints or body segments at rest. The tester grips bony prominences and avoids stimulating touch (pressure) receptors that provide the patient with additional information (e.g., grip laterally to move the hallux up/down). The tester moves the patient's extremity/joint through the range of motion and then holds it in a static position. The patient is asked to describe the position or duplicate it with the contralateral extremity. Proprioception is intact in individuals with cerebellar ataxia but is impaired in individuals with sensory ataxia (lesions in peripheral sensory nerves, dorsal roots, dorsal columns of the spinal cord, or medial lemnisci).

9. **List some of the special neurologic tests and explain their clinical importance.**

TEST	DESCRIPTION	RESPONSE	CLINICAL IMPORTANCE
Abdominal reflex	Upper or lower abdominal musculature is gently stroked	A normal response is motion of umbilicus toward stroking. An abnormal response (or positive test) is reduced or absent motion.	Positive test indicates upper motor neuron damage or involvement of pertinent spinal level reflexes (T7-9; upper abdominal region; T11-12, lower abdominal region)
Babinski sign (extensor plantar)	Plantar surface of foot is stroked with key or fingernail in a sweeping motion from heel and lateral border toward ball of foot	A normal response is flexion of the hallux. An abnormal response (or positive test) is extension of the hallux, with or without fanning of other toes.	Positive test indicates upper motor neuron lesion
Bulbocavernous reflex	Dorsum of penis is tapped	A normal response is retraction of bulbocavernous portion of penis and contraction of anal sphincter. An abnormal response (or positive test) is absent retraction or contraction.	Positive test indicates damage to pudendal nerve, sacral autonomic efferent nerves, or upper motor neuron
Clonus	Typically tested at the ankle by applying a quick, passive stretch into dorsiflexion	A normal response is no oscillation of the joint. An abnormal response (or positive test) is rhythmic oscillation of a joint.	Positive test indicates an upper motor neuron pathology
Finger to nose	Patient extends finger away from face and then toward nose, and repeats this movement	A normal response is performing the movement smoothly, correctly estimating distances and location. An abnormal response (or positive test) is the inability to perform the movement smoothly and inability to estimate distances and location (overshooting or undershooting).	Positive test possibly indicates cerebellar dysfunction (asynergy)
Hoffman sign	Distal phalanx of second, third, or fourth digits of the hand are subjected to rapid, gentle stroking	A normal response is no flexion of the thumb distal interphalangeal joint. An abnormal response (or positive test) is reflexive flexion of thumb distal interpharangeal joint or distal interpharangeal joint of any other finger not struck.	Positive test indicates upper motor neuron lesion
Inverted supinator reflex	With the patient's arm slightly pronated and relaxed, quickly tap near the styloid process of the radius at the brachioradialis tendon attachment	A normal response is wrist pronation and/or elbow flexion. An abnormal response (or positive test) is finger flexion and/or elbow extension.	Positive test indicates potential cervical myelopathy (C5-6)

Continued

TEST	DESCRIPTION	RESPONSE	CLINICAL IMPORTANCE
Oppenheim reflex	Stroke the anterior border of the tibia in a downward manner with reflex hammer or thumbnail	A normal response is no reaction. An abnormal response (or positive test) is the presence of a Babinski sign.	Positive test indicates upper motor neuron lesion
Rapidly alternating movements	Patient performs rapid forearm pronation and supination or ankle plantar flexion and dorsiflexion	A normal response is the ability to perform the movement. An abnormal response (or positive test) is the inability to perform the movement (dysdiadochokinesia).	Positive test indicates ipsilateral cerebellar dysfunction, especially lateral hemispheres
Romberg sign	Patient stands with feet close together and then closes eyes	A normal response is no loss of balance. An abnormal response (or positive test) is increased sway, stepping, or falling.	Positive test indicates dorsal (sensory) column disease or pathology (e.g., cervical spondylosis, tumor, tabes dorsalis) or peripheral neuropathy; unsteady with feet together and eyes open or closed indicates central nervous system dysfunction (e.g., cerebellar ataxia, vestibular disorder)
Tactile extinction	Apply random single and double simultaneous stimuli (e.g., touch the patient's left hand followed by touching both the left hand and right face)	A normal response is the ability to detect the stimuli correctly. An abnormal response (or positive test) is the inability to detect a stimulus only in the presence of another stimulus.	Positive test is typically associated with parietal lobe pathology; occasionally due to frontal lobe pathology; may involve either right or left hemisphere
Tandem gait	Patient walks in a straight line while touching the heel of one foot to the toe of the other	A normal response is task performance without unsteadiness and without deviation from the line. An abnormal response (or positive test) is unsteadiness and deviation from the line.	Positive test indicates potential truncal ataxia due to cerebellar vermis pathology; rule out peripheral neuropathy

10. Define referred pain and radicular pain.

- **Referred pain**—pain (constant, poorly localized or diffuse, aching) at a site removed from the source of involvement; possibly caused by irritation of a nerve root or by tissue supplied by the same nerve root because of the shared sensory distribution of spinal nerves receiving afferent pain fibers from different regions of the body or different tissues that also receive afferent input.
  - **Somatic referred pain**—pain perceived in a region topographically displaced from the region of the pain source. Pain can be referred to abdominal region, extremities, head, neck, trunk, pelvic region, and groin. Examples include C5 facet pain referred into the ipsilateral upper arm or hip pain referred into the medial thigh and/or knee.
  - **Visceral referred pain**—pain related to internal organs. Visceral pain is not perceived locally. Viscera have multilevel innervation, and the central pathways of visceral pain are poorly organized. When the painful

stimuli arise in visceral receptors, the brain is unable to distinguish visceral signals from the more common signals that arise from somatic receptors. This results in pain being interpreted as coming from the somatic regions rather than the viscera (e.g., cardiac ischemia referring to the chest, cervical spine, left shoulder; liver referring pain to the right upper abdominal quadrant, right side of lumbar spine, right shoulder, right side of cervical spine).

- **Radicular pain**—a specific type of referred pain that is felt in a dermatome, myotome, or sclerotome of an involved peripheral nerve root. Compression of the C5 nerve root may affect sensation on the anterior shoulder. Patients commonly describe radicular pain as sharp, shooting, band-like, electric, or zinging.

11. What is a "burner" or "stinger"?

A burner or a stinger is a traction or compression injury to a cervical nerve root or brachial plexus trunk. Often the injury involves the C5 or C6 nerve root or upper trunk of the brachial plexus, with burning, numbness, tingling, or weakness in the distribution of the involved root or trunk. The mechanism of injury can involve distraction of the shoulder girdle from the neck, either through excessive shoulder depression or through forced hyperlateral flexion of the neck. Forced oblique hyperextension of the neck may also cause ipsilateral compression injuries of the cervical nerve roots or upper brachial plexus trunks.

12. How accurate is reflex, sensory, and muscle strength testing in the diagnosis of cervical radiculopathy?

The testing accuracy of reflexes, sensation, and muscle strength in the diagnosis of cervical radiculopathy is considered fair. Side-to-side reflex changes and muscle weakness associated with cervical radiculopathy agree with surgical findings about 77% of the time, while sensory loss correlates approximately 65% of the time. The combination of segmental hyporeflex, dermatomal sensory loss, and myotomal weakness is most specific (99%) for predicting cervical root disease. Myotomal weakness is the most accurate single variable predictor of cervical radiculopathy (81% accuracy).

13. What is the best strength test to determine weakness of the quadriceps in patients with known L3-4 radiculopathy?

In L3 and L4 radiculopathy, unilateral quadriceps weakness is best detected by a single leg sit-to-stand test (knee fully extended and without ground contact, examiner can hold patient's hands for balance aid). The next best method is a standard knee extension manual muscle test.

14. How valuable are the Achilles tendon reflex and the Hoffmann reflex to detect L5/S1 radiculopathy?

The Achilles tendon reflex and the Hoffmann reflex (H-reflex) are not valuable to detect L5 radiculopathy. They are, however, more valuable to rule in S1 radiculopathy. The H-reflex (electrically stimulated) is more specific (91%) than sensitive (50%) when evaluating S1 radiculopathy. The Achilles tendon jerk is also more specific (90%) than sensitive (32%) when evaluating S1 radiculopathy.

15. What is a syrinx?

A syrinx (Latin, "tube") is a neuroglial cell–lined, fluid-filled cavity ("syringomyelia" in the spinal cord; "syringobulbia" in the brain stem) possibly due to an accumulation of cerebrospinal fluid, genetic malformations, or the proliferation and subsequent regression of embryonic cell nests. A syrinx within the central canal interrupts the decussating spinothalamic tract fibers resulting in bilateral loss of pain and temperature sensations around the level of the lesion. A syrinx that extends laterally into the lateral funiculus of the spinal cord involves the lateral corticospinal pathway resulting in ipsilateral upper motor neuron signs and symptoms. Involvement of neural regions that mediate esophageal and gastrointestinal reflexes will result in gastrointestinal disturbances (e.g., nausea, emesis, eating disturbances, weight loss). Given associated joint arthropathy, syringomyelia is the second most common cause of a Charcot joint.

16. What is Horner syndrome?

Horner syndrome involves an interruption of sympathetic nervous system innervation to the head and face usually caused by a brainstem lesion. Signs and symptoms include miosis (constricted pupil from uncompensated parasympathetic nervous system input to pupil), ptosis (eyelid drooping from lost sympathetic innervation of the levator palpebrae superioris tarsal muscle), enophthalmos (eyeball appears to be sunken into socket), anhidrosis (absence of sweat production on affected side of face), and flushing (increased superficial blood flow on affected side of face). Although rare, clinicians in an orthopaedic setting may experience treating a patient with Horner syndrome. Cases reported in the literature include post clavicle fracture, status post cervical fusion anterolateral approach, post interscalene brachial plexus block, status post rotator cuff repair surgery, and status post cervical myelopathy revision surgery.

17. **Differentiate common symptoms associated with vestibular disorders.**
    - **Dizziness**—vague sensation of whirling, lightheadedness, faintness, or unsteadiness.
    - **Vertigo**—the perception of movement, either of the self or surrounding objects (has a rotational, spinning component); typically associated with unilateralvestibular hypofunction (UVH), benign paroxysmal positional vertigo (BPPV), or a unilateral central (brainstem) lesion affecting the vestibular nuclei.
    - **Lightheadedness**—a feeling of imminent fainting typically due to nonvestibular disorders (e.g., orthostatic hypotension, hypoglycemia, anxiety, panic disorder).
    - **Dysequilibrium**—the sensation of being off balance and may be indicative of bilateral vestibular hypofunction (BVH), chronic UVH, diminished lower extremity somatosensation, brainstem/vestibular cortex lesion, or cerebellar and motor pathway lesions.
    - **Oscillopsia**—visual instability with head movements; images appear to move or bounce; may experience blurring or diplopia; can occur with vestibular hypofunction in which the vestibulo-ocular reflex (VOR) is diminished (VOR maintains stability of images on the retina during head movements).

18. **What is benign paroxysmal positional vertigo (BPPV)?**
    BPPV, a biomechanical disorder, is the most common peripheral vestibular pathology. Symptoms include nystagmus and vertigo with head position changes, dysequilibrium, and occasionally nausea. BPPV is theoretically caused by dislodged otoconia in the semicircular canals in which the otoconia becomes adhered to the cupula (cupulolithiasis) or floats freely (canalithiasis). Canalithiasis of the posterior semicircular canal is the most common form of BPPV. A diagnosis of posterior semicircular canal BPPV is indicated when a patient reports vertigo provoked by head position changes (relative to gravity) and the presence of characteristic nystagmus provoked by the Dix-Hallpike maneuver upon physical examination.

19. **What is the most common positional test to examine BPPV?**
    The Dix-Hallpike test is used to examine for BPPV due to involvement of the anterior or posterior semicircular canals. The patient sits in long sitting with the head rotated 45 degrees toward the side being tested (the side the patient reports symptoms). The patient can place their hands over their chest or hold on to the examiner's elbows. The patient is moved to a supine position with the head extended 20 degrees below horizontal while maintaining the 45 degrees rotation for 60 seconds. The patient is assisted to long sitting while maintaining the 45 degrees rotation.

20. **What is the best intervention for BPPV?**
    BPPV due to canalithiasis or cupulolithiasis is treated using the Canalith Repositioning Maneuver (Epley/Modified Epley Maneuver), which involves moving the patient's head through a sequence of four positions to move the otoconia out; movements depend on side and canal affected. BPPV due to cupulolithiasis is sometimes treated using the Liberatory (Semont) maneuver (rapidly moving the patient through positions in order to dislodge the otoconia). Brandt-Daroff exercises can also be used if the patient cannot tolerate the Canalith Repositing Maneuver for BPPV and involve 5 to 20 repetitions, two to three sets per day (the patient moves from sitting to sidelying with the head rotated 45 degrees toward the ceiling, the patient remains in this position for 30 seconds or until the vertigo stops, returns to sitting, repeats on the other side).

21. **What are typical symptom profiles for various vestibular related disorders?**

	BPPV	NEURITIS (E.G., VESTIBULAR NERVE)	MENIERE'S DISEASE	FISTULA (E.G., PERILYMPH FISTULA)	NERVE COMPRES- SION
Vertigo	+	+	+	+	+
Nystagmus	+	+	+	+	+
Nausea	–/+	+	+	–	+
Symptoms	Vertigo, nausea, emesis, diaphoresis, nystagmus	Acute onset	Fullness of ear, hearing loss, tinnitus	Loud tinnitus	Frequent attacks, tinnitus
Duration of symptoms	30 seconds–2 minutes	48–72 hours	20 minutes–24 hours	Seconds	Seconds minutes

22. **What are differential diagnosis considerations for dizziness and vestibular-type symptoms based on duration of symptoms?**

DURATION	DIAGNOSIS CONSIDERATIONS
1–5 seconds	BPPV, seizures
Seconds to minutes	BPPV, cardiac or cardiovascular event, panic disorder
Minutes to hours	Meniere's disease, migraine, panic disorder
Days to weeks	Migraine, stroke and other structural central nervous system lesions, vestibular neuritis/labyrinthitis, drug reactions
Months to years	Stroke and other structural central nervous system lesions, fluctuating vestibular disorder, multisensory dysequilibrium, ototoxicity, psychiatric disorders, persistent postural perceptual dizziness (3PD)

23. **How can a clinician determine if a patient has chronic neuropathic pain?**
Chronic neuropathic pain involves reactive processes of sensory neurons and immune cells, each leading to distinct forms of hypersensitivity. Patients typically present with allodynia, cold hypersensitivity, and nonmechanical patterns or symptoms. A score >12 points on the S-LANSS (Self Reported - Leeds Assessment of Neuropathic Symptoms and Signs) suggests pain of predominantly neuropathic origin. The S-LANSS scale correctly identified 75% of pain types when self-completed and 80% when used in interview format. Sensitivity for self-completed S-LANSS scores ranges from 74% to 78%.

24. **What is cauda equina syndrome?**
Cauda equina syndrome is associated with a large, space-occupying lesion within the canal of the lumbosacral spine that may be related to damage of the distal bundle of nerve roots (cauda equina) from direct mechanical compression and venous congestion or ischemia. Patients in their 40s and 50s are at highest risk and symptoms include acute onset of low back pain, unilateral or bilateral lower extremity pain and/or sensory changes/loss, urinary retention, saddle anesthesia, and bowel incontinence. Though rare, early detection of this medical emergency is important because the prognosis significantly decreases if surgical intervention is not performed within 48 hours.

Bibliography

Bennett, M. I., Smith, B. H., Torrance, N., & Potter, J. (2005). The S-LANSS score for identifying pain of predominantly neuropathic origin: validation for use in clinical and postal research. *Journal of Pain, 6*(3), 149–158.

Bhattacharyya, M. D., Gubbels, S., Schwartz, S., et al. (2017). Clinical practice guideline: Paroxysmal positional vertigo (update). *Otolaryngology—Head and Neck Surgery, 156,* S1–S47.

Bulut, T., Tahta, M., Sener, U., & Sener, M. (2018). Inter- and intra-tester reliability of sensibility testing in healthy individuals. *Journal of Plastic Surgery and Hand Surgery, 52*(3), 189–192.

Cobos, E. J., Nickerson, C. A., Gao, F., et al. (2018). Mechanistic differences in neuropathic pain modalities revealed by correlating behavior with global expression profiling. *Cell Reports, 22*(5), 1301–1312.

Fell, D. W., Lunnen, K. Y., & Rauk, R. P. (2018). *Lifespan neurorehabilitation: A patient-centered approach from examination to intervention and outcomes* (ed 1). Philadelphia: F. A. Davis Company.

Feinberg, J. H. (2000). Burners and stingers. *Physical Medicine and Rehabilitation Clinics of North America, 11,* 771–784.

Gerhardsson, L., & Hagberg, M. (2019). Vibration induced injuries in hands in long-term vibration exposed workers. *Journal of Occupational Medicine and Toxicology, 14,* 21.

Gilroy, J. (Ed.), (2000). *Basic neurology* (ed 3). New York: McGraw-Hill.

Lance, J. W. (2002). The Babinski sign. *Journal of Neurology, Neurosurgery and Psychiatry, 73,* 360–362.

Larsen, D., Kegelmeyer, D., Buford, J., et al. (2016). *Neurologic rehabilitation: Neuroscience and neuroplasticity in physical therapy practice* (ed 1). McGraw-Hill Education/Medical.

Lundy-Eckman, L. (2018). *Neuroscience: fundamentals for rehabilitation* (ed 5). St. Louis: Elsevier Saunders.

Meng, X., Deng, Y., Dai, Z., & Meng, Z. (2020). COVID-19 and anosmia: A review based on up-to-date knowledge. *American Journal of Otolaryngology, 41*(5), 102581.

Milhorat, T. H. (2000). Classification of syringomyelia. *Neurosurgical Focus, 8,* 1–6.

Peters, E. W., Bienfait, H. M. E., de Visser, M., & de Haan, R. J. (2003). The reliability of assessment of vibration sense. *Acta Neurologica Scandinavica, 107,* 293–298.

Rainville, J., Jouve, C., Finno, M., & Limke, J. (2003). Comparison of four tests of quadriceps strength in L3 or L4 radiculopathies. *Spine, 28,* 2466–2471.

Rico, R. E., & Jonkman, E. J. (1982). Measurement of the Achilles tendon reflex for the diagnosis of lumbosacral root compression syndromes. *Journal of Neurology, Neurosurgery and Psychiatry, 45,* 791–795.

Ropper, A. H., Samuels, M. A., Klein, J. P., & Prasad, S. (2019). *Adam's and Victor's principles of neurology* (11th ed.). New York: McGraw-Hill.
Rozental, T. D., Beredjiklian, P. K., Guyette, T. M., & Weiland, A. J. (2000). Intra- and interobserver reliability of sensibility testing in asymptomatic individuals. *Annals of Plastic Surgery, 44*, 605–609.
Shy, M. E., Frohman, E. M., So, Y. T., et al. (1996). Quantitative sensory testing: Report of the Therapeutics and Technology Assessment Subcommittee of the American Academy of Neurology. *Neurology, 60*, 898–904. 2003.
Waxman, S. G. (1996). *Correlative neuroanatomy* (ed 23). Stamford, CT: Appleton & Lange.

CHAPTER 18 QUESTIONS

1. **Which of the following statements is true when testing the oculomotor nerve?**
   a. The therapist performs the Weber test using a tuning fork to assess if the patient hears the sound fairly equally bilaterally.
   b. The therapist assesses the gag reflex.
   c. The therapist assesses sensation of the face by gently touching different portions of the face using a cotton wisp.
   d. The therapist assesses smooth and symmetrical eye movements and reproduction of diplopia by moving a pen in an "H" pattern.

Rationale: To assess the oculomotor nerve, test for eye movements. The most common method is using a finger or pen and moving in a "H" pattern. Assess for not only smooth and symmetrical eye movements but also ask the patient if any symptoms are reproduced including nausea, diplopia, dizziness, or headaches. The Weber test is used to assess the vestibulocochlear nerve. Testing the gag reflex assesses the glossopharyngeal nerve. Sensory testing of the face assesses the trigeminal nerve.

2. **A 40-year-old healthy male presents to your clinic with complaints of dizziness. His dizziness lasts between 1 to 2 minutes and often causes nausea, sweating, and emesis. He denies any hearing loss or headaches. Based on this information, which of the following is the most likely cause of his symptoms?**
   a. Benign paroxysmal positional vertigo
   b. Meniere's disease
   c. Cervicogenic dizziness
   d. Temporal arteritis

Rationale: Benign paroxysmal positional vertigo (BPPV) is most commonly associated with dizziness lasting between 30 seconds to 2 minutes. Associated symptoms include nausea, sweating, and vomiting. Dizziness from Meniere's disease can last 20 minutes to 24 hours. Patients with cervicogenic dizziness typically have dizziness with cervical range of motion or in sustained postures such as upper cervical extension. Typically, there are associated headaches and not nausea, sweating, or vomiting with cervicogenic dizziness. Temporal arteritis would cause severe unilateral or bilateral headaches.

3. **A 52-year-old female patient presents to your clinic with chronic cervical and right upper extremity pain from a whiplash-associated injury. Which of the following would most likely indicate signs of chronic neuropathic pain?**
   a. S-LANSS less than 10, paresthesia, and dizziness
   b. S-LANSS greater than 12, allodynia, and cold hypersensitivity
   c. S-LANSS less than 10, allodynia, and painful cervical range of motion
   d. S-LANSS greater than 12, painful cervical range of motion, and paresthesia

Rationale: Chronic neuropathic pain is typically associated with allodynia, cold hypersensitivity, and nonmechanical patterns or symptoms. The S-LANSS is an outcome measure aimed to identify pain of predominantly neuropathic origin. A score greater than 12 points suggests neuropathic pain.

CLINICAL RESEARCH AND DATA ANALYSIS

CHAPTER 19

F.B. Underwood, PT, PhD, ECS

1. **What is research?**
   Research is a controlled, systematic approach to obtain an answer to a question. Experimental research involves the manipulation of a variable and measurement of the effects of this manipulation. Nonexperimental research does not manipulate the environment but may describe the relationship between different variables, obtain information about opinions or policies, or describe current practice. Basic research is generally thought of as laboratory-based research, in which the researcher has control over nearly all aspects of the environment and subjects. Clinical or applied research usually uses entire, intact organisms in a more natural environment.

2. **What are variables?**
   Variables are measurements or phenomena that can assume more than one value or more than one category. A categorical or discrete variable is one that can assume only certain values and often is qualitative (no quantity or numerical value implied). Continuous variables are ones that can assume a wide range of possible values and are usually quantitative in nature.

3. **Define independent variable and dependent variable.**
   - Independent variable—the variable that is manipulated by the researcher
   - Dependent variable—the variable that is measured by the researcher

   Independent variables often are qualitative, and dependent variables usually are quantitative. The different permutations of the independent variable are called levels. To be an independent variable, there must be at least two levels; if some aspect of the research has only one possible value or category, it is a constant.

4. **Describe other types of variables.**
   Extraneous (also called nuisance or confounding) variables are phenomena that are not of interest to the researcher but may have an effect on the value of the dependent variable. Extraneous variables must be controlled as much as possible, usually by holding some aspect of the research constant. A covariate is a phenomenon that affects the dependent variable and is not of interest to the researcher, but that the researcher is unable to control.

5. **How accurate are measurements?**
   The observed measurement of any phenomenon is composed of a true score and error. Error may be systematic, in which case all scores are increased or decreased by a constant amount, or random. Systematic error generally is the result of using the measurement instrument incorrectly, improper calibration of the instrument, or operator bias. Random error is precisely that—random. Even if the true score is constant, and there is no systematic error, repeated measurements of a phenomenon do not produce identical scores. It is generally assumed that the effects of all of the sources of random error cancel each other, such that the measured score is the best estimate of the true score. If the true score is constant, repeating the measurement and calculating an average score may be a better estimate of the true score. If the true score is labile or is altered as a consequence of the measurement, repeated measurements may reduce the accuracy of the measurement.

6. **Define measurement reliability.**
   Reliability is related to consistency or repeatability. In the absence of a change in the true score, how similar are repeated measurements of the same phenomenon? Intra-rater reliability is a measure of how consistent an individual is at measuring a constant phenomenon, inter-rater reliability refers to how consistent different individuals are at measuring the same phenomenon, and instrument reliability pertains to the tool used to obtain the measurement. If a measurement cannot be performed reliably, it is difficult to ascribe changes in the dependent variable to the effects of the independent variable, rather than measurement error.

7. **Describe statistical procedures used to estimate reliability.**
   The intraclass correlation coefficient (ICC), which is based on an analysis of variance (ANOVA) statistical procedure, is a popular means of estimating reliability. A means of measuring absolute concordance is the kappa statistic. In the past, a Pearson or Spearman correlation procedure often was used to estimate reliability; these procedures are insufficient as measures of reliability because they measure covariance, not agreement.

8. **Define measurement validity.**
   It is an indication of whether the measurement is an accurate representation of the phenomenon of interest. Some clinical measurements have obvious validity. For example, using a goniometer to measure the angle between two bones with the joint as the axis is generally accepted as a valid indication of the status of the tissue that limits motion at that joint. For other measurements, the relationship between what is measured and what is inferred from the measurement is more tenuous. To establish the validity of a clinical test, a more direct measurement that is considered a gold standard is established. If acceptable numbers of patients with a positive Lachman test have anterior cruciate ligament tears and those without tears have a negative Lachman test, the Lachman test is considered a valid test for anterior cruciate ligament integrity. There is no universal definition of acceptable numbers; this is left to the researcher to defend and the clinician to accept or reject.

9. **What is a research design?**
   A research design is a plan or structure of the means used to answer the research question or to gather the information for a nonexperimental study. There are three basic designs for experimental research:
   A. A completely randomized design uses a single independent variable and assigns different groups of subjects to each level of the independent variable. Because each subject receives only one type of treatment, this design is also called a between-subjects design. If the independent variable is the type of brace and there are three levels (ie, three different braces are being used), then an individual subject would be measured while using only one of the three braces.
   B. A repeated measures design uses a single independent variable and measures each subject under all levels of the independent variable. If the independent variable is the dosage of a drug and levels are 200, 400, and 600 mg/day, then each subject would be measured while taking each of the three dosages. In this example, an appropriate wash-out period would be used between each dosage.
   C. A factorial design uses two or more independent variables. A completely randomized factorial design is one in which all of the independent variables are independent factors, meaning an individual subject is measured under only one condition. If the two independent variables are type of brace and dosage of a drug, and there are three levels of each variable, then nine groups of subjects would be studied. A within-subjects factorial design measures each subject in all levels of all variables. Using the brace and dosage variables, each subject would be measured with each brace and dosage (eg, brace A and 200 mg, brace A and 400 mg, brace A and 600 mg, and the same for brace B and brace C). A mixed factorial design uses at least one independent factor and at least one repeated factor. If subjects are assigned to only one brace, but are measured with all three drug dosages, the design is mixed.

10. **Which descriptive statistics are most useful for describing a set of data?**
    It depends on the data. If the data are distributed normally, the three measures of central tendency are equal; in this case, the mean is most often used to describe the typical performance. If there are a few scores at one extreme or the other in the set of data, the median is considered the best measure of central tendency. For example, in the data set 2, 4, 5, 7, 83, the mean is 20.2, and the median is 5; 5 is more descriptive of the typical score than 20.2. The standard deviation (or variance) is the most descriptive value for the variability of a data set that is distributed normally, and minimum-maximum may be the best measure of variability in data sets that are best described with the median.

11. **Are the terms normal distribution, bell curve, and gaussian distribution equivalent?**
    Yes, in that all three terms refer to the shape of a frequency histogram constructed using the scores from any measurement that is the sum of a true score and multiple, small, independent sources of error. Nearly any physiologic or anatomic parameter that is measured in a large group of individuals falls into a normal distribution. For example, suppose the maximal aerobic capacity is measured in 500 individuals selected at random. The scores are counted and grouped into increments of 5 (eg, the number of subjects with a maximal aerobic capacity of 0 to 5, 6 to 10, 11 to 15), and the results are used to construct a bar plot or frequency histogram with the increments on the x-axis and the number of individuals in each bin on the y-axis. If the average value was 31, and the standard deviation was 6, the resulting plot might look like figure. Most scores were near the mean of 31, with fewer scores at each extreme. For example, the number of scores in the 6 to 10 range is approximately equal to the number of scores in the 51 to 55 range. In a perfectly normal distribution, 68% of the scores will be found within one standard deviation of the mean; in this example, 340 of the 500 scores should be between 25 and 37 (31 ± 6), 95% of the scores will be within two standard deviations of the mean, and 99% of the scores will be within three standard deviations of the mean.

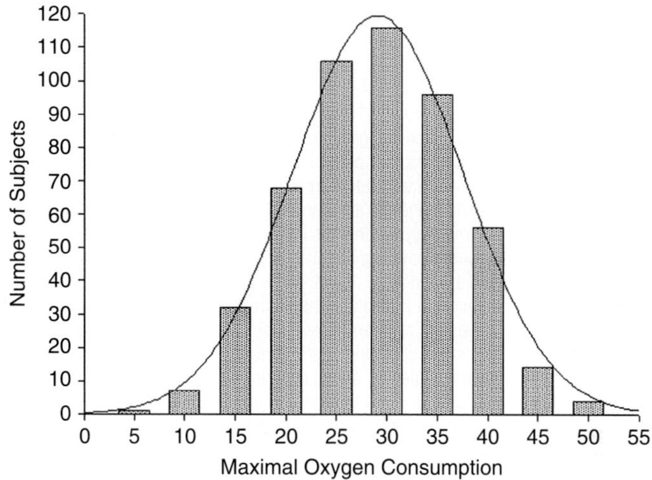

12. **Are there distributions other than a normal distribution?**
Yes, especially with small samples, skewed distributions are possible. A skewed distribution results when there are a few extreme scores at one end or the other of the distribution. For example, if most of the scores are low, but there are a few high scores, the distribution might be similar to figure. This distribution is skewed to the right by the few extremely high scores. If there are a few extremely low scores, the distribution is skewed to the left. The direction of the skew is determined by drawing (or imagining) a line connecting the top of each bar in the histogram and stating to which side of the plot the tail extends.

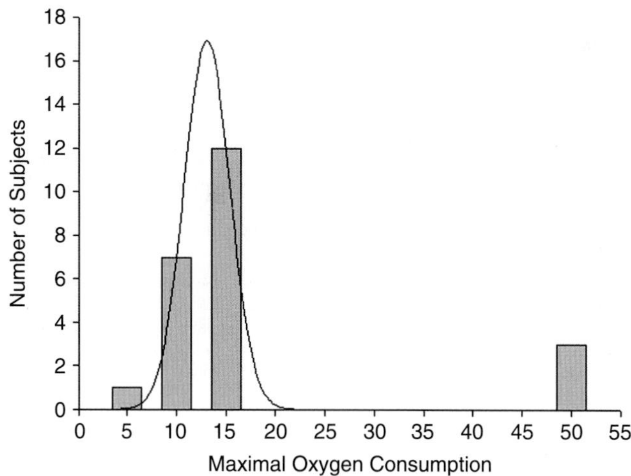

13. **Can the same concepts be used with a skewed distribution; that is, are 68% of the scores within one standard deviation of the mean?**
No. These values hold true only for a normal distribution. In the case of a skewed distribution, the median is a better descriptor of the typical score, and the minimum-maximum better describes the variability in the set of data.

14. **What are inferential statistics?**
When data are collected, the researcher needs to determine the probability of obtaining a particular set of scores by chance alone. The procedures used to calculate this probability are called inferential statistics and are the heart of testing an experimental hypothesis. There are different procedures used based on the research design, the nature of the research question (what the researcher is trying to answer), and the nature of the data.

15. **Describe the fundamental concept of inferential statistics.**
In the simplest case, consider a randomized design, with a single independent variable having two levels and a single dependent variable. Suppose a researcher posed the following question: What is the effect of adding neural glide techniques for the median nerve to the standard treatment for patients with carpal tunnel syndrome? The independent variable is treatment, and the levels are standard and neural glide. The dependent variable could be number of days until the patient is free of symptoms for 10 consecutive days. A sample of patients with carpal tunnel syndrome is selected at random from the population of patients with carpal tunnel syndrome, and the patients in the sample are assigned at random to one of the two treatment levels. Because the patients have been selected at random from the population, and then assigned at random to one of the two treatment groups, it is a reasonable assumption that the mean and standard deviation for the dependent variable would be the same for both treatment groups if there is no effect of adding neural glide to the standard treatment. All of the subjects are treated until the criterion for discharge is met (ie, free of symptoms for 10 consecutive days), and the data are summarized. If the standard group recovered in an average of 40 days, with a standard deviation of 7 days, and the neural glide group recovered in 32 days, with a standard deviation of 6 days, did the treatment work? There is a difference in the average days to recovery, but is that difference large enough to conclude that it was due to the neural glide, or could it be attributed to chance alone? Perhaps the subjects in the neural glide group did not have as severe compression of the median nerve at the beginning of the study and recovered more quickly despite the neural glide. The essence of inferential hypothesis testing is to answer the following question: What is the probability of having obtained a difference in days to recovery of this magnitude as a result of random factors? If this probability is low enough, the researcher can conclude that the treatment had a beneficial effect and should become a part of standard practice.

16. **How is the correct statistical test chosen?**
The short answer is that it depends on the question being asked:
- If the desire is to learn about the association between two variables (eg, the relationship between thigh girth and knee extensor force), a correlation coefficient should be calculated.
- If the question concerns prediction (eg, if a patient has knee range of motion of 5 to 60 degrees on the second postoperative day, how many days will the patient likely remain in the hospital?), a regression analysis is appropriate.
- If the question is whether a treatment has an effect (eg, does spinal traction reduce the signs and symptoms of a lumbosacral root compression?), a chi-square, analysis of variance (ANOVA), or t-test, which is a special case of the ANOVA, is appropriate.

However, because there are different types of data and different types of restrictions placed upon the testing, the answer is more complicated. There are four levels of data: nominal, ordinal, interval, and ratio. Information measured on a nominal scale results in a name only; that is, it does not imply a quantity. Left versus right, red versus blue, and "improved" versus "unchanged" are examples of nominal data. If a numeral is assigned to information on a nominal scale, a quantity is not implied; if red is coded 1 and blue is coded 2, it does not mean that blue is twice as much as red.

An ordinal scale implies a rank order, with some quantitative value. The person who finishes a race first receives the number 1, meaning this person finished the race in a shorter time than the second-place finisher. However, the amount of time between first and second place is not likely the same as the amount of time between fifth and sixth place.

For statistical purposes, there are no meaningful differences between an interval and a ratio scale; both imply not only a rank order but also an equivalence between points on the scale. The difference between 80 and 95 is the same as the difference between 25 and 40; in both cases, it is 15. The primary difference between these two scales of measurement is that for an interval scale, the value of zero is a construct and negative values are possible, whereas for a ratio scale, the value of zero is natural and negative values are not possible. The variable temperature is an example of a phenomenon that could be measured on either an interval or a ratio scale. If on the Celsius scale, it is interval, and if on the Kelvin scale, it is ratio.

For a correlation study, a Spearman rho (for Spearman, who developed the procedure, and rank order) is used for ordinal data. A Pearson correlation coefficient is calculated for interval data. In both cases, the coefficient can vary between −1.00 and +1.00. A value of zero means that there is no correlation, and a value of 1.00 signifies the correlation is perfect. If the sign is +, the value of one variable increases as the other increases. If the sign is −, the value of one variable decreases as the other increases.

For experimental studies, those designed to determine if there is a difference, a chi-square is computed for data that are nominal. There is some disagreement regarding the appropriate analysis when the data meet the definition of ordinal or interval. It is almost universally agreed that to perform a traditional ANOVA, the sets of data should have a normal distribution, and the variance of the sets of data should be similar (the definition of similar is usually lacking; a rule of thumb is that the variance of one set should be no more than twice the other set). There are formal tests that can be used to determine whether the data are normally distributed, and whether the variances are equal; these are beyond the scope of this book and are generally of little or no interest to the clinician. Some authors further state that the data must meet the definition of interval or ratio data; in fact, some researchers ignore the more important requirements of normal distribution and equality of variance and claim that the tests are robust enough that any data on an interval or ratio scale can be analyzed with a traditional ANOVA. However, the scale of the data was not an issue when the traditional ANOVA approach was developed. Therefore if the data are normally distributed, and the variances are equal, then a traditional ANOVA is appropriate, regardless of the scale of the data. Often, especially with the small sample sizes usually used in rehabilitation research, the two requirements of normal distribution and equality of variance are not met, even with ratio data, and a traditional ANOVA is inappropriate.

If the question is whether two groups differ on the dependent variable, and the data are normally distributed with equal variances, a t-test is appropriate. The t-test is a special case of the ANOVA, developed to make the calculations easier. With software, it is just as easy to use an ANOVA because the information is the same. If there are more than two levels of a single independent variable, or if there is more than one independent variable, the ANOVA can be extended to handle the variables. The type of ANOVA performed is often referred to by the number of rows and columns that are required to represent all of the permutations of the independent variables. A $2 \times 3 \times 2$ ANOVA means that there were three independent variables (because there are three numerals), two of the independent variables had two levels, and the third variable had three levels (the value of the numerals). The exception is a 1×4 ANOVA, which has only one independent variable, with four levels; if the value of one of the numerals is 1, it cannot represent a variable (because, by definition, variables have more than one possible value). If the data are not normally distributed, or the variances are not equal, a nonparametric equivalent is appropriate.

17. **Differentiate between parametric and nonparametric statistical procedures.**
Parametric statistical procedures are performed on data that have a normal distribution, such as the distribution observed in a population. Nonparametric procedures are performed on data that do not have a normal distribution, that is, a skewed distribution, as often is observed in a sample. Parametric procedures include the ANOVA and t-test, and nonparametric procedures include the chi-square, Kruskal-Wallis, and Spearman rho. As mentioned earlier, some authors add the requirement that the data have the characteristics of an interval or ratio scale in order to conduct parametric procedures, but this is debatable. Nonparametric procedures are often regarded as second-class procedures, used only when the data are extremely skewed. However, nonparametric procedures are nearly as powerful as their parametric equivalents when the data are normally distributed, and more powerful than parametric procedures when the data are skewed. Because of the small sample sizes typically used in orthopaedic and rehabilitation research, nonparametric procedures should likely be used more often.

18. **How is the appropriate type of statistical analysis determined?**
See table.

Samples Used			
PURPOSE OF ANALYSIS	**NATURE OF DISTRIBUTION**	**INDEPENDENT**	**RELATED**
Show a difference	Normal	ANOVA	Repeated measure ANOVA
	Skewed	Chi-square for frequency; Mann-Whitney or Kruskal-Wallis	McNemar's for frequency; Wilcoxon signed rank
Determine degree of association	Normal	Pearson or linear regression	Pearson or linear regression
	Skewed	Contingency coefficient for frequency; Spearman rho	Contingency coefficient for frequency; Spearman rho

19. **Other than intuition and clinical experience, how can the best clinical tests be identified?**
The performance of clinical tests (eg, straight-leg raise, Lachman test, shoulder impingement tests) can be measured in many ways, some more enlightening than others. The point of a clinical test is to sort patients into two basic categories: those who truly have the disorder and those who truly do not have the disorder. Depending on the situation, disease, dysfunction, or pathology can be substituted for the term disorder.

It is often difficult or hazardous to know with absolute certainty whether a disorder is present. For example, the definitive test for a ruptured anterior cruciate ligament (ACL) is direct visualization of the ligament, with an arthrotomy, arthroscopy, or, potentially, MRI. Obviously, it would be unreasonably hazardous to subject all patients with a clinical history suggestive of an ACL rupture to a surgical procedure, and MRI is expensive. These definitive tests are considered gold standards against which the results of a less invasive or less expensive test are compared.

The typical approach to establishing the performance of a clinical test is to conduct both the clinical test and the definitive test (gold standard) on a group of patients, some of whom have the disorder and some of whom are free of the disorder. Specific values are then calculated, and the clinician can determine how confident one can be in the results of the test. The clinical test is not always what is typically considered a test: It can be a specific question asked during the patient interview (such as "Did you hear a pop before your knee gave way?"), or it can be a combination of tests and interview information, such as whether the straight-leg raise is positive and the patient has pain radiating from the back to the buttock and down the posterior thigh.

20. What is meant by sensitivity, specificity, positive predictive value, and negative predictive value?

These terms are used to describe the usefulness of the clinical tests described above. It is easiest to comprehend these values if a 2 × 2 table is constructed, with the results of the definitive test entered in the columns, and the results of the clinical test entered in the rows. A study conducted by Roach et al. can illustrate the calculation and use of these values. Among other variables, the researchers determined the usefulness of asking patients with degenerative disk disease (DDD) and low back pain whether they also had pain radiating down the lower member; this was the clinical test used to predict the presence of spinal stenosis (the target disorder). Out of 17 patients with the target disorder (spinal stenosis), 16 had a positive clinical test (that is, they had pain radiating down the lower member). Out of 89 patients with DDD and low back pain but without the target disorder, 70 had pain radiating down the lower member. Table illustrates how to calculate the values.

Reality				
		STENOSIS	NO STENOSIS	ROW TOTAL
Radiating leg pain	Positive	a=16	b=70	a+b=86
	Negative	c=1	d=19	c+d=20
Column total		a+b=21	b+d=89	a+b+c+d=106

Sensitivity is the proportion of patients with a disorder who also have a positive clinical test; it is the probability of having a true positive test. It is calculated by dividing the number of patients with the target disorder and a positive test by the number of patients with the target disorder: Sensitivity $= a \div (a + c)$. Using the example above, $16 \div (16 + 1) = 0.94$. This means that of 100 patients with stenosis, 94 will have pain radiating down the lower member.

Specificity is the proportion of patients without the disorder who also have a negative clinical test; it is the probability of having a true negative test. It is calculated by dividing the number of patients without the target disorder and a negative test by the number of patients without the target disorder: Specificity $= d \div (d + b)$. Thus $19 \div (19 + 70) = 0.21$. This means that of 100 patients with DDD but without stenosis, only 21 will not have pain radiating down the lower member.

Sensitivity and specificity deal with reality; they are based on knowing for certain whether the target disorder is present. The reason clinicians use a clinical test in the first place is because they are trying to determine whether the target disorder is present; reality usually is unknown.

21. Do other performance characteristics depend on a knowledge of reality?

No. Positive predictive values (PPVs) and negative predictive values (NPVs) deal with the situation of having a patient and the results of a clinical test. This is the usual situation that confronts a clinician.

PPV is the proportion of patients with a positive clinical test who also have the target disorder. It is calculated by dividing the number of patients with a positive clinical test and the target disorder by the total number of patients with a positive clinical test: PPV $= a \div (a + b) = 16 \div (16 + 70) = 0.19$. This means that of 100 people with pain radiating down the lower member, only 19 will have stenosis.

NPV is the proportion of patients with a negative clinical test who also do not have the target disorder. It is calculated by dividing the number of patients with a negative clinical test and free of the target disorder by the total number of patients with a negative clinical test: NPV $= d \div (d + c) = 19 \div (19 + 1) = 0.95$. This means that of 100 people without pain radiating down the lower member, 95 will not have stenosis.

22. **What is the principal drawback to the PPV and NPV?**
These values change with changes in the prevalence of the target disorder; if the target disorder is uncommon, there are many more false-positive results, and the PPV goes down. Because the sensitivity and specificity deal with reality, they are not affected by changes in the prevalence of the target disorder.

23. **Is there a way to combine the best characteristics of sensitivity, specificity, PPV, and NPV?**
Yes; likelihood ratios are often considered a useful approach for clinical decision making. Likelihood ratios are expressed as odds and are calculated from values used to calculate sensitivity and specificity. The likelihood ratio of a positive test (LR+) is the quotient of the sensitivity and the complement of the specificity, ie, the sensitivity divided by 1 minus the specificity. In the example above, the LR+ is 0.94 ÷ (1 – 0.21), or 1.19. This means that the odds of a patient with the target disorder (ie, stenosis) having a positive test (ie, radiating leg pain) are 1.19 times greater than those for a patient without the target disorder. Another way of viewing a LR+ value is that it gives the odds that a patient with the target disorder would be expected to have a positive test. A likelihood ratio of 1.00 is of no value; a patient with a positive test is equally likely to have the target disorder as not.
The likelihood ratio of a negative test (LR–) is the quotient of the complement of the sensitivity and the specificity, ie, 1 minus the sensitivity divided by the specificity. In this example, the LR– is (1 – 0.94) ÷ 0.21 = 0.29. This means that the odds of a patient with the target disorder (stenosis) and a positive test are only 29% as great as those of a patient without the target disorder. An alternative way of viewing the LR– is to determine the inverse of the LR– (or divide the specificity by the complement of the sensitivity) and use this value to decide how much more likely an individual without the target disorder is to have a negative test than an individual with the target disorder. The reciprocal of 0.29 is 3.5 (or, 0.21 ÷ [1 – 0.94] = 3.5); therefore an individual without stenosis has odds 3.5 times greater of having a negative test than an individual with stenosis. Either approach is appropriate, but some clinicians find the second method more intuitive. An LR– value of 1.00 is equivalent to flipping a coin to determine the meaning of a negative test.

24. **Define the terms prevalence and incidence.**
Prevalence is the proportion of a population who has a particular disorder or condition at a specific point in time. If in a population of 233,658 there are 253 individuals with carpal tunnel syndrome (CTS), the prevalence of CTS is 253 ÷ 233,658 = 0.0010828. Because prevalence typically is a small number, it usually is multiplied by an appropriate constant and expressed as the number of cases per 1000 or 10,000. In this example, the prevalence of CTS would be about 1 per 1000.
Incidence is the rate of development of new cases of a disorder in a particular at-risk population over a given period of time. As with prevalence, the value usually is small and is multiplied by an appropriate constant and expressed as the number of cases per the constant for a given period of time. If a new manufacturing plant opens and employs 2355 people, and 89 people develop CTS during the calendar year from January 1, 1999, to December 31, 1999, the incidence of CTS is (89 ÷ 2355) × 1000 = 38 cases for that 1-year period. One difficulty in calculating incidence is in determining the denominator; it is unlikely that there will be 2355 people employed by the plant on January 1 and December 31. If the population is not constant, the size of the population at some point is selected to represent the size for the entire time period; usually, it is the midpoint of the time period, that is, July 1, 1999, in our example. Another difficulty is in defining the at-risk population. If one is determining the incidence of pregnancy, obviously males, premenarche girls, and postmenopausal women would not be included in the denominator. In the manufacturing plant that employs 2355 people, it may be that only the 985 people who work with impact tools are at risk for CTS.

25. **Discuss risk ratios and odds ratios.**
These are used to determine how likely it is that an individual with a particular risk factor will or will not develop a disease. The calculation of these ratios is similar to the calculation of likelihood ratios, PPVs, and NPVs. A risk ratio is calculated by dividing the incidence for the disorder for one group by the incidence for the disorder for another group; the two groups are considered to be at risk or not at risk. For example, if the manufacturing plant employs 2355 people and 985 of the employees use impact tools, the following question could be asked: "What is the risk of an employee who uses impact tools developing carpal tunnel syndrome (CTS) as compared to an employee who does not use impact tools?" Table illustrates how to construct a 2 × 2 table to assist in calculating these values.

Developed CTS During 1999				
		YES	**NO**	**ROW TOTAL**
Impact tool use?	Yes	a=297	b=688	a+b=985
	No	c=43	d=1327	c+d=1370
Column total		a+c=340	b+d=2015	a+b+c+d=2355

The incidence (expressed as a proportion) of CTS in the at-risk group is a ÷ (a + b) = 297 ÷ 985 = 0.30, and the incidence of CTS in the not-at-risk group is c ÷ (c + d) = 43 ÷ 1370 = 0.03. The risk ratio is then [a ÷ (a + b)] ÷ [c ÷ (c + d)] = 0.30 ÷ 0.03 = 10. An individual who uses impact tools is 10 times more likely to develop CTS as compared to an individual who does not use impact tools. As with PPVs and NPVs, which also are calculated using the data in the rows of the table, the risk ratio is changed easily by changes in the prevalence of the condition; the more rare the disorder, the higher the risk ratio.

An odds ratio is calculated using the information in the columns of the table, and similar to sensitivity and specificity, the odds ratio is not changed by changes in prevalence. The odds that someone with CTS uses impact tools is a ÷ c = 297 ÷ 43 = 6.9. The odds that someone without CTS uses impact tools is b ÷ d = 688 ÷ 1327 = 0.52. The odds ratio is (a ÷ c) ÷ (b ÷ d) = 6.9 ÷ 0.52 = 13.3, which means that someone with CTS is 13.3 times more likely to use impact tools.

26. A clinical test has a sensitivity of 0.94 and a specificity of 0.90. If your patient has a positive test result, what is the probability that she truly has the disease?

The answer is an unequivocal "It depends." The base rate or prevalence of the disease in your patient's population must be considered, as it will have a large effect on the answer.

Suppose the prevalence of the disease is 1%. If we test 500 people from this population, we expect that 5 people will have the disease. Given the sensitivity and specificity for the test, we can calculate the number of true positives, false positives (the value of interest here), true negatives, and false negatives.

Table provides the values given a prevalence of 1%.

		Disease		
		PRESENT	**ABSENT**	**TOTAL**
Test Result	Positive	A = 4.7	B = 49.5	54.2
	Negative	C = 0.3	D = 445.5	445.8
	Total	5	495	500

Given the prevalence, there will be 5 people who have the disease. Sensitivity is A/(A + C), so we know that 0.94 = A/5, and A therefore is 4.7 and C is 0.3 (the values will typically be rounded to whole numbers, but for this illustration we will retain the fractional cases). We also know that 495 people will not have the disease, and Specificity is D/(D + B), so 0.90 = D/495, and D is 445.5, leaving 49.5 in cell B. Therefore, the probability that your patient who has a positive result from the test has the disease is 4.7/54.2 = 0.087 or 8.7%.

Now suppose the prevalence is 23%. Using the same process, the probability that a patient who has a positive test has the disease is 108.1/146.6 = 0.737 or 73.7% as shown in table.

		Disease		
		PRESENT	**ABSENT**	**TOTAL**
Test Result	Positive	A = 108.1	B = 38.5	146.6
	Negative	C = 6.9	D = 346.5	353.4
	Total	115.0	385.0	500

The take-home message from this exercise is that knowing the base rate of the target disorder is essential in interpreting the test result.

27. Discuss how a clinician can judge the effectiveness of a treatment or prevention program.

One approach to assessing treatment effectiveness is by using relative risk reduction (RRR), absolute risk reduction (ARR), and the number needed to treat (NNT) estimates. To illustrate the use of these concepts, consider the effectiveness of an educational program (a back school) for the reduction of the incidence of low back pain (LBP) in an industrial setting. The fundamental question is: Does a back school reduce the rate of LBP, and if so, is it cost-effective? Because a history of LBP before attending the back school is likely to have an impact on the development of LBP during the study period, people enrolled in the study would need to be divided into those with and those without a history of LBP. After completing the back school, the subjects would be followed for a period of time, and the number of cases of LBP that occur among the subjects with and without a history of LBP would be recorded for subjects who had attended and who had not attended the back school. The incidence data in table can be used to calculate the RRR, ARR, and NNT values.

		Incidence of LBA (As a Proportion)		*RRR*	*ARR*	*NNT*
		CONTROL (C), NO BACK SCHOOL ATTENDANCE	**EXPERIMENTAL €, BACK SCHOOL**	**C-E/C**	**C-E**	**1/C-E**
Prior history of LBP	Yes	0.43	0.17	0.61	0.26	4
	No	0.13	0.06	0.54	0.07	14

The RRR values of 0.61 and 0.54 signify that the risk of developing LBP is reduced by 61% and 54% among individuals with a prior history of LBP and individuals without a prior history of LBP, respectively. What is missing from the RRR is the fact that the ARR for individuals without a history of LBP is relatively trivial. The reciprocal of the ARR yields a value that is potentially useful; the NNT is the number of people who would have to attend the back school to prevent an episode of LBP in one person. Therefore four people with a prior history of LBP should be sent to the back school to prevent the development of LBP in one person. Of the people who do not have a history of LBP, 14 need to attend the back school to prevent LBP in 1 member of this group. If the decision were made based solely on the RRR, everyone should attend back school. By assessing the NNT values, the decision might be to send anyone with a prior history of LBP to the back school but not the people without a history of LBP.

28. A researcher conducts a comprehensive meta-analysis comparing Oswestry scores of patients after 2 weeks of intervention for acute low back pain. The treatments compared were spinal manipulation versus education and walking as tolerated. Figure provides the results of the research. Based on this figure, answer the following questions. What is this type of plot called?

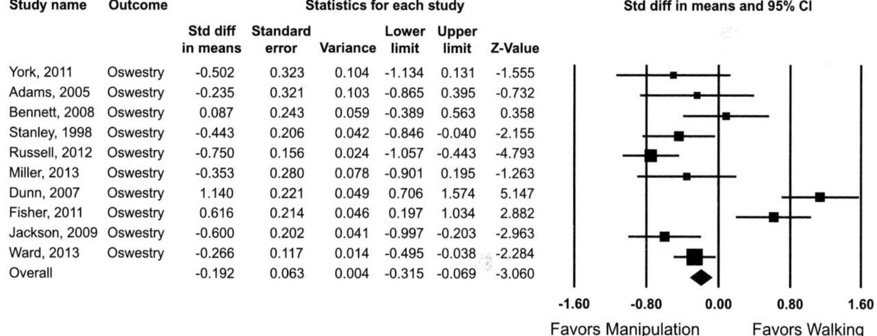

Study name	Outcome	Std diff in means	Standard error	Variance	Lower limit	Upper limit	Z-Value
York, 2011	Oswestry	-0.502	0.323	0.104	-1.134	0.131	-1.555
Adams, 2005	Oswestry	-0.235	0.321	0.103	-0.865	0.395	-0.732
Bennett, 2008	Oswestry	0.087	0.243	0.059	-0.389	0.563	0.358
Stanley, 1998	Oswestry	-0.443	0.206	0.042	-0.846	-0.040	-2.155
Russell, 2012	Oswestry	-0.750	0.156	0.024	-1.057	-0.443	-4.793
Miller, 2013	Oswestry	-0.353	0.280	0.078	-0.901	0.195	-1.263
Dunn, 2007	Oswestry	1.140	0.221	0.049	0.706	1.574	5.147
Fisher, 2011	Oswestry	0.616	0.214	0.046	0.197	1.034	2.882
Jackson, 2009	Oswestry	-0.600	0.202	0.041	-0.997	-0.203	-2.963
Ward, 2013	Oswestry	-0.266	0.117	0.014	-0.495	-0.038	-2.284
Overall		-0.192	0.063	0.004	-0.315	-0.069	-3.060

A forest plot.

29. Of the 10 studies that met the inclusion criteria for the study, how many resulted in a statistically significant difference between the treatment groups, which treatment was favored, and what is the basis for your determination of statistical significance?

Six reported a statistically significant difference (Stanley, Russell, Jackson, and Ward favored manipulation, whereas Dunn and Fisher favored walking). If the line representing the 95% confidence interval does not include a standardized difference between the means of 0, the difference is statistically significant at an alpha level of 0.05.

30. Was the overall analysis statistically significant? How do you know the answer from the figure alone?

Yes, there was a statistically significant difference overall, in favor of manipulation. This is demonstrated by the diamond symbol which does not include the value of zero difference.

31. **Which study had the most subjects? How can you tell?**
Ward (2013) had the most subjects based on the size of the symbol representing the standardized difference in means and 95% CI for that study. The symbol size is proportional to the sample size in a forest plot.

32. **What is the difference between linear regression and logistic regression?**
Linear regression uses one or more predictor variables (sometimes called "independent variables") to estimate the value of a predicted variable (sometimes called the "dependent variable") when the predicted variable is a continuous variable. Logistic regression is fundamentally the same concept, except the predicted variable is a categorical variable.

33. **Describe a situation where linear regression would be helpful.**
Suppose you wanted to provide a better prognosis for patients beginning treatment for chronic neck pain. You select the Neck Pain and Disability Scale (NPAD, scored on a 0 to 100 scale) as the outcome measure. Based on a thorough review of the evidence, you determine that you will measure five variables at the beginning of treatment and determine the NPAD score again after 3 weeks of treatment. After collecting data from a sample of patients, you then create a regression equation using the five predictor variables to estimate the final NPAD score of the sample. This equation could then be used for patients in the future to estimate the NPAD score after 3 weeks of treatment.

34. **What does a linear regression equation include?**

The general form for the regression equation is $\hat{y} = m_1x_1 + m_2x_2 + ...m_xx_x + b \pm error$

The ŷ is the estimated value of the predicted variable (read as "y hat"), the "m" is the slope of the regression line for each predictor variable, the "x" is the value of the predictor variable, "*b*" is the y-axis intercept (a constant), and "error" is the standard error of the estimate. Suppose in the NPAD example above, age in years, duration of symptoms in weeks, and whether litigation was pending were found to be meaningful predictors of the final NPAD score. The final equation could be

$$NPAD = 0.87(age) + 1.43(duration) + 3.55(litigation) + 3.3 \pm 4$$

To then calculate the estimated final NPAD score, you would multiply the patient's age in years by 0.87, add the product of the duration of symptoms in weeks by 1.43, then add the product of the value of the litigation variable times 3.55, and add 3.3. The actual value will be within $\pm$ 8 points for 95% of your patients, assuming the patients are similar to those who constituted the sample used to derive the equation.

35. **How can you multiply 3.55 times the litigation variable?**
Litigation is a categorical variable and must be coded as 0 or 1. In this case, if litigation was pending, the value of 1 is assigned, so litigation adds 3.55 to the predicted score. If litigation is not pending, it is coded as a 0, and that term drops from the equation.

36. **Describe a situation where logistic regression would be helpful.**
Basically the same situation as for linear regression, but the predicted variable is categorical instead of continuous. Suppose you wanted to predict whether patients who were undergoing a total hip arthroplasty would be able to be discharged to home or would need to be transferred to a facility for further rehabilitation. This is a categorical variable ("home" or "not home") and could be coded as 0 for "not home" and 1 for "home." Obviously, the outcome could be coded 1 for "not home" and 0 for "home," but the key is that the logistic regression equation will predict the status coded as "1." A logistic regression equation can be used just as a linear regression equation, but the value predicted is the probability of group membership in the group coded as "1." So, if the value of the equation is 0.83 and "home" was coded as group "1," then the probability that this patient will be discharged to home is 0.83.

37. **Is this how logistic regression equations are typically used?**
No. Instead, the results of the equation are expressed in odds ratios, usually called "Exp(B)." Suppose in the discharge environment example, a researcher reports that one predictor variable was "comorbidities" and was coded as 0 if "none" and 1 if "present" (so a categorical predictor of a categorical result), and the Exp(B) for that variable is 7.3. The predicted membership was in the group "not home." This means that if comorbidities are present, the odds of being discharged "not home" are 7.3-fold greater than if the patient does not have comorbidities. Remember, the odds ratio helps adjust the odds of the outcome, not the probability.

38. **Does the same process hold true for continuous predictor variables?**
Fundamentally, yes, but with a very important distinction. If the predictor variable is continuous, the Exp(B) gives the change in odds of membership in the group coded as "1" for each unit change in the predictor variable. Suppose in the discharge environment example one predictor variable was the preoperative 6-minute walk distance measured in meters, and the Exp(B) for this variable is 0.93. Typically, an Odds Ratio of 0.93 is considered a trivial, unimportant value, but in this case, it means that for each additional meter walked in this test, the odds of being in the group discharged "not home" are only 0.93 as large as an individual who walked only 1 meter less.

39. **Describe the approach to probability proposed by Thomas Bayes.**
Bayesian statistics is a general term used to describe an approach to probability proposed by Thomas Bayes in the mid-18th century. Because of the complexity of the computations and the development of other approaches to data (now called "classical statistics"), the method did not gain widespread use until the 1950s with the development of computers. The essential element of Bayesian statistics is that the probability of an event can be best estimated when the baseline probability is adjusted when new information becomes available. The terms commonly used are "prior" for the baseline probability, "likelihood" for the new information, and "posterior" for the final probability statement.

40. **What is Bayes's Theorem?**

$$p\left(A \mid B\right) = p\left(B \mid A\right)\frac{pA}{pB}$$

p(A|B) is the probability of the event A if the evidence is present, p(B|A) is the probability of the evidence being present *if* the outcome (the event) also occurs, pA is the probability of the event given no additional evidence, and pB is the probability of the evidence being present irrespective of the outcome.

41. **How can Bayes's Theorem be applied to clinical practice?**
The most obvious example is in the use of a diagnostic test. Suppose the data in table were collected from a sample of patients.

		Truth about Disease		
		PRESENT	**ABSENT**	**TOTAL**
Test result	Positive	30	4	34
	Negative	7	24	31
		37	28	65

p(A) is the probability of the disease being present before any knowledge of the test result is obtained. Here, this value is 37/65 = 0.569, and is the same as the prevalence of the disease.

p(B) is the probability of the evidence being present irrespective of the disease. Here, this value is the proportion of positive test results, 34/65 = 0.523.

p(B|A) is the probability of the evidence being present if the outcome is also positive, 30/37 = 0.811, and this is the same as the Sensitivity of the test.

Solving this equation gives a value of 0.882 and is the probability of the disease being present given a positive test result. From a diagnostic perspective, this is the same as the posttest probability and will be the same result if one calculates the Sensitivity, Specificity, and Likelihood ratios.

42. **Are there other uses for a Bayesian approach?**
Yes, this approach can be used for inferential analysis of events (categorical data) from a randomized controlled trial. Although there are passionate proponents for the Bayesian approach and equally passionate proponents for classical analysis, the two approaches complement each other and may well be best used together. In many respects, the Bayesian approach more closely mimics the day-to-day process of making any decision. Given a situation where one must make a decision, the probability of a desired outcome or result constantly changes as a result of additional information.

BIBLIOGRAPHY

Field, A. (2018). *Discovering statistics using SPSS* (5th ed.). Los Angeles: Sage.

Glantz, S. A. (2011). *Primer of biostatistics* (7th ed.). New York: McGraw-Hill.

Keppel, G. (1991). *Design and analysis: a researcher's handbook* (3rd ed.). Englewood Cliffs, NJ: Prentice Hall.

Norman, G. R., & Streiner, D. L. (2014). *Biostatistics: The bare essentials* (4th ed.). Shelton, CT: People's Medical Publishing House.

Osborne, J. W. (2015). *Best practices in logistic regression.* Los Angeles: Sage.

Roach, K. E., Brown, M. D., Albin, R. D., Delaney, K. G., Lipprandi, H. M., & Rangelli, D. (1997). The sensitivity and specificity of pain response to activity and position in categorizing patients with low back pain. *Physical Therapy, 77*, 730–738.

Sackett, D. L., Haynes, R. B., Guyatt, G. H., & Tugwell, P. (1991). *Clinical epidemiology: a basic science for clinical medicine* (2nd ed.). Boston, MA: Little Brown.

Wijeysundera, D. N., Austin, P. C., Hux, J. E., Beattie, W. S., & Laupacia, A. (2009). Bayesian statistical inference enhances the intepretation of contemporary randomized controlled trials. *Journal of Clinical Epidemiology, 62*, 13–21.

CHAPTER 19 QUESTIONS

1. **Given the following set of data, which measure of central tendency BEST describes the data, and why is that the best measure?**
   12, 10, 12, 14, 11, 12, 13, 2, 10, 12, 9, 12
   a. Mean, because the data are a normal distribution
   b. Median, because the data are skewed to the left
   c. Median, because the data are skewed to the right
   d. Mode, because there are several identical values in the data

2. **You are examining a patient with shoulder pain. After obtaining a history and asking the patient about her symptoms, you suspect she has a labral tear. You recently read a report of a clinical test for labral tears of the shoulder, and the researchers calculated a positive likelihood ratio (LR+) of 3.22. The result of this clinical test for this patient is positive. What does this mean?**
   a. The posttest probability of her having a labral tear are 3.22 times greater than the pretest probability.
   b. The posttest odds of her having a labral tear are 3.22 times greater than the pretest odds.
   c. The odds in favor of her having a labral tear are 3.22:1.
   d. The probability of her not having a labral tear is the reciprocal of 3.22, or 0.31.

3. **What type of analysis will allow you to identify which variables can be used to predict whether a patient who is treated with manual therapy will return to work within 8 weeks following the initiation of treatment?**
   a. Analysis of variance (ANOVA)
   b. Multiple linear regression
   c. Logistic regression
   d. Chi-square

CONCUSSION MANAGEMENT

B.J. Lee, PT, DPT, LAT, FAAOMPT, SCS, OCS, CSCS, USAW

EPIDEMIOLOGY

1. **What is a concussion and how do they occur?**
   A concussion is a mild traumatic brain injury induced by biomechanical forces. These forces result in a complex pathophysiological process that can occur due to a direct blow to the head or an indirect blow with an impact on the body. These forces can be due to coup contrecoup movements of the brain within the skull causing stress and strain to the brain tissue, vasculature, and the neural elements. The neuronal injuries caused by the rotational and linear shear forces from the acceleration and deceleration of the brain within the skull results in diffuse axonal injury. This leads to a neurometabolic crisis with shifts in ionic concentrations, the release of excitatory amino acids, an increase in brain-glucose metabolism, and decreased cerebral blood flow. Typically, concussions result in neuropathological changes without concomitant structural abnormalities seen upon imaging.

2. **How often and when do concussions occur and who is most at risk?**
   The CDC estimates that between 1.6 and 3.8 million sports-related concussions occur each year in the United States. The incidence of concussion is higher in competition than in practice. Sports with the highest risk of concussion are American football, female and male soccer, wrestling, and female basketball. Of these sports, American football accounts for the highest frequency of concussions. Although there may be sport- or reporting-dependent differences, concussions occur more frequently in females than males. Younger athletes have a higher incidence than older athletes and athletes with a history of prior concussion are at increased risk for a future concussion.

3. **What is the typical recovery trajectory after sport-related concussion?**
   Adults tend to recover within 10 to 14 days after injury and children tend to recover within 4 weeks of the injury. Recovery outside of these time frames is termed prolonged or persistent symptoms.

4. **What are the most common symptoms after concussion?**
   The most common symptoms after concussion can be divided into four main categories including somatic, cognitive, affective, and sleep-related symptoms. Common somatic symptoms are headache, nausea, vomiting, sensitivity to light, sensitivity to noise, visual problems, fatigue, feeling dazed, dizziness, and balance problems. Common cognitive symptoms are fogginess, feeling slowed down, delayed responses, difficulty concentrating, forgetfulness, repeating things, decreased academic performance, confusion, and amnesia. Common affective symptoms are irritability, sadness, depression, personality changes, anxiety, panic, feeling more emotional, and feeling apathetic. Common sleep-related symptoms are drowsiness, sleeping more, sleeping less, difficulty falling asleep, difficulty staying asleep, and not feeling rested.

5. **What is prolonged recovery? And who is most at risk?**
   Prolonged recovery or persistent symptoms is defined as clinical recovery following concussion that falls outside of the previously defined time frames for adults and children. Risk factors for prolonged recovery include dizziness at the time of injury, history of depression or anxiety, history of learning disorders/ADHD, delayed removal from play at time of initial injury, history of migraines, mental status changes at time of injury, history of prior concussions, higher total number of symptoms at time of injury, the tendency to somatization of the individual, the presence of sleep disturbances after injury, and negative expectations of recovery. Further, risk factors are sex, with females tending to take longer to recover than males, and age at time of injury, with younger athletes taking longer to recover than their older athlete counterparts.

ACUTE MANAGEMENT AND DIAGNOSIS

6. **What are the emergent conditions to be aware of and how can they be identified at the time of injury?**
   - **Second impact syndrome**
     For athletes who have experienced a prior head injury, one of the most concerning risks if they return to play too soon is a rare but potentially lethal injury called second impact syndrome (SIS). SIS occurs when the brain swells when an athlete incurs a second concussion prior to complete resolution of a prior concussion. The brain loses its ability to auto-regulate intracranial and cerebral perfusion pressure leading to severe edema and possible herniation. The best way to prevent SIS from occurring is a proper return-to-play progression after full symptom resolution of the athlete.

- **Cervical spine injuries**
  1. Fracture
     a. Canadian C-spine Rules
        i. Figure 20.1
     b. Jefferson fracture test
  2. Alar ligament rupture
     a. Alar ligament test
  3. Transverse ligament rupture
     a. Sharp-Purser test
     b. Transverse ligament test
  4. Vertebral artery disruption
     a. Vertebral artery test
- **Signs and Symptoms for Immediate Referral**
  Some of the signs and symptoms that would indicate a need for immediate referral to another provider are an abnormal cranial nerve exam, a rapid deterioration in presentation, an abnormal pupillary response upon examination, convulsions, seizures or tonic posturing, recurrent nausea and vomiting, weakness in the extremities, severe neck pain, the inability to be aroused, and significant confusion, agitation, and restlessness.

7. **What are some of the tools utilized on the sideline to help identify a concussion and how are they used?**
   Since concussion can result in many different signs and symptoms, sideline assessment of concussion needs to be comprehensive. Using any test in isolation is not recommended as no testing to date has been identified to be sensitive enough independently. Thus, each program and healthcare team need to work together to create a battery of testing items for their assessment.

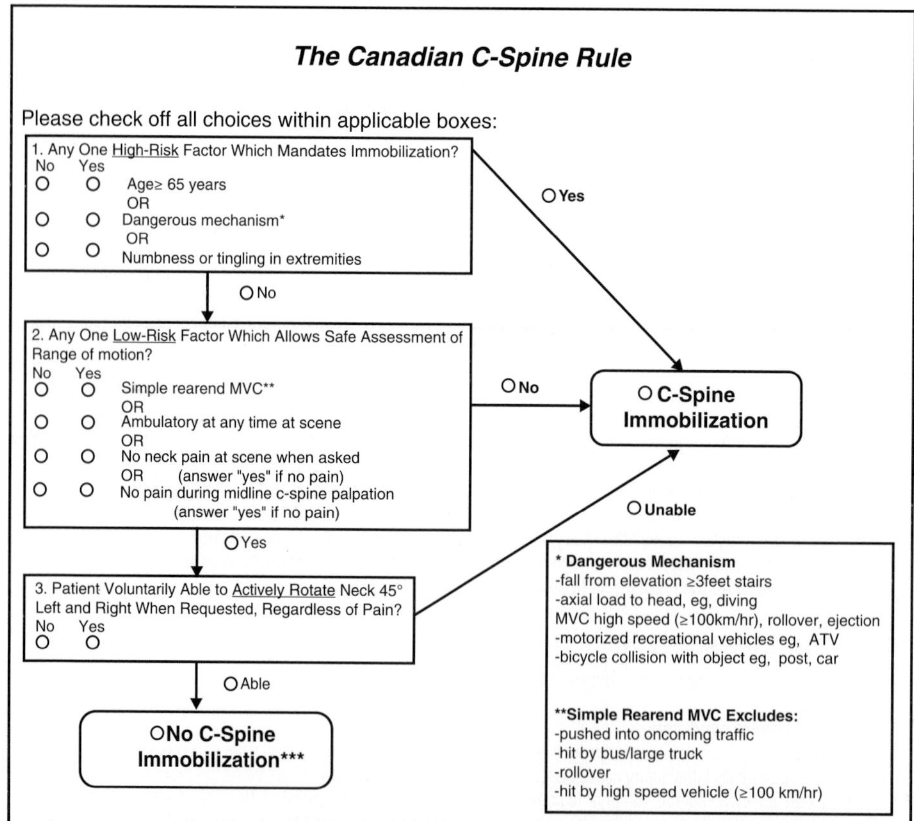

Figure 20.1 Canadian C-spine rules. *C-Spine*, Cervical spine, *MVC*, motor vehicle crash. (Vaillancourt C, Charette M, Kasaboski A, et al. (2011). Evaluation of the safety of C-spine clearance by paramedics: design and methodology. *BMC Emerg Med* 11, 1. https://doi.org/10.1186/1471-227X-11-1.)

- Sport Concussion Assessment Tool (SCAT5)

The Sport Concussion Assessment Tool—5th Edition (SCAT5) is a standardized tool utilized by healthcare providers to evaluate an athlete aged 13 and older for concussion. This test is often utilized on the sidelines and takes approximately 10 minutes to complete. The SCAT5 consists of the following basic components:

- Red flags identification
- Glasgow Coma Scale (GCS)—Scoring system to describe the level of consciousness of the athlete
- Symptom Evaluation through the Post-Concussion Symptom Scale (PCSS)
- Cognitive assessment including immediate memory, concentration, and delayed recall
- Cervical screen to rule out fractures (Canadian C-Spine Rules)
- Neurological screen that includes assessment of movements, eye movements, balance, and coordination
- Balance assessment—modified Balance Error Scoring System (mBESS) test utilizing three stances (Romberg, single leg stance, tandem) on firm surface only
- King-Devick Test

The King-Devick test is a quick sideline assessment utilized to assess a combination of saccadic and smooth pursuit oculomotor movements. The test is usually administered on a series of cards. The first card is an example card, followed by three cards with progressive increasing difficulty. The cards consist of numbers arrayed in rows and the athlete is asked to read the numbers out loud while the examiner times them. Their time is compared to baseline or normative data based on age group and gender. Although this test is a quick tool, it has poor sensitivity (60%) and specificity (39%). Therefore, this test should not be used in isolation to determine the presence of a concussion but can be a helpful addition to a comprehensive battery of tests.

- Visual Tracking devices

More in-depth oculomotor and vestibular assessment may be warranted on the sideline. However, most visual exams may add too much time to be easily and efficiently implemented in a sideline setting. Further, results may be vague due to lack of symptom reporting with testing and unreliable objective assessment of visual deviations. Thus, electronic devices are starting to be implemented that objectively track pupillary movement with camera capture systems and provide immediate objective data on the athletes' status. This technology is an emerging area for research, but overall accessibility is limited due to cost.

- Balance tests

The most used assessment is the Balance Error Scoring System (BESS). A modified version of this test is also a part of the SCAT5 assessment. The BESS test contains six testing conditions total in three positions (Romberg, single leg, and tandem), each performed on firm and foam surface. The athlete is asked to balance in each condition with their eyes closed and hands on their hips for 20 seconds. The examiner counts the number of errors the athlete makes during this time frame. Errors include opening eyes, lifting hands off hips, stepping, stumbling, or falling out of position, lifting forefoot or heel, abducting hip by more than 30 degrees, or failing to return to test position in more than 5 seconds if they fall out of position.

Other testing devices are starting to be implemented to objectively test the amount of sway an athlete has during a balance task using a phone or portable electronic device with an accelerometer utilized for measurement.

It is important to note that baseline testing with any method of balance testing is important for a true comparison and to make an informed decision after a potential concussive injury.

EXAMINATION/EVALUATION

General

8. What are the four impairment-based diagnostic categories identified by the Concussion Clinical Practice Guideline (CPG)?

The Concussion CPG have identified four categories of impairments that must be assessed. They are cervical, vestibulo-oculomotor impairments, autonomic/exertional tolerance impairments, and motor function impairments.

9. What are other identifiable clinical profiles that may require assessment and treatment?

Other clinical profiles associated with concussion are anxiety/mood disorders and cognitive disorders. Symptoms and deficits in these profiles may require referral to other health care providers for effective management.

10. What tests and measures are often utilized to assess each diagnostic category outlined by the CPG and additional clinical profiles?

- Cervical
  1. Active range of motion
  2. Passive range of motion
  3. Joint mobility
  4. Special tests
  5. Cervicogenic dizziness test
  6. Reproduction of symptoms
- Vestibulo-oculomotor Impairments

1. Vestibulo-Ocular Motor Screen (VOMS)
   Assesses the vestibular and oculomotor systems across five domains in different directions: horizontal and vertical smooth pursuit, horizontal saccades, vertical saccades, vergence, horizontal vestibular ocular reflex (VOR), vertical VOR, horizontal VOR cancellation.
2. Head thrust test
   Assess impairments in the VOR
3. Dynamic visual acuity test
   Assess impairments in the VOR
4. School bus test
   Assess static visual alignment
5. Frenzel tests
   Assess for the presence of benign paroxysmal positional vertigo (BPPV) and/or nystagmus
6. BPPV tests
   a. Posterior canal
      i. Dix-Hallpike test
   b. Horizontal canal
      ii. Log roll test

- Autonomic/Exertional Tolerance Impairments
  1. Buffalo Concussion Treadmill Test
  2. Buffalo Concussion Bike Test
- Motor Function Impairments
  1. Balance/postural control impairments
     BESS test
     Sway balance test
  2. Dual/multitasking impairments
     Most assessments of dual/multitasking impairments require the use of a lab. No clinical assessments have been identified to date.
  3. Delayed motor reaction time
     Often tested with neurocognitive assessments
  4. Motor coordination
     To date, no tests have been validated to assess for deficits in motor coordination after concussion.
- Anxiety/Mood
  Evaluation for the presence of anxiety/mood-related changes after concussion may include clinical interview, symptom-reporting outcome measure, neurocognitive testing, and/or psychological evaluation.
- Cognitive
  Neurocognitive tests are often utilized to measure dimensions such as visuomotor response timing, visual search, sustained attention, encoding, verbal working memory, spatial working memory, and visuospatial working memory. Some of the tests that are often utilized are the ImPACT, AxomSports, CNS Viital Signs, and C3 Logic assessment.

FUNCTIONAL OUTCOME TOOLS

11. What are some of the functional outcome tools (FOTs) used to examine patients after sport-related concussion?

Many of the FOTs utilized during concussion management are not concussion specific but related to many of the symptoms that may be present after the injury. The selection of which tool to use may be based on ease of use and symptoms present in the athlete in front of you.

1. PCSS—The Post-Concussion Symptom Scale is a 22-item scale
2. Rivermead Post-Concussion Symptom Questionnaire
3. DHI—Dizziness Handicap Inventory
4. DGI/Modified DGI—Dynamic Gait Index
5. VRBQ—Vestibular Rehabilitation Benefits Questionnaire
6. NDI—Neck Disability Index
7. Sleep functional outcome tools—utilization of general sleep FOTs or of concussion-specific forms such as the Sleep and Concussion Questionnaire (SCQ), which is in the process of being validated.

ASSESSMENT/PROGNOSIS

12. What sign/symptom is the strongest predictor of a slower recovery progression?

The strongest predictor of a slower recovery time is the severity of an athletes' initial symptoms in the first few days following injury.

13. How do you interpret the results of BPPV testing and deduce which treatment to implement?

1. Dix-Hallpike test: Assesses the posterior canal on the ipsilateral side and anterior canal on contralateral side
   a) Canalithiasis: Nystagmus lasting <60 seconds
      (1) Right Side Test:
         (a) Posterior canal—Nystagmus up and torsional towards the right
         (b) Anterior canal—Nystagmus down and torsional towards the right
      (2) Left Side Test:
         (a) Posterior canal—Nystagmus up and torsional towards the left
         (b) Anterior canal—Nystagmus down and torsional towards the left
   b) Cupulolithiasis: Persistent nystagmus lasting >60 seconds
         (a) Same nystagmus directions as above
2. Log roll test: Assesses the horizontal canals
   a) Canalithiasis:
      (1) Right Side Test:
         (a) Geotrophic nystagmus (beats towards the ground bilaterally; when right horizontal canal is the involved side, nystagmus beats stronger to the right when the head is turned to the right than when it beats to the left when the head is turned to the left)
      (2) Left Side Test:
         (a) Geotrophic nystagmus (beats towards the ground bilaterally; when left horizontal canal is the involved side, nystagmus beats stronger to the left when the head is turned to the left than when it beats to the right when the head is turned to the right)
   b) Cupulolithiasis:
      (1) Right Side Test:
         (a) Ageotrophic nystagmus (beats away from the ground bilaterally; when right horizontal canal is the involved side, nystagmus beats stronger to the left when the head is turned to the right than when it beats to the right when the head is turned to the left)
      (2) Left Side Test:
         (a) Ageotrophic nystagmus (beats away from the ground bilaterally; when left horizontal canal is the involved side, nystagmus beats stronger to the right when the head is turned to the left than when it beats to the left when the head is turned to the right)

14. Under what conditions is it considered appropriate for an athlete who continues to have a headache to return to play if that is the only persistent symptom?

Athletes with a history of migraines whose headaches have returned to prior baseline frequency and intensity.

- Athletes whose only remaining symptom after prolonged recovery is a headache that is being medically managed by the lead physician and cleared by an appropriate healthcare provider such as the physician.

INTERVENTIONS

15. How long should athletes rest after their injury?

Historically, athletes were instructed to rest until they were symptom free, at which time they could initiate a return-to-play progression. However, research suggests that the prolonged period of inactivity can lead to worsening symptoms and prolonged recovery. It is now suggested that after a concussion athletes rest at most for 24 to 48 hours prior to beginning subsymptomatic exercise.

16. At what intensity should athletes begin a graded exercise program after sustaining a concussion?

After implementing either the Buffalo Concussion Treadmill test or the Buffalo Concussion Bike test, it is recommended that the athlete do 30 minutes of exercise each day. This includes a 5-minute warm-up, followed by 20 minutes of cardiovascular exercise (walking or biking) at 80% of the heart rate at which symptom onset occurred during testing, then a 5-minute cool down. If heart rate assessment is not available at the time of testing, use approximately 80% of the rating of perceived exertion at which symptom onset occurred during testing. If neither heart rate nor rating of perceived exertion can be used, athletes should be instructed to implement exercise at a subsymptom threshold. Delaying the start of physical activity after concussion can be detrimental to recovery and lead to prolonged recovery time.

17. What is the recommended volume prescription of vestibular and oculomotor exercises to promote adaptation and habituation in an athlete with vestibulo-oculomotor impairments after concussion?

When prescribing vestibular and oculomotor exercises as part of an home exercise program, the goal is to work up to three sets of 45 seconds performed three to five times a day. If symptoms arise after one set, the athlete should wait until symptoms subside prior to beginning the next set. Repetition is important for habituation and adaptation to occur. If an athlete does not tolerate 45 seconds of an exercise, starting with a smaller volume and gradually increasing over time is permissible.

18. **What is the role of nutrition in recovery and treatment after concussion?**
Currently, there is no evidence of specific nutrition recommendations that help prevent the occurrence of concussion nor the speed of recovery after concussion. However, certain vitamins and minerals may help create a conducive environment for healing such as omega-3 fatty acids, vitamin C, vitamin D, magnesium, and zinc. Keeping a healthy diet can also help with an overall improved setting for promoting recovery. Caution is warranted with supplements such as caffeine. If athletes consumed caffeine prior to injury, cutting off or significantly reducing intake from the typical amount after injury may contribute to headaches due to withdrawal. In this instance, caffeine amounts may need to be reduced but not completely removed. For athletes who did not normally consume caffeine prior to injury, it may not be beneficial to add it into their diet during recovery.

MEDICAL MANAGEMENT

19. **What are the 11 Rs in concussion management according to the Berlin Guidelines?**
    i. Recognize
    ii. Remove
    iii. Re-evaluate
    iv. Rest
    v. Rehabilitation
    vi. Refer
    vii. Recovery
    viii. Return to sport
    ix. Reconsider
    x. Residual effects/sequelae
    xi. Risk reduction

20. **What is the role of imaging in the medical management of concussion?**
As most concussions are nonstructural in nature, traditional imaging such as x-ray, CT scans, and MRI are not frequently obtained. X-rays and CT scans are utilized when someone does not pass the Canadian C-Spine rules and a fracture or bony abnormality is suspected. A traditional MRI can be utilized if a vascular disruption or ligament tear is suspected in and around the head and neck. Functional MRIs (fMRI) measure brain connectivity and blood flow and are indicative of neurovascular coupling. Alterations in neural activity and connectivity are often detected after concussion with fMRI; however, their cost and lack of accessibility limit their usefulness. Diffusor Tensor Imaging (DTI) measures the directional diffusion patterns of water in the brain, which is an indirect measure of white matter structure. DTI can be used to measure chronic changes and disease in cerebral white matter and is an area of emerging research in terms of chronic traumatic encephalopathy (CTE) and long-term neurocognitive changes.

21. **What medications are recommended and often prescribed by the appropriate medical provider after concussion?**
Currently, there are no medications that have been approved by the FDA for treatment of concussion and no medications have been shown to improve recovery time. Some non-FDA-approved pharmacological treatments that are utilized to treat specific symptoms are included below:
    1. Emotional disruptions
        a. Selective serotonin reuptake inhibitors (SSRIs)
    2. Somatic symptoms-headache
        a. Pain reliever such as Tylenol
        b. Nonsteroidal anti-inflammatory drugs (NSAIDs)
        c. Tricyclic antidepressants such as Amitriptyline
        d. Beta-Blockers such as Propranolol
        e. Sphenopalatine ganglion (SPG) block
    3. Cognitive symptoms
        a. Neurostimulants such as amantadine and methylphenidate
    4. Sleep symptoms
        a. Melatonin-over the counter
        b. Trazodone
    5. Vitamins and minerals
        a. Fish oil-omega 3 fatty acids, specifically EPA and DHA, increase the fluidity of cell membranes, enhance cerebral blood flow, and reduce inflammation
        b. Vitamin D-deficiency may exacerbate inflammatory damage and behavioral impairment following brain injury

22. **What is the process for return to learn after concussion?**
There is limited research currently on the best process for student athletes to return to the classroom. Activities such as testing, group work, taking notes, reading, watching videos, and the lights and sounds of the environment

Table 20.1 Return to Learn

STAGE	RETURN TO LEARN	PROGRESS WHEN:
1	No formal school attendance: No tests, quizzes, or homework if increases symptoms Limited screen time (TV, phone, computer, etc.) based on symptom provocation	Little to no sensitivity to light and sound Able to read or look at screen for 10 mins without increased symptoms
2	Modified class schedule with restrictions: No tests, quizzes, or homework if increases symptoms Provide copies of notes and lectures if needed Hall pass to avoid busy times in between classes Sunglasses and other aids may be needed to assist in class participation Some social integration based on symptom tolerance	Overall decrease in symptoms Symptoms not increased with classes Able to attend at least ½ day of class each day of the week
3	Modified class schedule without restrictions: Tests, quizzes, and homework PRN with potential accommodations for time, etc. Decrease use of aids such as sunglasses or hat in class Progress social integration volume and settings	Neurocognitive test scores have normalized No symptoms with full workload during half-day class schedule
4	Full academic participation and load with restrictions: Tests, quizzes, and homework with accommodations PRN No use of aids such as sunglasses, hat, etc.	Asymptomatic with academic workload Able to tolerate full day of school No need for accommodations to complete academic tasks
5	Full academic participation with no restrictions	

PRN, When necessary.
To note, RTL process can be occurring simultaneously as RTP process; however, a student-athlete cannot return to play while unable to fully return to school.
Adapted from McCrory et al., 2017, *Consensus Statement on Concussion in Sport; Parachute Canadian Guideline on Concussion.*

of a classroom can all increase a student's symptoms as they attempt to return to school after a concussive injury. Similar to early integration into subsymptomatic exercise, students returning to the classroom should be able to return as soon as they are able to tolerate about 30 minutes of cognitive activity at home without significant symptom exacerbation. Once they can meet these criteria to return to school, modifications can be implemented to help students stay at a subsymptomatic level throughout the day. Such techniques may include sunglasses for light sensitivity, earplugs for loud noises, extended time for tests and assignments, frequent breaks, working in the library, extra tutoring, or review sessions, etc. For those students with prolonged symptoms, an educational action plan, such as a 504 plan, may need to be implemented with the assistance of the medical team and teachers. It is important to remember that student athletes are students first, and a return-to-learn progression should be completed prior to full return to play, though the two progressions may advance simultaneously under the supervision of the appropriate medical provider. Table 20.1 demonstrates one proposed return to learn model.

23. **How should an athlete return to play (RTP) after a concussion?**
Once an athlete is symptom free, they can begin a general 6-step return to play (RTP) process outlined in table lines in Table 20.2. Research now supports early participation in a subsymptomatic aerobic exercise program to help promote recovery and a quicker RTP. Further, it has been suggested that the RTP process be better defined with the use of target heart rates to define each stage and criteria for progression. Table 20.3 demonstrates an example of a progression that initiates an early subsymptomatic aerobic exercise program and progressions in the first few phases based on heart rate. Although the six-step process is widely accepted, each RTP plan should be individualized and sport specific. Athletes who experience prolonged symptoms may require alterations and a longer RTP progression. The final decision on allowing an athlete to RTP should be made by the designated healthcare provider and each state differs on which healthcare providers are eligible to make this decision.

TEAM-BASED MANAGEMENT

24. **Identify some of the healthcare providers and other team members who may be involved in the management of an athlete after sport-related concussion**
    a. Doctor
    b. Athletic trainer
    c. Physical therapist

Table 20.2 General RTP Progression

STAGE	EXERCISE RECOMMENDATION	OBJECTIVE
i. No activity	Symptom limited activity (physical and cognitive rest)	Recovery
ii. Light aerobic exercise	Aerobic exercise at <70% Max HR (mode: cycling, walking, swimming, sport specific) No resistance training	Gradual increase in HR
iii. Sport-specific exercise	Sport-specific noncontact drills No head impact activities	Add increased movement and sport participation
iv. Noncontact training drills	Progression to complex sport-specific drills with increased cognitive load Add resistance training	Add cognitive load and complexity to exercise
v. Full-contact practice	Return to normal practice after medical clearance by appropriate healthcare professional	Increase participation and confidence in sport participation
vi. Return to play	Full game or game simulation participation	

RTP, Return to play, HR, heart rate.
Adapted from McCrory P, Meeuwisse W, Dvorak J, Aubry M, Bailes J, Broglio S, Davis, GA. Consensus statement on concussion in sport—the 5th international conference on concussion in sport held in Berlin, October 2016. *Br J Sports Med.* 2017.

Table 20.3 RTP Progression With HR Guidelines

STAGE	EXERCISE RECOMMENDATION	ACTIVITIES
i. Target heart rate: <60% of max exertion	10–15 min of cardio exercise Low stimulus environment No impact activities Balance, vestibular, and cervical treatment (PRN) Limit head movement/ position change Limit concentration activities	Very light aerobic conditioning Sub-max strengthening ROM/Stretching Very low-level balance activities
ii. Target heart rate: <70% of max exertion	20–30 min of cardio exercise; exercise in gym areas Use various exercise equipment Some positional changes and head movement Low-level concentration activities	Moderate aerobic conditioning Lightweight strength exercise Stretching Low-level balance activities
iii. Target heart rate: <80% of max exertion	Use any environment for exercise (indoor, outdoor) Integrate strength and conditioning Balance/proprioceptive exercise Incorporate concentration challenges	Moderately aggressive aerobic exercise All forms of strength exercise (80% max) Impact activities running, plyometrics (no contact) Challenging proprio-balance activities
iv. Noncontact training drills	Avoid contact activity	Noncontact physical training
v. Target heart rate: <90% of max exertion	Resume aggressive aerobic and resistance training in all environments	Aggressive strength exercise Impact activities/plyometrics Sports-specific training activities

Table 20.3 RTP Progression With HR Guidelines

STAGE	EXERCISE RECOMMENDATION	ACTIVITIES
vi. Full-contact practice	Initiate contact activities as appropriate to sport activity Full exertion for sport	Resume full physical training activities with contact Continue aggressive strength/ conditioning exercise Sport-specific activities
vii. Return to play	Full game or game simulation participation	

RTP, Return to play, HR, heart rate, ROM, range of motion.
Adapted from Collins M, Learish S, Lovell M, et al. (2008) UPMC Sports Medicine Concussion Program Guidelines for Post-Concussion Rehab.

d. Speech language pathologist
e. Occupational therapist
f. Sports phycologist
g. Neuropsychologist
h. Ophthalmologist, neuro-ophthalmologist
i. Ear, nose, throat specialist
j. Audiologist

OUTCOMES

Dual/Multitasking

25. **What differences are seen in the ability to dual/multitask after concussion?**
After concussion there are often differences in walking gait with dual task assessments compared to healthy controls. Some of these differences include: increased medial-lateral sway with walking, decreased overall gait speed, the presence of a more conservative gait pattern, deviations in inter-joint coordination and in turning gait. All of these findings occurred with walking. Assessment of differences has not been evaluated with sport-specific tasks such as running to date.

Future Injury Risk

26. **What is the relationship between concussions and lower extremity injuries in athletes after returning to play?**
There is a significant increase in lower extremity injury risk after returning to play from a concussion with an increased odds ratio of 1.6 to 2.9 times increased risk compared to athletes who have not sustained a concussion. This increased risk of future injury continues to persist even when prior lower extremity injury is accounted for. Further, this increase in injury risk has been found to be higher in reserves compared to starters and males compared to females, though the latter could be due to sport participation stratification. Further, athletes who have sustained multiple concussions are at a further increased risk compared to athletes who have only sustained one concussion and those who have never sustained a concussion. Injuries vary from muscle strains, ligament sprains, to tears. The window of susceptibility has been found to be at least 1 year out from initial concussion. Current motor control and RTP testing criteria lack sensitivity to be able to detect why this increased risk is occurring. This could have implications in long-term prognosis and may require alterations in the traditional return to play progression. No current research has been conducted looking into the relationship between concussion and other types of injuries to date.

Long-term Neurocognitive Changes

27. **What is chronic traumatic encephalopathy (CTE) and what is its relationship to concussion?**
CTE is a progressive degenerative disease of the brain found in athletes (and others) with a history of repetitive brain trauma, including symptomatic concussions as well as asymptomatic subconcussive hits to the head. CTE has been known to affect boxers since the 1920s. However, recent reports have been published of neuropathologically confirmed CTE in retired professional football players and other athletes who have a history of repetitive brain trauma. This trauma triggers progressive degeneration of the brain tissue, specifically the build-up of an abnormal protein called tau in the frontal and temporal lobes. These changes in the brain can begin months, years, or even decades after the last brain trauma or the end of active athletic involvement. The brain degeneration is associated with memory loss, confusion, impaired judgment, impulse control problems,

aggression, depression, and, eventually, progressive dementia. CTE can only be diagnosed postmortem through brain biopsy. CTE has been primarily linked with subconcussive hits and the years of exposure to contact sports rather than to a history of multiple concussions. Currently, there are no supported interventions that can be implemented to prevent the development of CTE.

Prevention

28. What can be utilized to prevent concussive injuries?

Currently, there are no specific interventions that can be definitively implemented to prevent concussions. There have been many proposed pieces of equipment that are advertised as preventative measures but lack evidence to support that claim. The primary role of helmets is to prevent skull fractures and intracranial hemorrhages. However, improperly fitted helmets may increase the risk of concussion. Mouthguards are utilized to decrease risk of dental and oral trauma. Neither can be considered preventative for concussion at this time based on research findings. Further equipment such as headbands to decrease impact with heading a ball and swim caps with mesh designed to decrease impact with hitting the head on the wall or bottom of the pool also lack efficacy at this time. The use of such equipment could potentially increase risk of concussion by creating a false sense of security from the injury and increasing risky behavior patterns of the athlete. There is emerging evidence that increasing cervical musculature strength may have a protective effect for concussions. Studies have found that there is an increased risk for concussion for athletes with smaller neck circumference, neck to head circumference ratio, and overall neck strength. For every 1-pound increase in neck strength the odds of sustaining a concussion have been found to decrease by 5%.

Bibliography

Alosco, M.L., Mez, J., Tripodis, Y., et al. (2018). Age of first exposure to tackle football and chronic traumatic encephalopathy. *Annals of Neurology, 83*(5), 886–901.

Asken, B. M., Bauer, R. M., Guskiewicz, K. M., et al. (2018). Immediate removal from activity after sport-related concussion is associated with shorter clinical recovery and less severe symptoms in collegiate student-athletes. *American Journal of Sports Medicine, 46*(6), 1465–1474.

Barrett, E. C., Mcburney, M. I., & Ciappio, E. D. (2014). ω-3 fatty acid supplementation as a potential therapeutic aid for the recovery from mild traumatic brain injury/concussion. *Advances in Nutrition, 5*(3), 268–277.

Beauchamp, K., Mutlak, H., Smith, W. R., Shoham, E., & Stahel, P. (2008). Pharmacology of traumatic brain injury: Where is the "golden bullet"? *Molecular Medicine, 14*, 731–740.

Bell, D. R., Guskiewicz, K. M., Clark, M. A., & Padua, D. A. (2011). Systematic review of the Balance Error Scoring System. *Sports Health, 3*(3), 287–295.

Bey, T., & Ostick, B. (2009). Second impact syndrome. *Western Journal of Emergency Medicine, 10*(1), 6–10.

Brent, D. A., & Max, J. (2017). Psychiatric sequelae of concussions. *Current Psychiatry Reports, 19*, 1–8.

Broglio, S. P., Collins, M. W., Williams, R. M., Mucha, A., & Kontos, A. P. (2015). Current and emerging rehabilitation for concussions: A review of the evidence. *Clinics in Sports Medicine, 34*(2), 213–231.

Buckley, T. A., Oldham, J. R., & Caccese, J. B. (2016). Postural control deficits identifying lingering post-concussion neurological deficits. *Journal of Sport and Health Science, 5*, 61–69.

Catena, R. D., van Donkelaar, P., & Chou, L. -S. (2006). Cognitive task effects on gait stability following concussion. *Experimental Brain Research, 176*, 23–31.

Chen, H. L., Lu, T. W., & Chou, L. S. (2015). Effect of concussion on inter-joint coordination during divided-attention gait. *Journal of Medical and Biological Engineering, 35*, 28–33.

Chen, J. K., Johnston, K. M., Petrides, M., & Ptitio, A. (2008). Neural substrates of symptoms of depression following concussion in male athletes with persisting post-concussion symptoms. *Archives of General Psychiatry, 65*(1), 81–89.

Chiu, S. L., Osternig, L., & Chou, L. S. (2013). Concussion induces gait inter-joint coordination variability under conditions of divided attention and obstacle crossing. *Gait & Posture, 38*, 717–722.

Chong, C. D., & Schwedt, T. J. (2018). Research imaging of brain structure and function after concussion. *Headache, 58*(6), 827–835.

Churchill, N. W., Hutchison, M. G., Richards, D., Leung, G., Graham, S. J., & Schweizer, T. A. (2017). The first week after concussion: Blood flow, brain function and white matter microstructure. *NeuroImage: Clinical, 14*, 480–489.

Clay, M. B., Glover, K. L., & Lowe, D. T. (2013). Epidemiology of concussion in sport: A literature review. *Journal of Chiropractic Medicine, 12*(4), 230–251.

Collins, M. W., Grindel, S. H., & Lovell, M. R. (1999). Relationship between concussion and neuropsychological performance in college football players. *JAMA, 282*(10), 964–970.

Collins, M. W., Kontos, A. P., Reynolds, E., Murawski, C. D., & Fu, F. H. (2014). A comprehensive, targeted approach to the clinical care of athletes following sport-related concussion. *Knee Surgery, Sports Traumatology, Arthroscopy, 22*, 235–246.

Collins, M. W., Lovell, M. R., Iverson, G. L., Ide, T., & Maroon, J. (2006). Examining concussion rates and return to play in high school football players wearing newer helmet technology: A three- year prospective cohort study. *Neurosurgery, 58*(2), 275–286.

Covassin, T., Swanik, C. B., & Sachs, M. L. (2003). Sex differences and the incidence of concussions among collegiate athletes. *Journal of Athletic Training, 38*, 238–244.

DeMatteo, C., Stazyk, K., Giglia, L., et al. (2015). A balanced protocol for return to school for children and youth following concussive injury. *Clinical Pediatrics, 54*, 783–792.

Echemendia, R. J., Meeuwisse, W., McCrory, P., et al. (2017). The Sport Concussion Assessment Tool 5th Edition (SCAT5): Background and rationale. *British Journal of Sports Medicine, 51*(11), 848–850.

Field, M., Collins, M. W., Lovell, M. R., & Maroon, J. (2003). Does age play a role in recovery from sports-related concussion? A comparison of high school and collegiate athletes. *Journal of Pediatrics, 142*, 546–553.

Fino, P. C., Becker, L. N., Fino, N. F., Griesemer, B., Goforth, M., & Brolinson, P. G. (2017). Effects of recent concussion and injury history on instantaneous relative risk of lower extremity injury in Division 1 collegiate athletes. *Clinical Journal of Sport Medicine, 29*(3), 218–223.

Fuller, G. W., Cross, M. J., Stokes, K. A., & Kemp, S. P. T. (2018). King-Devick concussion test performs poorly as a screening tool in elite rugby union players: A prospective cohort study of two screening tests versus a clinical reference standard. *British Journal of Sports Medicine, 53*(24), 1526–1532.

Galetta, K. M., Morganroth, J., Moehringer, N., et al. (2015). Adding vision to concussion testing: a prospective study of sideline testing in youth and collegiate athletes. *Journal of Neuro-Ophthalmology, 35*, 235–241.

Gilbert, F. C., Burdette, G. T., Joyner, A. B., Llewellyn, T. A., & Buckley, T. A. (2016). Association between concussion and lower extremity injuries in collegiate athletes. *Sports Health, 8*(6), 561–567.

Guskiewicz, K. M., McCrea, M., Marshall, S. W., et al. (2003). Cumulative effects associated with recurrent concussion in collegiate football players: The NCAA Concussion Study. *JAMA, 290*, 2549–2555.

Guskiewicz, K., Teel, E., & McCrea, M. (2014). Concussion: Key stakeholders and multidisciplinary participation in making sports safe. *Neurosurgery, 75*(4), S113–S118.

Halstead, M. E., McAvoy, K., Devore, C. D., Carl, R., Lee, M., & Logan, K. (2013). Return to learning following concussion. *American Academy of Pediatrics, 132*(5), 948–957.

Harada, G. K., Rugg, C. M., Arshi, A., Vail, J., & Hame, S. L. (2019). Multiple concussions increase odds and rate of lower extremity injury in National Collegiate Athletic Association athletes after return to play. *The American Journal of Sports Medicine, 47*(13), 3256–3262.

Harmon, K. G., Drezner, J. A., Gammons, M., et al. (2013). American Medical Society for Sports Medicine position statement: Concussion in sport. *British Journal of Sports Medicine, 47*(1), 15–26.

Henry, L. C., Elbin, R. J., Collins, M. W., Marchetti, G., & Kantos, A. P. (2016). Examining recovery trajectories after sport related concussion with a multimodal clinical assessment approach. *Neurosurgery, 78*, 232–241.

Herman, D. C., Jones, D., Harrison, A., et al. (2017). Concussion may increase the risk of subsequent lower extremity musculoskeletal injury in collegiate athletes. *Sports Medicine, 47*(5), 1003–1010.

Hornibrook, J. (2011). Benign paroxysmal positional vertigo (BPPV): History, pathophysiology, office treatment and future directions. *International Journal of Otolaryngology, 2011*, 1–13.

Institute of Medicine (IOM) and National Research Council (NRC), (2014). *Sports-related concussions in youth: Improving the science, changing the culture.* Washington, DC: The National Academies Press.

Kirkwood, M. W., Yeates, K. O., & Wilson, P. E. (2006). Pediatric sport-related concussion: A review of the clinical management of an oft-neglected population. *Pediatrics, 117*(4), 1359–1371.

Langlois, J. A., Rutland-Brown, W., & Wald, M. M. (2006). The epidemiology and impact of traumatic brain injury: A brief overview. *Journal of Head Trauma Rehabilitation, 21*(5), 375–378.

Lau, B., Lovell, M. R., Collins, M. W., & Pardini, J. (2009). Neurocognitive and symptom predictors of recovery in high school athletes. *Clinical Journal of Sport Medicine, 19*, 216–221.

Lincoln, A., Caswell, S. V., Almquist, J. L., Dunn, R. E., Norris, J. B., & Hinton, R. Y. (2011). The American Journal of Sports Medicine trends in concussion incidence in high school sports: A prospective 11-year study. *American Journal of Sports Medicine, 39*(5), 958–963.

Lovell, M. R., Collins, M. W., Iverson, G. L., et al. (2003). Recovery from mild concussion in high school athletes. *Journal of Neurosurgery, 98*, 296–301.

Lovell, M. R., Iverson, G. L., Collins, M. W., et al. (2006). Measurement of symptoms following sports-related concussion: Reliability and normative data for the Post-Concussion Scale. *Applied Neuropsychology, 13*(3), 166–174.

Marar, M., McIlvain, N. M., Fields, S. K., & Comstock, R. D. (2012). Epidemiology of concussions among United States high school athletes in 20 sports. *American Journal of Sports Medicine, 40*(4), 747–755.

McCrory, P., Meeuwisse, W., Dvorak, J., et al. (2017). Consensus statement on concussion in sport—the 5th international conference on concussion in sport held in Berlin, October 2016. *British Journal of Sports Medicine, 51*(11), 838–847.

Meehan, W. P., Mannix, R. C., Stracciolini, A., Elbin, R. J., & Collins, M. W. (2013). Symptom severity predicts prolonged recovery after sport-related concussion, but age and amnesia do not. *Journal of Pediatrics, 163*(3), 721–725.

Parachute, (2017). *Canadian Guideline on Concussion in Sport.* Toronto: Parachute.

Parker, T. M., Osternig, L. R., van Donkelaar, P., & Chou, L. -S. (2008). Balance control during gait in athletes and non-athletes following concussion. *Medical Engineering & Physics, 30*, 959–967.

Quatman-Yates, C. C., Hunter-Giordano, A., Shimamura, K. K., et al. (2020). Physical therapy evaluation and treatment after concussion/mild traumatic brain injury. *Journal of Orthopaedic and Sports Physical Therapy, 50*(4), CPG1–CPG73.

Samadani, U., Li, M., Qian, M., Laska, E., & Ritlop, R. (2015). Sensitivity and specificity of an eye movement tracking-based biomarker for concussion. *Concussion, 2015*, CNC3.

Sandel, N., Reynolds, E., Cohen, P. E., Gillie, B. L., & Kontos, A. P. (2017). Anxiety and mood clinical profile following sport-related concussion: From risk factors to treatment. *Sport, Exercise, and Performance Psychology, 6*(3), 304–323.

Scrimgeour, A. G., & Condlin, M. L. (2014). Nutritional treatment for traumatic brain injury. *Journal of Neurotrauma, 31*(11), 989–999.

Stein, T. D., Alvarez, V. E., & McKee, A. C. (2015). Concussion in chronic traumatic encephalopathy. *Current Pain and Headache Reports, 19*(10), 47.

Stone, S., Lee, B., Garrison, J. C., Blueitt, D., & Creed, K. (2016). Sex differences in time to return-to-play progression after sport-related concussion. *Sports Health, 9*(1), 41–44.

The Sport Concussion Assessment Tool 5th Edition (SCAT5). (2017). Background and rationale. *British Journal of Sports Medicine, 51*, 848–850.

Thomas, D. G., Apps, J. N., & Hoffman, R. G. (2015). Benefits of strict rest after acute concussion: A randomized controlled trial. *Pediatrics, 135*(2), 213–223.

Toccalino, D., Wiseman-Hakes, C., & Zalai, D. M. (2021). Preliminary validation of the sleep and concussion questionnaire as an outcome measure for sleep following brain injury. *Brain Injury, 35*(7), 743–750.

Toledo, E., Lebel, A., Becerra, L., et al. (2012). The young brain and concussion: Imaging as a biomarker for diagnosis and prognosis. *Neuroscience & Biobehavioral Reviews, 36*, 1510–1531.

Vaillancourt, C., Charette, M., Kasaboski, A., Maloney, J., Wells, G., & Stiell, I. (2011). Evaluation of the safety of C-spine clearance by paramedics: Design and methodology. *BMC Emergency Medicine*, *11*, 1.

Wing, B. H., Tucker, B. J., Fong, A. K., & Allen, M. D. (2017). Developing the standard of care for post-concussion treatment: Neuroimaging-guided rehabilitation of neurovascular coupling. *The Open Neuroimaging Journal*, *11*, 58–71.

Zhu, D., Covassin, T., Nogle, S., et al. (2015). A potential biomarker in sports-related concussion: Brain functional connectivity alteration of the default-mode network measured with longitudinal resting-state fMRI over thirty days. *Journal of Neurotrauma*, *32*, 327–341.

CHAPTER 20 QUESTIONS

1. **Which of the following have been identified as risk factors for prolonged recovery after concussion?**
   a. A history of depression
   b. Younger age
   c. Delayed removal from play
   d. Dizziness
   e. All of the above

2. **At what intensity should the home exercises protocol be set from the Buffalo Concussion Treadmill or Bike test?**
   a. 60%
   b. 70%
   c. 80%
   d. 90%

3. **_______ test is used to assess for Benign Paroxysmal Positional Vertigo (BPPV) of the posterior canal, and _______ test is used to assess for BPPV of the horizontal canal.**
   a. Epley, Dix-Hallpike
   b. Dix-Hallpike, Log Roll
   c. Log-Roll, BBQ Roll
   d. Dix-Hallpike, BBQ roll

4. **True or False: Lower extremity injury risk after concussion is only increased in the first 90 days following RTP.**

5. **True or False: When an athlete has already had one concussion, you can expect them to present similarly for any subsequent concussions.**

DIFFERENTIAL DIAGNOSIS AND CLINICAL REASONING

F.D. Pociask, PT, PhD, OCS, FAAOMPT and J.R. Krauss, PhD, PT, OCS, FAAOMPT

CHAPTER 21

1. **What is a diagnosis, and what is a differential diagnosis?**

   A diagnosis is a named category of specific clinical data that labels a condition and provides characteristics of the condition when communicated to health care professionals. A differential diagnosis is a list of possible diagnoses generated from the patient interview and physical examination, listed in order of likelihood from the most likely to the least likely. In general terms, in the context of physical therapy (APTA, 2001) the diagnosis is used to identify "the impact of a condition on function at the level of the system and at the level of the whole person."

2. **What are examples of impairments that a physical therapist might diagnose?**
   - Impaired posture
   - Impaired gait/locomotion
   - Impaired range of motion
   - Impaired muscle performance
   - Impaired motor function
   - Impaired joint mobility
   - Impaired neural function

3. **What are characteristics of visceral symptoms?**
   - Location—unilateral or bilateral; poorly localized in terms of specific organ or system (eg, angina).
   - Quality—knifelike, boring, deep bone pain, deep aching, cutting, moderate to severe, and/or perceived from the inside out.
   - Character—symptoms often unrelieved by rest, changes in position, and interventions that would typically affect musculoskeletal disorders. Associated symptoms that do not occur with musculoskeletal disorders can be identified via a careful review of systems.
   - Quantity or severity—typically related to exacerbating factors and varies based on organ/organ system and status of disease processes (eg, dull to sharp or mild to severe).
   - Onset—recent or sudden but does not typically present as being chronically observed (ie, insidious onset often without an attributable mechanism).
   - Duration and frequency—constant or intermittent based on organ/system and attributing factors, gradually progressive, cyclical, or symptom may come in waves.
   - Aggravating factors—differ based on involved organ/system and status of disease processes (eg, fatty foods will typically aggravate a gallbladder disorder).
   - Relieving factors—differ based on involved organ/system and status of disease processes. A specific strategy such as rest may initially relieve symptoms (ie, pain), but there is typically a recurring progression of increasing frequency, intensity, and/or duration of symptoms.
   - Client's perception of the symptom—should be expected to vary among patients and will be influenced by cognitive, affective, cultural, socioeconomic, and environmental factors. For example, patients may self-diagnose, select unwise self-treatments, or perceive certain symptoms, such as coughing, sweating, or diarrhea as normal and not symptoms of illness.

4. **What are somatic disorders?**

   Somatic disorders are musculoskeletal syndromes in which symptoms are caused by nociceptive stimulation of pain-sensitive structures. The origin of somatic pain is mechanical and/or chemical stimulation of nerve endings. Somatic pain may be either localized to a body region and/or referred to other body regions. Somatic pain and somatic referred pain are typically static, aching in quality, and difficult to point-localize.

5. **What are characteristics of somatic symptoms?**
   - Location—typically unilateral and described as presenting in one joint or in one body region; somatic referred pain may or may not be present.
   - Quality—achy, deep, sharp, pulling, sore, stiff, and/or cramping pain.
   - Character—local tenderness or pain that is attributable to an activity or underlying pathology (eg, pain exacerbated by overhead activities with secondary impingement tendinosis; morning stiffness with osteoarthritis).
   - Quantity or severity—mild to severe.
   - Onset—sudden or gradual: sudden associated with acute overload stresses and macrotrauma, and gradual associated with chronic overloading stresses and repetitive microtrauma.
   - Duration and frequency—intermittent to constant: usually intermittent with varying intensity based on activity and/or position with mechanical disorders; constant with acute inflammatory disorders. Symptoms may present as chronologically observed, characterized by asymptomatic periods with exacerbations or progressively exacerbated symptoms attributed to causal factors or progression of the underlying disorder.
   - Aggravating factors—symptoms are typically exacerbated with specific movement, activities, loading, etc., and the degree of exacerbation is a function of attributing factors or progression of the underlying disorder.
   - Relieving factors—relieving factors are typically a function of identifying and managing aggravating factors (eg, activity modification, rest, pacing, therapeutic interventions, improved self-management, eliminating attributing factors, positioning, and relative rest).

6. **What are radicular disorders?**
   A radicular disorder is a neurogenic disorder in which signs and/or symptoms are caused by damage or irritation of the spinal nerves or spinal nerve roots. The origin of signs and symptoms is mechanical and/or chemical and is attributable to a block in conduction rather than stimulation of nerve endings. Radicular disorders produce lower motor neuron lesion signs and symptoms, which include muscle weakness, atrophy, hyporeflexia, and sensory changes such as paresthesia and/or numbness. A block in conduction itself does not necessarily cause pain in either the spine or the corresponding extremity, but radicular disorders typically occur concurrently with somatic pain disorders.

7. **What is a key characteristic of radicular symptoms?**
   Radicular pain is described as shooting or lacerating and is typically felt in a relatively narrow band about 4 cm wide; it is often combined with other radicular symptoms such as tingling, numbness, and burning sensations.

8. **What is the difference between radicular referred symptoms and somatic referred pain accompanying a radicular disorder?**
   Radicular symptoms result from a block in conduction rather than nociceptive stimulation of pain-sensitive structures (eg, the spinal nerve, nerve root, and DRG). Radicular symptoms are typically referred to the distribution supplied by the involved spinal nerve or nerve root, but this assumption must take into consideration the following:
   1. The distribution of radicular symptoms is not always distinctive.
   2. Radicular pain from a given nerve root does not always follow a consistent distribution.
   3. All radicular disorders do not result in referred pain.
   4. Radicular symptoms do not always extend to the distal portion of the involved dermatome.

   Somatic referred pain is generated by either mechanical or chemical irritation of somatic structures, such as the dural lining on the nerve root or the epineurium of the spinal nerve. Like radicular referred pain, somatic referred pain is felt in body regions separate from the irritated structures (eg, lumbar facet arthrosis can refer pain into the leg).

SCREENING FOR SYSTEMIC INVOLVEMENT

9. **Why do physical therapists need to screen for systemic involvement?**
   Physical therapists screen for systemic or non–physical therapy involvement because many visceral (ie, organ or organ system) diseases mimic orthopedic symptoms. For example, Jarvik and Deyo (2002) reported that among patients with low back pain being seen in ambulatory primary care clinics, 4% will have osteoporosis-related fractures, 2% will have spondylolisthesis (ie, forward displacement of a vertebral body) or spondylolysis (ie, fracture of a portion of the vertebra, which may lead to spondylolisthesis), 2% will have visceral disease, 0.7% will have cancer, and 0.5% will have infections. Given the possibility of such disorders, the clinician must promptly screen patients at risk for such medical conditions and make the appropriate referrals.

10. **List common body systems and aggregates of signs/symptoms that may indicate systemic involvement.**

General
- Adenopathy
- Appetite
- Chills
- Diaphoresis
- Edema
- Fatigue
- Fever
- Injuries
- Light-headedness
- Weakness
- Weight loss

Allergic
- Allergic rhinitis
- Asthma
- Bee sting
- Food
- Hay fever
- Seasonal

Breasts
- Asymmetry
- Discharge
- Gynecomastia
- Implants
- Mass
- Tenderness

Cardiopulmonary
- COPD
- Cough
- Cyanosis
- Dyspnea
- Expectoration
- Hemoptysis
- Hypertension
- Infarction
- Infections
- Murmur
- Orthopnea PND
- Palpitations
- Rheumatic fever
- Syncope
- TB skin test
- Tuberculosis
- Wheezing asthma

Endocrine/Metabolic
- Change in physical features
- Diabetes
- Goiter
- Hot/cold intolerance
- Irradiation exposure
- Lipid disorder

ENT
- Epistaxis
- Hearing loss
- Infections
- Tinnitus
- Vertigo
- Voice change

Eye
- Acuity
- Cataracts
- Diplopia
- Glasses/contacts
- Glaucoma
- Infections
- Pain
- Scotoma
- Visual fields

Gastrointestinal
- Blood
- Bowel habits
- Dysphagia
- Gas
- Hemorrhoids
- Hernia
- Jaundice
- Nausea
- Pain
- Pancreatitis
- Stones
- Ulcer history
- Vomiting

Genitourinary
- Contraceptive measures
- Discharge
- Infections
- Infertility
- Lesions
- Mass
- Pain
- Pelvic floor dysfunction
- Sexual dysfunction and disorders
- STDs and related conditions

Hematologic
- Anemia
- Bleeding
- Bruising
- Leukemia
- Sickle cell
- Transfusions

Integument (skin)
- Cyanosis
- Danger Signs (ABCDE's)
- Edema
- Erythema
- Exudate
- Jaundice
- Lesions
- Pallor
- Siccus
- Vascularity or bruising
- Widespread color changes

Integument (nails)
- Abnormal color, shape or contour
- Brittle or splitting
- Clubbing

Musculoskeletal Pain
- Arthritis
- Deformity
- Stiffness
- Weakness

Neurologic
- Gait
- Head trauma
- Headache pain
- Paresis/paralysis
- Paresthesia
- Seizures
- Speech
- Tremors
- Unconsciousness

Peripheral Vascular
- Claudication
- Raynaud's
- Thrombophlebitis
- Ulcers
- Varicosities

Mental health
- Anxiety
- Depression
- Treatment
- Neurobiologic disorder (NBD)
- Shy/sensitive
- Irritable/irate
- Nervous/worry
- Fearful
- Crying often

Renal
- Colic/calculi
- Dysuria
- Frequency
- Hematuria
- Incontinence
- Infections
- Nephritis
- Nocturia
- Proteinuria
- Pyuria
- Stream
- Urgency

11. **What are examples of common "red flags" that typically require physician referral and further investigation?**
- Anorexia
- Back and abdominal pain at the same level
- Bilateral symptoms
- Changes in mental status
- Chills

- Constipation
- Diaphoresis (excessive perspiration)
- Diarrhea
- Dyspnea (breathlessness at rest or after mild exertion)
- Early satiety (feeling full after eating)
- Elevated body temperature
- Fecal or urinary incontinence (inability to control bowels or urine)
- Frequency (increased urination)
- Headaches, dizziness, fainting, or falling
- Hematuria (blood in the urine)
- Insidious onset with progression of symptoms
- Melena (blood in feces)
- Nausea
- Night sweats
- Nocturia
- Obvious change in a wart or mole
- Pain at night
- Pain that forces a patient to curl up into fetal position
- Pain unrelieved by recumbency
- Painless weakness of muscles: more often proximal but may occur distally
- Poor or delayed healing
- Sacral pain without history of injury
- Skin lesions
- Thickening of a lump
- Unexplained weight loss
- Unusual bleeding, bruising, or discharge
- Unusual vital signs
- Urgency (sudden need to urinate)
- Visual disturbances
- Vomiting
- Weakness and/or fatigue
- Weight loss/gain without explanation

CARDIOVASCULAR

12. **True or false: Pain referral patterns associated with myocardial infarction (MI) are the same for men and women.**

    False. Symptoms of MI do not always follow the classic pattern, especially in women. Women may experience pain referred into the right shoulder in addition to shortness of breath, sometimes occurring in the middle of the night, and chronic, unexpected fatigue.

13. **What are silent heart attacks, and who do they commonly affect?**

    Silent attacks (ie, painless infarction without acute symptoms) are more common among nonwhites, older adults (>75 years), smokers, and adults with diabetes, presumably because of reduced sensitivity to pain.

14. **For myocardial infarctions associated with a blood clot, what time frame for the administration of medications that dissolve clots, promote vasodilation, and reduce infarct size is considered the most crucial?**

    Administration of medication within the first 70 minutes after the onset of symptoms is associated with improved outcomes.

15. What are typical pain referral patterns for the heart?

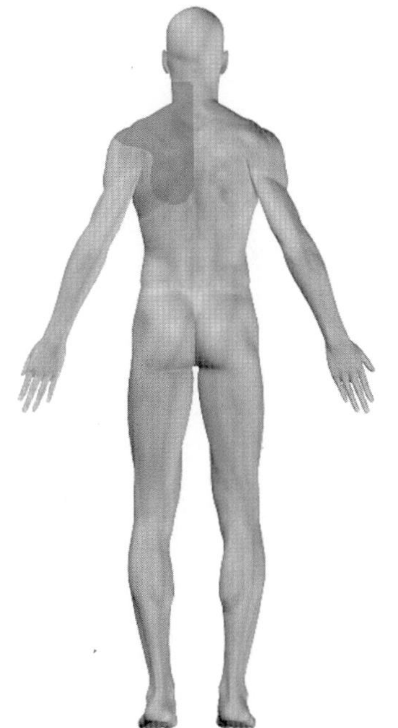

Angina pectoris.

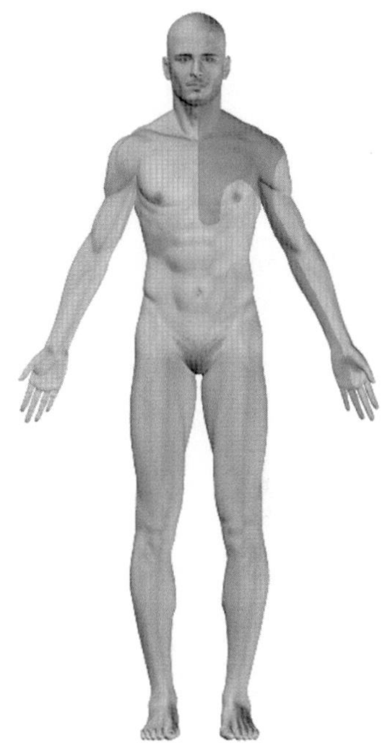

Angina pectoris.

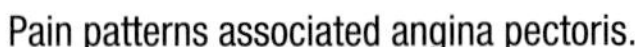

Pain patterns associated angina pectoris.

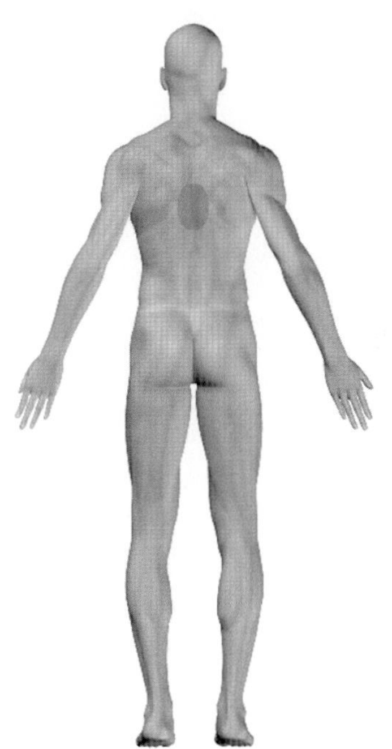

Myocardial infarction.

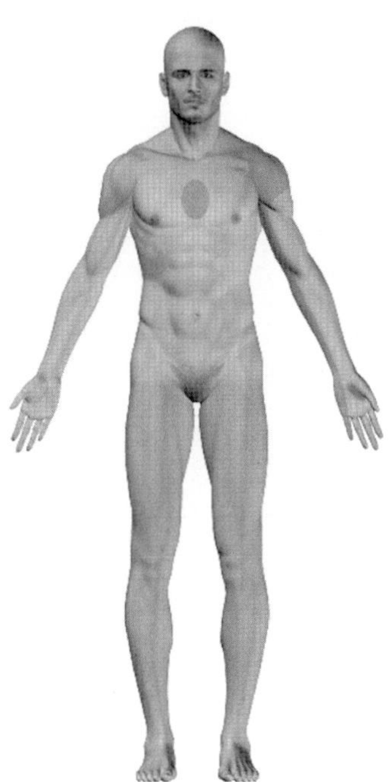

Myocardial infarction.

Pain patterns associated myocardial infarction.

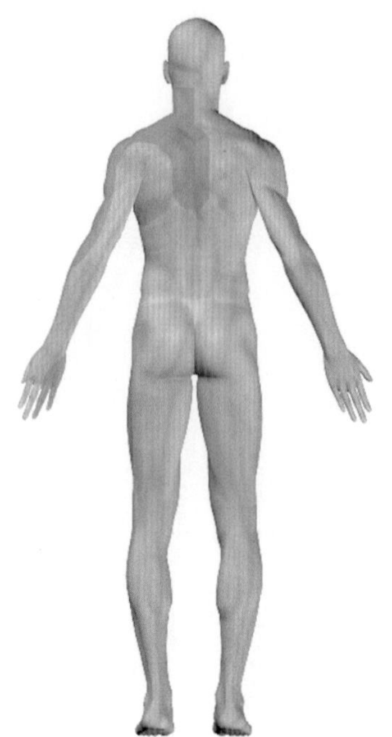

Pericarditis.

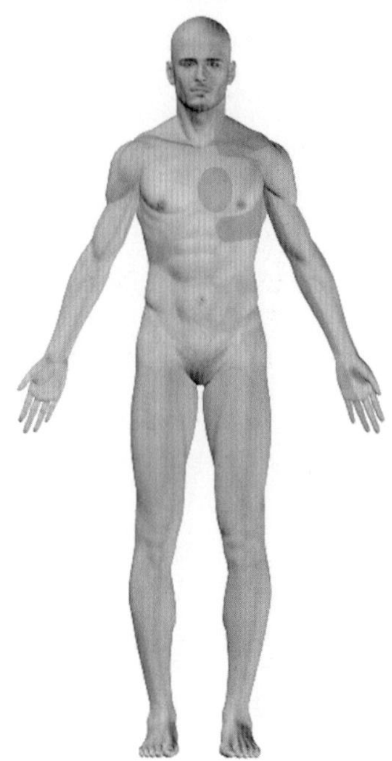

Pericarditis.

Pain patterns associated pericarditis.

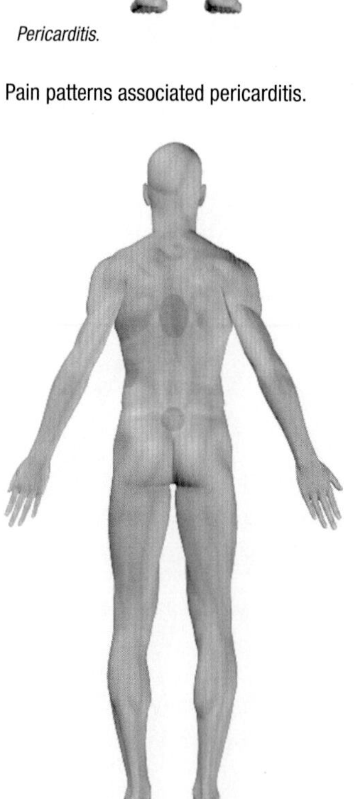

Dissecting aortic aneurysm.

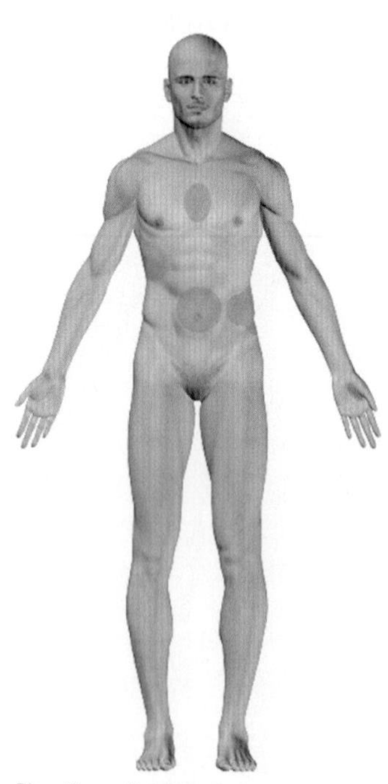

Dissecting aortic aneurysm.

Pain patterns associated dissecting aortic aneurysm.

16. **What signs and symptoms are commonly associated with cardiac pathology?**
    - There is a sudden sensation of pressure in the chest that occasionally radiates into the arms, throat, neck, and back.
    - Pain is constant, lasting 30 minutes to hours.
    - Pain may be accompanied by shortness of breath, pallor, and profuse perspiration.
    - Angina pectoralis has similar symptoms to an MI. However, angina pectoralis is less severe, does not last for hours (ie, rarely more than 5 minutes), and is relieved by cessation of all activity and administration of nitrates.
    - Symptoms of MI do not always follow the classic pattern, especially in women.
    - Two major symptoms in women are shortness of breath, sometimes occurring in the middle of the night, and chronic, unexpected fatigue.
    - A typical presentation may include continuous pain in the midthoracic spine or interscapular area, neck and shoulder pain, stomach or abdominal pain, nausea, unexplained anxiety, or heartburn that is not altered by antacids.
    - Silent attacks (painless infarction without acute symptoms) are more common among nonwhites, older adults (>75 years), smokers, and adults with diabetes (men and women), presumably because of reduced sensitivity to pain.
    - Nausea and vomiting may occur because of reflex stimulation of vomiting centers by pain fibers.
    - Fever may develop in the first 24 hours and persist for 1 week because of inflammatory activity within the myocardium.
    - Myocarditis and endocarditis do not produce chest pain but rather chest tightness with breathlessness.

17. **What are cardiac red flags?**
    Pain in the chest lasting longer than 30 minutes, shortness of breath with exertion or when sleeping, increased fatigue, nausea, vomiting, nonproductive cough, nocturia, changes in skin color (eg, blue or ashen), and onset of pain in the early morning hours are all cardiac red flags.

18. **What subjective questions should be asked when cardiac dysfunction is suspected?**
    - The presence of cardiac red flags.
    - Questions about pain, regarding the onset, location, and character of the pain.
    - Additional information regarding dietary habits, cigarette or alcohol use, and exercise habits.
    - Questions regarding the use of prescription, over-the-counter, or street drugs, especially antihypertensive medications, β-blockers, calcium channel blockers, digoxin, diuretics, and aspirin/anticoagulants.

19. **List common musculoskeletal disorders that mimic cardiovascular pain patterns.**
    Cervical radiculopathy (C8), ulnar nerve injuries, rotator cuff disorders, upper thoracic dysfunction, pectoralis major strain, subacromial bursitis, acromioclavicular arthritis, and temporomandibular (TM) joint pain mimic cardiovascular pain patterns.

PULMONARY

20. **Describe the clinical signs and symptoms of acute pleuritis.**
    Sharp, stabbing substernal pain, especially with exertion, pleural rub on auscultation, and referred upper trapezius and interscapular pain are symptoms of acute pleuritis.

21. **How does pulmonary function change with obstructive and restrictive pulmonary disorders?**
    - Restrictive—normal expiratory airflow, decreased vital capacity, decreased total lung capacity, decreased residual volume, and decreased $PaCO_2$
    - Obstructive—reduced airflow with/without changes in vital capacity, increased total lung capacity, increased residual volume, and increased $PaCO_2$

22. **What are typical pain referral patterns for the lungs?**
    Primary pain is typically noted over the midchest or involved lung and is often greater anterior as opposed to posterior. Referred pain may be noted in the neck, upper trapezius muscles, proximal shoulders, T1/C8 dermatome, along the ribs, and in the upper abdomen.

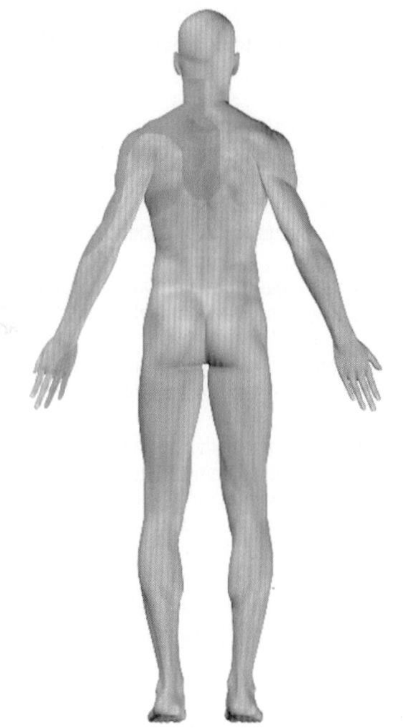

Pleuritis.

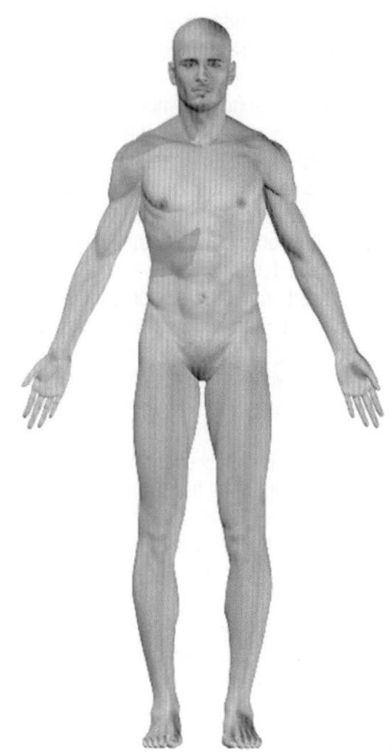

Pleuritis.

Pain patterns associated with pleuritis.

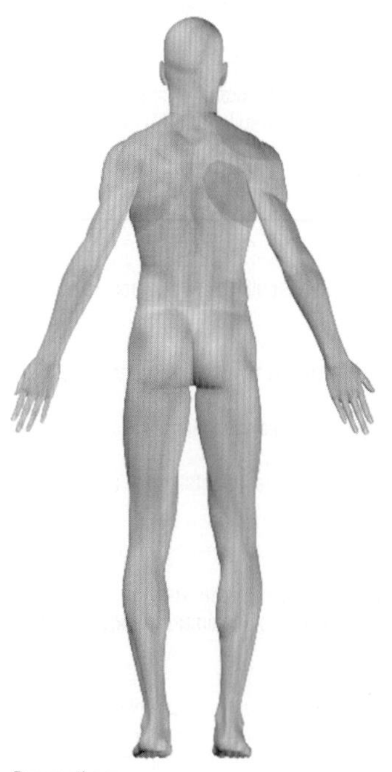

Pneumothorax.

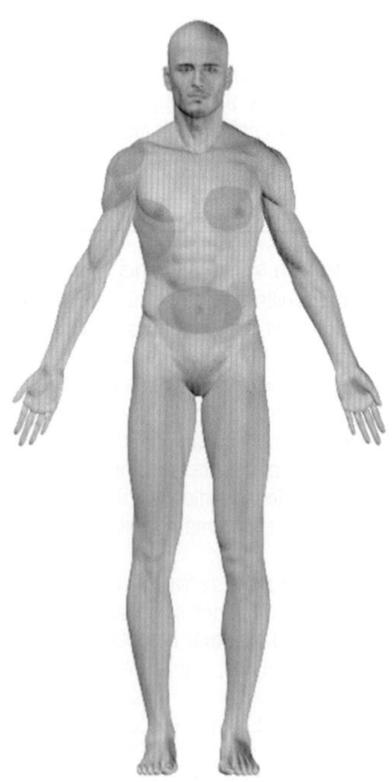

Pneumothorax.

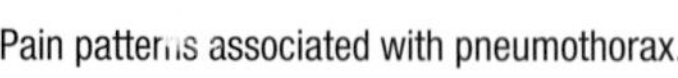

Pain patterns associated with pneumothorax.

23. **What signs and symptoms are commonly associated with pulmonary pathology?**
    - Cough—continuous coughing, possibly indicating an acute or chronic pathology (eg, respiratory tract infection, allergies, bronchitis, emphysema, COPD, lung cancer), time of day cough (eg, environmental exposure to an irritant), night cough (eg, sinusitis or allergies), and early morning cough (eg, bronchial inflammation secondary to smoking).
    - Sputum, including color and odor—clear to white sputum (eg, cold [viral infection] and bronchitis), purulent yellow or green sputum (eg, bacterial infections), reddish-brown sputum (eg, tuberculosis and pneumonia), and pink-foamy sputum (eg, pulmonary edema).
    - Hemoptysis or blood derived from the lungs or bronchial tubes may result from a large number of conditions (eg, pneumonia, infections, cancer, trauma).
    - Shortness of breath without physical exertion or with minimal physical exertion (eg, bronchitis, emphysema, pneumonia, pulmonary embolism, pleurisy, pneumothorax).
    - Cyanosis (eg, respiratory acidosis, chronic bronchitis, pneumonia, cystic fibrosis).
    - Chest pain that occurs with breathing (eg, pneumonia, pleurisy, lung cancer).
    - Changes in respiratory rate or breathing patterns (eg, acute and chronic bronchitis, respiratory acidosis, emphysema).
    - Change in normal breath sounds (eg, asthma, bronchitis, pneumonia, emphysema, pleurisy, lung cancer, and bronchiectasis).
    - Chest cavity deformities or compensatory breathing patterns (eg, a barrel chest deformity and use of accessory muscle of respiration are indicative of emphysema).
    - General undiagnosed symptoms of dizziness, fainting, fever, shortness of breath without exertion, cyanosis, night sweats, tachycardia, especially with a positive pulmonary history.

24. **What are pulmonary red flags?**
    - Central nervous system symptoms.
    - Change in normal breath sounds, especially wheezing.
    - Hemoptysis, especially with a long-term history of smoking.
    - Pain increased by recumbency or during sleep, especially if disturbing sleep.
    - Persistent undiagnosed cough.
    - Recurrent pulmonary infections.
    - Sharp pain with breathing, especially on inhalation.
    - Signs or symptoms of DVT.
    - Signs or symptoms of insufficient oxygenation or increased carbon dioxide levels.
    - Splinting used to reduce pain.
    - Sudden, sharp chest pain with or without trauma combined with changes in respiratory rate, diminished but rapid pulse rate, diminished blood pressure, and changes in respiratory rate.
    - Undiagnosed neck, shoulder, chest, and arm pain.
    - Unexplained hoarseness of voice and/or difficulty swallowing.
    - Unexplained upper extremity weakness.
    - Unexplained weight loss or gain, especially sudden.
    - Undiagnosed symptoms of dizziness, fainting, fever, shortness of breath without exertion, cyanosis, night sweats, tachycardia, especially when occurring in a cluster and in combination with specific pulmonary signs and symptoms.

25. **What subjective questions should be asked when pulmonary dysfunction is suspected?**
    - Presence of red flags as previously described.
    - Age (ie, >35-year-old female/>40-year-old male).
    - History of respiratory tract infections, cough, sputum, hemoptysis, dyspnea, infection, fever, chills
    - History of smoking.
    - History of exposure to environmental contaminants.
    - Personal and family history of cancer.
    - History of pain exacerbated by inhalation or exhalation (eg, breathing, coughing).
    - History of pain that is provoked or alleviated by lying on one side (eg, sleeping).
    - History of general self-care and medical management (eg, last TB test, last chest x-ray, immunizations).

26. **List common musculoskeletal disorders that mimic pulmonary pain patterns.**
    Musculoskeletal disorders mimicking pulmonary pain patterns include cervical radiculopathy (C8, T1), cervical and upper thoracic dysfunction (eg, arthrosis and spondylosis), rotator cuff disorders, acromioclavicular arthritis, and regional muscle dysfunction (eg, pectoralis major strain, intercostal muscle strain, trigger points).

INTEGUMENTARY

27. **What signs and symptoms are commonly associated with integumentary system pathology?**
    - Changes in a pigmented mole or benign tumor may indicate a possible malignancy.
    - Cyanosis (ie, dark bluish or purplish discoloration of the integument and mucous membranes) may indicate hypoxia or hematologic pathology.
    - Edema, if generalized, may indicate cardiovascular, pulmonary, or renal dysfunction; localized edema may indicate infection, inflammation, or sudden change in pressure (ie, compartment syndrome). If edema is unilateral, consider a local or peripheral cause; if bilateral, consider a central disorder (eg, congestive heart failure and renal dysfunction).
    - Hyperthermia may indicate localized or systemic infection, inflammation, thermal injury; hyperthyroidism or fever is generalized.
    - Hypothermia may indicate arterial insufficiency or shock.
    - Jaundice (ie, yellowish discoloration of skin and sclera) may indicate liver disease or hemolytic pathology.
    - Paleness of the skin may indicate arterial insufficiency, anemia, or shock.
    - Redness of the skin may indicate fever, local infection, local inflammation, carbon monoxide poisoning, or polycythemia.
    - Unexplained skin lesions may indicate infection, allergic reaction, parasitic infection, thermal injury, herpes, fungal infection, cancer, or neoplasm.

28. **What are integumentary system red flags?**
    - Sudden enlargement of an existing mole or benign tumor (ie, evolving changes).
    - New areas of involvement or spreading of an existing mole or benign tumor.
    - Sudden change in color of an existing mole or benign tumor.
    - Formation of an irregular border or butterfly appearance to a new or previously existing mole or benign tumor.
    - A previously flat mole becomes elevated or raised, especially with irregular borders or notching.
    - Irregular or clumping of colors across a new or existing mole or benign tumor (ie, nonuniform browns and blacks mixed with reds, blues, and/or whites).
    - Unexpected, especially sudden, changes, such as scaling, flaking, drainage, itching, redness, swelling, warmth, point tenderness, or bleeding.

29. **List common nail abnormalities of nails and probable causes.**

POSSIBLE NAIL CHARACTERISTICS	SUSPECTED ETIOLOGY
Brown band around nail plate	Addison's disease
Red nail bed	Carbon monoxide poisoning
Red lunula	Cardiac failure
Brown discoloration of distal 1/3 of nail plate	Chronic renal insufficiency
Clubbing of nails and distal finger/toes	Congenital chronic cyanotic heart disease, emphysema, cystic fibrosis, and/or chronic bronchitis
Blue nail bed	Cyanosis and/or hemorrhage
Absence or underdeveloped nail beds	Hereditary onycho-osteodysplasia
Yellow nail bed	Jaundice
White lines and/or white spots	Leukonychia
Cuticle darkening and/or dark streaks	Melanoma
Brown or yellow nail plate	Onychomycosis
White nail plate	Onychomycosis (superficial)
Yellow nail plate and bed and/or nail dystrophy	Psoriasis
Yellow nail plate	Tetracycline
Brittle nails and/or splitting of nail beds	Thyroid disease

30. **What subjective questions should be asked when integumentary system pathology is suspected?**
    - Presence of any red flags as previously described.
    - History of drug or topical agent use and self-care.
    - History of allergies.
    - History of circulatory or vasospastic disorders.
    - History of endocrine disorders (eg, thyroid disease or diabetes).
    - History of applicable environmental factors (eg, exposure to radiation or x-rays, living conditions, dietary habits, occupations, leisure activities, travel, emotional stress; especially changes that occurred before or during identification of possible integumentary involvement).
    - History of applicable genetic factors (eg, family history, gender, age, race).
    - History of gynecologic factors (eg, pregnancy, menstruation, birth control pills).

31. **What is the integumentary presentation of herpes zoster (shingles)?**
    Symptoms of shingles include vesicular eruptions and neuralgic pain in the cutaneous distributions supplied by peripheral nerves.

32. **Describe the signs and symptoms of dysvascular and neuropathic foot ulcer.**

DYSVASCULAR FOOT ULCER	NEUROPATHIC FOOT ULCER
• Lesions are painful	• Lesions are painless
• Irregularly shaped	• Circular in shape
• Multifocal	• Develop over bony plantar regions
• Located on toes	• Can be associated with callous formation
• Located over nonplantar areas	• Tend to be clean and nonnecrotic
• Lesions are typically necrotic	• Ulcer regions are warm and pink
• Ulcer regions are typically cool and pale	

33. **What are the key characteristics of cellulitis?**
    Cellulitis is clinically observed as a spreading erythematous inflammation of the subcutaneous tissue and deep dermis characterized by warmth, reddening, edema, tenderness, or pain in the infected area of the skin. Additional features may include small and large fluid-filled blisters and thickening and pitting of the skin.

GASTROINTESTINAL

34. **What is the most common intraabdominal disease referring pain to the musculoskeletal system?**
    It is ulceration or infection of the mucosal lining of the GI tract.

35. **How quickly do drug-induced symptoms occur in the GI tract?**
    Although some medications (eg, NSAIDs, digitalis, and antibiotics) may result in immediate symptoms in patients, it is not uncommon for symptoms to occur as long as 6 to 8 weeks after exposure.

36. **What are typical pain patterns for GI pathologies?**
    Pain of GI origin can mimic primary musculoskeletal lesions. Referral locations may include shoulder, neck, sternum, scapular regions, mid back, low back, hip, pelvis, and the sacrum.

37. **What signs and symptoms are commonly associated with esophageal pathologies?**
    Diseases affecting the esophagus can cause the following symptoms: 1) dysphagia (sensation of food catching in the throat), 2) odynophagia (pain with swallowing), and 3) a burning sensation beginning at the xiphoid and radiating to the neck and throat (heartburn).

    Causes of dysphagia include stricture, inflammation, neurologic conditions (such as stroke, Alzheimer's disease, and Parkinson's disease), drug side effects, and space-occupying lesions. Causes of odynophagia include inflammation, spasm, and viral or fungal infection. Esophageal pain is reported as sharp, knifelike, stabbing, strong, and burning.

38. **What signs and symptoms are commonly associated with stomach and duodenal pathologies?**
Stomach and duodenal pathologies (peptic ulcers, stomach carcinoma, and Kaposi's sarcoma) may be associated with early satiety, melena (ie, dark, tarry stools), and symptoms associated with eating. Pain is typically described as aching, burning, gnawing, and cramp-like. It ranges from mild to severe in intensity and typically comes in waves.

39. **What signs and symptoms are commonly associated with small intestine pathologies?**
Small intestine pain is described as moderate to severe cramping pain, is intermittent in duration, and may be associated with nausea, fever, and diarrhea. Pain relief may not occur after defecation or passing gas.

40. **What signs and symptoms are commonly associated with large intestine and colon pathologies?**
Large intestine and colon pain is described as a cramping pain, dull in intensity, and steady in duration; it may be associated with bloody diarrhea, increased urgency, or constipation. Pain relief may occur after defecation or passing gas.

41. **What signs and symptoms are commonly associated with pancreatic pathologies?**
Pancreatic pain is described as a severe, constant pain of sudden onset that is burning or gnawing in quality. Associated signs and symptoms include sudden weight loss, jaundice, nausea and vomiting, light-colored stools, weakness, fever, constipation, flatulence, and tachycardia; it may or may not be related to digestive activities.

42. **What subjective questions should be asked when GI pathology is suspected?**
- Presence of any red flags as previously described.
- History of drug or topical agent use, including self-care.
- History of previous gastric or peptic ulcer.

43. **What are GI red flags?**
- Difficulty swallowing.
- Pain when swallowing.
- Pain associated with eating (immediately or 2 to 3 hours post ingestion).
- Changes in frequency and ease of defecation.
- Changes in coloration of stools.
- Decreased appetite.
- Sudden weight loss.
- Vomiting.
- Gnawing, burning pain.
- Migratory arthralgias.
- Decreased immune response.

44. **List common musculoskeletal disorders that mimic GI disorders.**
Sports hernia, adductor strain/tear, lumbar disc disease, lumbar facet arthrosis, and symptomatic thoracic movement impairment are all common musculoskeletal disorders mimicking GI disorders.

45. **What is the McBurney point, and what is its significance?**
It is a point midway between the umbilicus and the right anterior-superior iliac spine used as a guide to locate the position of the appendix. The McBurney point is the most common site of maximum tenderness in acute appendicitis, which is typically determined by the pressure of one finger.

46. **What is Blumberg's sign, and what is its significance?**
Blumberg's sign, also known as rebound tenderness, is a clinical sign of peritonitis, where pain is reported upon the removal of pressure rather than application of pressure to the abdomen.

47. **List the structures contained in each of the four abdominal quadrants.**

RIGHT UPPER QUADRANT	LEFT UPPER QUADRANT
• Ascending colon (superior portion) • Duodenum • Gallbladder • Liver (right lobe) • Pancreas (head) • Right colic (hepatic) flexure • Right kidney • Right suprarenal gland • Stomach (pylorus) • Transverse colon (right half)	• Descending colon (superior portion) • Jejunum and proximal ileum • Left colic (hepatic) flexure • Left kidney • Left suprarenal gland • Liver (left lobe) • Pancreas (body and tail portions) • Spleen • Stomach • Transverse colon (left half)
RIGHT LOWER QUADRANT	**LEFT LOWER QUADRANT**
• Ascending colon (inferior portion) • Cecum • Ileum • Right ovary • Right spermatic cord (abdominal portion) • Right ureter (abdominal portion) • Right uterine tube • Urinary bladder (only when full) • Uterus (only when enlarged) • Vermiform appendix • Renal	• Descending colon (inferior portion) • Left ovary • Left spermatic cord (abdominal portion) • Left ureter (abdominal portion) • Left uterine tube • Sigmoid colon • Urinary bladder (only when full) • Uterus (if enlarged)

RENAL

48. **List the common signs and symptoms associated with chronic renal failure.**

Uremia, dizziness, headaches, heart failure, hypertension, ischemic lower extremity pain, muscle cramps, edema, peripheral neuropathy, weakness, decreased endurance, decreased heart rate, and decreased blood pressure and hypotension, among others.

49. **What is the costovertebral angle, and what is its significance?**

The costovertebral angle is the angle formed on either side of the vertebral column between the last rib and the lumbar vertebrae. Tenderness in this region is indicative of renal disease, and it is a potential site for unintended encroachment on the pleural cavity during surgery.

50. **What are the two most common urinary tract infections?**

- Cystitis—inflammation and infection of the bladder.
- Pyelonephritis—inflammation and infection of one or both kidneys.

51. **What is a key feature that typically distinguishes a radicular disorder from renal pain?**

Renal pain is rarely influenced by changes in spinal posture or movements of the spine.

52. **List common clinically observable signs and symptoms of chronic renal disease.**

Hyperpigmentation, bruising, itching, paleness/anemia, redness of the eyes, shortness of breath, uremic breath, tremors, footdrop, weakness/altered movement patterns, decreased ability to concentrate, lethargy, irritability, and impaired judgment.

53. **What are typical pain patterns for renal pathologies?**

Primary pain is typically noted in a T10 to L1 distribution, in the groin and genital regions. Pain is predominantly in the anterior, lateral, and posterior subcostal regions and posteriorly in the area of the lower costovertebral articulations. Referred pain may include the abdomen, lumbar "back belt," and ipsilateral shoulder.

54. **What signs and symptoms are commonly associated with renal pathologies?**

- Bladder and urethra—sharp and localized upper pelvic, lower abdominal, and back pain; painful spasms of the anal sphincter; involuntary straining and an urgent need to empty the bowel with minimal passage of urine or fecal matter; urinary urgency and burning pain with urination.

- Ureter—severe unilateral or bilateral costovertebral angle pain, painful spasms of the anal sphincter, involuntary straining, and an urgent need to empty the bowel with minimal passage of urine or fecal matter, malaise, vomiting, nausea, abdominal distention, kidney/ureter tenderness, abnormal tenderness, and pain in a T10 to L1 distribution; a lesion outside of the ureter may be provoked with an active contraction of the iliopsoas muscle.
- Kidney—pain in the posterior subcostal region and in the area of the costovertebral articulations, posterior to lateral referred pain into the abdominal region and groin (usually unilateral), malaise, fever, chills, frequent urination, possible blood in urine, nausea and vomiting, abdominal spasms, abnormal tenderness, and pain in a T9 to T10 distribution.

55. What are renal red flags?

- Abdominal muscle spasms.
- Abdominal splinting.
- Abnormal tenderness and pain in a T9 to L1 distribution.
- Blood in urine (eg, brown or red) or clouding of urine.
- Changes in sexual function or pain during intercourse.
- Changes in urinary patterns and/or urine flow.
- Costovertebral angle pain.
- Decreased or absent urination.
- Dependent edema (ie, moderate to significant).
- Fever and chills.
- Genital discharge.
- Genital lesions.
- Headaches.
- Low back and abdominal pain at the same level.
- Malaise.
- Masses, lesions, or swelling.
- Nausea and vomiting.
- Pain with urination.
- Proximal lateral thigh and/or lower lateral trunk pain.
- Shortness of breath.
- Shoulder pain (ie, usually with ipsilateral kidney problems).
- Tenesmus.

56. What subjective questions should be asked when renal pathology is suspected?

- Presence of red flags as previously described.
- Past medical and surgical history (eg, kidney stones, bladder stones, infections, abdominal injuries, hernias, history of cancer, abdominal surgery, all applicable interventions and outcomes).
- History of abdominal pain (eg, primary and referred pain, influence of movement and position on pain and referred pain).
- History of proximal lateral thigh and/or lower lateral trunk pain (eg, suspect kidney or ureter).
- History of upper pelvic and lower abdominal pain (eg, suspect bladder and/or urethra).
- History of changes in bowel/bladder function (eg, increased frequency of urination, suspect infection; decreased flow or trouble initiating flow, suspect urethral obstruction; decreased diameter of flow, suspect urethral obstruction; feeling of bladder fullness after urination, suspect bladder disorder or enlarged prostate; burning pain during or after urination, suspect sexually transmitted disease or lower urinary tract infection; loss of control, suspect incontinence).
- History of nutritional/dietary changes.
- History of relevant associated symptoms (eg, fatigue, nausea, vomiting, vaginal or penile discharge, changes in menstrual cycle and sexual habits as applicable).

57. List common musculoskeletal disorders that mimic renal disorders.

Common musculoskeletal disorders that mimic renal disorders include lower thoracic or lumbar plexus radiculopathy, lumbar and lower thoracic dysfunction (eg, arthrosis, spondylosis, and costal/costovertebral), regional muscle dysfunction (eg, adductor strain), central nervous system disease, meralgia paresthesia, and trauma.

HEPATIC AND BILIARY

58. **What musculoskeletal signs or symptoms may be associated with hepatic and biliary dysfunction?**
Bilateral carpal tunnel syndrome accompanied by bilateral tarsal tunnel syndrome is a musculoskeletal sign associated with hepatic and biliary dysfunction.

59. **What are typical pain patterns of the hepatic and biliary systems?**
Pain associated with the liver, gallbladder, and the common bile duct is typically located in the midepigastric or right upper quadrant of the abdomen. Musculoskeletal pain referred from the hepatic and biliary systems may be located in the right shoulder, upper trapezius, or right scapular area or between the scapulae.

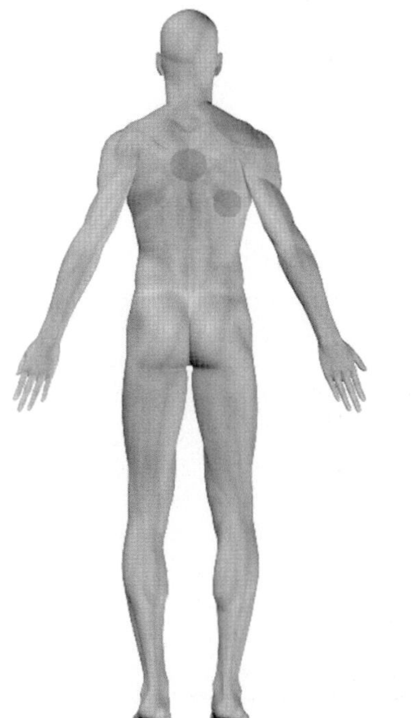

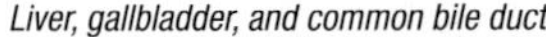

Liver, gallbladder, and common bile duct.

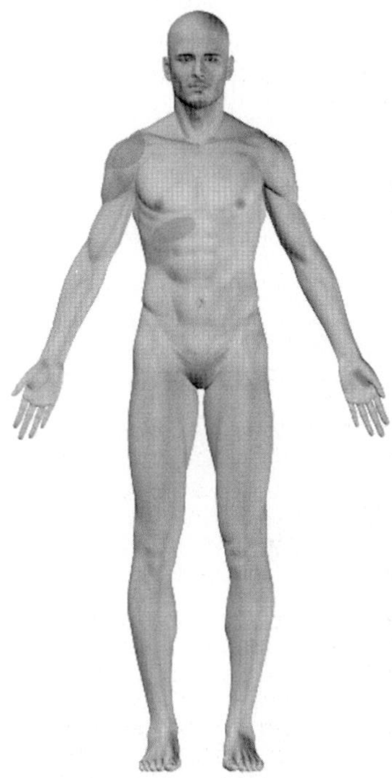

Liver, gallbladder, and common bile duct.

Pain patterns associated with the liver, gallbladder, and common bile duct pain (ie, upper right quadrant) and referred pain patterns (ie, shoulder and scapular regions).

60. **What signs and symptoms are commonly associated with hepatic and biliary system pathologies?**
In addition to the musculoskeletal pain referral patterns listed previously, patients experiencing hepatic or biliary dysfunction may also demonstrate changes in skin color, as well as neurologic symptoms. Skin changes include yellowing of the skin or sclera of the eyes (ie, jaundice), pallor, and orange or green skin. Neurologic signs and symptoms include confusion, sleep disturbances, muscle tremors, hyperactive reflexes, and asterixis (ie, a flapping tremor where the patient is unable to maintain wrist extension with forward flexion of the arms).

61. **What are hepatic and biliary system red flags?**
    - Anorexia, nausea, and vomiting.
    - Arthralgias.
    - Dark urine and light-colored or clay-colored feces.
    - Edema and oliguria (reduced urine secretion in relation to fluid intake).
    - Excessive belching.
    - Extreme fatigue.

- Gynecomastia.
- Neurologic symptoms (confusion, sleep disturbances, muscle tremors, hyperactive reflexes, asterixis, bilateral carpal/tarsal tunnel syndrome).
- Painful abdominal bloating.
- Pallor, yellowing of the eyes or skin.
- Right upper quadrant abdominal pain.
- Sense of fullness in the abdomen.
- Skin changes (jaundice, bruising, spider angioma, palmar erythema).

62. **What subjective questions should be asked when hepatic and biliary system pathology is suspected?**
    - Presence of any red flags as previously described.
    - Recent changes in bowel and bladder habits.
    - Exposure to needles (including injection, drug use, acupuncture, tattooing, ear or body piercing, recent operative procedure, hemodialysis), exposure to certain chemicals or medications, severe alcoholism, and fever.

63. **List common musculoskeletal disorders that mimic hepatic and biliary disorders.**
    Musculoskeletal conditions that may mimic hepatic and biliary pain patterns include symptomatic midthoracic hypomobility, rotator cuff dysfunction, and subacromial/deltoid bursitis.

HEMATOLOGY

64. **List the common disorders of erythrocytes, leukocytes, and platelets.**

ERYTHROCYTES	LEUKOCYTES	PLATELETS
• Anemia • Aplastic anemia • Hemorrhagic anemia • Hypochromic (iron deficiency) anemia • Leukopenia • Megaloblastic anemia • Pernicious anemia • Polycythemia • Sickle cell anemia	• Leukemia • Leukocytosis • Thrombocytopenia	• Thrombocytosis • Thrombocytopenia

65. **List the signs and symptoms of polycythemia (ie, increased red blood cell mass).**
    History of headaches, blurred vision, dizziness, fainting, altered mentation, feeling of fullness in the head, altered sensation in the distal extremities, malaise, fatigue, weight loss, easy or unexplained bruising, cyanosis, digital clubbing, and hypertension.

66. **List the common disorders or conditions that elevate red blood cell levels.**
    Alcoholism, burns, chronic pulmonary disease (eg, fibrosis), dehydration (eg, vomiting and diarrhea, burns, or use of diuretics), diminished blood-oxygen tension, heart disease (eg, cor pulmonale and congenital), liver disease, renal disease, smoking, and exposure to carbon monoxide.

67. **List the signs and symptoms of leukocytosis (increased white blood cell count).**
    Signs and/or symptoms consistent with local or systemic infection (eg, fever) and inflammation or trauma.

68. **List the common disorders or conditions that elevate white blood cell levels.**
    Burns, cancer, immune system responses (eg, lupus, rheumatoid arthritis), infections, inflammatory responses (eg, tissue damage), kidney failure, leukemia, lymphoma, malnutrition, multiple myeloma, removal of the spleen, stress (eg, emotional, physical), and tuberculosis.

69. **List the signs and symptoms of anemia (decreased red blood cell levels).**
    Pale skin and nails, shortness of breath with little to no exertion (based on degree), heart palpitation, and increased pulse rate; with severe anemia, fatigue, decreased diastolic blood pressure, and changes in mentation.

70. **List the common disorders or conditions that lower red blood cell levels.**
Addison's disease, anemia (eg, blood loss, hemorrhage, pernicious, sickle cell), bone marrow disease, bowel disease, colon cancer, excessive menstrual bleeding, hemolysis, kidney disease, lead poisoning, leukemia, malnutrition, multiple myeloma, stomach ulcers, and vitamin and/or mineral deficiencies (eg, B12, B6, folic acid, iron).

71. **List the signs and symptoms of leukopenia (decreased white blood cell levels).**
Cough, sore throat, fever, chills, swelling, ulceration of the mucous membranes, increased frequency of urination, painful urination, and persistent infections.

72. **List the common disorders or conditions that lower white blood cell levels.**
Alcoholism, aplastic anemia, autoimmune/collagen-vascular diseases (eg, lupus, AIDS), bone marrow failure, Cushing's syndrome, disorders of the spleen, infections, liver disease, radiation exposure or exposure to toxic chemicals (eg, chemotherapy), tumors, and viral infections.

73. **What are the hematologic red flags?**
- Evidence of platelet disorders (eg, bleeding with minor to no trauma, multiple petechiae, purpura, severe bruising, nosebleeds, hematemesis, blood in urine or stool, dark tarry stool, excessive menstrual bleeding; especially when undiagnosed, sudden, and/or unexplained).
- Evidence of anemia, especially in the presence of CNS, and cardiopulmonary manifestations.
- Undiagnosed muscle and joint pain in patients with a history of hemophilia.
- Undiagnosed variations in hematologic values.

74. **What subjective information should be obtained when hematologic pathologies are suspected?**
- Presence of any red flags as previously described.
- History of anemia (eg, excessive bruising or blood loss).
- Medical history including dental procedures (eg, blood transfusion, hemophilia, hepatitis, genetic, major trauma, cancer).
- Laboratory tests (eg, hematocrit, platelet count, hemoglobin concentration).
- Surgical history (eg, transplant surgery, oral surgery, major surgeries).
- History of radiation exposure or exposure to toxic chemicals (eg, chemotherapy, industrial gases).
- Integumentary changes as described in this chapter including bruising, petechia, purpura visible through the epidermis, widespread color changes, itching, body temperature, mobility, and turgor.

75. **List three early signs and symptoms of anemia.**
Difficult or labored breathing, weakness, and fatigue.

ENDOCRINE AND METABOLIC DISORDERS

76. **What are two primary life-threatening metabolic conditions that can develop if uncontrolled or untreated diabetes mellitus progresses to a state of severe hyperglycemia?**
- Diabetic ketoacidosis.
- Hyperglycemic, hyperosmolar, nonketotic coma (HHNC).

77. **What two patient types may exhibit orthostatic hypotension because of slight dehydration, especially when intense exercise increases the core body temperature?**
Athletes and normal adults.

78. **What signs and symptoms are commonly associated with endocrine system pathologies?**
Neuromusculoskeletal signs and symptoms include muscle weakness, myalgia and fatigue, bilateral carpal tunnel syndrome, periarthritis, chondrocalcinosis, spondyloarthropathy, osteoarthritis, hand stiffness, and pain.

79. **What are the endocrine system red flags?**
Diabetes insipidus
- Confusion.
- Increased frequency of urination (polyuria, nocturia).

Syndrome of Inappropriate Antidiuretic Hormone Secretion (SIADH)
- Excessive weight gain or loss.
- Edema.
- Headache, seizures, and muscle cramps.
- Vomiting/diarrhea.

Addison's disease
- Dark pigmentation of the skin, mucous membranes, and scars.
- Hypotension.
- Fatigue that improves with rest.
- Arthralgias.
- Tendon calcification.
- Hypoglycemia.

Cushing's syndrome
- Moon face.
- Cervicodorsal fat pad.
- Protuberant abdomen with accumulation of fatty tissue and stretch marks.
- Muscle wasting and weakness.
- Kyphosis and back pain secondary to bone loss.
- Easy bruising.
- Emotional disturbances.
- Diabetes mellitus, slow wound healing.
- In women: masculinizing effects.

Goiter (enlarged thyroid)
- Increased neck size.
- Hoarseness.
- Difficulty breathing and swallowing.

Hyperthyroidism
- Proximal weakness, primarily of pelvic girdle and thigh muscles.
- <50% of adults over 70: tachycardia, fatigue, and weight loss.
- <50 years of age: tachycardia, hyperactive reflexes, increased sweating, heat intolerance, fatigue, tremor, nervousness, polydipsia, weakness, increased appetite, dyspnea, and weight loss.
- Musculoskeletal symptoms including chronic periarthritis, pain and decreased ROM, periarticular and tendinous calcification.

Hypothyroidism
- Headaches, excessive fatigue, and drowsiness.
- Hoarseness and thick, slurred speech.
- Intolerance to cold.
- Weight gain.
- Dryness of skin.
- Nails become increasingly thin and brittle.
- Menses become irregular.
- Myxedema: nonpitting boggy edema around the eyes, hands, feet, and supraclavicular fossae.
- Synovial thickening and joint effusion.

Thyroid cancers
- New onset of hoarseness, hemoptysis, elevated blood pressure.

80. What red flags are associated with metabolic disorders?

Metabolic acidosis
- Headache, drowsiness, lethargy.
- Nausea, vomiting, diarrhea.
- Muscle twitching.
- Convulsions, coma (if severe).
- Rapid, deep breathing (hyperventilation).

Metabolic alkalosis
- Nausea, prolonged vomiting, diarrhea.
- Confusion, irritability, agitation, restlessness.
- Muscle twitching, cramping, weakness.
- Paresthesias.
- Convulsions, eventual coma.
- Slow, shallow breathing.

Gout
- Joint pain and swelling (especially the first metatarsal joint).
- Fever and chills, redness.
- Malaise.

Hemochromatosis
- Arthropathy, arthralgias, myalgias.
- Progressive weakness.
- Bilateral pitting edema (lower extremities).
- Vague abdominal pain.
- Hypogonadism (lack of menstrual periods, impotence).
- Congestive heart failure.
- Hyperpigmentation of the skin (gray/blue or yellow).
- Loss of body hair.
- Diabetes mellitus.

Osteoporosis
- Episodic back pain, kyphosis (Dowager's hump).
- Decreased activity tolerance.
- Early satiety.

Osteomalacia
- Bone pain, skeletal deformities, fractures.
- Myalgia, severe muscle weakness.

Paget's disease
- Headache and dizziness.
- Periosteal tenderness, bone fractures, vertebral compression and collapse, deformity (eg, bowing of long bones, increased size and abnormal contour of clavicles, osteoarthritis of adjacent joint, acetabular protrusion, and head enlargement).
- Compression neuropathy (eg, spinal stenosis, paresis, paraplegia, and muscle weakness).
- Decreased auditory acuity.

81. **What subjective information should be obtained when endocrine system pathology is suspected?**
    - Presence of any red flags as previously described.
    - Medication use, including use of insulin or cortisol, or excessive use of antacids.
    - Slow wound healing.
    - Family history of osteoporosis.
    - Increase in collar size (eg, goiter growth), difficulty in breathing or swallowing.

82. **List common musculoskeletal disorders that mimic endocrine system disorders.**
    Periarthritis and calcific tendinitis of the shoulder is common in endocrine clients and must be ruled out from other musculoskeletal disorders such as rotator cuff dysfunction, rotator cuff tears, slap lesions, labral tears, and subacromial/subdeltoid bursitis.

IMMUNOLOGIC

83. **What are the four principal classifications of immunologic disorders?**
    The four principal classifications are immunodeficiency, hypersensitivity, autoimmunity, and immunoproliferative disorders.

84. **Name the only disease known to directly attack the human immune system.**
    AIDS (acquired immunodeficiency syndrome).

85. **How are hypersensitivity disorders classified?**
    Hypersensitivity disorders are grouped into four types: type I anaphylactic hypersensitivity (allergies), type II hypersensitivity (cytolytic or cytotoxic), type III hypersensitivity (immune complex), and type IV hypersensitivity (cell-mediated or delayed).

86. **What neurologic disorders may be associated with immune system dysfunction?**
    Myasthenia gravis, Guillain-Barré syndrome, and multiple sclerosis are neurologic disorders associated with immune system dysfunction.

87. **List examples of autoimmune disorders.**
    Examples of autoimmune disorders are fibromyalgia syndrome, rheumatoid arthritis, systemic lupus erythematosus, scleroderma, spondyloarthropathy, Reiter syndrome, psoriatic arthritis, Lyme disease, and bacterial arthritis.

88. **What signs and symptoms are commonly associated with pathologies of the immunologic system?**

Acquired immunodeficiency syndrome (AIDS)

- Early signs and symptoms include fever, night sweats, fatigue, headache, minor oral infections, cough, shortness of breath, and skin changes (eg, rash, nail bed changes, dry skin).
- Advanced signs and symptoms include Kaposi's sarcoma and the presence of opportunistic diseases (eg, TB, pneumonia, lymphoma, thrush, herpes 1 and 2).

Hypersensitivity disorders

- Signs and symptoms may be as minor as sinus drainage to as severe as coma or death of the patient.
- Additional signs and symptoms include nausea, prolonged vomiting, and diarrhea; confusion, irritability, agitation, and restlessness; muscle twitching, cramping, and weakness; paresthesias; convulsions and eventual coma; slow, shallow breathing.

Neurologic disorders

- Signs and symptoms of myasthenia gravis include muscle fatigability and proximal muscle weakness aggravated with exertion, respiratory failure, ptosis, diplopia, dysarthria, and bulbar involvement (eg, alteration in voice quality, dysphagia, nasal regurgitation, choking).
- Signs and symptoms of Guillain-Barré syndrome include muscle weakness (eg, bilateral, progressing from the legs to the arms, to the chest and neck), diminished deep tendon reflexes, paresthesias, fever, malaise, and nausea.
- Signs and symptoms of multiple sclerosis include optic neuritis leading to unilateral visual impairment, paresthesia, nystagmus, spasticity or hyperreflexia leading to ataxia or unsteadiness, vertigo, fatigue, muscle weakness, and bowel and bladder dysfunction. Positive Babinski's sign, positive Lhermitte's sign, and absent abdominal reflex are also present.

Autoimmune disorders

- Signs and symptoms of fibromyalgia syndrome include fatigue, depression, anxiety, short-term memory loss, decreased attention span, headaches, nocturnal bruxism, myalgia, tender points of palpation, tendinitis, bursitis, morning stiffness, low back pain, subjective swelling, and irritable bowel and bladder symptoms.
- Signs and symptoms of rheumatoid arthritis include swelling in one or more joints, early morning stiffness, recurring joint pain or tenderness, impaired joint motion, joint redness and warmth, unexplained weight loss, and fever or weakness.
- Signs and symptoms of systemic lupus erythematosus include constitutional symptoms, arthralgia, arthritis, skin rashes, anemia, pulmonary and renal disorders, CNS signs and symptoms, hair loss, and mouth, nose, or vaginal ulcers.
- Signs and symptoms of systemic scleroderma include calcinosis (ie, abnormal deposition of calcium salts in tissues, particularly over bony prominences), Raynaud's phenomenon, dysphagia, heartburn, hardening and shrinking of the toes and fingers, and formation of spider-like hemangiomas in the face and hands.
- Signs and symptoms of spondyloarthropathy include back pain with insidious onset; first episode occurs before age 30, episodes of pain last for months, and pain intensifies with rest and decreases with movement.
- Signs and symptoms of ankylosing spondylitis include:
  - Early signs and symptoms—intermittent low-grade fever, fatigue, anemia, anorexia, painful limited spinal motion, loss of spinal motion, and inflammation of the iris (iritis or iridocyclitis).
  - Advanced signs and symptoms—constant low back pain, ankylosis of the SI joints and spine, muscle wasting in the shoulder and pelvic girdles, marked cervical kyphosis, decreased chest expansion, and arthritis in the extremity joints.
- Signs and symptoms of Reiter syndrome include polyarthritis, SI/low back pain, heel pain, plantar fasciitis, low-grade fever, urethritis, which precede other symptoms by 1 to 2 weeks, and bilateral conjunctivitis and iritis.
- Signs and symptoms of psoriatic arthritis include fever, fatigue, dystrophic nail bed changes, polyarthritis, psoriasis, and sore, swollen fingers.
- Signs and symptoms of Lyme disease include rash, flu-like symptoms, migratory musculoskeletal pain, severe headaches, numbness, weakness and pain in the extremities, and poor motor coordination.
- Signs and symptoms of bacterial arthritis include fever and chills, rapid onset of monoarticular involvement (eg, knees and shoulders are most frequent), joint inflammatory symptoms/signs, restricted motion, local tenosynovitis, and skin lesions near the involved joint.

89. **What are the immunologic red flags?**

In addition to the signs and symptoms described previously, the following red flags should be screened:

- Development of neurologic symptoms 1 to 3 weeks after an injection (eg, Guillain-Barré syndrome).
- New onset of inflammatory joint pain postoperatively, especially if accompanied by extraarticular signs and symptoms such as rash, diarrhea, urethritis, mouth ulcers, and raised skin patches.
- Joint pain preceded or accompanied by skin rash or lesions.
- Generalized weakness.
- Nail bed changes (eg, dystrophic nail changes associated with psoriasis, atrophy of the fingertips, calcific nodules, digital cyanosis, and tightening of the skin associated with scleroderma).

90. **What are other musculoskeletal causes of pain that must be differentially diagnosed from an immunologic disorder?**
Because of the multisystem effect of immunologic disorders, it is important that a complete health history is performed to identify if musculoskeletal signs and symptoms are attributable to a mechanical origin, or whether other sources should be investigated. Close cooperation and appropriate co-management with the referring physician are crucial for the proper management of musculoskeletal cases with suspicious origins.

91. **What are signs of opioid abuse?**
Signs of opioid abuse include the following: inability to control opioid use, uncontrollable cravings, drowsiness, changes in sleep habits, weight loss, frequent flu-like symptoms, decreased libido, lack of hygiene, changes in exercise habits, isolation from family or friends, stealing from family, friends or businesses, new financial difficulties.

CLINICAL REASONING

92. **Why do errors in clinical reasoning occur?**
It is well documented that human beings are for the most part noncritical thinkers and that we are prone to deductive and inductive errors in reasoning (ie, judgment errors). Additionally, the cognitive limitation of human working memory leads us to access simpler rather than more complex cognitive or problem-solving strategies (ie, shortcuts in reasoning). In actuality, it is likely that the combination of judgment errors and reliance on shortcuts in reasoning (eg, heuristics or clinical prediction rules) is what leads to most errors in clinical reasoning.
However, errors will vary based on the difficulty of the patient case, knowledge of content and context, strategy selection, experience, and integration and interpretation of pertinent patient information.

93. **Do knowledge, efficiency of data collection, and data interpretation improve with experience?**
No. Literature suggests that inadequate knowledge and imprecise data collection improve with increasing clinical experience, but data integration and interpretation do not.

94. **What is deductive reasoning?**
Deductive reasoning involves reaching a conclusion based on evidence. Deductive reasoning combines two or more pieces of evidence to reach a conclusion.

95. **What are examples of deductive reasoning errors?**
Illogical or poor reasoning, persistence of beliefs despite empirical data to the contrary, rationalizing, justifying, and using biases and heuristics to assess information are examples of deductive reasoning errors.

96. **What is inductive reasoning?**
Inductive reasoning uses specific pieces of evidence (ie, more than one example) to draw conclusions that are probably, but not necessarily, true (eg, generalizations, cause and effect, and analogies).

97. **What are examples of inductive reasoning errors?**
Examples include overconfidence in validity of beliefs, confusion of opinion or anecdotal evidence with truth, overestimation of knowledge, and basing a decision on personal interests.

98. **What is iterative hypothesis testing?**
Iterative hypothesis testing, as described by Kasper and Harrison, is a process used by medical practitioners to increase the efficiency of the interview process. During this process interview questions are used to confirm or refute the evolving diagnostic hypothesis. Iterative hypothesis testing uses specific questions to probe patient answers. Iterative hypothesis testing does not replace a systematic, thorough, and complete history of present illness, past medical history, review of systems, family history, and the physical examination. Iterative hypothesis testing represents a pattern of application of inductive and deductive reasoning.

99. **Provide an example of iterative hypothesis testing.**
The patient presents with a referral that states: "lumbar pain, evaluate and treat." Therapist: "What are you here for today?" Patient: "I have a pinched nerve in my back." Therapist: "Who was the doctor who diagnosed you with this condition?" Patient: "It was not my doctor." Therapist: "I am not certain if I understand; how did you determine that you have a pinched nerve in your back?" Patient: "About a year ago my neighbor had the same pain that I am having and he had a pinched nerve in his back." In this example, if the therapist did not test the hypothesis, a serious error could have occurred (ie, generating a diagnosis based on the patient's perception of illness).

100. **List common errors or biases in clinical reasoning and a potential consequence of the error or bias.**

ERROR OR BIAS	POSSIBLE CONSEQUENCE(S)
Faulty hypotheses testing and clinical reasoning skills	Making clinical decisions based on illogical or faulty reasoning processes or using more simplistic rather than more complex cognitive problem-solving strategies
Confusions between deductive and inductive logic	Deductive reasoning errors or drawing conclusions that go beyond the information contained in the premises (eg, Correct: If "A" then "B"; "A" therefore "B," Incorrect: If "A" then "B," therefore, if "B" then "A"). Inductive reasoning errors or generalizations based on specific observations that are not based on deductive reasoning (eg, All "A" are "B" ≠ All "B" are "A")
Confusing covariance with causality	Presuming that two or more factors are causally related when two factors have been found to co-vary
Errors in detecting variance	Making a judgment about the relationship of two factors without understanding how the two factors co-vary with one another
Causal reasoning errors	Assuming a causal relationship establishes proof and failing to recognize unknown factors and processes
Confusing temporal and causal succession (ie, assuming that there is a causal connection based only on temporal sequence)	Establishing erroneous causal relationships. Assuming a causal connection or that one event occurred because of another, when in fact one event merely occurred after another
Over-reliance on clinical prediction rules and heuristics (ie, shortcuts in reasoning)	Failure to identify the correct disease process, two or more independent disease processes, and/or the implications of comorbidities (eg, making clinical decisions based on choosing the simplest diagnoses capable of explaining the patient's signs and symptoms)
Confirmation bias (ie, emphasizing or validating information that supports the clinicians favored hypotheses while negating information that does not)	Failure to identify or address competing diagnoses and limiting examination to tests and measures to those that confirm the suspected diagnoses while ignoring evidence and testing that might disconfirm it. Confirmation bias likely represents one of the greatest single sources of error
Persistence of resilient beliefs	Making a diagnosis and/or setting a course of action despite empirical data to the contrary
Adding pragmatic inferences	Making diagnostic assumptions that result in misdiagnoses or faulty clinical decisions
Broad generalizations (ie, applying a general statement or rule too broadly)	Forming inferences or assumptions that do not apply to a specific patient case, event, pathology, etc.
Failure to sample enough information	Basing clinical decisions on generalizations and limited data and discontinuing the search for additional diagnoses after anticipated diagnoses are made
Erroneous integration and interpretation of data	Failure to synthesize and integrate clinical information deleteriously impacts all aspects of the clinical reasoning process. The ability to synthesize and integrate clinical information is the foremost distinguishing feature of a diagnostic expert.
Generating a diagnosis based on availability or recall	Overestimating the probability of a diagnosis and generating a false sense of frequency
Generating a diagnosis based on similarity or pattern recognition	Neglecting the prevalence of competing diagnoses based on weak and incomplete similarities, as opposed to hypothetical deductive reasoning

ERROR OR BIAS	POSSIBLE CONSEQUENCE(S)
Generating a diagnosis based on the patient's perception of illness	A type of confirmation bias in which the clinician seeks to validate a self-reported patient diagnosis
Considering too few diagnoses or hypotheses	Artificially or prematurely limiting the number of plausible diagnoses
Faulty or insufficient knowledge or skill base	Making clinical decisions based on omissions that stem from a lack of knowledge or omitting more beneficial interventions secondary to lack of knowledge and/or skill
Selecting a course of action based on outcomes	Selecting less beneficial interventions in place of potentially more beneficial interventions secondary to emphasizing adverse effects, cost, time, availability, etc.
Selecting a course of action based on treatment-driven practice patterns	Selecting interventions based on a narrow and often ineffectual or less effective range of treatment options as opposed to selecting interventions based upon a comprehensive examination, evaluation, and differential diagnosis
Selecting a course of action based on omission	Basing clinical decisions on desired or expected outcomes rather than logic and evidence supporting clinical decisions
Considering too few interventions	Choosing the same intervention when there are additional and potentially more effective alternative options available

101. What are the ultimate consequences of clinical decision-making errors?

Consequences range from little to none (eg, in cases where patient conditions are self-limiting and intervention selections are conservative) to potentially catastrophic (eg, in cases where emergent medical conditions are present or developing and appropriate intervention is not provided).

102. What are some examples from within the literature of evidence-based practices that may lead to errors in clinical reasoning?

The use of shortcuts in reasoning (eg, heuristics and clinical prediction rules) to select interventions for the treatment of conditions such as low back pain may lead to errors in clinical reasoning.

Bibliography

American Physical Therapy Association. (2001). Guide to Physical Therapist Practice. Second Edition. American Physical Therapy Association. *Physical Therapy, 81*(1), 9–746.

Bickley, L. S., Szilagyi, P. G., Hoffman, R. M., & Soriano, R. P. (2022). *Bates' guide to physical examination and history taking.* Philadelphia: Lippincott Williams & Wilkins.

Bordage, G. (1999). Why did I miss the diagnosis? Some cognitive explanations and educational implications. *Academic Medicine, 74*(10 Suppl), S138–143.

Croskerry, P. (2009). Clinical cognition and diagnostic error: applications of a dual process model of reasoning. *Advances in Health Sciences Education, 14*(Suppl 1), 27–35.

Crupi, V., & Elia, F. (2017). Understanding and improving decisions in clinical medicine (I): reasoning, heuristics, and error. *Internal and Emergency Medicine, 12*(5), 689–691.

Elstein, A. S. (1999). Heuristics and biases: selected errors in clinical reasoning. *Academic Medicine, 74*(7), 791–794.

Featherston, R., Downie, L. E., Vogel, A. P., Galvin, K. L., & Kumar, S. (2020). Decision making biases in the allied health professions: a systematic scoping review. *PLoS ONE, 15*, e0240716.

Friedman, M. H., Connell, K. J., Olthoff, A. J., Sinacore, J. M., & Bordage, G. (1998). Medical student errors in making a diagnosis. *Academic Medicine, 73*(10 Suppl), S19–21.

Goodman, C. C., Heick, J., & Lazaro, R. T. (2018). *Differential diagnosis for physical therapists: screening for referral.* St. Louis, MO: Elsevier.

Groves, M., O'Rourke, P., & Alexander, H. (2003a). The clinical reasoning characteristics of diagnostic experts. *Medical Teacher, 25*(3), 308–313.

Groves, M., O'Rourke, P., & Alexander, H. (2003b). Clinical reasoning: the relative contribution of identification, interpretation and hypothesis errors to misdiagnosis. *Medical Teacher, 25*(6), 621–625.

Gruppen, L. D. (2017). Clinical reasoning: defining it, teaching it, assessing it, studying it. *The Western Journal of Emergency Medicine, 18*(1), 4–7.

Hayes, M. M., Chatterjee, S., & Schwartzstein, R. M. (2017). Critical thinking in critical care: five strategies to improve teaching and learning in the intensive care unit. *Annals of the American Thoracic Society, 14*(4), 569–575.

Higgs, J., & Jones, M. A. (2000). *Clinical reasoning in the health professions.* Boston, MA: Butterworth-Heinemann.

Holloway, P. J. (2000). Inductive vs deductive reasoning. *British Dental Journal, 188*(12), 643–644.

Jameson, L. J., Fauci, A. S., Kasper, D. L., Hauser, S. L., Longo, D. L., & Loscalzo, J. (2018). *Harrison's principles of internal medicine.* New York, NY: McGraw-Hill.

Jarvik, J. G., & Deyo, R. A. (2002). Diagnostic evaluation of low back pain with emphasis on imaging. *Annals of Internal Medicine, 137*(7), 586–597.
Jarvis, C. (2020). *Physical examination and health assessment.* St. Louis, MO: Elsevier Inc.
Kempainen, R. R., Migeon, M. B., & Wolf, F. M. (2003). Understanding our mistakes: a primer on errors in clinical reasoning. *Medical Teacher, 25*(2), 177–181.
Leppink, J., & Heuvel, A. (2015). The evolution of cognitive load theory and its application to medical education. *Perspectives on Medical Education, 4*(3), 119–127.
McMahon, S., Koltzenburg, M., Tracey, I., & Turk, D. C. (2013). *Wall & Melzack's textbook of pain: Expert consult.* Philadelphia, PA: Elsevier/Saunders.
MedlinePlus. (2018). Skin conditions. Retrieved February 5, 2022, from https://medlineplus.gov/skinconditions.html#summary.
Moore, K. L., Dalley, A. F., & Agur, A. M. R. (2014). *Clinically oriented anatomy.* Philadelphia, PA: Wolters Kluwer/Lippincott Williams & Wilkins Health.
National Institutes of HealthNational Institutes of Health. (2014). Skin conditions. Retrieved January 3, 2014 from http://www.nlm.nih.gov/medlineplus/skinconditions.html.
Round, A. (2001). Introduction to clinical reasoning. *Journal of Evaluation in Clinical Practice, 7*(2), 109–117.
Royce, C. S., Hayes, M. M., & Schwartzstein, R. M. (2019). Teaching critical thinking: a case for instruction in cognitive biases to reduce diagnostic errors and improve patient safety. *Academic Medicine, 94*(2), 187–194.
Seidel, H. M., Stewart, R. W., Ball, J. W., Dains, J. E., Flynn, J. A., & Solomon, B. S. (2011). *Mosby's guide to physical examination.* St. Louis, MO: Mosby/Elsevier.
WebMD. (2020). Complete blood count (CBC). Retrieved February 5, 2022, from http://www.webmd.com/a-to-z-guides/complete-blood-count-cbc.
Willis, W. D., Jr. (1985). The pain system. The neural basis of nociceptive transmission in the mammalian nervous system. *Pain Headache, 8*, 1–346.

CHAPTER 21 QUESTIONS

1. **Select the interview question that BEST reflects screening for pulmonary red flags.**
   a. Do you experience unusual sweating, a fever, or chills at night?
   b. Have you experienced any unexplained weight loss or weight gain?
   c. Is your pain brought on or exacerbated by shoulder movements?
   d. Is your pain brought on or exacerbated by inhalation, exhalation, or coughing?

2. **During an integumentary examination, a physical therapist documents pathological clubbing of the patient's nails and distal fingers. Which of the following conditions is MOST likely present?**
   a. Chronic cyanotic heart disease
   b. Chronic anemia
   c. Thyroid disease
   d. Chronic renal insufficiency

3. **Your patient reports changes in appetite, darkened stools, and aching, burning, and cramping when eating. Which of the following conditions are most likely associated with these signs and symptoms?**
   a. Pancreatic cancer
   b. Colon cancer
   c. Stomach ulcer
   d. Appendicitis

4. **A 64-year-old is referred to physical therapy with a diagnosis of right knee osteoarthritis and complaints of right knee pain, swelling, and antalgic gait. During the examination, the patient demonstrates shortness of breath, wheezing, and the use of accessory muscles for respiration. The patient also reports that he does not tolerate supine positioning. Which of the following conditions is MOST likely present?**
   a. Acute bronchitis
   b. Chronic emphysema
   c. Pneumonia
   d. Weakness of respiratory muscles

5. A 52-year-old is referred to a physical therapy clinic with a diagnosis of left shoulder primary impingement tendinosis and physical therapy examination and radiologic findings are consistent with this diagnosis. A thorough medical screening reveals associated symptoms of fatigue, as well as an increased appetite, thirst, and urination over the past 3 to 6 months. Additional information includes: height = 5′10″ and weight = 320 lb; HDL cholesterol level = 30 mg/dl and triglyceride level = 450 mg/dl. Which of the following conditions is MOST likely present?
   a. Cardiovascular disease
   b. Hypothyroidism
   c. Renal disease
   d. Type 2 diabetes

6. A 54-year-old male is referred to a physical therapy clinic with a diagnosis of left ulnar neuropathy. He reports symptoms in the left lateral neck, left superior chest, and along the medial arm and reports symptoms increase with UE exercise and ambulation. He reports that symptoms are achy in quality and intense at times. Which test or measure will provide the most useful diagnostic information for this case?
   a. Observation of active motion
   b. Vital signs
   c. Tests of neural function
   d. Palpation of the nerve at the ulnar groove

CHAPTER 22

SPECIAL TESTS FOR MEDICAL SCREENING

M.E. Lonnemann, PT, DPT, OCS, FAAOMPT and A. Burke-Doe, PT, MPT, PhD

1. **Why is medical screening necessary?**
Performing a medical screen is an important step in making a physical therapy diagnosis and promoting a healthy population. Medical screening assists the physical therapist in identifying risks or problems beyond our expertise and scope of practice. Screening helps in determining whether patient referral to another practitioner is needed. When screening, if findings are suspicious or require diagnostic skills or equipment outside of the physical therapy scope of practice, a medical referral is warranted. By gathering information from the patient intake form, history, and the physical examination the therapist can determine whether a medical condition is present and not yet diagnosed, if a medical condition exists and is clinically stable, or if an existing clinical condition is medically unstable. Intake forms often include personal goals and aspirations, demographics, medical history, medications or complementary alternatives, health habits and behaviors, such as tobacco use, alcohol use, diet, physical activity, nutrition, sleep, hearing, functional activity, emotional status, integumentary status, pain, vision, body mass, mental functions, sensation, balance, and aerobic capacity.
The therapist uses screening tools such as red and yellow flag findings to recognize potential serious disorders. The therapist may be screening for visceral diseases, cancer, infections, fracture, and vascular disorders and can communicate with the physician regarding a list or pattern of signs and symptoms that have caused concern. Our role does not include suggesting the presence of a specific disease. The therapist is also screening based on population health such as pediatric, adult, or the aging population, which may have individualized tests and measures such as developmental milestones and fall history that should be addressed.

2. **When positive screening results are found, what are the red flags versus the yellow flags?**
Flags can be categorized into two areas. Clinical Flags and Psychosocial Flags.
Red-flag findings are signs or symptoms of serious pathology or conditions that may require immediate medical attention and are of particular concern that physical therapy should not be the primary provider of service. They are typically indicative of nonmechanical (nonneuromusculoskeletal) conditions or pathologies of visceral origin. Examples may include fever, night sweats, unexplained weight loss, unremitting night pain, bladder and bowel incontinence, saddle anesthesia, and previous or visual disturbances. Pathologies may include cauda equina syndrome, fracture, tumor, history of cancer.
Orange-flag findings include psychiatric symptoms, depression, personality disorder.
Yellow-flag findings can be grouped into two subcategories. Some describe yellow flags as potential confounding variables that may be cautionary warnings regarding the patient's condition. They suggest that the physical therapist take pause and monitor the influence of these findings on the patient's condition. Examples include dizziness, abnormal sensation patterns, fainting, progressive weakness, and circulatory or skin changes.
Yellow flags have also been described as unhelpful beliefs, appraisals, and judgement about a condition or injury. These may include unusual emotional responses, distress about not meeting criteria for diagnosis of mental disorder, worry, fear, and anxiety that may lead to pain behaviors where individuals avoid activities due to pain or potential for reinjury.
Blue flags are related to the individual's perception about work and ability to improve.

3. **A therapist screens systemic origins of a patient's signs and symptoms by considering pain referral, patient history, and clinical presentation. What are the most common sites of pain referral from a systemic disease?**
Pain from systemic disease is most often referred to the chest, back, shoulder, scapula, pelvis, hip, groin, and sacroiliac (SI) joint, with the back and shoulder being the most common within this group.

4. **Therapists must be aware of certain pathologies and their associated sites of pain referral. List the sites of referral and their associated pathologies.**

PAIN REFERRAL SITE	COMMON PATHOLOGY
Head, face, and TMJ Meningitis	
Primary brain tumor	
Subarachnoid hemorrhage	
Cervical and shoulder Metastatic lesions (leukemia, Hodgkin's disease)	
Cervical bone tumors	
Cervical cord tumors	
Pancoast's tumor	
Esophageal cancer	
Thyroid cancer	
Myocardial infarction	
Cervical ligamentous instabilities (possible cord compromise)	
Cervical and shoulder peripheral entrapment neuropathies	
Thoracic spine and ribs	Myocardial infarction
Unstable angina	
Stable angina	
Pericarditis	
Pulmonary embolus	
Pleurisy	
Pneumothorax	
Pneumonia	
Cholecystitis	
Peptic ulcer	
Pyelonephritis	
Nephrolithiasis	
Spinal fracture	
Metastatic lesions	
Pancreatic cancer	
Breast cancer	
Multiple myeloma	
Lumbar spine Multiple myeloma	
Primary bone tumors	
Neurogenic tumors (sacrum)	
Prostate cancer	
Testicular cancer	
Colorectal cancer	

Continued

PAIN REFERRAL SITE	COMMON PATHOLOGY
Back-related infection (osteomyelitis)	
Cauda equina syndrome	
Spinal fracture	
Abdominal aneurysm	
Lymphoma	
Endocarditis	
Myocarditis	
Acute pyelonephritis	
Perinephritic abscess	
Nephrolithiasis	
Ureteral colic (kidney stones)	
Urinary tract infection	
Dialysis (first-use syndrome)	
Renal tumors	
Obstruction (neoplasm)	
Irritable bowel syndrome	
Crohn's disease	
Diverticular disease	
Pancreatic disease	
Appendicitis	
Retroversion of the uterus	
Uterine fibroids	
Ovarian cysts	
Endometriosis	
Pelvic inflammatory disease (PID)	
Incest/sexual assault	
Rectocele, cystocele	
Uterine prolapse	
Pelvis, hip, and thigh colon cancer	
Pathologic fracture of the femoral neck	
Osteonecrosis of the femoral head	
Legg-Calvé-Perthes disease	
Slipped capita femoral epiphysis	
Metastasis	
Osteoid osteoma	
Chondrosarcoma	
Giant cell tumor	

PAIN REFERRAL SITE	COMMON PATHOLOGY
Ewing's sarcoma	
Arterial insufficiency	
Abdominal aortic aneurysm	
Avascular necrosis	
Kidney (renal) impairment; kidney stones	
Urinary tract infection	
Testicular cancer	
Abdominal or peritoneal inflammation (psoas abscess)	
Ankylosing spondylitis	
Appendicitis	
Crohn's disease; ulcerative colitis	
Diverticulitis	
Osteomyelitis (upper femur)	
PID	
Reiter's syndrome	
Inflammatory arthritis (RA, SLE, seronegative arthropathies, gout)	
Septic hip bursitis	
Tuberculosis	
Osteomalacia, osteoporosis	
Gaucher's disease	
Paget's disease	
Hemochromatosis	
Hemophilia	
Ectopic pregnancy	
Femoral artery catheterization	
Knee, leg, ankle, or foot	Peripheral arterial occlusive disease
Deep vein thrombosis	
Compartment syndrome	
Septic arthritis	
Cellulitis	

5. **List the organs and their respective locations in the abdominal quadrants.**

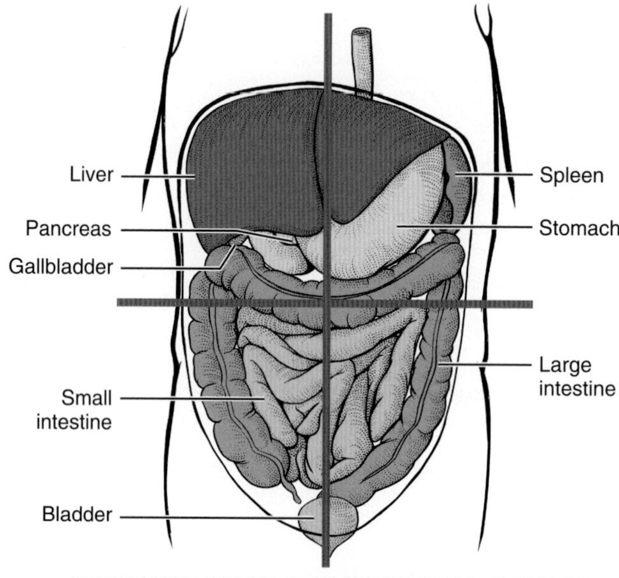

ANTERIOR VIEW OF ABDOMINAL CAVITY

(*From Goodman CC, Snyder TEK.* Differential Diagnosis for Physical Therapists: Screening for Referral, *6e, 2017, St. Louis, Elsevier, Inc.*)

- Right upper quadrant: gallbladder, liver, pancreas, and right kidney
- Left upper quadrant: spleen and stomach
- Right lower quadrant (RLQ): small intestine, appendix, and large intestine
- Left lower quadrant (LLQ): small and large intestine
- Central lower quadrant: bladder

6. **What are the components of the physical examination in the abdominal region when screening for visceral disorders?**

The components of the physical examination of the abdominal region are inspection, auscultation, percussion, and palpation. Inspection is the process of visually looking at the body for symmetry, alignment, skin color, and scars present. Auscultation follows inspection during examination of the abdominal region. Auscultation is performed to listen for bowel sounds. Normal bowel sounds are made by movement of the intestines as food and liquid pass through. Bowel sounds occur frequently, on the order of every 2 to 5 seconds, although there is a lot of variability. Palpation in the abdominal region is usually deep palpation (firm pressure) and is used to assess for tenderness and presence of visceral organs. Percussion is used to determine the size, shape, and density of tissue using sound. Direct percussion is performed using the examiner's fingers to tap directly on the surface of the body. Indirect percussion requires the middle finger of the examiner's nondominant hand to be positioned against the patient's skin and for the examiner to strike above or below the IP joint of the third digit with the dominant hand.

Blunt percussion using the examiner's border of the fifth metacarpal (ulnar border) with the hand in a fist is performed when assessing kidneys. The examiner listens for sounds that can range from tympani to a flat sound based on the tissue.

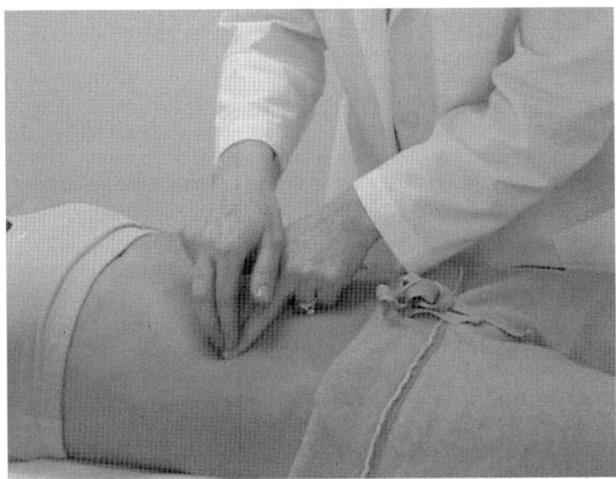

(*From Boissonnault WG.* Examination in Physical Therapy Examination: Screening for Medical Disease, *2e, New York, 1995, Churchill Livingstone.*)

7. **What types of percussive sounds can be heard in the body?**

   Percussion is used to detect changes in the density of an organ. Tissue density can range from high to low with percussive sounds ranging from flat, dull, resonant, hyperresonant, and tympanic. A dull sound indicates the presence of a solid mass under the surface such as the heart. A more resonant (vibrating) sound indicates hollow air-containing structures, such as the lungs and the hollow viscera of the abdomen. Tissues can also have abnormal fluid or a mass altering the typical sound heard in that anatomic location. In addition to producing different notes, percussion can also produce different sensations in the fingers, such as vibration.

8. **What are the specific qualities elicited by palpation?**

Texture	The surface characteristics of the skin and hair are noted (brittle, coarse, thick, thin, roughened, or smooth)
Moisture	Assess the moisture content of the skin, hair, and mucous membranes; are they moist and supple or dry and cracked?
Skin temperature	Palpate the head, face, trunk, arms, hands, legs, and feet to assess the local skin temperature and the distribution of heat
Characteristics of masses	When a mass or enlarged organ is discovered, record its size, shape, consistency, mobility, surface regularity, and presence or absence of expansile or transmitted pulsation
Precordial cardiac thrust	Palpate the precordium (portions of the body over heart and lower chest) for signs of heart action
Crepitus	During examination of the bones, joints, tendon sheaths, pleura, and subcutaneous tissue, feel for crepitation
Tenderness	Discomfort or pain on palpation of accessible tissues and over major organs should be noted; how much pressure is required to induce the uncomfortable sensation?
Thrills	Palpate the precordium for thrills; if bruits (abnormal sounds) are heard in the major arteries, palpate them for thrills
Vocal fremitus	Palpation of vocal vibrations through the chest wall provides important information about the underlying pleura and lung

9. **Describe the special tests for palpation and percussion of the liver in an adult.**
The adult liver is normally not palpable below the right anterior inferior costovertebral margin (acute angle created between the vertebral column and the twelfth rib).
With percussion of the liver, the examiner begins at a point lateral to the umbilicus at the midclavicular line and percusses using a technique with the nondominant hand's second or third digits as the "dummy fingers" and the dominant second and third digits to perform the percussion from the point lateral to the umbilicus in a superior direction. The test is positive if the liver spans greater than 10 cm.
To palpate for hepatomegaly the examiner uses the tips of the fingers with two hands inferior to the ribs in the midclavicular line. The examiner palpates for the liver to descend with inspiration.

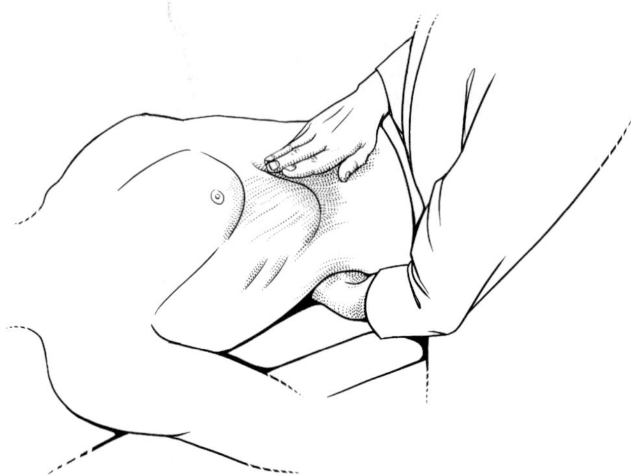

(*From Goodman CC, Snyder TEK.* Differential Diagnosis for Physical Therapists: Screening for Referral, *5e, 2013, St. Louis, Elsevier, Inc.*)

10. **How strong is the evidence to support the tests for palpation and percussion of the liver?**
There is minimal evidence to support the use of palpation and percussion of the liver for hepatomegaly.

11. **What is Murphy's sign and how is it performed?**
Murphy's sign is a test for cholecystitis. This test is performed with the patient in the supine position and the examiner placing his or her hands on the right upper abdominal quadrant at the inferior costal margin. The patient inspires and the examiner palpates deeply in the subcostal region with the fingertips. The test is considered positive if pain is perceived during inspiration or the patient stops inspiration because of discomfort.

12. **Name and describe palpation and percussion tests to assess for splenomegaly.**
Nixon's percussion test is performed with the patient in right side lying. The examiner percusses the posterior axillary line from the distal end of the lung to the middle anterior costal margin. This test is positive when dullness extends over 8 cm above the costal margin, with normal being 6 to 8 cm. Castell's percussion test is performed with the patient in the supine position. The examiner places his or her fingers over the eighth or ninth intercostal space, in line with the left anterior axillary line, and performs percussion during normal breathing and at full inspiration. The test is positive if dullness is noted during full inspiration.
Palpation of the spleen is performed through a bimanual palpation technique. The examiner stands on the patient's right side and reaches over to lift the left rib cage with the left hand. The right hand then palpates the costal margin and underneath the ribs to feel the spleen. The test is positive if the examiner is able to palpate the enlarged spleen. Middleton's maneuver is another test described with the patient lying supine with the examiner on the left side of the patient. The examiner stands at the patient's left shoulder and palpates the spleen under the left costal margin by flexing the fingers and palpating for the spleen while the patient inspires.

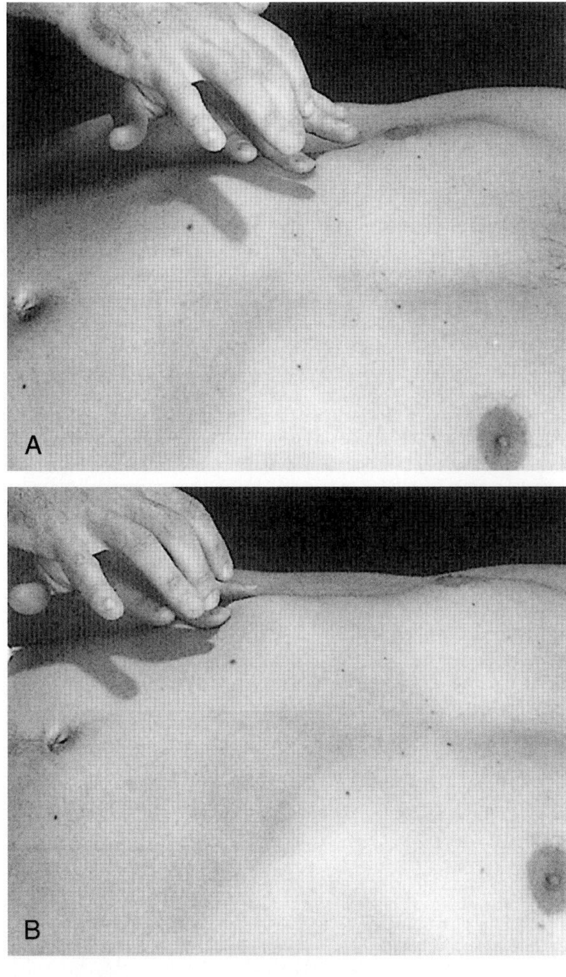

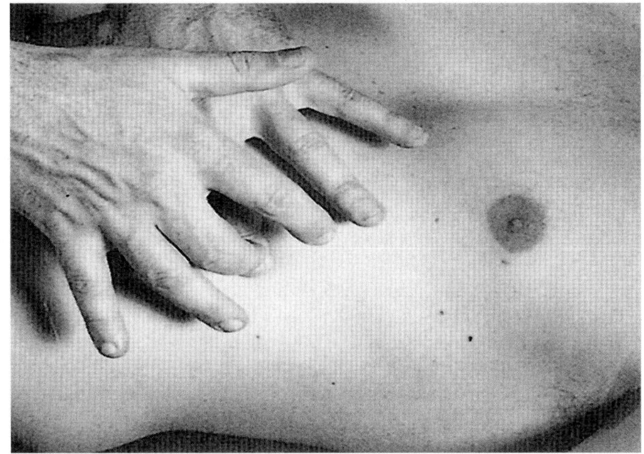

(*From Boissonnault WG.* Examination in Physical Therapy Examination: Screening for Medical Disease, *2e, New York, 1995, Churchill Livingstone.*)

13. In isolation, palpation and percussion tests for splenomegaly have minimal evidence to support their use and predictive value. When palpation and percussion are performed together does the evidence support the use of these tests?

There is moderate evidence to support the use of percussion and palpation tests of the spleen together. Sullivan and Williams (1976) reported sensitivity at 88% and specificity at 83% with a positive likelihood ratio of 5.18 and negative likelihood ratio of 14. Barkun et al. (1991) reported 46% sensitivity and 97% specificity with a positive likelihood ratio of 15.33 (greater than 10 alters posttest probability of a diagnosis to a moderate degree) and a negative likelihood ratio of 0.56.

14. Name and describe palpation and percussion tests to assess for the kidney.

Murphy's percussion test is also known as costovertebral angle tenderness (CVAT) or Murphy's punch sign and is used to rule out kidney involvement or pseudorenal pain. When performing this percussion test the patient can either be in prone or sitting. The examiner places one hand over the costovertebral angle (CVA) of the patient's back. Next, the examiner provides a percussive thump with the other hand, allowing the kidney to vibrate. A positive test is noted by either costovertebral tenderness or reproduction of back/flank pain signaling a red flag for renal involvement. If the patient experiences no pain after the thump is performed, then renal involvement is ruled out.

Palpation of the kidney is performed on the right side of the patient in supine position on a hard surface. The kidney is lifted by one hand in the CVA between the twelfth rib and the vertebral column. The patient then takes a deep breath; this causes the kidney to descend. As the patient inhales the anterior hand is pushed firmly and deeply beneath the costal margin in an effort to trap the kidney. When successful, the anterior hand can palpate the size, shape, and consistency of the organ as it slips back into normal position. The left kidney is usually not palpable because of its position beneath the bowel.

The diagnostic accuracy of this test is unknown as it appears to have not been tested.

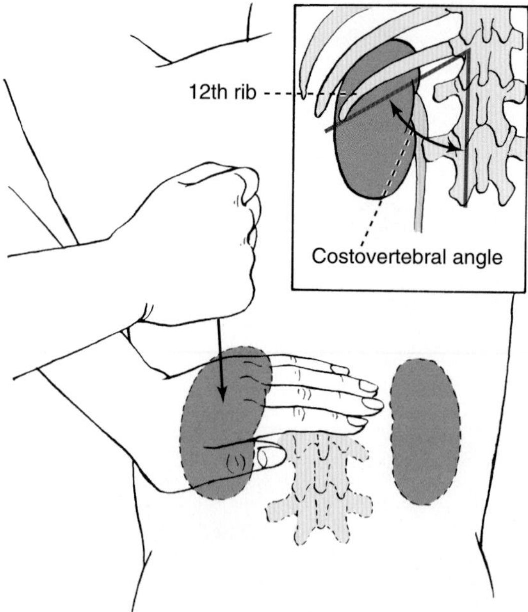

(From Black JM, Matassarin-Jacobs E, editors. Luckmann and Sorensen's Medical-Surgical Nursing, ed 4, 1993, Philadelphia, WB Saunders.)

15. **What structure(s) would be involved if a patient has a positive Murphy's percussion test, and how confident can a therapist be in the predictive value of this test?**
Murphy's percussion test is performed to assess for costovertebral tenderness and kidney involvement. The therapist uses the ulnar border (fifth metacarpal) of the fist to thump over the twelfth rib at the CVA with the patient either in sitting or prone position. The test is positive if pain is reproduced in the subcostal region, flank, or lateral aspect of the abdomen.

16. **What are the clinical findings related to appendicitis and the medical screens that would be utilized?**
    a. Discomfort and sharp pain in the RLQ of the abdominal area
    b. Abdominal tenderness and guarding of the RLQ
    c. McBurney point tenderness
    d. Tip of twelfth rib tenderness
    e. Pain in the belly button without trauma
    f. Right low back pain (LBP) without trauma and insidious onset
    g. Difficulty standing straight
    h. Psoas sign
    i. Obturator sign
    j. Rovsing sign (pain in RLQ reproduced with rebound testing of the LLQ)
    k. Increased heart rate and temperature
    l. Alvarado's score >6

17. **Where is McBurney's point and what does tenderness to palpation of this area indicate?**
McBurney's point is located in the RLQ of the abdomen, midway between the umbilicus and the anterior superior iliac spine (ASIS). Rebound tenderness or Blumberg's sign (examiner palpates deeply and then releases quickly) in this area would indicate appendicitis. Researchers have found tenderness to be more sensitive and Blumberg's sign to be more specific.

18. **What is Alvarado's score and what diagnostic utility does it have?**
Alvarado's score assesses the components of a physical examination for acute appendicitis. Alvarado's score determines the probability of a patient having acute appendicitis based on six clinical examinations and two laboratory tests. If the patient reports the following, he or she receives one or two points for each. The total score is then calculated out of 10.

Scores <5 were less likely to be acute appendicitis, and scores >6 were more likely. Sensitivity measures were recorded as high as 97% with a negative LR of 0.09 and QUADAS score of 9. When using a cutoff of >7, the specificity has been shown to be 100%.

EXAMINATION/TEST	SCORE
The patient reports that pain migrated from epigastric region to right lower quadrant	1
The patient reports anorexia 1	
The patient reports nausea and vomiting	1
The patient has tenderness in the right lower quadrant	2
Positive Blumberg's sign (rebound tenderness) over McBurney's point	1
Fever 1	
Leukocytosis 2	
Shift to left (white count shifts to left)	1
Total Score	10

19. **What are the clinical signs and causes of an iliopsoas (liacus or psoas) abscess, and what tests can be used to screen for this disorder?**

Signs and symptoms include fever, night sweats, pain; LBP, lower abdominal, pelvic, or anterior hip pain (medial thigh or groin); and sometimes knee pain, antalgic gait, pain, and swelling with palpation. Unilateral involvement can be associated with appendicitis, but it can be bilateral with generalized peritonitis. These abscesses are often associated with appendicitis, diverticulitis, Crohn's disease, kidney infection, or vertebral osteomyelitis status post lumbar spine surgery.

Screening tests for the psoas include the following:

- Heel tap—involves a gentle tap to the heel of the involved side.
- Hop test—ask the patient to hop on the involved lower extremity.
- Iliopsoas muscle test—the patient is in the supine position with both lower extremities relaxed.
- The examiner flexes the hip with the knee extended as in a straight leg raise. The examiner places resistance on the thigh to create an isometric hip flexion contraction. Pain is assessed as the patient resists this force with comparison to the uninvolved side. The test is positive if pain is reproduced in the lower quadrant.
- Palpation of the iliopsoas—the patient is in a supine position with the hips and knees flexed and supported at a 90-degree angle. The examiner slowly presses the pads of the fingers into the abdomen in a caudal and medial direction at approximately one-third the distance from the ASIS toward the umbilicus. The therapist can isolate the location by asking the patient to initiate hip flexion to help isolate the muscle and avoid palpating the bowel. A positive test is pain reproduction in the lower quadrant or abdomen.

20. **In addition to the iliopsoas muscle, what muscle test might be painful in the presence of appendicitis or peritonitis, and how would you test for involvement?**

Either of these conditions can irritate the obturator muscle and produce RLQ pain when performing an isometric-resistant contraction of the obturator. The test is performed with the patient in a supine position. The examiner performs active assistive hip and knee flexion to 90 degrees. In that position, the hip is rotated internally and externally. The examiner assesses for a painful response in the RLQ.

21. **What is the normal size of the aorta?**

The abdominal aorta lies slightly to the left of the midline of the body. A normal abdominal aorta is usually less than 3 cm wide. If the patient can relax, the abdomen should be deeply palpated a few centimeters above the umbilicus, slightly left of the midline, to detect an expansile pulse indicating a widened aorta.

22. **Describe the palpation and auscultation techniques to assess for an abdominal aortic aneurysm, and discuss the findings that indicate a positive test.**

The patient is in a supine position. The therapist applies pressure underneath the left side of the xiphoid process. With the pads of the fingers, gently apply a posterior pressure to assess for a pulse, gradually move inferior until a pulse is felt. In the area that the pulse is strongest, the therapist uses two index fingers over the spot where it is the strongest and then moves the fingers apart until the pulse is no longer felt. Move the fingers back in to feel the outer borders of the pulse, and judge the distance the fingers are apart. This process is repeated until the therapist reaches the umbilicus at which the bifurcation of the aorta into the common iliac arteries occurs. Obesity, voluntary guarding, and firm musculature limit the sensitivity of the examination.

Auscultation of the aorta is performed with a stethoscope over the area of the blood vessel. No abnormal sound should be present, such as a whooshing sound or strong pulse that would indicate a bruit. Aneurysms >5 cm in diameter have a high risk of rupture and should be considered for elective surgery; physical examination is only 75% sensitive for detecting aneurysms of this size.

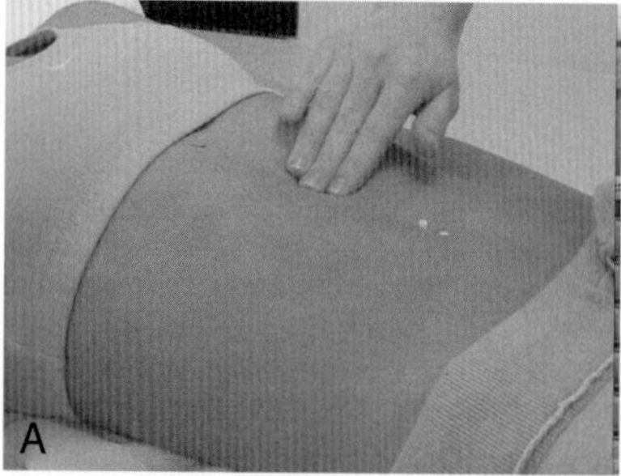

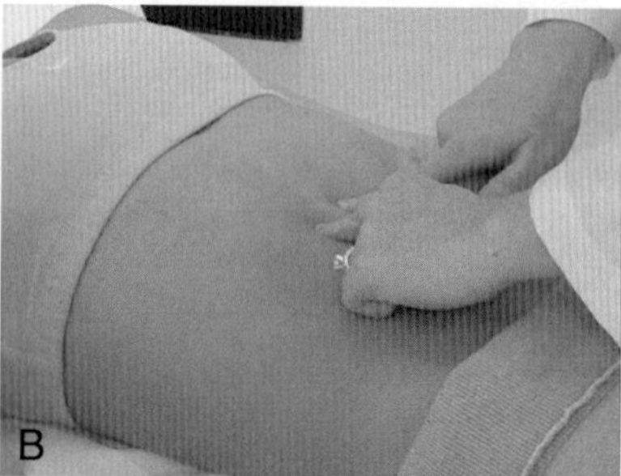

23. **What are Well's criteria for a pulmonary embolism? How confident are you in using this test?**

Clinical signs and symptoms of DVT (pain with palpation of the deep veins and leg swelling at a minimum)	+ 3.0
Pulmonary embolism is as likely or more likely than an alternative diagnosis	+ 3.0
Pulse >100	+ 1.5
Previous history of DVT or PE + 1.5	
Immobilization or major surgery in the past 4 weeks	+ 1.5
Hemoptysis	+ 1.0
Active cancer with ongoing treatment or within the past 6 months + 1.0	
A score less than or equal to 4; PE is unlikely, a score >4; PE is likely	

This test has demonstrated higher sensitivity overall than specificity in the studies scoring >10 QUADAS score, ranging from sensitivity of .89 to .93 and specificity of .65 to .98.

24. **List the Framingham criteria for heart failure.**

Major criteria
1. Paroxysmal nocturnal dyspnea or orthopnea
2. Neck vein distention
3. Rales
4. Cardiomegaly
5. Acute pulmonary edema
6. S3 gallop
7. Hepatojugular reflex

Minor criteria
1. Ankle edema
2. Nocturnal cough
3. Dyspnea on exertion
4. Hepatomegaly
5. Pleural effusion
6. Tachycardia (>120 beats per minute)

Heart failure is diagnosed by having two major criteria present or one major criterion with two minor.

25. **When should a therapist auscultate for bowel sounds, and what are the normal findings?**

Normal sounds are a result of peristaltic activity and consist of clicks and gurgles. Some abnormal bowel sounds are:
- High-pitched tinkling—usually from tension of air/fluid in a loop of dilated bowel. This suggests obstruction.
- Rushes—if located in one area, usually are caused by air/fluid being forced through a small partially occluded lumen. This suggests partial obstruction, especially if associated with concurrent abdominal activity.
- Hyperactive—sometimes normal, but if combined with abdominal complaints can indicate early obstruction or a GI bleed.
- Hypoactive or absent bowel sounds—sometimes normal, but combined with complaints can indicate paralytic ileus (a halt in peristaltic activity as a result of extreme irritation from obstructive peritonitis or unknown reasons). Bowel sounds cannot be said to be absent unless they are not heard after listening for 3 minutes.

26. **Which test uses a tuning fork to assess for fractures, and how confident can you be that they are accurate?**

Several tests have been described for assessment of fractures with a tuning fork. The Barford test for fracture assessment has been described for the screening of hip or femoral fractures. With this test the patient lies in a supine position, and the examiner places a stethoscope on the pubic symphysis or at the distal end of the femur. The examiner strikes the tuning fork and places it on the patella of the involved lower extremity. The test is considered positive if the examiner hears that the sound is muffled through the involved lower extremity compared with the uninvolved.

The sensitivities for this test have ranged in the low 80 s to low 90 s. However, the negative likelihood ratios reported are 0.4 and higher. The QUADAS scores were 8 and higher. With this likelihood ratio, there is still a 40% chance that the patient could have a fracture. In summary, there is moderate but not strong evidence to support the use of these tests.

Bibliography

Alvarado, A. (1986). A practical score for the early diagnosis of acute appendicitis. *Annals of Emergency Medicine, 15*, 557–564.

Bache, J. B., & Cross, A. B. (1984). The Barford test. A useful diagnostic sign in fractures of the femoral neck. *Practitioner, 228*, 305–308.

Barkun, A. N., Camus, M., Green, L., et al. (1991). The bedside assessment of splenic enlargement. *American Journal of Medicine, 91*, 512–518.

Boissonnault, W. (2011). *Primary care for the physical therapist* (2nd ed.). St. Louis: W.B. Saunders Company.

Cook, C., & Hegedus, E. (2012). *Orthopedic physical examination tests: An evidence-based approach* (2nd ed.). Upper Saddle River, NJ: Pearson.

Dutton, M. (2012). Differential diagnosis. In M. Dutton (Ed.), *Dutton's orthopaedic examination, evaluation, and intervention* (3rd ed.). New York: McGraw-Hill.

Goodman, C. (2013). *Differential diagnosis for physical therapists: Screening for referral* (5th ed.). St. Louis: W.B. Saunders Company.

LeBlond, R. F., Brown, D. D., Suneja, M., et al. (2014). The chest: Chest wall, pulmonary, and cardiovascular systems; The breasts. In R. F. LeBlond, D. D. Brown, M. Suneja, & J. F. Szot (Eds.), *DeGowin's diagnostic examination* (10th ed.). New York: McGraw-Hill.

Magee, D. J. (2008). *Orthopedic physical assessment* (5th ed.). St. Louis: W.B. Saunders Company.

Memon, A. A., Vohra, L. M., Khaliq, T., et al. (2009). Diagnostic accuracy of Alvarado score in the diagnosis of acute appendicitis. *Pakistan Journal of Medical Sciences, 25*, 118–121.

Meng, M. V., Tanagho, E. A., Maxwell, V., & Emil, A. (2013). Physical examination of the genitourinary tract. In J. W. McAninch & T. F. Lue (Eds.), *Smith and Tanagho's general urology* (18th ed.). New York: McGraw-Hill.

Misurya, R. K., Khare, A., Mallick, A., et al. (1987). Use of tuning fork in diagnostic auscultation of fractures. *Injury, 18*, 63–64.

Penaloza, A., Melto, C., Duchy, E., et al. (2007). Assessment of pretest probability of pulmonary embolism in the emergency department by physicians using the Wells model. *Thrombosis Research, 12*, 173–179.

Sullivan, S., & Williams, R. (1976). Reliability of clinical techniques for detecting splenic enlargement. *British Medical Journal, 2*, 1043–1044.

Tamayo, S. G., Rickman, L. S., Mathews, W. C., et al. (1993). Examiner dependence on physical diagnostic tests for the detection of splenomegaly: A prospective study with multiple observers. *Journal of General Internal Medicine, 8*, 69–75.

Underwood, H. Physiopedia: The Flag System. https://www.physio-pedia.com/index.php?title=The_Flag_System&utm_source=physiopedia&utm_medium=search&utm_campaign=ongoing_internal

Walsh, R.A., O'Rourke, R.A., Shaver, J.A., et al. The history, physical examination, and cardiac auscultation. In V. Fuster, R. A. Walsh, R. A. Harrington, V. Fuster, R. A. Walsh, & R. A. Harrington (Eds.), *Hurst's the heart* (13th ed.). New York: McGraw-Hill.

Wells, P. S., Ginsberg, J. S., Anderson, D. R., et al. (1998). Use of a clinical model for safe management of patients with suspected pulmonary embolism. *Annals of Internal Medicine, 129*, 997–1005.

Wilder, R. P., Vincent, H. K., Stewart, J., et al. (2009). Clinical use of tuning forks to identify running-related stress fractures. *Athletic Training and Sports Health Care, 1*, 12–18.

CHAPTER 22 QUESTIONS

1. **Which of the following tests would be the best predictor to determine whether a patient has appendicitis?**
   a. Iliopsoas muscle test
   b. + McBurney's point
   c. Alvarado's score >6
   d. Heel test

2. **You are evaluating a 34-year-old female for LBP. She reports that in the past 2 days she has been nauseous to the point of vomiting and has had chills. She relates to significant PMH. You take her temperature and note she has a low-grade fever. Which of the following tests would be most indicated, in addition to lumbar ROM and pain assessment?**
   a. Auscultation of bowel sounds
   b. Murphy's sign
   c. Iliopsoas muscle test
   d. Murphy's percussion test

3. **You are evaluating a mildly obese 53-year-old female who was referred to you for evaluation of the thoracic region. She relates she has had intermittent mid-thoracic pain, right greater than left for 3 weeks. She now has acute onset of right upper quadrant pain after a work luncheon celebrating the retirement of a colleague. What special test would be most indicated given this patient's history?**
   a. Murphy's sign
   b. Assessment for splenomegaly
   c. McBurney's point assessment
   d. Percussion of the abdomen

PEDIATRIC ORTHOPAEDIC PHYSICAL THERAPY

E. Ennis, PT, EdD, PCS

CHAPTER 23

1. **List the common developmental milestones.**
   - Rolls prone to supine: 4 months
   - Rolls supine to prone: 6 months
   - Sits alone: 6 to 7 months
   - Creeps/crawls: 9 months
   - Pulls to stand: 9 to 10 months
   - Cruises: 10 months
   - Walks well: 12 to 14 months
   - Climbs up steps with railing, marking time: 2 years
   - Jumps: 2 years
   - Down steps with railing marking time: 3 years
   - Hops: 4 years
   - Skips: 5 years

2. **Describe the normal progression of lower extremity alignment in children.**
   - Newborns: varus knees
   - 18 months: straight knees
   - 2.5 years: valgus knees
   - 4 to 6 years: normal alignment

3. **When do children develop an adult gait pattern?**
   Gait laboratory studies show that the normal pattern of adult gait is established at age 3, although heel strike is seen as early as 18 months. A stable pattern in the adult mode is present by age 7, but stride length continues to increase with increases in height and leg length.

4. **What lower extremity changes normally occur with growth?**
   Femoral anteversion decreases from 30 to 40 degrees at birth to 8 to 15 degrees at maturity, whereas tibial rotation increases from 5 degrees of external rotation to 15 degrees at skeletal maturity.

5. **What are growing pains?**
   Although not well defined, growing pains are nonspecific intermittent pains usually occurring at night but often coming and going. They can be in the quads, calves, or other muscle groups and usually occur during growth spurts. Growing pains were originally named due to the thought that bones grew faster than muscles stretched. However, current theory relates more to the pain being caused by excessive muscle use during the day rather than being related to growth. Growing pains have been more likely to occur in children with lower pain thresholds or hypermobility, but can occur in boys or girls and should be gone in the morning.

6. **Name the standardized tests commonly used in pediatric physical therapy. When are they useful?**

TOOL	AREAS EVALUATED	AGES EVALUATED	TYPE OF TOOL	STRENGTHS
Denver (DDDST II)	Motor, cognitive, language, social, and adaptive	1 week–6.5 years	Screen	Quick and easy to learn
Alberta	Gross Motor	Birth–18 months	Screen	Observational
Peabody (PDMS III)	Gross and fine motor	1–72 months	Evaluation	Allows for emerging skills

Continued

TOOL	AREAS EVALUATED	AGES EVALUATED	TYPE OF TOOL	STRENGTHS
Bayley IV	Motor, cognitive, language, social, and adaptive	1–42 months	Global Developmental Evaluation	Considered gold standard
Movement assessment battery for children (MABC-2)	Motor, dexterity, and balance	3–16 years	Evaluation (screen also available)	Good for evaluation of milder movement disorders
Bruininks-Oseretsky II	Gross and fine motor, bilateral coordination	4–21 years	Evaluation	Tests bilateral coordination and balance
Pediatric evaluation of disability inventory (PEDI) and PEDI-CAT	Functional activities	6 months–7.5 years (functional level; not chronological age)	Evaluation	Assesses functional skills in children with motor and cognitive disabilities
Gross motor function measure (GMFM 66 and 88)	Motor skills	5 months–16 years	Evaluation	Used to document progress in children with CP and Down's syndrome
Test of infant motor performance (TIMP)	Motor skills	32 weeks' gestation–4 months	Evaluation	Standardized tool to evaluate early motor skills in infants; can be used preterm
Miller first step	Motor, cognitive, language, social, and adaptive	2 years 9 months–6 years 2 months	Screen	Identify children at risk

7. **How early can children benefit from using a wheelchair or powered mobility?**
If a child is not going to be ambulatory, or mobility will be significantly delayed, wheeled mobility should be explored early to provide some movement opportunities for the child and allow inclusion in family and community activities. If a child will have the ability to self-propel in the future, he or she should be started with a manual chair and not a stroller-type seating system. For children who will not self-propel, a chair with adequate support and necessary modifications would be appropriate. Some children may need a power chair but not if the home has insufficient space to make it useful. Children as young as 18 months of age can be competent, independent users of powered mobility. One consistent movement, such as an eye blink or wrist twitch, and some amount of cognitive ability are all that is needed for power mobility to be attempted. Current research looking at the link between mobility and cognition indicates that early simple power mobility as young as 6 to 9 months old can assist children with motor delays to improve exploration and increase curiosity and problem solving. For any seating system, consulting with a therapist with specialized skills in seating and mobility is advised.

8. **What is the role of physical therapy for children with torticollis?**
Children with congenital muscular torticollis demonstrate decreased cervical range of motion in rotation to the same side and lateral flexion to the opposite side of the tight sternocleidomastoid muscle (SCM). It will generally be present as a result of in utero positioning, or postdelivery positioning in a reclined position before the development of head control, allowing the head to tip to one side. Cervical restriction patterns other than the aforementioned pattern may suggest other skeletal or neurologic issues and should be referred for further evaluation. Radiologic assessment should be considered if any atypical presentation is noted to rule out other pathologies like Klippel-Feil syndrome. Often, as a result of the head positioning, shortening of the trunk on the same side as the tightness leads to decreased use of the opposite side of the trunk. Prone positioning often results

in hiking of the same side hip with weight shifting away from that side. Treatment for torticollis ranges from aggressive stretching, bracing, and positioning to encouraging active motion and using vision to align the head and body. However, active movement and positioning appear to be the most successful, especially in children with positional torticollis or muscular torticollis. Torticollis with palpable sternomastoid tumor is the most resistant to treatment. Early age at initiation of treatment is also associated with positive results from conservative treatment. The Academy of Pediatric Physical Therapy issued a clinical practice guideline update in 2018 with referral patterns, classification and treatment strategies, and ratings of the evidence on various treatment techniques. The CPG can be found here: https://pediatricapta.org/clinical-practice-guidelines/Congenital-Muscular-Torticollis.cfm

9. **What is deformational plagiocephaly?**

Deformational plagiocephaly is a flattening of the skull, causing asymmetry in alignment of the ears, orbits, or jaw if the flattening is on one side, or elongation of the skull if the flattening is centrally located. It is often accompanied by torticollis, and generally one is the cause of the other. Once evaluation has determined that the change in shape is not caused by premature fusion of the sutures (craniosynostosis), the head shape may benefit from remolding using molding helmets or bands. Helmets or bands are generally worn 23 hours a day, for 3 to 6 months, and are fabricated by orthotists. Referral for the helmet should occur at or before 5 months of age, as the use of a helmet is most effective before 1 year of age. Cranial measurements can be used to assess progress and determine the need for a helmet; often these are done digitally at the orthotist's office. Helmets are an FDA-approved device and must be made by certified professionals. Physical therapy intervention has been shown to be superior to education on positioning and is recommended for children over 7 weeks of age in the clinical practice guideline developed by the American Academy of Neurosurgeons. The Plagiocephaly Severity Scale (PSS) developed by Children's Hospital Atlanta can be used to guide referral and has some positioning recommendations based on age and measurements.

10. **Is developmental dysplasia of the hip (DDH) the same as congenital dislocation of the hip (CDH)?**

Yes. DDH used to be called CDH, but the newer terminology better describes its dynamic nature. DDH refers to a wide spectrum of hip abnormalities, ranging from complete dislocation of the femoral head to mild acetabular abnormality or laxity of the hip. It is more common in females, in children with a family history of the disorder, and in first-born children. Breech births, decreased uterine space, metatarsus adductus, and torticollis are also associated with DDH. Screening done early in the first week of life shows a higher incidence of DDH than screening later in the first week, indicating some level of spontaneous resolution without treatment.

11. **Describe the classic tests used to evaluate DDH.**

- Ortolani sign—the child is supine, and the examiner grasps the flexed thigh with thumbs on the inner thigh and fingers on the greater trochanters. As the hip is abducted and the greater trochanter is elevated, a clunk is felt, indicating that the hip is reduced. This test is less sensitive after 2 months of age; mnemonic: Ortolani's = out to in.
- Barlow's test—begin this test the same as the Ortolani procedure; adduct the flexed hip and gently push the thigh posteriorly, testing for dislocation. This test is also less sensitive after 2 months of age because of muscular development.
- Galeazzi sign or Allis sign—a test of apparent thigh length. The patient lies supine with hips and knees flexed to 90 degrees. In a positive test, one knee is higher than the other, indicative of subluxation/dislocation on that side. The results will not be accurate if bilateral DDH is present.
- Ultrasound is also used to diagnose DDH, but studies have shown no increase in effective diagnosis using ultrasound versus clinical diagnosis.

12. **How is DDH treated?**

Infants with DDH who are under 6 months of age usually are treated with the Pavlik harness. Previous treatments included double or triple diapering, but this has not been shown to be any more effective than no treatment. Treatment for older children varies with age. In children younger than 1.5 years, reduction probably will be attempted (with or without prior traction), and older children usually need open surgical reduction, possibly with proximal femoral shortening and a pelvic osteotomy (such as the Salter's or Pemberton's procedure). Patients who are not corrected in childhood tend to have a high incidence of osteoarthritis and need for surgical intervention later. The American Academy of Orthopedic Surgeons has a clinical practice guideline for infants under 6 months of age to manage with bracing on the web here https://www.aaos.org/pddhcpg; however, altered positioning and its impact on infant development is not addressed in these guidelines and can be addressed through a consult with PT.

13. **What is the role of physical therapy in the treatment of DDH?**

Although the harness is in place, the therapist can be a resource for positioning that fosters development, such as an adapted prone position. Otherwise, the child remains in supine with hips in flexion, external rotation, and abduction, which limit the development of head control and trunk activity. Occasionally, physical therapy will be requested for a child just out of a harness, because of difficulty with prone positioning and active hip extension after prolonged positioning in hip flexion and external rotation. This can limit the development of rolling and transitions in sitting, as well as movement in prone. If an older child is referred, pool therapy or kicking-out exercises in a warm bathtub at home are excellent choices for treatment. Tricycles and bicycles with adjustable seat heights are also helpful for increasing hip range of motion (ROM) and weight bearing. If a child is treated after age 6, the gluteus medius and maximus have worked at a mechanical disadvantage for a long period and the child may walk with an abductor lurch or trunk shift. Such walking habits are hard to break without the use of visual feedback (e.g., walking toward a mirror) but may also be addressed well in an aquatic environment where fear of falling is reduced.

14. **What are the various types and causes of clubfoot?**
   a. Positional—a normal foot that was held in an abnormal position in utero. The bony alignment is normal, and the foot is usually corrected by stretching or a short course of casting.
   b. Teratologic—associated with neurologic disorders such as spina bifida.
   c. Syndromic—associated with an overall genetic syndrome such as arthrogryposis. Both teratologic and syndromic clubfeet almost always require surgery as definitive treatment, although casting does help stretch the soft tissues in preparation for surgery.
   d. Congenital—present with abnormal bony deformity at birth but not associated with any neuromuscular causes or syndromes.

15. **What are the components of a clubfoot (talipes equinovarus)?**
   - Hindfoot varus and equinus
   - Supination/adduction of the forefoot
   - Medial and plantar rotation of the talus

   This can be seen either unilaterally or bilaterally. Usually this is accompanied by altered muscle tone or length, depending on the amount of deformity and age of the child.

16. **How are physical therapists involved in treating children with congenital clubfoot?**
   The best treatment begins as close to birth as possible and consists of repositioning of the foot, either manually or surgically, followed by casting. Forced dorsiflexion by serial casting must be avoided as a rocker-bottom foot may develop. However, splinting in ankle-foot orthosis (AFO), or taping, especially if the infant is in the neonatal intensive care unit with other issues, can be used to gain range of motion and improve positioning. Ponseti's technique of manipulation and casting, followed by Achilles tenotomy, if needed, has shown up to 90% success, reducing the need for surgical correction. After surgery or casting/bracing, the physical therapist may be involved in teaching postoperative exercises to maintain or regain ROM and to regain strength in the muscles of the calf and foot. The French physical therapy method includes surgical lengthening, physical therapy for range of motion and muscle stimulation, and rigid and elastic taping for positioning. Occasionally a combination of methods is needed to address a significant deformity. The Dutch Orthopedic Association published a clinical practice guideline in 2017 (https://www.ncbi.nlm.nih.gov/pmc/articles/PMC5434600/) for children treated within 6 months of birth, mostly detailing medical management. However, there is evidence to show delay in motor skill development related to clubfoot; therefore, therapy is needed to address these delays as well.

17. **What is brachial plexus palsy (BPP) in infants?**
   BPP is the term commonly used to describe injury to the brachial plexus during birth. Larger infants (such as those born to mothers with gestational diabetes) are at greater risk, as are breech and assisted (forceps or vacuum) deliveries. Erb's palsy (C5, C6) or waiter's tip deformity has the best prognosis, followed by Klumpke's palsy (C8–T1); complete plexus palsy has the worst prognosis. Several types of nerve injuries can occur, from traction injuries to rupture of the axon with sheath intact, to complete neuronal rupture, and prognosis will also depend on the type of neuronal injury. Occasionally, a clavicle fracture accompanies the injury and should be ruled out.

18. **How is BPP treated?**
   Approximately 80% to 90% of children recover spontaneously, but there are indicators for a better prognosis. Traction injuries tend to recover over time, whereas avulsion injuries are less responsive. If movement is not regained in the first 4 months, the child should be referred for further evaluation and possible surgical intervention. Initial therapy involvement includes positioning to decrease further stretch on the shoulder and prone-supported weight-bearing activities to stimulate muscle activity. Therapy can also minimize the likelihood of a contracture when the muscles recover to whatever level they can reach. Stimulation of muscle activity can help to diagnose return in an injured nerve and is a very important part of the process. However, return of nerve function can often be accompanied by paresthesias, which can be upsetting to the child and the parents or caregivers. These paresthesias and the pain response that accompanies them should be noted as a typical part of the return of function and worked through with firm touch and deep pressure, as light touch can be noxious.

19. **What actions can be taken to make a baby move its arms to test for BPP?**
   Tactile stimulation along the muscles, stimulation of the grasp reflex, vibration, and sharp/dull testing should produce active movement in innervated muscles. The Moro test (dropping the child backward suddenly in a

controlled fashion) is occasionally seen but can cause additional tension on the shoulder and should generally be avoided. If movement does not return after 1 to 2 weeks, EMGs are often used to determine the extent of injury.

20. **Can physical therapy to reduce spasticity improve function in children with cerebral palsy?**
No scientific evidence indicates that physical therapy can reduce spasticity over the long term. Therapy techniques such as global warmth, deep pressure, and prolonged stretch have been shown to be effective in the short term; however, significant spasticity often needs to be addressed to improve functional independence. Generally, underneath the stiffness caused by the spasticity is a weak muscle. Evidence has shown that therapy to strengthen spastic muscles has a positive effect on strength and does not negatively influence spasticity. Typical growth and development can also cause changes that shorten spastic muscles and can cause loss of function. This can be addressed by physical therapy.

21. **What are some methods of addressing spasticity medically?**
Of the various medical treatments for spasticity reduction, the easiest to use is an oral agent such as diazepam (Valium) or oral baclofen. The dosage needed to cross the blood-brain barrier for effectiveness, however, may make the child sleepy or have other unwanted side effects. Baclofen delivered intrathecally from a battery-powered pump has helped some children who are severely limited by spasticity and tends to have more of an impact on legs than arms. This method allows a much lower dose to be administered, reducing the side effects with orally administered medications. For children with more localized issues, intramuscular injection of botulinum toxin type A (Botox) prevents the presynaptic release of acetylcholine at the nerve-muscle junction. The effects of Botox are short-lived, between 2 and 6 months, but allow for strengthening of antagonists to reduce the influence of the spastic muscle on the child's movement, allowing for improved function.

22. **What is Gowers' sign or maneuver?**
Children with significant proximal hip/pelvic girdle weakness and lack of core strength use Gowers' maneuver to stand up from the floor. The child rolls prone, gets onto the hands and knees, extends the knees, and uses the hands to "walk up" the legs until the erect position is achieved. Gowers' maneuver is not normal. Suspect a muscular dystrophy (most commonly Duchenne's disease in males) and refer the child to the appropriate physician immediately. Another classic sign of Duchenne's is the pseudohypertrophy of the calves.

23. **Define osteochondritis dissecans (OCD).**
OCD is a necrotic bone lesion with no known cause that may affect subchondral bone and adjacent articular cartilage. It is seen most commonly in the knee (in the intercondylar region of the medial femoral condyle). The ankle and elbow are other areas that may be affected. Lesions are staged 1 through 4, with stage 1 being a small area of compression and stage 4 having a displaced loose body. Generally boys are more affected than girls, but the gap is decreasing, as is the age of onset, because of an increase in participation in impact activities and intense sports engagement by both genders. Adult onset is often thought to be an unresolved childhood form but can appear as a new lesion.

24. **What tests are useful for the diagnosis of OCD?**
The Wilson test may be useful to diagnose OCD of the knee. With the knee flexed to 90 degrees, the tibia is rotated medially. The knee is extended passively, and medial tibial rotation is maintained. Pain is detected at about 30 degrees of knee flexion and relieved by lateral tibial rotation. However, there are no studies on the reliability or validity of this test, and it is often negative on an existing lesion. X-rays are also not noted to be useful because of nonspecific results. MRI and MRA tend to have better predictive value, and generally a combination of evaluative techniques is used.

25. **How is OCD treated?**
Activity restriction for 6 weeks to 6 months with nonweight-bearing for 6 weeks is common. Children with open epiphyseal plates tend to respond well to 2 to 3 months of casting, immobilization, or unloader bracing. Isometric exercises are indicated during casting, progressing to active exercise to regain full ROM when the cast is removed, and finally to resisted strength training and return to full activity. If a loose fragment is present or if the subchondral bone is involved, surgery (usually arthroscopic) is indicated. A 2010 clinical practice guideline from the American Academy of Orthopedic Surgeons (https://www.aaos.org/quality/quality-programs/lower-extremity-programs/osteochondritis-dissecans/) has consensus support for surgical intervention, especially in symptomatic patients with unstable lesions, and often it is recommended with stable lesions as well, even in cases of skeletal immaturity, but a lack of consensus on what type of surgical intervention. A recent review of the literature was inconclusive regarding the role of conservative treatment in cases with stable lesions.

26. **What is Osgood-Schlatter disease?**
Osgood-Schlatter disease involves enlargement and microfractures of the apophysis of the tibial tubercle (where the quadriceps inserts) and is commonly seen in young, highly active adolescent males who are going through

a rapid growth spurt. Males are typically affected from ages 13 to 14, whereas girls more often have symptoms from the age of 11 or 12. The tibial tubercle is usually prominent and tender. The pain is worsened by squatting, jumping, or kneeling and often appears in sports that highlight or emphasize these activities. Given the increase in female participation in similar sports, the ratio of boys to girls is decreasing.

27. **How is Osgood-Schlatter disease treated?**
Treatment is directed at relief of symptoms with heat or ice massage, changes in activity, use of knee pads, and administration of antiinflammatory medication. The condition usually resolves once the tibial tubercle apophysis fuses. Although the problem is being treated, flexibility and isometric strengthening exercises for the quadriceps and hamstring muscles may help. Sometimes a separate ossicle (small bone) develops under the patellar tendon and may need to be removed surgically. Splinting is rarely indicated but has been used in situations where the condition does not resolve. Generally, corticosteroid use is contraindicated and surgery should be avoided in cases of skeletal immaturity.

28. **What is Legg-Calvé-Perthes (LCP) disease?**
LCP disease is idiopathic avascular necrosis (probably episodic) of the femoral head. It is seen most often in children aged 4 to 12 and affects boys more often than girls (4:1). The disease is bilateral in approximately 12% of cases. The hip progresses from synovitis to an avascular stage, to fragmentation, to reossification, and finally heals within approximately 18 to 24 months following reossification. The Stulberg classification system has been used to discuss resulting deformities of the femoral head and neck, with corresponding prognoses. Levels I and II tend to resolve well, level II has additional onset of hip symptoms in adulthood, and levels IV and V will often show additional onset of symptoms in their twenties.

29. **How is LCP disease treated?**
Treatment usually consists of maintaining or regaining hip ROM, especially abduction, to keep the deformable involved segment of the femoral head contained within the acetabulum. Generally, surgery is avoided in children under age 8, as they are still investigating the benefits of surgery for this age group. Unweighting using crutches, limiting impact activities, and use of antiinflammatory medications are typically used. Bracing in an abducted and internally rotated position and osteotomy are other options. However, bracing has not been shown to be effective, and some studies show that children over the age of 8 at onset with more significant presentations do better with surgical intervention. After age 11, conventional surgical interventions do not appear to be as effective. The International Perthes Study Group (https://perthesdisease.org/) is currently investigating various factors involved in the treatment of LCP disease, such as surgical versus nonsurgical treatment in children under age 8, effectiveness of weight-bearing versus nonweight-bearing in children 8 to 11, and various surgical interventions for children over the age of 11.

30. **What type of individual is most likely to suffer from a slipped capital femoral epiphysis (SCFE)?**
Obese adolescent males, ages 10 to 16, are most likely to have a "slip" or displacement of the capital (i.e., head or proximal) femoral epiphysis. Incidence in the United States is 10.8 per 100,000, versus 2 per 100,000 globally, and may be bilateral in as many as 60% of cases, although severity is not always symmetric. They present with limping and pain in the distal thigh or knee. Because of this symptom, the diagnosis is often incorrect as a result of isolated evaluation of the knee. The condition is more prevalent in cases of obesity but also has a link to race, with higher incidence in African American males. Bilateral conditions tend to present more in children with endocrine disorders or in those younger than 10 years old. Slips can be acute or chronic, and patients have limited hip ROM, especially internal rotation. Patients with chronic slips may show shortening of the involved leg. Gait can be waddling in nature with a laterally rotated leg.

31. **Describe the treatment for SCFE.**
Generally, once diagnosed, consensus is surgical treatment is necessary. A stable SCFE is generally treated with a single screw pinning, and an unstable SCFE will use reduction, decompression, and internal fixation for successful resolution. In some situations, pinning of the noninvolved hip is considered due to the risk in some children of a bilateral presentation in the future. Postoperative physical therapy involves regaining hip ROM, strengthening the lower extremity, especially the hip abductors, and protected partial weight-bearing with crutches. Partial weight-bearing is suggested (even if minimal) because nonweight-bearing requires the use of hip muscles to maintain the leg in the air and puts more stress on the hip than resting the foot on the floor. Chondrolysis and avascular necrosis (AVN) are potential late complications.

32. **What conditions can affect the young baseball pitcher?**
Repetitive stress may cause epiphysiolysis at the proximal humerus (little league shoulder) or stress the medial epicondyle apophysis (little league elbow). Studies have emerged showing that young pitchers who throw more than 100 innings in a season are at higher risk of shoulder and elbow injuries, although types of pitches do not

seem to correlate with increased injury. The link to mechanics, including trunk rotation and other factors, is also emerging in the literature, and education programs for coaches are increasing in popularity as the prevalence of club sports has skyrocketed in the past 10 years. Thus, the recommendations from American Sports Medicine Institute (ASMI) for preventing injuries in youth baseball pitchers are:

- Watch and respond to signs of fatigue (such as decreased ball velocity, decreased accuracy, upright trunk during pitching, dropped elbow during pitching, or increased time between pitches). If a youth pitcher complains of fatigue or looks fatigued, let him rest from pitching and other throwing.
- Avoid curveball throwing in the young pitcher.
- No overhead throwing of any kind for at least 2 to 3 months per year (4 months is preferred). No competitive baseball pitching for at least 4 months per year.
- Do not pitch more than 100 innings in games in any calendar year.
- Follow limits for pitch counts and days of rest.

ASMI also discourages the use of radar guns and pitching on multiple teams in a season to protect the developing pitcher.

33. What is a pectus excavatum (funnel chest) indicative of in a child?

Pectus excavatum is the most common chest wall deformity in children, occurring in 1 of every 400 newborns with male predominance (male-to-female ratio of 3:1). This is a depression of the sternum, and its etiology is generally unknown, although it is often seen in children with cardiopulmonary or hypermobility issues and can be thought to be caused by atypical bone and cartilage formation in the sternal area. In these children, depression of the sternum is generally related to poor muscle tone and respiratory insufficiency. Overuse of the diaphragm without support from the lower abdomen generates increased negative pressure in the chest cavity; the flexible joint in this complex is the sternocostal area, which gets pulled in. Abdominal support providing compression in the lower trunk to improve the effectiveness of the diaphragm could help to decrease the pectus. Strengthening of core muscles, including the rectus and obliques, provides the same effect without the need for external support. In cases of severe excavatum, surgery may be indicated to reduce compression on the chest cavity. The Nuss procedure is one procedure used to correct the sternal position.

34. What is nursemaid's elbow?

Also referred to as pulled elbow, temper tantrum elbow, or supermarket elbow, nursemaid's elbow is subluxation of the radial head from the annular ligament. The mechanism of injury is usually a traction force on the arm, often seen when children are swung by the hands or an arm is jerked rapidly. This tends to occur in children younger than 6 as the annular ligament thickens and provides more protection as they age. Radiographs showing displacement of 3 mm or more from the capitellum suggest subluxation. Reduction is achieved with supination followed by elbow flexion. Recurrence rates vary from 5% to 39%, depending on the amount of instability at the annular ligament, as this is occasionally torn.

35. How do growth plate injuries in children occur?

Children who have not reached skeletal maturity are at risk for several types of fractures, including avulsions and green stick fractures, secondary to imbalance of muscles from growth or overtraining, or heavy impact use of joints. Growth plate injuries most often occur in lower leg, distal forearm, and fingers and require immediate attention as they can impact further development of the bones. There is also a growing incidence of growth plate injury following ACL repair in the youth with skeletal immaturity. These findings make it critical to educate parents, athletes, and coaches regarding flexibility, balanced use of muscle groups, and risks of overtraining. It also encourages a critical decision-making process for using surgical correction of ACL pathology in the young athlete.

36. What is the occurrence of scoliosis in youth?

Scoliosis, or a lateral curvature of the spine of more than 10 degrees, has various causes that are present at different ages. Infantile scoliosis of idiopathic cause presents in children from birth to 3 years old. Current prevalence literature discusses a rate of 2% to 3% in the adolescent population, where rapid growth and muscle imbalances can be a cause. Neuromuscular scoliosis can present in cases where asymmetric tone is present. Treatment varies between idiopathic causes and neuromuscular causes. In children with idiopathic scoliosis with less than a 25-degree curve, aggressive exercise to address muscle imbalances can help to decrease curvature. Between 25 degrees and 40 degrees, bracing is recommended, but controversy exists over the use of rigid bracing versus dynamic bracing. It should also be noted that bracing does not reverse the curve but halts progression in up to 80% of cases. Greater than 40 degrees, candidates are generally referred for surgical correction. In cases of neurogenic scoliosis, surgical correction may be indicated, but the underlying neurologic cause needs to be addressed as well. Otherwise, pseudoarthrosis above or below the surgical rods may develop. The International Scientific Society on Scoliosis Orthopedic and Rehabilitation Treatment (SOSORT) has updated its clinical practice guidelines as of 2016 and they can be accessed here: https://scoliosisjournal.biomedcentral.com/articles/10.1186/s13013-017-0145-8

37. **What is Sever's disease?**
Also known as calcaneal apophysitis, Sever's disease can appear in children between the ages of 8 and 15 and is characterized by pain in the posterior and inferior region of the heel. It generally appears in children who are either overweight or very active. The literature is inconclusive regarding effectiveness of treatment, but strategies vary from relative rest, to heel cups, to over-the-counter insert orthotics and taping. Shoe changes may be necessary to control this condition. Stretching of the lower limbs (all muscle groups—easy on gastroc and soleus) can help to unload the insertion of the gastroc.

38. **What is Blount's disease (tibia varum)?**
Blount's disease is diagnosed as early onset or late onset, depending on age of presentation (before or after the age of 4). It is generally diagnosed in children who have had excessive early weight-bearing, are obese, or have metabolic disorders. Some studies indicate a higher incidence in children of African American descent or in females; there is a difference in early versus late-onset presentation. Late-onset groups have more of a distal femoral component, and early-onset groups show more proximal tibial varus and internal rotation. Treatment generally involves observation with alignment correction, if needed, bracing, if needed, and surgical intervention as a last resort. However, some information shows improved outcomes if surgical correction of severe Blount's is used before age 4.

39. **What is metatarsus adductus?**
Metatarsus adductus is one of the most common foot abnormalities in young children, with an incidence of 1 to 2 per 1000, with a coincidence of hip dysplasia in 10% of children. Generally, this is a flexible deformity that resolves but needs to be monitored as persistent presentation can cause concerns with regard to gait. There is some evidence of benefit to stretching, taping, and shoe modification depending on the cause and presentation.

40. **What is flexible pes planus?**
Pes planus presents in approximately 14% of the population and is usually flexible. In a nonweight-bearing position the foot presents as if it has a normal arch. However, in a weight-bearing position the foot appears flat, and if the child is asked to rise up on his or her toes, an arch is noted. Parents and grandparents worry that the child has flat feet and want to get rigid shoes. Generally, a normal arch will develop later in childhood, and asymptomatic presentations do not need treatment. If symptoms are present (i.e., pain, difficulty with gait and balance) consider an arch support or supportive shoe to decrease the medial collapse. However, going above the ankle changes gait mechanics and should be avoided if possible.

41. **What are two common causes of rigid pes planus?**
    - Vertical talus (convex pes valgus)—a rare condition for which the exact cause is unknown; however, it is commonly associated with neuromuscular disease in children (usually with atypical tone or connective tissue disorders). It presents as a rocker bottom foot, and nonsurgical interventions such as casting, bracing, stretching, and exercise are viable options. However, most cases require surgical correction of the deformity.
    - Tarsal coalition (peroneal spastic flatfoot)—very rare and is an atypical fusion of the calcaneus to either the navicular or the talus. Although tarsal coalition is often present at birth, children typically do not show signs of the disorder until early adolescence. The foot may become stiff and painful, and in some cases the individual may report recurrent episodes of ankle sprains. If nonsurgical approaches such as rest, orthotics, casts, and injections do not relieve the patient's symptoms, then surgery is required to release the fusion.

42. **Are orthotics useful for the correction of foot/gait deviations in children?**
As children learn to walk, their foot position changes as a result of movement exploration that encourages strengthening in the muscles of the foot. For example, standing at furniture and rotating causes a supination moment in the same side foot, helping to strengthen the muscles of the medial arch. In general, putting shoes on children learning to walk alters gait mechanics and shifts the use of muscles from the foot to the hip and knee, increasing stance phase time. Therefore, a general recommendation is to allow children learning to walk to do so without shoes. Still, some children continue to demonstrate excessive pronation, leading to external rotation of the feet to increase the base of support. For these children, continuing to walk with feet in this position could lengthen the medial structures, causing further damage not only to soft tissue but to bony development. There is support for orthotics, using the minimal amount needed to achieve correction, in these cases. Too much support will alter mechanics, but minimal support may allow correction with minimal changes to mechanics and prevent further damage.

43. **What are the considerations for prosthetic use in children with limb deformities or amputation?**
Historically, children with lower extremity limb deficiencies were provided with prosthetics once they were of age to be up and walking and, generally, were given a locked knee prosthetic until age 4 to 5. However, current trends encourage early use of a prosthetic for the lower extremity with a functional knee, even during crawling and pulling to stand phases. Less compensatory strategies are noted in these children, leading to fewer deviations

as mobility improves. Initiation of upper extremity prosthetic use will vary depending on the function of the residual limb. Children are encouraged to use both hands as early as 6 months old, and delays in development, cognition, and exploration can occur. If minimal function is available in the residual upper extremity, prosthetic use should begin early, with modifications as needed. In a recently printed guideline in the Journal of the Pediatric Orthopaedic Society of North America, recommendations include use of upper extremity prostheses when sitting balance has been achieved and lower extremity prostheses when pulling to stand is emerging.

44. What is arthrogryposis multiplex congenita (AMC)?

AMC is a descriptive diagnosis that covers multiple disorders of multiple nonprogressive contractures that are present at birth, in specific upper and lower extremity patterns. This disorder occurs in 1 of every 3000 to 6000 live births, and there is evidence of anterior horn cell involvement as well as fetal akinesis. Generally, there are neurogenic, myogenic, and/or periarticular factors involved in the various diagnoses. Usually there is no effect on cognition, but the contractures in multiple joints are significant and can sway function dramatically. Therefore, early multidisciplinary intervention is indicated to reduce contracture, improve joint integrity, address mobility, and provide adaptive equipment as needed. This support will help to improve the participation of the child in daily routines and community activities. An update on diagnosis and treatment was published in the *Archives of Medical Science* (https://www.ncbi.nlm.nih.gov/pmc/articles/PMC4754365/) in 2016.

45. What is osteogenesis imperfecta (OI)?

OI is a genetic condition that affects bone and connective tissue, resulting in extreme fragility of bones in 1 of every 10,000 individuals. There are five groups, each with multiple types, related to number, location, and type of fracture, which can occur with or without impact, as well as inheritance pattern. An update published in *Frontiers in Endocrinology* in 2020 details the various advances in medical and surgical management. Therapists need to balance therapy to address these concerns with the risk of fracture and the consequences. However, use of aquatic therapy for strengthening in an unweighted environment can be beneficial.

BIBLIOGRAPHY

American Academy of Neurological Surgeons. Scoliosis. https://www.aans.org/en/Patients/Neurosurgical-Conditions-and-Treatments/Scoliosis. Accessed September 30, 2021.

American Academy of Orthopaedic Surgeons. (2014). Detection and nonoperative management of pediatric developmental dysplasia of the hip in infants up to six months of age. https://www.aaos.org/globalassets/quality-and-practice-resources/pddh/pediatric-developmental-dysplasia-hip-clinical-practice-guideline-4-23-19.pdf

American Academy of Orthopaedic Surgeons. (2010). Evidence-based clinical practice guideline of the diagnosis and treatment of osteochondritis dissecans. https://www.aaos.org/globalassets/quality-and-practice-resources/osteochondritis-dissecans/osteochondritis-dissecan-clinical-practice-guideline.pdf

American Sports Medicine, Institute. (2013). Position Statement for Adolescent Baseball Players. https://asmi.org/position-statement-for-adolescent-baseball-pitchers/.

Aprato, A., Conti, A., Bertolo, F., & Massè, A. (2019). Slipped capital femoral epiphysis: Current management strategies. *Orthopedic Research and Reviews, 11*, 47–54.

Besselaar, A. T., Sakkers, R. J. B., Schuppers, H. A., et al. (2017). Guideline on the diagnosis and treatment of primary idiopathic clubfoot. *Acta Orthopaedica, 88*(3), 305–309.

Caine, D., Purcell, L., & Maffulli, N. (2014). The child and adolescent athlete: A review of three potentially serious injuries. *BMC Sports Science, Medicine and Rehabilitation, 6*(1), 22.

Carr, J. B., 2nd, Yang, S., & Lather, L. A. (2016). Pediatric pes planus: A state-of-the-art review. *Pediatrics, 137*(3), e20151230.

Dalal, A., Pimentel-Tejeda, A., & Kim, A. (2011). Literature review of metatarsus adductus in children. *NYCPM, 20*, 24–29.

DiFiori, J. P. (2010). Evaluation of overuse injuries in children and adolescents. *Current Sports Medicine Reports, 9*(6), 372–378.

Dimeglio, A., & Canavese, F. (2012). The French functional physical therapy method for the treatment of congenital clubfoot. *Journal of Pediatric Orthopaedics B, 21*(1), 28–39.

Effgen, S. K. (2013). *Meeting the physical therapy needs of children* (2nd ed.). Philadelphia: FA Davis.

Garcia, N. L., McMulkin, M. L., Tompkins, B. J., Caskey, P. M., Mader, S. L., & Baird, G. O. (2011). Gross motor development in babies with treated idiopathic clubfoot. *Pediatric Physical Therapy, 23*(4), 347–352.

Hall, M., Cummings, D. R., Welling, I. E., Jr., et al. (2020). Essentials of pediatric prosthetics. *Journal of Pediatric Orthopedic Society of North America, 2*(3), 1–15.

James, A. M., Williams, C. M., & Haines, T. P. (2012). Effectiveness of interventions in reducing pain and maintaining physical activity in children and adolescents with calcaneal apophysitis (Sever's disease): A systematic review. *Journal of Foot and Ankle Research, 6*(1), 1–13.

Joseph, B. (2015). Management of Perthes' disease. *Indian Journal of Orthopaedics, 49*(1), 10–16.

Janoyer, M. (2019). Blount disease. *Orthopaedics & Traumatology: Surgery & Research, 105*(1S), S111–S121.

Kepler, C. K., Bogner, E. A., Hammoud, S., Malcolmson, G., Potter, H. G., & Green, D. W. (2011). Zone of injury of the medial patellofemoral ligament after acute patellar dislocation in children and adolescents. *American Journal of Sports Medicine, 39*(7), 1444–1449.

Kowalczyk, B., & Feluś, J. (2016). Arthrogryposis: An update on clinical aspects, etiology, and treatment strategies. *Archives of Medical Science, 12*(1), 10–24.

Maffulli, N., Longo, U. G., Gougoulias, N., Loppini, M., & Denaro, V. (2010a). Long-term health outcomes of youth sports injuries. *British Journal of Sports Medicine, 44*(1), 21–25.

Maffulli, N., Longo, U. G., Spiezia, F., & Denaro, V. (2010b). Sports injuries in young athletes: Long-term outcome and prevention strategies. *The Physician and Sportsmedicine, 38*(2), 29–34.

Mirtz, T. A., Chandler, J. P., & Eyers, C. M. (2011). The effects of physical activity on the epiphyseal growth plates: A review of the literature on normal physiology and clinical implications. *Journal of Clinical Medicine Research, 3*(1), 1.
Negrini, S., Donzelli, S., Aulisa, A. G., et al. (2018). 2016 SOSORT guidelines: Orthopaedic and rehabilitation treatment of idiopathic scoliosis during growth. *Scoliosis and Spinal Disorders, 13,* 3.
Palisano, R., Orlin, M., & Schreiber, J. (2018). *Campbell's physical therapy for children* (5th ed.). St. Louis, MO: Elsevier.
Paterno, M. V., Prokop, T. R., & Schmitt, L. C. (2014). Physical therapy management of patients with osteochondritis dissecans: A comprehensive review. *Clinics in Sports Medicine, 33*(2), 353–374.
Pathirana, S., Champion, D., Jaaniste, T., Yee, A., & Chapman, C. (2011). Somatosensory test responses in children with growing pains. *Journal of Pain Research, 4,* 393.
Ralston, S. H., & Gaston, M. S. (2020). Management of osteogenesis imperfecta. *Frontiers in Endocrinology, 10,* 924.
Rome, K., Ashford, R. L., & Evans, A. M. (2010). Non-surgical interventions for paediatric pes planus. *Cochrane Database of Systematic Reviews, 7,* CD006311.
Ross, C. G., & Shore, S. (2011). The effect of gross motor therapy and orthotic intervention in children with hypotonia and flexible flatfeet. *Journal of Prosthetics and Orthotics, 23*(3), 149–154.
Sabharwal, S. (2015). Blount disease: An update. *Orthopedic Clinics of North America, 46*(1), 37–47.
Siebenrock, K. A., Behning, A., Mamisch, T. C., & Schwab, J. M. (2013). Growth plate alteration precedes cam-type deformity in elite basketball players. *Clinical Orthopaedics and Related Research, 471*(4), 1084–1091.
Smith, J. M., & Varacallo, M. (2023). Sever disease: In: StatPearls [Internet]. Treasure Island (FL): StatPearls Publishing.
Wegener, C., Hunt, A. E., Vanwanseele, B., Burns, J., & Smith, R. M. (2011). Effect of children's shoes on gait: A systematic review and meta-analysis. *Journal of Foot and Ankle Research, 4,* 3.
Whitmore, A. (2013). Osgood-Schlatter disease. *Journal of the American Academy of Physician Assistants, 26*(10), 51–52.
Yang, J. S., Bogunovic, L., & Wright, R. W. (2014). Nonoperative treatment of osteochondritis dissecans of the knee. *Clinics in Sports Medicine, 33*(2), 295–304.
Yoo, W. J., Kocher, M. S., & Micheli, L. J. (2011). Growth plate disturbance after transphyseal reconstruction of the anterior cruciate ligament in skeletally immature adolescent patients: An MR imaging study. *Journal of Pediatric Orthopaedics, 31*(6), 691–696.

CHAPTER 23 QUESTIONS

1. Which of the following interventions will BEST benefit a child born with a vertical talus and rigid pes planus?
   a. Corrective shoe wear
   b. Joint mobilizations
   c. Corrective surgery
   d. Orthotics

2. You are evaluating a 5-year-old for a right lower extremity concern that requires her to remain nonweight-bearing. You notice that she is fairly impulsive and easily distracted. Upon evaluation, you notice some mild coordination issues. What would be the appropriate assistive device to request for this child?
   a. Lofstrand crutches
   b. Axillary crutches
   c. Walker
   d. Wheelchair

3. You receive a referral for a 3-month-old infant and notice that he has a head tilt to the left with some right rotation. His head shape is symmetrical, but he has some muscle tightness on the left side of his neck and difficulty holding his head in midline. You feel this child has:
   a. Typical torticollis and would benefit from treatment
   b. Atypical torticollis and would benefit from radiological evaluation
   c. Plagiocephaly and would benefit from referral for orthosis
   d. Hypotonia and would benefit from referral to neurology

4. You are evaluating an 8-year-old boy with some clumsiness and poor trunk control. During evaluation, you note that he stands up by walking his hands up his legs. Your first thought regarding diagnosis should be:
   a. Cerebral palsy
   b. Osgood-Schlatter disease
   c. Slipped capita femoral epiphysis
   d. Duchenne's muscular dystrophy

5. All of the following affect boys more than girls except:
   a. Osteochondritis dissecans
   b. Legg-Calvé-Perthes
   c. Slipped capita femoral epiphysis
   d. Nursemaid's elbow

PELVIC HEALTH PHYSICAL THERAPY

P.M. King, PT, PhD, FAAOMPT and M.L. Bowman, PT, DPT, WCS

ANATOMY AND PHYSIOLOGY

1. **Describe the anatomical structure of the pelvic floor muscles.**
   The pelvic floor refers to the pelvic diaphragm, which arises from the posterior superior pubic rami, inner ischial spines, and obturator fascia. The fibers of the pelvic diaphragm insert around the vaginal and rectal openings at the perineal body. Pelvic floor muscle refers to the levator ani, which is comprised of three separate muscles: iliococcygeus, pubococcygeus, and the puborectalis. A fourth muscle known as the coccygeus is also part of the pelvic floor but is not considered one of the muscles that make up the levator ani. The pelvic floor creates a sling support for the internal organs and openings for the urethra, vagina, and anus.

2. **What are the anatomical connections of the pelvic floor muscles with the sacroiliac joints and hips?**
   The pelvic floor muscles have bony attachments along the pubic rami, ischium, sacrum, and coccyx. The iliococcygeus, which is the most lateral of the levator ani muscles, has a fascial attachment to the obturator internus.

3. **Describe the functional relationships of the pelvic floor muscles (PFM).**
   The pelvic floor muscles close off the bony inlet of the pelvis, support the contents of the pelvic cavity, and provide compressive forces to prevent incontinence. The muscles also relax to allow for evacuation of the bowel and voiding urine. The PFM assists in the stability of the spine and is often referred to in clinical practice as "the floor of the core." The PFM function synergistically with the abdominal muscles to alternately support and relax the abdomen and the floor of the pelvis.

4. **Describe the primary sources of innervation, motor and sensory, for the pelvic floor area.**
   The pudendal nerve that originates from S2-4 provides motor innervation to the PFM and the external anal sphincter and sensory innervation to the external genitalia. Sensory innervation to the pelvic floor is also provided via the ilioinguinal, iliohypogastric, and genitofemoral nerves.

   The iliohypogastric and ilioinguinal nerves arise from the anterior/ventral ramus of the L1 spinal nerve root. The iliohypogastric nerve supplies both motor and sensory innervation to the abdominal muscles, as well as sensory innervation to the skin of the posterolateral gluteal and suprapubic regions.

   The ilioinguinal nerve provides sensory innervation to the skin of the upper and medial part of the thigh and emerges as the anterior scrotal nerve in males and the anterior labial nerve in females. In males the ilioinguinal nerves serve the skin at the root of the penis and upper part of the scrotum. In females they serve the skin covering the external genitalia, specifically the mons pubis and the labia majora.

   The genitofemoral nerve originates from L 1-2 concluding as two branches, the genital and femoral. In males the genital branch supplies the cremaster and scrotal skin. In females, the genital branch innervates the skin of the mons pons and labia majora. The femoral branch innervates skin of the anterior and medial side of the thigh including the femoral triangle. Iliohypogastric, ilioinguinal, and genitofemoral nerves all have anatomical proximity to the iliopsoas and abdominal muscles along their routes, creating opportunities for entrapment or irritation with changes in muscle tone, length, and function.

   The lateral femoral cutaneous nerve, which derives from L2-3 nerve roots, supplies sensory innervation to the lateral thigh. Although not technically a part of the pelvic floor, the hip and lateral thigh are associated functionally with the pelvis, hip, and abdomen and may contribute to symptoms and functional changes in the area.

5. **What is the fast twitch/slow twitch fibers make-up of the pelvic floor musculature?**
   The levator ani is comprised of approximately 70% fast-twitch fibers and 30% slow-twitch fibers. There is an increased density of fast-twitch (type II) fibers distributed in the periurethral and perianal areas.

PELVIC HEALTH CONDITIONS AND DIFFERENTIAL DIAGNOSIS

6. **List some examples of pelvic health conditions and/or wellness needs that can be managed at least in part by orthopaedic physical therapy.**
   Pregnancy-related low back pain; preparation for labor and delivery; postpartum rehabilitation; diastasis recti; postprostatectomy rehabilitation; incontinence (urinary and fecal); pelvic organ prolapse; pelvic pain (includes a

variety of complaints and diagnoses); painful menstruation; irritable bowel syndrome; constipation; pelvic hernias; and sexual dysfunction.

7. **Are there pelvic health issues throughout the lifespan appropriate for physical therapy management?**
Yes. Incontinence is often an issue in childhood. Painful conditions and abnormalities of menstruation may begin in childhood and/or adolescence and extend throughout much of the lifespan. Sexual abuse and assault are a strong correlate of pelvic pain that afflicts many in childhood, adolescence, adulthood, and late life. Incontinence often appears after childbearing, thus being an issue for young and mid-life females. Changes that occur in menopause increase risk for pelvic pain, incontinence, and pelvic organ prolapse for older females. In particular, older females are at risk for painful sexual intercourse (dyspareunia) and bleeding with intercourse associated with vaginal tissue thinning. Risk for incontinence, both fecal and urinary, increases with aging in both males and females. Prostate function changes with aging for males and simultaneously the effects of aging on musculoskeletal tissues reduce the support provided to the pelvic organs by the pelvic floor. Prostate surgeries and related interventions often present opportunities for physical therapy interventions for pelvic health for men as they age. Sexual dysfunction for males and females may occur throughout the lifespan and be associated with musculoskeletal impairments and functional changes in the pelvis, hips, and spine.

8. **Are pelvic health issues predominately issues of concern for females?**
Pelvic health issues can affect individuals of any sex or gender, but they are more commonly associated with females due to the unique anatomical structures and reproductive organs that females have. However, it's important to recognize that pelvic health issues can impact anyone with a pelvis, regardless of their biological sex or gender identity.
Some common pelvic health issues that can affect individuals of any sex or gender include Incontinence (Urinary or Fecal), Pelvic Pain, Pelvic Organ Prolapse, Sexual Dysfunction, Bowel Issues, Pelvic Floor Dysfunction. It is important to remember to approach pelvic health issues with sensitivity and respect for an individual's gender identity and specific health needs. Additionally, some individuals may require specialized care related to gender-affirming surgeries or hormone therapy, which can impact pelvic health in unique ways. Therefore, pelvic health is a concern for all individuals and tailored to each person's specific needs.

9. **What is meralgia paresthetica and how does physical therapy contribute to management of the condition?**
Meralgia paresthetica refers to a sensory mononeuropathy of the lateral femoral cutaneous nerve as it exits the pelvis and enters the lower extremity. Entrapment likely occurs as the nerve passes around the anterior superior iliac spine or through the inguinal ligament. This condition often occurs during pregnancy as a result of mechanical changes related to increased intraabdominal pressure; the occurrence of meralgia paresthetica can also be related to increased lumbar lordosis or can occur after delivery from prolonged positioning in the lithotomy position during delivery. Symptoms typically include anesthesia, paresthesia, or allodynia on the anterolateral thigh that may be exacerbated by prolonged standing but may also be aggravated by sitting. Deep palpation along the inguinal ligament may reproduce these symptoms. Unique to this condition is an absence of motor deficits.
Physical therapy intervention for meralgia paresthetica may include nerve sliding and flossing, and soft tissue techniques to release and relax medial and anterior thigh soft tissue are utilized to address factors contributing to lateral femoral cutaneous nerve entrapment. Treatment of pelvic and sacroiliac (SI) dysfunction, abdominal stabilization exercises, and transverse abdominus training can also decrease pain and improve function. Modification of activities of daily living, including avoiding exacerbating activities such as prolonged standing or restrictive clothing, or belts that may contribute to symptoms, is also warranted. Abdominal support that lifts the gravid abdomen off the inguinal area can often relieve symptoms.

PELVIC PAIN

10. **How is "pelvic pain" defined in pelvic health practice?**
In orthopaedic physical therapy practice "pelvic pain" is usually associated with sacroiliac related pain, which is primarily located in the posterior pelvis. In pelvic health practice, pelvic pain refers to pain occurring predominantly in the abdomen, usually in the lower abdomen, and often extended to or primarily located in the external genitalia and/or pelvic floor. Pelvic pain may be acute or chronic, with chronic pelvic pain (CPP) diagnosed after 6 months of unresolved symptoms. Pelvic pain in females is often comorbid with low back pain; however, pelvic pain may not be reported during the physical therapy intake unless patients are specifically asked about the condition or related symptom as a part of the history and interview. The differing pain locations, and the tendency to interpret abdominal pain as visceral or reproductive, often preclude patients from making connections between the two types of pain and instead report perceived "female" problems as relevant comorbidities when seeking physical therapy care for low back pain.

11. **What body systems commonly contribute to pelvic pain?**
The urologic, genitourinary, gastrointestinal, musculoskeletal, and reproductive systems all may contribute to symptoms of pelvic pain. Due to their shared patterns of innervation, referred pain complicates symptom investigation and diagnosis. Knowledge of signs and symptoms associated with each of these systems is important in the differential diagnosis process. Multisystems are often involved, particularly in cases of chronic pelvic pain. The tissues and organs of the reproductive, urogenital, gastrointestinal, and musculoskeletal systems associated with pelvic pain are all innervated by the same spinal nerve roots, principally the thoracic and sacral spinal levels as well as from the same autonomic nerve plexuses, which complicates the clinical interpretation of pain patterns. Through the process of neurophysiologic convergence, signals from each separate body system involved in pelvic pain can alter function and pain perception in tissues and structures in the other systems. The neurophysiologic connections between these key systems involved in pelvic pain limit the efficacy of treatment approaches that narrowly examine one body system. Fragmented, specialty, or system-specific approaches to pelvic pain may contribute to lengthy periods of care seeking and are thought to contribute in many cases to the development of chronic pelvic pain.

12. **Name conditions of the urologic, genitourinary, gastrointestinal, musculoskeletal, and reproductive systems commonly associated with pelvic pain.**
Reproductive: dyspareunia, pelvic inflammatory disease (PID), endometriosis, dysmenorrhea, uterine fibroids, pelvic organ prolapse
Gastrointestinal: irritable bowel, constipation, incontinence (fecal), hemorrhoids, rectocele, bowel obstructions, bowel adhesions
Urologic: urinary tract infections (UTI), cystocele, interstitial cystitis (IC)
Genitourinary: vulvodynia, vulvar vestibulitis
Musculoskeletal: pelvic hernias, diastasis recti, pelvic floor muscle tension, PFM trigger points, abdominal trigger points, PFM weakness, core muscle weakness

13. **Does pelvic pain occur in both males and females?**
Yes. The prevalence rate of pelvic pain for females worldwide is 26% and 15% for males. The actual prevalence is likely much higher than reported in prevalence studies in both females and males. Pelvic pain is thought to be generally underreported due to the sensitive nature of the anatomical location of the pain and its frequent association with sexual dysfunction and problems with bowel and bladder function, which people may be hesitant to report on surveys or even discuss with health care practitioners.

14. **Does the etiology of pelvic pain differ between males and females?**
Pelvic pain is generally assumed to be associated with the reproductive or urogenital systems by both practitioners and both males and females experiencing it. Unless the symptoms are strongly associated with bladder function, most females first seek health care from gynecologists or other specialists in reproductive health. Prostatitis is often assumed to be the primary etiology of male pelvic pain; however, reports indicate pelvic pain in men is directly related to actual prostatitis in as few as 5% of cases. Faulty diagnosis of prostatitis has occurred in up to 95% of cases, in part due to lack of lab studies to support the presence of infection or inflammation. Prostatitis and/or postprostatectomy are, however, two of the most common reasons males are referred to physical therapy for pelvic health treatments. Male pelvic pain is strongly associated with physical injuries related to sports and occupation with pudendal neuralgia apparently responsible for many cases of male pelvic pain initially assumed to be prostate related. Pudendal neuralgia is also common in females. Pudendal neuralgia may occur because of injury during vaginal births with recovery from the injury usually occurring within 3 months.

15. **Do the location, signs, and symptoms of pelvic pain vary between males and females?**
Pain location is essentially the same, with the lower abdomen, rectum, bladder, reproductive organs, and genitalia being the affected areas. Few differences in pain severity or type are explained by gender or sex. Both males and females may experience impaired sexual function, with erectile dysfunction and ejaculation disorders being primary complaints among males and both superficial (entrance) and deep dyspareunia being associated with pelvic pain in females. Sexual violence and abuse is a strong correlate of pelvic pain for males and females. Studies find there is variance in the location, type, and functional changes associated with pelvic pain between male and female victims of sexual violence and/or abuse with males more likely to develop gastrointestinal conditions and females more likely to report genital, sexual, and reproductive issues.

16. **What are common temporal patterns associated with complaints of pelvic pain?**
Pelvic pain may be acute (lasting 1 month or less), recurrent (reoccurring in some type of pattern), or chronic or persistent (lasting 3 months or more by some definitions and 6 months or more by others). Recurrent pelvic pain may be either cyclic, as in the case of painful menstrual periods (dysmenorrhea), or episodic, as in the case of pain associated with sexual intercourse (dyspareunia).

17. **What are the most common musculoskeletal impairments and conditions that contribute to pelvic pain?**
Weakness and length tension issues of the core muscles, including the pelvic floor, are the most common musculoskeletal impairment associated with pelvic pain. Associated with muscle weakness and imbalance of the core, physical therapists report impairments in joint and soft tissue mobility in the hips and spine. Abdominal and pelvic hernias, myofascial trigger points; pelvic floor muscle tension; pelvic floor muscle wasting, pelvic floor muscle strain; peripheral nerve entrapments, sacroiliac dysfunction, hip stiffness, levator ani syndrome; and coccydynia are all reported correlates of pelvic pain. Dysfunctional breathing patterns are also common among individuals with pelvic pain and instruction in diaphragmatic breathing in conjunction with core and pelvic muscle training is often a key aspect of the musculoskeletal therapeutic exercise plan utilized to address pelvic pain. A typical pattern of faulty posture associated with chronic pelvic pain has been successfully utilized in physical therapy to address musculoskeletal factors contributing to abdominal and pelvic floor pain.

18. a. **How are mental health, violence, and abuse associated with pelvic pain?**
Women with chronic or persistent pelvic pain are much more likely than other women to have been exposed to violence or abuse (physical or sexual and particularly childhood sexual abuse), to have a history of sexually transmitted diseases, and to be diagnosed with depression and/or anxiety, including posttraumatic stress syndrome.

    b. **How does the correlation of violence, abuse, depression, and anxiety with pelvic pain impact physical therapy examination and treatment?**
Because of the strong correlation between violence, abuse, depression, and anxiety with pelvic pain, it's important for physical therapists to always include screening questions in the examination. If screening reveals these comorbidities, referrals to colleagues in mental health or other psychosocial services may be appropriate and facilitate achievement of best outcomes to care. Modifications to the physical therapy intervention may also be appropriate to accommodate related issues such as touch sensitivity and issues with energy, endurance, trust, and concentration.

19. **An orthopedic physical therapist is seeing a postmenopausal female patient who is complaining of lower back pain that is worse later in the day after she has been standing for long periods of time. The medical history includes a hysterectomy 5 years ago. Why is it important for the physical therapist to screen this patient for pelvic floor muscle dysfunction?**
Low back pain after prolonged standing is a common symptom of pelvic organ prolapse. Identification of this significant condition will indicate either the inclusion intervention to address PFM weakness and/or referrals to other health professionals. In addition, the pelvic floor contributes to the stability of the spine and functions as part of the core. The assessment of pelvic floor muscle function and performance is key to the development of a comprehensive exercise program to improve the function and stability of the spine and trunk.

20. **Why is back pain common in pregnancy?**
The biomechanical changes in posture and the center of gravity that occur during pregnancy stress the spine, pelvis, and hips. The hormones relaxin and progesterone relax muscles and loosen ligaments and joints, especially in the pelvic area, which combined with the extra weight and body changes in pregnancy all contribute to the development of back pain that usually worsens as the pregnancy progresses.

PREGNANCY

21. **If a pregnant woman is referred to physical therapy for adhesive capsulitis, is it important to address her blood pressure as a part of the physical therapy examination and ongoing treatment?**
Blood pressure should be routinely monitored in pregnant patients at the first visit and at each subsequent visit if there is a history of preexisting hypertension. Blood pressure should also be monitored if there is a sudden increase in edema, persistent headache, or if the patient expresses concern about her blood pressure. Blood pressure should also be monitored when beginning any new aerobic exercise routine.

22. **How does blood pressure change over the course of pregnancy?**
Women who are pregnant may have a slightly elevated blood pressure in the first and third trimesters and often have a normal drop in blood pressure during the second trimester. All medical decisions and diagnoses are made based on the relative change from baseline at the beginning of pregnancy. Any change in pressure greater than 15 mmHg is significant and should result in the patient's immediate referral to her obstetric provider.

23. **Is a blood pressure of 142/84 at the initial evaluation a concern if the woman is 10 weeks pregnant?**
Women who are pregnant may have a slightly elevated blood pressure in the first and third trimesters (10 weeks is within the 1st trimester). 142/84 is not a significant concern unless it is a variation of 15 mmHg from the baseline at the beginning of pregnancy.

24. **Does body position impact blood pressure in pregnant women?**
Yes, blood pressure readings during the second and third trimesters may be higher in sitting due to increased weight on the vena cava from the enlarged uterus. Blood pressure readings may be reduced in left side lying as this diminishes the weight on the vena cava. Checking the blood pressure with the patient in left side lying after the first trimester will provide the most accurate reading.

25. **What position ought to be avoided by pregnant females during exercises and why?**
After the first trimester, supine and hook lying positions ought to be avoided for both exercise and for prolonged periods of rest. After the first trimester, cardiac output is reduced by 25% to 30% when lying supine and 10% to 15% in sitting due to positional changes of the enlarged uterus. The patient may experience supine hypotension, which is also known as inferior vena cava syndrome. Symptoms are experienced in up to 11% of pregnant women and include dizziness and light-headedness that may occur as a result of changes in heart rate, mean arterial pressure, and cardiac output.

26. **What is the best position to minimize and/or prevent symptoms of inferior vena cava syndrome (supine hypotension)?**
The left lateral recumbent position has been shown to allow maximum blood flow. If supine position is necessary for clinical examination, minimized time in that position to 3 to 4 minutes is recommended.

27. **A patient who is 8 weeks postpartum is working with an orthopedic physical therapist to determine the best exercise routine to minimize her chronic low back pain as she returns to her prepregnancy fitness level. The therapist notices a dome-shaped bulge in the abdomen just above the umbilicus when performing muscle testing of trunk flexion.**

   a. **What is the most probable cause of this bulge?**
   The patient has a condition known as diastasis recti abdominis (DRA). DRA is a separation of the fascial midline connection of the right and left rectus abdominis muscle bellies at the linea alba. It often occurs in pregnancy due to the mechanical stress of the enlarging uterus and weakening of connective tissue from hormonal influences. It may also occur during labor and delivery. It is not a tear but a separation and is most common at or above the umbilicus although it can occur below. DRA gradually decreases after delivery but often does not return to normal and remains significant in 39% of those affected for many years after delivery.

   b. **How can the therapist objectively measure the DRA?**
   DRA can be measured clinically with palpation above, below, and at the level of the umbilicus. It can also be measured using a tape measure or caliper technique. The gold standard for measuring DRA is ultrasound imaging. When using palpation to assess DRA, the patient is positioned in hook lying and asked to perform a head lift while the clinician palpates along the midline 2.5 to 4.5 cm above the superior border of the umbilicus, 2.5 to 4.5 below the inferior border of the umbilicus, and at the umbilicus. Separation is measured by the number of finger widths filling the separation and is considered significant if greater than two finger widths.

   c. **Are there musculoskeletal or other implications of the DRA the therapist should consider?**
   DRA decreases abdominal muscle function and can contribute to abdominal, pelvic girdle, and low back pain. It may negatively affect load transfer of the pelvic girdle, further contributing to low back and pelvic girdle pain during pregnancy and postpartum. It may also be a contributing factor in urinary incontinence, fecal incontinence, pelvic organ prolapse, and pelvic pain. DRA that is present long standing should be considered as a contributing factor with any woman complaining of back, pelvic girdle, or hip pain.

28. **What specific exercises can be prescribed to reduce a diastasis recti abdominis (DRA)?**
Transverse abdominis activation through a "drawing in of the abdomen" may be helpful. Pelvic floor exercises (Kegels) have also been found to have some benefits. Patients should be taught to manually approximate the rectus abdominis muscles bellies while performing head lifts or partial curl ups. In cases of significant DRA, use of an abdominal compression brace or binder may be helpful to minimize the bulging during activities that aggravate the condition.

29. **An orthopedic physical therapist is seeing a patient who is 32 weeks pregnant with a diagnosis of lower back and hip pain. The patient has not made progress despite the therapist's therapeutic interventions and reports that her hip pain has become worse with walking.**

   a. **What is a rare condition seen in pregnancy that could be the cause of the hip pain?**
   Transient osteoporosis is a rare condition in pregnancy that causes temporary bone loss often affecting the hip and resulting in significant pain and disability. The onset of pain from transient osteoporosis of the hip is most common in the third trimester, usually resulting in antalgic gait or inability to bear weight.

b. **Can transient osteoporosis during pregnancy affect areas other than the hip?**
Yes, osteoporosis of the spine has also been reported in pregnancy resulting in back pain. Changes in height related to a compression fracture are rare but possible.

c. **How is transient osteoporosis during pregnancy diagnosed?**
The diagnosis is one of exclusion. A confirmed diagnosis can be made postpartum with medical imaging. Preexisting osteopenia has been shown to predispose pregnant women to this condition.

d. **What goals are appropriate for physical therapy management of transient osteoporosis during pregnancy?**
Treatment is aimed at preserving joint integrity and minimizing disability.

30. **How might the anatomic or physiologic changes associated with pregnancy contribute to the following signs and symptoms?**

a. **Loss of balance, especially when going down the steps.**
The center of gravity moves forward secondary to the enlarging breasts and uterus and may result in increased loss of balance and elevated fall risk.

b. **Increased lumbar lordotic curve and anteriorly tilted pelvis.**
As the uterus enlarges and moves out of the abdominal cavity, the abdominal muscles become stretched, and the back muscles may become shortened resulting in shortened iliopsoas and weakness of the gluteal and hamstring muscles

c. **The patient presents with a "waddle" gait pattern.**
Trunk rotation is limited as the uterus enlarges and moves out of the pelvic cavity. The rib cage expands to accommodate an increase in oxygen demand resulting in hypomobility of the costochondral and costovertebral joints restricting spinal rotation.

31. **What pregnancy-related changes could be contributing to the following complaints?**

a. **Sharp pelvic girdle pain when transferring in and out of bed.**
Global joint laxity occurs throughout the pregnancy due to hormonal changes. Asymmetrical laxity of the sacroiliac joint and/or the pubic symphysis may result in pain with movements of the hip and pelvis.

b. **Pain around the pubic symphysis, worsened by weight bearing.**
The pubic symphysis begins to widen during the 10th to 12th week of pregnancy. Separation up to 6 mm is considered normal. Separations greater than 1 cm are considered pubic diastasis and often result in pain and disability.

c. **Complaint of numbness in both hands at night.**
Increased body fluid and plasma levels may result in increased soft tissue edema and can contribute to median nerve compression resulting in pregnancy-related carpal tunnel syndrome.

d. **Paresthesia and allodynia along the anterolateral thigh that is aggravated by prolonged sitting or standing.**
Increased intraabdominal pressure along with an increased lordosis may lead to entrapment of the lateral femoral cutaneous nerve as it passes through the inguinal ligament resulting in a condition known as meralgia paresthetica.

32. **A patient who is 26 weeks' gestation in an uncomplicated pregnancy is being seen by an orthopedic therapist for discharge having successfully completed a episode of care for low back pain. The therapist is providing the patient with aerobic exercise guidelines to be performed in addition to the home exercises to prevent the recurrence of the low back pain. What are the general guidelines for a safe and effective exercise regimen for this patient?**
An exercise program with a goal of moderate-intensity exercise for at least 20 to 30 minutes per day on most or all days of the week should be developed with the patient. The patient should gradually progress exercises to prepregnancy duration if she was an exerciser prior to the pregnancy. However, high intensity or prolonged exercise for more than 45 minutes can lead to hypoglycemia. Therefore, the patient should be advised to assure adequate caloric intake before exercise or limit the intensity or length of the exercise session. Prolonged exercise should be performed with minimal exposure to avoid excessive elevation of core body temperature.

33. **What recommendations are appropriate for a physical therapist to provide the patient in question 32 for monitoring the intensity of the exercise?**
Because blunted and normal heart rate responses have been reported in pregnant women, the use of ratings of perceived exertion may be a more effective tool to monitor intensity. For moderate intensity, a Borg rating of perceived exertion scale of 13–14 (somewhat hard) should be recommended. The patient could also utilize the "talk test." If she can carry on a conversation while exercising, she is most likely not overexerting herself.

34. **What warning signs are important to share with pregnant patients/clients that indicate it is time to stop exercising?**
Exercise ought to be discontinued for any of the following warning signs:
- Vaginal bleeding
- Abdominal pain
- Regular painful contractions
- Amniotic fluid leakage
- Dyspnea before exertion
- Dizziness
- Headache
- Chest pain
- Muscle weakness affecting balance
- Calf pain or swelling

MENSTRUAL CYCLE AND MENOPAUSE

35. **Define "delayed menarche" and explain why it is relevant to the practice of orthopedic physical therapy.**
Delayed menarche is lack of menstruation by the age of 16. Studies have shown that there is a strong association between delayed menarche and increased risk of scoliosis and stress fractures with females involved in high-impact sports (runners, ballet dancers).

36. **Describe oligomenorrhea and amenorrhea, including causative factors and the relevance to physical therapy practice.**
Oligomenorrhea is scanty menstruation that can occur with a sudden weight loss of 10 lb with no regard to the woman's original weight. Amenorrhea is an abnormal cessation of the menses for 3 or more months after menarche has already started
Causative factors that are relevant to history, screening, and referral in physical therapy practice include:
- Strong emotional disturbance
- Exercise induced—increased endorphins inhibiting hypothalamic function
- Pathologic secondary to disease process
- Dietary—severe weight loss or gain. Typically, menses cease when a young woman loses weight to the point at which she is about 85% of her ideal body weight for age and height. Women and girls with a history of anorexia nervosa and/or long-standing amenorrhea are hypoestrogenic and at high risk for osteopenia/osteoporosis

PELVIC ORGAN PROLAPSE

37. **How common is pelvic organ prolapse among postmenopausal women?**
Pelvic organ prolapse affects up to 50% of postmenopausal women. It is a condition that worsens over time if not treated and may not be recognized by the patient without screening and examination by a health care provider.

38. **Is it possible for physical therapists to screen for pelvic organ prolapse?**
Screening of pelvic organ prolapse may be done through the patient's history as there are several common etiologies including pregnancy and childbirth, early onset of menopause, previous hysterectomy, chronic constipation, obesity, smoker's cough, and history of heavy lifting. The patient interview may also provide an opportunity to ask questions that could help screen for prolapse. The patient may complain of heaviness or dullness in the pelvis and might report feeling a lump in their vagina. Women with prolapse often experience urinary and bowel symptoms including frequent UTIs, incontinence, and constipation. Pelvic organ prolapse occurs when there is a weakness in the supporting structures of the pelvic diaphragm and pelvic floor muscles allowing the pelvic viscera to descend into the urogenital, anatomical defect.

39. **Can a physical therapist diagnose a pelvic organ prolapse?**
Pelvic organ prolapse diagnosis is confirmed through a pelvic exam by a physician or nurse practitioner or a physical therapist with special training in pelvic health.

40. Are there precautions the therapist should take if pelvic organ prolapse is suspected?
Yes, the patient should avoid exercises that create increased intraabdominal pressures, Valsalva maneuvers, and breath holding. Heavy lifting and squatting can increase pelvic descent and worsen the prolapse.

41. If the therapist suspects the patient has a prolapse, should the patient be referred to another provider?
Symptomatic prolapse should be evaluated by a medical provider. If the patient has symptoms of UTI, medical screening is recommended.

42. What interventions can physical therapists use to address pelvic organ prolapse?
Interventions for prolapse are centered around improving the function of the pelvic floor muscles in addition to the synergistic muscles to the pelvic floor including the transverses abdominis, lumbar multifidus, and the respiratory diaphragm. There is also evidence that strengthening the deep hip external rotator muscles, specifically the obturator internus, may improve strength in the pelvic floor muscles due to its close proximity. Interventions should include exercises to improve strength, endurance, and coordination of the musculature. Patients should also be provided instructions on activity modification to limit activities that increase downward descent of the pelvis such as heavy lifting and straining.

INCONTINENCE

43. How common is incontinence?
Urinary incontinence affects 40% of females over the age of 30 and 31% of males over 65 years old. Stress incontinence specifically is reported to impact 37% to 42% of females. Male urinary incontinence post TURP occurs among 10% to 17% of males undergoing the procedure with some studies showing that 30% to 40% are still incontinent a year after the surgery. Fecal incontinence is reported to impact 7% of females and 5% of males with increases up to 10% after the age of 60.

44. What is the most common type of urinary incontinence related to muscle weakness?
Stress urinary incontinence is primarily a result of weakness in the pelvic floor muscles and is defined as the complaint of any involuntary loss of urine on effort or physical exertion (eg, sporting activities) or on sneezing or coughing.

45. What are the other common types of urinary incontinence (in addition to stress incontinence)?
Urge incontinence and mixed urinary incontinence are the other common types of urinary incontinence. Urge incontinence is defined as the involuntary loss of urine accompanied by or immediately preceded by urgency. It is caused by uninhibited bladder contractions along with closure and support deficits that may be related to pelvic floor muscle dysfunction. It is sometimes referred to as overactive bladder syndrome. Mixed urinary incontinence is a combination of both stress and urge incontinence.

46. Based upon the American College of Physicians clinical guidelines, should physical therapists understand the role of pelvic muscle function in treating incontinence for female patients and be able to effectively instruct patients in proper exercises?
Yes, based on the following recommendations, physical therapists should have knowledge of pelvic muscle function related to urinary incontinence and be able to instruct patients in proper exercises.

Recommendation 1: First-line treatment with pelvic floor muscle training in women with stress UI. (Grade: strong recommendation, high-quality evidence)

Recommendation 2: Bladder training in women with urgency UI. (Grade: weak recommendation, low-quality evidence)

Recommendation 3: Pelvic floor muscle training with bladder training in women with mixed UI. (Grade: strong recommendation, high-quality evidence)

Recommendation 4: Against treatment with systemic pharmacology therapy for stress UI. (Grade: strong recommendation, high-quality evidence)

Recommendation 5: Pharmacologic treatment in women with urgency UI if bladder training was unsuccessful. (Grade: strong recommendation, high quality of evidence)

Recommendation 6: Weight loss and exercise for obese women with UI. (Grade: strong recommendation, moderate-quality evidence)

47. When should an orthopedic physical therapist refer a patient with incontinence to a pelvic health physical therapist?
An orthopedic physical therapist should refer a patient with urinary incontinence to a pelvic health physical therapist under any of the following conditions:

Symptoms do not improve with basic PFM exercises

Symptoms become worse with PFM exercises

Urinary incontinence is complicated by fecal incontinence and/or pelvic pain/pelvic muscle spasms
Inability of the patient to contract the pelvic floor muscle or inability to understand how to contract the pelvic floor with basic instructions
Uncertainty of the treating physical therapist
Patient's apprehension

MALE PELVIC HEALTH

48. Why is it important for orthopaedic physical therapists to screen for urinary incontinence in males who are 12 months or more postprostatectomy? What questions can be utilized to accomplish this screening?

It is important for orthopaedic physical therapists to screen for urinary incontinence in male patients with history of prostatectomy no matter how long ago the surgery occurred. The incidence of residual incontinence 12 months after surgery ranges greatly in published reports with rates ranging between 40% to 95%. Most males continuing to experience urinary incontinence for that length of time post surgery are usually managing it with pads, and often without having had the benefit of physical therapy intervention.

The questions below are recommended for use in this screening:

- Do you leak or dribble urine?
- Do you need to urinate frequently (more than every 2 hours)?
- Is your sleep interrupted from having to urinate during the night?

For each question, ask about the longevity of the symptom to determine if it is new or residual incontinence related to the surgical history.

49. What therapeutic exercises can be incorporated into the physical therapy plan of care to address postprostatectomy urinary incontinence?

PFM strengthening exercises are suggested to improve incontinence after prostate surgery. PFM contraction may improve the strength of the external urethral sphincter during periods of increased abdominal pressure such as bending, lifting, and squatting as well as improve the muscle performance of the PFM. Exercises to improve strength and activation of the transverse abdominis ought to be performed as well due to their facilitatory role of the pelvic floor muscle. Improving muscle performance of the transverse abdominis also serves to reduce abdominal pressure on the pelvic floor and the bladder. Exercises targeting awareness and endurance of the diaphragm also ought to be included due to the synergistic actions of the diaphragm, transverse abdominis, and PFM.

50. In addition to urinary incontinence, what are other possible complications of a prostatectomy?

Frequency and urgency of micturition, poor urinary stream, poor urinary stream, and erectile dysfunction.

51. Pelvic floor pain syndrome of a musculoskeletal origin (pelvic floor muscle tension/spasms) can cause pain in the pelvic floor and groin in males and females. What common activities may exacerbate symptoms in a male with this condition?

Abdominal strengthening exercises and deep leg squat exercises often aggravate pelvic floor pain. Pelvic floor muscle pain often intensifies with sitting for greater than 20 minutes.

52. How might a male with pelvic floor pain of musculoskeletal origin describe his symptoms?

Males suffering from pelvic floor pain syndrome of a musculoskeletal origin will often describe their symptoms as feeling like they are "sitting on a block of wood" or that they are "sitting on a golf ball". They will often relate the feeling directly to the perineum.

53. In addition to the pain described in question 50, what are other common complaints associated with chronic pelvic floor pain syndrome in males?

- Urinary pain or frequent urination
- Rectal pain after a bowel movement
- Constipation
- Ejaculatory pain
- Weak erection
- Premature ejaculation

54. Males may be reluctant to discuss many of these symptoms; how might the physical therapist approach asking the pertinent questions?

The NIH-Chronic Prostatitis Symptom Index (NIH-CPSI) can be used as an "ice breaker." Start with questions about symptoms and progress to questions about urinary, bowel, and sexual health. Often, men will be relieved that someone has finally asked about these symptoms.

55. What other musculoskeletal areas ought to be included in the physical examination of males with complaints of pain in the pelvic floor and groin areas?

- Lumbar spine as many men with chronic pelvic pain often have concomitant LBP
- Abdominal, paraspinal, and thigh muscles as trigger points may also be found in many of these muscles even if not directly involved with the pelvis
- Hip muscles as obturator internus and psoas dysfunction are often involved when there is pelvic floor muscle pain
- Diaphragm, rib cage, lower thoracic, and breathing—men with pelvic pain often have dysfunctional breathing mechanics including habitual breath-holding with lifting/straining and poor excursion of the diaphragm

56. An adult male seeking physical therapy care for an acute low back strain after working in his garden has a medical history significant for robotic prostatectomy 6 months ago. Why is it important to screen this patient for urinary incontinence?

Urinary incontinence is common immediately following prostate surgery. Persistent urinary incontinence beyond 6 weeks is also common, reported in up to 40% of cases. Persistent postoperative urinary incontinence may indicate pelvic muscle dysfunction that may respond to physical therapy intervention. So, no matter the length of time since a prostatectomy, it is important to screen for urinary incontinence in males with that history who are seeking orthopedic physical therapy even for seemingly unrelated conditions. Screening for UI in these cases assures a comprehensive picture of the patient's health and function is established and that an appropriate physical therapy plan of care, including referrals to pelvic health physical therapy specialists, is employed.

PHYSICAL THERAPIST EXAMINATION OF THE PELVIC FLOOR

57. Can the pelvic floor muscle be assessed by an orthopedic physical therapist who has not had specific training in internal palpation of the pelvic floor muscles?

While the preferred method recommended by the APTA Pelvic Health Academy for pelvic muscle strength testing is by internal palpation, the patient's ability to contract and relax the muscle can be palpated by external palpation. Palpation occurs with the patient's side lying. The therapist palpates just medial to the ischial tuberosity in the space of the ischiorectal fossa at the ischial spine. Patients are instructed to contract the muscle as if trying to prevent urination or passing gas without using the gluteal or hip abductor muscles. The patient should also be instructed to avoid holding their breath. When the patient correctly contracts the muscle, the therapist will feel the muscle lift into their finger. The muscle should be palpated bilaterally with the right muscle palpated with the patient in left side lying and the left muscle in right side lying. Timing the sustained contraction without breath-holding or accessory muscle activation (glutes/adductors) as well as the number of quick contractions in 10 seconds allows for objective measurement without internal palpation. When instructing a patient in doing pelvic floor muscle exercises, therapist should educate the patient on the optimum methods and positions to perform these exercises.

PELVIC FLOOR MUSCLE EXERCISE INSTRUCTION

58. Why are patients instructed NOT to sit on the toilet and stop and start the flow of urine as a method of exercising the muscle?

Micturition is a coordinated physiological response of the autonomic and somatic nervous systems requiring both reflexive activation of the detrusor and coordinated control of the skeletal muscles of the pelvic floor. For normal bladder emptying, the parasympathetic nervous system signals the detrusor muscle to contract. However, the skeletal muscles must relax so that urethral pressure decreases adequately for the flow of urine. Once this process begins, an active contraction of the pelvic floor will signal the sympathetic nervous system to diminish the activation of the detrusor muscle and contract the smooth muscles in the internal urethral sphincter, which in essence "confuses the bladder." For normal neuromuscular function during micturition, the bladder should be allowed to empty after voiding has been voluntarily initiated.

59. Why is it best to instruct patients to avoid activation of the gluteal and hip adductor muscles when performing pelvic floor muscle exercises?

The gluteal and hip adductor muscles are considered accessory muscles of the pelvic floor. When there is dysfunction in the pelvic floor muscles, these muscles will often attempt to compensate but are not effective in creating closure or adequate support of the pelvic contents. Co-contraction of the gluteal and hip adductor muscles with the pelvic floor is not effective in strengthening the pelvic floor muscle but rather may diminish the activation and awareness of the pelvic floor muscle during rehab efforts.

60. Why are patients discouraged from breath holding during pelvic floor muscle exercises?

The diaphragm is a synergistic muscle to the pelvic floor; when a patient holds their breath, the diaphragm isometric contraction will activate the pelvic floor muscle. During normal activation of the pelvic floor for support and closure, it must work independently of the diaphragm to allow for normal respiration. Secondly, during inhale, the diaphragm moves caudally. When the pelvic floor is contracted, it moves cephalic. If the patient inhales and holds the breath, which is a common substitution seen when the pelvic muscle is weak, the pelvic floor muscle will have to contract against the downward force of the diaphragm. Teaching the patient to breathe normally as they perform pelvic floor muscle exercises will prevent this.

61. **What common errors are made when trying to contract the pelvic floor muscles? What observation may be noted by the physical therapist?**

EXERCISE ERROR	THERAPIST OBSERVATION
Contraction of outer abdominal muscles instead of the pelvic floor muscles	The person is curving the back or starts the attempt to contract by pulling the stomach inwards. Note that a small "hollowing" of the stomach can be seen in a correct contraction with co-contraction of the transverse abdominal muscle
Contraction of hip adductor muscles instead of the pelvic floor muscles	The muscles of the inner thigh can be observed contracting or the person squeezes knees together
Contraction of the gluteal muscles instead of the pelvic floor muscles	The person is pressing the buttocks together or lifting the bottom from the treatment surface; in sitting, the person appears to get "taller"
Stop breathing	The person closes their mouth and holds their breath
Enhanced inhaling	The person takes a deep inspiration often accompanied by contraction of the abdominal muscles trying to "lift up" the pelvic floor by inspiration

62. **Is internal palpation necessary for a physical therapist to utilize to instruct patients in pelvic floor exercise?**

No. As noted in the response to question 58, training in internal exam and treatment of the pelvic floor is ideal; however, physical therapists are able to instruct patients in PFM exercise and evaluate progress using external palpation, patient reports of symptoms and function, and functional scales as well as other clinical measures to assess exercise performance and response to treatment. The synergistic actions of the pelvic floor and transverse abdominis can be utilized in conjunction with coordination with breathing (contracting both on exhale, relaxing both on inhale) to facilitate PFM contraction with or without external palpation by the therapist. Likewise, manual release of the PFM can be accomplished externally through contact medial to the ischial tuberosity with the patient positioned in sidelying in a 90-90 hip and knee flexed position. This technique is commonly utilized by orthopaedic manual physical therapists in the management of sacroiliac problems and is effective in the passive release of myofascial tension in the pelvic floor.

Bibliography

Ahangari, A. (2014). Prevalence of chronic pelvic pain among women: an updated review. *Pain Physician*, *17*(2), E141–147.

Alappattu, M., Neville, C., Beneciuk, J., & Bishop, M. (2016). Urinary incontinence symptoms and impact on quality of life in patients seeking outpatient physical therapy services. *Physiotherapy Theory and Practice*, *32*(2), 107–112.

Andrews, J., Reynolds, W.S., Likis, F.E., Sathe, N.A., & Jerome, R.N. (2012). Noncyclic chronic pelvic pain therapies for women: comparative effectiveness. Comparative Effectiveness Review No. 41. (Prepared by the Vanderbilt Evidence-based Practice Center under Contract No. 290-2007-10065-I.) AHRQ Publication No. 11(12)-EHC088-EF. Rockville, MD: Agency for Healthcare Research and Quality.

Antolak, S. J., Hough, D. M., Pawlina, W., & Spinner, R. J. (2002). Anatomical basis of chronic pelvic pain syndrome: the ischial spine and pudendal nerve entrapment. *Medical Hypotheses*, *59*(3), 349–353.

Avers, D. (2019). Testing the muscles of the trunk and pelvic floor. In M. Brown (Ed.), *Daniels and Worthingham's muscle testing: techniques of manual examination and performance testing*. St. Louis, MO: Elsevier.

Baker, P. K. (1993). Musculoskeletal origins of chronic pelvic pain. *Obstetrics and Gynecology North America*, *20*, 719–742.

Benjamin, D. R., van de Water, A. T. M., & Peiris, C. L. (2014). Effects of exercise on diastasis of the rectus abdominis muscle in the antenatal and postnatal periods: a systematic review. *Physiotherapy*, *100*(1), 1–8.

Berg-Poppe, P., Hauer, M., Jones, C., Munger, M., & Wethor, C. (2022). Use of exercise in the management of postpartum diastasis recti: a systematic review. *Journal of Women's Health Physical Therapy*, *46*(1), 35–47.

Berkley, K. (2005). A life of pelvic pain. *Physiology and Behavior*, *86*(30), 272–280.

Berkley, K. (2005). Chronic pelvic pain: pathogenic mechanisms, treatment innovations and research implications. In *Neural mechanisms of pelvic pain: viscero-visceral interactions and reproductive status*. Bethesda: National Institute of Health.

Boissonnault, J. S. (2002). Modifying labor and delivery positions for women with spine and pelvic ring dysfunction. *Journal of Women's Health Physical Therapy*, *26*(2), 9–13.

Boissonnault, W. G., & Boissonnault, J. S. (2005). Transient osteoporosis of the hip associated with pregnancy. *Journal of Women's Health Physical Therapy*, *29*(3), 33–39.

Boxer, S., & Jones, S. (1997). Intra-rater reliability of rectus abdominis diastasis measurement using dial calipers. *Australian Journal of Physiotherapy, 43*(2), 109–114.

Bø, K., Berghmans, B., Mørkved, S., & Kampen, M. V. (2015). Measurement of pelvic floor muscle function and strength and pelvic organ prolapse. In *Evidence-based physical therapy for the pelvic floor: bridging science and clinical practice* (pp. 47–48) (2nd ed.). Edinburgh: Churchill Livingstone.

Bø, K., Berghmans, B., Mørkved, S., & Kampen, M. V. (2015). Pelvic floor and exercise science. In *Evidence-based physical therapy for the pelvic floor: bridging science and clinical practice* (pp. 111–128) (2nd ed.). Edinburgh: Churchill Livingstone.

Cassidy, T., Fortin, A., Kaczmer, S., Shumaker, J. T. L., Szeto, J., & Madill, S. J. (2017). Relationship between back pain and urinary incontinence in the Canadian population. *Physical Therapy, 97*(4), 449–454.

Cherkasky, C. J., & Moalli, P. A. (2016). Role of pelvic floor in lower urinary tract function. *Autonomic Neuroscience, 200*, 43–48.

Drossman, D. A., Leserman, J., Nachman, G., et al. (1990). Sexual and physical abuse in women with functional or organic gastrointestinal disorders. *Annals of Internal Medicine, 113*(11), 828–894.

Drossman, D. A. (1995). Sexual and physical abuse and gastrointestinal illness. *Scandinavian Journal of Gastroenterology, 30*(sup208), 90–96.

Farmer, M. A. (2020). Pathophysiology of pain. In *Female sexual pain disorders: evaluation and management* (pp. 15–30). Wiley-Blackwell.

Fricke, A., Lark, S. D., Fink, P. W., Mundel, T., & Shultz, S. P. (2021). Exercise interventions to improve pelvic floor muscle functioning in older women with urinary incontinence: a systematic review. *Journal of Women's Health Physical Therapy, 45*(3), 115–125.

Gorniak, G., & Conrad, W. (2015). An anatomical and functional perspective of the pelvic floor and urogenital organ support system. *Journal of Women's Health Physical Therapy, 39*(2), 65–82.

Gorniak, G., & King, P. M. (2016). The peripheral neuroanatomy of the pelvic floor. *Journal of Women's Health Physical Therapy, 40*(1), 3–14.

Gorniak, G., & William, C. (2018). *Human anatomy synopsis: pelvic girdle and lower.* Bookboon.com.

Grace, V., & Zondervan, K. (2006). Chronic pelvic pain in women in New Zealand: Comparative well-being, comorbidity, and impact on work and other activities. *Health Care for Women International, 27*(7), 585–599.

Haggerty, C. L., Peipert, J. F., Weitzen, S., et al. (2005). Predictors of chronic pelvic pain in an urban population of women with symptoms and signs of pelvic inflammatory disease. *Sexually Transmitted Diseases, 32*(5), 293–299.

Harlow, B. L., & Stewart, E. G. (2003). A population-based assessment of chronic unexplained vulvar pain: have we underestimated the prevalence of vulvadynia? *Journal of American Medical Women's Association, 589*(2), 82–88.

Harm-Ernandes, I., Boyle, V., Hartmann, D., et al. (2021). Assessment of the pelvic floor and associated musculoskeletal system: guide for medical practitioners. *Female Pelvic Medicine & Reconstructive Surgery, 27*(12), 711–718.

Harrop, G., Katon, W., Walker, W. E., Holm, L., Russo, J., & Hickok, L. (1988). The association between chronic pelvic pain, psychiatric diagnoses, and childhood sexual abuse. *Obstetrics and Gynecology, 71*, 589–593.

Hartigan, E., McAuley, J. A., Lawrence, M., et al. (2020). Hip angles, joint moments, and muscle activity during gait in women with and without self-reported stress urinary incontinence. *Journal of Women's Health Physical Therapy, 44*(3), 107–116.

Heim, C., Ehlert, U., Hanker, J. P., & Hellhammer, D. H. (1998). Abuse-related posttraumatic stress disorder and alterations of the hypothalamic-pituitary-adrenal axis in women with chronic pelvic pain. *Psychosomatic Medicine, 60*(3), 309–318.

Heim, C., Ehlert, U., Hanker, J. P., & Hellhammer, D. H. (1999). Psychological and endocrine correlates of chronic pelvic pain associated with adhesions. *Journal of Psychosomatic Obstetrics & Gynecology, 20*(1), 11–20.

Herschorn, S. (2004). Female pelvic floor anatomy: the pelvic floor, supporting structures, and pelvic organs. *Reviews in Urology, Suppl 5*, S2–S10.

Herschorn, S. (2011). Female pelvic floor anatomy: the pelvic floor, supporting structures, and pelvic organs. *Reviews in Urology, 20*, 1895–1905.

Howard, F. M., Perry, C. P., Carter, J. E., & El-Minawi, A. M. (2000). Dyspareunia. In *Pelvic Pain: Diagnosis and Management* (pp. 112–121). Philadelphia, PA: Lippincott Williams & Wilkins.

Howard, F. M., Perry, C. P., Carter, J. E., & El-Minawi, A. M. (2000). Hernias. In *Pelvic pain: diagnosis and management.* Philadelphia, PA: Lippincott Williams & Wilkins.

Howard, F. M., Perry, C. P., Carter, J. E., & El-Minawi, A. M. (2000). Pelvic floor relaxation disorders. In *Pelvic pain: diagnosis and management.* Philadelphia, PA: Lippincott Williams & Wilkins.

Jamieson, D. J., & Steege, J. F. (1997). The association of sexual abuse with pelvic pain complaints in a primary care population. *American Journal of Obstetrics and Gynecology, 177*(6), 1408–1412.

Johnson, K. T., Williams, P. G., & Hill, A. J. (2021). The importance of information: prenatal education surrounding birth-related pelvic floor trauma mitigates symptom-related distress. *Journal of Women's Health Physical Therapy, 46*(2), 62–72.

Jordre, B., & Schweinle, W. (2014). Comparing resisted hip rotation with pelvic floor muscle training in women with stress urinary incontinence. *Journal of Women's Health Physical Therapy, 38*(2), 81–89.

Kasitinon, D., Kelly, B., Price, T. L., Chhabra, A., & Scott, K. M. (2020). Pudendal nerve injuries in sports and exercise: a case series of pudendal neuropathies from squats. *Journal of Women's Health Physical Therapy, 45*(1), 3–9.

King, P. M. (2006). Psychosocial factors associated with menopause. *Journal of Women's Health Physical Therapy, 30*(3), 13–17.

Kotarinos, R. K., & Kotarinos, E. (2014). The past, present and future of pop and physical therapy. *Current Obstetrics and Gynecology Reports, 3*(3), 180–185.

LaCross, J. A., Borello-France, D., Marchetti, G. F., Turner, R., & George, S. (2022). Physical therapy management of functional constipation in adults: a 2021 evidence-based clinical practice guideline from the American Physical Therapy Association's Academy of Pelvic Health Physical Therapy. *Journal of Women's Health Physical Therapy, 46*(3), 147–153.

Lamvu, G., Carrillo, J., & Rapkin, A. (2021). Chronic pelvic pain in women: a review. *JAMA, 325*(23), 2381–2391.

Latthe, P., Mignini, L., Gray, R., Hills, R., & Khan, K. (2006). Factors predisposing women to chronic pelvic pain: systematic review. *BMJ, 332*(7544), 749–755.

Livingston, B. P. (2016). Anatomy and neural control of the lower urinary tract and pelvic floor. *Topics in Geriatric Rehabilitation, 32*(4), 280–294.

Lukban, J., Whitmore, K., Kellogg-Spadt, S., Bologna, R., Lesher, A., & Fletcher, E. (2001). The effect of manual physical therapy in patients diagnosed with interstitial cystitis, high-tone pelvic floor dysfunction, and sacroiliac dysfunction. *Urology, 57*(6), 121–122.

Mathias, S. (1996). Chronic pelvic pain: prevalence, health-related quality of life, and economic correlates. *Obstetrics & Gynecology, 87*(3), 321–327.
Milios, J. E., Ackland, T. R., & Green, D. J. (2019). Pelvic floor muscle training in radical prostatectomy: A randomized controlled trial of the impacts on pelvic floor muscle function and urinary incontinence. *BMC Urology, 19*(1), 116.
Nassar, K., & Janani, S. (2020). Transient osteoporosis of hip during pregnancy. *International Journal of Clinical Rheumatology, 15*(6), 175–177.
Physical activity and exercise during pregnancy and the postpartum period, (2020). *Obstetrics & Gynecology, 135*(4), 178–188.
Price, N., Dawood, R., & Jackson, S. R. (2010). Pelvic floor exercise for urinary incontinence: a systematic literature review. *Maturitas, 67*(4), 309–315.
Rosier, P. (2019). Contemporary diagnosis of lower urinary tract dysfunction. F1000Research, 8, F1000 Faculty Rev-644. https://doi.org/10.12688/f1000research.16120.1.
Saunders, K. (2017). Recent advances in understanding pelvic-floor tissue of women with and without pelvic organ prolapse: considerations for physical therapists. *Physical Therapy, 97*(4), 455–463.
Simonds, A. H., Abraham, K., & Spitznagle, T. (2022). Clinical practice guidelines for pelvic girdle pain in the postpartum population. *Journal of Women's Health Physical Therapy, 46*(1). https://doi.org/10.1097/jwh.0000000000000236.
Singla, N., & Singla, A. K. (2014). Post-prostatectomy incontinence: etiology, evaluation, and Management. *Türk Üroloji Dergisi/Turkish Journal of Urology, 40*(1), 1–8.
Siqueira-Campos, V. M., de Deus, M. S., Poli-Neto, O. B., Rosa-e-Silva, J. C., de Deus, J. M., & Conde, D. M. (2022). Current challenges in the management of chronic pelvic pain in women: from bench to bedside. *International Journal of Women's Health, 14*, 225–244.
Steege, J. F., Metzger, D. A., & Levy, B. S. (1998). Musculoskeletal problems. In *Chronic pelvic pain: an integrated approach*. Philadelphia, PA: Saunders.
Van Alstyne, L. S., Harrington, K. L., & Haskvitz, E. M. (2010). Physical therapist management of chronic prostatitis/chronic pelvic pain syndrome. *Physical Therapy, 90*(12), 1795–1806.
Verit, F. F., Verit, A., & Yeni, E. (2006). The prevalence of sexual dysfunction and associated risk factors in women with chronic pelvic pain: a cross-sectional study. *Archives of Gynecology and Obstetrics, 274*(5), 297–302.
Wei, J. T., & De Lancey, J. O. (2004). Functional anatomy of the pelvic floor and lower urinary tract. *Clinical Obstetrics and Gynecology, 47*(1), 3–17.

CHAPTER 24 QUESTIONS

1. **An orthopedic physical therapist is seeing a patient for low back pain who is in the 24th week of pregnancy. The therapist plans to prescribe posterior pelvic tilts and hamstring stretches as part of her home exercise program. What positions are best to avoid during these exercises?**
   a. There are no position restrictions at this point in the pregnancy.
   b. Prone position is to be avoided due to the size of the abdomen.
   c. Left side lying must be avoided due to vena cava issues.
   d. Supine and hook lying are to be avoided due to vena cava issues.

2. **The following is true of diastasis rectus abdominus (DRA):**
   a. It only occurs in females.
   b. It is a decrease in the width of the linea alba that requires imaging to assess.
   c. Clinical exam for DRA with palpation is recommended.
   d. DRA, once in place, will not change but PT can help manage the issue.

3. **An orthopedic physical therapist is seeing a patient who is 32 weeks pregnant with a diagnosis of lower back and hip pain. The patient has not made progress despite the therapist's therapeutic interventions and reports that her hip pain has become worse with walking. Which of the following is a likely cause of the hip pain?**
   a. Transient osteoporosis
   b. Diastasis recti abdominis
   c. Interstitial cystitis
   d. She is carrying twins

4. **How is transient osteoporosis during pregnancy diagnosed?**
   a. Hip scour test
   b. Marching test
   c. The diagnosis is one of primarily exclusion during pregnancy
   d. Palpation and diagnostic ultrasound

5. **Which of the following are signs a pregnant women should stop exercising?**
   a. Vaginal bleeding
   b. Abdominal pain
   c. Dyspnea before exertion
   d. Dizziness
   e. All of the above

6. **During the health history portion of the physical therapy examination, if pelvic pain is identified, which of the following approaches would be best in completing the examination?**
   a. Screen the reproductive first for both males and females, add gastrointestinal and urologic screening at a later visit if reproductive is negative and the patient does not respond well to the physical therapy plan of care
   b. Screen reproductive, genitourinary, gastrointestinal, and urologic systems for indicators of medical referral
   c. Screen all body systems known to contribute to pelvic pain; if any other than musculoskeletal are positive, do not treat the patient, only refer and do so immediately
   d. It is unnecessary to screen any systems other than musculoskeletal before beginning physical therapy treatment. If the patient does not respond in a reasonable time, then add these screenings to determine if a referral may be useful

INTERVENTIONAL PAIN MANAGEMENT

S.K. Young, MD and J. Placzek, MD, PT

1. **What is the cost of chronic pain?**
   The economic cost secondary to lost productivity and health care expenses for all chronic pain approaches $635 billion annually in the United States.

2. **How does acute pain become chronic pain?**
   Acute pain can progress into chronic pain when there is repeated and/or continuous nerve stimulation that precipitates a series of altered pain pathways, resulting in central sensitization. Central sensitization causes recruitment of previously subthreshold synaptic inputs to nociceptive neurons, resulting in pain hypersensitivity to innocuous stimulation. There is also believed to be some degree of genetic priming by which some people have brain circuitry and dysregulation of glial function that predisposes them to more easily transitioning from acute pain to chronic pain.

3. **Can chronic pain be prevented?**
   The quality of acute pain management is an important factor in the subsequent development or prevention of chronic pain. Persistent postsurgical pain may be seen in patients in whom lower doses of analgesics were initially prescribed, resulting in ineffective analgesia in the early postoperative days. Nerve block and spinal analgesic techniques can hasten the rehabilitation of orthopedic patients. Patients receiving multimodal analgesia that includes spinal local anesthetics and spinal opiates have improved health-related quality-of-life measures for months after surgery compared with patients receiving intravenous analgesic regimens.

4. **Define preemptive analgesia.**
   Preemptive analgesia is a treatment that is initiated before and in some cases during a medical procedure to reduce the physiological consequences of nociception caused by the procedure and to prevent the ensuing cascade of events that could lead to the development of chronic pain.

5. **How does the response of the central nervous system contribute to the genesis of chronic pain?**
   High-intensity noxious stimulation alters central processing of afferent neural information. Studies elucidating the mechanisms for central hypersensitivity have documented a host of neurochemical changes, including enhancement of dorsal horn neuronal activity after repetitive C-fiber barrage (wind-up); receptive field expansion with decreased dorsal horn threshold, resulting in both temporal and spatial summation; and increases in immediate gene and dynorphin expression. Resultant increases in the synthesis of nitric oxide (NO), a highly diffusible gas that freely disperses to surrounding regions of the spinal cord, induce a positive feedback cycle with clinical pain on light touch (allodynia). Spinal cord sensitization leads to increased sensitivity in wide areas surrounding the site of injury (secondary hyperalgesia). This sensitivity interferes with movement and rehabilitation. Further, considerable evidence supports a heritable basis for some neurologic conditions, including neuropathic pain. Susceptible people may be predisposed to the development of chronic pain after trauma, especially in the presence of unrelieved acute pain, where spinal mechanisms (including constitutive cyclooxygenase-2 pathways) participate in the development of a "memory" for pain.

6. **If no pain relief is obtained by sympathetic block, can the diagnosis still be sympathetically maintained pain?**
   Sympathetically maintained pain (SMP) retains clinical utility for its therapeutic implications. It applies to a multitude of posttraumatic pain conditions with both burning pain and allodynia, which are, by definition, relieved by sympathetic block. Dystrophic changes, neural injury, and vasomotor or sudomotor changes are often present but are not required for the diagnosis. CRPS may be either sympathetically maintained (SMP) or sympathetically independent (SIP).

7. **Is chronic neuropathic pain peripheral or central in origin?**
   Neural injury can alter the tonic level of conduction from the dorsal root ganglia and thus sensitize the nociceptors subserving the cutaneous distributions of the affected nerve root. The spread of sensitization to areas surrounding the injury appears to be mediated in part via wide dynamic range (WDR) neurons in the spinal cord. WDR neurons also appear to be the mediators of SMP. Sensitization of WDR neurons in the spinal cord is termed *wind-up*. Any low-threshold myelinated mechanoreceptor afferent activity converging on the same WDR neurons results

in an exaggerated response, such as allodynia. Continuous pain results from sympathetic efferent sensitization of the peripheral sensory receptors, which in turn produces tonic firing of the low-threshold myelinated mechanoreceptors, projecting onto previously sensitized WDR neurons. Thus a painful cycle involving both peripheral and central components maintains neuropathic pain.

8. **Why do muscles ache?**
Although muscle pain and deep hyperalgesia are associated with a number of conditions as secondary phenomena, they may also be the primary source of pain. Primary nociceptors from muscle tissue are nerve fibers that, unlike rapidly transmitting "sharp" pain pathways, transmit afferent information slowly, thus giving rise to dull, aching pain. A-delta polymodal nociceptors responding to mechanical stimulation (group III) and unmyelinated C-fibers responding to ischemia and chemical stimuli (group IV) give rise to poorly localized, cramping muscle pain. The referred pain from muscle likely represents the extensive involvement of reflex mechanisms in the central nervous system. Hyperalgesia caused by central sensitization may result from activation of *N*-methyl-D-aspartate (NMDA) or other mechanisms of modulation of central synaptic processing.

9. **How do trigger points differ from chronic muscle tenderness secondary to fibromyalgia?**
Histologic changes associated with trigger points include atrophy of type II muscle fibers, a characteristic "moth-eaten" appearance of type I fibers, and segmental muscle fiber necrosis. Some investigators have noted elastic projections constricting affected muscle fibers. Lipid and glycogen deposition and abnormal mitochondrial accumulations are seen and result in muscular bands that are often clinically palpable. Pain from deep somatic structures is typically dull and diffuse. The ability to localize precise trigger areas decreases with increasing tissue depth. Diffusion and radiation can be indicators of severity. Muscle spasm and tenderness in zones of reference (as distinguished from trigger points) often appear at sites distant from the lesion.

10. **What causes a trigger point and why are they painful?**
After damage to the t-tubule system, stored calcium ions are released into the area of injury. Adenosine triphosphate (ATP) may activate the actin-myosin contractile mechanism focally in the absence of action potentials. A palpable band of electrically silent muscle may result. With calcium reuptake limited, unabated focal contractile activity persists. High levels of metabolic activity, documented by ATP depletion, produce the "hot spots" seen on infrared thermography. Further, because ATP is required for the calcium pump to retrieve calcium into the sarcoplasmic reticulum, depletion of ATP further enhances calcium availability and thus perpetuates contractile activity. Accumulation of metabolic byproducts results in local acidosis, which sensitizes adjacent nociceptors. Likewise, increased calcium may act as a second messenger to induce nociceptive neuronal hypersensitivity. Increased vascular permeability, local vasoconstriction, and reduced tissue oxygenation also contribute to the elaboration of algesic substances, which sensitize peripheral nociceptors. In addition, sensitized dorsal horn cells may cause enlargement of the receptive field, resulting in spreading dysesthesia.

11. **How can trigger points induce sympathetic overactivity?**
Sensitized muscle nociceptors may evoke sympathetic hyperactivity. Sympathetic activation may sensitize nociceptors, inducing cyclical reflex mechanisms. The progression from acute posttraumatic muscular pain to chronic myofascial pain probably involves peripheral sensitization of high-threshold mechanoreceptors, recruitment of low-threshold mechanoreceptors, and central sensitization of dorsal horn neurons. Increased sensitivity of muscle vasculature to sympathetic transmitter substances may contribute. Clinically, persistence of trigger point activity can result in sympathetically mediated vasomotor changes. In such cases, sympathetic blockade can assist the manipulative therapy.

12. **What measures are effective in treating a trigger point?**
Perpetuation of trigger point activity can be expected until the integrity of the sarcoplasmic reticulum is reestablished or the band is physically lengthened to prevent further interaction of the actin-myosin complex. If the taut muscular band comprising the trigger point can be stretched effectively without inducing reflexive contraction secondary to pain, the reparative process is facilitated. Additionally, the application of ischemic compression, acupuncture, acupressure, dry-needling, relaxation, and EMG biofeedback can be employed.

13. **Are trigger point injections effective?**
Yes, infiltration with local anesthetic (trigger point injection) relieves pain, relaxes muscles (by blocking ongoing reflex activity), and physically flushes away excessive extracellular calcium, hydrogen ions, and algesic substances. Relaxation and electromyogram biofeedback should be considered adjunctive measures.

14. **How can trigger point injections abolish pain at sites distal to the injection?**
Afferent pain signals secondary to activation of nociceptors enter the spinal cord through the dorsal root, where communication via internuncial neurons leads to hyperactivity in the anterior and anterolateral horn cells. Hyperactivity results in efferent traffic, causing intensified muscle spasm, vasoconstriction, and referred pain.

Neural blockade interrupts this reflex arc. Resultant alterations in central nervous system processing of input from the receptive field may be responsible for the spreading tenderness after injury. This response is terminated by local anesthetic application.

15. **Should nerve blocks be used to facilitate physical therapy in patients with chronic pain?**
Neural blockade immediately before manipulation of the spine enhances the efficacy of treatment used either alone or sequentially. Medial branch nerve blocks may allow improved manipulation by prevention of reflex muscle spasm and guarding during treatment. Precision in blockade is essential to avoid total sensory loss, which may permit dangerous overstretching of the tissues. Widespread nonspecific blockade may permit stretch beyond safe limits. Careful and specific physical interventions within the physiologic range, combined with blockade limited to specific target elements, are designed to minimize such risks.

16. **What circumstances require the application of regional local anesthetic blockade?**
Somatic regional block is used when multiple trigger points in a contiguous region make individual injections impractical or when simultaneous antisympathetic effect is required to increase blood flow or reduce sympathetic activity. Regional sympathetic blockade blocks perpetuating sympathetic activity and improves microcirculation, thus decreasing focal ischemia.

17. **Discuss the role of sympathetic blocks.**
Sympathetic block, by definition, relieves the pain of SMP. Although repeated sympathetic blockade may reduce or permanently eliminate clinical findings, most neuropathic pains are not sympathetically maintained. In fact, not even all cases of CRPS type I are amenable to sympathectomy. However, when a positive response from sympathetic blockade is obtained, the effect of the block often significantly outlasts the action of the local anesthetic, especially when repeated. Of interest, neural blockade distal to the sympathetic chain is also effective in reducing SMP, presumably because neurogenic block of the affected receptive field reduces the low-threshold mechanoreceptor activity that is stimulated by sympathetic outflow. With time, the plasticity of the central nervous system permits enhanced transmission over previously quiescent pathways. Enhanced transmission contributes to the clinical impression that, in the most chronic cases, peripheral measures are ineffective.

18. **Which medications are appropriate for chronic pain?**
Medications for chronic pain are administered by oral, topical/transdermal, IV regional, intraspinal, and nerve-blocking techniques. The oral route is by far the most common.

AGENT	INDICATION	MECHANISM
Tricyclic antidepressants	Neuropathic pain, depression, myofascial pain	Multiple, including central inhibition of 5-HT and NE reuptake
Anticonvulsants		
Gabapentin (Neurontin)	Neuropathic pain	Multiple, including NA channel inhibition, reduced spontaneous depolarization
Clonazepam (Klonopin)	Neuropathic pain, panic attacks, anxiety states	GABA agonist
Capsaicinoids (eg, capsaicin [Zostrix])	Neuropathic pain after severe nerve injury	Depletion of substance P
Muscle relaxants (eg, baclofen [Lioresal]	Spasticity after spinal cord injury; myofascial component	GABA agonist
NMDA receptor antagonists (eg, ketamine [Ketalar])	Posttraumatic, myofascial neuropathic pain; opioid tolerance	Glutamate receptor antagonism
Local anesthetic derivatives (eg, mexiletine [Mexitil])	Neuropathic pain with C-fiber hyperactivity, neural injury or neuroma with mechanical hypersensitivity, allodynia	Na channel blockade, reduce spontaneous depolarization
Antihypertensives (eg, clonidine [Catapres TTS])	Neuropathic pain with hyperpathia/ allodynia	α_2-adrenergic agonist

Continued

AGENT	INDICATION	MECHANISM
Opioids (eg, oxycodone [Oxycontin])	Nociceptive pain uncontrolled by other measures in patients at low psychological risk for addiction	Opiate receptor agonists
Nonsteroidal antiinflammatory drugs (eg, celecoxib [Celebrex])	Neuropathic and myofascial pain	Cyclooxygenase inhibition blocks prostaglandin synthesis

5-HT, 5-Hydroxytryptamine; *NE*, norepinephrine; *Na*, sodium; *GABA*, gamma-aminobutyric acid.

19. **Discuss the role of epidural steroids in management of chronic back pain.**
Epidural steroid injections are an option for short-term relief of radicular pain after failure of conservative treatment and as a means of avoiding surgery. In a randomized, controlled trial, the transforaminal epidural steroid injections have been reported to eliminate the need for surgery in 50% of patients with radicular pain originating from one or two spinal levels. Evidence-based meta-analysis of epidural steroid injections for treatment of chronic low back pain yields conflicting results. Although the Oxford group reported efficacy with an NNT of 7.3 for greater than 75% relief at up to 60 days and an NNT of 13 for greater than 50% relief at up to 12 months, the Cochrane group found no such evidence.

20. **Discuss the utility of epidural opioids for analgesia.**
Epidural administration of opioids allows for more direct interaction with the opioid receptor in the substantia gelatinosa of the spinal cord, which lowers the dose needed to obtain analgesia. This lowered dose results in less supraspinal side effects. Because there is still systemic absorption, sedation, respiratory depression, and other opioid side effects are still possible. Using more lipophilic opioids, such as fentanyl, results in less dermatomal spread, shorter duration of action, and higher systemic absorption. Use of more hydrophilic opioids, such as morphine, is conversely associated with longer duration or action, more rostral spread, and delayed respiratory depression.

21. **Do continuous analgesic infusions prevent early recognition of posttraumatic compartment syndromes?**
The pain associated with acute compartment syndrome typically breaks through properly regulated analgesia during brachial plexus infusion or lumbar epidural infusion. Furthermore, if weakness develops during the infusion, the local anesthetic can be withheld to facilitate prompt assessment.

22. **What is complex regional pain syndrome (CRPS)?**
CRPS, previously known as reflex sympathetic dystrophy, is a syndrome characterized by pain, vasomotor instability, trophic changes, bony changes, and sensory changes.

23. **What is the difference between CRPS types I and II?**
When there is no clear nerve injury, this is defined as CRPS type I (formerly reflex sympathetic dystrophy). If there is a specific nerve injury, this is classified as CRPS type II (formerly causalgia). CRPS is a clinical diagnosis with a constellation of symptoms and physical exam findings including pain out of proportion to the initial injury, limited range of motion, allodynia, change in skin temperature and/or color, swelling, abnormal sweating, and abnormal nail or hair growth.

24. **What is the treatment for CRPS II?**
CRPS type II should be treated by decompression of the involved nerve and a postoperative therapy program.

25. **What is the treatment for CRPS type I?**
Physical therapy is the most important treatment for CRPS. There are multiple medications used to treat the pain and other symptoms of CRPS including NSAIDs, neuropathic agents (gabapentin, pregabalin, duloxetine), topical anesthetics, corticosteroids, opioids, and ketamine. Sympathetic nerve blocks can provide temporary symptom improvement. For patients that do not respond to these more conservative treatments, spinal cord stimulation and dorsal root ganglion stimulation devices are the long-term treatment of choice.

26. **Can corticosteroids interfere with healing?**
The timing of therapeutic intervention affects the quality of the reparative process. Corticosteroid administration in the first 2 weeks can inhibit prostaglandin synthesis, thus interfering with the initial proliferative phases of healing. Corticosteroids should be used with caution in acute strains and only when the joint is to be placed at rest. Furthermore, corticosteroid-induced fluid retention may contribute to tissue swelling. This effect may be most

damaging after crush or blunt trauma to an extremity, where additional swelling may predispose to development of a compartment syndrome.

27. **What is the indication for the radiofrequency ablation (RFA) procedure?**
Facet joint arthropathy/arthritis is a common cause of axial low back and neck pain, without radicular symptoms. The facet joints of the spine are innervated by paired medial branches of the posterior ramus of the spinal nerve. This procedure uses high-frequency electrical current to create a thermal lesion within the medial branch nerve that disrupts nociceptive pain signals. The RFA procedure is indicated for patients with greater than 3 months of axial low back pain without radiculopathy that does not respond to conservative therapies such as NSAIDs and physical therapy.

28. **What is neuromodulation?**
Neuromodulation is technology that acts directly on nerves. It is the alteration, or modulation, of neural activity by delivering electrical or pharmaceutical agents directly to the target area. Neuromodulation is used to treat a variety of diseases including headaches, tremors, spinal cord damage, ischemic disorders, and urinary incontinence. The most frequent use of this technology is to treat chronic pain. For chronic pain, spinal cord stimulators (SCS), dorsal root ganglion stimulators (DRG), and intrathecal pumps are the most commonly used neuromodulation devices. SCS is frequently used for patients who have persistent low back pain and neuropathic pain in the extremities following spine surgery. DRG is indicated for CRPS of the lower limbs.

29. **What drug can be used to manage acute pain in patients with opioid dependence or tolerance?**
Ketamine therapy may be considered in acute pain management for patients who are opioid tolerant or opioid dependent and are presenting for surgery or acute exacerbation of chronic pain. Patients with an increased risk of opioid-related respiratory depression, such as patients with obstructive sleep apnea, may also benefit.

30. **What are the symptoms of opioid withdrawal?**
Opioid withdrawal can start shortly after administering an opioid antagonist or several hours after the last dose of a short-acting opioid. Symptoms typically peak around 24 to 48 hours. Symptoms include elevated heart rate, sweating, difficulty sitting still, dilated pupils, joint/muscle aches, rhinorrhea, lacrimation, diarrhea, vomiting, gross tremor, frequent yawning, and gooseflesh.

31. **What substance, if found on urine toxicology testing, would indicate illicit opioid use?**
6-monoacetylmorphine (6-MAM) is a unique metabolite of heroin and is not found in any commercially available prescription opioids, and thus indicates illicit opioid use. Morphine, hydrocodone, oxycodone, codeine, hydromorphone, and oxymorphone are all prescription opioids. The presence of these substances alone does not necessarily indicate illicit opioid use.

Bibliography

Bigos, S., Bowyer, O.R., Braen, G.R., et al. (1994). *Acute low back problems in adults, clinical practice guideline No. 14.* AHCPR Publication No. 95-0642, Rockville, MD: Agency for Health Care Policy and Research, U.S. Department of Health and Human Services.

Boersma, K., Linton, S., Overmeer, T., Jansson, M., Vlaeyen, J., & de Jong, J. (2004). Lowering fear-avoidance and enhancing function through exposure in vivo: a multiple baseline study across six patients with back pain. *Pain, 108*, 8–16.

Capdevila, X., Barthelet, Y., Biboulet, P., Ryckwaert, Y., Rubenovitch, J., & d'Athis, F. (1999). Effects of perioperative analgesic techniques on the surgical outcome and duration of rehabilitation after major knee surgery. *Anesthesiology, 91*, 8–15.

Carli, F., Mayo, N., Klubien, K., Schricker, T., Trudel, J., & Belliveau, P. (2002). Epidural analgesia enhances functional exercise capacity and health-related quality of life after colonic surgery. *Anesthesiology, 97*, 540–549.

Cherkin, D. C., Sherman, K. J., Deyo, R. A., & Shekelle, P. G. (2003). A review of the evidence for the effectiveness, safety, and cost of acupuncture, massage therapy, and spinal manipulation for back pain. *Ann Intern Med, 138*, 898–906.

Dreyfus, P., Michaelsen, M., & Horn, M. (1995). MUJA: Manipulation under joint anesthesia/analgesia: A treatment approach for recalcitrant low back pain of synovial joint origin. *Journal of Manipulative and Physiological Therapeutics, 18*, 537–546.

Elias, M. (2000). Cervical sympathetic and stellate ganglion blocks. *Pain Physician, 3*(3), 294–304.

Esposito, M. F., Malayil, R., Hanes, M., & Deer, T. (2019). Unique characteristics of the dorsal root ganglion as a target for neuromodulation. *Pain Med, 20*(Supplement_1), S23–30.

Gam, A. N., Warming, S., Larsen, L. H., et al. (1998). Treatment of myofascial trigger-points with ultrasound combined with massage and exercise: a randomized controlled trial. *Pain, 77*, 73–79.

Hartrick, C. T. (1995). Managing the difficult pain patient. In P. P. Raj & D. Niv (Eds.), *Management of pain: a world perspective* (pp. 330–334). Bologna, Italy: Moduzzi.

Hartrick, C. T. (1998). Pain due to trauma including sports injuries. *Pain Digest, 8*, 237–259.

Hartrick, C. T. (1998). Screening instruments predict long-term response to epidural steroids. *Journal of Contemporary Neurology, 3*, 1–6.

Hartrick, C. T. (2004). Multimodal postoperative pain management. *Am J Health Syst Pharm, 61*, S4–S10.

Hartrick, C. T., Kovan, J. P., & Naismith, P. (2004). Outcome prediction following sympathetic block for complex regional pain syndrome. *Pain Practice, 4*, 222–228.

Kapural, L., & Mekhail, N. (2001). Radiofrequency ablation for chronic pain control. *Curr Pain Headache Rep, 5*(6), 517–525.

Kemler, M. A., & Furnee, C. A. (2002). Economic evaluation of spinal cord stimulation for chronic reflex sympathetic dystrophy. *Neurology, 59*, 1203–1209.
Nelemans, P. J., de Bie, R. A., de Vet, H. C., & Sturmans, F. (2001). Injection therapy for subacute and chronic benign low back pain. *Spine, 26*, 501–515. (*Cochrane Database Syst Rev* 2:CD001824, 2000).
Nelson, L., Aspergren, D., & Bova, C. (1997). The use of epidural steroid injection and manipulation on patients with chronic low back pain. *J Manip Physiol Ther, 20*, 263–266.
Pauza, K. J., Howell, S., Dreyfuss, P., Peloza, J. H., Dawson, K., & Bogduk, N. (2004). A randomized, placebo-controlled trial of intradiscal electrothermal therapy for the treatment of discogenic low back pain. *Spine J, 4*, 27–35.
Peppin, J. F., Passik, S. D., Couto, J. E., et al. (2012). Recommendations for urine drug monitoring as a component of opioid therapy in the treatment of chronic pain. *Pain Med, 13*(7), 886–896.
Placzek, J. D., Boyer, M. I., Gelberman, R. H., Sopp, B., & Goldfarb, C. A. (2005). Nerve decompression for complex regional pain syndrome type II following upper extremity surgery. *J Hand Surg Am, 30*(1), 69–74.
Polatin, P. B., Cox, B., Gatchel, R. J., & Mayer, T. G. (1997). A prospective study of Waddell signs in patients with chronic low back pain. *Spine, 22*, 1618–1621.
Riew, K., Yin, Y., Gilula, L., et al. (2000). The effect of nerve-root injections on the need for operative treatment of lumbar radicular pain. A prospective, randomized, controlled, double- blind study. *J Bone Joint Surg Am, 82*, 1589–1593.
Wesson, D. R., & Ling, W. (2003). The clinical opiate withdrawal scale (COWS). *J Psychoact Drugs, 35*(2), 253–259.

CHAPTER 25 QUESTIONS

1. **Corticosteroids can interfere with the healing process by:**
   a. Increasing DNA synthesis
   b. Interrupting the initial proliferative phase of healing
   c. Stimulating mitosis
   d. Increasing fibrosis

2. **Which of the following is an indication for the radiofrequency ablation (RFA) procedure?**
   a. Radiculopathy
   b. Axial back/neck pain greater than 3 months
   c. A patient that responds positively to physical therapy
   d. Opioid dependence

3. **Chronic regional pain syndrome:**
   a. Is self-limiting and leaves no permanent disability
   b. Type II is treated by nerve decompression and therapy
   c. Can result in joint laxity
   d. Results in increased cortical density

4. **Which of the following drugs can be used to manage acute pain in patients with opioid dependence or tolerance?**
   a. Ketamine
   b. Zostrix
   c. Klonopin
   d. Neurontin

CERVICOGENIC HEADACHE

E. Sigman, PT, DPT, OCS

1. **How can it be determined that a patient with headache is appropriate for physical therapy?**
   The International Headache Classification describes all known headache disorders (Oelsen et al., 2018). The classification is comprised of three parts. The first part describes primary headaches, the second part describes secondary headaches, and the third part describes neuropathies, facial pain, and other headaches. Primary headaches are not associated with demonstratable organic disease or structural neurology abnormality and typically associated with a normal clinical exam. Common examples of primary headache diagnoses are: migraine headache (MH), tension-type headache (TTH), and cluster headache. Secondary headaches are caused by an underlying condition or disease and typically associated with an abnormal clinical exam. While cervicogenic headache (CGH) is an example of a secondary headache, it's important to recognize that many secondary headache disorders are serious and can be life threatening.

2. **What serious secondary headache disorders should a physical therapist be aware of and how would you screen for them?**
   Examples of more serious secondary headache disorders, include (but are not limited to) headache due to: cranial or cervical vascular disorder, meningitis, cervical fracture, upper cervical instability, lesions of the posterior fossa, and meningioma. While it is estimated that only 18% of persons with headache have a secondary headache disorder, it's important to be able to appropriately screen these patients as many secondary headaches are not appropriate for physical therapy (Do et al., 2019). Clinicians can use the mnemonic, SNOOP10 to help with screening (Do et al., 2019):
   S: Systemic symptoms including fever
   N: History of neoplasm
   N: Neurologic deficit or dysfunction
   O: Onset of headache is sudden or abrupt. Time to maximum headache intensity is <1 minute.
   O: Older age (>50 y/o). Onset of new headache occurred over the age of 50. Patients over the age of 50 tend to have a higher incidence of headaches due to a serious secondary cause compared to younger patients.
   P: Pattern change. A headache with a different pattern compared to the patient's known previous history of headaches.
   P: Positional headache. A headache occurring immediately/within seconds of assuming an upright position and resolving quickly after lying supine can be suggestive of a cerebrospinal fluid (CSF) leak.
   P: Precipitated by sneezing, coughing/Valsalva, or exercise. These headaches can be due to a Chiari malformation, brain metastases, subdural hematomas, issues related to abnormal CSF pressure, infection, vascular disease, etc.
   P: Papilledema. Papilledema is optic disc swelling that physical therapists are unable to measure in the clinic but often associated with disorders that increase intracranial pressure. This is included in this mnemonic because this screening tool was initially developed for practitioners who would be able to measure this clinically.
   P: Progressive headache or atypical headache presentations.
   P: Pregnancy or puerperium. A new onset of headache can affect up to 5% of women and tends to happen more in the third trimester. This could be due to hormone changes, use of epidurals, or hypercoagulability.
   P: Painful eye with autonomic features. While this could be a feature of cluster headache (which is a primary headache disorder), the prevalence of cluster headache is so low that all patients with these features should be referred for neuroimaging to rule out a structural lesion as the cause of these symptoms.
   P: Posttraumatic onset of headache
   P: Pathology of the immune system such as HIV. Headache is the most common pain problem in patients with HIV.
   P: Painkiller overuse or new drug at onset of headache. Medication overuse headache is the most common secondary headache disorder and requires management by a physician.
   The presence of any of these features should warrant further evaluation and, in many cases, referral (Do et al., 2019).

3. **List the competing diagnoses for cervicogenic headache.**
   - Chiari I malformation
   - Lesions of the posterior fossa
   - Dissecting aneurysms of the vertebral or internal carotid arteries
   - Meningitis
   - Herpes zoster

- Paroxysmal hemicrania
- Hemicrania continua
- C2 neuralgia
- Occipital neuralgia
- Syringomyelia
- Temporomandibular joint dysfunction (TMD)
- Neck-tongue syndrome
- Headache attributed to whiplash injury
- Posttraumatic headache
- Cervical fracture
- Upper cervical instability
- Myofascial pain syndrome
- Headache attributed to craniocervical dystonia
- Migraine headache
- Tension-type headache

4. **What is the prevalence of CGH and other common headache disorders?**
   The prevalence of CGH in the general population has been estimated to be between 0.4% and 2.5% but can reach as high as 20% in people with chronic headaches (ie, more than 15 headache days in a month for 3 consecutive months) (Biondi 2005). The incidence of CGH increases to 54.3% in persons with a recent history of cervical injury (Haldeman & Dagenais, 2001). Globally, 11% of the adult population has an active headache disorder with 42% being TTH and 11% being MH (Stovner et al., 2007). Of note, 75% of patients with MH also fulfill the diagnostic criteria for CGH (Haldeman & Dagenais, 2001).

5. **Describe the clinical presentation of common headache diagnoses that also present with neck pain (from the International Headache Classification).**

	MIGRAINE WITHOUT AURA	TENSION-TYPE	CERVICOGENIC (Sjaastad et al., 1998)	OCCIPITAL NEURALGIA
Frequency	Variable	Variable	Variable	Variable
Duration	4–72 hours	30 min–7 days	Variable (ranges from several hours to several weeks)	Continuous during an attack
Location	Unilateral (40% bilateral)	Bilateral	Unilateral, cervical spine, and/or occipital region. Starts in the cervical spine.	Distribution of the greater, lesser and/or third occipital nerves; unilateral or bilateral; pain may radiate up the head toward the eye; neck pain is common
Description	Pulsating	Pressing/tightening; "band like"; nonpulsating	Dull ache that radiates from cervical spine to the head/face. Nonthrobbing, nonlancinating	Paroxysmal stabbing or shooting pain with or without persistent aching between attacks
Intensity	Moderate to severe	Mild to moderate	Mild to moderate	Moderate to severe
Effect of routine physical activity	Aggravated by or cause avoidance of routine physical activity	Not aggravated by routine physical activity	Not aggravated by routine physical activity	Not aggravated by routine physical activity
Nausea or vomiting	Yes	No	No	No

	MIGRAINE WITHOUT AURA	TENSION-TYPE	CERVICOGENIC (Sjaastad et al., 1998)	OCCIPITAL NEURALGIA
Photophobia or phonophobia	One or both	No more than one	No	No
Additional features	Neck pain is common. There can be a presence of aura. Can have lacrimation and rhinorrhea	Pericranial tenderness and neck pain is common	Can be associated with history of cervical trauma. Cervical pain precedes/causes headache. Demonstration of clinical signs that implicate that the source of pain is in the cervical region and/or abolition of headache after a diagnostic blockade in the cervical spine	Tenderness over the scalp by the affected nerve. Diminished sensation in the affected area. Pain is eased temporarily by local anesthetic block of the nerve

From Oelsen, J., Bendtsen, L., Goadsby, P., et al. (2018). The International Classification of Headache Disorders (3rd edition) *Cephalgia* (38, pp. 1–211)

Diagnostic Criteria for Cervicogenic Headache according to the International Headache Classification (ICHD-3) (Oelsen et al., 2018):

A: Any headache fulfilling criterion C

B: Clinical and/or imaging evidence of a disorder or lesion within the cervical spine or soft tissues of the neck known to cause headache

C: Evidence of causation demonstrated by at least two of the following:

- headache has developed in temporal relation to the onset of the cervical disorder or appearance of the lesion
- headache has significantly improved or resolved in parallel with improvement in, or resolution of, the cervical disorder or lesion
- cervical range of motion is reduced, and headache is made significantly worse by provocative maneuvers
- headache is abolished following diagnostic blockade of a cervical structure or its nerve supply

D: Not better accounted for by another ICHD-3 diagnosis

Other diagnostic criteria and considerations:

- Common symptoms include: unilateral neck pain with associated headache and/or the headache is triggered or aggravated by cervical spine sustained positions/postures and/or movements (Blanpied et al., 2017).
- Exam findings:
  - Positive cervical flexion rotation test (CFRT) to the affected side (Blanpied et al., 2017; Howard et al., 2015; Rubio-Ochoa et al., 2016).
  - Pain reproduction and joint restriction noted with passive accessory intervertebral movement to all cervical spine segments cranial to C4, with the most common affected segment being C1-2 (Blanpied et al., 2017; Howard et al., 2015; Rubio-Ochoa et al., 2016).
  - Limited cervical spine range of motion (ROM) (Blanpied et al., 2017; Howard et al., 2015; Rubio-Ochoa et al., 2016).
  - Endurance and strength deficits of the cervical spine extensors and flexors (Blanpied et al., 2017; Howard et al., 2015).

6. **Discuss the neuroanatomic basis for cervicogenic headache.**

Dysfunction in the cervical spine can be perceived as headache due to the convergence of cervical (C1-3) and trigeminal afferent fibers in the brainstem within the trigeminocervical nucleus (Bogduk, 2001; Bogduk & Govind, 2009). In addition to the interaction of these afferents in the trigeminocervical nucleus, trigeminal and cervical afferents also overlap in the spinal cord. There have been cases observed, where the trigeminal nerve extends as far down as C4, highlighting the importance of considering all cervical spine segments cranial to C4 when investigating CGH (Bogduk, 2001). When primary afferents from different regions of the body converge in the central nervous system, it allows activity in one afferent to contribute to pain perception in another body region (Bogduk, 2001). In this case, when there is activity in the cervical spine afferents, it can cause pain perception in the head and face.

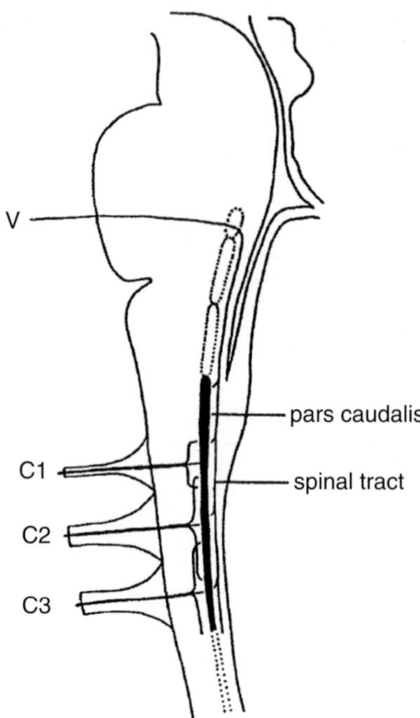

Trigeminocervical nucleus. (*From Bogduk N. (1994). Cervical causes of headache and dizziness. In Grieve's Modern Manual of Therapy (pp 317–331), Edinburgh: Churchill Livingstone.*)

7. **Which structures provide afferent information to the trigeminocervical nucleus?**
   Structures include:
   - The zygapophyseal joints, ligaments, and posterior cervical muscles associated with cervical spine segments above C4 (Bogduk, 2001)
   - The nerve roots from C1-3 (Bogduk, 2001)
   - The upper portion of the vertebral artery
   - The temporomandibular joint
   - The posterior cranial fossa/upper spinal cord dura mater (Haldeman & Dagenais, 2001)
   - Cranial nerves V, VII, IX, and X.

8. **Describe the myofascial structures of the neck that can contribute to headache and the pathoanatomical mechanism behind their pain referral patterns.**
   The muscles that can refer pain to the head include: the muscles of mastication (specifically masseter and temporalis), upper trapezius, sternocleidomastoid, splenius capitis, and the suboccipitals (Simons et al., 1999). Muscle nociceptors can be excited in response to mechanical, thermal, or chemical stimuli. This excitation triggers the release of histamine, prostaglandins, and serotonin, which further decreases the threshold for further stimulation to cause pain (Fernández-de-Las-Peñas, 2015). The reason these muscles can cause pain in the head (in addition to the convergence of these afferents with trigeminal afferents in the trigeminocervical nucleus as outlined above) is due to the close proximity of the spinal accessory nerve afferents to the upper cervical spine afferents in the spinal cord (Fernández-de-Las-Peñas, 2015).

9. **What do cervical radiographs show in patients with headache?**
   For CGH, conventional radiographic studies either demonstrated no abnormalities or no difference when comparing patients with CGH to healthy controls (Bogduk & Govind, 2009).

10. **What is the gold standard for diagnosis of cervical headache?**
    Controlled diagnostic facet blocks at C2-3 and C3-4 can be used to determine a source of pain in patients with suspected CGH (Bogduk & Govind, 2009; Getsoian et al., 2020). Facet blocks typically use lidocaine 2% and bupivacaine 0.5% (Getsoian et al., 2020). Some studies state that a positive blockade results in complete relief

of headache while others determine success as at least a 70% reduction in headache (Bogduk & Govind, 2009; Getsoian et al., 2020). While these blockades can be useful in the diagnosis of CGH, studies report no long-lasting therapeutic effect or even remission of pain when these facet blocks are used as treatment.

11. **What manual therapy interventions are useful in the treatment of CGH?**
Physical therapy treatment of CGH should be multidimensional and focused on addressing the patient's participation and functional goals, and decreasing headache frequency. The physical examination and relevant impairments discovered should be addressed with specific interventions. When cervical spine zygapophyseal joint dysfunction is found, there is good evidence to support the use of cervical spine manipulation/mobilization. Cervical spine manipulation has demonstrated a significant reduction in the frequency and intensity of headache in the short and long term (Haldeman & Dagenais, 2001; Chaibi & Russell, 2012; Jull et al., 2002; Posadzki & Ernst, 2011). Cervical spine manipulation/mobilization has also been shown to decrease the consumption of medication (Chaibi & Russell, 2012). Thoracic spine manipulation might be considered, particularly for patients who might not consent to or be appropriate for cervical spine mobilization/manipulation as patients who have received thoracic spine manipulation have demonstrated a significant decrease in neck pain (Cleland et al., 2005).

12. **What therapeutic exercises have been shown to be beneficial in the treatment of CGH?**
Deep neck flexor endurance training has demonstrated a significant reduction in the frequency and intensity of headache in patients with CGH at 3, 6, and 12 months. Endurance training of the serratus anterior and lower trapezius has resulted in similar clinical improvements to improved deep neck flexor endurance (Jull et al., 2002).

13. **Are there predictors of responsiveness to physical therapy treatment on cervicogenic headache?**
No. Jull and Stanton evaluated the locus of control in patients with CGH using the Headache-Specific Locus of Control (HSLC). They initially sought to determine the effectiveness of physical therapy treatment on the HSLC score. Later, they looked to find if there were any variables that would shed light on predictors of responsiveness to physical therapy management of CGH and they did not find a consistent or significant pattern of predictors (Stanton & Jull, 2003).

14. **What other medical management has been shown to be effective in the treatment of CGH?**
   - Radiofrequency neurotomy (Bogduk & Govind, 2009)
   - Anesthetic blockades of zygapophyseal joints C2-3 and C3-4 (Bogduk & Govind, 2009)

15. **What do systematic reviews reveal regarding the management of cervicogenic headache with physical therapy and/or manual therapies?**
The majority of systematic reviews investigating the role of physical therapy in the management of CGH are largely focused on manual therapy, specifically spinal manipulation. In these reviews, spinal manipulation has been found to be effective in the management of cervicogenic headaches with regard to reducing headache intensity, frequency, duration, and neck pain (Chaibi & Russell, 2012; Posadzki & Ernst, 2011; Fernandez et al., 2020). There is one systematic review that demonstrated the most effective intervention was a *combination* of mobilization, manipulation, and cervicoscapular strengthening exercises (Racicki et al., 2013).

Bibliography

Biondi, D. M. (2005). Cervicogenic headache: a review of diagnostic and treatment strategies. *Journal of the American Osteopathic Association, 105*(4 Suppl 2), 16S–22S.

Blanpied, P. R., Gross, A. R., Elliott, J. M., et al. (2017). Neck pain: revision 2017. *Journal of Orthopaedic & Sports Physical Therapy, 47*(7), A1–A83.

Bogduk, N. (2001). Cervicogenic headache: anatomic basis and pathophysiologic mechanisms. *Current Pain and Headache Reports, 5*(4), 382–386.

Bogduk, N., & Govind, J. (2009). Cervicogenic headache: an assessment of the evidence on clinical diagnosis, invasive tests, and treatment. *Lancet Neurology, 8*(10), 959–968.

Chaibi, A., & Russell, M. B. (2012). Manual therapies for cervicogenic headache: a systematic review. *Journal of Headache and Pain, 13*(5), 351–359.

Cleland, J. A., Childs, J. D., McRae, M., Palmer, J. A., & Stowell, T. (2005). Immediate effects of thoracic manipulation in patients with neck pain: a randomized clinical trial. *Manual Therapy, 10*(2), 127–135.

Do, T. P., Remmers, A., Schytz, H. W., et al. (2019). Red and orange flags for secondary headaches in clinical practice: SNNOOP10 list. *Neurology, 92*(3), 134–144.

Fernandez, M., Moore, C., Tan, J., et al. (2020). Spinal manipulation for the management of cervicogenic headache: a systematic review and meta-analysis. *European Journal of Pain, 24*(9), 1687–1702.

Fernández-de-Las-Peñas, C. (2015). Myofascial head pain. *Current Pain and Headache Reports, 19*(7), 28.

Getsoian, S. L., Gulati, S. M., Okpareke, I., Nee, R. J., & Jull, G. A. (2020). Validation of a clinical examination to differentiate a cervicogenic source of headache: a diagnostic prediction model using controlled diagnostic blocks. *BMJ Open, 10*(5), e035245.

Haldeman, S., & Dagenais, S. (2001). Cervicogenic headaches: a critical review. *Spine Journal, 1*(1), 31–46.

Howard, P. D., Behrns, W., Martino, M. D., DiMambro, A., McIntyre, K., & Shurer, C. (2015). Manual examination in the diagnosis of cervicogenic headache: a systematic literature review. *Journal of Manual & Manipulative Therapy, 23*(4), 210–218.

Jull, G., Trott, P., Potter, H., et al. (2002). A randomized controlled trial of exercise and manipulative therapy for cervicogenic headache. *Spine (Phila Pa 1976), 27*(17), 1835–1843; discussion 1843.

Oelsen, J., Bendtsen, L., Goadsby, P., et al. (2018). The International Classification of Headache Disorders (3rd edition) *Cephalgia* (38, pp. 1–211)

Posadzki, P., & Ernst, E. (2011). Spinal manipulations for cervicogenic headaches: a systematic review of randomized clinical trials. *Headache, 51*(7), 1132–1139.

Racicki, S., Gerwin, S., Diclaudio, S., Reinmann, S., & Donaldson, M. (2013). Conservative physical therapy management for the treatment of cervicogenic headache: a systematic review. *Journal of Manual and Manipulative Therapy, 21*(2), 113–124.

Rubio-Ochoa, J., Benítez-Martínez, J., Lluch, E., Santacruz-Zaragozá, S., Gómez-Contreras, P., & Cook, C. E. (2016). Physical examination tests for screening and diagnosis of cervicogenic headache: a systematic review. *Manual Therapy, 21*, 35–40.

Simons, D. G., Travell, J. G., & Simons, L. S. (1999). *Myofascial pain and dysfunction: the trigger point manual:* (vol 1). Lippincott Williams & Wilkins.

Sjaastad, O., Fredriksen, T. A., & Pfaffenrath, V. (1998). Cervicogenic headache: diagnostic criteria. The Cervicogenic Headache International Study Group. *Headache, 38*(6), 442–445.

Stanton, W. R., & Jull, G. A. (2003). Cervicogenic headache: locus of control and success of treatment. *Headache, 43*(9), 956–961.

Stovner, L., Hagen, K., Jensen, R., et al. (2007). The global burden of headache: a documentation of headache prevalence and disability worldwide. *Cephalalgia, 27*(3), 193–210.

CHAPTER 26 QUESTIONS

1. Which structure does not interact with the trigeminocervical nucleus?
   a. Cranial nerve III
   b. Cranial nerve V
   c. Cranial nerve VII
   d. Cranial nerve IX

2. Which muscle can refer pain to the head?
   a. Levator scapula
   b. Rhomboid major
   c. Anterior scalene
   d. Upper trapezius

3. Which headache disorder presents with nausea?
   a. CGH
   b. Migraine
   c. Tension
   d. Occipital Neuralgia

THE NEUROSCIENCE OF PAIN AND TREATMENT

D. Rico, PT, DPT and N. Maiers, PT

1. **What is the definition of pain?**

   The International Association for the Study of Pain recently published an updated definition of pain. The updated definition describes pain as an unpleasant sensory and emotional experience associated with or resembling that associated with actual or potential tissue damage.

   Alternatively, pain has been described as an output of the brain that is produced whenever the brain concludes that body tissue is in danger and action is required.

2. **Are nociception and pain the same?**

   No. Pain and nociception are different phenomena. Nociception is a result of the activation of sensory neurons in response to noxious-level mechanical, thermal, or chemical stimuli. Nociception is an input whereas pain is considered an output of the brain.

3. **Which areas of the brain are involved in the experience of pain?**

   Several areas of the brain play a role in processing an experience of pain. When occupied by processing pain, these areas may struggle to execute their other functions.
   - Premotor/motor cortex (organize and prepare movements)
   - Cingulate cortex (concentration, focus)
   - The prefrontal cortex (problem-solving, memory)
   - Amygdala (fear, addiction)
   - Sensory cortex (sensory discrimination)
   - Hypothalamus/thalamus (stress response, autonomic regulation, motivation)
   - Cerebellum (movement, cognition)
   - Hippocampus (memory, spatial recognition, fear conditioning)

4. **What is a neuromatrix and how does it relate to pain?**

   The collective activation within the various regions of the brain during an experience of pain represents an individual's pain neuromatrix. Cognitive, sensory, and affective regions of the brain work together to determine the perception of threat and if any behavioral response would be beneficial given the unique circumstances.

   For example, imagine you are stepping off the edge of a curb to walk across the street and you catch your toe and sprain your ankle. Most of the time this would result in the experience of pain as sensory signaling from the periphery would be interpreted by the brain indicating the potential for tissue damage in the ankle.

   Now imagine you are stepping off the edge of a curb to walk across the street, you catch your toe and sprain your ankle, but out of the corner of your eye you see a bus speeding toward you. Will the ankle hurt?

   Within that moment, a neuromatrix representing a variety of regions of the brain will be activated to determine which is a greater threat, ankle sprain or speeding bus. Most likely, the greater threat will be determined to be the speeding bus, so instead of producing pain to bring your awareness to the ankle, your neuromatrix will opt for the behavioral response of running out of the way of the bus.

   Once the perceived threat of the bus is removed, it's quite reasonable that the ankle will begin to hurt.

   In even the simplest experiences of pain, complex networks of the brain are being activated to determine the most optimal response.

5. **Which factors influence the experience of pain?**

   Many factors can influence the experience of pain. The primary domains contributing to the experience of pain are nociceptive input, peripheral neuropathy, central nociplastic change, emotional dysregulation, maladaptive cognitions, socio-environmental context, and sensorimotor disintegration.

6. **What are the three primary classifications of pain?**
   - Nociceptive dominant—pain associated with activation of nociceptors due to actual or threatened damage to nonneural tissues.
   - Peripheral neurogenic dominant—pain associated with a lesion or disease of the peripheral nervous system.
   - Central sensitization dominant—pain associated with increased responsiveness of normal and subthreshold afferent input within the central nervous system.

7. **What are the subjective and objective characteristics of nociceptive dominant pain?**
   Patients with the following signs and symptoms are considered 100x more likely to have a predominantly nociceptive mechanism of pain.
   Subjective:
   - Intermittent, sharp pain with aggravation
   - Dull ache or throbbing at rest
   - Mechanical nature to aggravating/easing factors
   - Pain proportional to injury/pathology
   - Pain localized to area of injury/pathology
   - Resolves in accordance with expected tissue healing times
   - Pain of recent onset

   Objective:
   - Clear, consistent, and proportionate mechanical/anatomical pattern of pain reproduction on movement or mechanical testing of target tissues
   - Localized pain on palpation
   - Absence of hyperalgesia or allodynia
   - Pain-relieving postures or movement patterns

   Example diagnoses commonly associated with nociceptive dominant pain
   - Muscle and ligament sprains
   - Fractures
   - Acute inflammatory conditions
   - Postsurgical
   - Repetitive overuse injuries

8. **What are the subjective and objective characteristics of peripheral neurogenic dominant pain?**
   Patients with the following signs and symptoms are considered 150x more likely to have a predominantly peripheral neuropathic mechanism of pain.
   Subjective:
   - Burning, shooting, sharp, or electric shock-like pain
   - History of nerve injury or pathology
   - Neurological symptoms (numbness, weakness, pins and needles)
   - Less responsive to simple analgesics, more responsive to antiepileptics/antidepressants
   - Severe and irritable pain
   - Mechanical pattern associated with loading/compression of neural tissue
   - Reports of spontaneous pain

   Objective:
   - Symptom provocation with tests that move/load/compress neural tissue (eg, neurodynamic tests—SLR)
   - Pain with palpation of neural tissues
   - Positive neurological findings (altered reflexes/sensation in a dermatomal distribution)
   - Hyperalgesia and/or allodynia

   Example diagnoses commonly associated with peripheral neurogenic dominant pain:
   - Cervical radiculopathy
   - Lumbar radiculopathy
   - Postherpetic neuralgia
   - Diabetic polyneuropathy
   - Peripheral nerve lesion

9. **What are the subjective and objective characteristics of central sensitization dominant pain?**
   Patients with the following signs and symptoms are considered 486x more likely to have a predominantly central sensitization mechanism of pain.
   Subjective:
   - Severe, irritable, unremitting pain disproportionate to the nature of the initial injury
   - Pain persists beyond expected tissue healing times
   - Widespread, nonanatomical pain distribution
   - Multiple, nonspecific aggravating/easing factors that are nonmechanical
   - Neurological type symptoms (burning, numbness, pins, and needles)
   - Sensitivity to sound, smell, hot, cold, or light touch
   - Association with psychosocial factors, maladaptive pain behaviors, and disturbed sleep

Objective:
- Disproportionate, inconsistent, nonmechanical pattern of pain provocation
- Hyperalgesia and allodynia
- Diffuse, nonanatomic areas of pain on palpation
- Positive identification of psychosocial factors (catastrophizing, fear avoidance, distress)

Example diagnoses commonly associated with central sensitization dominant pain:
- Chronic low back pain
- Chronic whiplash associated disorder
- Fibromyalgia
- Chronic headache
- Chronic fatigue syndrome

10. Which biological processes contribute to central sensitization?

Several biological processes play a role in the development of central sensitization. The persistent firing of C-fibers from the periphery, such as that which can occur from unresolved inflammation, can create a caustic environment in the dorsal horn of the spinal cord. This can result in the death of inhibitory interneurons at the spinal cord which decreases gating from the periphery. The development of C-fiber retraction and A-fiber infiltration at spinal levels contribute to allodynia. Upregulation of second-order neurons results in increased firing toward the brain. Synapsing from other spinal levels contributes to the experience of spreading and mirror pains. Decreased endogenous mechanisms can contribute to hyperalgesia and allodynia.

11. Which cognitions have a strong association with the persistence of pain?

Fear and catastrophization are two key cognitions related to the persistence of pain. Fear is defined as a distressing negative sensation induced by a perceived threat. Catastrophization is defined as the inability to foresee anything other than the worst possible outcome, however unlikely. The fear-avoidance model of pain presents the association between maladaptive cognitions and the persistence of pain. (See the figure below.)

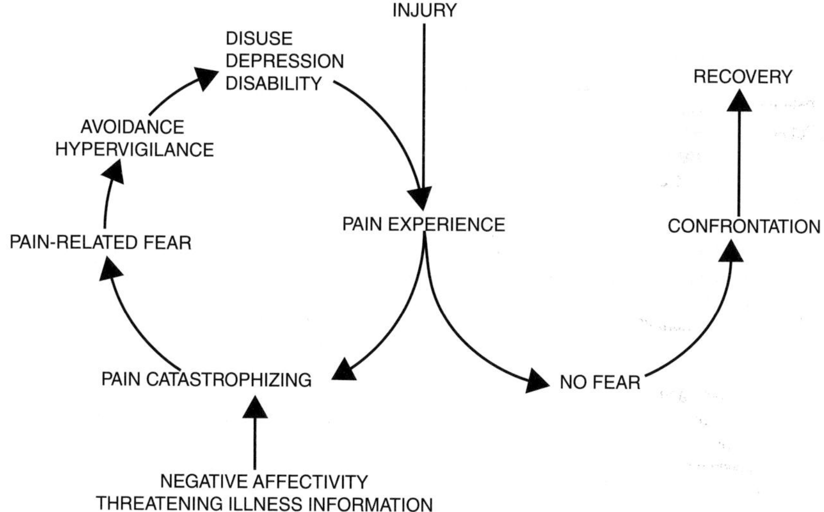

12. What other factors strongly influence someone's pain?

The environment and context in which an individual experiences pain have a significant influence on the experience of pain. Generally, the more stress a person is experiencing the more likely they will experience pain, for example, a car accident and whiplash-associated disorder. In addition to environmental and contextual factors, high severity acute pain can contribute to the development of chronic pain. The mature organism model presents the relationship between inputs and outputs associated with the experience of pain. (See the Figure below.)

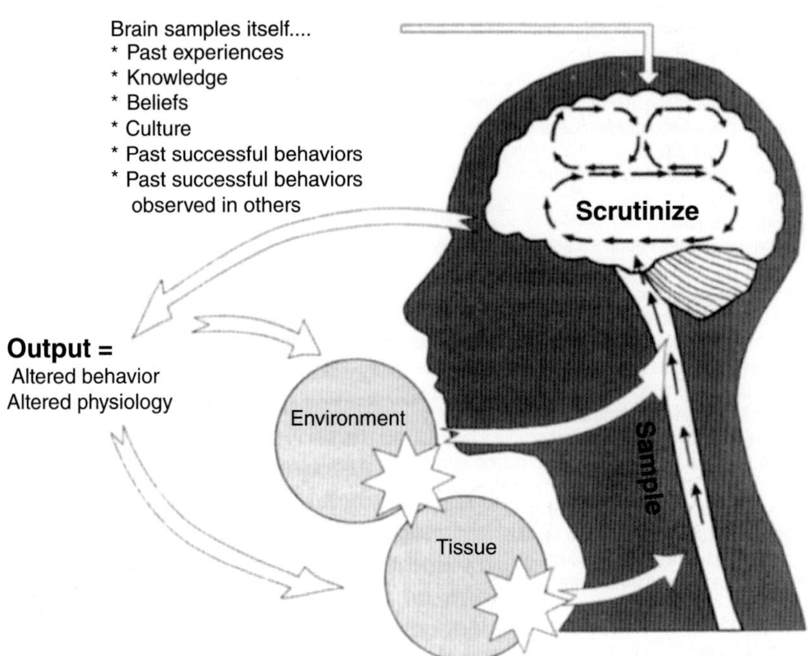

13. What are the four main pillars traditionally used to treat chronic pain without interventional medicine?

1. Pain neuroscience education
2. Patient goal setting
3. Improving sleep quality
4. Movement/aerobic exercise

14. What is pain neuroscience education (PNE)?

The first pain education study was published in 2002 by Lorimer Moseley. Over the last 20 years, a growing body of strong evidence shows PNE is effective at improving kinesiophobia, decreasing pain catastrophization, and helping the patient develop more active coping strategies. PNE has also been shown to be effective in improving function and movement as well as decreasing health care costs through improving a patient's self-efficacy through self-limiting the number of health care visits. While the majority of the research has focused on chronic pain, this treatment strategy is shown to be effective at reducing fear and catastrophization during preoperative education and with acute pain.

PNE reconceptualizes a patient's understanding of their pain experience. There are various names in the literature referring to PNE: therapeutic neuroscience education (TNE), explain pain, pain biology education, and pain neurophysiology education. While many people believe their pain is solely due to biomechanical causes, PNE teaches the patient to have a deeper biopsychosocial understanding of their pain. Research has shown PNE is most effective when combined with another therapy. Examples include but are not limited to movement, aerobic exercise, manual therapy, and meditation. Pain education uses metaphors and nonthreatening language to deemphasize biomechanical causes for someone's pain while emphasizing the neurophysiology and biology of pain.

15. Why is patient goal setting so important in treating chronic pain?

Many patients who suffer from chronic pain are controlled and limited by their pain. Their goal is to get rid of their pain before engaging in movement or exercise. Having patients explore what is meaningful to them and what would they like to do again despite the pain helps the patient shift the focus from pain reduction toward meaningful function.

Patient-centered goals are created by the patient and based on what the patient would like to do again/do better if they did not have pain. Patient-centered goals usually require guidance from the physical therapist. Having patients think about and write their own goals gives insight into what is important to the patient, allowing for a more cognitive-targeted progression of exercises.

An example of this would be that a patient reports they would like to play with their grandchildren on the floor. The therapist and patient collectively come up with the long-term patient-centered goal: "I will be able to sit down on the floor and play with my grandchildren for 30 minutes in 2 months." Short-term patient-centered goal: "I will be able to sit on the floor for 3 minutes without a flare in my symptoms."

The other significant objective here is to help the patient experience success. As the patient experiences functional progress through achieving their short-term goals it will also improve their self-efficacy.

16. **Why is improving the sleep quality so important in treating chronic pain?**
Sleep deprivation increases the sensitivity of the nervous system, impairs the endogenous opioid system, and induces low-grade inflammation. We know that pain can disrupt sleep but poor sleep can also increase the pain experience. Nearly 90% of people who suffer from chronic pain have insomnia. As a part of the therapist's intake, asking a patient how quickly they fall asleep, how many hours they sleep, and if they wake during the night can be used to screen for insomnia. The Insomnia Severity Index is a useful screening tool to help the therapist understand the patient's quality of sleep. Encouraging good sleep hygiene, cognitive-behavioral therapy (CBT), teaching relaxation techniques, and tracking daily sleep patterns are effective treatments to improve sleep. Sleep hygiene is a series of behavioral practices to help a person sleep. The two most effective practices are maintaining a consistent bedtime and wake time and reserving the bedroom for sleeping and sexual activity. Other sleep hygiene practices include refraining from stimulants (ie, caffeine or nicotine), refraining from drinking alcohol, limiting or avoiding napping during the day, and avoiding the consumption of large amounts of food and beverages, particularly spicy food, 2 to 4 hours before bedtime.

17. **Why are movement and aerobic exercise so important in treating chronic pain?**
Exercise-induced hypoalgesia (reduction in pain sensitivity) can occur with moderate aerobic and submaximal isometric and/or resistance exercise. Exercise promotes descending inhibition and other inhibitory mechanisms acting on the nervous system. When combined with PNE, which addresses patient fears and catastrophizing regarding exercise, movement becomes a powerful tool to treat pain. Ask the patient about their thoughts on the exercise prescribed; do they feel it would help them or hurt them? Then specifically address the patient's concerns about the prescribed exercise and teach them the effects of exercise on pain.

18. **How should a therapist prescribe exercise to reduce pain?**
Graded exposure and graded activity approaches have both been shown to be effective at improving function and pain. These approaches teach the patient it is not the movement that is causing the pain but a maladaptive nervous system. Many patients with chronic pain tend to overdo (boom-bust) or underdo (if it hurts, don't do it) activity. For example, a typical boom-bust cycle may be on days they feel relatively good, they try and get everything done they can before the pain increases (boom). Later, they are exhausted, hurt more, and regret what they had done earlier (bust). They train their nervous system to become more sensitive to movement. The next time they feel relatively good, the nervous system busts with less activity (cannot do as much as the last time) and with more pain. Other patients will under do activity. They never move enough to improve their functional movement or quality of life. Usually out of fear, these patients will stay away from activities they believe will flare their symptoms. As a result, they never train their nervous system to become less sensitive. Graded exposure retrains the nervous system through repeated exposure by breaking activities into smaller portions and gradually pushing into a patient's discomfort.

19. **How does language impact pain?**
Fear-provoking language has been shown to have a nocebo effect on people and can increase a pain experience. For example, in a sham headache-inducing study, 53% of the subjects reported a headache when they were told they may experience a headache. Clinicians should avoid language that increases threat levels in patients experiencing pain. The use of words such as "rip," "rupture," "torn," "wear and tear," "degeneration," or sayings such as "that looks bad" or "you have an instability" have been found to increase a patient's level of anxiety and pain. Even using the word "pain" or warning someone of pain, such as, "you may hurt later," increases someone's pain experience and anxiety levels. Conversely, positive framing of movement and avoiding biomechanical explanations of why someone hurts can have significant positive effects on a person's clinical outcome and pain levels.

20. **What are common screening tools and outcome measures utilized to measure pain?**
There are many tools in research and in clinical practice to help establish a patient's pain level, psychosocial aspects, and function. The following is an abbreviated list of measures validated for objectifying the various biopsychosocial aspects of an individual's pain experience.
    a. NPRS (Numeric Pain Rating Scale)—0–10 rating. Zero (meaning no pain) and ten (meaning the worst possible pain). This is arguably the most commonly utilized way of measuring a person's pain.
    b. Fear-avoidance Beliefs Questionnaire (FABQ), Tampa Scale of Kinesiophobia (TSK), and the Pain Catastrophization Scale (PCS)—all measure a person's level of fear and their pain.
    c. PROMIS—Patient-Reported Outcomes Measurement Information System from the U.S. Department of Health and Human Services measures physical, mental, and social aspects of pain.

d. Patient Health Questionnaires (PHQ-2 or PHQ-9)—either a 2 or 9 question form addressing the presence of depression since many patients who have chronic pain suffer from depression. A PHQ-2 score of 2 or higher and/or a PHQ-9 score of 10 or higher indicates the presence of depression.
e. Neck Disability Index (NDI), Oswestry Disability Index (ODI), Disabilities of the Arm, Shoulder and Hand (DASH), Lower Extremity Functional Scale (LEFS)—all measure a patient's function specific to the area of pain and self-perceived level of improvement.
f. Global Rating of Change (GROC) is a self-report scale of the individual's perceived level of improvement.

Bibliography

Gifford, L. (1998). Pain, the tissues and the nervous system. *Physiotherapy, 84*(1), 27–36.

Levis, B., Sun, Y., He, C., et al. (2020). Accuracy of the PHQ-2 alone and in combination with the PHQ-9 for screening to detect major depression: systematic review and meta-analysis. *JAMA, 323*(22), 2290–2300.

Louw, A., Zimney, K., Puentedura, E. J., & Diener, I. (2016). The efficacy of pain neuroscience education on musculoskeletal pain: a systematic review of the literature. *Physiotherapy: Theory and Practice, 32*(5), 332–355.

Mairesse, O., Neu, D., Cagnie, B., et al. (2018). Sleep disturbances in chronic pain: neurobiology, assessment, and treatment in physical therapist practice. *Physical Therapy, 98*(5), 1–11.

Moseley, G. L. (2003). A pain neuromatrix approach to patients with chronic pain. *Manual Therapy, 8*(3), 130–140.

Nijs, J., Lahousse, A., Kapreli, E., et al. (2021). Nociplastic pain criteria or recognition of central sensitization? Pain phenotyping in the past, present and future. *Journal of Clinical Medicine, 10*(15), 3203.

Nijs, J., Lluch Girbés, E., Lundberg, M., Malfliet, A., & Sterling, M. (2015). Exercise therapy for chronic musculoskeletal pain: innovation by altering pain memories. *Manual Therapy, 20*(1), 216–220.

Nijs, J., Wijma, A. J., Willaert, W., et al. (2020). Integrating motivational interviewing in pain neuroscience education for people with chronic pain: a practical guide for clinicians. *Physical Therapy, 100*(5), 846–859.

Perl, E. R. (1996). Cutaneous polymodal receptors: characteristics and plasticity. *Progress in Brain Research, 113*, 21–37.

Puentedura, E. J., & Louw, A. (2012). A neuroscience approach to managing athletes with low back pain. *Physical Therapy in Sport, 13*(3), 123–133.

Raja, S. N., Carr, D. B., Cohen, M., et al. (2020). The revised International Association for the Study of Pain definition of pain: concepts, challenges, and compromises. *Pain, 161*(9), 1976–1982.

Smart, K. M., Blake, C., Staines, A., Thacker, M., & Doody, C. (2012). Mechanisms-based classifications of musculoskeletal pain: Part 1 of 3: Symptoms and signs of central sensitisation in patients with low back (+/– leg) pain. *Manual Therapy, 17*, 336–344.

Smart, K. M., Blake, C., Staines, A., Thacker, M., & Doody, C. (2012). Mechanisms-based classifications of musculoskeletal pain: Part 2 of 3: Symptoms and signs of peripheral neuropathic pain in patients with low back (+/– leg) pain. *Manual Therapy, 17*, 345–351.

Smart, K. M., Blake, C., Staines, A., Thacker, M., & Doody, C. (2012). Mechanisms-based classifications of musculoskeletal pain: Part 3 of 3: Symptoms and signs of nociceptive pain in patients with low back (+/– leg) pain. *Manual Therapy, 17*, 352–357.

Stewart, M., & Loftus, S. (2018). Sticks and stones: the impact of language in musculoskeletal rehabilitation. *Journal of Orthopaedic & Sports Physical Therapy, 48*(7), 519–522.

Sullivan, M. J. L. (2009). *The pain catastrophizing scale.* Montreal, Quebec.

Vlaeyen, J. W. S., Crombez, G., & Linton, S. J. (2016). The fear-avoidance model of pain. *Pain, 157*(8), 1588–1589.

Walton, D. M., & Elliott, J. M. (2018). A new clinical model for facilitating the development of pattern recognition skills in clinical pain assessment. *Musculoskeletal Science & Practice, 36*, 17–24.

CHAPTER 27 QUESTIONS

1. What are the three main classifications of pain?
   a. Nociceptive, neuropathic, and central sensitization
   b. Nociplastic, nociceptive, and central sensitization
   c. Acute, subacute, and chronic
   d. Maladaptive, trauma, and neuropathic

2. Which of the following is considered a pillar traditionally used for treating chronic pain?
   a. Mental health
   b. Sleep quality
   c. Physical strength
   d. Flexibility

2. Clinicians can increase someone's pain experience by _______
   a. Telling a patient they have a torn rotator cuff muscle
   b. Placing them in a warm environment
   c. Surrounding them with family members during treatment
   d. Having them perform submaximal isometric exercises

ANATOMY MNEMONICS

M.T. Bee, PhD and J.P. Owens, BAppSci (Sport Science)

1. **What is a mnemonic?**
   Named after Mnemosyne, the Greek goddess of memory, mnemonics simply means "memory aid." It is a learning device in which we relate a collection of hard facts to a known word, sequence of letters or numbers, or a rhyme in an effort to recall facts accurately and sequentially. Mnemonics can also be images, movements, or expressions. Mnemonics are also be correlated for higher recall scores during testing, retention of information, application of knowledge, and improved clinical reasoning.

2. **Can I make up my own mnemonics?**
   Yes. You have a poetic license to construct your own mnemonics based on things you encounter in your own life. You can improve the effectiveness of a mnemonic when you associate it with vivid colorful images, sounds, smells, humor, rude rhymes, and symbols.

3. **Should one SIT Still to learn the rotator cuff muscles?**
   Using the initials SIT S helps us remember the four rotator cuff muscles: supraspinatus, infraspinatus, teres minor, and subscapularis. Expanding on this, consider the phrase: "Great minds SIT Less Still." This helps us remember that muscles inserting into the GREATer tubercle (from superior to inferior) are the supraspinatus, infraspinatus, and teres minor. Inserting into the LESSer tubercle is the subscapularis muscle.

4. **What do beans, spinning, and IQ have to do with the sciatic foramina?**
   Consider both the greater and lesser sciatic foramina that are bounded by ligaments and sciatic notches on the hip bone. These two important openings allow for the passageway of many structures that are traveling between the pelvis and the lower limb. To help remember the multitude of structures passing through, consider these terms and phrases:
   - Passing through the lesser foramen is PINTO. This stands for Pudendal nerve, Internal pudendal vessels, Nerve to obturator internus and superior gemellus, and Tendon of Obturator internus.
   - Passing through the greater foramen is SPIN Pause SPIN.
     - SPIN stands for Superior gluteal vessels and nerve, Piriformis muscle, Inferior gluteal vessels and nerve, and the Nerve to obturator internus and superior gemellus.
     - "Pause" represents the Posterior femoral cutaneous nerve.
     - The second term SPIN: Sciatic nerve, Pudendal nerve, Internal pudendal vessels, and Nerve to quadratus femoris and inferior gemellus.
   - An additional acronym helps when remembering a subset of these structures. "POPS IQ" has initials for each of the nerves passing through the greater sciatic foramen and lying inferior to the piriformis muscle, namely: Posterior femoral cutaneous nerve, nerve to Obturator internus and superior gemellus, Pudendal nerve, Sciatic nerve, Inferior gluteal nerve, nerve to Quadratus femoris and inferior gemellus.

5. **How does a technological device remind us of the thoracoacromial trunk branches?**
   We are all familiar with an I-PAD, but let's consider a C-PAD. This mnemonic helps when remembering the branches of the thoracoacromial trunk. The thoracoacromial trunk, commonly referred to as the TA trunk, is the second branch of the axillary artery. It courses a short distance and gives off its four branches: Clavicular, Pectoral, Acromial, and Deltoid.

6. **What does B + B = A mean?**
   This formula describes the fact that, although there is a defined point where the axillary artery becomes the brachial artery (lower border of teres major), no such similar landmark exists at a point where the axillary vein begins. The origin and termination of blood vessels in a limb are always based on blood flow; therefore veins will begin distally and terminate proximally. Wherever the basilic vein (B) joins a brachial vein (B), the axillary vein (A) begins.

7. **How can the arrangement of structures in the cubital fossa be remembered?**
   This triangular fossa on the anterior surface of the elbow is bounded by the brachioradialis, pronator teres, and a line through the humeral epicondyles. Within this fossa from lateral to medial are TAN:
   - T—Tendon of biceps brachii as it inserts into the radius
   - A—Artery, specifically the termination of the brachial artery before it bifurcates into the radial and ulnar arteries
   - N—Nerve, the median nerve, which within the fossa gives rise to the anterior interosseous nerve

The direction from lateral to medial, if forgotten, is recalled easily because the tendon and artery are both palpable, and feeling them will indicate the direction. The most medial structure is the median nerve; this is a common site for stimulating the median nerve in nerve conduction studies relative to carpal tunnel syndrome.

8. **What is the area code for carpal country?**
The number ("area code") 921 reminds us of the carpal canal contents:
   - 9 tendons—four tendons from flexor digitorum profundus and four tendons from flexor digitorum superficialis, plus the single tendon from flexor pollicis longus.
   - 2 bursae—one large bursa called the ulnar bursa surrounds the eight digitorum tendons and is sometimes called the common synovial sheath. The smaller radial bursa surrounds only the flexor pollicis longus. Bursae are small fascial sacs elongated over tendons to minimize friction when the tendons slide.
   - 1 nerve—median nerve; this nerve is compressed in carpal tunnel syndrome.

9. **Is it true that a risqué mnemonic relates to the carpal bones?**
The mnemonic is:
   - Some Lovers Try Positions That They Can't Handle

   The carpal bones are arranged in two rows of four bones each.
   - In the proximal row, from lateral to medial they are: Scaphoid, Lunate, Triquetrum (or triangular), Pisiform.
   - In the distal row, from lateral to medial they are: Trapezium, Trapezoid, Capitate, Hamate.
     - It's also helpful to remember the rhyme that: "By the thumb, is the trapezium."

10. **How can you remember the contents of the femoral triangle?**
To remember the contents of the femoral triangle and the orientation use NAVEL. Starting from medial to lateral, the femoral triangle contents consist of a femoral Nerve, femoral Artery, femoral Vein, Empty space, and Lymph nodes.

11. **How can you remember the spinal nerve root innervation for the pelvic floor?**
S2, S3, and S4 keep pee and poop off the floor. The pudendal nerve is also supplied by the spinal nerve roots S2–S4.

12. **Is LARP a radio station in California?**
LARP refers to the twisting of the right and left vagus nerves as they course onto the esophagus after passing the heart. The anterior and posterior vagal trunks come from the left and right vagus nerves, respectively. Thus LARP, or Left Anterior Right Posterior, refers to the fact that the left vagus nerve primarily forms the anterior vagal trunk, while that right vagus nerve primarily forms the posterior vagal trunk.

13. **What does the formula S + S = P mean?**
The large portal vein that carries nutrient-rich blood from the intestines to the liver is formed by two veins that both begin with "S." Hence this formula states that when the splenic vein joins the superior mesenteric vein, the portal vein is formed.

14. **How does the spelling of the word SCALP help us understand its layers?**
SCALP can be used to remember the scalp's five layers, which from superficial to deep are:
   - Skin—covered with hairs, with follicles that extend to deeper layers.
   - Close subcutaneous tissue—called "close" because of its tightness and the fact that it binds skin to the aponeurosis.
   - Aponeurosis, specifically the galea aponeurotica—a flat tendon between the frontalis muscle in the forehead and the occipitalis muscle posteriorly (the term epicranius can be used for this entire layer).
   - Loose subaponeurotic layer—layer of loose connective tissue that allows for the first three layers to move as a group. It is also called the "dangerous layer" because infections can spread through it.
   - Pericranium—the periosteum on the outside of the cranial bone.

15. **Is there an easy way to remember the terminal branches of the facial nerve?**
Two Zebras Bit My Chin. The five terminal branches of the facial nerve originate from the facial plexus embedded within the parotid gland:
   - Temporal—to muscles of the eye and forehead
   - Zygomatic—to muscles of the eye and upper lip
   - Buccal—to muscles of the cheek and upper lip
   - Marginal mandibular—to muscles of the lower lip
   - Cervical—to the neck muscle, platysma

16. **What can help me remember the cranial nerves?**
Oh, Oh, Oh, To Touch And Feel Very Good Velvet, AH! This is a classic mnemonic for the 12 cranial nerves. Here are roman numerals, names, and the general function of each nerve:
I. Olfactory, sensory to the nasal mucosa as smell
II. Optic, sensory to the eye as vision
III. Oculomotor, motor to the eye
IV. Trochlear, motor to the superior oblique muscle
V. Trigeminal, both sensory to the head through its three divisions (ophthalmic, maxillary, and mandibular) and motor to the muscles of mastication
VI. Abducent, motor to the lateral rectus muscle
VII. Facial, both motor to the muscles of facial expression and sensory for tongue, in addition to parasympathetic to the head
VIII. Vestibulocochlear (or auditory or acoustic), sensory for balance and hearing
IX. Glossopharyngeal, both sensory to the tongue and motor to the stylopharyngeus
X. Vagus, both sensory and motor, as well as parasympathetic to head, neck, thorax, and abdomen
XI. Accessory (or spinal accessory), motor to trapezius and sternocleidomastoid muscles
XII. Hypoglossal, motor to the tongue

Regarding fiber content, the 12 cranial nerves follow the saying, with S = sensory, M = motor, and B = both sensory and motor (again, the capital letters are the 12 nerves in sequence): Some Say Marry Money, But My Brother Says Big Brains Matter More (Some—Olfactory-Sensory, Says—Optic-Sensory, Marry—Oculomotor-Motor, etc.).

17. **What is the formula for remembering the nerve supply to the seven muscles of the orbit?**
The formula for cranial nerve supply to the muscles that move the eyeball is: LR6(SO4)3

The lateral rectus (LR) is supplied by CN VI—abducens; the superior oblique (SO) by CN IV—trochlear; and the remaining five muscles (superior rectus, medial rectus, inferior rectus, inferior oblique, and levator labii superioris) by CN III—oculomotor.

18. **Are there any slick mnemonics for the back muscles?**
Not slick, but SLIC. The largest deep back muscle that is concerned with posture is termed the erector spinae or sacrospinalis. This muscle consists of three longitudinal columns of muscle that, from medial to lateral, are the Spinalis, Longissimus, and IlioCostalis. Or another one is (from lateral to medial) "I Like Spaghetti," IlioCostalis, Longissimus, and Spinalis.

19. **Is poetry ever used to assist in the recall of anatomic facts?**
On occasion, mnemonics can be in the form of poems. The intervertebral discs that separate vertebral bodies help bind the vertebral canal as well. Each disc consists of the outer, tough fibrous annulus fibrosus and the inner, semigelatinous nucleus pulposus. Hence the poem:
Said the nucleus pulposus to the annulus fibrosus,
"Why do you hold me so tight?"
"If I didn't, you would fall into the vertebral canal,
And then you would be out of sight."

20. **What does the phrase "say grace before tea" stand for?**
The pes anserina ("foot of the goose") on the medial side of the knee is formed by three tendons that insert from anterior to posterior in this order: sartorius, gracilis, and semitendinosus. This arrangement can be recalled by the letters in the mnemonic Say Grace before Tea for Sartorius, Gracilis, and semiTendinosus. That is the order in which they insert proximally to distally as well as superficial to deep. "Before" reminds us that there is a bursa situated deep to the pes anserina and can be upset by muscle imbalances or direct trauma to the area.

21. **Who are Tom, Dick, and A Very Nervous Harry?**
On the medial side of the ankle lies the flexor retinaculum, which with the tarsal bones form the tarsal tunnel. Through this tunnel will pass three tendons (tibialis posterior, flexor digitorum longus, and the flexor hallucis longus), vessels (posterior tibial artery and veins) and a nerve (tibial nerve). The order of these structures can be recalled by the phrase "Tom, Dick, and A Very Nervous Harry." The association from anterior to posterior is Tibialis posterior, flexor Digitorum longus, posterior tibial Artery and Vein, tibial Nerve, and flexor Hallucis longus, respectively.

22. **What are the major branches of the brachial plexus from lateral to medial? Remember, "MAR-MU."**
- Musculocutaneous
- Axillary

- Radial
- Median
- Ulnar

23. **What nerve roots comprise the long thoracic nerve that innervates the serratus anterior?**
SALT 57 (Serratus Anterior Long Thoracic C5–C7). Or C5, C6, C7 raise your arms to heaven. A patient with damage to the long thoracic nerve may present with winged scapula and difficulty raising the upper limb on the affected side above the horizontal plane.

24. **What nerve roots comprise the thoracodorsal nerve that innervates the latissimus dorsi?**
TOUCH DOWN 68 (Thoracodorsal C6–C8).

25. **What is the innervation of the pectoral muscles? Remember, "lateral is less and medial is more."**
The lateral pectoral nerve innervates the pectoralis major only, and the medial pectoral nerve innervates both the pectoralis major and pectoralis minor, thus "lateral is less and medial is more." Remember, these are named for the cord of the brachial plexus from which they are derived.

26. **How do you remember the actions that peroneal (fibular) and tibial nerve injury drive? Remember "PED and TIP."**
   - PED - **P**eroneal (Fibular)—**E**verts and **D**orsiflexes; loss = foot drop
   - TIP - **T**ibial—**I**nverts and **P**lantar flexes; loss = cannot walk on TIP toes

27. **What is the relationship of the suprascapular artery and nerve at the suprascapular notch?**
The suprascapular notch lies on the superior surface of the scapula. Connecting both edges of the notch is the transverse scapular ligament, that appears like a bridge. To help remember the structures that pass over and under the ligament, we consider our armed forces. The Army (artery) travels over the bridge, while the Navy (nerve) travels under.

28. **What is a refreshing way to remember the formation of the brachial plexus?**
Real Therapists Drink Cold Beer.
This phrase corresponds with Rami, Trunks, Divisions, Cords, Branches.
Rami:
Ventral rami of C5, C6, C7, C8, and T1 contribute to the brachial plexus.
Trunks:
C5 and C6 join to form the upper trunk.
C7 stays by itself and forms the middle trunk.
C8 and T1 come together and form the lower trunk.
Divisions:
Each of the three trunks gives off an anterior and posterior division.
Anterior division of the upper trunk and the anterior division of the middle trunk form the lateral cord.
Posterior divisions of all trunks form the posterior cord.
Anterior division of the lower trunk continues and forms the medial cord.
Cords:
The lateral, posterior, and medial cords are named in relationship to the axillary artery.
For example, the posterior cord is located posterior to the axillary artery.
Branches:
Branches of the brachial plexus are classified as supraclavicular and infraclavicular.
Supraclavicular branches arise off the roots and trunks.
Infraclavicular branches arise off the cords.

29. **Who is hungry for a triple decker adductor sandwich?**
The triple decker adductor sandwich reminds us about the arrangement of the three adductor muscles and the two nerve branches passing between them in the medial thigh. Just like two layers of turkey between three slices of bread in a sandwich, the two branches of the obturator course between three of the adductor muscles. The obturator nerve divides into anterior and posterior branches proximal to the obturator foramen that course between the adductor muscles in the following order, anterior to posterior:
Adductor Longus—most superficial muscle
Anterior branch of obturator nerve
Adductor Brevis—middle muscle
Posterior branch of obturator nerve
Adductor Magnus—deepest muscle

30. **Remember the actions of palmar and dorsal interossei of the hand and foot.**
    Palmar interossei ADDuct = PAD
    Dorsal interossei ABDuct = DAB

31. **Feeling lost (or LeST) learning the superficial muscles in the upper back?**
    There are five superficial back muscles: trapezius, latissimus dorsi, levator scapula, rhomboid major, and rhomboid minor. All of these originate from the spinous processes, except for one: levator scapula. If we consider the word LeST, it helps us remember that the Levator Scapula originates from the Transverse processes. Specifically, it arises from the transverse processes of cervical vertebrae 1–4.

32. **Remember Achilles only had one weak spot.**
    S1 is the level that is tested with an Achilles tendon reflex test.

33. **What is the military saying for shoulder muscles?**
    "Lady between two majors." "Lady" is actually "lati" because we are referring to latissimus dorsi. The majors are pectoralis major and teres major muscles. The proximal end of the humerus presents crests for its two tubercles, the greater and lesser. Inserting onto the crest of the greater tubercle is the pectoralis major. Inserting onto the crest of the lesser tubercle is the teres major. Latissimus dorsi inserts into the intertubercular groove between the two tubercles and their crests, hence "lady" (lati) between two majors–one lady inserting into the depression, between two majors. The depression is named the bicipital groove or intertubercular sulcus.

34. **Why would one DAP the meninges?**
    DAP reminds us of the meninges that surround the brain and spinal cord. From external to internal, they are the Dura mater, Arachnoid, and Pia mater. Don't forget that the term "mater" not matter, means "mother" and "dura" means "tough" so this outermost meninx (singular for meninges) is translated to be the "tough mother."

BIBLIOGRAPHY

Amey, L., Donald, K. J., & Teodorczuk, A. (2017). Teaching clinical reasoning to medical students. *British Journal of Hospital Medicine*, *78*(7), 399–401.

Mackler, H. (1955). Mnemonics in physical therapy. *Physical Therapy Reviews*, *35*(3), 135.

Meyer, A. J., Armson, A., Losco, C. D., et al. (2015). Factors influencing student performance on the carpal bone test as a preliminary evaluation of anatomical knowledge retention. *Anatomical Sciences Education*, *8*(2), 133–139.

Stalder, D.R. (2005). Learning and motivational benefits of acronym use in introductory psychology. *Teaching of Psychology*, 32(4), 222–228. https://doi.org/10.1207/s15328023top3204_3

Putnam, A. L. (2015). Mnemonics in education: Current research and applications. *Translational Issues in Psychological Science*, *1*(2), 130–139.

Thompson, M., Johansen, D., Stoner, R., et al. (2017). Comparative effectiveness of a mnemonic-use approach vs. self-study to interpret a lateral chest X-ray. *Advances in Physiology Education*, *41*(4), 518–521.

CHAPTER 28 QUESTIONS

1. **What nerve roots innervate the serratus anterior?**
    a. C4, C5, C6
    b. C5, C6, C7
    c. C6, C7, C8
    d. C7, C8, T1

2. **What is the action of the palmar interossei?**
    a. Adduction
    b. Abduction
    c. Opposition
    d. Circumduction

3. **The spinal level evaluated by the Achilles reflex is?**
    a. L3
    b. L4
    c. L5
    d. S1

CHAPTER 29

NUTRITION

D. Burd, MEd, RD

1. What are the dietary guidelines for Americans?

Concerned by the escalating incidence of obesity and related health issues in the United States, the Department of Agriculture and the Department of Health and Human Services created a set of recommendations designed to promote general health. These recommendations may be applied to anyone in the general population. Adoption of these guidelines hopefully will improve overall health by promoting healthy body weight, reducing the incidence of type 2 diabetes, and reducing the risk of cardiovascular disease. Major guidelines include:

1. Follow a healthy dietary pattern at every stage of life
   - First 6 months
     Preferably breastfeed exclusively for the first 6 months of life. If breastfeeding is not an option, then iron-fortified formula should be given to the infant.
   - 6 months – 1 year
     Breast milk and/or iron-fortified formula should be continued. Nutrient-dense complementary foods should be introduced in reasonable portions. Foods known to cause allergies may also be introduced at this time.
   - 12 months through older adulthood
     A nutrient-dense diet should be selected to help meet nutrient needs, maintain a healthy body weight, and reduce the risk of chronic diseases.
2. Customize and enjoy nutrient-dense food and beverage choices to reflect personal preferences, cultural tradition, and budgetary considerations.
3. Focus on meeting food group needs with nutrient-dense foods and beverages, and stay within calorie limits. Food groups include
   - Vegetables—Choose colorful vegetables such as red, green, orange, or yellow. Starchy vegetables such as beans, potatoes, lentils, and corn are good options as well. Fresh, frozen, and many canned vegetables are healthy choices.
   - Fruit—Choose a variety of whole fruits. Frozen fruits and fruits canned in juice or water are good options.
   - Grains – Choose cereals (ie, oats), breads (ie, wheat), pasta, rice, beans, and starchy vegetables. Half of the grain servings should come from whole grain sources, daily.
   - Dairy—Choose low-fat or reduced-fat dairy products. Fortified, dairy-free alternatives are acceptable.
   - Protein—Choose lean meats as a protein source. Eggs, beans, lentils, seafood, nut seeds, and soy are acceptable alternatives.
   - Oils—Choose vegetable oils (corn, canola, soybean, safflower, or sunflower) as the primary fat source. Seafood and nuts may also be a healthy source of oil.
4. Limit foods and beverages higher in added sugars, saturated fat, and sodium, and limit alcoholic beverages.
   - Reduce sodium intake to less than 2300 mg/day (1 teaspoon) in children and adults.
   - Reduce intake of foods containing saturated fat to less than 10% of the total calorie intake per day in children over the age of two and adults.
   - Reduce added sugars to less than 10% of total calories/day in children over the age of 2 and adults. Sugar-sweetened beverages are high in simple sugar and should not be given to children under the age of 2.
   - If alcohol is consumed it should be consumed in moderation. Moderation defined as one alcoholic beverage for females and two alcoholic beverages for males per day.

2. Describe the Ornish low-fat diet. What does it claim to do?

The Ornish diet is a vegetarian (lacto-ovo) diet based mainly on vegetables, fruits, whole grains, and beans. No animal products are eaten except moderate amounts of egg whites and nonfat dairy. It consists of 10% fat, mainly polyunsaturated fat, and monounsaturated fat; 70% to 75% carbohydrates, mainly complex; 15% to 20% protein; and 5 mg cholesterol per day. According to Dr. Ornish, people lose weight on his diet for several reasons: (1) it takes more calories to metabolize complex carbohydrates than simple carbohydrates; (2) metabolic rate may increase on the diet; and (3) people consume fewer calories when eating complex carbohydrates because they are more filling. Meat and animal products contain protein, but they also contain saturated fats and cholesterol. Ornish claims that his diet is the most effective diet for lowering cholesterol, preventing heart disease, reducing symptoms of type 2 diabetes, and decreasing the risk of developing many cancers.

3. What are the possible problems that may result from being on a very low-fat diet?

Very low-fat diets (approximately 16 g fat, 10% of calories from fat) may lead to insufficient amounts of essential fatty acids. Individuals with low HDL, high triglyceride, and high insulin levels may have these abnormalities amplified with these types of diets. Some studies have found these diets to be low in vitamins E, B_{12}, and zinc, but these reports are inconsistent.

4. **Briefly describe the ketogenic (keto) diet. What does it claim to do?**
The keto diet was originally used to manage uncontrolled seizures in individuals with epilepsy. The keto diet is a modified version of the Atkins diet, which is traditionally a low-carbohydrate, high-protein, high-fat diet. The purpose of the diet is to switch the type of fuel your body uses. By limiting carbohydrates, the body is forced to use ketones that come from fat, thus promoting weight loss through ketosis. The most restrictive stage limits carbohydrate consumption to 20 grams per day with a maintenance goal of 45 grams of carbohydrate, 75 grams of protein, and 165 grams of fat per day. Most nutritionists recommend about 300 grams of carbohydrate/day. There is no differentiation in the keto diet between choosing leaner proteins versus high-fat proteins and heart-healthy (poly and monounsaturated) fats versus saturated fats. The diet does not restrict protein, fat, or calories, but many dieters have suppressed appetite due to ketosis and decrease their caloric intake, thus producing weight loss.

5. **According to most traditional nutritional professionals, why do high-protein and high-fat diets cause weight loss?**
Fewer calories are consumed on high-protein and high-fat diets because proteins and fats are more filling than simple carbohydrates. The fewer calories you consume, the more weight you lose. Much of the initial weight loss is from water loss from natriuresis. Additional water loss occurs when glycogen is converted to glucose. This conversion of glycogen to glucose must occur to maintain serum blood glucose levels. In subsequent weeks, weight loss is from body fat, at a rate of 1 to 2 lbs per week. This rate is similar to that obtained with other types of low-calorie diets.

6. **What are the possible side effects of a high-protein, high-fat diet?**
Some authors report few side effects of a high-protein, high-fat diet, although others report several significant side effects. The following side effects have been reported by some authors: High-protein, high-fat diets cause the liver and kidneys to work harder to metabolize and excrete excessive nitrogen. This may result in organ failure. Excessive water loss may result in dehydration and orthostatic hypotension. Dosage of certain medications may need to be adjusted to compensate for diuresis. There may be an increased risk of osteoporosis caused by calcium loss that occurs with excess water loss. Evidence suggests that high-protein/high saturated fat diets are associated with certain cancers and heart disease. There is an increased risk for micronutrient deficiencies such as selenium, magnesium, phosphorus, vitamin B complex, and vitamin C. Due to the low fiber content of the diet, constipation may become an issue. There is also the possibility of a lack of focus and mood swings due to limited glucose that is available to the brain. Endurance athletes may also experience difficulties due to the lowered glycogen stores.

7. **Is there a difference in the adherence rates between keto (Atkins), Ornish, and Weight Watchers?**
Not many studies have compared adherence rates of various diets. Dansinger et al. have shown no significant difference in the adherence rates of the more extreme keto and Ornish diets compared with the moderate Weight Watchers diet after 1 year, but that there was a trend toward better adherence in the moderate diet. The average adherence rate for all of the diets combined was only 58%. This rather low adherence rate is the major problem for lack of long-term success with all of these diets.

8. **When would the recommendation for bariatric surgery be appropriate?**
Bariatric surgery promotes rapid weight loss in individuals who have been unsuccessful in weight loss attempts and who are morbidly obese (body mass index [BMI] > 40). Individuals with a BMI of 35 or greater with comorbidities such as type 2 diabetes, hypertension, heart disease, or sleep apnea would also be candidates for surgery. The gastric bypass procedure entails stapling off the stomach to a one quarter cup pouch and attaching the jejunum to the pouch. The lap band procedure places a plastic ring around the stomach making it smaller. Two thirds of the stomach is surgically removed in the gastric sleeve procedure. In each case stomach capacity is significantly reduced, resulting in limited calorie intake. Weight loss may be significant during the first year after the surgery. Potential complications would include hernia risk, numerous vitamin and mineral deficiencies, and malnutrition due to malabsorption.

9. **What does a typical American diet consist of?**
A typical American diet consists of 35% fat, 50% carbohydrates, and 15% protein.

10. **What type of diet is most effective for long-term weight loss?**
There are widely varying opinions on which diet is most effective for long-term weight loss. Most scientifically controlled studies indicate diets that reduce caloric intake are most effective for long-term weight loss and body

fat reduction regardless of the macronutrient composition. Dansinger et al. found no significant difference in weight loss after 1 year between individuals on the Atkins (keto), Ornish, or Weight Watchers diets. Weight loss will occur if the number of calories consumed is less than the number of calories expended. For most people the caloric deficit should be about 1000 kcal per day. If physical activity is not increased a diet of approximately 1400–1500 kcal/day seems to be optimal.

11. **Why lower sodium intake?**
Research has shown that sodium consumption increases fluid retention in the body. This added fluid increases blood pressure resulting in damaged blood vessel walls. The damage promotes atherosclerosis leading to a heart attack or stroke. Recommended sodium intake is 1500 to 2300 mg/day. One teaspoon of salt contains 2300 mg of sodium. The average adult's consumption is well above the recommendation. Incorporating more fresh foods in the diet; eating out less often; not adding salt during cooking or at the table; and cutting back on processed foods will lower sodium intake.

12. **Does soy protein decrease the risk of developing cardiovascular disease?**
A meta-analysis concluded that consumption of soy protein in place of animal protein significantly lowers blood levels of total cholesterol, LDL, and triglycerides without affecting HDL. This is especially true in subjects with baseline cholesterol levels greater than 240 mg/dL. The FDA has approved labeling of food that contains greater than 6.25 g of soy protein per serving stating that these foods reduce the risk of heart disease, assuming an intake of 25 g of soy protein daily. The FDA further recommends at risk individuals also consume a diet that is low in saturated fat and cholesterol.

13. **Do antioxidant supplements decrease the risk of developing cardiovascular disease?**
There is insufficient evidence for recommending the use of antioxidant supplements for decreasing the risk of developing cardiovascular disease. A longitudinal study by Jun et al., in the *Journal of the American College of Cardiology*, published in 2020 indicates that consuming a diet containing antioxidants may decrease an individual's risk for cardiovascular disease. A diet high in antioxidants would include fruits and vegetables that are red, yellow, green, and blue in color as well as whole grains.

14. **Does folic acid, vitamin B6, and vitamin B12 decrease the risk of developing cardiovascular disease?**
Preliminary data in ongoing clinical trials indicate that vitamins B6, B12, and folic acid may reduce the risk of cardiovascular disease in those individuals with high homocysteine levels. The amino acid homocysteine is inflammatory, causing blood clots to form in heart vessels. The vitamins lower the homocysteine levels in the body, thus reducing inflammation and the risk for clots. Clinical trials are ongoing.

15. **Do omega-3 fatty acids alter mortality rate, incidence of cardiovascular events, or cancer?**
There has been debate over the past 20 plus years as to whether or not omega-3 fatty acid supplements reduce the risk of cardiac events. Most physicians encourage patients to eat a healthy diet and include dietary sources of omega-3 such as salmon or flax seed. Recent clinical trials have demonstrated a benefit of adding omega-3 fatty acid supplement daily, to reduce serum triglyceride values, the number of heart attacks, strokes, and stenting procedures.
Omega-3 fatty acids may also play a role in the management of a cancer diagnosis by reducing inflammation in those individuals who have developed cancer cachexia. There is ongoing research looking at the potential benefits of managing other cancer complications with omega-3 fatty acids.

16. **Do folate supplements decrease the incidence of neural tube defects?**
Yes, there is a significant reduction in the incidence of neural tube defects when folate supplements are taken before and during the first 2 months of pregnancy.

17. **Do folic acid supplements with or without vitamin B12 supplements improve cognitive function or mood?**
Although studies are limited, there is no evidence that folic acid with or without vitamin B_{12} improves cognitive function or mood in normal or cognitively impaired older adults. Folic acid with vitamin B_{12} has been shown to reduce serum levels of the amino acid homocysteine. Elevated homocysteine has been linked to an increased risk of developing dementia.

18. **What are the health benefits of adding fiber to the diet?**
There are two forms of fiber that provide significant health benefits when incorporated into the diet. The first, insoluble fiber, promotes bowel regularity. It keeps water in the colon thus reducing the risk of constipation and diverticulitis. Found in whole grains, bran, brown rice, and the peelings of fruit and vegetables, it initially creates a sense of fullness (satiety). Feeling full should reduce total caloric intake and insoluble fiber may facilitate the

weight loss process. The second, soluble fiber, promotes heart health by lowering cholesterol. The soluble fiber binds with dietary cholesterol in the gastrointestinal tract and it is eliminated through solid waste thus reducing serum cholesterol values. Found in oats, flax seed, and fresh, frozen, or canned fruit, it also creates a sense of satiety. It too may play a role in weight reduction. Adults should incorporate 25 to 38 g of fiber (soluble and insoluble) into their daily diet.

19. **Do calcium supplements increase bone density in postmenopausal women?**
Calcium supplements appear to increase bone density between 1.6% and 2%. There is a trend toward reduction in vertebral fractures associated with this increase, but the evidence is not clear regarding a reduction in nonvertebral fractures. It is always best to get calcium from dietary sources.

20. **A Mediterranean diet may be helpful in managing which medical condition?**
To promote heart health and reduce the risk of cardiovascular disease many health care providers recommend the Mediterranean diet. Consumption of fresh fruits, fresh vegetables, and whole grains is the centerpiece of the diet. Red meat and high-fat dairy are limited, but seafood is encouraged. Nuts are a daily source of protein and fat. Food preparation utilizes olive or canola oil along with spices in place of salt. Baking, broiling, and grilling are preferred cooking techniques. Red wine consumption, a component of the diet, has also demonstrated heart health benefits.
For the past several years the Mediterranean diet has been consistently recommended as the best diet to promote weight loss.

21. **How should the daily recommended percentages of carbohydrate, fat, and protein intake be altered during heavy training?**
In a training athlete, the percentage of carbohydrates should be higher (>50% of total calories), the percentage of fats should be lower, and the percentage of protein should be the same as for a sedentary person. Carbohydrates are the primary nutrient used during prolonged, moderate-to-high intensity exercise.

22. **Should athletes consume additional protein when they are in training?**
The current recommended daily allowance for protein in sedentary people is 0.8 gm protein/kg body weight per day. Several investigators have shown that athletes require more protein. Recommended amounts range from 1.2–1.8 gm/kg of body weight per day for aerobic and resistance training athletes. Vegetarians should consume 1.3–1.8 gm/kg of body weight/day. People just beginning an exercise program should use the upper end of this range. Because the average North American diet consists of 1.9 gm/kg per day, additional protein usually is not necessary.

23. **Does carbohydrate consumption affect the amount of muscle growth?**
Yes, carbohydrate consumption causes an increase in the release of insulin, which stimulates muscle synthesis. Testosterone levels, which also stimulate muscle synthesis, appear to be highest when the ratio of carbohydrate to protein intake is 4:1. Maximal muscle growth seems to occur when protein intake is 1.7–1.8 gm protein/kg body weight a day, energy intake is sufficient to prevent weight loss, and carbohydrate intake is 60% to 65% of nutrient intake. Consuming a carbohydrate with protein beverage (chocolate milk) after resistance exercise may enhance recovery or reduce muscle breakdown.

24. **What is the primary factor that determines whether carbohydrates, fats, or proteins are metabolized during a bout of exercise?**
The availability of oxygen is the main factor that determines whether fats or carbohydrates are metabolized. The more limited the supply of oxygen, the more carbohydrates will be metabolized. Less oxygen is needed for carbohydrate metabolism than for fat metabolism. More calories per liter of oxygen are produced from carbohydrates, and oxidation of carbohydrates occurs more quickly. Therefore, during high intensity exercise carbohydrates are the prominent fuel source. As exercise intensity decreases, oxygen becomes more readily available, carbohydrate metabolism decreases, and fat metabolism increases. However, duration of exercise also contributes to the type of fuel used. The longer the duration of exercise, the greater the contribution of fat. Under normal circumstances proteins provide only 5% to 10% of the fuel source during exercise. The contribution is directly proportional to the intensity and duration of exercise. The increase in protein utilization with prolonged exercise seems to be related to glycogen stores. As glycogen stores are depleted, the body depends more on protein for energy production.

25. **Do creatine supplements improve an athlete's performance?**
Most studies agree that creatine supplements are beneficial for short-duration, repetitive bursts of intense exercise. There are various recommendations regarding loading dose, maintenance dose, and length of supplementation. The International Society of Sports Nutrition suggests a loading phase of 0.3 gm/kg per day for 5 to 7 days and a maintenance dose of 0.03 gm/kg per day. There are no dosing recommendations for children

or adolescents. Kreider has shown that short-term creatine supplementation (15–25 gm/day for 5 to 7 days) improves maximal power and strength by 5% to 15%, work performed during sets of maximal effort muscle contractions by 5% to 15%, single-effort sprint performance by 1% to 5%, and work performed during repetitive sprint performance by 5% to 15%. Long-term supplementation (15–25 gm/day for 5–7 days and 2–25 gm/day for 7–84 days) also results in significantly greater gains in strength, sprint performance, and fat-free mass. Creatine supplements do not appear to improve longer-duration, aerobic exercise performance.

26. **What are the side effects of creatine supplementation?**

Documented side effects with the use of creatine supplements vary widely in the literature. The safety and efficacy of creatine supplements has not been determined in children and adolescents. More research is needed to determine the long-term effects of creatine supplement usage.

The most common side effect cited would be weight gain due to an increase in intracellular water volume. As a result of the weight gain, an individual may experience muscle cramps, dehydration, and an increased susceptibility to heat illness. There have also been concerns expressed about compromised renal function and potential hepatic injury with creatine supplement usage.

Bibliography

Atkins, R. C. (1992). *New diet revolution.* New York, NY: Avon Books.
Berning, J. R., & Steen, S. N. (1998). *Nutrition for sport and exercise* (2nd ed.). Gaithersburg, MD: Aspen.
Blackburn, G. L., Phillips, J. C., & Morreale, S. (2001). Physician's guide to popular low carbohydrate weight-loss diets. *Cleveland Clinic Journal of Medicine, 68,* 761–778.
Butts, J., Jacobs, B., & Silvis, M. (2018). Creatine use in sports. *Sports Health, 10*(1), 31–34.
CDC National Center for Disease Control and Prevention. (2017). Get the Facts: Sodium and the Dietary Guidelines. www.cdc.gov.
Daller, J. (2021). Bariatric surgery. Dept. of Surgery, Crozer-Chester Medical Center, Chester, PA, review provided by Vermed Healthcare Network. Also reviewed by A.D.A.M. Health Solutions Inc, Ebix, Inc., editorial team, Zieve, D., Slon, S., and Wang, N.
Dansinger, M. L., Gleason, J. A., Griffith, J. L., Selker, H. P., & Schaefer, E. J. (2005). Comparison of the Atkins, Ornish, Weight Watchers, and Zone diets for weight loss and heart disease. *JAMA, 293*(1), 43–53.
Estruch, R., & Ros, E. (2020). The role of the Mediterranean diet on weight loss and obesity-related diseases. *Review Endocrine Metabolic Disorders, 21*(3), 315–327.
Freedman, M. R., King, J., & Kennedy, E. (2001). Popular diets: a scientific review, executive summary. *Obesity Research, 9,* 1S–5S.
Freitas, R. D., & Campos, M. M. (2019). Protective effects of omega-3 fatty acids in cancer related complications. *Nutrients, 11*(5), 945.
Kelley-Hedgespeth, A. (2021). *Omega-3 fatty acids & the heart: new evidence, more questions.* Heart Health, Harvard Health Publishing. Harvard Medical School.
Li, J., Hoon Lee, D., Hu, J., et al. (2020). Dietary inflammatory potential & risk of cardiovascular disease among men & women in the U.S. *Journal of the American College of Cardiology, 76*(19), 2181–2193.
Lumley, J., Watson, L., Watson, M., & Bower, C. (2001). Periconceptional supplementation with folate and multivitamins for preventing neural tube defects. *The Cochrane Database of Systematic Reviews, 3,* CD001056.
Malouf, R., Grimley Evans, J., & Areosa Sastre, A. (2003). Folic acid with or without vitamin B_{12} for cognition and dementia. *The Cochrane Database of Systematic Reviews, 4,* CD004514.
Mayo Clinic Staff. (2020). Dietary fiber: Essential for a healthy diet. Healthy Lifestyle Nutrition and Healthy Eating. https://www.mayoclinic.org/healthy-lifestyle/nutrition-and-healthy-eating/in-depth/fiber/art-20043983
Mayo Clinic Staff. (2021). Folate. https://www.mayoclinic.org/drugs-supplements-folate/art-20364625
Mechanick, J. I., Apovian, C., Brethauer, S., et al. (2020). Clinical practice guidelines for the perioperative nutrition, metabolic, and nonsurgical support of patients undergoing bariatric procedures. *Endocrine Practice, 25*(12), 1346–1359.
Medline Plus. (2021). Gastric bypass surgery. U.S. National Library of Medicine.
NIH. (2018). Calcium and vitamin D important at every age. NIH Osteoporosis and Related Bone Diseases National Resource Center.
Ornish, D. (1990). *Dr. Dean Ornish's program for reversing heart disease.* New York, NY: Ballantine Books.
Robergs, R. A., & Roberts, S. O. (1997). *Exercise physiology: exercise, performance, and clinical applications.* St. Louis: Mosby.
Stein, K. (2000). High-protein, low-carbohydrate diets: do they work? *Journal of the American Dietetic Association, 100,* 760–761.
Tello, M. (2018). *Calcium, vitamin D and fractures.* Harvard Health Publishing, Harvard School of Medicine.
U.S. Department of Agriculture and U.S. Department of Health and Human Services. (2020). *Dietary guidelines for Americans* (9th ed.). Washington DC: U.S. Government Printing Office.
Volek, J. S. (2000). Enhancing exercise performance: nutritional implications. In W. Garrett & D. T. Kirkendall (Eds.), *Exercise in sport science* (pp. 471–485). Philadelphia, PA: Williams and Wilkins.
Wheeler, K. B., & Lombardo, J. A. (1999). Nutritional Aspects of Exercise. Philadelphia, PA: W.B. Saunders.
Zieve, D. (2012a). Gastric bypass surgery. Medline Plus.
Zieve, D. (2012b). Gastric lap band. Medline Plus.

CHAPTER 29 QUESTIONS

1. **Which of the following is a potential health benefit attributed to adding soluble fiber to the diet?**
   a. Improvement in gout symptoms
   b. Improved kidney function
   c. Reduced serum sodium levels
   d. Reduced serum cholesterol levels

2. Adherence to a Mediterranean diet would incorporate which of the following fats in the diet?
   a. Butter
   b. Olive oil
   c. Corn oil
   d. Coconut oil

3. An individual engaged in heavy training for an endurance event should increase the percentage of which nutrient in his/her diet?
   a. Carbohydrate
   b. Cholesterol
   c. Fat
   d. Protein

CHAPTER 30

DRY NEEDLING

K.R. Maywhort, PT, DPT and E.D. Zylstra, PT, DPT

1. **What is dry needling?**
Dry needling is defined by Federation of State Boards of Physical Therapy as a skilled technique performed by a physical therapist using filiform needles to penetrate the skin and/or underlying tissues to affect change in body structures and functions for the evaluation and management of neuromusculoskeletal conditions, pain, movement impairment, and disability. It is a treatment approach used worldwide by many types of practitioners including physical therapists, physicians, physician assistants, nurse practitioners, chiropractors, acupuncturists, and some occupational therapists and athletic trainers for neural health and recruitment, muscle facilitation, muscle recovery, flexibility, performance, and connective tissue dysfunction.

2. **How does dry needling differ from wet needling?**
Dry needling and wet needling differ primarily in the type of needle used and whether or not an injectate is introduced. Dry needling utilizes a solid filament needle to stimulate neuromuscular tissue, where wet needling utilizes a hollow hypodermic needle to inject pain relievers, corticosteroids, or Botox into neuromuscular tissue. Needles utilized for dry needling are typically much smaller than hypodermic needles and are referred to in terms of diameter and length rather than "gauge." They are solid rather than hollow and have a rounded rather than the beveled, cutting-edge tip of a hypodermic needle and so are generally more comfortable and carry less risk of introducing infection.

3. **What is the difference between dry needling and acupuncture?**
This is quite likely one of the most frequently asked questions. The discussion of "acupuncture" here will refer to acupuncture as a procedure, skill, or intervention, not to acupuncture as a profession. While the tool used for acupuncture and dry needling is the same (solid filament needle), acupuncture by an Oriental medicine practitioner and dry needling by a physical therapist are distinctly different. State boards who regulate licensure of healthcare professionals categorically define dry needling and acupuncture as distinctly different.
The defining difference between acupuncture and dry needling lies in exam, assessment, and reasoning behind the application of the needle (ie, where to place needles and why). An exam by practitioners trained in acupuncture would intend to make a diagnosis related to a patient's life force, or "qi" (pronounced "chee"), via an extensive subjective and screen of organ systems, and examination of the tongue and pulse. The practitioner would then insert needles into specific acupoints that lie along meridians (channels) of the body through which the life force, or "qi," flows. The overall goal of placement of these needles would be to restore normal flow of the life force. In contrast, dry needling revolves around a practitioner using a thin filiform needle to penetrate the skin and underlying tissues for the management of neuromusculoskeletal conditions, pain, movement impairments, and disability. Although these two practices are distinctly different, research suggests there is correlation between acupuncture and trigger points (approximately 20%).

4. **What is the proposed mechanism of dry needling?**
Dry needling has been thought by many to be primarily a trigger point therapy. We know it to be an intervention that creates a neurophysiologic reset through biomechanical, biochemical, and bioelectric effects on local tissue, the motor end plate, the dorsal horn, and the central nervous system.
Following a local twitch response, the muscle fiber length-tension relationship is changed, allowing the muscle to perform more effectively. There is also a complex biochemical response with a shift in pH and changes in concentrations of neurotransmitters, cytokines, chemokines, and immune markers that altogether impact nociception, inflammation, vascularity, and neural transmission. Biochemical changes are observed in local tissue as well as remotely including in the motor end plate and the dorsal horn.
Supraspinal changes are also seen with activation of descending pain modulatory system and intracortical inhibition. With the addition of electrical stim through needles (percutaneous electrical stimulation) there is additional cortical drive.

5. **Is dry needling synonymous with "trigger point therapy"?**
No. A trigger point is defined as a taut band of skeletal muscle/fascia that is painful upon compression, producing recognizable pain, referred symptoms, motor dysfunction, and/or autonomic phenomena. It is at its core a somatic pain referral pattern from muscle. Dry needling is one of many different approaches for the treatment of a trigger point and its pain referral pattern but applications of dry needling go well beyond this singular purpose with documented physiologic effects on far more than muscle alone.

6. **What is a local twitch response (LTR)?**
LTR is a reflexive, spinal cord–mediated muscle response to mechanical input. It is characterized by a brief localized contraction of "banded" muscle fibers. The LTR appears as a quick twitch or dimpling of the skin overlying the banded muscle fibers. Placement of a monofilament needle precisely into an identifiable dense (often sensitive) area within a banded muscle and then moving it in and out of the target tissue (pistoning) stimulates the LTR. It can alternatively be elicited electrically through the use of electrical stimulation.

7. **Is the LTR necessary for a therapeutic response?**
It is hypothesized that an LTR is what generates biochemical and supraspinal changes to decrease pain and improve function. However, repetitive elicitation of LTR has been correlated with increased posttreatment soreness. Increased soreness with increased number of LTRs elicited can be explained in that pistoning creates disruption of local muscle, connective tissue, the motor end plate, and axons with inflammatory and repair phases to follow. However, placing the needle strategically where an LTR is elicited and then utilizing electrical stimulation through the needle to elicit subsequent LTRs can produce the therapeutic benefit of the LTR without significant tissue disruption.

8. **Is there evidence to support the use of dry needling?**
There is a growing body of literature surrounding the practice of dry needling. The overall quality of the evidence is considered low to moderate. The evidence suggests that dry needling performed by physical therapists is more effective than no treatment or sham treatments at reducing pain. Multiple clinical trials and systematic reviews have been published supporting its use for spasticity, fibromyalgia, low back pain, hip osteoarthritis, knee pain, plantar fasciitis/heel pain, neck pain, temporomandibular dysfunction, tension-type headache, shoulder pain, lateral epicondylalgia, generalized musculoskeletal conditions, tendinopathy, flexibility, and performance.

9. **Is dry needling safe?**
The main risks identified with dry needling include infection, and neural or visceral compromise. In the hands of a skilled practitioner who is knowledgeable in anatomy, physiology, and differential diagnosis dry needling has proven to be safe. While there do exist case reports of significant adverse events such as infection, pneumothorax, radial nerve injury, and spinal epidural hematoma, it should be noted that these are very rare.
   - Significant adverse events (AEs) such as infection, pneumothorax, and neural compromise are documented to occur with an incidence rate of <0.04% to <0.1%.
   - Minor AEs such as mild bleeding bruising and pain after treatment are more common with an incidence rate of 36.7%.
   - Uncommon AEs include aggravation of symptoms (0.88%), drowsiness (0.26%), headache (0.14%), and nausea (0.13%). Rare AEs were fatigue (0.04%), altered emotions (0.04%), shaking, itching, claustrophobia, and numbness, all 0.01%.

10. **What types of supplies are required to perform dry needling?**
Required supplies include:
    - Sterile, single-use solid filiform needles of varying lengths and diameters. As the length increases so should the diameter for improved needle control. Appropriate lengths vary from 30 to 135 mm in length and 0.20 to 0.40 in diameter.
    - Isopropyl alcohol, alcohol swab, or antiviral/antibacterial for skin preparation
    - Firm-fitting treatment gloves
    - Sharps container for disposal of used needles
    - Recommended: electrical stimulation unit that has the capacity to modulate frequency and pulse width to apply electrical stimulation through needles (percutaneous electrical stimulation)

11. **Describe a general protocol when performing dry needling.**
When performing dry needling the clinician must have solid clinical reasoning. This includes a thorough examination, identification of the severity, irritability, nature, stage, and stability (SINSS) of a dysfunction, and development of a working diagnosis as this will drive the placement of needles and the dosing (ie, how many needles, duration of indwelling needles, use, and parameters of electrical stimulation through needles). It also includes identification of key exam findings that will be used for test/re-test measures to assess effectiveness of the intervention. The procedure is as follows:
    a. Determine absence of contraindications
    b. Perform examination, develop working diagnosis, plan intervention
    c. Obtain written and verbal consent with disclosure of potential adverse effects that should include risk of infection, neural compromise, and pneumothorax. Written consent must be on file. Verbal consent should be gained and documented at every visit
    d. Adherence to standards of universal precautions and Center for Disease Control guidelines (ie, donning of gloves, cleaning of skin, and use of single-use filiform needles)

e. Identification of target tissue (use of palpation to identify a dense area in banded muscle or bony landmarks to be used as target)
f. Direct needle to target tissue or to a bony backdrop with goal of eliciting a twitch response when target is within a muscle. Various techniques exist (piston motion, placement without use of piston motion, etc.) and are at the discretion of the practitioner
g. Application of electrical stimulation through needle (optional)
h. Removal and proper disposal of needle; check patient for adverse effects
i. Reevaluation of the patient's impairments to determine effect of needling
j. Introduction of other necessary therapeutic interventions such as manual therapy, therapeutic exercise, or modalities that would be indicated to further reduce the patient's impairments and improve function. Dry needling is effectively coupled with adjunctive therapies to enhance long-term carryover.

12. **What are the precautions to dry needling?**
    - Needle phobia/aversion
    - Significant cognitive impairment
    - Communication barrier
    - History of traumatic or spontaneous pneumothorax
    - Hyperalgesia or allodynia
    - Local skin lesions or infections
    - Compromised immune system
    - Metal allergies
    - Abnormal bleeding tendency
    - Vascular disease
    - Over any implant
    - Area of laminectomy

13. **What are the absolute contraindications to dry needling?**
    - Consent denied by patient
    - Inadequate knowledge of the practitioner (lack of training or proper training)
    - Compromised equipment
    - First trimester of pregnancy
    - Scalp area of infants
    - Nipples, umbilicus, and external genitalia
    - Uncontrolled anticoagulant usage
    - Local infection, skin lesion, or active tumor
    - Occipital region with Arnold-Chiari malformation
    - Over a cardiac pacemaker

Bibliography

Berrigan, W. A., Whitehair, C. L., & Zorowitz, R. D. (2019). Acute spinal epidural hematoma as a complication of dry needling: a case report. *PM & R, 11*(3), 313–316.

Botelho, L., Angoleri, L., Zortea, M., et al. (2018). Insights about the neuroplasticity state on the effect of intramuscular electrical stimulation in pain and disability associated with chronic myofascial pain syndrome (MPS): a double-blind, randomized, sham-controlled trial. *Frontiers in Human Neuroscience, 12*, 388.

Boyce, D., Wempe, H., Campbell, C., et al. (2020). Adverse events associated with therapeutic dry needling. *International Journal of Sports Physical Therapy, 15*(1), 103–113.

Brady, S., McEvoy, J., Dommerholt, J., & Doody, C. (2014). Adverse events following trigger point dry needling: a prospective survey of chartered physiotherapists. *Journal of Manual and Manipulative Therapy, 22*(3), 134–140.

Bron, C., Dommerholt, J., Stegenga, B., Wensing, M., & Oostendorp, R. A. B. (2011). High prevalence of shoulder girdle muscles with myofascial trigger points in patients with shoulder pain. *BMC Musculoskeletal Disorders, 12*, 139.

Cagnie, B., Dewitte, V., Barbe, T., Timmermans, F., Delrue, N., & Meeus, M. (2013). Physiologic effects of dry needling. *Current Pain and Headache Reports, 17*(8), 348.

Caramagno, J., Adrian, L., Mueller, L., & Purl, J. (2015). Analysis of competencies for dry needling by physical therapists. Human Resouces Research Organization, 1–49.

Chen, J. T., Chung, K. C., Hou, C. R., Kuan, T. S., Chen, S. M., & Hong, C. Z. (2001). Inhibitory effect of dry needling on the spontaneous electrical activity recorded from myofascial trigger spots of rabbit skeletal muscle. *American Journal of Physical Medicine & Rehabilitation, 80*(10), 729–735.

Cotchett, M. P., Landorf, K. B., Munteanu, S. E., & Raspovic, A. (2011). Effectiveness of trigger point dry needling for plantar heel pain: study protocol for a randomised controlled trial. *Journal of Foot and Ankle Research, 4*(1), 5.

Dembowski, S. C., Westrick, R. B., Zylstra, E., & Johnson, M. R. (2013). Treatment of hamstring strain in a collegiate pole-vaulter integrating dry needling with an eccentric training program: a resident's case report. *International Journal of Sports Physical Therapy, 8*(3), 328–339.

Fernández-de-Las-Peñas, C., & Nijs, J. (2019). Trigger point dry needling for the treatment of myofascial pain syndrome: current perspectives within a pain neuroscience paradigm. *Journal of Pain Research, 12*, 1899–1911.

Gafarov, G. A. (2020). Acupuncture research methods. *Journal of Applied Biotechnology and Bioengineering, 7*(6), 276–278.

Ge, H. Y., Fernández-de-Las-Peñas, C., & Yue, S. W. (2011). Myofascial trigger points: spontaneous electrical activity and its consequences for pain induction and propagation. *Chinese Medicine, 6*, 13.
González-Iglesias, J., Cleland, J. A., del Rosario Gutierrez-Vega, M., & Fernández-de-las-Peñas, C. (2011). Multimodal management of lateral epicondylalgia in rock climbers: A prospective case series. *Journal of Manipulative and Physiological Therapeutics, 34*(9), 635–642.
Gonzalez-Perez, L. M., Infante-Cossio, P., Granados-Nuñez, M., & Urresti-Lopez, F. J. (2012). Multimodal management of lateral epicondylalgia in rock climbers: a prospective case series. *Medicina Oral Patologia Oral Cirugia Bucal, 17*(5), e781–e785.
Hsieh, Y. L., Yang, S. A., Yang, C. C., & Chou, L. W. (2012). Dry needling at myofascial trigger spots of rabbit skeletal muscles modulates the biochemicals associated with pain, inflammation, and hypoxia. *Evidence-Based Complementary and Alternative Medicine, 2012*, 342165.
Huguenin, L., Brukner, P. D., McCrory, P., et al. (2005). Effect of dry needling of gluteal muscles on straight leg raise: a randomised, placebo controlled, double blind trial. *British Journal of Sports Medicine, 39*(2), 84–90.
Kubo, K., Yajima, H., Takayama, M., Ikebukuro, T., Mizoguchi, H., & Takakura, N. (2010). Effects of acupuncture and heating on blood volume and oxygen saturation of human Achilles tendon in vivo. *European Journal of Applied Physiology, 109*(3), 545–550.
Lee, J.-H., Lee, H., & Jo, D.-J. (2011). An acute cervical epidural hematoma as a complication of dry needling. *Spine, 36*(13), E891–E893.
Lu, Z., Briley, A., Zhou, P., & Li, S. (2020). Are there trigger points in the spastic muscles? Electromyographical evidence of dry needling effects on spastic finger flexors in chronic stroke. *Frontiers in Neurology, 11*, 78.
Mason, J. S., Tansey, K. A., & Westrick, R. B. (2014). Treatment of subacute posterior knee pain in an adolescent ballet dancer utilizing trigger point dry needling: a case report. *International Journal of Sports Physical Therapy, 9*(1), 116–124.
McPartland, J. M. (2004). Travell trigger points—molecular and osteopathic perspectives. *The Journal of the American Osteopathic Association, 104*, 244–249.
McShane, J. M., Shah, V. N., & Nazarian, L. N. (2008). Sonographically guided percutaneous needle tenotomy for treatment of common extensor tendinosis in the elbow: is a corticosteroid necessary? *Journal of Ultrasound in Medicine, 27*(8), 1137–1144.
Meng, F., Ge, H. Y., Wang, Y. H., & Tue, S. W. (2015). Afferent fibers are involved in the pathology of central changes in the spinal dorsal horn associated with myofascial trigger spots in rats. *Experimental Brain Research, 233*(11), 3133–3143.
Moseley, G. L. (2003). A pain neuromatrix approach to patients with chronic pain. *Manual Therapy, 8*(3), 130–140.
Niddam, D. M., Chan, R. C., Lee, S. H., Yeh, T. C., & Hsieh, J. C. (2007). Central modulation of pain evoked from myofascial trigger point. *Clinical Journal of Pain, 23*, 440–448.
Niddam, D. M., Chan, R. C., Lee, S. H., Yeh, T. C., & Hsieh, J. C. (2008). Central representation of hyperalgesia from myofascial trigger point. *Neuroimage, 39*, 1299–1306.
Osborne, N. J., & Gatt, I. T. (2010). Management of shoulder injuries using dry needling in elite volleyball players. *Acupuncture in Medicine, 28*(1), 42–45.
Patel, N., Patel, M., & Poustinchian, B. (2019). Dry needling–induced pneumothorax. *Journal of Osteopathic Medicine, 119*(1), 59–62.
Rha, D., Shin, J. C., Kim, Y.-K., et al. (2011). Detecting local twitch responses of myofascial trigger points in the lower-back muscles using ultrasonography. *Archives of Physical Medicine and Rehabilitation, 92*(10), 1576–1580. e1.
Sciotti, V. M., Mittak, V. L., DiMarco, L., et al. (2001). Clinical precision of myofascial trigger point location in the trapezius muscle. *Pain, 93*(3), 259–266.
Shah, J. P., Danoff, J. V., Desai, M. J., et al. (2008). Biochemicals associated with pain and inflammation are elevated in sites near to and remote from active myofascial trigger points. *Archives of Physical Medicine and Rehabilitation, 89*, 16–23.
Shah, J. P., & Gilliams, E. A. (2008). Uncovering the biochemical milieu of myofascial trigger points using in vivo microdialysis: an application of muscle pain concepts to myofascial pain syndrome. *Journal of Bodywork and Movement Therapies, 12*, 371–384.
Sikdar, S., Shah, J. P., Gebreab, T., et al. (2009). Novel applications of ultrasound technology to visualize and characterize myofascial trigger points and surrounding soft tissue. *Archives of Physical Medicine and Rehabilitation, 90*(11), 1829–1838.
Suputtitada, A. (2016). Myofascial pain syndrome and sensitization. Physical Medicine and Rehabilitation Research, 1(4), 71–79.
Tekin, L., Akarsu, S., Durmuş, O., Cakar, E., Dinçer, U., & Kıralp, M. Z. (2013). The effect of dry needling in the treatment of myofascial pain syndrome: a randomized double-blinded placebo-controlled trial. *Clinical Rheumatology, 32*(3), 309–315.
Tough, E. A., White, A. R., Cummings, T. M., Richards, S. H., & Campbell, J. L. (2009). Acupuncture and dry needling in the management of myofascial trigger point pain: a systematic review and meta-analysis of randomised controlled trials. *European Journal of Pain, 13*(1), 3–10.
Travell, J. G., & Simons, D. G. (1983). *Myofascial pain and dysfunction: the trigger point manual.* Baltimore, MD: Williams & Wilkins.
Valdes, V. (2019). Dry needling in physical therapy practice: adverse events. *International Journal of Physical Therapy & Rehabilitation, 5*(2), 1–9.
Westrick, R. B., Zylstra, E., Issa, T., Miller, J. M., & Gerber, J. P. (2012). Evaluation and treatment of musculoskeletal chest wall pain in a military athlete. *International Journal of Sports Physical Therapy, 7*(3), 323–332.
Ziaeifar, M., Arab, A. M., Karimi, N., & Nourbakhsh, M. R. (2014). The effect of dry needling on pain, pressure pain threshold and disability in patients with a myofascial trigger point in the upper trapezius muscle. *Journal of Bodywork and Movement Therapies, 18*(2), 298–305.

CHAPTER 30 QUESTIONS

1. **All of the following are contraindications to dry needling except:**
   a. First trimester of pregnancy
   b. Consent denied by patient
   c. Acute injury
   d. Radicular symptoms

2. **Your patient asks you whether dry needling is the same as acupuncture. Your best response is:**
   a. Dry needling and acupuncture are similar in the tool used to provide the intervention.
   b. Dry needling and acupuncture are similar in the thought process behind where to place needles.
   c. Dry needling and acupuncture are similar in the overall intended goal of the treatment.
   d. Dry needling and acupuncture are not differentiated in the perspective of many state boards.

3. **Which of the following is a proposed mechanism of dry needling?**
   a. Improve the flow of electrons and protons along the nerve pathway
   b. Biochemical changes in the dorsal horn changes causing change in neural transmission
   c. Intercranial blood flow is increased
   d. Spinal cord fluid viscosity improves allowing for greater prostaglandin release

EXERCISE IN AGING AND DISEASE

CHAPTER 31

J. Hanks, PT, PhD, DPT, CLT, Certified DN

1. **Summarize the critical demographics of aging in America and the effects on health care.**
Functional declines, physical disability, and greater use of health care resources are associated with aging. Health care costs are higher per capita among older Americans than any other age group. Older adults comprise the fastest growing segment of the US population. Projections are that by 2060, the US population aged 65 and older will be more than 98 million, comprising nearly a quarter of the population. The number of persons 85 years and older is expected to triple in the same time frame. By 2060, the older population will be more ethnically and racially diverse. A larger proportional growth is anticipated among foreign-born than native-born in all age groups, with the most pronounced increase in persons aged 65 and older. In the 65 years and older age group, the native population is expected to increase 77% and the foreign-born population is expected to increase over 300%. The working-age population (18–64 years) is projected to decrease from 62% to 57% of the total population in the same time frame. The old-age dependency ratio is projected to be 41, meaning there will be 41 people aged 65 years and older per every 100 people in the working age population. Due to the high projected enrollment growth, Medicare expects a 7.6% per year spending increase over the years 2019 to 2028.

2. **Summarize the health status of older adults.**
More than 85% of older adults have at least one chronic illness and more than 56% have multiple chronic conditions. Leading causes of death among persons older than 65 regardless of race and sex are cancer, heart disease, chronic lower respiratory disease, diabetes, cerebrovascular disease, accidents, chronic liver disease, kidney disease, septicemia, Alzheimer's disease, influenza, and pneumonia. The prevalence of hypertension among older adults contributes to preventable mortality and morbidity as well as early disability.

3. **What is the importance of fall risk assessment in older adults? What factors are associated with an increased incidence of falls?**
Falls are the leading cause of injury among older adults with one in three adults over 65 years and one in two adults 80 years or older reporting a fall each year. Persons aged 85 years or older were more likely to report a fall or fall-related injury than those of younger ages. A multifactorial fall risk assessment should be conducted on all persons who report falling in the previous year or on those who have gait and lower extremity muscle strength or balance abnormalities. The Centers for Disease Control and Prevention Injury Center "STEADI (Stopping Elderly Accident, Deaths and Injuries), Preventing Falls in Older Patients—A Provider Tool Kit" is an assessment and intervention tool that includes questionnaires, screening tools, falls risk, and appraisal. Risk factors associated with falls include lower extremity muscle weakness, gait and balance impairments, impaired vision, variable blood pressure, poor vision, cognitive impairment, psychoactive medications or polypharmacy, footwear or foot problems, and environmental hazards.

4. **Can exercise reduce the risk of falling?**
Exercise as a single intervention can decrease risk for falls by 21% in community-dwelling older adults, with larger effects found with exercise that challenges balance and the completion of exercise more than 3 hours per week. However, multifaceted treatment approaches are typically used and may be more effective than exercise alone. Individual and group exercise programs that include balance, coordination, and gait and strength training have been shown to reduce falls among community-dwelling older people and frail older adults. Training programs longer than
12 weeks are most effective. Caution should be used when initiating exercise among sedentary older persons with limited mobility, as exercise could increase fall rate.

5. **What medications are associated with increased risk of falling?**
Antidepressants and sedatives are most strongly linked to increased risk of falls, but cardiovascular drugs to control hypertension and arrhythmias are also implicated. A significant number of falls are associated with postural hypotension, an adverse side effect of many cardiovascular medications.

6. **What is orthostatic (postural) hypotension, and what are common signs and symptoms?**
Orthostatic hypotension is defined as a drop in systolic blood pressure of ≥20 mm Hg or a drop in diastolic blood pressure of 10 mm Hg with a concurrent rise in pulse rate within 3 minutes of moving from supine or sitting to a standing position. Associated signs and symptoms include dizziness, lightheadedness, blurred vision, and syncope or fainting. Orthostatic hypotension has been associated with increased falls among older adults.

7. **Describe physical therapy interventions for orthostatic hypotension.**
Treatment strategies include progressive elevation of the head of the bed, progressive sitting on the side of the bed while performing active leg exercises, and deep breathing. Abdominal compressions and leg muscle pumping may also improve orthostatic hypotension. The use of lower extremity elastic stockings during physical activity and elevating the head of the bed by 5 to 20 degrees during sleep is recommended.

8. **Describe the musculoskeletal effects of aging.**
Sarcopenia is an age-related loss of muscle mass, strength, and function. Contributing factors include decreased type II muscle fiber size and number, insulin resistance, inactivity, obesity, hormonal changes, inadequate protein consumption, and a lack of resistance exercise. Each decade after the age of 50, approximately 8% of muscle mass is lost until age 70, at which time the loss accelerates to an approximate 15% loss per decade. Joint capsules and ligaments stiffen with age. By the seventh decade, joint motion may decrease 20% to 30% and can affect mobility. These musculoskeletal effects may lead to functional declines, frailty, and ultimately, loss of independent living. Bone mass declines with age regardless of sex, with the highest rates of loss occurring in postmenopausal women. Estrogen deficiency plays a role in reduced bone formation and increased bone loss in men and women.

9. **What causes frailty in older adults?**
Sarcopenia is a major contributor to frailty, a common syndrome particularly among persons older than 80 years of age. Frailty is associated with an increased risk of falling, disability, and death. Although there is disagreement regarding the definition of frailty, many consider a person frail when two or more of the following factors are present: unintended weight loss of 10 poungs or more in a year, extreme exhaustion, muscle weakness, reduced gait speed, and low physical activity level. A vicious cycle of inactivity and functional decline ensues among persons who are frail because a high percentage of energy reserves are used to perform simple activities. A multidisciplinary treatment approach that includes progressive resistance exercise and functional training has been shown to be of particular benefit.

10. **What muscle groups are often weak in older adults?**
In general, trunk and lower extremity muscles are affected to a greater extent than upper extremity muscles. With inactivity, the postural antigravity muscles such as the quadriceps, gluteals, erector spinae, and gastrocnemius-soleus are affected the most. These muscle groups are important for upright posture, locomotion, and functional independence. Furthermore, men tend to demonstrate a greater rate of decline in muscle function.

11. **What musculoskeletal effects of aging can be reversed or attenuated with exercise?**
Exercise positively affects flexibility, strength, power, and muscle mass in older adults. The age-related decline in bone mass may be offset by weight-bearing endurance and resistance exercise. Bone-loading forces should be moderate to high to affect bone mineral density. In postmenopausal women, hormone therapy may be necessary to prevent osteoporosis, even among those who are physically active.

12. **Summarize the recommended protocol for strength and power training in older adults.**
For muscle adaptations to occur with strength training, an intensity of 60% to 80% of the muscle's maximum force-generating capacity (one repetition maximum [1-RM]) is recommended. The 1-RM threshold is considered the workload that can be lifted only once through the full range of motion while using excellent form. Percentages of the 1-RM can be determined using a rate of perceived exertion (RPE) scale or by determining the maximum number of repetitions achieved by an exercising muscle at near failure (demonstrated by a decline in form or lack of full motion for the last one to two repetitions). A maximum repetition capacity of 15 (RPE of fairly light to moderately hard) equates to a 60% overload stimulus, and an 80% workload equates to a maximum repetition capacity of 10 (RPE of hard to very hard). Emphasis should be placed on strengthening the major muscle groups, especially those of the hips, trunk, and lower extremities. Each major muscle group should be exercised two to three times a week with 1 to 2 days of rest before the next workout of the same muscle group. Strength gains can be achieved with a single set of repetitions per exercise maneuver, with greater strength gains realized with higher numbers of sets. Power training (generating muscle force quickly) should be incorporated into the resistance training routine once an individual can complete two sets of 10 to 15 maximum repetitions of an exercise maneuver. The concentric phase of an exercise should be performed quickly, and the eccentric phase performed more slowly. The power training component should progress from 20% to 60% of the 1-RM.

13. **When is exercise or exercise testing not recommended in older adults?**
According to the American College of Sports Medicine (ACSM), exercise and/or exercise testing is not recommended if there are recent changes in an ECG suggesting myocardial ischemia, an acute cardiac event such as myocardial infarction, pulmonary embolism, severe aortic stenosis, symptomatic heart failure, or an aortic aneurysm. Other contraindications include severe shortness of breath, infection or inflammation of the heart, or any systemic infection.

14. **When is heavy resistance training not recommended in older adults?**
    Resistance training is contraindicated in older adults with unstable medical conditions because of the risk of dangerously high blood pressure, particularly associated with the Valsalva maneuver. Absolute and relative contraindications include unstable coronary heart disease, decompensated heart failure, uncontrolled arrhythmias, severe pulmonary hypertension, symptomatic and severe aortic stenosis, cardiac inflammation, uncontrolled hypertension, aortic dissection, Marfan syndrome, diabetic retinopathy, and musculoskeletal limitations.

15. **Summarize the recommendations for strength training in older adults with hypertension.**
    Resting systolic and diastolic blood pressure ≥160 mm Hg and diastolic blood pressure ≥100 mm Hg are relative contraindications to a resistance training program. Resistance should be of low to moderate weight load or 30% to 60% of one repetition maximum. The rate of perceived exertion should not be higher than 11 to 13 (fairly light to somewhat hard) on the 20-point Borg scale. Static hand-gripping and breath holding should be avoided. Increase resistance with each exercise only after 12 to 15 repetitions can be comfortably performed. Prolonged cool down after strength training is recommended to decrease risk for hypotensive reaction to quick cessation of activity. Exercise should be discontinued with the onset of abnormal signs or symptoms such as dizziness, unusual shortness of breath, angina-type discomfort, abnormal heart rhythm, cold sweat, confusion, excessive fatigue, or incoordination.

16. **Summarize the recommendations for aerobic exercise in older adults.**
    Physical/aerobic activity is recommended at a moderate exertion level 5 days a week. Older adults who are deconditioned should start at lower intensity levels and may need to exercise several times a day in 10-minute bouts to reach recommended exercise time frames. However, any level or amount of activity is better than remaining sedentary. A progressive increase in time and/or intensity is necessary for improvement in aerobic fitness. Walking is one of the best types of aerobic activities for older adults because it is functional, provides weight-bearing stimulus to the lower extremities, and requires no special equipment. Unusual shortness of breath, angina-type discomfort, abnormal heart rhythm, cold sweat, confusion, excessive fatigue, or incoordination are contraindications to aerobic exercise. In persons with significant loss of muscle mass, a muscle strengthening program should be implemented before an aerobic training program.

17. **Can older adults improve aerobic capacity with endurance training?**
    Yes; improvements are similar to that in younger adults. The amount of improvement in aerobic capacity depends on baseline fitness level and training intensity. Greater health benefits occur with a combination of moderate and vigorous-intensity activity.

18. **Can exercise improve functional outcomes in older adults?**
    Exercise can improve lower extremity strength, power, and walking speed. Rising from a chair, the ability to climb steps, and cross the street are improved with high-velocity resistance training. An increase in walking speed has also been associated with a decreased risk of mortality in older adults. Balance training can yield improvements of 16% to 42% compared to balance measures at baseline, decreasing risk of falls in elderly adults.

19. **Can exercise reduce mortality and increase life expectancy?**
    Moderate and vigorous physical activity has been associated with reduced all-cause mortality with greater relative risk reductions occurring with more vigorous exercise.

    Compared with inactive individuals, those who exercise a minimum of 15 minutes per day or 90 minutes per week have a 3-year longer life expectancy. Furthermore, inactive individuals demonstrate a hazard ratio of ~1.6 compared to active individuals.

20. **What are the primary risk factors for cardiovascular disease? Why is this information important to orthopedic specialists?**
    Risk factors for cardiovascular disease include elevated blood pressure, smoking, obesity, inadequate physical activity, diabetes, and elevated levels of fat (cholesterol and triglyceride) in the blood. These risk factors can be influenced by lifestyle and diet modifications. Other risk factors include age, male gender, and a positive family history of cardiovascular disease. If the patient experiences pain above the waist that commences with activity and is relieved by rest, cardiac disease should be considered until ruled out. Patients with a primary diagnosis of orthopedic dysfunction should be screened for cardiovascular risk factors if exercise is a planned intervention.

21. **What are appropriate cardiovascular responses to aerobic or dynamic exercise?**
    Heart rate and systolic and mean arterial blood pressure rise, and diastolic blood pressure remains the same, or falls slightly, with increasing workload. Failure of systolic blood pressure to rise with increasing workloads, or a drop >20 mmHg may indicate a decrease in cardiac output and correlate with myocardial ischemia or left ventricular dysfunction.

22. **How should a person taking beta-blocker (β-blocker) medications be monitored during exercise?**
Beta-blockers decrease the workload of the heart by decreasing heart rate and contractility and thus blood pressure at rest. During exercise, β-blockers blunt the heart rate and blood pressure responses; thus, heart rate and blood pressure measurements during exercise may not be a true measure of exercise effort. Patient symptoms and rating of perceived exertion are more helpful in evaluating tolerance to exercise. An exercise performance test is needed to prescribe exercise accurately. Calculating a target heart rate from the age-predicted maximal heart rate is inappropriate in patients taking β-blockers.

23. **How should a person with a pacemaker or implantable cardioverter defibrillator (ICD) be monitored during exercise?**
Warm-up and cool-down periods should be longer for people with fixed-rate pacemakers and exercise intensity must be monitored by methods other than pulse counting (eg, patient symptoms, rating of perceived exertion, and blood pressure measurements). Rate-responsive pacemakers adapt the pacing rate to physical activity demands. Moderate to high intensity exercise has been shown to be a safe and effective way to improve cardiopulmonary outcomes without adverse events in those with an implantable cardioverter defibrillator or cardiac resynchronization pacemaker. Abnormal exercise response or unusual symptoms such as dyspnea, dizziness, or syncope should be reported immediately to a physician.

24. **How can general musculoskeletal chest pain be distinguished from cardiac ischemic pain?**
The diffuse burning, squeezing, or crushing chest pain caused by cardiovascular disease should be differentiated from the more specific sharp, localized, stabbing, or burning chest pain of musculoskeletal origin. Musculoskeletal chest pain is generally unaffected by nitroglycerin, is accompanied by muscle and joint soreness, or tenderness to palpation and is not associated with electrocardiographic changes or constitutional symptoms. Cardiac chest pain (angina) is relieved by nitroglycerin and is associated with diaphoresis, shortness of breath, nausea, and/or ST-segment changes on the ECG. Anginal chest pain may occur anywhere above the waist, commence with exertion, and decrease with rest.

25. **Can a patient experience a heart attack without the usual symptoms?**
Yes. Typical symptoms of myocardial infarction are chest, jaw, or arm pain described as dull, heavy, tight, squeezing, or crushing. Atypical symptoms include indigestion-like pain, epigastric pain, and back pain. Associated features, such as nausea, vomiting, sweating, and dyspnea may occur. Sometimes people have no pain during an episode of critical loss of blood flow to the heart (ie, silent ischemia) but may complain of shortness of breath, weakness, fatigue, exhaustion, or flu-like symptoms. Persons with diabetes are at higher risk of silent ischemia because of the autonomic neuropathy associated with the disease.

26. **What are the exercise recommendations for patients with heart failure (HF)?**
In the past, physical activity was restricted for patients with HF. However, recent studies have shown that exercise training can improve activity tolerance, symptoms, and quality of life without adversely affecting ventricular function. Exercise guidelines for persons with HF are difficult to implement because the patient's condition often fluctuates, but exercise can be done safely in selected patients. Patients should be assessed thoroughly before exercise and vital signs and symptoms should be closely monitored during exercise. A relative contraindication for exercise is uncompensated HF. Exercise can be initiated in patients with compensated HF, determined clinically by the ability to speak comfortably with a respiratory rate <30 breaths per minute, less than moderate fatigue, crackles in less than half of the lungs, and a resting heart rate of less than 120 beats per minute. Exercise should be modified or terminated if the patient demonstrates extreme shortness of breath, marked fatigue, abnormal hemodynamic responses, development of abnormal heart sounds, arrhythmias, increase in pulmonary crackles, or evidence of myocardial ischemia. Because patients with HF are generally deconditioned, a low level of effort may be sufficient to induce positive physiological changes. Short walking sessions can be progressed to longer, less frequent bouts of activity. Dynamic light resistance training can improve muscle strength and endurance without adversely affecting left ventricular function.

27. **What types of exercises are recommended for patients with chronic primary or secondary pulmonary disease?**
Persons with pulmonary disease may benefit from an individually tailored program of breathing exercises, coughing techniques, cardiopulmonary endurance training, strength training (including high intensity interval training), flexibility, respiratory muscle training, and relaxation exercises/techniques. Other components should include airway clearance techniques, ventilatory strategies, energy conservation, and patient education. Exercise training in persons with pulmonary disease may not directly improve lung function but may reduce hospital admissions and mortality and improve quality of life and function, particularly following acute exacerbations.

28. What types of exercises are recommended for people with osteoporosis?

Recommendations include moderate intensity weight-bearing aerobic exercise performed 3 to 5 days a week. Resistance training should be done 2 to 3 days a week and should include 8 to 12 repetitions of exercises of the major muscle groups. Exercise should emphasize hip and trunk stabilizing muscles, avoiding spinal flexion. While high-impact loading and abrupt, ballistic movements should be avoided, high intensity interval resistance training may be efficacious and without adverse events when highly supervised.

29. What are the most common causes of sport injuries in the older athlete?

Acute muscle injuries and overuse injuries in the lower extremities are the most common causes of sport injuries, particularly if the older adult suddenly increases the amount of physical activity involving repetitive movement. Older adult athletes performing a novel sport are at higher risk for injury than younger persons.

Bibliography

Alswyan, A., Liberato, A., & Dougherty, C. (2018). A systematic review of exercise training in patients with cardiac implantable devices. *Journal of Cardiopulmonary Rehabilitation and Prevention, 38*(2), 70–84.

American College of Sports Medicine Position Stand. (1998). Exercise and physical activity for older adults. *Medicine & Science in Sports & Exercise, 30*(6), 992–1008.

Ardeljan, A., & Hurezeanu, R. (2021). Sarcopenia. *StatPearls [Internet] Treasure Island (FL).* StatPearls Publishing.

Bromfield, S., Ngameni, C., & Colantonio, L. (2017). Blood pressure, antihypertensive polypharmacy, frailty, and risk for serious fall injuries among older treated adults with hypertension. *Hypertension, 70*(2), 259–266.

Cadore, E., Rodríguez-Mañas, L., Sinclair, A., & Izquierdo, M. (2013). Effects of different exercise interventions on risk of falls, gait ability, and balance in physically frail older adults: a systematic review. *Rejuvenation Research, 16*(2), 105–114.

Centers for Disease Control and Prevention. National Center for Health Statistics. (2015). Percent of U.S. adults 55 and over with chronic conditions. https://www.cdc.gov/nchs/health_policy/adult_chronic_conditions.htm. Accessed March 3, 2022.

Centers for Disease Control and Prevention. (2015). Deaths, percent of total deaths, and death rates for the 15 leading causes of death in 5-year age groups, by race and sex: United States, 1999–2015. In: System NVS, ed: Centers for Disease Control and Statistics.

Centers for Disease Control and Prevention. (2021a). Physical activity is essential to healthy aging. https://www.cdc.gov/physicalactivity/basics/older_adults/index.htm. Accessed February 22, 2022.

Centers for Disease Control and Prevention. (2021b). STEADI: Stopping elderly accidents, deaths and injuries. Centers for Disease Control and Prevention. https://www.cdc.gov/steadi/. Accessed February 24, 2022.

Centers for Medicare and Medicaid Services. (2021). National Health Expenditure Data: Fact Sheet. https://www.cms.gov/Research-Statistics-Data-and-Systems/Statistics-Trends-and-Reports/NationalHealthExpendData/NHE-Fact-Sheet. Accessed February 20, 2022.

Colby, S., & Ortman, J. (2014). Projections of the size and composition of the U.S. population: 2014 to 2060: Current population reports. Report Number P-25-1143. United States Census Bureau. https://www.census.gov/library/publications/2015/demo/p25-1143.html. Accessed March 2, 2022.

Ditroilo, M., Forte, R., Benelli, P., Gambarara, D., & De Vito, G. (2010). Effects of age and limb dominance on upper and lower limb muscle function in healthy males and females aged 40–80 years. *Journal of Sports Sciences, 28*(6), 667–677.

Ferry, A., Anand, A., Strachan, F., et al. (2019). Presenting symptoms in men and women diagnosed with myocardial infarction using sex-specific criteria. *Journal of the American Heart Association, 8*(17), e012307.

Fragala, M., Cadore, E., Dorgo, S., et al. (2019). Resistance training for older adults: position statement from the National Strength and Conditioning Association. *Journal of Strength & Conditioning Research, 33*(8), 2019–2052.

Francula-Zaninovic, S., & Nola, I. (2018). Management of measurable variable cardiovascular disease' risk factors. *Current Cardiology Reviews, 14*(3), 153–163.

Gao, M., Huang, Y., Wang, Q., Liu, K., & Sun, G. (2022). Effects of high-intensity interval training on pulmonary function and exercise capacity in individuals with chronic obstructive pulmonary disease: a meta-analysis and systematic review. *Advances in Therapy, 39*(1), 94–116.

Goodman, C., Heick, J., & Lazaro, R. (2018). *Differential diagnosis for physical therapists: screening for referral* (6th ed.). St. Louis, MO: Elsevier.

Hilfiker, R., Meichtry, A., Eicher, M., et al. (2018). Exercise and other non-pharmaceutical interventions for cancer-related fatigue in patients during or after cancer treatment: a systematic review incorporating an indirect-comparisons meta-analysis. *British Journal of Sports Medicine, 52*(10), 651–658.

Hillegass, E. (2016). *Essentials of cardiopulmonary physical therapy* (4th ed.). Elsevier.

Juraschek, S., Simpson, L., Davis, B., Beach, J., Ishak, A., & Mukamal, K. (2019). Effects of antihypertensive class on falls, syncope, and orthostatic hypotension in older adults: the ALLHAT Trial. *Hypertension, 74*(4), 1033–1040.

Levin, V., Jiang, X., & Kagan, R. (2018). Estrogen therapy for osteoporosis in the modern era. *Osteoporosis International, 29*(5), 1049–1055.

Liguori, G. (2021). *ACSM's guidelines for exercise testing and prescription* (11th ed.). Wolters Kluwer Health.

Logan, A., Freeman, J., & Pooler, J. (2020). Effectiveness of non-pharmacological interventions to treat orthostatic hypotension in elderly people and people with a neurological condition: a systematic review. *JBI Evidence Synthesis, 18*(12), 2556–2617.

Lopez, P., Pinto, R., Radaelli, R., et al. (2018). Benefits of resistance training in physically frail elderly: a systematic review. *Aging Clinical and Experimental Research, 30*(8), 889–899.

Marcum, Z., Perera, S., Thorpe, J., et al. (2016). Antidepressant use and recurrent falls in community-dwelling older adults: findings from the Health ABC Study. *Annals of Pharmacotherapy, 50*(7), 525–533.

Mills, P., Fung, C., Travlos, A., & Krassioukov, A. (2015). Nonpharmacologic management of orthostatic hypotension: a systematic review. *Archives of Physical Medicine and Rehabilitation, 96*(2), 366–375.e6.

Moreland, B., Kakara, R., & Henry, A. (2020). Trends in nonfatal falls and fall-related injuries among adults aged ≥65 years—United States, 2012–2018. *Morbidity and Mortality Weekly Report, 69*, 875–881.

Palmer, K., Bowles, K., Paton, M., Jepson, M., & Lane, R. (2018). Chronic heart failure and exercise rehabilitation: a systematic review and meta-analysis. *Archives of Physical Medicine and Rehabilitation, 99*(12), 2570–2582.

Panel on Prevention of Falls in Older Persons, American Geriatrics Society and British Geriatrics Society. (2011). Summary of the Updated American Geriatrics Society/British Geriatrics Society clinical practice guideline for prevention of falls in older persons. *Journal of the American Geriatrics Society, 59*(1), 148–157.

Phelan, E., & Ritchey, K. (2018). Fall prevention in community-dwelling older adults. *Annals of Internal Medicine, 169*(11), 81–96.

Seppala, L., van de Glind, E., Daams, J. G., et al. (2018). Fall-risk-increasing drugs: a systematic review and meta-analysis: III. Others. *Journal of the American Medical Directors Association, 19*(4), 372.e371–372.e378.

Sherrington, C., Michaleff, Z. A., Fairhall, N., et al. (2017). Exercise to prevent falls in older adults: an updated systematic review and meta-analysis. *British Journal of Sports Medicine, 51*(24), 1750–1758.

Shoemaker, M., Dias, K., Lefebvre, K., Heick, J., & Collins, S. (2020). Physical therapist clinical practice guideline for the management of individuals with heart failure. *Physical Therapy, 100*(1), 14–43.

Stringhini, S., Carmeli, C., Jokela, M., et al. (2017). Socioeconomic status and the 25 × 25 risk factors as determinants of premature mortality: a multicohort study and meta-analysis of 1·7 million men and women. *Lancet, 389*(10075), 1229–1237.

Thomas, E., Battaglia, G., Patti, A., et al. (2019). Physical activity programs for balance and fall prevention in elderly: a systematic review. *Medicine (Baltimore), 98*(27), e16218.

United States Census Bureau. Projections of the population by sex and selected age groups for the United States: 2015 to 2060. https://www.census.gov/data/tables/2014/demo/popproj/2014-summary-tables.html. Accessed March 4, 2022.

Vespa, J., Medina, L., & Armstrong, D. (2020). Demographic turning points for the United States: population projections for 2020 to 2060. Report number P25-1144. United States Census Bureau. https://www.census.gov/library/publications/2020/demo/p25-1144.html. Accessed March 2, 2022.

Walston, J., Buta, B., & Xue, Q. (2018). Frailty screening and interventions: considerations for clinical practice. *Clinics in Geriatric Medicine, 34*(1), 25–38.

Watson, S., Weeks, B., Weis, L., Harding, A., Horan, S., & Beck, B. (2018). High-intensity resistance and impact training improves bone mineral density and physical function in postmenopausal women with osteopenia and osteoporosis: The LIFTMOR Randomized Controlled Trial. *Journal of Bone and Mineral Research, 33*(2), 211–220.

Whelton, P., Carey, R. M., Aranow, W. S., et al. (2018). 2017 ACC/AHA/AAPA/ABC/ACPM/AGS/APhA/ASH/ASPC/NMA/PCNA Guideline for the Prevention, Detection, Evaluation, and Management of High Blood Pressure in Adults: a report of the American College of Cardiology/American Heart Association Task Force on Clinical Practice Guidelines. *Hypertension, 71*(6), e13–e115.

Yu, S., Khow, K., Jadczak, A., & Visvanathan, R. (2016). Clinical screening tools for sarcopenia and its management. *Current Gerontology and Geriatric Research, 2016*, 5978523.

CHAPTER 31 QUESTIONS

1. **It is estimated that by 2060, the percentage of the US population aged 65 and older will be:**
   a. 5%
   b. 10 %
   c. 25% of the population
   d. 50% of the population

2. **The leading causes of death among persons aged 65 and older are:**
   a. Heart disease and cancer
   b. Cancer and chronic obstructive pulmonary disease
   c. Stroke and heart disease
   d. Alzheimer's disease and pneumonia

3. **The ACSM recommends that older adults should participate in aerobic exercise training at a moderate intensity of:**
   a. 1 day a week
   b. 2 days a week
   c. 3 days a week
   d. At least 5 days a week

ORTHOPAEDIC RADIOLOGY

K.A. Brindle, MS, MDs and T.J. Brindle, PT, PhD, AT-R

CHAPTER 32

1. **Is x-ray imaging dangerous?**

   In general, x-ray imaging is not dangerous. Radiation exposure from a single x-ray of an extremity is 0.01 millisievert (mSv), from a chest x-ray is 0.02 mSv, and from a lumbar spine/pelvic x-ray is 1.3 mSv. To put this in context, most people are exposed to a certain amount of radiation in the environment each day; an extremity x-ray is equivalent to one half day of exposure, whereas chest and lumbar spine/pelvic x-rays are equivalent to 1 and 65 days of exposure, respectively.

2. **How is an x-ray different from an arthrogram?**

   An arthrogram is an x-ray with a contrast material to examine soft tissue structure. The contrast material is commonly radiopaque iodine or gadolinium and is injected into the joint, typically to determine whether there is disruption of the joint capsule, thus evaluating the soft tissue structure of the joint.

3. **What are the ABCs of reading a radiograph?**

   - A—Alignment: view the joint surfaces for congruency and alignment. For example, the shoulder, a ball-and-socket joint, should demonstrate the ball of the humeral head aligned within the cup of the glenoid fossa. Deviation from this normal anatomic alignment could indicate a minor subluxation or a major dislocation.
   - B—Bone density: observe the general bone density and look for distinct cortical edges. A loss of the distinct cortical edges may indicate loss of bone mass. Next, observe the local bone density. Look for areas of increased density that would indicate sclerosis. Also, observe texture abnormalities of the bone. When the mineralization of a bone is changed, the trabeculae can appear thin, delicate, coarsened, fluffy, or smudged.
   - C—Cartilage: although cartilage is not directly seen on an x-ray, inspecting the region in which cartilage lies can indicate possible problems with cartilage. Narrowed joint space (the area between articulating bones) can indicate arthritis, whereas widened joint space can be indicative of joint effusion or a genetic/metabolic condition such as acromegaly or chondrocalcinosis.
   - S—Soft tissue: typically swelling can be observed with an x-ray but is a nonspecific finding. Other soft tissue findings can be the presence of gas following surgery or trauma, calcification, and an abnormal soft tissue mass such as a hematoma, abscess, or tumor.

4. **How many views are typically ordered to diagnose injuries?**

   The minimum number of films needed is usually two—the anteroposterior (AP) view and the lateral view. More often three views are obtained. An oblique view is often included because bones that overlap in either an AP or a lateral view can mask subtle fracture lines.

5. **What is computed axial tomography (CAT/CT) scanning?**

   CT scans, also called CAT scans, were developed jointly in 1972 by Sir Godfrey Newbold Hounsfield in the United Kingdom and Dr. Allan Cormack in the United States and are based on mathematical reconstruction of multiple axial slices of x-rays surrounding the body part to be imaged. CT scans provide between 200 and 300 shades of gray compared with x-rays, which produce 20 to 30 shades of gray. All images are collected in the axial plane and then mathematically reconstructed to provide other views, such as coronal, sagittal, or 3D images.

6. **How does magnetic resonance imaging (MRI) work?**

   An MRI image is based on tissue response to multiple magnetic fields. The magnetic field knocks the tissue off its aligned position, which then responds based on its water content or, more specifically, hydrogen ion concentration. In other words, it is a matter of lining up the molecules (B0) and then knocking them down (B1).

   The image is generated by how fast tissue responds to being knocked down. The time it takes to return to the upright position generates the T1 signal, also called the spin-lattice relaxation time, and the time it takes to return to moving at its natural frequency generates the T2 signal, or the spin-spin relaxation time.

7. **What are the characteristics of the T1 image?**

   T1-weighted images show fat and blood as white, muscle tissue as gray, and edema, tumors, and cerebrospinal fluid (CSF) as black.

8. **What are the characteristics of a T2 image?**
T2-weighted images show CSF, edema, and tumors as white, muscle as gray, and fat, cartilage, and tendons as black.

9. **Is exposure to the magnetic fields during MRI dangerous?**
Magnetic fields of 1.5 and 3T are generally not thought to be dangerous because of the relatively short exposure time experienced by patients. However, it is unknown at what exposure level (intensity or duration) magnetic fields become dangerous. Therefore in relatively healthy populations the only contraindication for MRI is pregnancy because of the unknown effects of magnetic fields on the developing fetus.

10. **Should people with metal implants or electronic implants be excluded from MRI?**
Metal implants can severely degrade an image, which renders MRI useless and warrants the use of other imaging studies for these types of patients. The farther away the metal is from the area being scanned, the less the effect. Therefore metal implants in the lower extremity should not affect MRI being conducted of the brain. Ferrous metal implants are considered a contraindication for MRI. Magnetic fields can also interfere with electronics and pose a risk to patients with electronic implants.

11. **What is an MRI arthrogram?**
It is similar to an x-ray and CT arthrogram, in that the contrast material (gadolinium) is injected to enhance the contrast between tissues.

12. **What is the most valuable MRI sequence for assessing pathology?**
A T2-weighted image is probably the most useful sequence to assess abnormalities on MRI. The reason for this is that fluid is bright and therefore stands out on T2-weighted images. Most pathologic processes (trauma, infection, tumors) lead to increased fluid content in tissues and therefore are bright on a T2-weighted image.

13. **Is MRI best for evaluating soft tissue injuries?**
Yes; however, there are circumstances where MRI might not be needed or warranted. In addition, multiple imaging planes increase scanning time and can cause patients to become claustrophobic. It is necessary for the radiologist to have an idea of what to look for so that the proper sequence can be conducted to image the correct anatomic region. For example, the ACL is best imaged in the sagittal plane where the full length of the ligament can be seen to assess its integrity.

14. **What is the appearance of a normal ligament or tendon on MRI?**
Both ligaments and tendons should be dark in all imaging sequences. Sometimes striations can be seen within these structures on MRI. The anterior cruciate ligament and the quadriceps and triceps tendons are examples where a striated appearance can be seen.

15. **What is positron emission tomography (PET) scanning?**
A PET scan is a diagnostic examination that is the acquisition of positrons from a radioactive substance administered to the patient. It is used most commonly to detect cancer and examine its effects by characterizing biochemical changes in the body. Patients are given a radioactive or tagged substance, usually glucose, before the examination. The tagged glucose will accumulate in areas representing biologic activity, differentiating it from areas that demonstrate greater uptake of glucose, such as a tumor. This is typically described as a hot spot. PET scans are also used to evaluate brain and heart function. Radiation doses are very small and short lived and will not affect normal body processes. Pregnant women should not undergo this type of study.

16. **What is a bone scan?**
A bone scan or scintigraphy involves the injection of a slightly radioactive tracer (technetium-99m) into a vein to evaluate biophysiologic aspects of bone and disease. Bone scans are helpful in identifying stress fractures very early, before the onset of architectural changes in the bone. They are also valuable for detecting bone infections, arthritis, metabolic disorders such as Paget's disease, and cancers that can spread to the bone. The amount of radioactive material is small and eliminated quickly. Complications are rare; however, pregnant women are not candidates for this procedure.

17. **When will a stress fracture become visible on a plain film? What is the typical appearance on radiographs?**

A stress fracture will not be visible on an x-ray film until approximately 7 to 14 days after the injury. Radiographic abnormalities can include a subtle thin radiolucent line through the cortex, a focal band of sclerosis, or periosteal cortical thickening. An example of a second metatarsal stress fracture is provided with plain film radiographs.

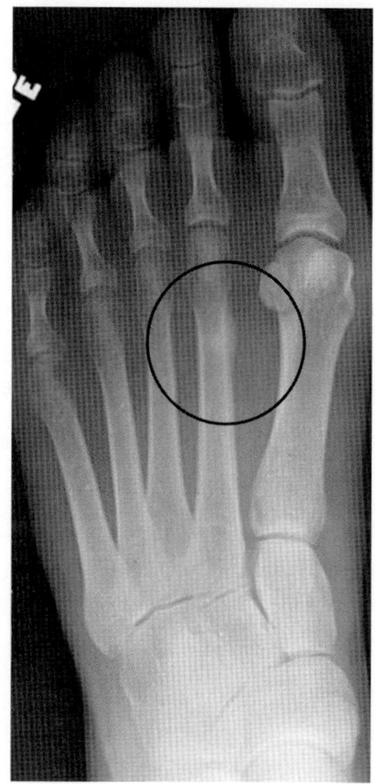

AP view of the foot demonstrates callus formation along the medial aspect of the distal second metatarsal, compatible with a healing stress fracture.

18. **Is osteoporosis detectable by x-ray imaging and, if so, what is its appearance?**

Yes, it is visible. However, it is visible only after a 30% to 50% loss of bone. Plain film radiographs typically show "picture framing," where the cortex is sharp but the trabeculae are decreased. The vertebral bodies appear as an "empty box," because of increased density of the vertebral endplates. The vertebral bodies also show concavity and will demonstrate compression fractures with more severe cases of osteoporosis. Compression fractures are typically viewed as a wedge-shaped deformity of the vertebral body with loss of vertebral body height.

19. **What are a delayed union and a nonunion?**

Delayed fracture healing occurs when healing is slower than expected (16–18 weeks), and nonunion occurs when healing is delayed for longer than 6 months. Nonunion fractures may be broadly classified as atrophic or hypertrophic. Atrophic nonunions typically require stabilization and bone grafting, whereas hypertrophic nonunions may require stabilization only.

20. **What is spondylolysis and how is it diagnosed radiographically?**

Spondylolysis is a bony defect in the pars interarticularis caused by a chronic stress fracture; it is typically seen at the L5 vertebra in adolescent athletes. With oblique plain film radiographs, a collar or radiolucency is seen around the pars interarticularis, reminiscent of a dog collar. Spondylolisthesis occurs with a bilateral pars interarticularis defect, and there is slippage of one vertebral body on another because of the loss of stability provided by the bony architecture.

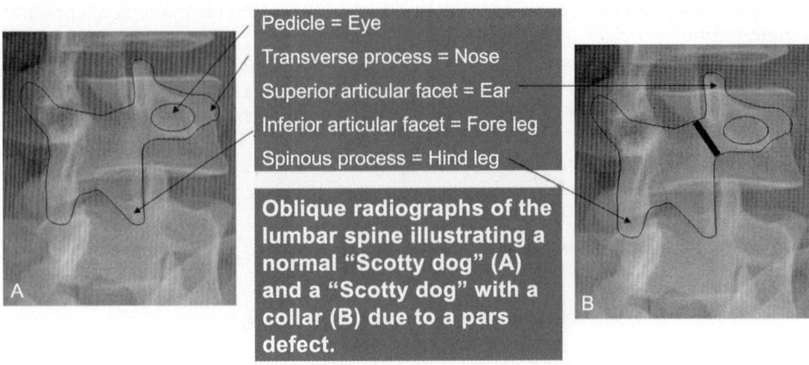

Oblique radiographs of the lumbar spine illustrating a normal "Scotty dog" (A) and a "Scotty dog" with a collar (B) due to a pars defect.

21. **How is scoliosis measured radiographically?**

It is measured on a posteroanterior (PA) film of the entire spine obtained with the patient in a standing position without wearing shoes. The standard method of measuring scoliosis uses the Cobb method. Lines are drawn along the superior endplate and the inferior endplate of the highest and lowest vertebrae involved in the curvature. The angle subtended by lines drawn perpendicular to these two lines forms the Cobb angle.

AP view of the thoracolumbar spine. The scoliosis in the lower spine is measured using the Cobb angle.

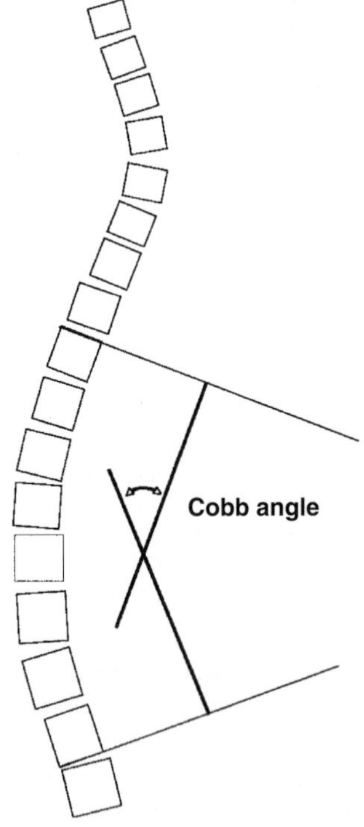

22. **How is alignment of the cervical spine evaluated?**
Three imaginary smooth curved lines can be drawn on a lateral view of the cervical spine to assess alignment. The lines are drawn along the anterior aspects of the vertebral bodies, the posterior aspects of the vertebral bodies, and the spinolaminar line. A fourth line can be drawn along the posterior aspects of the C2 to C7 spinous processes, though even in normal patients this line may not be smooth and contiguous. In the setting of trauma, any malalignment of the first three lines should be considered evidence of fracture or ligamentous injury.

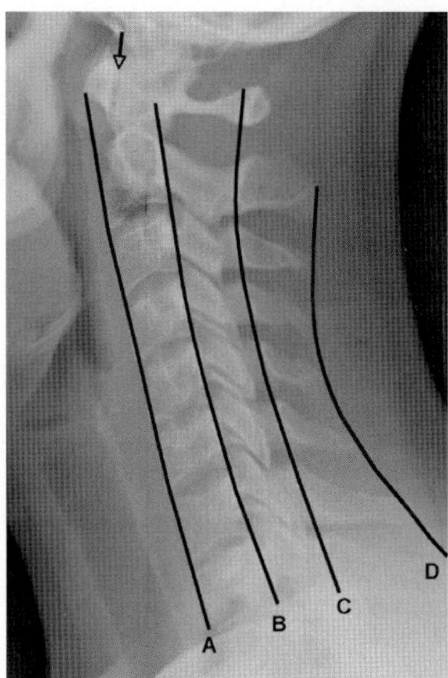

Lateral view of the cervical spine depicting the **(A)** anterior spinal line, **(B)** posterior spinal line, **(C)** spinolaminar line, and **(D)** spinous process line. Note the predental space (*arrow*). It is normal in this adult patient, measuring less than 3 mm.

23. **When is the predental space considered abnormal?**
The predental space (or atlantodental interval) is the space between the odontoid process and the anterior aspect of the ring of C1 (see arrow from figure 22 above). It is evaluated on the lateral radiograph of the cervical spine. The predental space is abnormal when it measures greater than 3 mm in adults and 5 mm in children. An increased atlantodental interval indicates atlantoaxial instability caused by rupture of the transverse ligament.

24. **What is the normal thickness of the prevertebral soft tissues in the cervical spine?**
Hematoma and edema of the soft tissues secondary to trauma can cause thickening of the soft tissues on the lateral radiograph of the cervical spine. Anterior to the C2 vertebral body, the soft tissues should not normally measure more than 7 mm. Anterior to C7, the prevertebral soft tissues can normally measure up to 22 mm.

25. **What is the most common vertebral fracture that can result in neurological symptoms, usually associated with high velocity trauma such as car accidents or falls from high places?**
Compression fractures between T10 and L2 are the most common fracture with high velocity trauma. This is due to the biomechanically rigid thoracic spine and the more mobile lumbar spine. Up to 25% of these fractures will include some neurological symptoms. With the conus medullaris around the L1 level, neurological symptoms (upper motor neuron injuries) are more common above the L1 level.

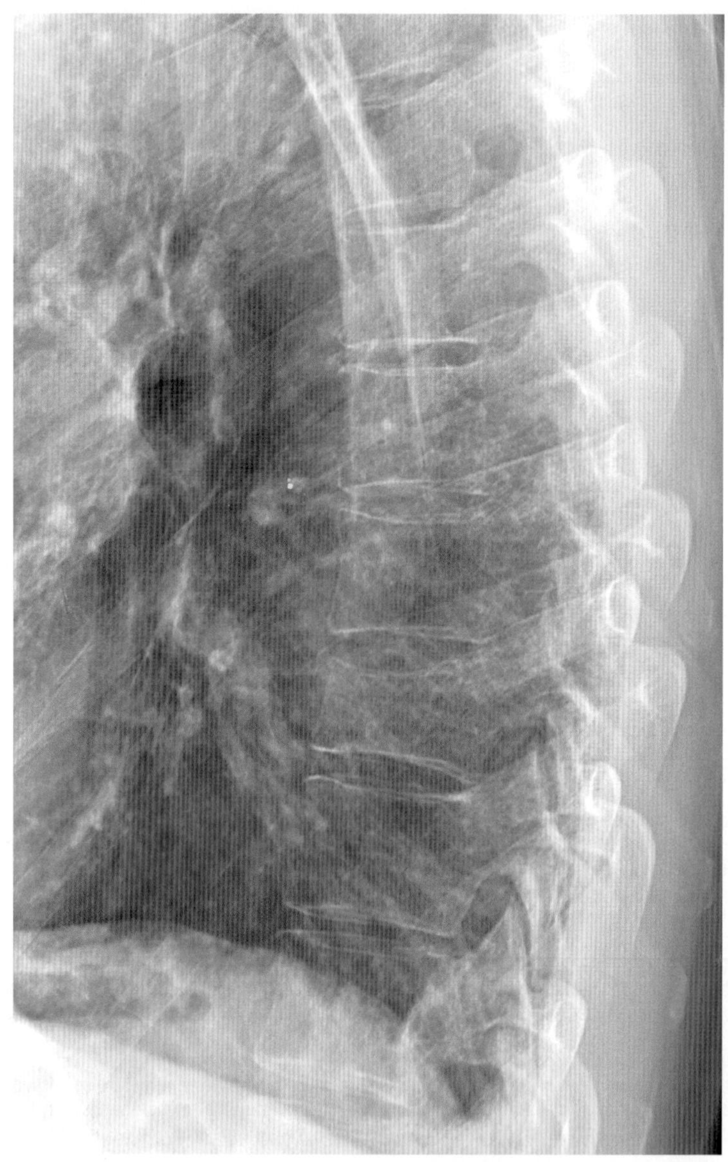

26. How does an anterior dislocation of the shoulder appear on a radiograph?

AP view of the shoulder in a patient with an anterior dislocation. Although the anterior location of the humeral head (*thin black arrow*) relative to the glenoid (*thick black arrow*) cannot be detected on this view, the position of the humeral head below the coracoid process (*thin white arrow*) and medial and inferior to the glenoid is classic for this type of dislocation.

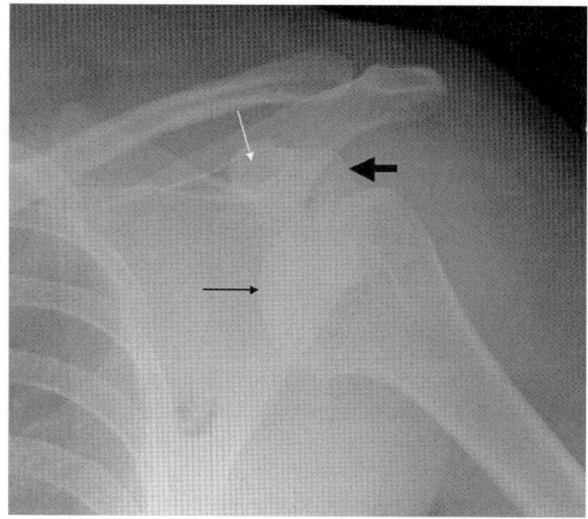

27. **What are the MRI findings of a shoulder dislocation?**
Hill-Sachs lesions of the humeral head are associated with as much as 75% of all shoulder dislocations and are an impaction of the humeral head on the glenoid as the humeral head tries to relocate into the glenoid fossa. Bankart tears occur when a piece of the labrum is torn off during an anterior shoulder dislocation. These lesions can also occur in up to 70% of anterior shoulder dislocations. Sometimes a bone chip from the glenoid rim is included, and this is called a bony Bankart lesion.

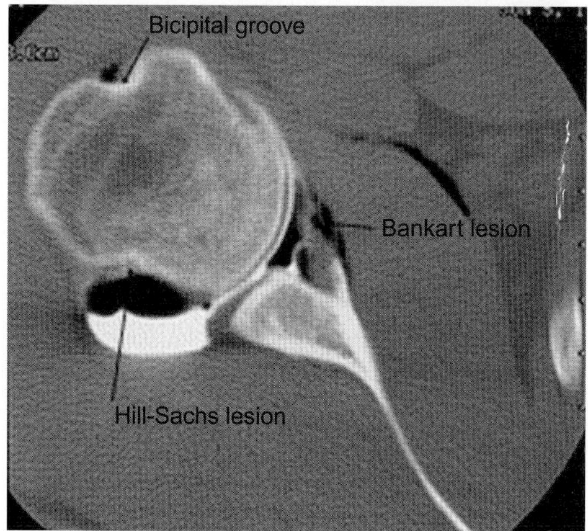

28. **What is the radiographic appearance of an acromioclavicular separation?**
Acromioclavicular separations can appear as a minimal disruption that requires conservative or severe treatment that could necessitate surgical intervention to restore normal anatomy. Minor A-C separations, such as grade I and II, demonstrate widening of the AC joint but normal coracoclavicular distance and are treated conservatively. More severe AC separations will have marked widening of both the AC and coraclavicular spaces. Right figure demonstrates grade III separation.

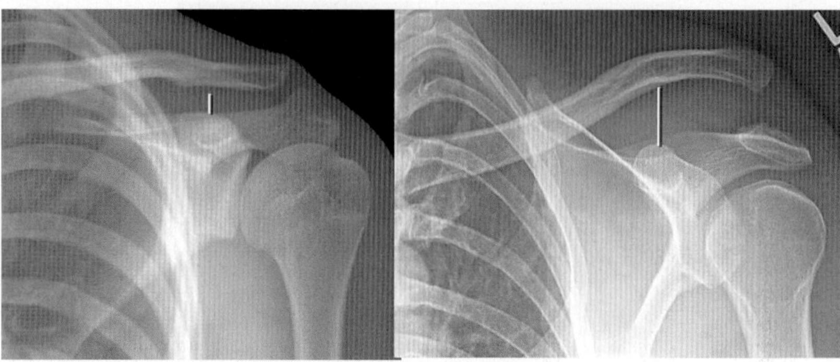

29. **How does a greater tuberosity fracture appear on MRI?**
Coronal oblique T1-weighted MRI of the shoulder. The subcutaneous fat and the fat in the bone marrow are normally white or high signal on a T1-weighted image. In the region of the greater tuberosity, there is a gray signal in the bone marrow with black lines running through it (*white arrows*). This is compatible with a fracture and surrounding bone marrow edema, confirming the finding seen on the previous x-ray. The black line below the fracture is the normal physeal remnant (*black arrows*). Note the normal supraspinatus muscle and tendon just above the humeral head (*open white arrows*).

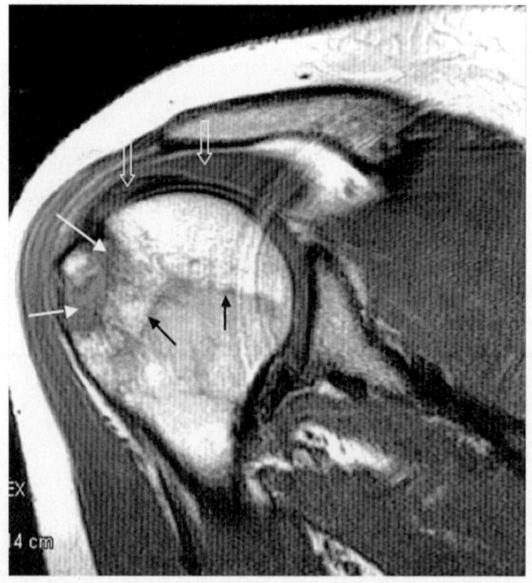

30. **What is the turtle neck sign?**
The turtle neck sign is indicative of a biceps tendon rupture and is when the tendon curls up after the rupture. The tendon can also retract linearly.

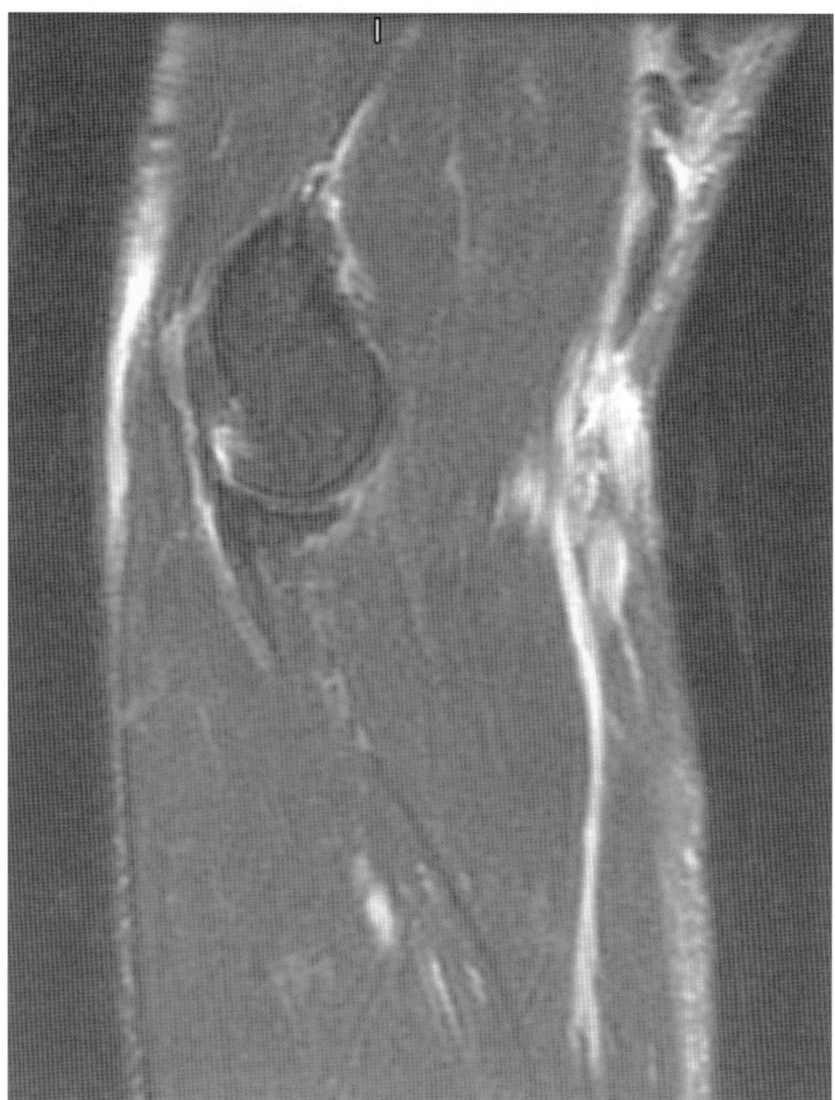

31. **What is ulnar variance?**

Ulnar variance refers to the position of the distal articular surface of the ulna relative to the radius. Ulna neutral exists when the radius and ulna are of equal length.

In this situation, 80% of the axial load across the wrist is transmitted through the radius and 20% through the ulna. Ulnar variance is negative if the articular surface of the ulna is proximal to that of the radius.

Positive ulnar variance exists when the ulna is longer than the radius. With negative ulnar variance, less stress is borne by the ulna; conversely, with positive ulnar variance, the stress borne by the distal ulna increases. Eighty percent of people are ±1 mm of ulnar neutral.

PA view of the wrist in a patient who is ulnar neutral. The radius and ulna are of equal length.

PA view of the wrist demonstrating negative ulnar variance. The ulna is shorter than the radius.

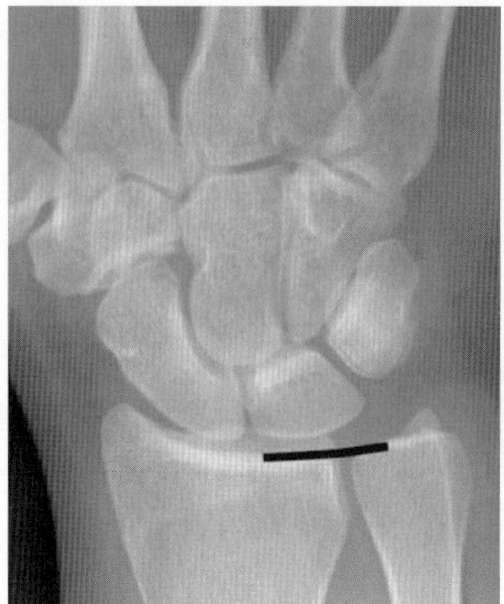

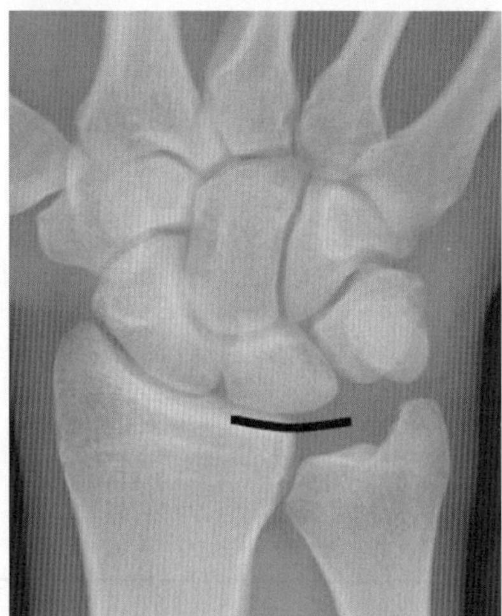

32. What are some of the common radiographic measurements made on wrist x-rays?
   - Scapholunate angle—the angle formed by lines drawn through the long axis of the scaphoid and the axis of the lunate on a lateral view of the wrist. In normal individuals the scapholunate angle measures between 30 and 60 degrees. Ligament injuries and fractures can lead to carpal collapse patterns that result in an abnormally increased or decreased scapholunate angle.
   - Capitolunate angle—the intersection of lines drawn through the long axis of the capitate and the axis of the lunate on a lateral x-ray. Normally the capitolunate angles measure less than 20 degrees. An increase in this angle can be seen with carpal instability.
   - Radial inclination—drawn on a PA view of the wrist. This is the angle formed by a line drawn perpendicular to the long axis of the radius and a line drawn from medial to lateral along the distal edge of the radius. Normal radial inclination is approximately 23 degrees.
   - Palmar tilt—drawn similar to the angle of radial inclination except on a lateral view of the wrist. The first line is perpendicular to the long axis of the radius. The second line extends along the distal aspect of the radius, bridging the volar and dorsal edges. A measurement of 10 to 15 degrees is considered normal.

   Lateral view of the wrist depicting the scapholunate angle. Line 1 is drawn along the long axis of the scaphoid while line 2 is drawn through the lunate. Normally, the angle measures between 30 and 60 degrees.

   Lateral view of the wrist depicting the capitolunate angle. Line 1 is drawn along the long axis of the capitate while line 2 is drawn through the lunate. Normally, the angle measures less than 20 degrees.

   PA view of the wrist demonstrating the normal angle of radial inclination.

   Lateral view of the wrist demonstrating normal volar tilt of the distal radius.

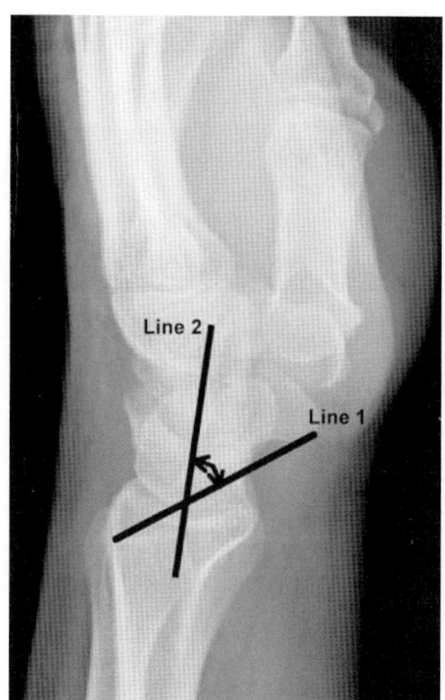
Line 2
Line 1

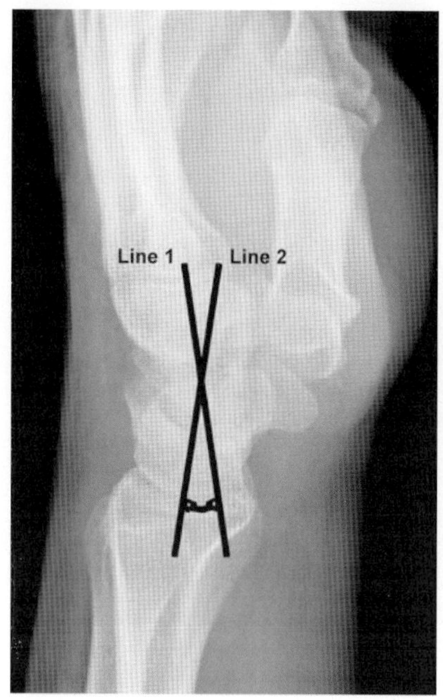
Line 1
Line 2

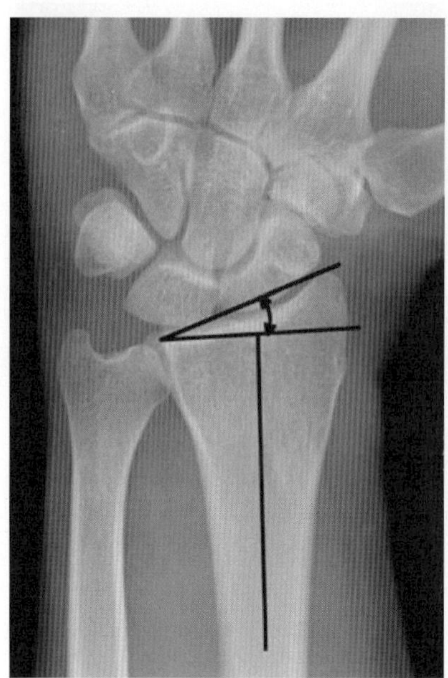

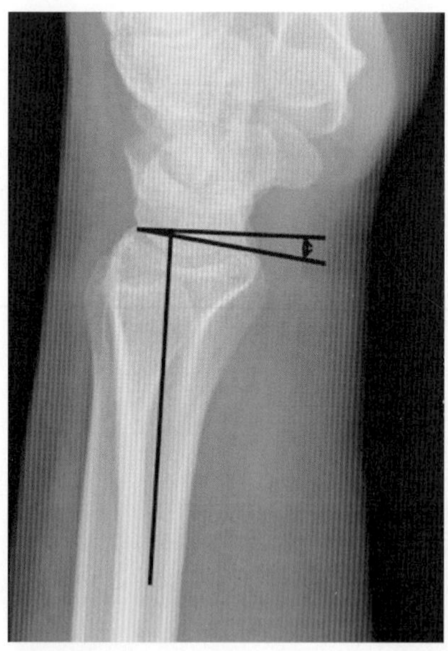

33. **What is the MRI appearance of a triangle fibrocartilage complex (TFCC) tear?**
Triangle fibrocartilage complex (TFCC) includes a cartilaginous disc and ligaments at the distal end of the ulna as it approximates the proximal carpals of the wrist. Tears can be classified as traumatic or degenerative and present with pain or discomfort ulnarly, near the styloid. Traumatic TFCC tears are associated with up to 50% of wrist dislocations and fractures. Note in the pictures a normal TFCC on the left and a TFCC tear indicated by fluid accumulation at the distal end of the ulna from a T2-weighted MRI.

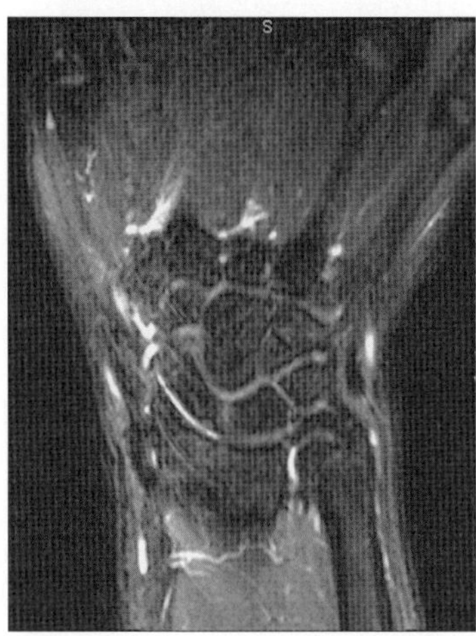

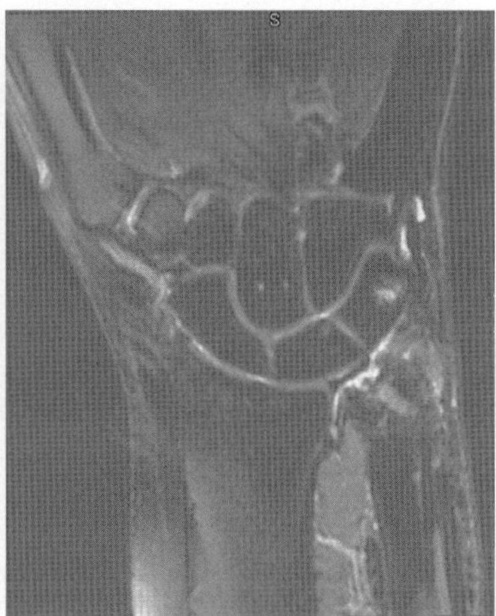

34. **What radiographic lines and angles can be used in the diagnosis of developmental dysplasia of the hip (DDH)?**
- Hilgenreiner's line—a horizontal line drawn through the triradiate cartilage
- Perkin's line—drawn vertically along the lateral rim of the acetabulum

The intersection of Hilgenreiner's line and Perkin's line divides the hip into four quadrants. The femoral head ossification center should normally be within the inner lower quadrant. With hip dislocation or DDH, the femoral ossific nucleus will be outside of this area.

- Shenton's line—smooth curved line drawn between the medial femoral neck and the superior portion of the obturator foramen; may be broken or discontinuous in DDH or hip dislocation.
- Acetabular index—a measure of the slope of the acetabular roof. The angle is formed by the intersection of Hilgenreiner's line with a line drawn through the lateral margin of the acetabular roof. It varies with age; at birth, the angle normally measures between 18 and 36 degrees. Acetabular dysplasia is suggested when the acetabular index is increased.
- Wiberg's center-edge angle (CE angle)—this angle is formed by a vertical line drawn superiorly from the center of the femoral head and a line drawn from the center of the femoral head to the lateral margin of the acetabular roof. It is an indication of acetabular depth. The CE angle is normal when it measures 20 to 40 degrees. The angle is decreased in dysplastic hips.

Anteroposterior view of a normal pediatric hip. Perkin's line, Hilgenreiner's line, Shenton's line, and the acetabular index are shown. Note that a major portion of the femoral head ossification center is located in the inner lower quadrant of the intersection of Perkin's and Hilgenreiner's lines.

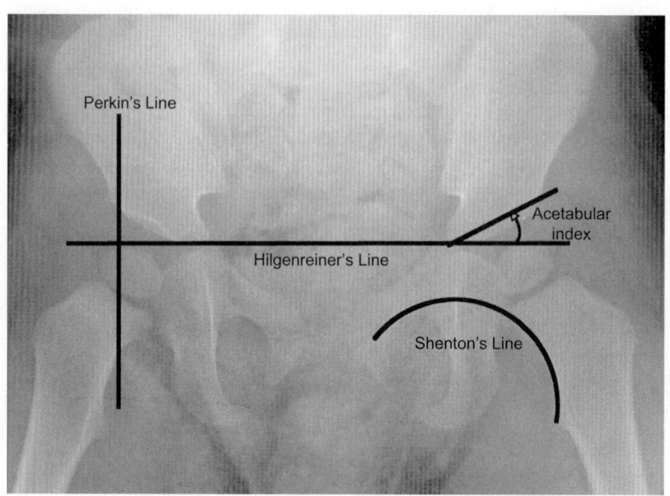

35. What is the femoral neck-shaft angle?

The femoral neck-shaft angle is the intersection of lines drawn through the axis of the femoral neck and femoral shaft. It measures approximately 150 degrees at birth and normally decreases with age. The neck-shaft angle measures 120 to 130 degrees in adults. A decrease in the neck-shaft angle is termed coxa vara, and an increase in this angle represents coxa valga.

AP view of an adult pelvis with a normal center-edge angle shown on the right and a normal neck-shaft angle on the left.

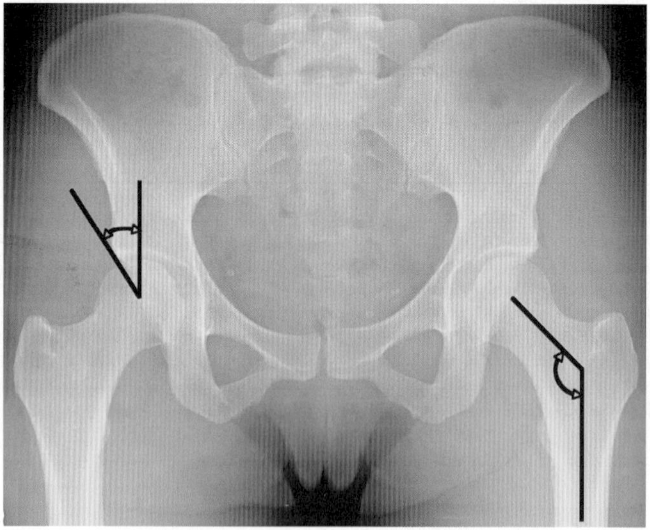

36. **How are hip fractures imaged and classified?**

Radiographs are the first-line modality to image hip fractures and these fractures are classified based on their relationship to the hip capsule. Intracapsular fractures include femoral neck fractures while fractures that are extracapsular generally include intertrochanteric and subtrochanteric fractures. Most of these fractures are due to falls, especially in elderly women.

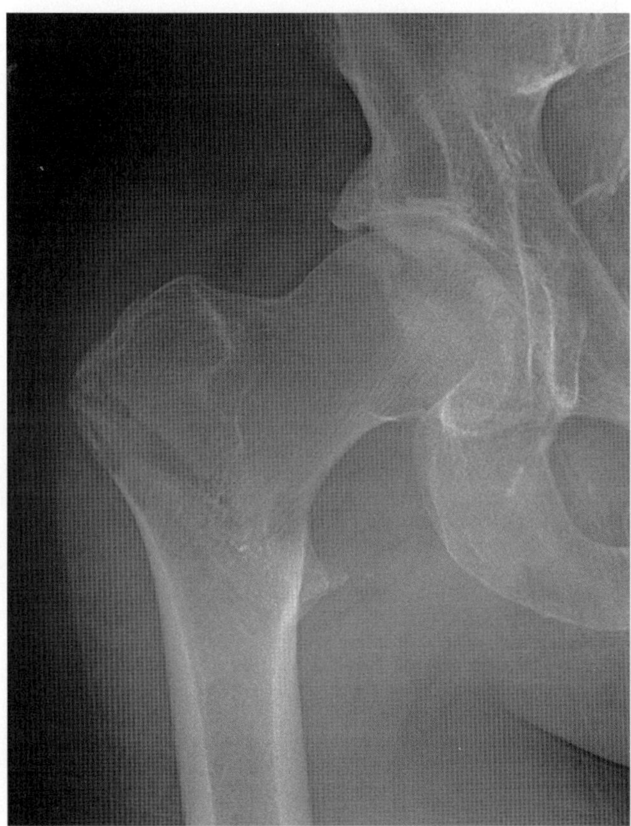

AP view of intertrochanteric femoral fracture

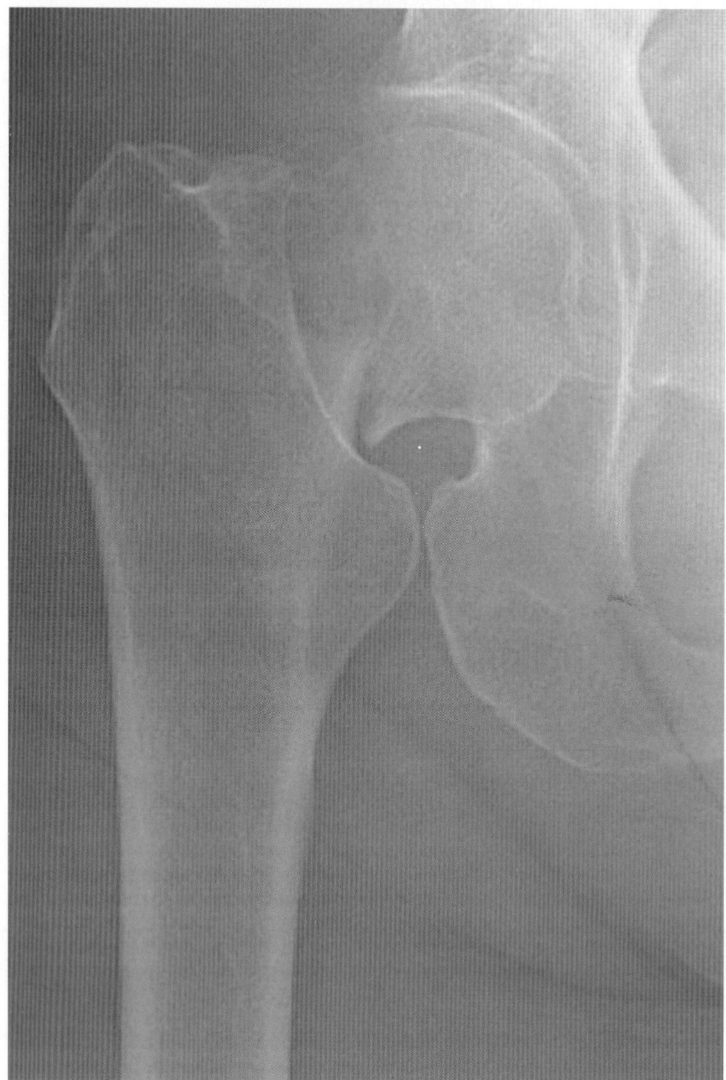

AP view of femoral neck fracture

37. What is femoroacetabular impingement (FAI)?

FAI is when the femoral head abuts the acetabulum. This is usually associated with repetitive hip loading in maximal flexion during adolescence. Deformities at the proximal femur (CAM-Type FAI) or acetabular overcoverage of the femoral head (pincer-type FAI) can result in FAI.

This patient with FAI has a "bump," otherwise known as a cam deformity at the anterolateral femoral head/neck junction.

In this patient with pincer-type FAI, the femoral head is deep within the joint and overcovered by the acetabulum.

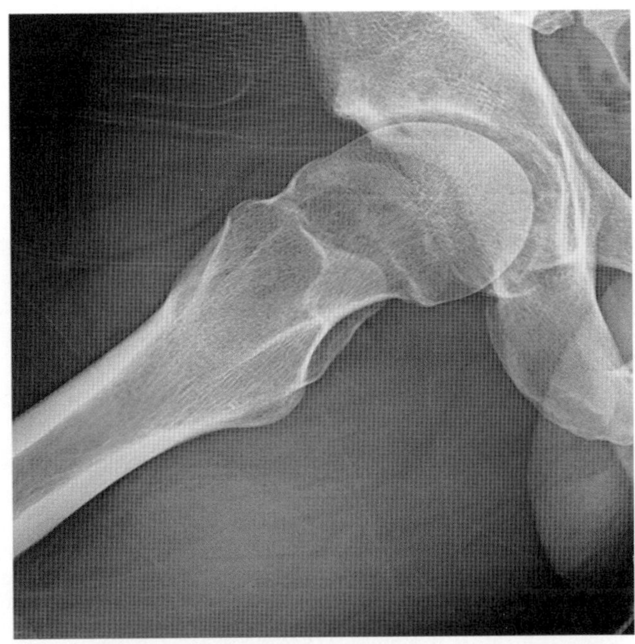

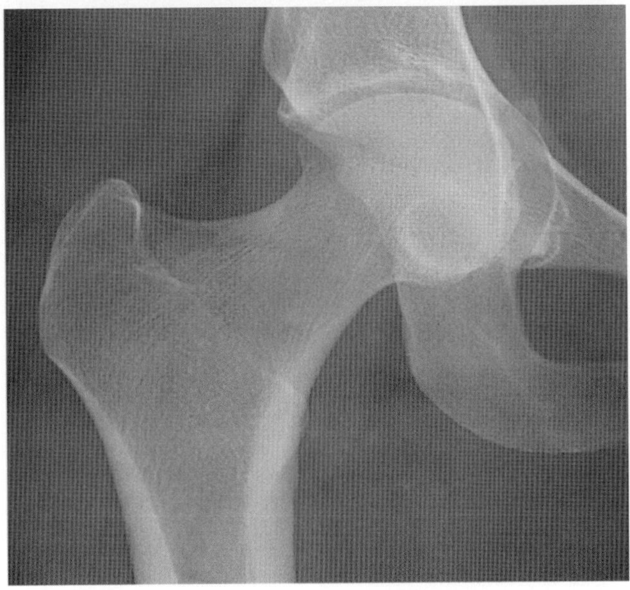

38. **What is the radiographic appearance of proper and improper total hip arthroplasty component positioning?**
With aging populations, hip arthroplasty ("total hip" or "hip replacement") is expected to rise for the foreseeable future. This procedure has been hailed as a major medical improvement over the past quarter century because of how it can restore pain-free lower extremity function. However, biomechanically correct placement of prostheses is necessary to restore function. Hip arthroplasty requires optimal placement of prosthetic components in order to maximize effectiveness. The acetabular cup should be anteverted 10 to 20 degrees and between 30 to 50 degrees of abduction in order to reduce the dislocation rate. Note the greater anteversion on the patient's left side (right side of image) compared with the contralateral side.

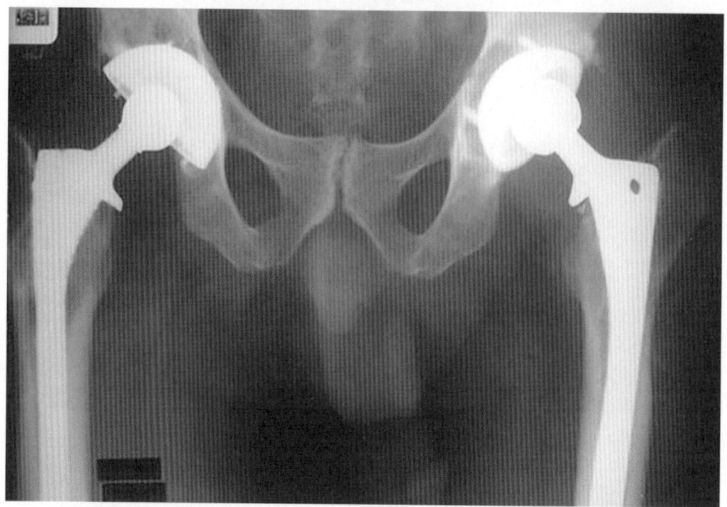

39. **What are the radiographic and MR appearances of avascular necrosis of the hip?**
Between 5% to 40% of hip dislocations can lead to avascular necrosis (AVN) of the femoral head. However, it may take 3 to 4 months to show up radiographically. MRI can help identify bony changes earlier than conventional radiographs. Note that in part **(A)** the MRI can detect early changes. Radiographically a "crescent sign" can be seen at the tip of the femoral head. As destruction of the bone ensues, the femoral head will collapse as a result of weight bearing **(B)**.

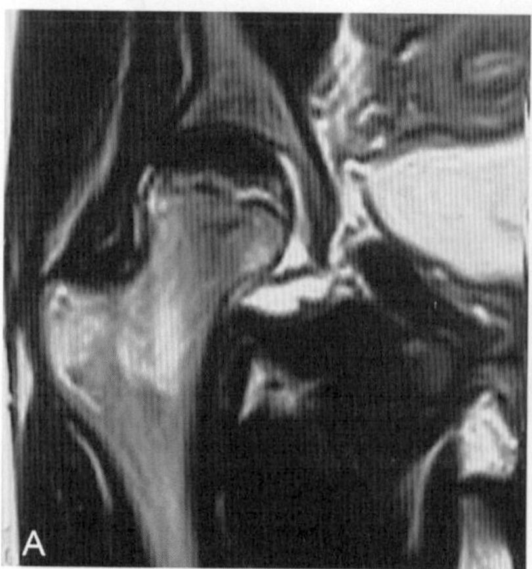

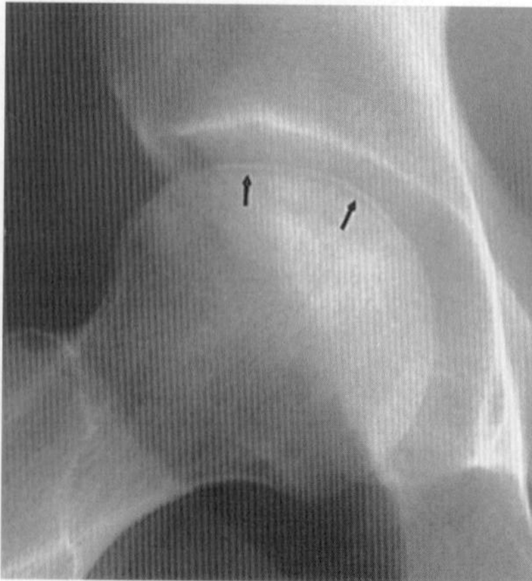

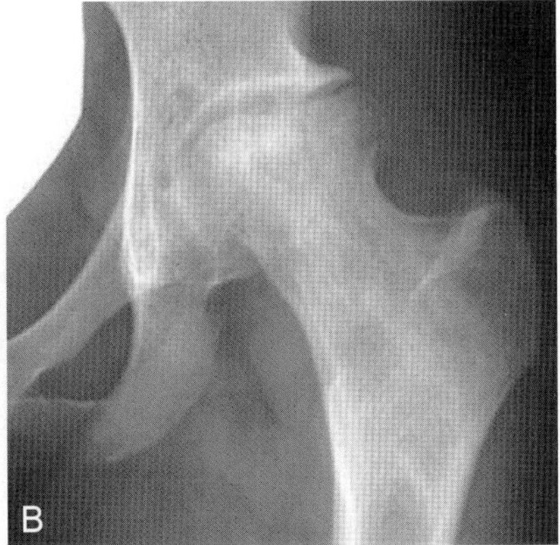

40. **What is patella alta and how is it diagnosed on radiographs?**
Patella alta is a condition in which the patella is more superiorly displaced than normal. This can be seen with clinical observations or can also be examined radiographically with the Insall-Salvati ratio. The Insall-Salvati ratio is measured with the knee flexed 30 degrees on a lateral knee radiograph and is calculated as the length of the patella over the length of the patella tendon. Normally, this ratio is 1; a 20% deviation indicates patella alta.

41. **What is a sulcus angle?**
The sulcus angle is used to quantify the angle of the femoral sulcus, in which the patella sits. The sulcus angle is generated from a Merchant's view radiograph, where the knee is flexed 30 degrees, and the image demonstrates the patella sitting in its femoral sulcus. The angle is defined by the highest and lowest points of the medial and lateral intercondylar sulci. A sulcus angle >140 degrees indicates a shallower intercondylar sulcus and is suggestive of patellofemoral problems.

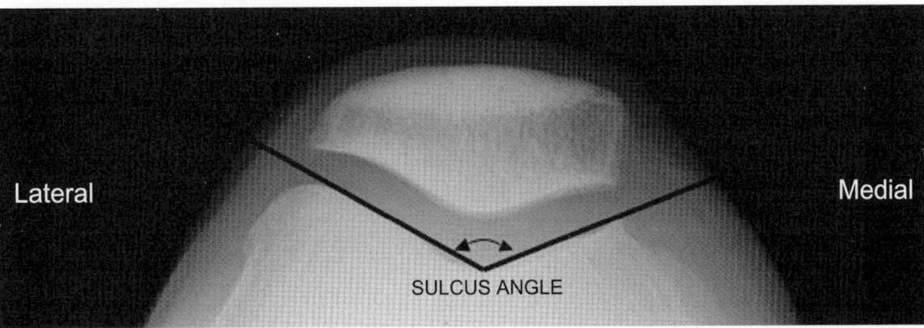

Merchant's view of the knee. The lateral facet of the patella is longer than the medial facet of the patella. Thus on this image, lateral is to the left and medial to the right. Measurement of the sulcus angle is demonstrated. In this patient it measures 130 degrees.

42. **How does an osteochondral lesion of the lateral femoral condyle appear on a radiograph?**
Tunnel view of the knee. There is deformity along the articular surface of the lateral femoral condyle (*thin white arrow*). There is a lucent defect with sclerosis (*increased whiteness*) in the surrounding bone. This is compatible with osteochondritis dissecans. A free fragment is seen in the notch (*thin black arrow*). Note that the physes are still open in this teenager.

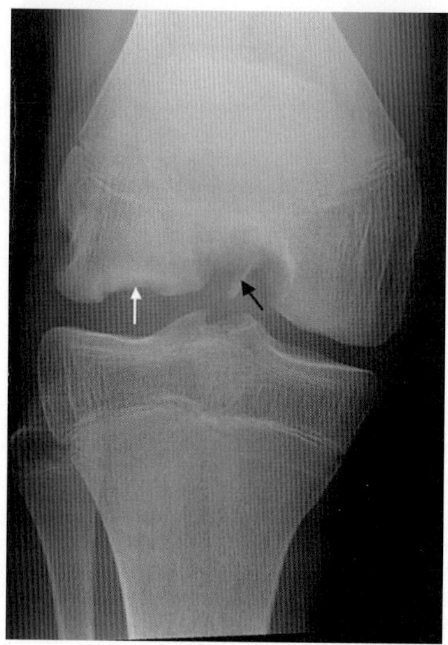

43. **What is the best method, to date, to quantify the degenerative knee joint disease or osteoarthritis?**
The Kellgren Lawrence Classification system ranges from 0 or normal to 4.
Grade 1—doubtful or minimal to no narrowing of joint space with possible osteophyte formation
Grade 2—possible joint narrowing of joint space with definite osteophyte formation
Grade 3—definite joint narrowing with moderate osteophyte formation, some sclerosis and possible bone deformity
Grade 4—severe joint narrowing, large osteophyte formation with patent sclerosis and bone deformity

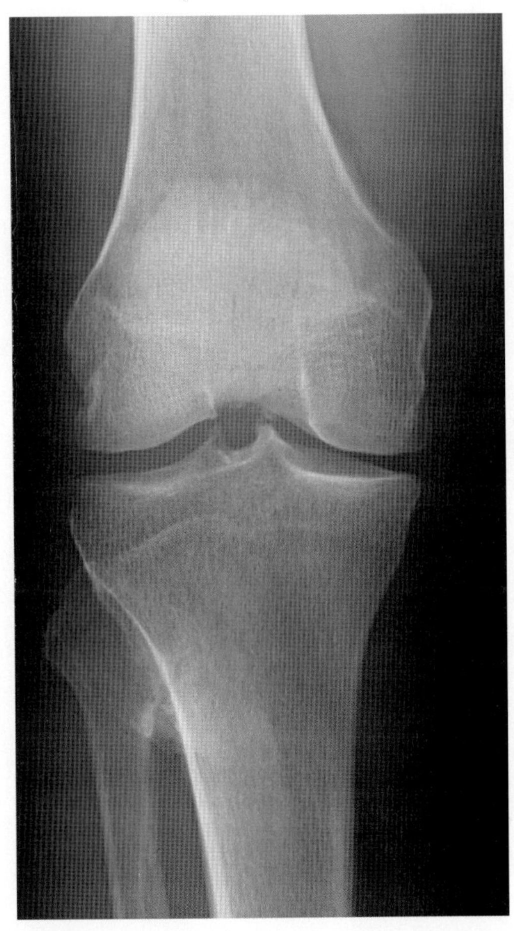

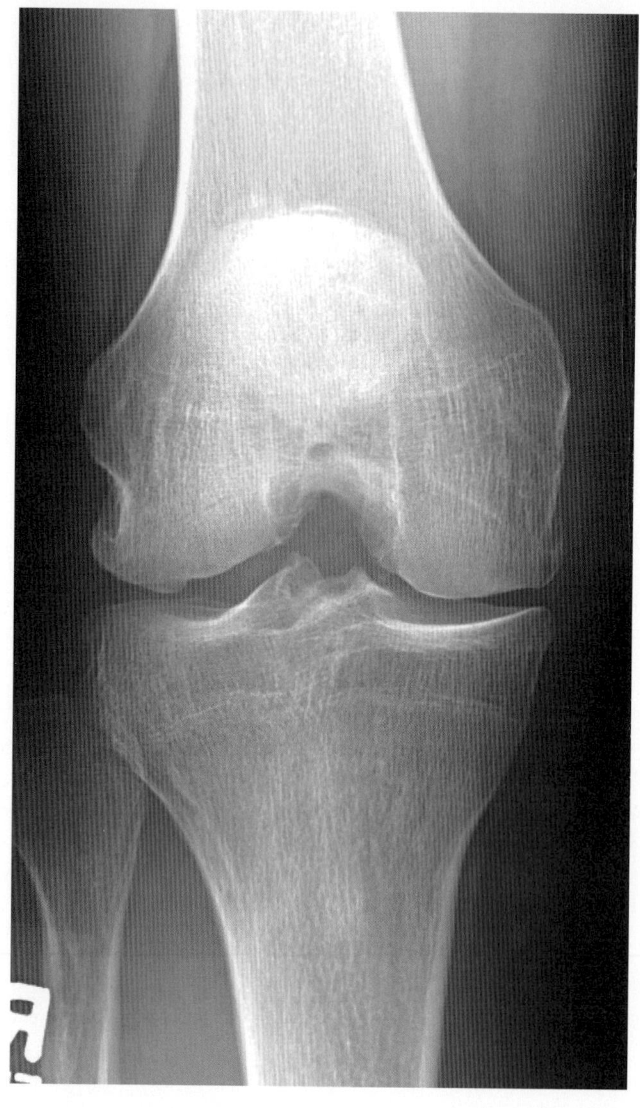

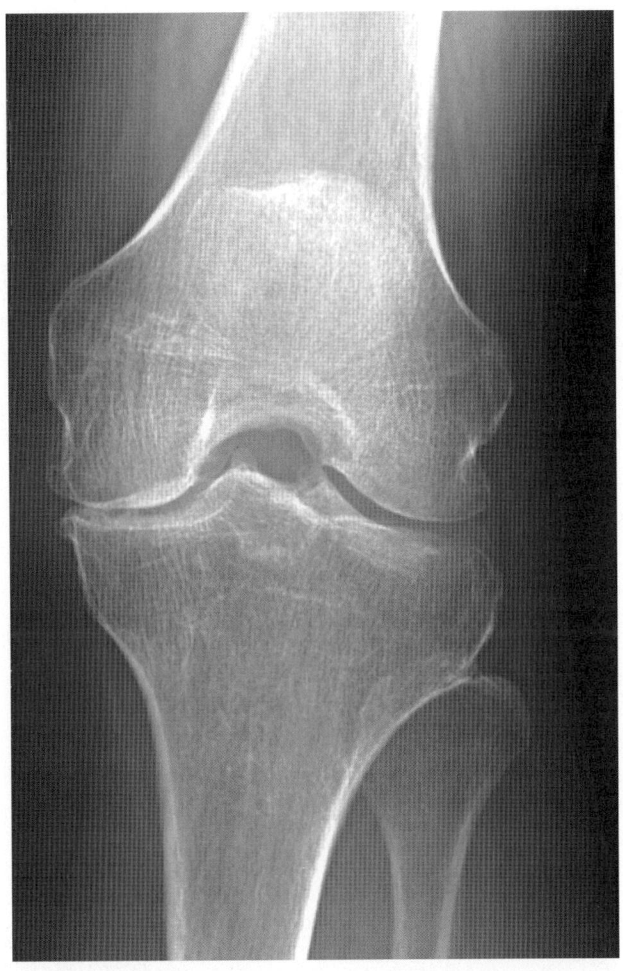

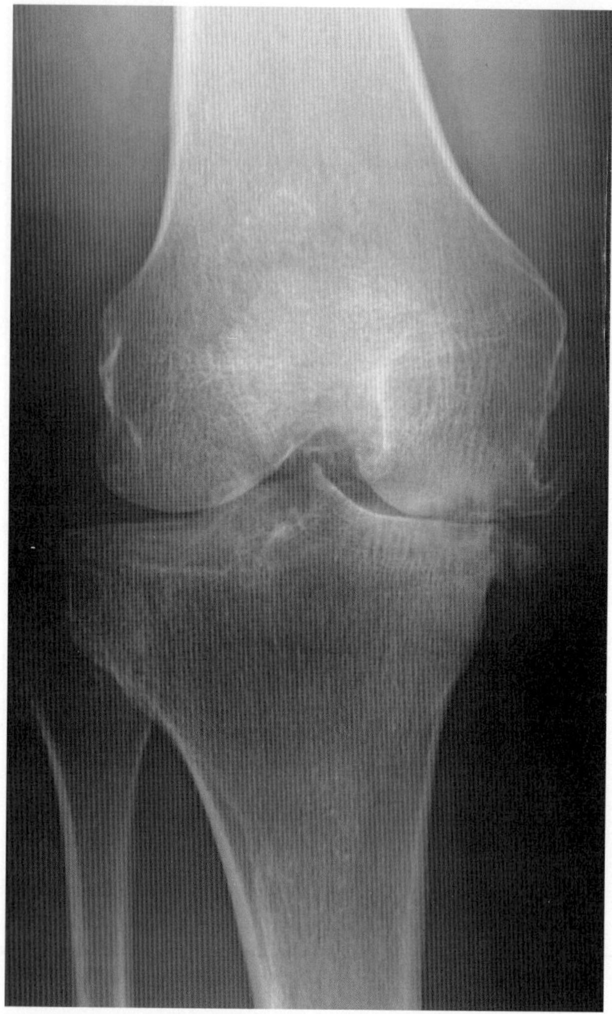

44. **How does a normal ACL appear on MRI?**

Sagittal proton density images demonstrating a normal ACL. A black signal is seen throughout the ACL as it extends from the femur to the proximal tibia (*white arrows*). The course of the ACL should parallel the posterior aspect of the intercondylar notch of the femur (*black arrows*). This is called Blumensaat's line. Note the normal gray cartilage at the anterior aspect of the distal femur (*open white arrow*).

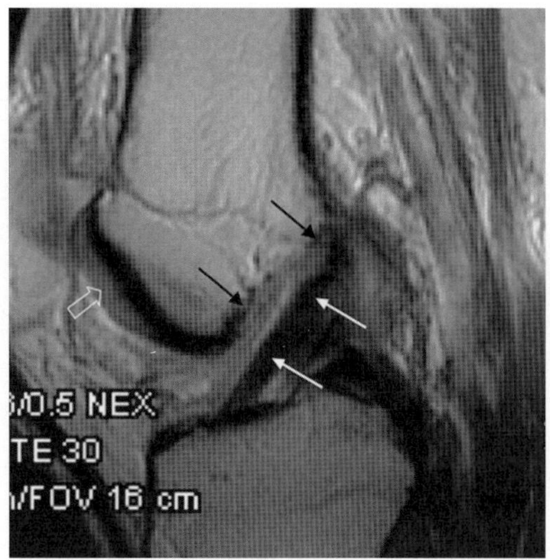

45. **How does a ruptured ACL appear on MRI?**
Sagittal proton density MRI of the knee. Normal tendons are black or low signal on MRI. Note the normal patella tendon anteriorly (*thin black arrows*). The posterior cruciate ligament (PCL) is also normal (*thin white arrows*). Only the inferior portion of the PCL is seen on this image. The anterior cruciate ligament (ACL) is abnormal. There is an amorphous intermediate or grayish signal where the normal ACL should be (*open white arrows*). Only the inferior aspect of the ACL contains the normal black signal.

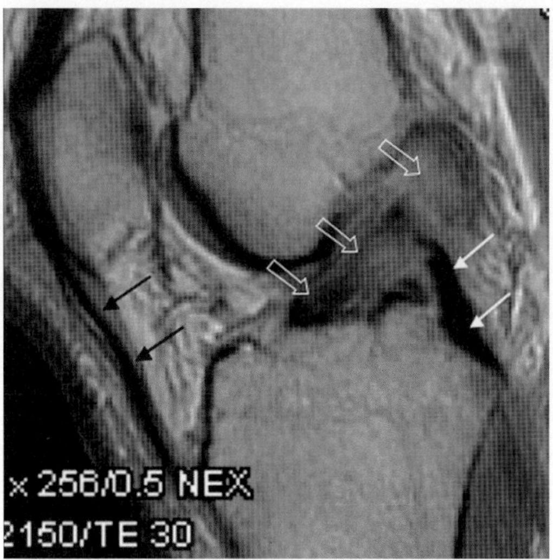

46. **What bones are affected by a trimalleolar fracture?**
A trimalleolar fracture includes a medial malleolar fracture and a posterior malleolar fracture at the distal tibia and a lateral malleolar fracture of the fibula.

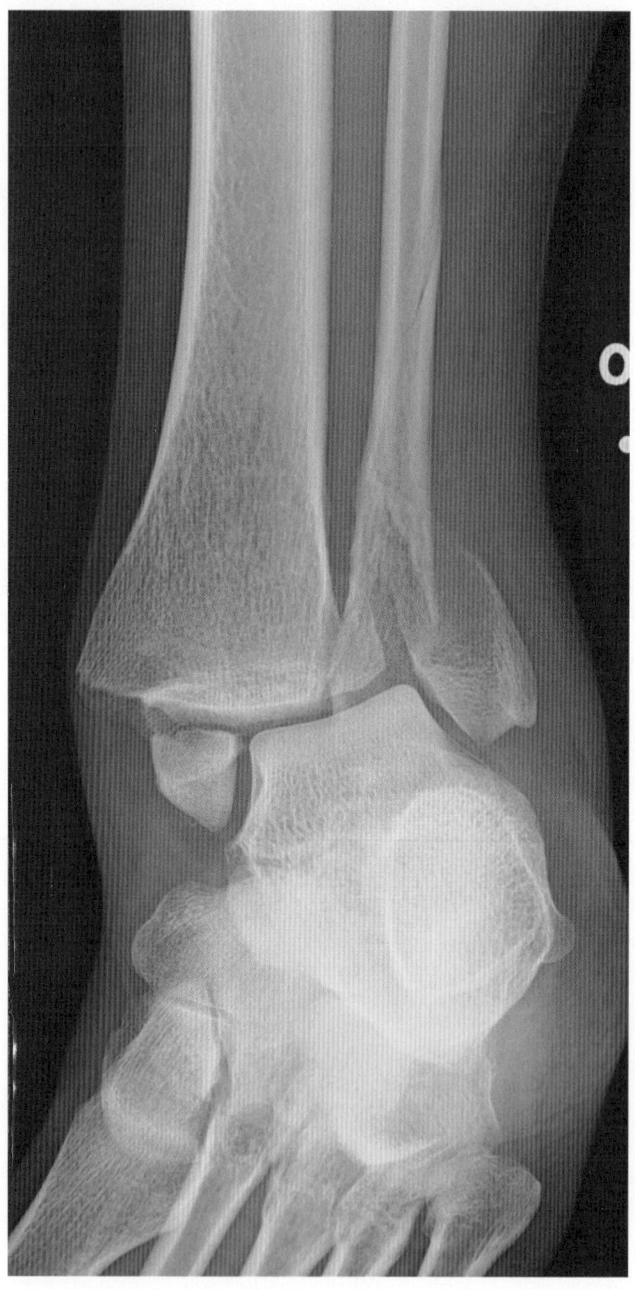

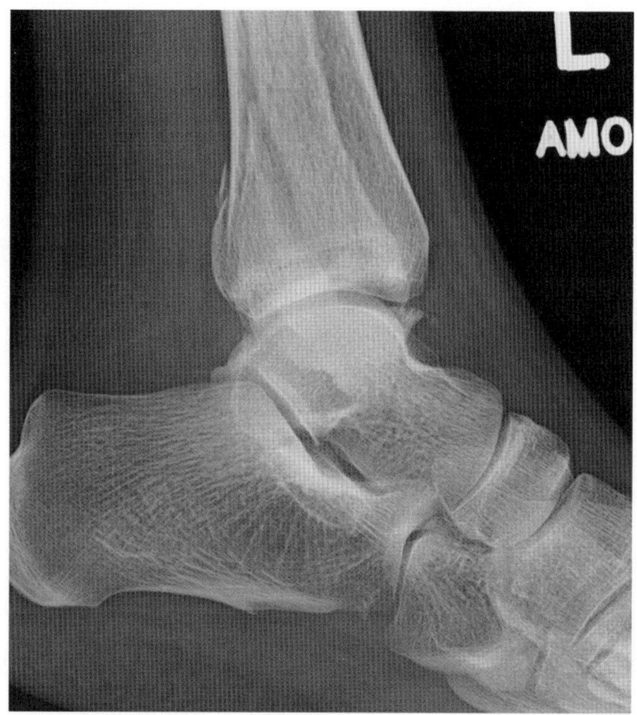

47. **What is the radiographic appearance of a Jones fracture?**
    Jones fracture is typically at the base of the fifth metatarsal and needs to be distinguished from the avulsion fracture and from the peroneus brevis, sometimes called the pseudo-Jones fracture. This injury usually occurs with landing on an inverted foot. Note the oblique view gives better visualization of the fracture at the base of the fifth metatarsal.

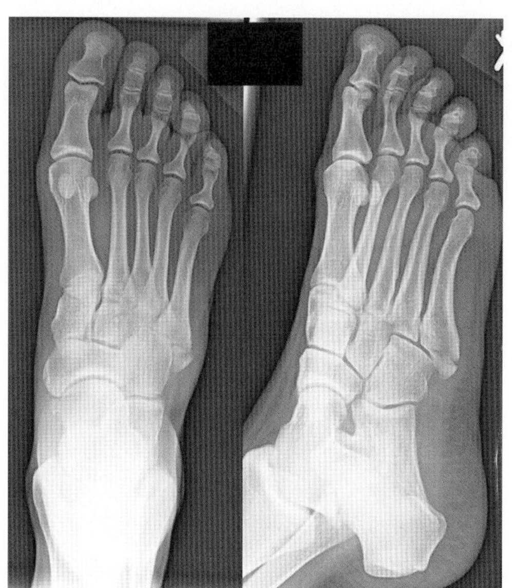

BIBLIOGRAPHY

Boonrod, A., Harasymczuk, M., Ramazanian, T., Boonrod, A., Smith, J., & O'Driscoll, S. W. (2022). The turtle neck sign: identification of severe retracted distal biceps tendon rupture. *Orthopaedic Journal of Sports Medicine, 10*(1), 23259671211065040.

Curry, T. S., Dowdey, J. E., & Murry, R. C. (1990). *Christensen's physics of diagnostic radiology* (4th ed.). Philadelphia, PA: Lea & Febiger.

Dwyer, A. J., John, B., Singh, S. A., & Mam, M. K. (2006). Complications after posterior dislocations of the hip. *International Orthopaedics, 30*(4), 224–227.

Fernandez-de Thomas, R.J. (2021) Thoracolumbar spin fracture, In: Stat Pearls Internet. Treasure Island, FL (Available from: https://www.ncbi.nlm.nih.gov/books/NBK562204/).

Hak, D. J., & Gautsch, T. L. (1995). A review of radiographic lines and angles used in orthopedics. *American Journal of Orthopedics, 24*, 590–601.

Halpern, B., Herring, S. A., Altchek, D., & Herzog, R. (1997). *Imaging in musculoskeletal and sports medicine.* Malden, MA: Blackwell.

Kaplan, P. A., Dussault, R., Helms, C. A., Anderson, M. W., & Major, N. M. (2001). *Musculoskeletal MRI.* Philadelphia, PA: WB Saunders.

Kohn, M. D., Sassoon, A. A., & Fernando, N. D. (2016). Classifications in brief: Kellgren-Lawrence classification of osteoarthritis. *Clinical Orthopaedics and Related Research, 474*(8), 1886–1893.

Larson, C. M., LaPrade, R. F., Floyd, E. R., McGaver, R. S., & Bedi, A. (2021). Acetabular rim disorders/pincer-type femoroacetabular impingement and hip arthroscopy. *Sports Medicine and Arthroscopy Review, 29*(1), 35–43.

Luhmann, S. J., Schootman, M., Gordon, J. E., & Wright, R. W. (2005). Magnetic resonance imaging of the knee in children and adolescents: its role in clinical decision-making. *Journal of Bone and Joint Surgery (American), 87*, 497–502.

Parker, M., & Johansen, A. (2006). Hip fracture. *BMJ, 333*(7557), 27–30.

Resnick, D. (2005). *Bone and joint imaging.* Philadelphia, PA: Elsevier Saunders.

Resnick, D., & Kang, H. F. (1997). *Internal derangement of joints.* Philadelphia, PA: WB Saunders.

Rogers, L. F. (2002). *Radiology of skeletal trauma.* New York, NY: Churchill Livingstone.

Widmer, K. T. (2007). Containment versus impingement: finding a compromise for cup placement in total hip arthroplasty. *International Orthopaedics, 31*(Sup 1), 29–33.

CHAPTER 32 QUESTIONS

1. Normal radiographic anatomy of the distal radius does not include:
   a. Dorsal tilt of 10 to 15 degrees
   b. Radial inclination of 23 degrees
   c. SL angle of 30 to 60 degrees
   d. ±1 mm of ulnar neutral variance

2. Normal femoral shaft angle in adult hips is approximately:
   a. 110 degrees
   b. 125 degrees
   c. 145 degrees
   d. 160 degrees

3. Characteristics of T_2 images include:
   a. Fat as white
   b. CSF as black
   c. Tendon as black
   d. Edema as black

BLOOD FLOW RESTRICTION TRAINING

J.G. Owens, MPT and S.D. Patterson, PhD

1. **What is blood flow restriction (BFR) training?**
   BFR is the application of a tourniquet to the proximal thigh or proximal arm to reduce arterial inflow and block venous outflow. The hypoxic environment created by BFR promotes muscle strength and hypertrophy adaptations at low loads.

2. **What are the indications for BFR?**
   Although exact clinical conditions most appropriate for BFR are still being studied, in general, it is used to improve muscle quantity and quality when high resistance loads are contraindicated such as postoperatively, after injury, with painful conditions, or in the elderly who are load intolerant.

3. **What are contraindications of BFR?**
   - Venous thromboembolism
   - Impaired circulation of vascular compromise
   - Extremities with a dialysis access
   - Acidosis
   - Sickle cell anemia
   - Extremity infection
   - Tumor distal to the tourniquet
   - Medications and supplements known to increase clotting risk
   - Increased intracranial pressure
   - Open soft tissue injuries
   - Severe crush injuries
   - Severe hypertension
   - Lymphectomies
   - Cancer
   - Skin grafts in which all bleeding points must be readily distinguished

4. **What are the mechanisms behind BFR?**
   Figure

   Local muscle hypoxia via application of a tourniquet to low load exercises appears to be the primary driver of increases in muscle strength and size associated with BFR. Increased muscle fiber recruitment inducing fatigue and metabolite accumulation have been proposed mechanisms. However, recent evidence has not found a direct correlation between the hormonal responses associated with BFR and changes in increased muscle strength and size. The physiologic rationale behind the adaptation seen with low load-BFR training may need to emphasize local skeletal muscle mechanisms that are like high load training compared to any systemic or acute hormonal pathways. Lending more credence to the notion that BFR is not a simple hormonal response but a physiological response very similar to high load training.

   Some suggested mechanisms include:

   Increased muscle fiber recruitment and fatigue
   - Muscle fiber recruitment is higher with BFR versus low load exercise resulting in more rapid muscle fatigue.

   Increased muscle protein synthesis (MPS)
   - After exercising at low loads with BFR, there is a significant increase in MPS that can drive muscle hypertrophy.

   Altered gene expression
   - Changes in gene expression have been measured after performing BFR. These include downregulation of myostatin, upregulation of vascular endothelial growth factor, and proliferation of myogenic and mesenchymal stem cells. However, when exploring 29 genes responsible for muscle adaptation after training with low load-BFR versus high load training, no difference was found in gene expression between the groups.

   Accumulation of muscle metabolites
   - The anaerobic environment created by BFR, via reduced blood flow and increased hypoxia, results in an accumulation of muscle metabolites that may serve as an anabolic signal for positive muscle adaptation.

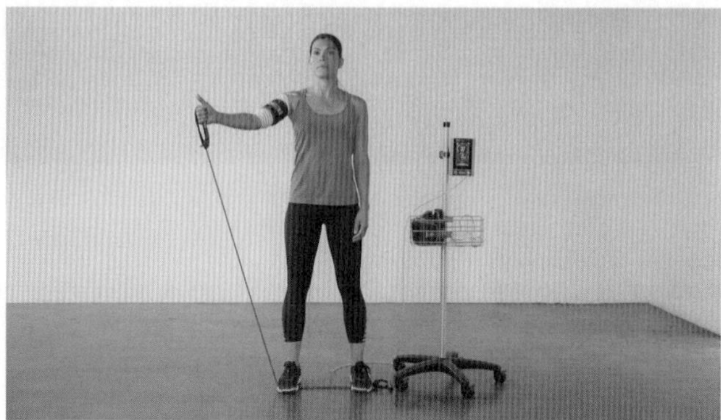

Low load exercise with blood flow restriction.

5. **Does the current evidence support BFR?**
Numerous systematic reviews and meta-analysis support BFR as an intervention with superior results for muscle strength and hypertrophy compared to low load exercise. These include healthy, elderly, and clinical populations. Outcome studies have demonstrated improvements in muscle strength and size when BFR is utilized with low load resistance exercise or low-level aerobic exercise compared to free-flow conditions following postoperative anterior cruciate ligament (ACL) surgeries, knee osteoarthritis, older adults at risk of sarcopenia, and inclusion body myositis. Additionally, compared to heavy loads used after ACL surgery BFR demonstrated similar increases in muscle size and strength, but also improved functional and self-reported outcomes.
Ongoing randomized trials are assessing the efficacy and safety of BFR in different clinical populations.

6. **Is BFR safe?**
In general, BFR appears safe, with very few adverse events reported in the literature. BFR does not appear to activate coagulation pathways. Anti-thrombolytic factors such as tissue plasminogen factor have been shown to increase after BFR. Hemodynamics such as heart rate and blood pressure are generally elevated during BFR more than low load exercise; however, these elevations are usually less than high load exercise.

7. **Have any adverse events been reported in individuals performing BFR?**
The most common adverse events related to the use of BFR are delayed onset muscle soreness (39.2%), numbness (18.5%), fainting/dizziness (14.6%), and bruising (13.1%).
There have been four cases of rhabdomyolysis, a serious condition that can be fatal and is generally the result of damaged muscle releasing metabolites into the system and overwhelming the kidneys, reported in the literature in individuals who have engaged in BFR. These cases may be explained by individuals who are unaccustomed to exercise, too much volume of exercise, or other preexisting conditions.

8. **How is BFR typically performed?**
The most common application of BFR is to combine it with low load resistance exercise. The recommended load is between 20% and 40% of a 1-repetition maximum. A set and repetition scheme of four sets of 30/15/15/15 reps with 30-second rest period between each set is often used. The tourniquet stays inflated during the exercise and rest periods; however, deflation during rest periods may be required if BFR is uncomfortable. When utilizing low loads, 20% to 30% 1RM, the frequency of BFR sessions typically only needs to be two to three sessions a week. However, when using very low or no loads with BFR, termed passive or cell swelling BFR, the frequency may need to increase to daily or twice daily to slow the muscle loss associated with disuse.

9. **What is the recommended pressure application during BFR?**
The pressure applied is based on 100% arterial occlusion termed limb occlusion pressure (LOP) and reduced to a range of 40% to 80% LOP during exercise.

10. **What patient characteristics determine LOP?**
The size of the limb, blood pressure, cuff width, laterality (left versus right limb), and body position all play roles in how much pressure will be needed to achieve LOP.

11. **Are there other applications for BFR besides low load exercise?**
BFR combined with low-level endurance exercises such as walking or cycling improved aerobic capacity, muscle strength, size, and functional outcomes. Passive BFR, the application of BFR without exercise, has demonstrated the ability to slow muscle and strength loss during periods of disuse. BFR combined with electrical stimulation has been shown to increase muscle strength, size, and vascular function.

12. **What changes occur to muscles proximal to the cuff (tourniquet) placement?**
Although not fully understood and data are still limited, improvements in muscle size and strength proximal to the tourniquet have been noted at the hip, shoulder, and pectoralis region. Theories behind these improvements include fatigue of muscle groups below the cuff driving more proximal muscle recruitment or a systemic effect from the increased anabolism associated with BFR.

13. **Has BFR been found to improve the cardiovascular system?**
In addition to muscle strength and hypertrophy, BFR has been found to promote angiogenesis and aerobic capacity.

14. **Can BFR exercise be used to reduce pain?**
Research suggests that BFR resistance exercise has an analgesic effect that can last for 24 hrs. This effect has been observed in healthy and multiple clinical conditions.

15. **BFR uses low loads, what impact does this play on the tendon?**
Previous research suggested there was no effect of BFR exercise on tendon adaptations; however, recent research suggests that BFR exercise may lead to changes in tendon stiffness and cross-sectional area.

16. **Does BFR fall within the scope of physical therapy practice, and what are the current practice requirements for physical therapists to perform BFR in the United States?**
The American Physical Therapy Association has determined that BFR falls within the professional scope of practice for a physical therapist. Currently, all 50-state practice acts within the United States allow physical therapists to perform BFR.

17. **What are the "pros and cons" of using elastic bands versus a "limb occlusion pressure device" in the administration of BFR?**
There are multiple options on the market to perform BFR. Tourniquets are medical devices listed in the FDA database. It is recommended clinicians utilize an FDA device for patient care. The FDA classified tourniquets as class I devices, the safest classification, once autoregulation (the ability of the cuff to adapt and maintain pressure based on limb movement) became available. Additionally, personalized tourniquet pressure and wider cuffs limits unnecessarily high pressures and pressure gradients that may cause muscle damage. Options on the market that do not meet these criteria are not suggested for clinical use.

18. **Is specialized training required to perform BFR?**
Scope of practice falls under three pillars, professional, jurisdictional, and personal. It is incumbent on clinicians to determine their knowledge in BFR for their personal scope of practice. If education in BFR and tourniquet use was not taught to them in school, then advanced continuing education is recommended.

Bibliography

Bowman, E. N., Elshaar, R., Milligan, H., et al. (2019). Proximal, distal, and contralateral effects of blood flow restriction training on the lower extremities: a randomized controlled trial. *Sports Health*, *11*, 149–156.

Centner, C., Lauber, B., Seynnes, O. R., et al. (2019). Low-load blood flow restriction training induces similar morphological and mechanical Achilles tendon adaptations compared to high-load resistance training. *Journal of Applied Physiology*, *127*, 1660–1667.

Clark, B. C., Manini, T. M., Hoffman, R. L., et al. (2011). Relative safety of 4 weeks of blood flow-restricted resistance exercise in young, healthy adults. *Scandinavian Journal of Medicine & Science in Sports*, *21*, 653–662.

Ellefsen, S., Hammarström, D., Strand, T. A., et al. (2015). Blood flow-restricted strength training displays high functional and biological efficacy in women: a within-subject comparison with high-load strength training. *American Journal of Physiology. Regulatory, Integrative and Comparative Physiology*, *309*, R767–779.

Formiga, M. F., Fay, R., Hutchinson, S., et al. (2020). Effect of aerobic exercise training with and without blood flow restriction on aerobic capacity in healthy young adults: a systematic review with meta-analysis. *International Journal of Sports Physical Therapy*, *15*(2), 175–187.

Fry, C. S., Glynn, E. L., Drummond, M. J., et al. (2010). Blood flow restriction exercise stimulates mTORC1 signaling and muscle protein synthesis in older men. *Journal of Applied Physiology*, *108*(5), 1199–1209.

Hughes, L., & Patterson, S. D. (2020). The effect of blood flow restriction exercise on exercise-induced hypoalgesia and endogenous opioid and endocannabinoid mechanisms of pain modulation. *Journal of Applied Physiology*, *128*(4), 914–924.

Jack, R. A., 2nd, Lambert, B. S., Hedt, C. A., et al. (2022). Blood flow restriction therapy preserves lower extremity bone and muscle mass after ACL reconstruction. *Sports Health*, *15*(3), 361–371.

Jørgensen, A. N., Jensen, K. Y., Nielsen, J. L., et al. (2021). Effects of blood-flow restricted resistance training on mechanical muscle function and thigh lean mass in sIBM patients. *Scandinavian Journal of Medicine & Science in Sports, 32*(2), 359–371.

Laurentino, G. C., Loenneke, J. P., Ugrinowitsch, C., et al. (2022). Blood-flow-restriction-training-induced hormonal response is not associated with gains in muscle size and strength. *Journal of Human Kinetics, 83*, 235–243.

Mattocks, K. T., Jessee, M. B., Mouser, J. G., et al. (2018). The application of blood flow restriction: lessons from the laboratory. *Current Sports Medicine Reports, 17*(4), 129–134.

McEwen, J. A., Owens, J. G., & Jeyasurya, J. (2018). Why is it crucial to use personalized occlusion pressures in blood flow restriction (BFR) rehabilitation? *Journal of Medical and Biological Engineering, 39*(3).

Nielsen, J. L., Aagaard, P., Bech, R. D., et al. (2012). Proliferation of myogenic stem cells in human skeletal muscle in response to low-load resistance training with blood flow restriction. *The Journal of Physiology, 590*(17), 4351–4361.

Ohta, H., Kurosawa, H., Ikeda, H., Iwase, Y., Satou, N., & Nakamura, S. (2003). Low-load resistance muscular training with moderate restriction of blood flow after anterior cruciate ligament reconstruction. *Acta Orthopaedica Scandinavica, 74*(1), 62–68.

Patterson, S., Hughes, L., Warmington, S., et al. (2019). Blood flow restriction exercise position stand: considerations of methodology, application and safety. *Frontiers in Physiology, 10*, 533.

Segal, N. A., Williams, G. N., Davis, M. C., Wallace, R. B., & Mikesky, A. E. (2015). Efficacy of blood flow–restricted, low-load resistance training in women with risk factors for symptomatic knee osteoarthritis. *PM&R, 7*(4), 376–384.

Slysz, J. T., Boston, M., King, R., Pignanelli, C., Power, G. A., & Burr, J. F. (2020). Blood flow restriction combined with electrical stimulation attenuates thigh muscle disuse atrophy. *Medicine and Science in Sports and Exercise, 53*(5), 1033–1040.

Takarada, Y., Nakamura, Y., Aruga, S., Onda, T., Miyazaki, S., & Ishii, N. (2000). Rapid increase in plasma growth hormone after low-intensity resistance exercise with vascular occlusion. *Journal of Applied Physiology, 88*(1), 61–65.

Thompson, K., Slysz, J. T., & Burr, J. F. (2017). Risks of exertional rhabdomyolysis with blood flow–restricted training: beyond the case report. *Clinical Journal of Sport Medicine, 28*(6), 491–492.

Zhao, Y., Lin, A., & Jiao, L. (2020). Eight weeks of resistance training with blood flow restriction improve cardiac function and vascular endothelial function in healthy young Asian males. *International Health, 13*(5), 471–479.

CHAPTER 33 QUESTIONS

1. **Which best describes the BFR mechanism responsible for muscular hypertrophy?**
   a. Rhabdomyolysis
   b. Increased muscle protein synthesis
   c. Opioid production
   d. Ketosis

2. **What is the recommended arterial limb occlusion pressure in the lower extremities when using BFR during exercise?**
   a. 100%
   b. 40% to 80%
   c. 10% to 20%
   d. 10%

3. **Which of the following is a contraindication of BFR?**
   a. Joint replacement
   b. Tendon repair
   c. Deep vein thrombosis
   d. Fracture distal to tourniquet

4. **The recommended rest period with low-load BFR resistance exercise is?**
   a. BFR does not use a rest period
   b. 2 minutes
   c. 30 seconds
   d. 4 minutes

RUNNING

E.T. Greenberg, PT, DPT, SCS and J. Tuori, PT, DPT

1. **What running-related injuries are most commonly seen in recreational runners?**
   Running-related injuries, commonly defined as pain that causes a restriction on running for at least seven days or three consecutive training sessions, have an estimated incidence of 7.7 per 1000 hours of training in recreational runners. Among this group, the injuries with the highest incidence are patellofemoral pain, Achilles tendinopathy, tibial bone stress injuries (BSIs), plantar heel pain, and iliotibial band syndrome. The knee, ankle, and lower leg are the most commonly injured areas in this population, with up to 70% of injuries occurring at or below the knee. The vast majority of running-related injuries are atraumatic, and therefore etiology is variable.
   How do injury patterns differ between:
   a. **Youth and masters runners?**
   b. **Male and female runners?**
   c. **Sprinters and long-distance runners?**
   a. Youth runners experience growth plate and bone injuries at much higher rates than older runners. These include BSIs to the tibia and metatarsals, and apophyseal injuries at the tibial tuberosity, inferior pole of the patella, and calcaneus. Muscle and tendon injuries are much more prevalent in masters runners. Achilles tendinopathy, proximal hamstring tendinopathy, and plantar heel pain are some of the most common injuries in this population.
   b. Knee injuries are the most common among male and female runners with a higher total proportion in females. Male runners experience a slightly higher proportion of foot/ankle and lower leg injuries, while female runners are more often injured at the hip. Patellofemoral pain and BSIs are more commonly seen in female runners, whereas Achilles tendinopathy and plantar heel pain are more common in male runners.
   c. Consistent with the proximal shift in demand with increased running speeds, sprinters experience acute hamstring and quadriceps strains at much higher rates than long-distance runners. Long-distance running injuries are more common at the knee, ankle, and lower leg, with Achilles tendinopathy, plantar heel pain, and patellofemoral pain.

2. **What is the strongest risk factor for the development of a running-related injury?**
   The strongest predictive factor for both general and specific running-related injuries is a history of previous injury. This has consistently been shown to be a strong nonmodifiable risk factor. Running-related injury etiology is thought to be a result of an imbalance between tissue capacity and tissue loading; if the load applied over a number of strides or running sessions exceeds the tolerance of the tissue, then injury occurs. Interestingly, there is a lack of evidence identifying training-related or biomechanical risk factors associated with the development of general running-related injuries across all populations. This is likely due to the multifaceted nature of injury development; some variables may be associated with specific injuries in specific running populations, but the association will be lost when analyzed as a homogenous group.

3. **What are the main differences between walking and running?**
   Walking consists of double and single limb phases of stance while running consists of single-limb support and a float phase, where neither limb is in contact with the support surface. In running, the runner's center of mass is at its greatest during the swing phase and lowest during midstance. In walking, the center of mass reaches its peak during midstance and at its lowest during initial contact (heel strike). Though the kinematic patterns are similar, running requires greater limb velocities and joint excursions compared to walking. Running has greater amplitudes of internal and external forces and rates of applied ground reaction force (GRF). The peak amplitude of the vertical GRF in walking and running increases with speed from approximately 1.0 to 1.5 times body weight and 2.0 to 2.9 times body weight, respectively. Additionally, strike patterns at initial contact are more variable with running, while in walking it is abnormal to contact the ground with anything other than the heel (Figure).

4. **What are the specific phases and key events of the running gait cycle?**
   Stance Phase: 40% of the running gait cycle is the stance phase where only one limb is in contact with the ground.
   - *Initial Contact:* The point in time where the reference limb makes contact with the support surface. The limb position at initial contact will differ depending on the runner's strike pattern.
   - *Absorption (Braking):* The first half of stance phase where the limb absorbs the ground reaction forces (GRFs) and terminates in midstance, the point at which the vertical GRF is at its greatest. This is also the point where the runner's center of mass is at its lowest and of peak dorsiflexion and knee flexion during stance phase.

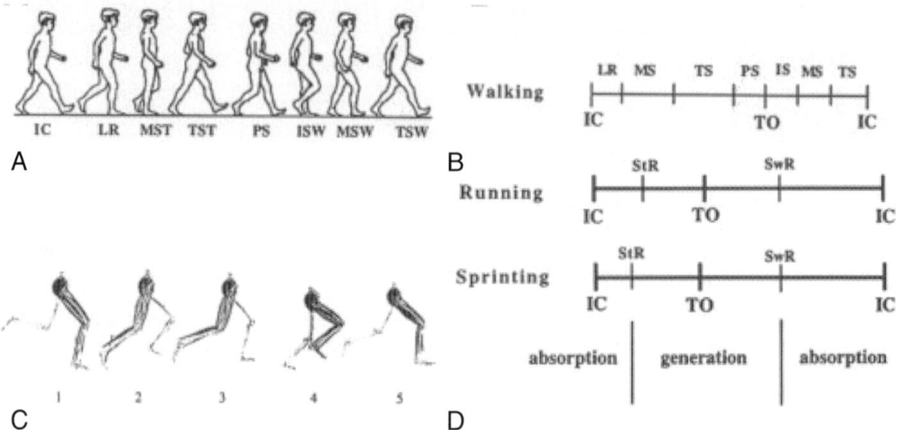

The gait cycle. (A) Walking figure. IC, initial contact; ISW, initial swing; LR, loading response; MST, midstance; MSW, midswing; PS, preswing; TST, terminal stance; TSW, terminal swing. (B) Walking gait cycle. IC, initial contact; LR, loading response; IS, initial swing; MS (first instance), midstance; MS (second instance), midswing; PS, preswing; TO, toe off; TS (first instance), terminal stance; TS (second instance), terminal swing. (C) Running figure. 1. Stance phase absorption. 2. Stance phase generation. 3. Swing phase generation. 4. Swing phase reversal. 5. Swing phase absorption. (D) Running gait cycle for running and sprinting. Absorption, from SwR through IC to StR; generation, from StR through TO to SwR. IC, initial contact; StR, stance phase reversal; SwR, swing phase reversal; TO, toe off. (Figure published in Dicharry, J. (2010). Kinematics and kinetics of gait: From lab to clinic. *Clinics in Sports Medicine, 29*(3), 347–364, originally from Novacheck, T. F. (1998). The biomechanics of running. *Gait Posture,* 7, 77–95; with permission.)

- *Propulsion:* The second half of stance phase where the hip and knee extend and propel the body forward. Stance phase terminated with toe-off, the last point in time where the foot is in contact with the support surface.

Swing: 60% of the gait cycle is when the reference limb is not in contact with the ground. Two periods of float, one at the start of swing and one at the end, together make up about half of the entire swing phase and is defined as when neither limb is in contact with the support surface. During the swing phase, the runner's center of mass reaches its greatest peak.

5. **What are the roles of the lower extremity musculature during the stance phase of the running gait cycle?**
At ground contact, the role of the lower extremity musculature is to attenuate GRFs in all three planes. Runners with a rearfoot strike (RFS) will have increased muscle activation of the tibialis anterior to eccentrically control plantarflexion at ground contact. Once a foot flat position is achieved, the posterior lower leg compartment muscles will eccentrically control foot pronation and ankle dorsiflexion as the runner progresses into midstance. Alternatively, runners with non-rearfoot strike (NRFS) patterns will rely on the posterior compartment much earlier, during early loading, to eccentrically control the absorption of GRFs. Concurrently, the quadriceps also work eccentrically at this time. The hamstrings concentrically assist to extend the hip to allow for the anterior progression of the runner's center of mass as they progress from early loading to midstance. At midstance, the musculotendinous structures of the calf, quadriceps, and distal hamstrings utilize the potential energy stored from the absorption phase and concentrically contract to propel the runner's center of mass forward. Simultaneously, the proximal hamstrings continue to concentrically extend the hip, continuing the center of mass forward progression. The hip flexors eccentrically contract, storing potential energy in preparation for limb advancement during swing phase.

6. **What are the roles of the lower extremity musculature during the swing phase of the running gait cycle?**
After toe-off, the elastic return of the hip flexors assists with concentric hip flexion. The hamstrings and tibialis anterior assist in ground clearance by flexing the knee and dorsiflexing the ankle, respectively. During mid-swing the hamstrings eccentrically control knee and hip flexion. The hamstrings, along with the gluteals, concentrically extend the hip as it prepares the limb for ground contact during late swing.

7. **What are the differences in the various foot strike patterns at initial contact?**
Despite recent claims, one foot strike is not more advantageous than another, but instead differs on the location of force attenuation during the absorption phase of stance. Most runners (~80% to 90%) have an RFS pattern. The remaining 10% to 20% of runners contact the ground in NRFS pattern. Compared to an NRFS pattern, an RFS pattern is associated with greater loading rates and loads incurred at the knee and hip, with less demands at the foot and ankle as the GRF passes posterior to the ankle joint. Conversely, an NRFS shifts the loads more distally and increases energy demands and stresses at the foot, ankle, and lower leg musculature as the vertical GRF is anterior to the axis of rotation of the ankle joint. Though peak vertical GRFs are similar, an RFS has an initial impact peak that reduces loads on the Achilles tendon but increases eccentric internal loads to the tibialis anterior muscle. This initial impact peak is diminished or absent in NRFS patterns, resulting in lower loading rates and collision forces; however, this increases loads to the forefoot structures, Achilles tendon, and superficial and deep posterior calf musculature. Running without shoes (unshod) may promote an NRFS pattern in habitual RFS runners.

8. **How is the gait cycle influenced as running speed increases?**
As running speed increases so do external and internal forces, joint velocities, and energy demands. Initial contact shifts more toward the forefoot and muscular demands shift more proximally. Time spent in swing and float phases increases, stance time decreases, and cycle time shortens (step rate increases). Though step rate increases, increases in step length contribute more to running speed increases.

9. **What are the equipment requirements to conduct a video-based clinical running gait evaluation?**
In order to perform a thorough clinical running evaluation, a treadmill with enough space around it (about 6 feet in each direction) is highly recommended. The treadmill should be stiff to limit excessive bouncing and be low profile to avoid any view obstructions. Three-dimensional motion analysis systems and force plates are becoming more readily available for clinical use; however, they are expensive, time intensive, and typically reserved for research purposes. Two-dimensional analysis can adequately provide clinicians with the needed kinematic information to assist in the assessment of running technique. A high-speed camera of at least 100 frames/second should be used and capture the runner at a minimum of two views, right angles to each other. Typically, posterior and lateral views are the most common and offer adequate information. A fixed camera location will improve the reliability of assessments while motion analysis software can assist with the observations and measurements of various temporospatial and kinematic measurements. To increase accuracy and reliability, markers (ie, a bright colored tape) can be placed at various anatomical landmarks. To avoid interference from clothing, the runner should wear tight-fitting clothing and markers should be placed directly on the skin whenever possible. Other instrumentation such as commercial-grade accelerometry, pressure sensor insoles, or a fitness watch can supplement two-dimensional video analysis.

10. **What metrics are considered reliable when performing a two-dimensional running evaluation?**
Strike pattern at initial contact and step rate have been considered reliable across raters of various levels of experience. Similarly, other sagittal plane metrics such as foot inclination angle, tibial inclination angle, knee flexion angle, and heel to center of mass (COM) distance at initial contact have been shown to be more reliable than measures in other planes of motion. Peak DF at midstance and COM vertical displacement should be more cautiously considered. Frontal plane measures of rearfoot position during various phases of gait and contralateral pelvic drop angle, hip adduction, and knee abduction at midstance (knee window) should be considered when observing a runner in a posterior view (Figure). However, due to the wide range of variability in normative measures, specific values should be used cautiously, and instead these metrics may benefit from a more qualitative assessment.

11. **What is the difference between overground running and running on the treadmill?**
Kinematically, running on a treadmill is very similar to running overground. While on a treadmill, runners tend to contact the ground with a flatter foot. From a temporospatial perspective running on a treadmill may result in smaller step lengths and greater step rates while running overground at the same speed. Kinetically, differences may exist in peak vertical GRFs and joint moments and power. Though a 1% treadmill grade (incline) most accurately reflects the energy demands of overground running, the incline will result in biomechanical changes and may not be appropriate for clinical gait analysis. Because treadmill speeds are fixed, running speeds on a treadmill should attempt to match the overground running pace.

12. **What is running gait retraining?**
Running gait retraining is a movement-specific intervention that aims to facilitate a change in running technique by targeting specific biomechanical variables. Typically, running gait retraining is implemented to manage running injuries, reduce the risk of injury, or to improve performance. Because of the multifactorial nature of running-related injuries, gait retraining should be included as a component of a comprehensive management plan and not used as an isolated intervention. Controversy exists whether running gait alterations should be implemented in

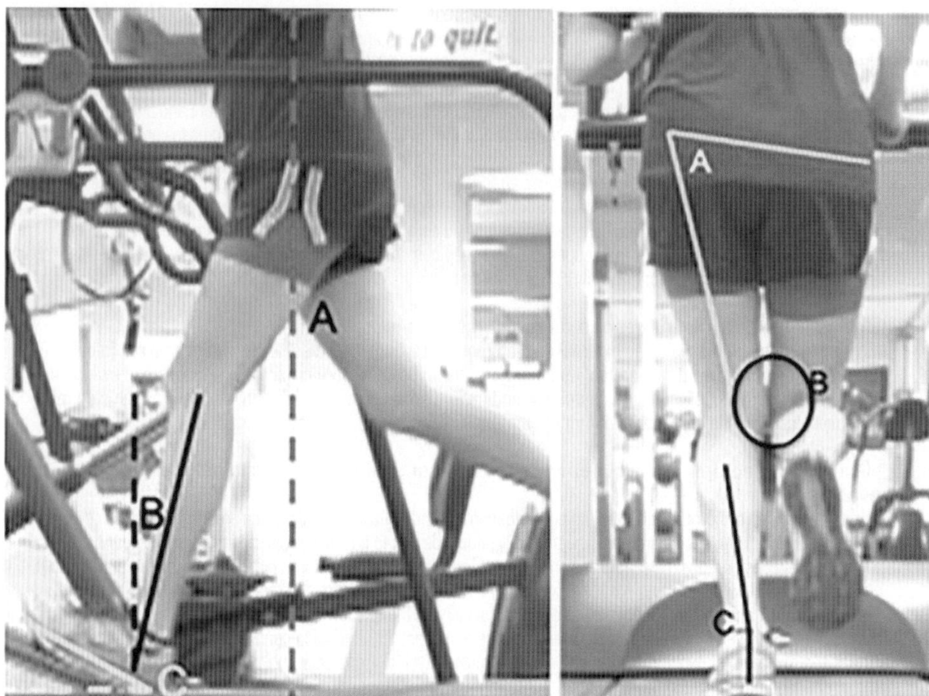

The left picture is a lateral view of a runner at initial contact. The relationship of the foot at initial contact to the center of mass (A), tibial inclination angle (B), and foot inclination angle (C) are pictured. The picture on the right is a posterior view of the same runner. Contralateral pelvic drop angle (A), knee window (B), and rearfoot angle (C) are highlighted.

healthy runners or reserved strictly following a running-related injury. Additionally, there is a lack of agreement whether changes in running technique should be considered a short-term symptom modification strategy or a more permanent running strategy.

13. **What principles of motor learning are important to consider when implementing a running gait retraining program?**
Gait retraining programs should be individualized and tailored to meet the needs of each runner. Principles of motor learning need to be considered to promote not only the performance of a task but, more importantly, the retainment (learning) of the task. Interventions should also be specific to a targeted movement goal and work within the runner's current capacity. Augmented feedback that is provided by an outside source is commonly utilized in the earlier stages to enhance the acquisition of a novel running technique. The systematic removal of augmented feedback is crucial to help a runner reach a point where they no longer rely on external feedback for task performance and instead develop an internal sensation of the desired running gait. Factors to consider when designing a running gait retraining program are outlined in Table.

14. **What is the role of increasing running step rate and how should it be prescribed and implemented?**
Increasing a preferred step rate by 5% to 10% can result in up to a 20% reduction in energy absorption at the knee and hip without affecting running efficiency and performance. More aggressive increases in step rates (>10%) may result in increased energy consumption and impair running performance. Because speed is the product of step rate and step length, an increase in step rate will result in a smaller step length when speed is held constant; as a result, the runner will contact the ground closer to their COM. Therefore, when implementing running step rate increases, it is important to keep running speed consistent within and across training sessions. The use of a metronome, fitness watch, or music with a beat matched to the prescribed step rate can all be utilized as augmented feedback to retrain step rate. Despite claims that 180 steps/min is the optimum step rate in runners, this has not been supported by the literature as preferred step rate is more of a function of speed, limb length, and running experience. However, step rates lower than 164 steps/min may be a risk factor for

Running Gait Retraining Motor Learning Strategies

VARIABLE	OPTIONS	DESCRIPTION
Practice Schedules	Massed	Minimal rest between running bouts within the same day
	Distributed	Practice sessions are spaced out with longer time between bouts (days or weeks apart)
	Constant	Running under the same condition (surface, speed, shoe wear, contextual factors)
	Variable	Running in a variety of settings (surface, shoe wear, contextual factors)
Type of Practice	Blocked	Running practice maintained without interruption from nonrunning activities (only running)
	Random	Running with contextual interference (other activities added within the running session)
Augmented Feedback Type	Verbal	Words used to reinforce the goal or quality of movement ("land softer," "contact on your heel")
	Auditory	Use of nonverbal auditory feedback to reinforce the goal or quality of movement (metronome, "beep," or other tone)
	Visual	Use of mirrors, video monitors, gestures, or other objects to reinforce the goal or quality of movement (running in front of mirror, real-time video, graphical representations of kinetics or kinematics, fitness watch screen)
	Haptic	Use of tactile sensations to reinforce the goal or quality of movement (vibratory sensors, sensory input from elastic tubing)
Focus of Attention	Internal Focus	Attention is directed to a particular limb, or body part, in an attempt to produce the desired movement (cues to run on forefoot, maintain a level pelvis, don't let knees touch each other)
	External Focus	Attention is directed at factors outside the body, like an implement, support surface, the trajectory of an object or a target. (Matching step rate to metronome to decrease knee loads, "run on hot coals" to promote forefoot contact, run without touching a line to widen step width)
Timing of Feedback	Concurrent	Feedback is given synchronously while running (real-time step rate data, watching a live video recording while running, mirror feedback)
	Terminal	Feedback offered at the end of trial or running session (watching a video recording following performance, data on a fitness watch viewed after a run)
Feedback Frequency	Constant	Feedback is given 100% of the run time (always running in front of a mirror or with a metronome)
	Faded	Feedback is systematically removed over time as performance changes or improves (progressive decreased use of a metronome and increasing run time without feedback)
	Bandwidth	Feedback that is given when a runner's performance falls outside a certain acceptable level of error (feedback is offered when outside a step rate of 170 to 182 steps/min, feedback offered when pelvic drops is greater than 7 degrees)
	Self-selected	Feedback is offered or given at the request of the runner (looking at a fitness watch at any time they want while running)

tibial BSIs in adolescent runners. Though meager increases in step rate will result in more loading cycles for a given distance, the decrease in cumulative loading parameters per step outweighs the loading increases, due more running cycles, when implemented in runners with high impact loading and low step rates. Conversely, step rate increases in runners with higher step rates can result in excessive cumulative loads due to the increase in loading cycles and be detrimental. Step rate manipulation can also affect frontal plane mechanics. Because of a decreased ground contact time per step and more efficient timing of gluteal musculature activation, small increases in step rate can also result in decreased peak hip adduction, knee abduction, contralateral pelvic drop, and foot pronation during stance.

15. **What methods can be implemented to retrain a runner with a narrow step width?**
A narrow step width (crossover mechanics), defined as crossing over the midline of the body at initial contact and through midstance, has been linked to variables associated with tibial BSIs and iliotibial band pain. Meager step width increases of only 5% of leg length have been shown to decrease stresses at the tibia and lateral knee. Strategies such as running without crossing over a line on the ground (ie, lane markers on a track or bike lane line on the side of the road) or a chalk line drawn down the center of the treadmill belt can assist with augmented feedback to increase step width.

16. **What are the benefits and pitfalls of directly retraining modifications in foot strike patterns in runners?**
Despite claims, there is no optimal foot strike pattern. Instead, different foot strike patterns alter the manner in which loads are absorbed and generated by the body. For instance, a runner with anterior knee pain may benefit from adapting to a forefoot strike to unload the knee. Conversely, someone with Achilles tendon pain may adapt a more rearfoot strike to unload the Achilles. However, transitioning a runner to a different strike pattern should be done gradually and be performed in conjunction with a strengthening program that prepares tissue to tolerate the shift in loads. The direct instruction to alter foot strike pattern may actually result in some negative consequences. The internal focus of attention of the task is not effective for long-term learnings, will constrain movement, and result in excessive limb stiffness. External focus of attention strategies and tasks such as increasing step rate, instructions to "land softly," or visual feedback to lower impact rates may be better options to facilitate a more forefoot contact.

17. **Does strength training assist in a change of running technique/biomechanics?**
Strength training is an important component of programs aimed to manage running injury, reduce injury risk, and enhance performance. Specific strength training interventions should target structures with inadequate load tolerance abilities (ie, weight-bearing exercises to promote osteogenesis and adaptation of osseous structures following a BSI) and accompany any gait retraining intervention to prepare body structures for the shift in load (ie, calf muscle training when transitioning to an NRFS pattern). However, strength training in isolation is not effective in influencing changes in running biomechanics and technique.

18. **True or False: A strength training program for runners should be limited to high-repetition, fatigue-resistant training to be more specific to the performance demands of distance running.**
False; though muscle adaptations can occur with lower intensity training, the time demands required for adaptation may not be as efficient as slow, high-intensity resistance training. Additionally, slow, high-intensity resistance training will increase load tolerance of a muscle as well as promote positive adaptations to inert tissues such as tendons, bones, and ligaments. Care should be taken to target the soleus muscle, as loading demands with running are greater than other lower extremity musculature.

19. **How does strength training affect running performance?**
Strength training has been shown to improve running economy by 2% to 8% in recreational and elite runners. This improvement in running economy (or the metabolic cost of running) has been associated with a 2% to 5% improvement in running performance. Strength training appears to have no effects on VO_{2max}, lactate threshold, or BMI; this indicates that while the mechanism by which it improves running performance is not fully understood, it is likely related to the improvements in running economy. The optimal strength training prescription varies based on the training age and goals of the runner, but common parameters investigated have been two to three sessions per week for 6 to >14 weeks. These sessions may consist of maximal strength training, explosive resistance training, plyometrics, and/or sprint training. Muscle hypertrophy and body mass changes are typically not seen across these strength training programs due to the volume of training; most exercises range from one to four sets of four to six repetitions, which is unlikely to stimulate significant muscle growth at two sessions per week, but still sufficient to develop strength and power characteristics.

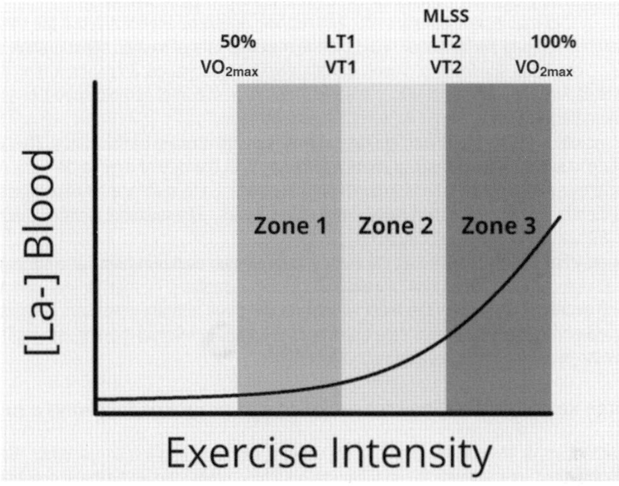

Running intensity training zones. La-, blood lactate. (Figure adapted from Seiler, S. (2010). What is best practice for training intensity and duration distribution in endurance athletes? *International Journal of Sports Physiology and Performance, 5*(3), 276–291.)

20. The majority of an elite runner's training is typically spent at what intensity?

Both three-zone and five-zone intensity models are commonly used to describe training intensity. These models are commonly centered around the lactate threshold, or first and second lactate turn points; below 2 mM blood lactate concentration is considered low intensity, and above 4 mM blood lactate concentration is considered high intensity, with a "threshold" zone in between (Figure).

The five-zone model further breaks down zones 1 and 3 into two separate zones, but these are not based on clearly defined physiological markers. Interestingly, elite runners tend to self-select training intensities that fall within zone 1 for 80% to 90% of their weekly training volume, depending on their discipline and time of season. The two most common types of training intensity distribution are described as polarized and pyramidal. In polarized training, the majority of weekly intensity is spent in zone 1, with the remainder in zone 3 and a very minimal amount in zone 2. In pyramidal training, the highest volume is still in zone 1, but with more training in zone 2 than in zone 3. Both of these intensity distributions have been shown to improve performance without a clearly defined "superior" approach.

21. What is the relative energy system contribution for each of the following running distances?

a. **5 km**
b. **800 m**
c. **1500 m**

Energy systems are commonly dichotomized into anaerobic and aerobic during exercise. While both systems are active concurrently, the relative energy contribution to exercise changes with duration and intensity. The first of two anaerobic systems commonly described is the phosphocreatine system. This is quick to act and to regenerate, typically depleted within 10 seconds of exercise. The second anaerobic metabolic pathway is the glycolytic system, which breaks down carbohydrates in the blood or stored in muscle to produce energy. This is the dominant energy system for bouts of exercise up to 2 minutes. The aerobic energy system involves the process of oxidative phosphorylation. This pathway uses oxygen and has the highest energy yield, but is the slowest to ramp up, becoming the dominant energy system past 2 minutes.

The 5-kilometer run has been shown to have a 90% to 95% aerobic energy system contribution, with the remainder a result of anaerobic systems. This is, of course, also dependent on the duration of the run; a world-class male runner completing the race in under 13 minutes will have a different relative contribution compared to a novice runner finishing the race in 30 minutes. Conversely, the 800-meter run demonstrates a 60% to 70% aerobic energy system contribution, with the remaining 30% to 40% dependent on the anaerobic systems. At nearly twice the distance, the 1500-meter run has been shown to have a 75% to 85% aerobic energy contribution. The differences in relative energy contribution for each race distance have implications on the training required to maximize performance.

22. What are the primary determinants of distance running performance?

The runner's VO_{2max}, maximal lactate steady state, and running economy are considered the three primary predictors of distance running performance. VO_{2max} is the maximal rate of oxygen consumption during exercise. While a high VO_{2max} has been shown to positively correlate with performance, it is not a strong predictor of performance in isolation. The velocity at VO_{2max}, also referred to as maximal aerobic speed, is estimated to be around the 3-kilometer race pace.

The maximal lactate steady state is also strongly correlated with running performance. This is the threshold at which steady state is achieved by balancing energy demands with the rate of oxygen delivery. Above this point, the anaerobic energy system contributions exponentially increase. Long-distance runners typically demonstrate higher maximal lactate steady states than middle-distance runners. The maximal lactate steady state is estimated to be 80% to 85% of the velocity at VO_{2max}.

Running economy has been described as the steady state oxygen cost of running at a submaximal pace. This value is the result of a complex interaction of metabolic, cardiopulmonary, biomechanical, and neuromuscular systems. Running economy is typically the most variable of the three primary predictors of distance running performance. Interventions such as endurance training, high-intensity interval training, strength training, and plyometrics have been shown to improve running economy.

23. What are some key considerations for return-to-run programs following a running-related injury?

The primary components of any training plan involve volume, intensity, and frequency. While there is not an established gold standard for returning to run following an injury, protocols will typically emphasize restoring some percentage of running volume and frequency prior to intensity; the rationale is that for many running-related injuries, cumulative load tolerance should be prioritized over peak load tolerance in order to successfully return to an activity that involves a significant amount of cumulative load. For many injuries, a symptom monitoring scale will be implemented, such that symptoms do not escalate to an intolerable level or remain worse for longer than 24 hours following the running session. This allows the initial prescription to be sustainable and progressive at a given frequency per week.

Several considerations must be made to gauge how conservative or accelerated a return-to-run program may start. These include but are not limited to the severity of the injury, the tissue type, how long the athlete has been away from running, the training age, the running goals, and the time until the next competition. For example, a novice runner returning to training after a 4-month layoff following a high-risk BSI should start at a much lower weekly dosage than a collegiate cross-country runner returning to training after resting for 2 weeks following an acute Achilles tendinopathy flare-up. Given the complexity involved, it is therefore not possible to provide a standardized return-to-run protocol for all runners.

24. What are the main goals of running footwear design?

Running footwear is constructed to increase comfort, improve performance, and to change biomechanical variables thought to be associated with injury risk. The assessment of comfort has traditionally been limited in practice, as it is related to many subjective variables. The RUN-CAT assessment tool was developed to create a comfort score by including heel cushion, forefoot cushion, shoe stability, and forefoot flexibility components. It has been theorized that a runner self-selecting a comfortable shoe will decrease the risk of injury, but this has yet to be thoroughly investigated.

The majority of running footwear research has been conducted in the area of performance. Increasing the longitudinal bending stiffness of a shoe has been shown to decrease the metabolic cost of running by reducing energy lost at the metatarsophalangeal joints. The effect of increasing midsole thickness has traditionally been difficult to differentiate from increasing the weight of the shoe, but newer technology has demonstrated that a lightweight, high stack shoe is beneficial for running economy at submaximal speeds.

Regarding biomechanical changes with footwear, there is evidence that motion control footwear can modestly reduce peak ankle eversion angle and vertical impact peak. There is no evidence that proximal mechanics or kinetics are affected by motion control footwear as compared to traditional footwear.

25. What are the different classifications of running shoes?

The traditional running shoe classifications can be separated into neutral, stability, and motion-control categories. These categories were originally thought to match the function and shape of the foot. Neutral shoes are designed with maximal cushioning properties with minimal frontal plane guidance. Motion-control shoes are constructed with increased medial support to limit rearfoot motion, specifically into pronation. Stability shoes have elements of both high cushioning and moderate medial support.

Minimalist footwear became an increasingly popular classification in the early 2000s. A consensus statement established the minimalist definition as "Footwear providing minimal interference with the natural movement of the foot due to its high flexibility, low heel to toe drop, weight and stack height, and the absence of motion control and stability devices." Minimalist shoes have been shown to decrease loading at the patellofemoral joint but increase loading at the ankle and metatarsophalangeal joints. As a result,

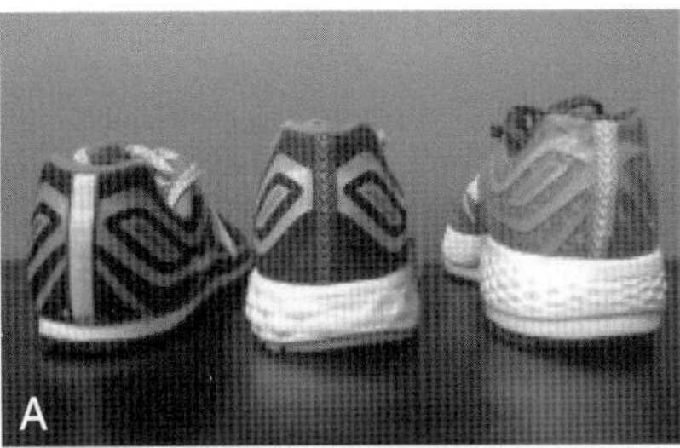

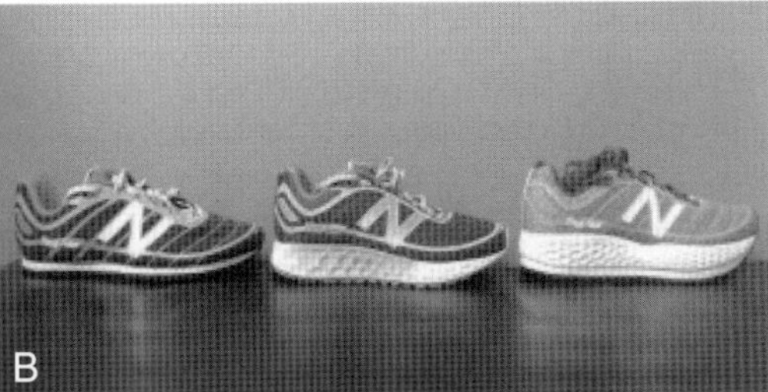

From left to right, a minimal, traditional, and maximal shoe from the back (A) and side (B) views. (Figure from Hannigan, J. J., & Pollard, C. D. (2021). Comparing walking biomechanics of older females in maximal, minimal, and traditional shoes. *Gait Posture, 83*, 245–249. doi:10.1016/j.gaitpost.2020.10.030; with permission.)

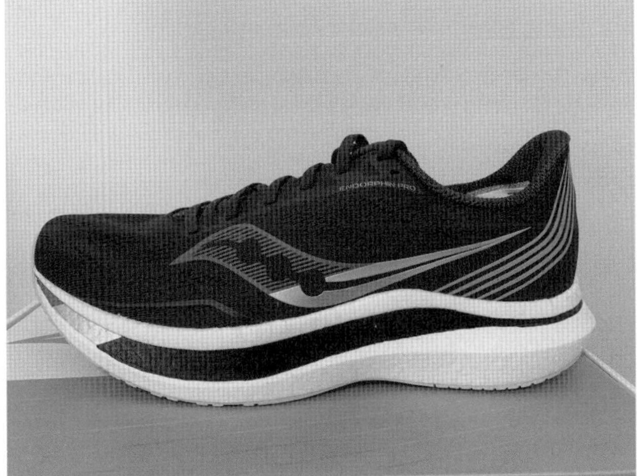

A "super shoe" with a notably high stack height and curved toe spring.

a runner who habitually wears traditional running shoes should be advised to gradually transition into a minimalist shoe if desired.

The maximalist footwear classification is relatively new, and consists of high stack, extremely cushioned shoes designed to provide shock absorption. Despite the popular claims, maximalist shoes have not been found to reduce impact forces; on the contrary, some studies have shown increased impact peaks, loading rates, and eversion moments when comparing maximalist to traditional running footwear. A comparison between traditional, minimalist, and maximalist shoes can be seen in Figure.

The most recent, and by far most controversial, category of running shoes developed are nicknamed "super shoes" (Figure). This category of footwear is designed to optimize distance running performance, and consists of a high stack, lightweight shoe with a curved carbon fiber plate embedded within the midsole. This combination of midsole components has been found to improve running economy compared to traditional marathon racing shoes and is thought to be a result of the interaction between a lightweight, energy-efficient foam and the stiffness of the carbon fiber plate. While not investigated thoroughly at this time, these shoes have consistently demonstrated a decreased metabolic cost of running at submaximal speeds, translating to an improvement in running performance.

26. How does loading change during running on a firm surface compared to a compliant surface?

Stiffness of the lower limb during running is a factor of the total force applied into the ground and the total vertical displacement of the joints in the limb. Stiffness is positively correlated with running economy, as the elastic return of energy from tendons decreases the metabolic cost of running. On a more compliant (softer) surface, lower limb stiffness is increased. This is thought to be a regulatory mechanism to maintain consistent support, as the total vertical displacement of the runner's center of mass does not seem to significantly change as stiffness increases.

Additionally, the metabolic cost of running decreases on more compliant surfaces. This is also related to the elastic property of the surface; a highly elastic and compliant surface will return more energy than a damping, yet compliant surface. Conversely, on a less compliant surface, stiffness in the lower limb will decrease, and more muscular effort is needed for cushioning. The compliant properties of footwear reduce metabolic cost, but this may be offset by the added weight to the limb by wearing a shoe; for each additional 100 grams in a shoe, the metabolic cost of running increases by around 1%. The most economical type of footwear is therefore both lightweight and compliant.

27. **True or false: Prescribing running shoes based on static arch height does not reduce the risk of developing a running-related injury.**
True; the idea of matching shoes of various degrees of stability with foot morphology has long been theorized to reduce injury risk by attenuating forces and reducing excessive foot pronation. Despite the fact that motion control footwear can reduce the peak ankle eversion angle by an average of 2 degrees during the stance phase, excessive foot pronation has not been found to be a risk factor for general running-related injuries. In a large meta-analysis of over 7000 military recruits, there was no difference in injury rates between matching shoe type to foot morphology and assigning a shoe at random.

28. **What effects do foot orthoses have on running biomechanics?**
Foot orthoses seem to have their largest effects on the kinetics at the foot and ankle. Rearfoot inversion moments are decreased in foot orthoses with a rearfoot posting. Lateral plantar pressure is typically increased in foot orthoses with medial or lateral posting. There is conflicting evidence on the effects of orthoses on loading rates and peak impact forces. Lower extremity kinematics do not appear to significantly change during running with foot orthoses, contrary to popular belief.

29. **What is one benefit of using modern wearable devices in the treatment of a tibial BSI? What is one downside?**
There has been a significant advancement in wearable technology in the past decade, resulting in more data available than ever before. Wearable devices are able to accurately report metrics such as step rate and stride length in real time, and alerts can be programmed for in-field feedback. Given the evidence that a low step rate is associated with a higher risk of BSIs in collegiate runners, an intervention to increase step rate and thereby decrease peak load per stride could be beneficial when returning to run following a tibial BSI. An increase in step rate is typically prescribed at 5% to 10% above preferred and can be reinforced with feedback from the wearable device. A downside to be aware of here is the potential for inappropriately using certain metrics as surrogate measures. For example, some wearable devices may report on peak tibial acceleration and represent this as bone stress. Peak tibial acceleration occurs at impact, but the largest amount of tibial compressive force occurs during midstance. Similarly, training load metrics may be derived from external loads like distance or time in the absence of internal loads such as heart rate or rating of perceived exertion. Training load is difficult to quantify and often requires the combination of an external and internal load to appropriately describe the effort of the session.

30. **Is there evidence for a "10% rule" to guide training load prescription?**
The traditional recommendation to avoid increasing weekly training volume by more than 10%, while sensible in nature, lacks evidence for use in both rehabilitation and injury risk reduction; no differences have been found in injury risk with weekly volume increases between 10% and 24% in recreational runners, although data are very limited. Practically, a major limitation of the "10% rule" is that it assumes that a spike in running volume is the largest contributor to injury development. No differences have been found in injury risk when comparing increases in weekly running volume versus running intensity in recreational runners. Another practical limitation of the "10% rule" is its use during very low- or high-volume baselines. For example, for a runner returning from injury logging 1 mile per week, it would take over 8 months to return to over 30 miles per week; this is likely more conservative than is necessary. Conversely, strictly adhering to the rule for a runner logging 70 miles per week could result in over a 30-mile increase across 4 weeks; for some runners at this volume, this could be problematic to achieve.

CASE STUDIES

Case Study One

Patient Description: 17-year-old cis-gendered male cross-country runner presents with a 1-month history of right lower leg pain. The pain began 2 weeks following a 10-day vacation where he decreased his normal running volume.

Chief Complaint: Localized pain to the posteromedial middle ⅓ of tibia

PMH: left tibial BSI 3 years ago

BMI: 21 lb/kg^2

Training History: He has been exclusively running competitively since he was 12 years old. Pain begins in the first 5 minutes of his run that increases throughout the duration of his run. Prior to the injury he was running 6 days/week and had a weekly running volume of 50 miles/week. Because of the pain, he recently reduced his training to 3 days a week and a volume of 15 miles/week. He also reports pain with walking following his training days.

Diagnostic Imaging: Bilateral plain radiographs were normal and unremarkable

Questions

31. What are the primary differential diagnoses?

a. Tibial stress fracture
   Indication: Past history of BSI to the contralateral limb, early specialization in running and lacks an appropriate osteogenic stimulus, insidious onset with a rapid spike in training load following a period of decreased training, high running volume, localized pain to posteromedial tibia that worsens throughout the run, pain with lower bone loads such as walking the following day after training.

b. Medial tibial stress syndrome
   Indication: Insidious onset with a rapid spike in training load following a period of decreased training, pain spans ⅓ of tibia along the posteromedial surface of the tibia, normal radiographs

c. Exercise-induced compartment syndrome
   Indication: Pain increases at a predictable time at the beginning of the run and continues throughout the run, normal radiographs

32. What other testing should be recommended?

Physical exam findings such as pain with palpation, hopping, and fulcrum stress test may all be useful, but are not specific. Resistive muscle testing may help distinguish a BSI from tendinopathy and exercise-induced compartment syndrome. With the high suspicion of BSI, specifically a stress fracture, MRI should be considered as it is the gold standard. Plain radiographs may not be sensitive enough to detect stress fractures in the early stages.

The term Relative Energy Deficiency in Sport (RED-S) has replaced "Female Athlete Triad," as individuals may not demonstrate all three factors in order to suffer negative health sequelae. More importantly, a relative energy deficiency resulting in poor bone health and other negative consequences is not reserved for females and needs to be considered in males with a history of chronic/multiple BSIs (Figure). Referral to other medical providers may be warranted for further diagnostic testing including bloodwork, bone mineral density testing, nutritional status and eating assessment, and psychological evaluation.

33. Assuming the most likely diagnosis, what acute load management strategies are appropriate at this point?

Given the likelihood of a tibial stress fracture, a period of unloading and relative rest is warranted to allow for bony healing. A short course (2–3 weeks) of protected weight-bearing with an assistive device, with or without the use of Controlled Ankle Motion (CAM) boot, may be necessary depending on the location, severity on imaging, and irritability. Other low load forms of exercise such as deep water running, upper body ergometer training, and strength training to proximal and contralateral lower limb musculature should be prescribed to maintain fitness levels. The tibia should be gradually exposed to incremental loads based on various factors including degree of bony healing on diagnostic imaging, physical exam objective measures, and pain levels. This includes the progressive weaning of the CAM boot and crutches to promote full weight-bearing and pain-free ambulation. BSIs tend not to fare well when even low levels of pain are permitted with activity. Soft tissue mobilization, muscle stretching, and joint mobilization can act as adjuncts to maintain mobility during the time of reduced activity.

34. What additional treatment interventions should be considered?

Patient education throughout the rehabilitation process will be the most important intervention. Stressing the importance of proper nutrition, sleep, and stress management will help create a positive environment to promote recovery and healing. Educating the runner on proper training habits and consistency can help monitor any fluctuations in acute workloads. The importance of incorporating start-stop and change of direction activities into training can help promote osteogenesis and overall bone health.

Once it is tolerated, weight-bearing exercise should be the mainstay treatment and initiated in a progressive manner. Total leg strengthening to help attenuate forces acting on the lower extremity should be performed with a focus on foot stability and control, triceps surae load tolerance, and proximal limb muscle performance. A jumping and hopping progression will assist in osteogenesis, increase load tolerance to GRF of greater magnitudes and rates, and train the elasticity of the stretch-shortening cycle.

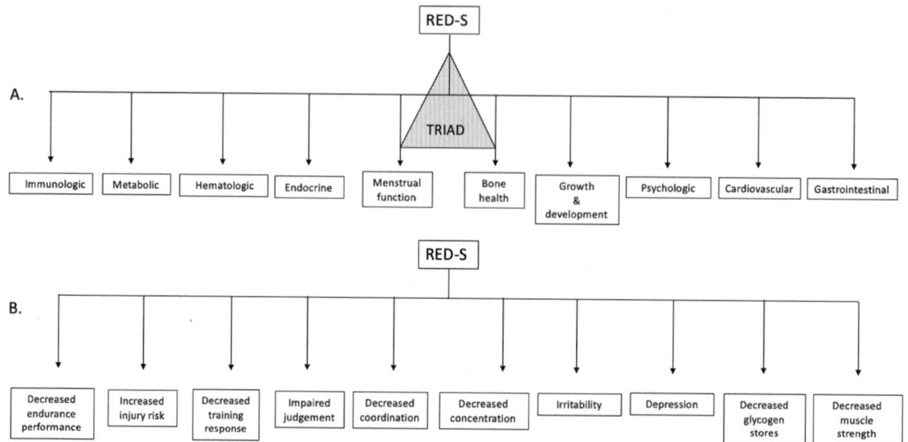

(A) Health consequences of relative energy deficiency in sports (RED-S) showing an expanded concept of the female athlete triad. (B) Potential performance (aerobic and anaerobic) consequences of RED-S. (Karenm, S. et al. (2021). The Female Athlete Triad/Relative Energy Deficiency in Sports. In The Female Athlete by Frank, R. Elsevier.)

35. **How would a return-to-run progression be structured for this patient?**

A running evaluation should be performed to identify any movement characteristics that may contribute to excessive tibial loads including low step rate, overstriding, or narrow step width. Gait retraining interventions directed at the movement dysfunction should occur in tandem with a progressive running program. The University of Wisconsin Running Injury and Recovery Index is a reliable and valid patient-reported outcome measure that can help assess progress and clinical decision-making throughout the rehabilitation process.

The program should start with a walk-run program to gradually load the tibia. Total run time should gradually increase over weeks with a gradual decline in walk time. Because of the running age and previous mileage of this current runner, his run progression may be more aggressive than an individual with less running experience but should be more conservative than others recovering from a non-BSI. A focus on increasing run duration and volume rather than intensity should be of initial focus. Rest days should separate run days in the early stages to allow for recovery and pain response monitoring. A run schedule should always be fluid in nature to account for response and rating of perceived exertion. In this case, a pain monitoring model can guide progression and should not permit any pain while running or on the following day after training. If a runner does experience concordant tibial pain, the athlete should cease running for that day, take at least 1 day off from running, and then resume at their previous run level when they did not experience any symptoms.

Case Study Two

Patient Description: A 55-year-old female Masters level runner presents with a 3-month history of posterior thigh and hip pain.

Chief Complaint: Localized buttock pain with occasional dull pain in the posterior thigh and hip

BMI: 25 lb/kg^2

Training History: She has been running recreationally for 3 years as a means of general activity. She has since decided to train for her first half-marathon. She has been progressively increasing her weekly running volume. Pain will begin early in her run, then decrease toward the end of the run. Her pain also seems to be greater during her shorter, high-intensity runs and more prevalent with walking the following morning. She notes an increase in buttock pain with forward bending and sitting.

Running Shoe: Maximalist running shoe

Diagnostic imaging: None

Questions

36. **What are the primary differential diagnoses?**
   a. Proximal hamstring tendinopathy
      Indication: Insidious onset, localized buttock pain, pain with bending and sitting, a recent increase in running volume, pain that "warms up," menopausal age
   b. Sacral BSI

Indication: Insidious onset, buttock pain, dull pain into posterior thigh, recent increase in running volume, pain increases linearly with intensity, menopausal age, female

c. Deep gluteal pain syndrome
Indication: Insidious onset, buttock and thigh pain, pain with bending and sitting

37. **What other testing should be recommended?**
Proximal hamstring tendinopathies are easily identified with magnetic resonance imaging. A sacral BSI may also be suspected because of the location and nature of onset (female >50 with a recent increase in training volume); an MRI would be the image of choice to rule this in or out. Pain provocation tests involving compression on the proximal hamstring tendon may increase the suspicion of a proximal hamstring tendinopathy given a positive concordant sign. These include the bent-knee stretch test, as well as any active loading of the hamstring in lengthened states (hip flexion and knee extension) such as a Romanian deadlift or straight-leg march.

38. **Assuming the most likely diagnosis, what acute load management strategies are appropriate at this point?**
Assuming the most likely diagnosis of proximal hamstring tendinopathy, the primary short-term goal in the management of this patient is to determine how much running can be tolerated without worsening the condition. While there is limited research on interventions for proximal hamstring tendinopathies, in Achilles tendinopathy it appears that equivocal outcomes can be achieved whether sports activities are stopped or continued using a pain threshold. The common recommendations are to stay below a score of 4/10 on the VAS and to have symptoms settled within 24 hours of the activity. The modifiable stressors, specifically of compressive hamstring tendon positions, should also be addressed. These may include limiting sitting time and avoiding hills/high-intensity training for a short period until tolerance is improved. Gait retraining strategies such as increasing running cadence may be attempted, as it will decrease stride length and hip flexion angle at initial contact.

A footwear change may be considered as an acute load management strategy in some cases, but with careful consideration. If this runner had recently switched to a maximalist shoe from something much lighter, it may be worth temporarily transitioning back into the lighter shoe to redistribute some load away from the hip and knee. It is largely not recommended to encourage a large change in footwear if someone is well-trained in a certain type, as the fast change in force distribution may result in a different injury.

39. **What additional treatment interventions should be considered?**
Initial hamstring loading interventions will be based on the clinical presentation and symptom irritability, but commonly involve avoiding loading the hamstring in compressive positions (increased hip flexion and anterior pelvic tilt). Resistance training exercises involving both hip extension and knee flexion are commonly prescribed to improve the local capacity of the hamstrings. It is also beneficial to address other kinetic chain impairments found, such as quadriceps or triceps surae strength deficits. The type of muscle contraction (isometric, concentric, eccentric) does not seem to matter as much in tendinopathy rehabilitation as the prescribed intensity, which should be progressive over the course of several months. Plyometric loading is commonly prescribed toward the end stages of rehabilitation, as is loading in compressive positions if needed for the athlete.

40. **How would a return-to-run progression be structured for this patient?**
If this runner required a longer period of running cessation, it would be practical to use a walk/run progression to initiate returning to run. This would typically be based on symptom irritability, as well as several other factors including her prior running volume and when her half-marathon is scheduled. Once a certain volume of easy continuous running is restored with symptoms well-managed, higher intensity running is often re-introduced. In this particular case, marathon-pace training will likely make up the bulk of her higher intensity work, as well as hill running if that is applicable to the half-marathon course. For the proximal hamstring tendon, hill training and speed work should be carefully re-introduced due to the increase in compressive loading.

BIBLIOGRAPHY

Agresta, C., & Brown, A. (2015). Gait retraining for injured and healthy runners using augmented feedback: A systematic literature review. *Journal of Orthopaedic & Sports Physical Therapy*, *45*(8), 576–584.

Barnes, K. R., & Kilding, A. E. (2015). Strategies to improve running economy. *Sports Medicine*, *45*(1), 37–56.

Bishop, C., Buckley, J. D., Esterman, A. E., & Arnold, J. B. (2020). The running shoe comfort assessment tool (RUN-CAT): Development and evaluation of a new multi-item assessment tool for evaluating the comfort of running footwear. *Journal of Sports Sciences*, *38*(18), 2100–2107.

Blagrove, R., & Hayes, P. R. (2021). *The science and practice of middle and long distance running training* (1st ed.). New York, NY: Routledge.

Blagrove, R. C., Howatson, G., & Hayes, P. R. (2018). Effects of strength training on the physiological determinants of middle- and long-distance running performance: A systematic review. *Sports Medicine*, *48*(5), 1117–1149.

Brughelli, M., Cronin, J., & Chaouachi, A. (2011). Effects of running velocity on running kinetics and kinematics. *Journal of Strength and Conditioning Research*, *25*(4), 933–939.

Ceyssens, L., Vanelderen, R., Barton, C., Malliaras, P., & Dingenen, B. (2019). Biomechanical risk factors associated with running-related injuries: A systematic review. *Sports Medicine*, *49*(7), 1095–1115.

Chan, Z. Y. S., Au, I. P. H., Lau, F. O. Y., Ching, E. C. K., Zhang, J. H., & Cheung, R. T. H. (2018). Does maximalist footwear lower impact loading during level ground and downhill running? *European Journal of Sport Science*, *18*(8), 1083–1089.

Damsted, C., Glad, S., Nielsen, R. O., Sorensen, H., & Malisoux, L. (2018). Is there evidence for an association between changes in training load and running-related injuries? A systematic review. *International Journal of Sports Physical Therapy, 13*(6), 931–942.

de Oliveira, F. C. L., Fredette, A., Echeverria, S. O., Batcho, C. S., & Roy, J. S. (2019). Validity and reliability of 2-dimensional video-based assessment to analyze foot strike pattern and step rate during running: A systematic review. *Sports Health, 11*(5), 409–415.

Esculier, J. F., Dubois, B., Dionne, C. E., Leblond, J., & Roy, J. S. (2015). A consensus definition and rating scale for minimalist shoes. *Journal of Foot and Ankle Research, 8*, 42.

Esculier, J. F., Silvini, T., Bouyer, L. J., & Roy, J. S. (2018). Video-based assessment of foot strike pattern and step rate is valid and reliable in runners with patellofemoral pain. *Physical Therapy in Sport, 29*, 108–112.

Fellin, R. E., Manal, K., & Davis, I. S. (2010). Comparison of lower extremity kinematic curves during overground and treadmill running. *Journal of Applied Biomechanics, 26*(4), 407–414.

Francis, P., Whatman, C., Sheerin, K., Hume, P., & Johnson, M. I. (2019). The proportion of lower limb running injuries by gender, anatomical location and specific pathology: A systematic review. *Journal of Sports Science and Medicine, 18*(1), 21–31.

Goom, T. S., Malliaras, P., Reiman, M. P., & Purdam, C. R. (2016). Proximal hamstring tendinopathy: Clinical aspects of assessment and management. *Journal of Orthopaedic & Sports Physical Therapy, 46*(6), 483–493.

Greenberg, E. T., Garcia, M. C., Galante, J., & Werner, W. G. (2022). Acute changes in sagittal plane kinematics while wearing a novel belt device during treadmill running. *Sports Biomechanics, 21*(6), 718–730.

Greenberg, E. T., Greenberg, S., & Brown-Budde, K. (2015). Biomechanics and gait analysis for stress fractures In T. Miller & C. Kaeding (Eds.), *Stress fractures in athletes.* Cham: Springer.

Hannigan, J. J., & Pollard, C. D. (2021). Comparing walking biomechanics of older females in maximal, minimal, and traditional shoes. *Gait & Posture, 83*, 245–249.

Heiderscheit, B. C., Chumanov, E. S., Michalski, M. P., Wille, C. M., & Ryan, M. B. (2011). Effects of step rate manipulation on joint mechanics during running. *Medicine & Science in Sports & Exercise, 43*(2), 296–302.

Heiderscheit, B., & McClinton, S. (2016). Evaluation and management of hip and pelvis injuries. *Physical Medicine and Rehabilitation Clinics of North America, 27*(1), 1–29.

Hoogkamer, W., Kipp, S., Frank, J. H., Farina, E. M., Luo, G., & Kram, R. (2018). A comparison of the energetic cost of running in marathon racing shoes. *Sports Medicine, 48*(4), 1009–1019.

Hoogkamer, W., Kipp, S., Spiering, B. A., & Kram, R. (2016). Altered running economy directly translates to altered distance-running performance. *Medicine & Science in Sports & Exercise, 48*(11), 2175–2180.

Hulme, A., Nielsen, R. O., Timpka, T., Verhagen, E., & Finch, C. (2017). Risk and protective factors for middle- and long-distance running-related injury. *Sports Medicine, 47*(5), 869–886.

Jones, A. M., & Doust, J. H. (1996). A 1% treadmill grade most accurately reflects the energetic cost of outdoor running. *Journal of Sports Sciences, 14*(4), 321–327.

Kenneally, M., Casado, A., & Santos-Concejero, J. (2018). The effect of periodization and training intensity distribution on middle- and long-distance running performance: A systematic review. *International Journal of Sports Physiology and Performance, 13*(9), 1114–1121.

Kerdok, A. E., Biewener, A. A., McMahon, T. A., Weyand, P. G., & Herr, H. M. (2002). Energetics and mechanics of human running on surfaces of different stiffnesses. *Journal of Applied Physiology (1985), 92*(2), 469–478.

Kliethermes, S. A., Stiffler-Joachim, M. R., Wille, C. M., Sanfilippo, J. L., Zavala, P., & Heiderscheit, B. C. (2021). Lower step rate is associated with a higher risk of bone stress injury: a prospective study of collegiate cross country runners. *British Journal of Sports Medicine, 55*(15), 851–856.

Kluitenberg, B., van Middelkoop, M., Diercks, R., & van der Worp, H. (2015). What are the differences in injury proportions between different populations of runners? A systematic review and meta-analysis. *Sports Medicine, 45*(8), 1143–1161.

Knapik, J. J., Trone, D. W., Tchandja, J., & Jones, B. H. (2014). Injury-reduction effectiveness of prescribing running shoes on the basis of foot arch height: Summary of military investigations. *Journal of Orthopaedic & Sports Physical Therapy, 44*(10), 805–812.

Koltun, K. J., Strock, N. C. A., Southmayd, E. A., Oneglia, A. P., Williams, N. I., & De Souza, M. J. (2019). Comparison of Female Athlete Triad Coalition and RED-S risk assessment tools. *Journal of Sports Sciences, 37*(21), 2433–2442.

Krabak, B. J., Snitily, B., & Milani, C. J. (2016). Running injuries during adolescence and childhood. *Physical Medicine and Rehabilitation Clinics of North America, 27*(1), 179–202.

Lambert, C., Reinert, N., Stahl, L., et al. (2020). Epidemiology of injuries in track and field athletes: A cross-sectional study of specific injuries based on time loss and reduction in sporting level. *The Physician and Sportsmedicine, 50*(1), 20–29.

Lee, S. J., & Hidler, J. (2008). Biomechanics of overground vs. treadmill walking in healthy individuals. *Journal of Applied Physiology (1985), 104*(3), 747–755.

Luedke, L. E., Heiderscheit, B. C., Williams, D. S., & Rauh, M. J. (2016). Influence of step rate on shin injury and anterior knee pain in high school runners. *Medicine & Science in Sports & Exercise, 48*(7), 1244–1250.

Malliaras, P., Barton, C. J., Reeves, N. D., & Langberg, H. (2013). Achilles and patellar tendinopathy loading programmes: A systematic review comparing clinical outcomes and identifying potential mechanisms for effectiveness. *Sports Medicine, 43*(4), 267–286.

McMillan, A., & Payne, C. (2008). Effect of foot orthoses on lower extremity kinetics during running: a systematic literature review. *Journal of Foot and Ankle Research, 1*(1), 13.

Meardon, S. A., Campbell, S., & Derrick, T. R. (2012). Step width alters iliotibial band strain during running. *Sports Biomechanics, 11*(4), 464–472.

Meardon, S. A., & Derrick, T. R. (2014). Effect of step width manipulation on tibial stress during running. *Journal of Biomechanics, 47*(11), 2738–2744.

Moore, I. S., & Willy, R. W. (2019). Use of wearables: Tracking and retraining in endurance runners. *Current Sports Medicine Reports, 18*(12), 437–444.

Mountjoy, M., Sundgot-Borgen, J. K., Burke, L. M., et al. (2018). IOC consensus statement on relative energy deficiency in sport (RED-S): 2018 update. *British Journal of Sports Medicine, 52*(11), 687–697.

Napier, C., & Lewis, A. (2020). *Science of Running: Analyze Your Technique, Prevent Injury, Revolutionize Your Training* (First American ed.). New York, NY: Dorling Kindersley.

Nelson, E. O., Kliethermes, S., & Heiderscheit, B. (2020). Construct validity and responsiveness of the University of Wisconsin Running Injury and Recovery Index. *Journal of Orthopaedic & Sports Physical Therapy, 50*(12), 702–710.

Nielsen, R. O., Buist, I., Parner, E. T., Nohr, E. A., Sorensen, H., Lind, M., & Rasmussen, S. (2014). Foot pronation is not associated with increased injury risk in novice runners wearing a neutral shoe: A 1-year prospective cohort study. *British Journal of Sports Medicine, 48*(6), 440–447.

Nigg, B. M., Baltich, J., Hoerzer, S., & Enders, H. (2015). Running shoes and running injuries: Mythbusting and a proposal for two new paradigms: "Preferred movement path" and "comfort filter". *British Journal of Sports Medicine, 49*(20), 1290–1294.

Nilsson, J., & Thorstensson, A. (1989). Ground reaction forces at different speeds of human walking and running. *Acta Physiologica Scandinavica, 136*(2), 217–227.

Novacheck, T. F. (1998). The biomechanics of running. *Gait & Posture, 7*(1), 77–95.

Paquette, M. R., Napier, C., Willy, R. W., & Stellingwerff, T. (2020). Moving beyond weekly "distance": Optimizing quantification of training load in runners. *Journal of Orthopaedic & Sports Physical Therapy, 50*(10), 564–569.

Pipkin, A., Kotecki, K., Hetzel, S., & Heiderscheit, B. (2016). Reliability of a qualitative video analysis for running. *Journal of Orthopaedic & Sports Physical Therapy, 46*(7), 556–561.

Ramskov, D., Rasmussen, S., Sorensen, H., Parner, E. T., Lind, M., & Nielsen, R. O. (2018). Run Clever—No difference in risk of injury when comparing progression in running volume and running intensity in recreational runners: A randomised trial. *BMJ Open Sport & Exercise Medicine, 4*(1), e000333.

Reinking, M. F., Dugan, L., Ripple, N., et al. (2018). Reliability of two-dimensional video-based running gait analysis. *International Journal of Sports Physical Therapy, 13*(3), 453–461.

Riley, P. O., Dicharry, J., Franz, J., Della Croce, U., Wilder, R. P., & Kerrigan, D. C. (2008). A kinematics and kinetic comparison of overground and treadmill running. *Medicine & Science in Sports & Exercise, 40*(6), 1093–1100.

Sandford, G. N., & Stellingwerff, T. (2019). "Question your categories": The misunderstood complexity of middle-distance running profiles with implications for research methods and application. *Frontiers in Sports and Active Living, 1*, 28.

Seiler, S. (2010). What is best practice for training intensity and duration distribution in endurance athletes? *International Journal of Sports Physiology and Performance, 5*(3), 276–291.

Sun, X., Lam, W. K., Zhang, X., Wang, J., & Fu, W. (2020). Systematic review of the role of footwear constructions in running biomechanics: Implications for running-related injury and performance. *Journal of Sports Science and Medicine, 19*(1), 20–37.

Tenforde, A. S., Borgstrom, H. E., Outerleys, J., & Davis, I. S. (2019). Is cadence related to leg length and load rate? *Journal of Orthopaedic & Sports Physical Therapy, 49*(4), 280–283.

Trowell, D., Vicenzino, B., Saunders, N., Fox, A., & Bonacci, J. (2020). Effect of strength training on biomechanical and neuromuscular variables in distance runners: A systematic review and meta-analysis. *Sports Medicine, 50*(1), 133–150.

Tung, K. D., Franz, J. R., & Kram, R. (2014). A test of the metabolic cost of cushioning hypothesis during unshod and shod running. *Medicine & Science in Sports & Exercise, 46*(2), 324–329.

van Gent, R. N., Siem, D., van Middelkoop, M., van Os, A. G., Bierma-Zeinstra, S. M., & Koes, B. W. (2007). Incidence and determinants of lower extremity running injuries in long distance runners: A systematic review. *British Journal of Sports Medicine, 41*(8), 469–480; discussion 480.

Videbaek, S., Bueno, A. M., Nielsen, R. O., & Rasmussen, S. (2015). Incidence of running-related injuries per 1000 h of running in different types of runners: A systematic review and meta-analysis. *Sports Medicine, 45*(7), 1017–1026.

Warden, S. J., Davis, I. S., & Fredericson, M. (2014). Management and prevention of bone stress injuries in long-distance runners. *Journal of Orthopaedic & Sports Physical Therapy, 44*(10), 749–765.

Wille, C. M., Lenhart, R. L., Wang, S., Thelen, D. G., & Heiderscheit, B. C. (2014). Ability of sagittal kinematic variables to estimate ground reaction forces and joint kinetics in running. *Journal of Orthopaedic & Sports Physical Therapy, 44*(10), 825–830.

Willy, R. W., Buchenic, L., Rogacki, K., Ackerman, J., Schmidt, A., & Willson, J. D. (2016). In-field gait retraining and mobile monitoring to address running biomechanics associated with tibial stress fracture. *Scandinavian Journal of Medicine & Science in Sports, 26*(2), 197–205.

Willy, R. W., & Davis, I. S. (2011). The effect of a hip-strengthening program on mechanics during running and during a single-leg squat. *Journal of Orthopaedic & Sports Physical Therapy, 41*(9), 625–632.

Willy, R. W., & Paquette, M. R. (2019). The physiology and biomechanics of the Master runner. *Sports Medicine and Arthroscopy Review, 27*(1), 15–21.

Wulf, G. (2007). *Attention and motor skill learning.* Champaign, IL: Human Kinetics.

CHAPTER 34 QUESTIONS

1. A 19-year old male runner presents with anterior knee pain. Running assessment reveals a preferred step rate of 165 steps/min. An increase in this runner's step rate at the same running speed will result in which of the following?
   a. Decreased overall work at the knee
   b. Decreased overall work at the ankle
   c. Greater foot inclination angle at ground contact
   d. Less vertical tibia orientation at ground contact

2. Which of the following statements is TRUE regarding running shoe wear?
   a. Evidence is limited supporting the use of static foot posture in running shoe prescription
   b. Motion control shoes are designed for runners with excessive lateral wear and hyper-pronated feet
   c. Runners with a high foot posture index should be prescribed a more cushioned shoe
   d. Shoe fit and comfort is not as important as the individual's running mechanics when prescribing shoes

3. In evaluating a patient's running mechanics, what view would best to assess peak knee flexion angle at midstance?
   a. Anterior view
   b. Lateral view
   c. Posterior view

4. What statement supports the decision to increase step rate in a runner with excessive vertical impact peaks and vertical loading rates?
   a. an increase to at least 180 steps/min is required to reduce loads at the hip and knee
   b. an increase of at least 15% preferred step rate is needed to significantly reduce knee loads
   c. an increase of 7.5% preferred step rate will decrease loads at the knee and hip
   d. an increase in 7.5% preferred step rate will decrease running economy

DIAGNOSTIC ULTRASOUND

H. Agustsson, PhD, DPT

1. **What is the physical basis of ultrasound imaging?**
   Ultrasound imaging is based on waves that are emitted from a transducer and subsequently reflected from the tissues back to the transducer. The creation and reception of these waves is as follows. When electrical charges are applied to the crystals in the transducer, there is deformation of the crystals, according to the reversed piezoelectric effect. This gives rise to a wavelike motion of the crystals with the same frequency as the applied current. This motion is the basis of the ultrasound beam that is transmitted in the soft tissues of the body. When waves are reflected back from the tissues this causes the crystals in the transducer to deform, creating electrical charges. The strength, location, and timing of these electrical charges are the data from which an image is constructed in the ultrasound unit.

2. **What information is used to produce the images?**
   Ultrasound images contain information about the reflective characteristics of body structures and the location of these structures. 1) The brightness of structures in an image is based on the strength of waves reflected from the tissues. The strength of the wave-signal is based on the reflective characteristics of the tissues (echogenicity). Tissues that reflect much energy and create a bright image are said to be hyperechoic and those that reflect small amounts of energy and create a dark image are called hypoechoic, or even anechoic if they return no signal. 2) The location of a structure is determined by which crystals along the longitudinal axis of the transducer's surface receive the reflected waves. 3) The depth of the structure is calculated based on the timing of the reflection of the sound. When imaging a superficial structure, the waves return more quickly to the transducer.

3. **How does ultrasound differ from other imaging modalities?**
   Ultrasound imaging is dynamic, and the interpretation typically takes place while scanning. This allows scanning to be modified in response to the findings, as well as allowing the application of physical examination techniques during imaging. Structures are often located by palpation in advance, but they may also be palpated through the ultrasound transducer.

4. **How is the ultrasound image displayed?**
   Ultrasound imaging displays cross-sectional images. However, the field of view is far smaller than for CT or MRI and, unlike CT and MRI, the slices are not necessarily in the orthogonal planes. The imaging plane is best described as being in the direction of the ultrasound beam, a direct continuation of the transducer. However, some ultrasound units are capable of extended field of view that displays a sequence of images and demonstrate structures that are longer than the long axis of the transducer.

5. **How are ultrasound images named?**
   Ultrasound images are not named according to the orthogonal planes, but relative to the structure of interest. Thus, when the transducer is aligned with the long axis of a tendon, this is called a longitudinal sonogram. When the transducer is applied across the tendon, that is a transverse sonogram (Figure).

6. **What is the value of diagnostic ultrasound imaging in current musculoskeletal care?**
   The use of ultrasound in the diagnosis of musculoskeletal problems is embraced by many health care professions. This is understandable due to its diagnostic accuracy for musculoskeletal soft tissue lesions, which is often comparable with, or superior to, magnetic resonance imaging (MRI). There are also substantial savings when MRI can be substituted with ultrasound. The development of smaller, more portable, and less expensive ultrasound units has furthermore increased its utilization. During the last 30 years, there has been a significant increase in the number of ultrasound scans, largely due to an increased number of scans by nonradiologist practitioners. At the same time, the proportion of scans performed by radiologists has fallen.

7. **What health care professionals employ musculoskeletal ultrasound?**
   In addition to radiologists, musculoskeletal ultrasound is used by nonradiologist health care professionals, such as rheumatologists, orthopedic surgeons, physical therapists, and chiropractors. Radiologists still have an advantage due to their extensive training, as well as their knowledge of other imaging techniques. The latter increases the likelihood of patients receiving optimal imaging for their conditions.

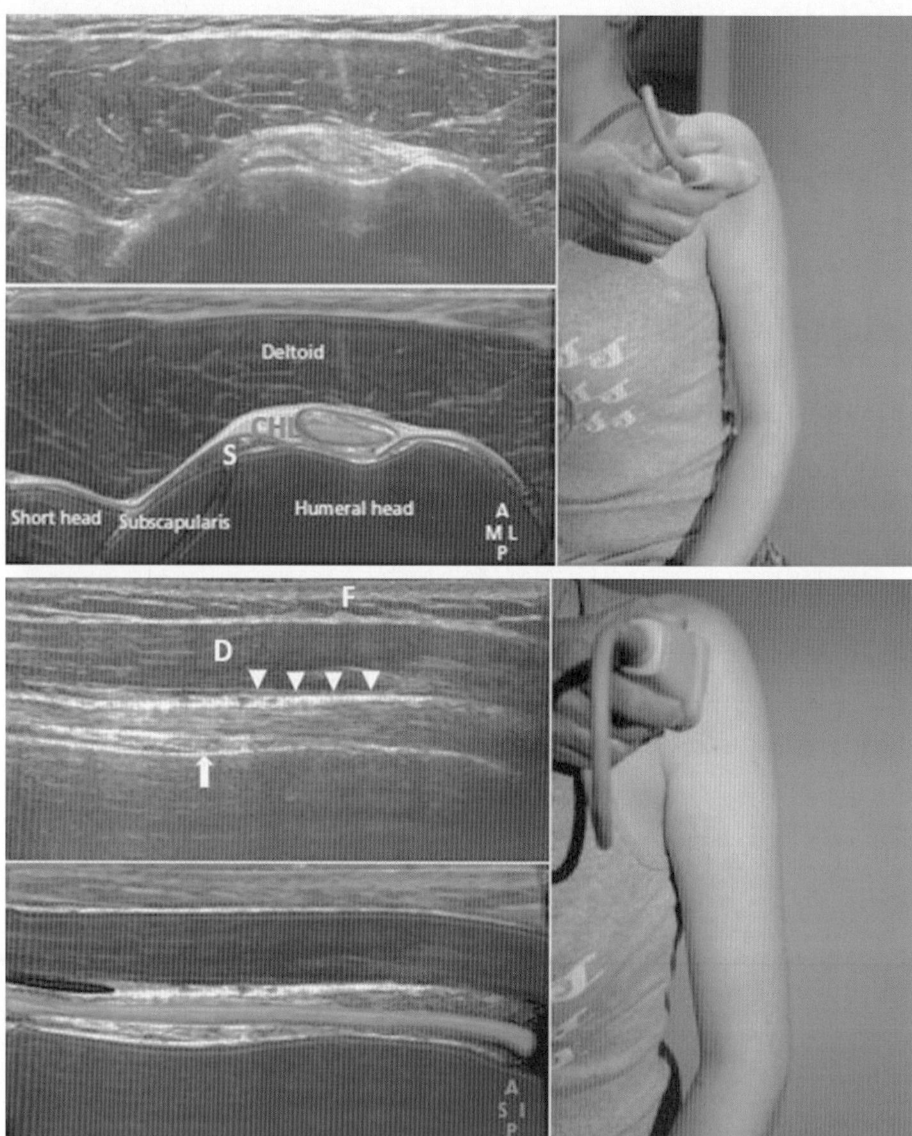

The top image shows a transverse view of the long head of biceps tendon in the bicipital groove of the humerus. Note the coracohumeral ligament (CHL) and the subscapularis tendon (S). The lower image shows a longitudinal view, with the tendon (arrowheads) against the cortical outline of the humerus (arrow). Superficial to it, the deltoid muscle (D) and subcutaneous fat (F). McNally. Chapter 1: Shoulder Joint, in Practical Musculoskeletal Ultrasound.

8. **What is point-of-care ultrasound?**
   The use of ultrasound by nonradiologists for augmenting the patient examination and improving treatments has been referred to as point-of-care ultrasound. This approach saves time for the clinician, as well as the patient since it allows initiating treatment earlier than would otherwise be possible. In addition to using diagnostic ultrasound to confirm the clinical diagnosis and for monitoring treatment outcomes, physical therapists have long used ultrasound to guide treatment interventions and improve their effectiveness.

9. **Can physical therapists use diagnostic ultrasound imaging in clinical practice?**
   Physical therapists can successfully use diagnostic ultrasound as a part of patient examination. The use of diagnostic ultrasound by physical therapists is not prohibited by state practice acts. Practice acts, if they mention

imaging at all, are primarily concerned with limiting the use of harmful radiation. Physical therapists have used ultrasound to evaluate tendinopathy, ligament integrity, and muscle injuries. However, it should be emphasized that extensive training is essential and without that you will not be able to perform accurate diagnostics. For the purposes of training, numerous seminars are available, and physical therapists can complete a musculoskeletal sonography certification, offered by the American Institute for Ultrasound in Medicine.

10. **What physical therapist skills help with ultrasound imaging?**
Physical therapists are well placed to become competent in diagnostic ultrasound of the musculoskeletal system. Patient-handling and examination skills, along with a solid foundation in anatomy, allow them to scan while using palpation to guide transducer placement. Furthermore, the therapist can improve the reliability of scanning by performing traction, ligament tests, and muscle contractions. This increases the diagnostic value of the examination while decreasing the influence of findings that may not be clinically relevant.

11. **What is rehabilitative ultrasound imaging?**
Rehabilitative ultrasound imaging has been used in the treatment of musculoskeletal pain and dysfunctions since the 1990s. Physical therapists have mostly used it as a form of biofeedback for the purpose of improving neuromuscular control, but rehabilitative ultrasound also involves the measurement of muscle length, thickness, and cross-sectional area.

12. **Can ultrasound reliably demonstrate muscle morphology?**
MRI has been the gold standard for morphological measurements. However, ultrasound imaging, which is less expensive and more readily available, has shown good correlation with MRI. Early studies by physical therapists used such measurements to demonstrate atrophy of the lumbar multifidus in patients with low back pain. This atrophy was found to be on the symptomatic side and at the involved spinal level. Changes in muscle morphology can also be followed over time, for example, before and after treatment with manual therapy or exercises.

13. **How does ultrasound display muscle function?**
Therapists and patients can view muscle contractions in terms of thickening of the muscle of interest during contraction versus during rest (Figure). As of now, there is inconclusive evidence of correlation between changes in muscle morphology as seen with ultrasound imaging and muscle activity detected with electromyography.

14. **How do physical therapists use ultrasound for biofeedback?**
The real-time view of muscle activity with ultrasound imaging allows the patient to understand how different strategies for engagement and coordination of muscle activity are working. This approach was employed in early studies on the role of the multifidus and transversus abdominis muscles in stabilization of the lumbar spine. These studies demonstrated that the activity of these muscles was decreased in the presence of low back pain and did not automatically reverse with the resolution of pain. The development of effective treatments to reduce the risk of recurrence of low back pain employed ultrasound biofeedback.

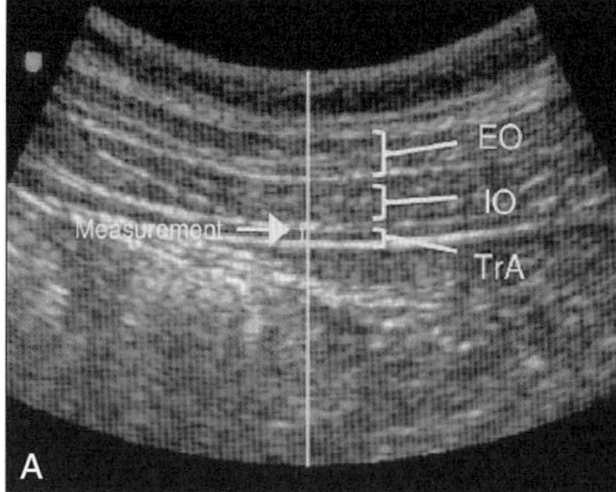

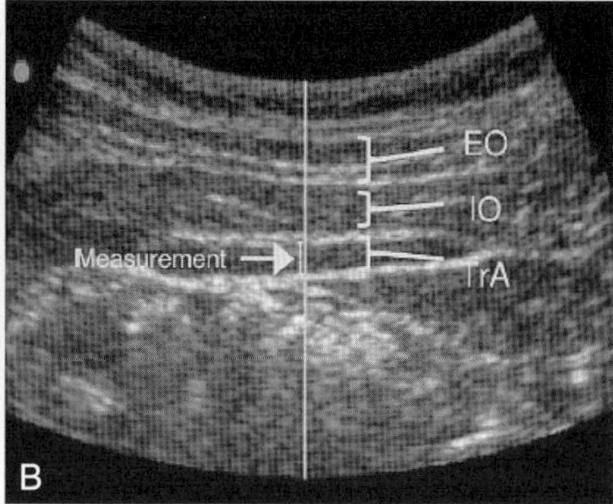

Ultrasound images of the transversus abdominis (TrA), internal oblique (IO), and external oblique (EO) muscles during rest (image A) and during an abdominal drawing-in maneuver (image B). Thickness measurements are made between the superficial and deep borders of the transversus abdominis muscle. The therapist also looks for changes in the position of the aponeuroses and other structures to which the muscle attaches. (Koppenhaver SL et al, Arch Phys Med Rehabil. 2009 Jan;90(1):87–94.)

15. **Can ultrasound assist in the treatment of pelvic floor dysfunction?**
    Pelvic floor dysfunctions such as urinary incontinence have been successfully treated with the help of ultrasound. Ultrasound imaging that displays the bladder through the anterior abdominal wall or from the perineum is used to evaluate the pelvic floor muscles. (Figure).

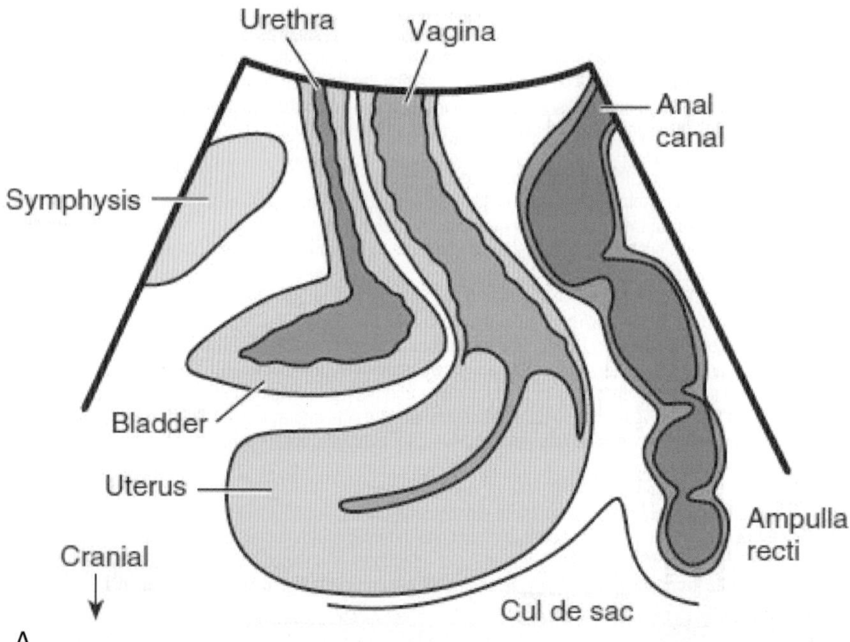

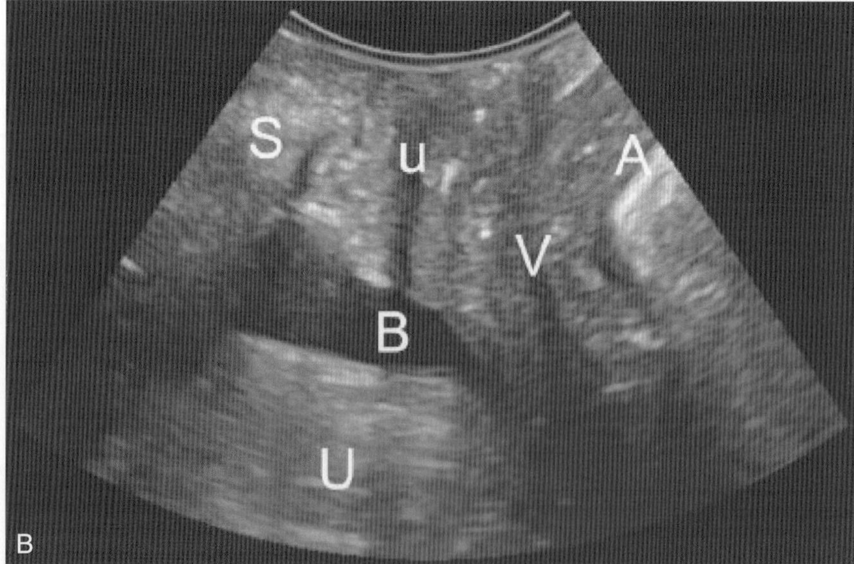

A schematic diagram (top image) and an ultrasound image (lower image) showing a midsagittal transperineal ultrasound. Anal canal (A), vagina (V), urethra (u), uterus (U), bladder (B), and symphysis pubis (S). The activity of the pelvic floor muscles is evaluated based on changes in the position of the bladder, which demonstrates how well the pelvic floor muscles are supporting the bladder during various maneuvers. Walters and Karram. Urogynecology and Reconstructive Pelvic Surgery, Ch. 13. (A from Dietz HP. Pelvic floor ultrasound: a review. *Am J Obstet Gynecol.* 2010;202:321. With permission.)

16. **Do physical therapists use interventional ultrasound?**
Physicians have used ultrasound to direct injections into tendons and joints and to guide biopsies, as well as for joint aspiration. In physical therapy, ultrasound used to guide dry needling of deeper structures is an example of interventional ultrasound (Figure). Ultrasound-guided dry needling may employ Doppler ultrasound in order to avoid blood vessels.

17. **Are there different types of ultrasound transducers?**
Musculoskeletal ultrasound typically uses straight (linear) transducers in order to display structures in correct proportions. The field of view equals the diameter of the transducer. But, for rehabilitative ultrasound of the paraspinal muscles and the lateral abdominal wall, as well as for pelvic and abdominal ultrasound, the transducer is curvilinear. The curvilinear transducer gives rise to a diverging beam that makes deeper structures appear larger (Figure). Transducers also vary in size. Smaller transducers, which are suitable for areas such as the fingers, have higher frequency that emphasizes superficial structures.

18. **What is the value of Doppler ultrasound?**
Doppler ultrasound is used to measure blood flow. It employs the Doppler effect where the velocity and direction of movement change the frequency of the reflected ultrasound waves. Greater flow velocity of blood cells toward the transducer is typically displayed with red color and lower velocity with blue. Doppler ultrasound can be used to identify vessel constriction, such as seen in arterial stenosis, because flow in a narrowed vessel is characterized by turbulence that shows up as a multitude of colors.

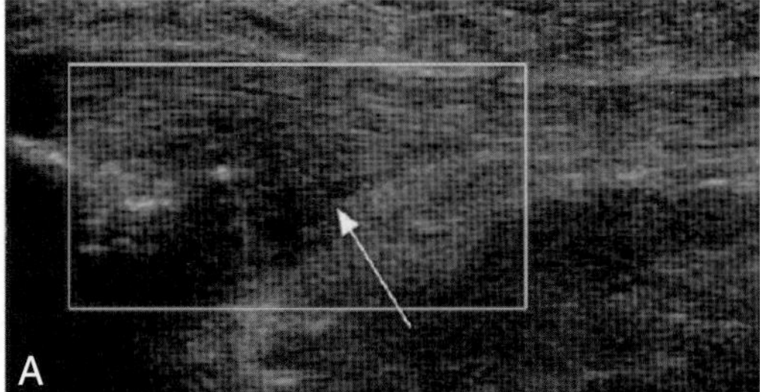

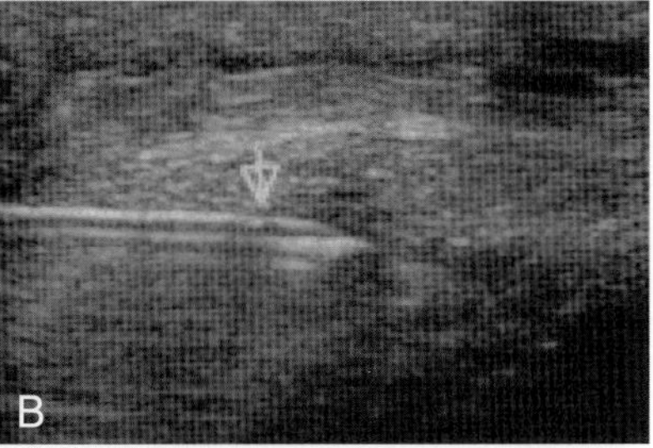

Image (A) shows a thickened dark area, signifying inflammation, at the inferior aspect of the patellar ligament (arrow). The open arrow in image (B) shows the position of the needle within the area of tendinitis during the dry needling. Davidson, Guided interventions in musculoskeletal ultrasound: what's the evidence? Clinical Radiology 66 (2011) 140e152.

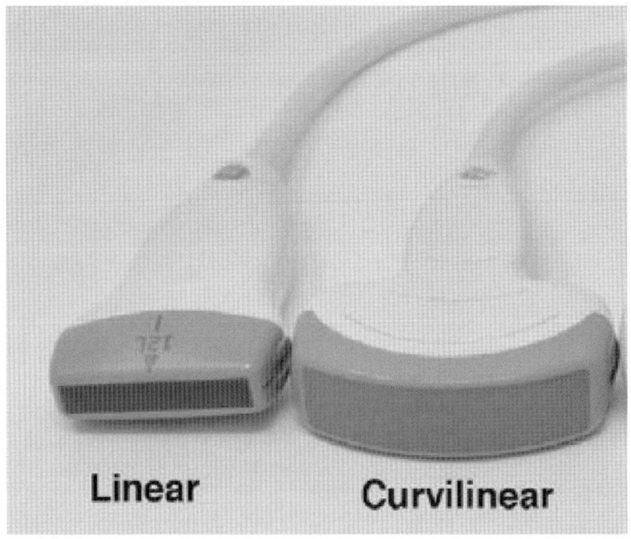

Linear vs. curvilinear transducers. (From pocus101.com; with permission.)

19. **Is power Doppler different from Doppler ultrasound?**
While Doppler ultrasound shows the direction and velocity of blood flow, it does not provide general information about the overall circulation in an area. However, power Doppler can demonstrate the volume of blood flow in an area without estimating its velocity. Power Doppler is widely used by rheumatologists because it shows changes in local blood flow associated with inflammation and synovial proliferation.

20. **What are the characteristics of ultrasound signals?**
The imaging characteristics of tissues mostly result from their echogenicity. Highly echogenic tissues, such as tendons and cortices of bones, render bright signals, typically described with reference to surrounding tissues. Thus, the infraspinatus tendon forming within the muscle is said to be hyperechoic relative to the surrounding muscle fibers. The reflective characteristics of surfaces and the interface between adjacent tissues are also important. Smooth tissue surfaces give rise to stronger signals as do interfaces between tissues with different echogenicity.
a) What is the signal from bone?
As with therapeutic ultrasound, ultrasound imaging does not penetrate bone. Thus, the interface between bone and soft tissue reflects all waves, resulting in a bright signal from the cortex, while subcortical bone appears as dark (Figure).
b) What is the signal from tendons and ligaments?
Tendons appear bright compared to fat and to muscle. They have a dotted appearance in the transverse sonogram but a distinct parallel fiber pattern in longitudinal sonograms (Figure). Ligaments are similarly bright and display a distinct fiber pattern, though with a smaller distance between fibers than seen in tendons.

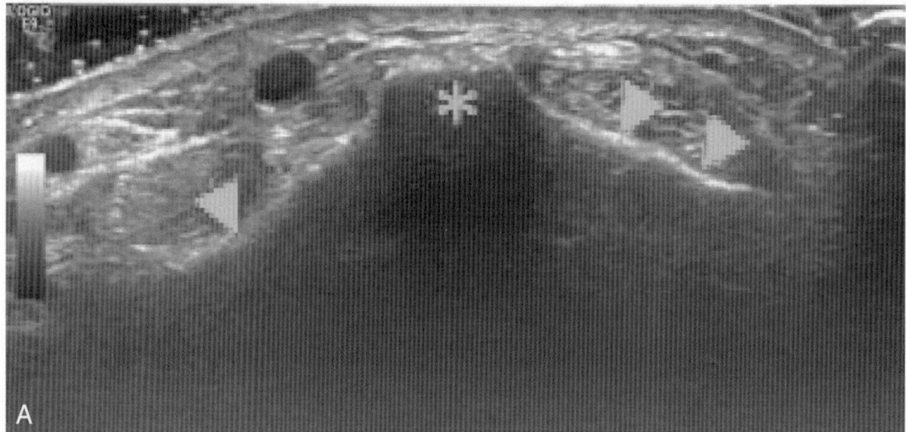

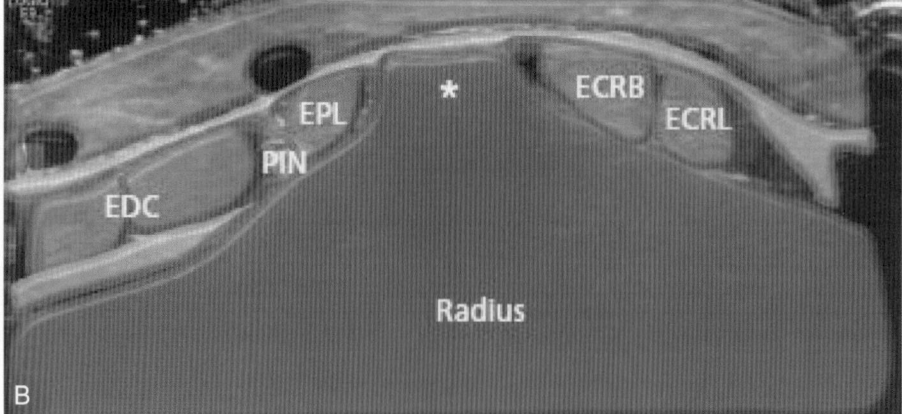

Transverse ultrasound of the dorsal distal forearm shows the bright cortical outline of the radius [arrows], including the Lister's tubercle [*]. Extensor digitorum communis (EDC), posterior interosseous nerve is missing in the captions (PIN), extensor pollicis longus (EPL), extensor carpi radialis brevis (ECRB), and extensor carpi radialis longus (ECRL). Practical Musculoskeletal Ultrasound – Ch 10 Forearm and Wrist.

c) What is the signal from muscles?
Overall, muscles are relatively dark when compared to tendons or surrounding fasciae. Between muscles, and within the muscle substance, there are fibroadipose septa that form bright lines (Figure). These septa group together muscle fibers into fascicles that are seen on ultrasound as dark bundles. The septa may be disrupted in case of muscle strains. The extent of this disruption differs according to the grade of the injury. Injuries are often associated with hematoma that gradually appear darker with time.

d) What is the signal from cartilage?
Fibrocartilage, such as found in the menisci of the knee, is fairly bright (Figure). However, hyaline cartilage is seen as a dark layer distinct from the bright cortical bone on either side (Figure). Therefore, hyaline cartilage thinning, or defects, can clearly be visualized with ultrasound imaging.

e) What is the signal from nerve?
Nerves appear darker than tendons but brighter than muscle. Like tendons, they have a longitudinal fiber pattern. Nerve compression, as in carpal tunnel syndrome, can be seen as flattening of the nerve at the point of compression, with swelling of the nerve proximal to the compression. The advantages of ultrasound for the evaluation of nerve injury relate to the high resolution and the ability to image the nerve throughout the extremity with added contributions from patient feedback.

f) What is the signal from bursa?
Bursae are displayed as dark lines between brighter structures, such as bones and ligaments, although they are difficult to see unless there is swelling. The walls of the bursa are not visible but, in case of chronic bursitis, the thickened walls of the bursa may appear bright.

21. What can degrade and distort the ultrasound image?
Certain conditions may lead to signal changes that result in loss of quality and accuracy. Such changes are known as artifacts. Some artifacts result from poor scanning technique, others cannot be avoided. Examples of artifacts

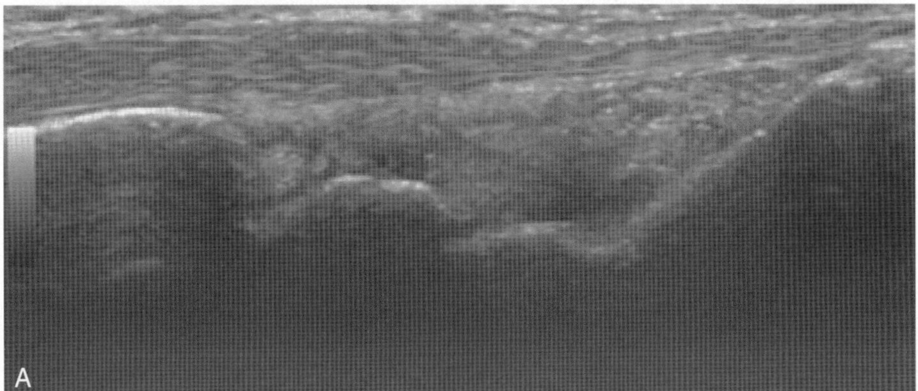

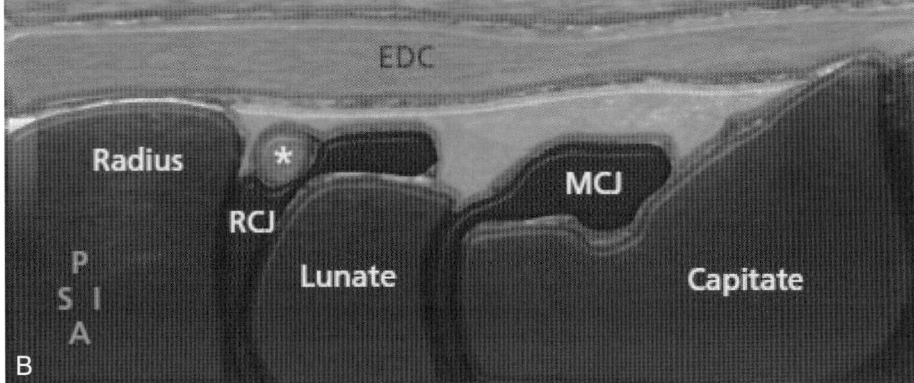

This long axis ultrasound of the radiocarpal and midcarpal joints shows the regular, longitudinal fiber pattern of the extensor digitorum tendon (EDC), the radiocarpal joint (RCJ and the midcarpal joint (MCJ). Practical Musculoskeletal Ultrasound – Ch 10 Forearm and Wrist.

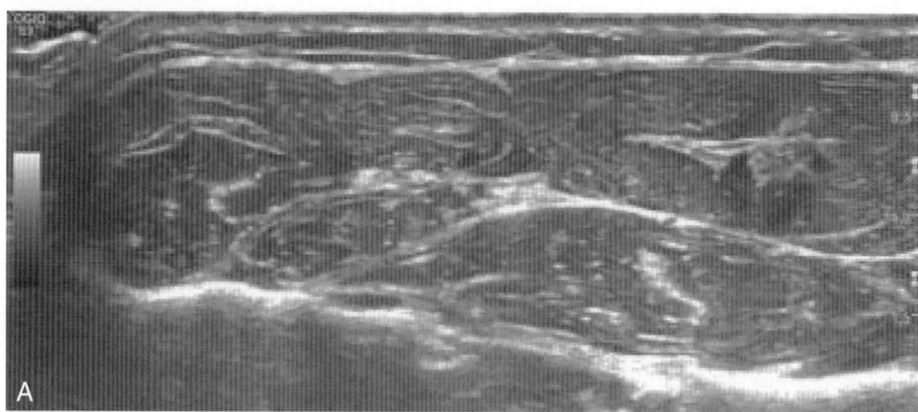

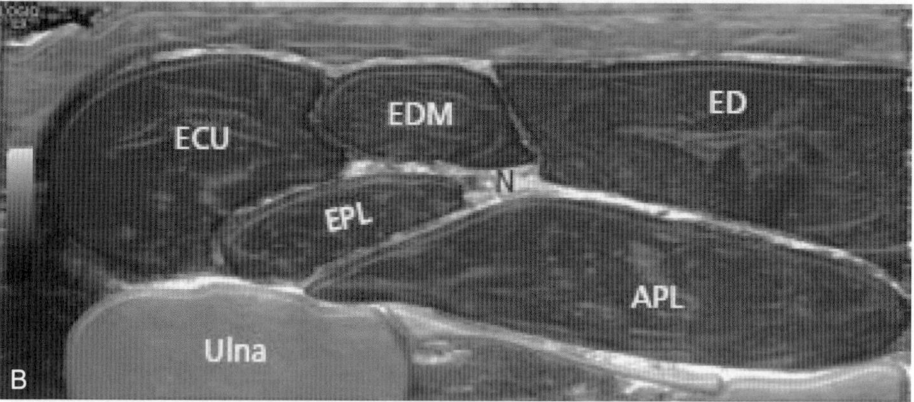

Transverse ultrasound of the of the dorsal musculature of the distal forearm. Note how muscles are enveloped in intermuscular septa. *APL*, Abductor pollicis longus; *ECU*, extensor carpi ulnaris; *ED*, extensor digitorum; *EDM*, extensor digiti minimi; *EPL*, extensor pollicis longus; *N*, posterior interosseous nerve. Practical Musculoskeletal Ultrasound – Ch 10 Forearm and Wrist.

include: 1) Anisotropy, when the fibers of tendons and ligaments that are normally bright appear dark if examined at certain angles (Figure). To avoid this, the beam must be at right angles to the tendon. A change in angulation of as little as five degrees during longitudinal ultrasound can change a tendon from bright to dark, so anisotropy can often be corrected with a slight tilt of the transducer. 2) Acoustic enhancement is when there is increased signal from tissues that lie deep to a structure that has limited absorption, such as the urinary bladder. 3) Acoustic shadowing is the opposite to enhancement. Areas that lie deep to structures with strong reflective characteristics show a decrease in the reflection of ultrasound waves and, therefore, appear dark. See the dark subcortical bone in Figure.

22. Compared to MRI, what are the advantages of diagnostic ultrasound?

Ultrasound and MRI are the most sensitive imaging methods for the diagnosis of musculoskeletal soft tissue lesions. The general advantages of ultrasound over MRI include lower cost, no associated health hazards, and the ability to use in the presence of metal. Thus, ultrasound is ideal for the evaluation of soft-tissue abnormalities that may appear near orthopedic hardware. Another advantage is the possibility of modifying the imaging process, while imaging, based on findings. Additionally, because ultrasound is not limited to orthogonal planes, it can follow structures from beginning to end. This is useful when imaging structures with complex orientation such as the tendons on the medial and lateral side of the ankle. For soft tissue diagnosis, ultrasound is just as accurate as MRI. Indeed, it provides greater resolution of the internal architecture of muscles, ligaments, and tendons. Additionally, ultrasound has advantages over other imaging modalities for the location of foreign bodies in soft tissues, such as wood splinters and glass. Foreign bodies will usually appear bright relative to the surrounding soft tissue.

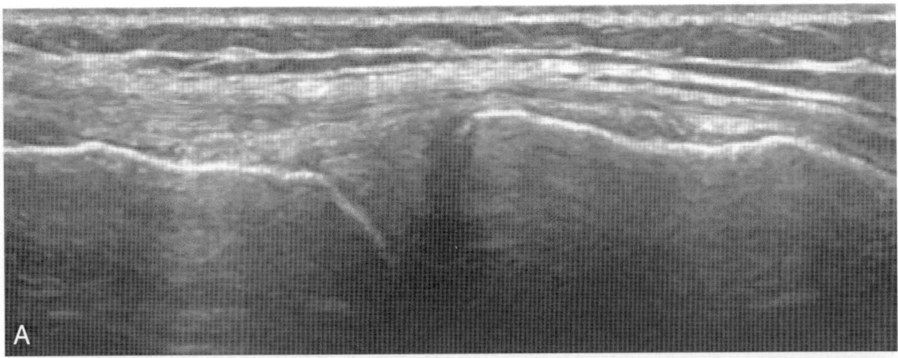

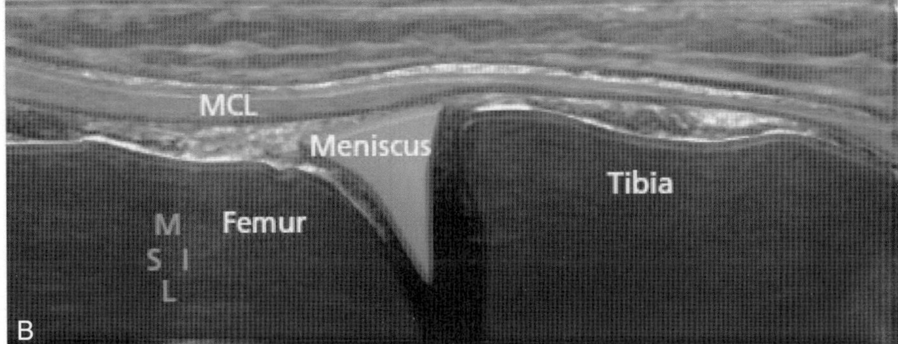

This longitudinal ultrasound of the medial aspect of the knee shows the medial meniscus deep to the medial collateral ligament (MCL). Hyaline cartilage is seen as a dark layer distinct from the tibia. Practical Musculoskeletal Ultrasound – Ch 21 Knee.

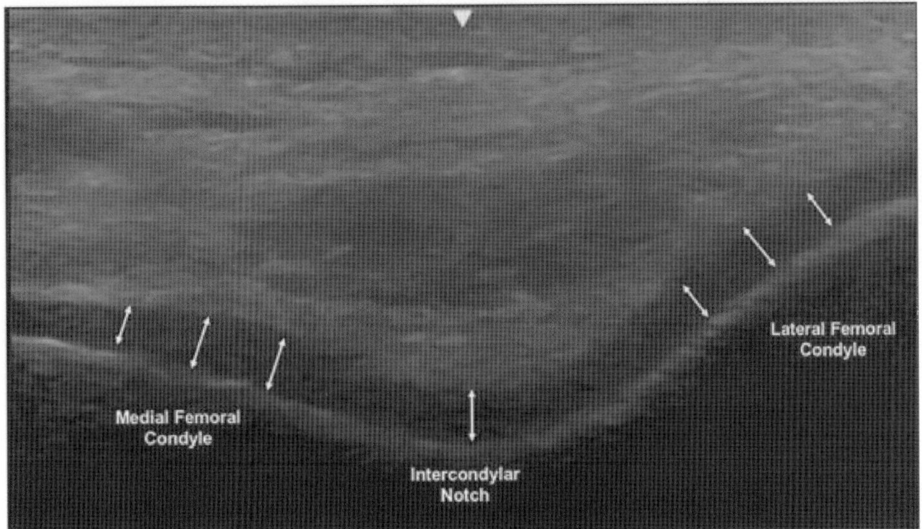

This transverse ultrasound of the patellar groove shows dark cartilage (double arrows) in contrast to the cortical outlines of the medial and lateral femoral condyles. Therefore, hyaline cartilage thinning, or defects, can clearly be visualized with ultrasound imaging. (Pamukoff, Montgomery et al. Gait & Posture, 2018;65:221–227.)

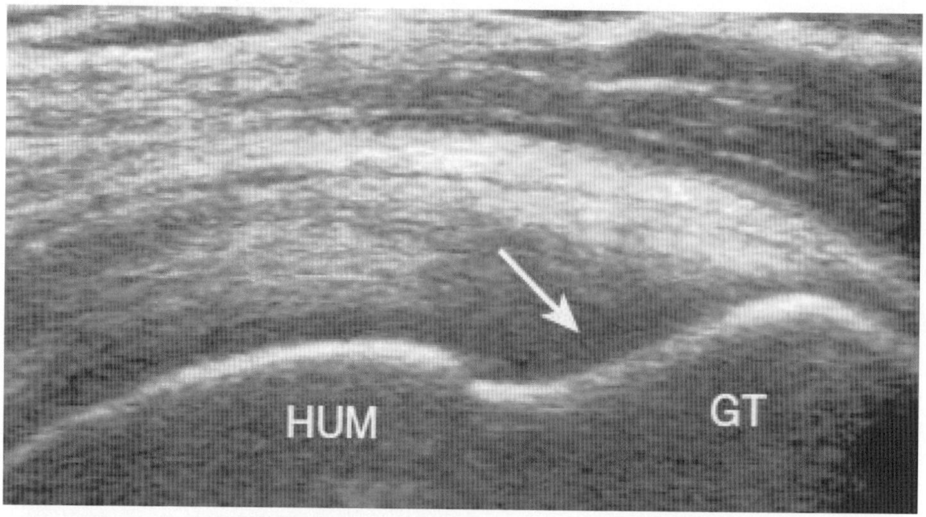

Anisotropy artifact [arrow] at the supraspinatus insertion on greater tuberosity [GT] of the humerus [HUM]. This falsely appears like a tear. Hill, Lavallee, Fowler. (Pfenninger and Fowler's Procedures for Primary Care, Chapter 171, 1140–1153.)

23. **What are the main limitations of ultrasound imaging?**
Ultrasound imaging has several limitations: 1) It is operator dependent compared to the other imaging methods. This may make it difficult to repeat a previous examination exactly. Still, interobserver reliability between experienced sonographers is fairly good. 2) The field of view in musculoskeletal ultrasound is limited, as the ultrasound beam has the same width as the diameter of the transducer. 3) Ultrasound does not penetrate cortical bone, so intraarticular structures are not well seen. Although ultrasound can evaluate some parts of cartilage, MRI offers a more complete evaluation. 4) Imaging obese patients may be associated with loss of image quality since fat absorbs the sound waves.

24. **Does ultrasound imaging have any adverse effects?**
Ultrasound imaging has no known adverse effects. Unlike therapeutic ultrasound that can lead to thermal damage under certain circumstances, the dose of ultrasound used for diagnostic imaging is too low to result in the build-up of heat or other physiological effects.

Bibliography

Boyles, R. E., Gorman, I., Pinto, D., & Ross, M. D. (2011). Physical therapist practice and the role of diagnostic imaging. *Journal of Orthopaedic & Sports Physical Therapy, 41*, 829–837.

Bureau, N. J., & Ziegler, D. (2016). Economics of musculoskeletal ultrasound. *Current Radiology Reports, 4*, 44.

Jacobson, J. A. (2009). Musculoskeletal ultrasound: focused impact on MRI. *American Journal of Roentgenology, 193*(3), 619–627.

Liu, F., Cheng, X., Dong, J., Zhou, D., Han, S., & Yang, Y. (2020). Comparison of MRI and MRA for the diagnosis of rotator cuff tears: a meta-analysis. *Medicine (Baltimore), 99*(12), e19579.

Whittaker, J. L., & Stokes, M. (2011). Ultrasound imaging and muscle function. *Journal of Orthopaedic & Sports Physical Therapy, 41*(8), 572–580.

CHAPTER 35 QUESTIONS

1. **You are treating Achilles tendinosis in a patient who recently had an ankle fracture that was treated with plates and screws. After 3 weeks of limited progress, you want additional information about the status of the tendon and recommend ultrasound imaging. What would be a reason for choosing ultrasound over magnetic resonance imaging (MRI)?**
   a. Ultrasound imaging has a bigger field of view.
   b. Ultrasound imaging is not contraindicated in the presence of orthopedic hardware.
   c. Ultrasound has better differential diagnosis capabilities.
   d. Ultrasound can provide information about the fracture healing in addition to the status of the tendon.

2. **Your patient has limited and painful shoulder rotation. Since there is history of a rotator cuff tear of the opposite shoulder, you are considering an imaging study. Your clinic acquired an ultrasound imaging unit last week and you took an ultrasound seminar over the weekend. Is there a reason you should not perform the ultrasound yourself?**
   a. It is probably prohibited by your state practice act.
   b. Like with therapeutic ultrasound, there is the risk of thermal injury next to the cortex of the humeral head.
   c. Ultrasound imaging is too expensive to be warranted for such a minor problem.
   d. You should not use ultrasound as a diagnostic tool without extensive training.

3. **You have been treating a patient with rheumatoid arthritis affecting the elbow. You want to understand the degree to which her loss of flexion is the result of synovial proliferation in the joint. Being a competent musculoskeletal sonographer, you conclude that the following would best serve your purpose:**
   a. Doppler ultrasound
   b. Interventional ultrasound
   c. Power Doppler ultrasound
   d. Standard radiography

CHAPTER 36

FUNCTIONAL ANATOMY OF THE SHOULDER

O. Oshikoya, MD, PharmD and J.M. Wiater, MD

1. Name the origins, insertions, innervation, and actions of all muscles that attach to the scapula.

There are 17 muscles attached to the scapula, and the following table summarizes their origins, insertions, innervation, and action.

MUSCLE	ORIGIN	INSERTION	INNERVATION	ACTION
Subscapularis	Subscapularis fossa	Lesser tuberosity of humerus	Upper and lower subscapular nerve	Glenohumeral head depressor; extension, adduction, and medial rotation of humerus
Supraspinatus	Supraspinatus fossa	Superior facet on greater tuberosity	Suprascapular nerve	Abduction, stabilization of glenohumeral joint
Infraspinatus	Infraspinatus fossa	Middle facet on greater tuberosity	Suprascapular nerve	Extension and external rotation
Teres minor	Superior part of lateral border of scapula	Inferior facet on greater tuberosity	Axillary nerve	Extension and external rotation
Teres major	Dorsal surface of inferior angle of scapula	Medial lip of intertubercular groove of humerus	Lower subscapular	Adducts and internally rotates arm
Serratus anterior	External surfaces of lateral parts of ribs 1–8	Anterior surface of medial border of scapula	Long thoracic nerve	Protracts and rotates scapula and holds it against thoracic wall
Deltoid	Lateral one third of clavicle, acromion, and spine of scapula	Deltoid tuberosity of humerus	Axillary nerve	Flexes, abducts, and extends arm
Trapezius	Spinous processes of cervical and thoracic vertebrae	Scapula and acromion	Spinal accessory nerve and branches of ansa cervicalis	Elevates, retracts, and rotates scapula
Levator scapula	Posterior tubercles of transverse processes of C1–C4 vertebrae	Superior part of medial border of scapula	Dorsal scapular nerve	Elevates scapula and tilts glenoid cavity inferiorly by rotating scapula

MUSCLE	ORIGIN	INSERTION	INNERVATION	ACTION
Rhomboids (major and minor)	Ligamentum nuchae and spinous processes of C7–T5	Medial border of scapula from level of spine to inferior angle	Dorsal scapular nerve	Retracts scapula and rotates it to depress glenoid cavity
Triceps	Superior one third of posterior and lateral surface of humerus, infraglenoid tubercle	Supraposterior surface of olecranon process of ulna and deep fascia of forearm	Radial nerve	Extends forearm at elbow; extension of arm at shoulder
Pectoralis minor	Ribs 3–5 near their costal cartilages	Medial border and superior surface of coracoid process of scapula	Medial pectoral nerve	Stabilizes scapula by drawing it inferiorly and anteriorly against thoracic wall
Coracobrachialis	Tip of coracoid process of scapula	Middle medial border of humerus	Musculocutaneous nerve	Horizontal flexion and adduction of humerus at shoulder
Biceps brachii	Tip of coracoid and supraglenoid tubercle of scapula	Tuberosity of radius and lacertus fibrosis	Musculocutaneous nerve	Supinates forearm and when supine flexes forearm
Omohyoid	Superior border of scapula and suprascapular ligament	Inferior border of hyoid bone	Ansa cervicalis	Functions in swallowing and phonation
Latissimus Dorsi	Spinous processes of T7-T12, thoracolumbar fascia, posterior third of iliac crest and inferior angle of the scapula	Intertubercular groove of the humerus	Thoracodorsal nerve (C6-C8)	Arm adduction, extension and internal rotation

2. **What is the normal scapulohumeral rhythm?**

   Normal scapulohumeral rhythm, as initially described by Codman in 1934, refers to the steady and continuous motion that occurs simultaneously at the scapulohumeral and scapulothoracic articulations during elevation of the arm. If the shoulder joint is abnormal, the scapula moves haltingly on the chest wall and not in concert with the glenohumeral joint. Although the relative motion of the glenohumeral joint to the scapulothoracic joint varies among individuals and at different ranges of the shoulder (1.25 to 1 to 4.3 to 1), the average is approximately 2 to 1.

3. **Describe the gliding movements at the shoulder.**

   During rotational motion of the shoulder, obligate translation of the humeral head is a result of the asymmetric tightening and loosening of the capsuloligamentous structures. Anterior translation of the humeral head occurs with forward elevation beyond 55 degrees, and posterior translation occurs with extension >35 degrees. Surgical tightening of the posterior capsule or rotator interval tissue results in increased obligate anterior translation during forward elevation. Conversely, excessively tight anterior instability repairs shift the humeral head and joint contact point posteriorly. These findings illustrate that capsular restriction in one direction can lead to instability in the opposite direction. During elevation the humeral head moves superiorly 3 mm early in elevation then rotates in place with little translation.

4. **How is glenohumeral joint stability maintained?**
Stability of the glenohumeral joint depends on both static and dynamic stabilizers of the shoulder joint. The static or passive stabilizers of the shoulder joint include the glenohumeral joint capsule and ligaments. These structures are normally lax during the mid-range of motion but tighten at the extremes of motion, serving as passive checkreins to excessive glenohumeral translation. The dynamic stabilizers include primarily the rotator cuff and deltoid muscles, although all glenohumeral muscles contribute to stability to some degree. The dynamic stabilizers make the greatest contribution to stability within the functional mid-range of motion by actively contracting and keeping the humeral head centered in the glenoid fossa, producing a concavity-compression effect. They lose their effectiveness as they are stretched beyond their functional length at the extremes of motion.

5. **Which structure is the most important static restraint to anterior glenohumeral translation in the 90-degree abducted-externally rotated position?**
Most traumatic shoulder dislocations are anterior and occur with the arm in the extreme abducted and externally rotated position. Cadaveric ligament-cutting studies have shown that different regions of the glenohumeral capsule and ligament complex are placed on stretch, depending on the position of the arm. The anterior band of the inferior glenohumeral ligament is the principal static restraint to the anterior translation of the humeral head with the arm in the 90-degree abducted-externally rotated position. The middle glenohumeral ligament is a significant restraint to anterior translation in the mid-range of shoulder elevation. The superior glenohumeral ligament appears to prevent excessive external rotation and inferior translation with the arm adducted at the side.

6. **What are the normal strength ratios of the shoulder?**
   - Internal to external rotation: 3 to 2
   - Adduction to abduction: 2 to 1
   - Extension to flexion: 5 to 4

   Women have approximately 45% to 65% of the shoulder strength of men.

7. **What are the four parts of the proximal humerus?**
The proximal humerus is composed of four distinct anatomic segments: (1) the shaft of the humerus, (2) the greater tuberosity, (3) the lesser tuberosity, and (4) the articular or head segment. These segments correspond to the four ossification centers of the proximal humerus. The shaft of the humerus connects with the proximal humerus at the surgical neck, just below the tuberosities. The anatomic neck is above the tuberosities, between the articular margin and the attachment of the articular capsule. The greater tuberosity has three facets for the attachment of the supraspinatus, infraspinatus, and teres minor muscles. The lesser tuberosity is the site of insertion of the subscapularis muscle. The four parts of the proximal humerus are common sites of fractures, especially in older patients with osteopenic bone, and form the basis for the Neer classification of proximal humerus fractures.

8. **What is the normal shape of the human glenoid?**
The normal anatomy of the bony glenoid is highly variable. The glenoid articular surface is often described as pear-shaped, with a larger diameter in the lower portion than in the upper portion. Although this is the most common shape seen, a cadaver study showed 29% of normal glenoids were ovoid in shape, with similar diameter in the upper and lower portions. Mean glenoid width is approximately 26.8 mm, with a normal range between 20 and 35 mm. Average glenoid height is 38 mm, with normal values ranging from 29.4 to 50.1 mm. Men typically have slightly larger glenoids than women in both of these dimensions. Inclination (or tilt) is the slope of the glenoid face in the superior-inferior direction. Average inclination is reported from −2.2 degrees (inferior tilt) to +4.2 degrees (superior tilt) but with normal ranges anywhere from −12 degrees to +15.8 degrees. Glenoid version is the direction of the glenoid surface in the anterior-posterior plane. Average glenoid version is about 2 degrees of retroversion, but normal version ranges between 12 degrees of anteversion and 14 degrees of retroversion.

9. **What is the rotator interval?**
The rotator interval, as originally described by Neer, is the capsular tissue in the interval between the subscapularis and supraspinatus tendons. The rotator interval is composed of parts of the supraspinatus and subscapularis tendons, the coracohumeral ligament, and the superior glenohumeral ligament. These structures contribute to stability of the shoulder by limiting inferior translation and external rotation with the arm adducted, as well as posterior translation when the arm is forward flexed, adducted, and internally rotated. The more medial part of the interval primarily limits inferior translation and to a lesser extent external rotation, although the lateral part of the interval primarily limits external rotation in the adducted arm. Pathologic rotator interval tissue can play a significant role in limiting motion, particularly external rotation, in the setting of adhesive capsulitis. At the

opposite end of the spectrum, deficient or attenuated rotator interval tissue may be associated with recurrent anteroinferior or multidirectional instability of the shoulder.

10. **What are the basic biomechanical functions of the rotator cuff?**
The rotator cuff acts to provide stability through force couples and aid in motion about the glenohumeral joint. The subscapularis, the strongest of the cuff muscles, makes up the anterior portion of this transverse force couple. This balances the posterior portion, made up of the supraspinatus, infraspinatus, and teres minor. The combined action of the anterior and posterior force couple creates compression of the humeral head into the glenoid and a humeral head–depressing effect that counteracts the superior pull of the deltoid muscle. Concavity compression refers to the stability obtained by compression of the humeral head into the concave glenoid fossa. This compressive load is primarily provided by dynamic muscle contraction of the rotator cuff muscles, enhancing glenohumeral stability during motion and maintaining proper position of the humeral head within the glenoid.

11. **Describe the anatomy of the supraspinatus tendon and its clinical significance.**
The supraspinatus muscle functions to initiate abduction and depress the humeral head against the upward pull of the deltoid. The muscle and tendon travel slightly obliquely from posterior to anterior, allowing it to contribute to external rotation as well. It has a broad attachment at the greater tuberosity, which is why supraspinatus strength testing is best performed in internal rotation, as this brings the tendon insertion into the plane of the scapula. There are two muscle bellies, anterior and posterior. The anterior muscle belly is larger and pulls through a smaller tendon area. Thus the anterior tendon stress is significantly greater than the posterior tendon stress, and rotator cuff tendon repairs should incorporate the anterior tendon whenever possible, as it acts as the primary contractile unit.

12. **What is the anatomy of the rotator cuff insertion?**

TENDON, SHAPE	SHAPE	MAXIMUM AVERAGE MEDIAL TO LATERAL, MM	MAXIMUM AVERAGE ANTERIOR TO POSTERIOR, MM
Supraspinatus	Triangular	6.9	12.6
Infraspinatus	Trapezoidal	10.2	32.7
Teres minor	Triangular	29	21
Subscapularis	Comma-shaped	40	20

13. **Describe the biomechanics after superior capsular reconstruction.**
In a healthy shoulder, the deltoid and rotator cuff muscles function to maintain balance around the glenohumeral joint. The rotator cuff serves as a dynamic stabilizer of the glenohumeral joint by resisting cranial migration of the humerus as a result of deltoid contraction. Disruption of the rotator cuff leads to imbalance across the glenohumeral joint due to alterations in the magnitude and direction of joint reactive forces. This manifests in the patient as difficulty with abduction and elevation of the arm. The superior capsule, which lies on the undersurface of the supraspinatus muscle, is believed to transmit force from the rotator cuff and aid in the stability of the glenohumeral joint. Rybalko et al. looked at the biomechanical effects of superior capsular reconstruction in a rotator cuff deficient shoulder. The authors found that superior capsular reconstruction (SCR) restores biomechanical properties of the shoulder including greater functional force at 0 degrees compared to cadavers with an irreparable, complete supraspinatus tear. Additionally, they found decreased superior migration similar to intact shoulders at 0 and 30 degrees of abduction and was not significantly different from intact shoulders at any angle. SCR did lead to decreased passive shoulder extension and increased abduction compared to the intact configuration. Overall arc of axial rotation was not different between the SCR and intact shoulder cadavers.

14. **What is the importance of teres minor?**
Teres minor has been referred to as the forgotten muscle of the rotator cuff. Teres minor becomes a key component in maintaining shoulder function when other rotator cuff tendons fail. Teres minor maintains a balanced glenohumeral joint and changes from an insignificant to the most significant external rotator in the setting of major rotator dysfunction. Imaging of teres minor in the setting of massive, irreparable rotator cuff tears demonstrate hypertrophy of the muscle belly, which serves as an indicator of the greater force necessary to counter balance the subscapularis in patients with supraspinatus and infraspinatus tendon tears.

15. **Describe the role of the long head of the biceps.**
Opinions vary considerably. Some investigators suggest that it is a vestigial structure, whereas others believe that it plays a crucial role in shoulder stability. Dynamic cadaveric and in vivo electromyographic studies have

shown that the long head of the biceps may contribute to anterior stability of the shoulder by decreasing translation of the humeral head and may have a humeral head–depressing effect in the presence of a large rotator cuff tear by restraining superior migration of the humeral head. Elbow flexion strength can decrease by as much as 30% after a tear of the long head of the biceps. Supination decreases by an average of 10% to 20%. Abduction strength may decrease 20% after a tear of the long head of the biceps secondary to the loss of its stabilizing function.

16. **What is the role of the bicipital groove in anterosuperior shoulder pain?**
The differential diagnosis of anterosuperior shoulder pain can include impingement syndrome, rotator cuff pathology, acromioclavicular joint pain, instability, and biceps tendon disease. Furthermore, there is a positive association between radiographic degenerative changes of the bicipital groove and anterosuperior shoulder pain. Studies have shown there is an increased incidence of bicipital tendon disease in patients with degenerative changes in the bicipital groove. These degenerative changes include stenosis and osteophyte formation, which has been correlated to biceps tendon disease via ultrasonography.

17. **Describe the most common variations of the labral origin of the biceps anchor.**
Forty to sixty percent of the biceps tendon origin is from the supraglenoid tubercle, although the remaining fibers originate from the superior glenoid labrum. There is considerable variability in the attachment to the superior labrum. The most common variation is an equal contribution of anterior and posterior labral attachment. The next most common is attachment, mostly posterior, but with a small contribution to the anterior labrum. The third most common variation consists of an entirely posterior attachment. Finally, the least common labral attachment is mostly anterior but with a small contribution to the posterior labrum.

18. **How do you differentiate normal labral variants from pathology?**
Use of contrast can aid in diagnosing a labral tear. Features of labral tear include lateral orientation of increased signal on oblique coronal images, irregular margins, increased depth of separation from the glenoid articular surface greater than 2 mm, extension posterior to the biceps tendon, and abnormal morphology or signal of the labrum. It is important to recognize the presence of a paralabral cyst as an initial indication of a labral tear. For SLAP (superior labrum anterior to posterior) tear, anteroposterior extension of high signal on axial images with concomitant anterosuperior labral tear is helpful in diagnosis.

19. **What are the different types of SLAP lesions?**
The description of SLAP lesions is based on the attachment of the biceps tendon.
- SLAP type I lesions are characterized by fraying without frank tearing of the superior portion of the glenoid labrum. The biceps tendon is intact
- SLAP type II lesions are characterized by fraying and stripping of the superior labrum and detachment of the biceps tendon from the glenoid labrum
- SLAP type III lesions are bucket-handle tears of the superior labrum with the central portion of the tear displaced into the joint. No involvement of the biceps tendon
- SLAP type IV lesions are bucket-handle tears of the superior labrum with extension into the biceps tendon
- SLAP type V lesions are anterior-inferior (Bankart) lesions with superior extension into the superior labrum and biceps tendon
- SLAP type VI lesions are flap tears, either anterior or posterior with separation of the biceps superiorly
- SLAP type VII lesions involve tearing of the superior labrum and biceps tendon separation that extends anteriorly to include the middle glenohumeral ligament
- SLAP type VIII lesions are superior labral tears with extensive posterior extension
- SLAP type IX lesions are superior tears with extensive anterior and posterior extension resulting in complete or near complete detachment of the labrum from the glenoid
- SLAP type X lesions are tears of the superior labrum with extension into the rotator cuff interval

20. **Define the borders of the quadrangular space, triangular space, and triangular interval. Which structures pass through them, respectively?**
The quadrangular space (also known as the quadrilateral space) is an anatomic interval formed by the shaft of the humerus laterally, the long head of the triceps medially, the teres minor muscle superiorly, and the teres major muscle inferiorly. The axillary nerve and the posterior humeral circumflex artery pass through this space from anterior to posterior.

The triangular space is an anatomic interval medial to the quadrangular space. Its borders are formed by the long head of the triceps laterally, the teres minor superiorly, and the teres major inferiorly. The circumflex scapular artery, a branch of the scapular artery, passes through the triangular space.

The triangular interval is inferior to the quadrangular space, bordered by the teres major superiorly, the long head of the triceps medially, and the lateral head of the triceps laterally. The radial nerve and profunda brachii artery pass through the triangular interval.

21. **Describe the three most common normal variations in anterior labral anatomy.**
The three most common variations are the following: (1) the presence of a sublabral foramen, defined as the sulcus between a well-developed anterosuperior portion of the labrum and glenoid articular cartilage; (2) the presence of a sublabral foramen and a cordlike middle glenohumeral ligament; (3) the complete absence of labral tissue at the anterosuperior aspect of the labrum in association with a cordlike middle glenohumeral ligament attached to the superior part of the labrum at the base of the biceps (Buford complex).

22. **What is a Bankart lesion?**
A Bankart lesion represents a lesion of the glenoid labrum corresponding to the detachment of the anchoring point of the anterior band of the inferior glenohumeral ligament and middle glenohumeral ligament from the glenoid rim. It is the result of a traumatic anterior dislocation of the glenohumeral joint. The injury can be of soft tissue, diagnosed as a labral tear at the anterior glenoid. There can also be fractures of the anterior lip of the glenoid, termed "bony Bankart" lesions.

23. **What is a HAGL lesion?**
A HAGL lesion represents an avulsion of the humeral attachment of the inferior glenohumeral ligament as a result of glenohumeral dislocation. This lesion can predispose patients to recurrence of anterior glenohumeral instability. The HAGL lesion is analogous to an avulsion of the glenoid attachment of the inferior glenohumeral ligament that often accompanies a labral tear or Bankart lesion.

24. **What is a Hill-Sachs lesion and how does it relate to recurrent anterior shoulder instability?**
A Hill-Sachs lesion represents an impression fracture of the posterolateral margin of the humeral head caused by impaction on the anteroinferior rim of the glenoid during an anterior shoulder dislocation. Hill-Sachs lesions are felt to become clinically important if they engage around the anterior rim of the glenoid at a position of function. Large Hill-Sachs lesions involving more than 30% of the humeral articular surface often contribute to recurrent shoulder instability. Smaller Hill-Sachs lesions can also contribute to recurrence when combined with anterior glenoid bone loss or Bankart lesions.

25. **What is the most common nerve injured after anterior shoulder dislocation?**
The most common nerve injury is most often a transient neuropraxia of the axillary nerve. The sensory function of the axillary nerve can be evaluated over the deltoid tuberosity. The motor examination of the axillary nerve can be challenging because of pain and limited range of motion in the dislocated shoulder.

26. **What is the biomechanical function of the clavicle?**
The clavicle attaches medially to the manubrium through the sternoclavicular articulation and laterally to the scapula through the acromioclavicular articulation and the coracoclavicular ligaments. The clavicle functions as a strut for the shoulder girdle, providing the only bony connection between the upper extremity and the axial skeleton. By maintaining the upper extremity away from the midline, the clavicle improves the biomechanical efficiency of the axiohumeral muscles. As a result, the muscles do not expend their energy pulling the shoulder medially but rather create motion at the glenohumeral joint.

27. **What are the normal motions of the clavicle?**
During full abduction of the arm, the clavicle rotates 50 degrees axially. This clavicular rotation permits the glenoid fossa to continue to elevate with increasing arm elevation. If the clavicle is prevented from rotating, arm abduction is limited to 120 degrees. With arm motion, the clavicle has also been noted to retract and elevate at the acromioclavicular joint with arm abduction in the scapular or coronal plane. Compared with the clavicle position at rest, its lateral elevation is estimated between 15 degrees and 20 degrees and posterior retraction approximately 30 degrees with arm motion. Clavicle depression and protraction are seen to lesser degrees with shoulder extension and adduction.

28. **Describe the origin, insertion, innervation, and function of the subclavius muscle.**
The subclavius muscle has a tendinous origin from the first rib and inserts on the inferior surface of the middle third of the clavicle. It receives innervation from the nerve to the subclavius, a branch of the superior trunk of the brachial plexus with contributions from C5 and C6. The function of the subclavius muscle is to stabilize the sternoclavicular joint during strenuous activity.

29. **Name the primary arterial supply to the humeral head.**
The arcuate artery, the terminal branch of the ascending branch of the anterior humeral circumflex artery, supplies most of the blood to the humeral head. This branch ascends the bicipital groove with the long head of the biceps tendon, entering the bone near the articular margin. The remainder of the blood supply to the head comes from branches of the posterior humeral circumflex artery and from branches within the rotator cuff tendon insertions.

The primary blood supply to the head has been debated after one study showed the posterior circumflex humeral artery to provide 64% of humeral head blood supply.

30. **What is the average proximal humerus articular version relative to the transepicondylar axis of the distal humerus?**
The proximal humeral articular surface is retroverted toward the face of the glenoid. The average proximal humerus retroversion is 30 degrees relative to the transepicondylar axis of the elbow.

31. **Describe the course of the suprascapular nerve.**
The suprascapular nerve arises from the upper trunk of the brachial plexus. It courses posteriorly to the suprascapular notch of the scapula, accompanied by the suprascapular artery. The nerve passes through the notch deep to the transverse scapular ligament, whereas the artery passes over the ligament. The suprascapular nerve then travels deep to the supraspinatus, which it innervates. Next, it passes through the spinoglenoid notch at the base of the spine of the scapula before it continues deep to the infraspinatus, which it also innervates. Articular sensory branches are given off to the acromioclavicular and glenohumeral joints along the course of the nerve. Compression of the suprascapular nerve can occur at the suprascapular or spinoglenoid notches, producing posterior shoulder pain and weakness.

32. **Which neurovascular structure is at greatest risk during anterior shoulder surgery? Describe the course and branches of this structure.**
The structure at greatest risk during this surgery is the axillary nerve, which traverses posteriorly from the posterior cord of the brachial plexus to innervate the deltoid and teres minor muscles, as well as the skin over the lateral aspect of the upper arm. With the posterior humeral circumflex artery, it passes below the inferior border of the subscapularis and travels along the inferior glenohumeral joint capsule, with which it is intimately associated. Although passing through the quadrangular space, the axillary nerve will divide into four branches—motor branches to the anterior and posterior portions of the deltoid muscle, a sensory branch (superior lateral brachial cutaneous nerve), and a motor branch to the teres minor muscle. Careless surgical dissection of the subscapularis or anterior/inferior capsule, as well as aggressive retraction, can result in injury to the axillary nerve or one of its branches.

33. **Which nerve lies superficial in the posterior cervical triangle and is susceptible to injury?**
Cranial nerve XI (spinal accessory nerve) travels through the posterior cervical triangle just below the cervical fascia. The posterior cervical triangle is bordered by the sternocleidomastoid anteriorly, the trapezius posteriorly, and the clavicle inferiorly. The spinal accessory nerve may be injured iatrogenically, most commonly during cervical lymph node biopsy, or by direct trauma. Injury to the spinal accessory nerve, which innervates the trapezius, leads to drooping of the shoulder, an asymmetric neckline, pain, and weakness in elevation of the arm.

34. **Which nerve injury leads to primary medial scapular winging?**
The direction of scapular winging is defined by the direction of the inferior angle of the scapula. Injury to the long thoracic nerve leads to paralysis of the serratus anterior muscle, which normally stabilizes the scapula laterally. Medial winging of the scapula results because the medial scapular stabilizers remain unopposed and the lateral border of the scapula is no longer closely held against the thoracic cage.

35. **Which nerve injuries lead to lateral scapular winging?**
Palsy of the spinal accessory nerve (cranial nerve XI) leads to weakness of the trapezius muscle, a medial scapular stabilizer. Injury to the dorsal scapular nerve leads to weakness of the rhomboid major and minor muscles, which also attach to the medial scapula. Weakness of medial muscles from injury to either of these nerves leads to lateral scapular winging. Weakness of the trapezius leads to more pronounced lateral winging than that seen with loss of the rhomboids.

36. **Describe the alterations of shoulder kinematics in symptomatic and asymptomatic shoulder patients.**
Global range of motion of the arm is the result of coordinated motion of the shoulder complex including the glenohumeral, scapulothoracic, sternoclavicular, and acromioclavicular joints. Normal shoulder kinematics relies on coordinated motion between the scapula and thorax through the clavicle via its sternoclavicular and acromioclavicular joints. Any disruption of this kinetic chain can lead to abnormal glenohumeral or scapulothoracic motion.

- In the setting of shoulder impingement, causes are related to intrinsic and extrinsic factors. Intrinsic etiology relates to underlying degenerative rotator cuff disease due to age-related degeneration within the tendons or repeated microtrauma. Extrinsic causes are related to mechanical compression of the tendon by external structures related to acromial shape or altered biomechanics of the shoulder complex during movements. In shoulder impingement, the scapula may demonstrate a decrease in lateral rotation and posterior tilt. There may be no or only a small amount of superior humeral translation contributing to the pathology.

- Stiff, painful shoulders also have altered kinematics compared to asymptomatic controls. Studies assessing patients with adhesive capsulitis demonstrate significant increase in scapular lateral rotation during arm elevation. Additionally, there is less scapular internal rotation in the setting of adhesive capsulitis or glenohumeral osteoarthritis. The lateral rotation increase is believed to be a compensatory mechanism to the limited glenohumeral range of motion. Capsular stiffness secondary to intraarticular problems is likely the origin of the scapular monobloc mobility during upper limb elevation. Furthermore, studies demonstrate a significant decrease in posterior tilt in patients with shoulder pain and restricted shoulder mobility.
- In patients with multidirectional instability, the shoulder experiences repetitive microtrauma superimposed on a congenitally lax joint capsule. Several studies demonstrate decrease in scapular lateral rotation and an increase in scapular internal rotation. Von Eisenhart-Rothe et al. assessed the simultaneous position of the humeral head in the glenoid and the glenoid in space in patients with multidirectional instability using 3D open MRI. Results showed humeral head antero-inferior decentering, decreased scapular lateral rotation, and increased scapular internal rotation during active or passive lateral arm elevation.

37. Describe the course of the musculocutaneous nerve.

The musculocutaneous nerve is a terminal branch of the lateral cord of the brachial plexus with contributions from C5, C6, and C7. It penetrates the muscle belly of the coracobrachialis, providing innervation through small motor branches. It then travels into the brachium between the brachialis and biceps brachii muscles, innervating both. Its terminal sensory branch emerges between the brachialis and brachioradialis muscles and travels into the forearm as the lateral antebrachial cutaneous nerve. This nerve provides sensation to the lateral aspect of the forearm.

38. Describe the basic structure of the brachial plexus.

The brachial plexus, which provides sensory and motor innervation to the upper extremity and shoulder girdle, receives contributions from spinal nerves C5–C8 and T1. Inconstant innervation is received from C3 and C4. The five roots from the ventral rami of C5–T1 coalesce to form three trunks (superior, middle, and inferior). The three trunks divide to produce three anterior and three posterior divisions. The divisions combine into the three cords of the brachial plexus (lateral, posterior, and medial). Finally, the cords end in the terminal branches, which are the musculocutaneous, axillary, radial, median, and ulnar nerves. A helpful mnemonic to remember the order of the components of the brachial plexus (roots, trunks, divisions, cords, branches) is Rod Taylor Drinks Cold Beer.

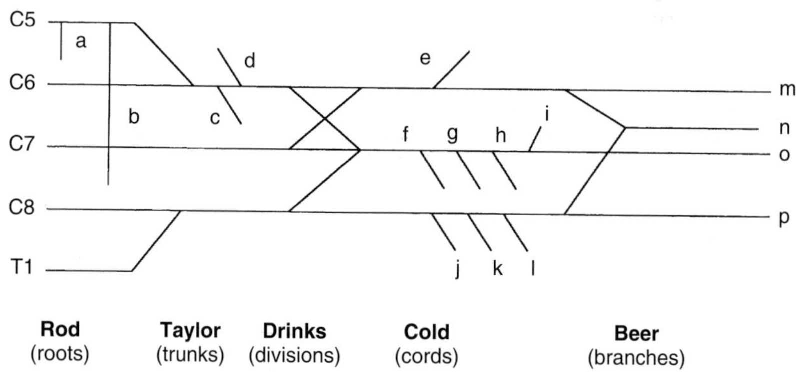

The brachial plexus. a, Dorsal scapular; b, long thoracic; c, suprascapular; d, nerve to subclavius; e, lateral pectoral; f, upper subscapular; g, thoracodorsal; h, lower subscapular; i, axillary; j, medial pectoral; k, medial brachial cutaneous; l, medial antebrachial cutaneous; m, musculocutaneous; n, median; o, radial; and p, ulnar.

39. Is there a relationship between glenoid inclination and rotator cuff tears/instability?

Yes. Preliminary studies have demonstrated that increasing superior inclination of the glenoid significantly reduces the amount of force required for superior humeral head migration. This suggests that more upward-facing glenoids may increase the risk for superior humeral translation, which has been shown to contribute to the development of rotator cuff disease. Increased glenoid retroversion has been shown to increase the risk for posterior instability.

40. Where is the center of rotation of the normal glenohumeral joint? Where is the center of rotation in the severely cuff-deficient glenohumeral joint?

The center of rotation in the normal glenohumeral joint is at the center of the humeral head at the mid-glenoid level. In a severely rotator cuff–deficient glenohumeral joint, the head of the humerus migrates superiorly and medially secondary to the unopposed pull of the deltoid and the loss of the humeral head–depressing function of the rotator cuff. As a result, the center of rotation migrates superiorly. When the humeral head is no longer centered in the glenoid cavity because of abnormal force couples and loss of the glenohumeral fulcrum, the deltoid is at a mechanical disadvantage and limited abduction results.

41. What are the glenoid erosion patterns typically seen in osteoarthritis and rotator cuff arthropathy?

The most common erosion pattern seen with primary osteoarthritis is posterior glenoid wear with a variable degree of posterior humeral head subluxation. Posterior glenoid wear in osteoarthritis is often accentuated by internal rotation contractures that develop with worsening disease. Posterior wear increases glenoid retroversion and, if severe, can lead to formation of a biconcave glenoid. Severe retroversion is usually secondary to glenoid dysplasia, which is often a deficient formation of the posterior and inferior glenoid. Central glenoid erosion can also occur with osteoarthritis but is more often seen with inflammatory arthritis.

Rotator cuff arthropathy is defined by worsening proximal humeral migration, which leads to superior glenoid erosion. The humeral head is no longer depressed by a functional rotator cuff, and the head eventually articulates superiorly with the acromion. Superior wear of the glenoid leads to increasing glenoid inclination/tilt.

42. What are the most frequently occurring anatomic variations of the coracoacromial (CA) ligament?

Variations include quadrangular (48%), Y shape (42%), broader lateral and thinner medial band, broad-banded (8%), and multiple bands (2%).

43. Are the acromial attachments of the coracoacromial ligament and anterior deltoid preserved during arthroscopic acromioplasty?

In most cases, the acromial attachment of the CA ligament is released during an arthroscopic acromioplasty, as it can be an impinging structure and often has calcification or enthesopathy within it, contributing to anterior acromial spur formation. Some surgeons attempt to preserve the anterior attachment of the ligament, as it has a role in static restraint of the glenohumeral joint. The overlying deltoid originating at the anterior part of the acromion is always left attached during acromioplasty by a bridge of tissue composed of periosteum and deltoid tendon.

44. Describe the anatomy of the pectoralis major tendon including the insertion and anatomy of the medial and lateral pectoral nerves as they relate to the insertion of the tendon.

The width of the insertion of the pectoralis major is approximately 6 cm. The insertion is broad on the undersurface of the tendon and small on the anterior surface. The sternal head spirals into its insertion to form the posterior lamina, and the clavicular head remains anterior as it inserts into the humerus to form the anterior lamina.

The medial pectoral nerve enters the pectoralis major approximately 12 cm from its lateral humeral insertion and 2 cm from its inferior edge. The lateral pectoral nerve inserts approximately 12.5 cm from its humeral insertion. The medial pectoral nerve's insertion into the pectoralis major is inferior to the lateral pectoral nerve's insertion. The lateral pectoral nerve passes medial to the pectoralis minor before entering the pectoralis major, whereas the medial pectoral nerve passes through or lateral to the pectoralis minor before entering the pectoralis major.

45. Describe the anatomy of the deltoid insertion.

The anterior, middle, and posterior deltoid muscle fibers enter into the deltoid insertion in a V-shaped tendinous confluence. This consists of a broad posterior band and a narrow separate anterior band. The anterior band accounts for approximately one fifth of the insertion. The insertion can be extremely close to the pectoralis major insertion and in some cases nearly opposed to each other. The average distance from the axillary nerve is approximately 5.6 cm anteriorly and 4.5 cm posteriorly.

46. What are the main stabilizers of the AC joint, and in which direction do they resist displacement?

The acromioclavicular ligament and joint capsule acts as a primary constraint for posterior displacement of the clavicle and posterior axial rotation. The conoid ligament plays a primary role in constraining anterior and superior rotation, as well as anterior and superior displacement of the clavicle. The trapezoid ligament contributes to constraint for both horizontal and vertical displacement primarily when the clavicle moves in axial compression toward the acromion.

47. **What direction is the most common with traumatic sternoclavicular dislocation? What direction is the most dangerous?**
Traumatic sternoclavicular joint dislocations are usually the result of high energy and can be either anterior or posterior. Anterior dislocations are far more common and much less dangerous. Posterior dislocations can potentially injure the mediastinal vessels and trachea, which can be life-threatening. These injuries require more urgent reduction and may require assistance from a cardiothoracic surgeon. It is also important to determine whether a medial clavicle physeal separation has occurred, rather than a joint dislocation. The medial physis (growth plate) of the clavicle is the last to fuse in the body, usually around 25 years of age.

Bibliography

American Academy of Orthopaedic Surgeons. (2002). *OKU shoulder and elbow 2.* Rosemont, CA: AAOS.
Ball, C. M., Steger, T., Galatz, L. M., & Yamaguchi, K. (2003). The posterior branch of the axillary nerve: An anatomic study. *Journal of Bone and Joint Surgery, 85*(8), 1497–1501.
Bankart, A. S. B. (1923). Recurrent or habitual dislocation of the shoulder joint. *BMJ, 2*, 1132–1133.
Chang, D., Mohana-Borges, A., Borso, M., & Chung, C. B. (2008). SLAP lesions: Anatomy, clinical presentation, MR imaging diagnosis and characterization. *European Journal of Radiology, 68*(1), 72–87.
Checroun, A. J., Hawkins, C., Kummer, F. J., & Zuckerman, J. D. (2002). Fit of current glenoid component designs: An anatomic cadaver study. *Journal of Shoulder and Elbow Surgery, 11*, 614–617.
Churchill, R. S., Brems, J. J., & Kotschi, H. (2001). Glenoid size, inclination, and version: An anatomic study. *Journal of Shoulder and Elbow Surgery, 10*, 327–332.
Clark, J. M., & Harryman, D. T., II. (1992). Tendons, ligaments and capsule of the rotator cuff. *Journal of Bone and Joint Surgery, 74*(5), 713–725.
Cole, B. J., & Warner, J. P. (1999). Anatomy, biomechanics, and pathophysiology of glenohumeral instability. In J. P. Iannotti & G. R. Williams (Eds.), *Disorders of the shoulder: Diagnosis and management* (pp. 207–232). Baltimore, MD: Lippincott Williams & Wilkins.
Flatow, E. L. (1998). Shoulder anatomy and biomechanics. In M. Post (Ed.), et al., *The shoulder: Operative technique* (pp. 1–42). Baltimore, MD: Williams & Wilkins.
Frank, R., Cvetanovich, G., Savin, D., & Romeo, A. (2018). Superior capsular reconstruction. *JBJS Reviews, 6*(7), e10.
Gerber, C., Schneeberger, A. G., & Vinh, T. S. (1990). The arterial vascularization of the humeral head: An anatomical study. *Journal of Bone and Joint Surgery (American), 72*(10), 1486–1494.
Harryman, D. T., II, Sidles, J. A., Clark, J. M., McQuade, K. J., Gibb, T. D., & Matsen, F. A., III (1990). Translation of the humeral head on the glenoid with passive glenohumeral motion. *Journal of Bone and Joint Surgery, 72*(9), 1334–1343.
Hettrich, C. M., Boraiah, S., Dyke, J. P., Neviaser, A., Helfet, D. L., & Lorich, D. G. (2010). Quantitative assessment of the vascularity of the proximal part of the humerus. *Journal of Bone and Joint Surgery (American), 92*(4), 943–948.
Hunt, J. L., Moore, R. J., & Krishnan, J. (2000). The fate of the coracoacromial ligament in arthroscopic acromioplasty: An anatomical study. *Journal of Shoulder and Elbow Surgery, 9*, 491–494.
Jost, B., Kocj, P. P., & Gerber, C. (2000). Anatomy and functional aspects of the rotator interval. *Journal of Shoulder and Elbow Surgery, 9*, 336–341.
Klepps, S. J., Goldfarb, C., Flatow, E., Galatz, L. M., & Yamaguchi, K. (2001). Anatomic evaluation of the subcoracoid pectoralis major transfer in human cadavers. *Journal of Shoulder and Elbow Surgery, 10*, 453–459.
Laing, P. G. (1956). The arterial supply of the adult humerus. *Journal of Bone and Joint Surgery, 38-A*(5), 1105–1116.
Lee, T. Q., Black, A. D., Tibone, J. E., & McMahon, P. J. (2001). Release of the coracoacromial ligament can lead to glenohumeral laxity: A biomechanical study. *Journal of Shoulder and Elbow Surgery, 10*(1), 68–72.
Lefèvre-Colau, M. -M., Nguyen, C., Palazoo, C., et al. (2018). Kinematic patterns in normal and degenerative shoulders. Part II: Review of 3-D scapular kinematic patterns in patients with shoulder pain, and clinical implications. *Annals of Physical and Rehabilitation Medicine, 61*(1), 46–53.
Ludewig, P. M., Behrens, S. A., Meyer, S. M., Spoden, S. M., & Wilson, L. A. (2004). Three-dimensional clavicular motion during arm elevation: Reliability and descriptive data. *The Journal of Orthopaedic and Sports Physical Therapy, 34*(3), 140–149.
Mallon, W. J., Brown, H. R., Vogler, J. B., & Martinez, S. (1992). Radiographic and geometric anatomy of the scapula. *Clinical Orthopaedics and Related Research, 277*, 142–154.
Neer, C. S., II. (1972). Anterior acromioplasty for the chronic impingement syndrome in the shoulder. *Journal of Bone and Joint Surgery, 54*(1), 41–50.
Pfahler, M., Branner, S., & Refior, H. J. (1999). The role of the bicipital groove in tendopathy of the long biceps tendon. *Journal of Shoulder and Elbow Surgery, 8*, 419–424.
Pieper, H., Radas, C. B., Krahl, H., & Blank, M. (1997). Anatomic variation of the coracoacromial ligament: A macroscopic and microscopic cadaveric study. *Journal of Shoulder and Elbow Surgery, 6*, 291–296.
Price, M. R., Tillett, E. D., & Acland, R. D. (2004). Determining the relationship of the axillary nerve to the shoulder joint capsule from an arthroscopic perspective. *Journal of Bone and Joint Surgery, 86*(10), 2135–2142.
Provencher, M. T., Midtgaard, K. S., Owens, B. D., & Tokish, J. M. (2021). Diagnosis and management of traumatic anterior shoulder instability. *Journal of the American Academy of Orthopaedic Surgeons, 29*(2), e51–e61.
Roh, M. S., Wang, V. M., April, E. W., Pollock, R. G., Bigliani, L. U., & Flatow, E. L. (2000). Anterior and posterior musculotendinous anatomy of the supraspinatus. *Journal of Shoulder and Elbow Surgery, 9*, 436–440.
Rybalko, D., Bobko, A., Amirouche, F., et al. (2020). Biomechanical effects of superior capsular reconstruction in a rotator cuff–deficient shoulder: a cadaveric study. *Journal of Shoulder and Elbow Surgery, 29*(10), 1959–1966.
Sarrafian, S. K. (1983). Gross and functional anatomy of the shoulder. *Clinical Orthopaedics, 173*, 11–19.
Turkel, S. J., Panio, M. W., Marshall, J. L., & Girgis, F. G. (1981). Stabilizing mechanisms preventing anterior dislocation of the glenohumeral joint. *Journal of Bone and Joint Surgery, 63*(8), 1208–1217.

Vangsness, C. T., Jr., Jorgenson, S. S., Watson, T., & Johnson, D. L. (1994). The origin of the long head of the biceps from the scapula and glenoid labrum. *Journal of Bone and Joint Surgery (British)*, *76*(6), 951–954.
Von Schroeder, H., Kuiper, S. D., & Botte, M. J. (2001). Osseous anatomy of the scapula. *Clinical Orthopaedics and Related Research*, *383*, 131–139.
von Eisenhart-Rothe, R., Matsen, F.A., Eckstein, F., Vogi, T., & Graichen, H. (2005). Pathomechanics in atraumatic shoulder instability: Scapular positioning correlates with humeral head centering. Clinical Orthopaedics and Related Research, 433, 82–89. In this issue.
Williams, M. D., Edwards, T. B., & Walch, G. (2018). Understanding the importance of the teres minor for shoulder function: Functional anatomy and pathology. *Journal of the American Academy of Orthopaedic Surgeons*, *26*(5), 150–161.
Wong, A. S., Gallo, L., Kuhn, J. E., Carpenter, J. E., & Hughes, R. E. (2003). The effect of glenoid inclination on superior humeral head migration. *Journal of Shoulder and Elbow Surgery*, *12*, 360–364.

CHAPTER 36 QUESTIONS

1. **The muscle with the largest medial to lateral tendinous insertion within the rotator cuff is?**
   a. Supraspinatus
   b. Infraspinatus
   c. Teres minor
   d. Subscapularis

2. **Which disease process is associated with increase in scapular lateral rotation and decrease in internal rotation?**
   a. Full thickness rotator cuff tear
   b. Adhesive capsulitis
   c. Impingement syndrome
   d. Multidirectional instability

3. **Lesion of which nerve leads to lateral winging of the scapula?**
   a. Long thoracic
   b. Dorsal scapular
   c. Spinal accessory
   d. Thoracodorsal

4. **In osteoarthritis of the shoulder, glenoid erosions are primarily**
   a. Anterior
   b. Posterior
   c. Central
   d. Superior

5. **The nerve derived from C5, C6, and C7 nerve roots is the**
   a. Axillary
   b. Thoracodorsal
   c. Lateral pectoral
   d. Long thoracic

6. **Which structure passes through the quadrangular space?**
   a. Circumflex scapular artery
   b. Radial nerve
   c. Posterior humeral circumflex artery
   d. Profunda brachii artery

SHOULDER IMPINGEMENT AND ROTATOR CUFF TEARS

D.A. Boyce, PT, EdD, OCS, ECS, J. Girard, DPT, DSc, OCS, FAAOMPT, and T.A. Brosky, Jr., PT, DHSc, SCS

CHAPTER 37

1. **What are the prevalence and natural history of rotator cuff disease?**
   Prevalence data deemed from cadaver investigations range from 7% to 40%. Recent MRI and ultrasound investigations of asymptomatic subjects demonstrated the prevalence of rotator cuff tears to range from 13% to 34%. The prevalence ranges from 51% to 54% in 60- to 80-year-old subjects. Patients with rotator cuff tear who are asymptomatic have a 51% chance of becoming symptomatic in the future.

2. **What are the three morphologic types of the acromion?**
   Bigliani classified the acromion according to its shape. Type I acromion is flat (17% incidence); type II (43% incidence) curves downward into the rotator cuff outlet; and type III (40% incidence) is hooked downward into the rotator cuff outlet. Of patients with rotator cuff tears, 70% have type III acromion, 27% have type II, and 3% have type I. Types II and III decrease the area of the rotator cuff outlet and can traumatize the superior surface of the rotator cuff tendons.

3. **Describe the coracoacromial arch and its clinical importance.**
   The coracoacromial arch consists of the coracoacromial ligament, which spans the distance between the coracoid and acromion of the scapula. The ligament provides a protective covering over the subacromial bursa and rotator cuff tendons and restricts excessive superior humeral head migration. Clinically, the coracoacromial ligament has been associated with rotator cuff pathology (especially in overhead athletes). During humeral elevation and internal rotation, the greater tuberosity and the attached rotator cuff tendons can be compressed against the arch. Repetitive compression may traumatize the rotator cuff tendons and lead to pathology. It has also been proposed that traction spurs can form within the coracoacromial ligament from the superior humeral head migration against the coracoacromial arch, producing type II and III acromion. Acromial traction spurs are similar to those that form at the attachment of the plantar fascia.

4. **Describe Neer's classification of rotator cuff pathology.**
   - Stage I—edema and hemorrhage. Patients usually are less than 25 years old and have pain with activity that often resolves with rest. The condition is reversible, and treatment is conservative (relative rest and medication).
   - Stage II—fibrosis and tendinitis. Patients typically are between 25 and 40 years old and experience recurrent pain with activity that does not always abate with rest. According to Neer, subacromial decompression should be considered if conservative treatment fails.
   - Stage III—bone spur and tendon rupture. Patients typically are older than 40 years and have a history of progressive disability that has led to a tear of the rotator cuff. Rotator cuff repair is advised.
   - Stage IV—cuff tear arthropathy. Patients typically are older than 60 years and have a history of progressive disability with a torn rotator cuff. Clinical management consists of rotator cuff repair, hemi-arthroplasty, or total shoulder replacement.

5. **What is a partial-thickness rotator cuff tear (tensile failure of the rotator cuff)?**
   The rotator cuff degenerates naturally with increasing age, especially after the third decade of life. Degeneration or tensile failure of the rotator cuff begins deep within the tissue near the undersurface attachment of the tuberosity. With time it may extend outward until it becomes a full-thickness tear. Partial-thickness tears of the rotator cuff also may occur on the bursal side of the cuff, most commonly near the insertion.

6. **Do partial-thickness tears heal or progress to full-thickness tears?**
   Partial-thickness tears attempt to heal, but in most instances they progress to full-thickness tears. Matsen describes why partial-thickness rotator cuff tears eventually progress to full-thickness tears:
   - Ruptured fibers can no longer sustain a load; thus increased loads are placed on neighboring fibers, making them more susceptible to rupture.
   - Disruption of the tendon fibers also disrupts local blood supply within the tendon, thus inducing ischemia.

- Disrupted tendon fibers are exposed to joint fluid, which has a lytic effect on tendons that impairs the healing process.
- When a tendon heals, the scar tissue that replaces the ruptured tendon fibers does not have the same tensile strength as the original tissue; thus it is at increased risk of failure.
- Once the tear becomes full thickness, loads that normally are distributed through the entire intact tendon often are transmitted at the torn margins of the rotator cuff tendon; this process produces a "zipper effect" and extends or unzips the tendon from the tuberosity.

7. **What is an undersurface rotator cuff tear?**
Undersurface rotator cuff tears are caused by rupture of the deep tissues of the rotator cuff that attach to the tuberosity. Undersurface tears, in fact, are partial-thickness tears of the rotator cuff on the articular surface. They can result from the natural degenerative process that affects the shoulder, but often are noted in younger overhead athletes. Undersurface tearing in overhead athletes is thought to result from repetitive eccentric tensile loading (ie, deceleration of the throwing arm).

8. **What is rotator cuff arthropathy?**
With massive tearing of the rotator cuff, cuff tendons slide off the humeral head. These tendons, which once served as humeral head depressors, now act as humeral head elevators and promote superior translation of the humeral head. The result is excessive wear and degeneration on both the humeral head and the undersurface of the acromion. If allowed to progress, the degeneration of the glenohumeral joint can become so significant and painful that a hemi-arthroplasty or total shoulder replacement is indicated. In severe cases of rotator cuff arthropathy, radiographs can aid in the diagnosis before surgery. Radiographs reveal sclerosis of the undersurface of the acromion ("eyebrow sign") secondary to prolonged bone-on-bone contact (humeral head in contact with undersurface of acromion) and cystic changes of the greater tuberosity.

9. **When are acromioplasty and subacromial decompression required? What are the two types?**
The typical patient requiring acromioplasty and decompression is between 25 and 40 years of age, experiences recurrent pain with activity that does not always abate with rest, and has failed conservative treatment (physical therapy, medications). The two types of acromioplasty and decompression are open and arthroscopic. Some surgeons believe that a more complete decompression is accomplished with the open technique. In addition, if a large rotator cuff tear is encountered during the open procedure, it can be repaired with relative ease, whereas arthroscopic repair of a large rotator cuff tear is difficult and technically demanding.

10. **Should the coracoacromial ligament be released during subacromial decompression?**
The coracoacromial ligament is a static stabilizer that limits superior humeral head translation. Release of the ligament contributes to increased superior humeral head migration and degenerative processes in shoulders with a massive rotator cuff tear. Thus some surgeons believe in retaining the coracoacromial ligament and preserving the arch to limit more severe superior humeral head migration, which may lead or contribute to rotator cuff arthropathy.

11. **What is the Mumford procedure?**
The Mumford procedure is an excision of the distal 2 cm of the clavicle. Mumford originally intended the surgery to provide pain relief for patients suffering from acromioclavicular dislocation. Distal clavicle excision often is performed during acromioplasty and subacromial decompression to allow even greater rotator cuff decompression. The acromioclavicular joint no longer exists, however; distal stability of the scapula is maintained through the intact costoclavicular ligaments (conoid and trapezoid).

12. **What are the primary rotator cuff exercises?**
The primary or "core" rotator cuff exercises involve the SITS muscles:
    - Supraspinatus—Full can exercise—Described as abduction in the plane of the scapula with the thumb pointing upward. Another form of this exercise is prone full can exercise scaption, in which the patient lies prone and performs scaption from 90 degrees of elevation to approximately 120 to 150 degrees.
    - Infraspinatus—External rotation can be performed in many different positions, such as standing or side-lying. It is advocated to place a small towel roll under the arm to maximize form, inhibit the posterior fibers of the deltoid, and isolate the rotator cuff muscles that externally rotate the glenohumeral joint. Higher-level exercises consist of prone external rotation at 90 degrees of abduction.
    - Teres minor—Prone extension with external rotation is preferred. The teres minor is also an external rotator but seems to have greater electromyographic activity when external rotation is combined with glenohumeral extension. The patient lies prone with the arm hanging off the table and then extends the shoulder level with the horizon while maintaining the shoulder in external rotation.

- Subscapularis—Internal rotation can be performed in standing with the arm adducted to the side. Higher-level exercises consist of internal rotation at 90 degrees of abduction and diagonal PNF patterns incorporating shoulder internal rotation.

Exercise of the SITS muscles alone does not include all muscles that contribute to optimal dynamic shoulder function. The therapist also should address the axioscapular (eg, serratus anterior) and the axiohumeral (eg, pectoralis major) muscle groups.

13. **What is the EMG activity of commonly used rotator cuff exercises?**
Supraspinatus—The full can, empty can, and prone full can exercises demonstrated a range of 62% to 67% of maximum voluntary contraction (MVC). However, the full can demonstrated the least amount of deltoid activity, thus placing more emphasis on the supraspinatus muscle. Prone scaption is considered an advanced exercise position and can induce shoulder pain more readily. Judgment must be exercised when prescribing this exercise.
Infraspinatus and Teres Minor—Side-lying external rotation results in the greatest EMG activity of the infraspinatus and teres minor (62%–67% MVC.)
Subscapularis—There is conflicting evidence regarding which exercise, internal rotation performed in standing with the arm adducted to the side or internal rotation at 90 degrees of abduction, produces the greatest EMG activity. However, internal rotation performed at 90 degrees of abduction may reduce large muscle activity of the pectoralis major and latissimus dorsi and isolate the subscapularis to a greater extent.

14. **What is primary rotator cuff impingement?**
Primary impingement is a mechanical impingement of the rotator cuff beneath the coracoacromial arch and typically results from subacromial overcrowding. Factors related to primary impingement involve abnormal structural characteristics (eg, congenital anomalies of the osseous structures of the acromioclavicular [AC] joint, coracoid process, or greater tuberosity of the humerus) or tendon thickening attributable to calcific deposits, trauma, or surgery.

15. **What is secondary rotator cuff impingement?**
Secondary rotator cuff impingement is a relative decrease in the subacromial space caused by microinstability of the glenohumeral joint or scapulothoracic instability. Attempts by the active restraints of the glenohumeral joint to compensate for the loss of the passive restraint function of the joint capsule and ligaments result in eventual fatigue and abnormal translation of the humeral head, leading to mechanical impingement of the rotator cuff by the coracoacromial arch.

16. **What is posterior (internal) impingement?**
Posterior impingement often is seen in overhead athletes, such as throwers, swimmers, and tennis players. It occurs when the arm is in an elevated and externally rotated position (similar to the cocking phase in throwing). The infraspinatus and supraspinatus muscles are pinched between the posterior superior aspect of the glenoid when the upper limb is in the cocked position. The lesion occurs on the undersurface rather than the bursal side of the rotator cuff. In addition, this form of impingement is thought to be associated with anterior instability.

17. **What are the typical age, gender, and occupation of patients with rotator cuff tears?**
The frequency of rotator cuff tears increases significantly with age. Tears become increasingly more common after the age of 40 years. Occupations or activities that predispose the rotator cuff to pathology require excessive and repetitive overhead motions. Sports that involve throwing or repetitive overhead motions (eg, baseball pitching, tennis, swimming) also have a high prevalence of rotator cuff injuries. However, most cuff defects have a degenerative etiology. Neer reported that 40% of patients with cuff defects never performed strenuous physical work, and many heavy laborers never developed cuff defects. Fifty percent of patients with rotator cuff tears had no recollection of shoulder trauma. A high incidence (70%) of rotator cuff defects occurs in sedentary people doing light work; two-thirds of cases occur in males.

18. **Do shoulder dislocations lead to rotator cuff tears?**
Rotator cuff tears may occur with anterior and inferior glenohumeral dislocations. The frequency of rotator cuff tears accompanying glenohumeral dislocations increases with advancing age and has been reported to exceed 30% in patients over 40 and 80% in patients over 60 years of age.

19. **What classification system is used to describe the extent or size of a rotator cuff tear?**
According to the grading system adopted by the American Academy of Orthopedic Surgeons, a small tear is <1 cm, a medium tear is 1 to 3 cm, a large tear is 3 to 5 cm, and a massive tear is >5 cm.

20. **Do full-thickness rotator cuff tears heal?**
No. Although primary healing of a full-thickness tear is unlikely, the results of nonoperative management of patients with full-thickness rotator cuff defects have demonstrated various degrees of improvement (33%–90%)

in pain and overall function. Partial-thickness tears may progress to full-thickness tears if left untreated, with deterioration in function over time.

21. **How accurate is a clinical examination of the shoulder in predicting rotator cuff pathology?**
The sensitivity of a clinical examination of the shoulder (which includes the use of various shoulder-special tests) is approximately 91% with a specificity of 75%. Data that assist in the specific diagnosis of a rotator cuff tear are age of the patient (>40 years), previous trauma (minor), and degenerative changes on radiologic examination. Thus a good clinical examination is accurate and more cost-effective than a battery of radiologic studies in diagnosing rotator cuff pathology.

22. **Describe the sensitivity and specificity of the various tests used in rotator cuff pathology.**

TEST	SENSITIVITY (%)	SPECIFICITY (%)
Neer impingement	78	58
Hawkin's-Kennedy	74	57
Cross-over	82	22.5
Painful arc sign	73.5	81.1
Drop-arm	21	92
Jobe/empty can	69	62
Lift-off sign	42	97
Internal rotation lag	97	96
External rotation lag	70	100
Drop arm	21	92
Yergason's	32	78
Speed's	38.3	83.3

23. **What clinical tests are most predictive for impingement or rotator cuff tear?**
Rotator Cuff Impingement
- According to Park, if the Hawkins-Kennedy impingement sign, the painful arc sign, and the infraspinatus muscle test are positive, there is a 95% probability of impingement syndrome.

Rotator Cuff Tear
- According to Park, if the painful arc sign, drop-arm sign, and infraspinatus muscle test are positive, there is a 91% probability of a full-thickness rotator cuff tear.
- According to Murrell and Walton, three simple tests are highly predictive of rotator cuff tear: supraspinatus weakness, weakness in external rotation, and impingement sign. When all three of these clinical tests are positive, or if two tests are positive and the patient is aged 60 or older, the individual has a 98% chance of having a rotator cuff tear. Furthermore, the investigators reported that any patient with a positive drop-arm sign also has a 98% chance of rotator cuff tear.

24. **How accurate is ultrasonography in diagnosing a rotator cuff tear?**
When performed by experienced clinicians, ultrasonography can reveal noninvasively and nonradiographically not only rotator cuff integrity but also the thickness and location of the tear(s). The diagnostic sensitivity and specificity for partial-thickness tears are .84% and .89%, respectively; for full-thickness, tears are .96% and .93%, respectively. When considering safety, cost, and accuracy, ultrasonography is considered a better option than MRI or MRI arthrogram.

25. **How accurate is MRI in determining a rotator cuff tear?**
Magnetic resonance imaging (MRI) is a commonly used method of diagnosing rotator cuff tears. Recent meta-analysis indicates an MRI's sensitivity and specificity for partial thickness is .67 % and .94%, respectively, and for full thickness tears .90% and .93%, respectively.

26. **Should a patient with a confirmed rotator cuff tear undergo physical therapy or surgery?**
Several studies have compared the outcomes of patients with confirmed rotator cuff tear that underwent surgical repair of the rotator cuff versus conservative physical therapy. Early surgical intervention is recommended in patients with rotator cuff disease who have greater than 12 months' duration of symptoms, severe functional impairment, or a confirmed rotator cuff tear greater than 1 cm. All other patients should undergo a minimum of 18 months of conservative management, including NSAIDs, physical therapy, and subacromial injection. Of these patients, 76% can anticipate a good or excellent result in 6 to 12 months. Of patients with impingement syndrome without rotator cuff tear, 85% will experience a good or excellent result with conservative management of at least 18 months. Failure of conservative treatment or worsening of symptoms may warrant a surgical consult.

27. **What are some of the common physical therapy interventions for shoulder (rotator cuff) pain, and are they effective?**
According to a Cochrane Database Systematic Review, the following statements can be made regarding common physical therapy interventions for shoulder (rotator cuff) pain:
- Exercise (rotator cuff) is effective in the short-term recovery in rotator cuff disease.
- Exercise (rotator cuff) has long-term benefits with respect to function.
- Exercise and nonthrust mobilization (posterior/inferior glide of glenohumeral joint) are more effective than exercise alone.
- Laser is not any more effective than placebo for rotator cuff tendinitis.
- Ultrasound is of no additional benefit than exercise (rotator cuff) alone.
- Manual therapy and exercise together are more effective than placebo.
- Inconclusive if manual therapy and exercise are more effective in improving function when compared to patients taking oral nonsteroidal antiinflammatory medications.

28. **Describe a typical rehabilitation protocol for patients that have undergone rotator cuff repair.**
There is no established consensus regarding rehabilitation protocols following a rotator cuff repair. In general, physical therapists support shorter immobilization times, earlier strengthening, and more frequent home exercises, whereas orthopedic surgeons prefer more of a conservative approach and time-based phase transitions. Rehabilitation after rotator cuff repair depends on many factors: size of the tear, quality of the tissue, method/type of surgical repair, age of the patient, chronicity of the condition, and occupation and/or desired activities. The typical acromioplasty and open cuff repair is followed by a short period of immobilization with or without an abduction pillow—1 to 6 weeks, depending on the size of the tear and quality of repair. Early passive motion exercises (flexion, abduction, external rotation), including pendulum exercises and pulleys, begin within the first few postoperative days to prevent adhesions and loss of motion. Scapulothoracic, cervical, and elbow, wrist, and hand range of motion (ROM) exercises should be incorporated immediately. Submaximal isometrics for shoulder internal/external rotators, flexors, and abductors may begin at 3 to 4 weeks. Active assisted ROM exercises should be progressed, delaying active abduction for up to 6 to 8 weeks. Care should be taken to ensure that exercises are performed in the scapular plane whenever possible. Full ROM should be restored by 8 to 10 weeks. Rhythmic stabilization of the scapulothoracic and glenohumeral joints is incorporated later and progresses as tolerated to promote dynamic stabilization. Strengthening typically progresses from supine to side-lying, sitting, and standing. Isotonic exercises via small handheld weights or elastic tubing typically begin in 4 to 6 weeks. Further progression and rehabilitation should be based on the needs of the individual patient.

29. **What are the expected ROM, strength, pain, and function of a patient with rotator cuff repair at 1 and 5 years?**
Problems with analyzing outcomes after rotator cuff repair are as a result of variable accuracy in describing preoperative functional levels, extent and location of the tears, tissue quality, follow-up schedule, and postoperative functional status. Cofield's investigations describing the outcomes of rotator cuff repair reported improvements in pain (averaging 87%) and patient overall satisfaction rates of 77%. Hawkins et al. reported pain relief in 86% of patients; 78% were able to perform activities of daily living (ADLs) above the level of the shoulder after repair compared with only 16% before repair. Neer et al. reported excellent (77%) or satisfactory (14%) results in 91% of patients (n = 233) after rotator cuff repair at an average follow-up of 4.6 years. Gore et al. reported subjective improvement in 95% of patients (n = 63), including significant pain relief and minimal to no limitations in ADL function at an average follow-up of 5.5 years. In the same series, flexion ROM averaged 126 degrees actively and 147 degrees passively. Matsen et al. reported that patients with intact repairs at 5-year follow-up averaged flexion of 132 degrees, external rotation (at 90 degrees of abduction) of 71 degrees, and functional internal rotation to T7. At least 12 months is required to restore strength after rotator cuff repair; the most significant increases are noted 6 to 12 months after surgery. Walker et al. reported that isokinetic abductor strength returned to 80% of normal (uninvolved shoulder) and external rotation to 90% of normal after 1 year. Rokito et al., reporting isokinetic torques after rotator cuff repair at 1 year, demonstrated side-to-side comparisons (involved/uninvolved) for flexion, abduction, and external rotation of 84%, 90%, and 91%, respectively. Brems

reported that the strength of the external rotators of the repaired shoulder was 71% of the uninvolved shoulder. Favorable outcomes are achieved in more than 75% of patients undergoing rotator cuff repair. However, some studies have reported satisfactory results in upward of 90% of patients.

30. **If a patient cannot attend formal physical therapy programs after surgical repair of the rotator cuff, is a standardized home program effective?**
The literature has indicated that a standardized home program (to include written and video instructions) for patients following rotator cuff repair resulted in favorable outcomes in regard to range of motion, strength, and patient-reported outcomes.

31. **What is the clinical outcome of a patient suffering structural failure of a rotator cuff repair?**
Jost et al. reported that patients who ruptured a repaired rotator cuff reported a subjective shoulder outcome score of approximately 75% of the uninvolved normal shoulder. Following structural failure of the rotator cuff, 55% of the subjects reported that they were very satisfied, 30% were satisfied, and 15% were disappointed with the outcome. These outcomes still persist 7 years after the ruptured a repaired rotator cuff was diagnosed.

32. **What are the options for management of an irreparable rotator cuff tear secondary to arthropathy?**
Because each patient has different levels of pain and functional disability, options for the management of arthropathy vary. Patients with mild degrees of pain usually are treated with analgesics and exercise programs to maintain levels of ADL function. Shoulder arthrodesis and total shoulder arthroplasty are options in severe cases.

Bibliography

Alqunaee, M., Galvin, R., & Fahey, T. (2012). Diagnostic accuracy of clinical tests for subacromial impingement syndrome: a systematic review and meta-analysis. *Archives of Physical Medicine and Rehabilitation, 93*(2), 229–236.

Baker, C.L., Jr., & Liu, S.H. (1993). Neurovascular injuries to the shoulder. *Journal of Orthopaedic and Sports Physical Therapy*, 18(1), 360–364.

Bartolozzi, A., Andreychik, D., & Ahmad, S. (1994). Determinants of outcome in the treatment of rotator cuff disease. *Clinical Orthopaedics and Related Research, 308*, 90–97.

Blanchard, T., Bearcroft, P. W., Constant, C. R., Griffin, D. R., & Dixon, A. K. (1999). Diagnostic and therapeutic impact of MRI and arthrography in the investigation of full-thickness rotator cuff tears. *European Radiology, 9*, 638–642.

Boublik, M., & Hawkins, R.J. (1993). Clinical examination of the shoulder complex. *Journal of Orthopaedic and Sports Physical Therapy*, 18(1), 379–385.

Brems, J. J. (1979). Digital muscle strength measurement in rotator cuff. *American Journal of Sports Medicine, 7*, 102–110.

Brotzman, S. B. (1996). Rehabilitation of the shoulder. In Jobe, F. W., et al. (Eds.), *Clinical orthopaedic rehabilitation* (pp. 91–141). St. Louis, MO: Mosby.

Cofield, R. H. (1985). Current concepts review: rotator cuff disease of the shoulder. *Journal of Bone and Joint Surgery, 67*(6), 974–979.

Gore, D. R., Murray, M. P., Sepic, S. B., & Gardner, G. M. (1986). Shoulder-muscle strength and range of motion following surgical repair of full-thickness rotator cuff tears. *Journal of Bone and Joint Surgery, 68*, 266–272.

Green, S., Buchbinder, R., & Hetrick, S. (2003). Physiotherapy interventions for shoulder pain. *Cochrane Database of Systematic Reviews, 2003*(2), CD004258.

Hawkins, R. J., Misamore, G. W., & Hobeika, P. E. (1985). Surgery of full thickness rotator cuff tears. *Journal of Bone and Joint Surgery, 67*(9), 1349–1355.

Hertel, R., Ballmer, F. T., Lombert, S. M., & Gerber, C. (1996). Lag signs in the diagnosis of rotator cuff rupture. *Journal of Shoulder and Elbow Surgery, 5*, 307–313.

Ho, C.P. (1993). Applied MRI anatomy of the shoulder. Journal of Orthopaedic and Sports Physical Therapy, 18(1), 351–359.

Holtby, R., & Razmjou, H. (2002). Validity of the supraspinatus test as a single clinical test in diagnosing patients with rotator cuff pathology. *The Journal of Orthopaedic and Sports Physical Therapy, 32*, 194–200.

Jost, B., Pfirrmann, C. W., Gerber, C., & Switzerland, Z. (2000). Clinical outcome after structural failure of rotator cuff repairs. *Journal of Bone and Joint Surgery, 82*(3), 304–314.

Kane, L. T., Lazarus, M. D., Namdari, S., Seitz, A. L., & Abboud, J. A. (2020). Comparing expert opinion within the care team regarding postoperative rehabilitation protocol following rotator cuff repair. *Journal of Shoulder and Elbow Surgery, 29*(9), e330–e337.

Lashgari, C., & Yamaguchi, K. (2002). Natural history and nonsurgical treatment of rotator cuff disorders. In T. Norris (Ed.), *OKU shoulder and elbow 2* (pp. 155–162). Rosemont, CA: AAOS.

Matsen F. A. et. al. (1994). Practical evaluation and management of the shoulder. Philadelphia: WB Saunders.

Neer, C. S., II, Flatow, E. L., & Lech, O. (1988). Tears of the rotator cuff: long-term results of anterior acromioplasty and repair, ASES 4th Meeting, Atlanta.

Park, H. B., Yokota, A., Gill, H. S., El Rassi, G., & McFarland, E. G. (2005). Diagnostic accuracy of clinical tests for the different degrees of subacromial impingement syndrome. *Journal of Bone and Joint Surgery, 87*(7), 1446–1455.

Pearsall, A. W., 4th, Bonsell, S., Heitman, R. J., Helsm, C. A., Osbahr, D., & Soeer, K. P. (2003). Radiographic findings associated with symptomatic rotator cuff tears. *Journal of Shoulder and Elbow Surgery, 12*, 122–127.

Reinold, M. M., Escamilla, R. F., & Wilk, K. E. (2009). Current concepts in the scientific and clinical rationale behind exercises for glenohumeral and scapulothoracic musculature. *Journal of Orthopaedic & Sports Physical Therapy, 39*(2), 105–117.

Rockwood, C. A., & Matsen, F. A. (1998). Rotator cuff. In *The shoulder* (pp. 755–839) (2nd ed.). Philadelphia, PA: WB Saunders.

Roddey, T. S., Olsen, S. L., Gartsman, G. M., Hanten, W. P., & Cook, K. F. (2002). A randomized controlled trial comparing 2 instructional approaches to home exercise instruction following arthroscopic full-thickness rotator cuff repair surgery. *Journal of Orthopaedic and Sports Physical Therapy, 32*, 548–559.

Rokito, A. S., Cuomo, F., Gallagher, M. A., & Zuckerman, J. D. (1999). Long-term functional outcome of repair of large and massive chronic tears of the rotator cuff. *Journal of Bone and Joint Surgery (American), 81*, 991–997.
Rokito, A. S., Zuckerman, J. D., Gallagher, M. A., & Cuomo, F. (1996). Strength after surgical repair of the rotator cuff. *Journal of Shoulder and Elbow Surgery, 5*, 12–17.
Roy, J. S., Braën, C., Leblond, J., et al. (2015). Diagnostic accuracy of ultrasonography, MRI and MR arthrography in the characterisation of rotator cuff disorders: a systematic review and meta-analysis. *British Journal of Sports Medicine, 49*(20), 1316–1328.
Smidt, G. L. (Ed.). (1993). Journal of Orthopaedic and Sports Physical Therapy (Special Issue), 18(1).
Smith, T. O., Back, T., Toms, A. P., & Hing, C. B. (2011). Diagnostic accuracy of ultrasound for rotator cuff tears in adults: a systematic review and meta-analysis. *Clinical Radiology, 66*(11), 1036–1048.
van Holsbeeck, E., DeRycke, J., Declercq, G., Martens, M., Verstreken, J., & Fabry, G. (1992). Subacromial impingement: open versus arthroscopic decompression. *Arthroscopy, 8*, 173–178.
Walker, S. W. et al. (1987). Isokinetic strength of the shoulder after repair of a torn rotator cuff. *Journal of Bone and Joint Surgery*, 69, 1041–1044.
Wilk, K. W. (Ed.). (1993). Journal of Orthopaedic and Sports Physical Therapy (Special Issue), 18(2).
Wilk, K. E., & Arrigo, C. (1993). Current concepts in the rehabilitation of the athletic shoulder. Journal of Orthopaedic and Sports Physical Therapy, 18(1), 365–378.

CHAPTER 37 QUESTIONS

1. A 55-year-old male reports right shoulder pain and weakness with overhead activities. Your upper quarter clearing examination rules out cervical radiculopathy. During the special testing portion of your examination, you find a painful arc sign, significant weakness and pain with shoulder external rotation MMT, and a positive drop arm sign. Which of the below conditions is MOST likely given your clinical examination findings?
   a. Rotator cuff impingement
   b. Rotator cuff tear
   c. SLAP lesion
   d. Biceps tendon rupture

   Rationale: The combination of the painful arc sign, drop-arm sign, and infraspinatus muscle test produced the best posttest probability (91%) for full-thickness rotator cuff tears.

2. A 23-year-old male pitcher reports right posterior shoulder pain with throwing. During your clinical examination, you note anterior capsular laxity and tenderness to palpation of the posterior lateral shoulder just below spine of the scapula. Additionally, you note a painful arc sign, weakness and pain with shoulder external rotation MMT, and a positive Hawkins-Kennedy impingement sign. Which of the below conditions is MOST likely given your clinical examination findings?
   a. Secondary rotator cuff impingement
   b. Rotator cuff tear
   c. Posterior impingement
   d. Multidirectional instability of the shoulder

   Rationale: Posterior impingement often is seen in overhead athletes, such as throwers, swimmers, and tennis players. It occurs when the arm is in an elevated and externally rotated position (similar to the cocking phase in throwing). The infraspinatus and supraspinatus muscles are pinched between the posterior superior aspect of the glenoid when the upper limb is in the cocked position. The lesion occurs on the undersurface rather than the bursal side of the rotator cuff. In addition, this form of impingement is thought to be associated with anterior instability. Combination of the Hawkins-Kennedy impingement sign, the painful arc sign, and the infraspinatus muscle test yielded the best posttest probability (95%) for any degree of impingement syndrome.

CHAPTER 38

SHOULDER INSTABILITY

M.L. Voight, PT, DHSc, OCS, SCS, ATC, FAPTA

1. **How do the size, shape, and orientation of the glenoid fossa affect glenohumeral joint stability?**
The glenoid cavity can be described as an irregularly shaped oval, much like an inverted comma. On the basis of studies conducted by Saha, the average height is 35 mm and the average width is 25 mm. Saha also demonstrated that in 75% of the specimens examined, the glenoid fossa was retroverted approximately 7 degrees. In the remaining 25%, the glenoid was anteverted from 2 to 10 degrees. The glenoid is also tilted from superomedial to inferolateral by an average of 15 degrees. The depth of the fossa is enhanced by the glenoid labrum, which can contribute up to 50% of the fossa's depth.

2. **Describe the passive stabilizing mechanisms for the glenohumeral joint.**
Passive stability is provided by the bony geometry, glenoid labrum, limited joint volume, negative intraarticular pressure, adhesion and cohesion, and capsuloligamentous structures. The glenohumeral joint has a slightly negative pressure of −4.0 mmHg, which creates a relative vacuum. As long as the relative vacuum effect is maintained, limited joint volume does not allow the joint surfaces to be easily distracted or subluxated.
The close match of the articular surfaces produces intermolecular forces of surface tension, cohesion, and adhesion, which provide continued coupling of the humerus to the glenoid. Adhesion refers to the attraction of unlike substances (joint fluid to bone), whereas cohesion refers to the attraction of like substances (joint fluid to joint fluid). In addition, the glenoid labrum deepens the fossa by 5 mm in an anteroposterior direction and by 9 mm in the superior and inferior direction.

3. **What are the primary static stabilizers of the glenohumeral joint?**
The superior, middle, and inferior glenohumeral ligaments provide anterior stability. With the arm in the adducted position, the superior glenohumeral and coracohumeral ligaments act in a suspensory role to resist inferior translation of the humeral head. As the arm is brought up into the mid-range of abduction, the middle glenohumeral ligament provides more of a stabilizing role. In addition, as the arm is abducted to 45 degrees and beyond, the anterior and posterior portions of the inferior glenohumeral ligament complex become the stabilizers to resist inferior translation. Above 90 degrees of abduction, the inferior glenohumeral ligament becomes the primary stabilizing function. The anterior band of the inferior glenohumeral ligament complex is the primary restraint to anterior translation at 90 degrees of abduction. Posterior stabilization of the glenohumeral joint with the arm at 90 degrees of abduction is provided primarily by the posterior band of the inferior glenohumeral ligament complex.

4. **Describe the mechanisms for achieving dynamic stability at the glenohumeral joint.**
Stability is achieved through three mechanisms: 1) joint compression of matching concave-convex surfaces as the muscles press the humeral head into the fossa; 2) synergistic, coordinated contraction of the rotator cuff muscles, acting to steer the humeral head into the glenoid in different positions of arm rotation; and 3) dynamization or tensioning of the glenohumeral ligaments through the direct attachment or blending of the rotator cuff tendons into the glenohumeral capsule and ligaments. In addition, the glenoid fossa has an upward, lateral, and forward orientation that serves as a shelf for the humeral head. This source of stability is provided by the normal muscle control of the scapular protractors. When these muscles (serratus anterior, upper trapezius) become weakened, dynamic stability may be lost and the humeral head may simply slide down and off the near vertical glenoid fossa.

5. **What is the most common direction and mechanism of injury causing shoulder instability?**
Subcoracoid anterior dislocation is the most common direction of dislocation. The most common mechanism of injury for anterior shoulder dislocation is an indirect force with the arm in an abducted, extended, and externally rotated position. The majority of dislocations results from trauma.

6. **What is the most common nerve injury after anterior shoulder dislocation?**
Injury to the axillary nerve has an overall incidence of approximately 30%. The risk of axillary nerve injury increases with age, duration of dislocation, and force of trauma. The most common type of axillary nerve injury is traction neurapraxia. Because the axillary nerve originates at the posterior cord of the brachial plexus and its anterior branch (humeral circumflex) wraps directly around the humeral wall in the area of the surgical neck, the nerve can be exposed to trauma. Anterior dislocation may cause traction to the portion of the axillary nerve lying in close relation to the capsular structures. Most patients respond to conservative treatment over 10 weeks.

7. **Describe the most common mechanism of posterior shoulder dislocation.**
A posterior dislocation results most commonly from axial loading of the arm in an adducted, flexed, and internally rotated position. The classic mechanism of injury is either a blow to the front of the shoulder or a fall onto the outstretched arm. Lesser tuberosity fractures are common and often cause the humeral head to become locked in the dislocated position. Posterior dislocations are less common than anterior and account for only 2% to 4% of all dislocations.

8. **Why is posterior shoulder dislocation more likely than anterior dislocation after electric shock or convulsive seizures?**
Electric shock and convulsive seizures can result in violent contracture of all muscle groups surrounding the shoulder girdle. The combined strength of the latissimus dorsi, pectoralis major, and subscapularis overwhelms the infraspinatus and teres minor muscles by virtue of greater muscle bulk. As a result, the stronger internal rotators simply overpower the relatively weaker external rotators, resulting in a posterior dislocation.

9. **What is multidirectional instability with atraumatic onset?**
Multidirectional instability is a symptomatic glenohumeral subluxation or dislocation in more than one direction. The basic pathologic changes of multidirectional instability include 1) a loose, redundant, or torn joint capsule; 2) a lax ligamentous mechanism; and 3) a weakened musculotendinous system.

10. **In describing shoulder instability, what is meant by the acronym TUBS?**
- T—Traumatic onset
- U—Unidirectional (anterior)
- B—Bankart lesion (usually present)
- S—Surgery (success rate with nonoperative treatment is >20%)

11. **What is meant by the acronym AMBRI in describing shoulder instability?**
- A—Atraumatic onset
- M—Multidirectional in nature
- B—Bilateral (usually)
- R—Rehabilitation (success with conservative treatment is usually >80%)
- I—Inferior capsular shift (procedure of choice if conservative treatment fails)

12. **What type of lesion is characterized by the acronym ALPSA?**
The ALPSA lesion as originally described by Neviaser stands for anterior labroligamentous periosteal sleeve avulsion. This will often accompany a traumatic anterior dislocation and is characterized by the labrum and periosteal sleeve of the anterior glenoid being avulsed and displaced medially.

13. **What type of lesion is characterized by the acronym HAGL?**
The HAGL lesion occurs with traumatic dislocation when the arm is forced into a hyperabducted position. The acronym stands for humeral avulsion of the glenohumeral ligament.

14. **Describe the load-shift test.**
The load-shift test allows evaluation of glenohumeral translation. A compressive axial load is applied to the humeral head to reduce it into the glenoid. This reduction is important because the humeral head may be resting in a subluxated position, which may give a false sense of the direction of the instability. Anterior and posterior forces then are placed on the proximal humerus, and the direction and degree of translation are determined.

15. **Describe the anterior release test.**
The patient is supine and the shoulder is placed in 90-degree abduction and 90-degree external rotation (ER) (apprehension position), during which a posterior-directed force is applied to the humeral head (anterior surface of shoulder). The posterior force is then released; if the patient experiences pain and apprehension, then the test is considered positive.

16. **What are the sensitivity and specificity values of commonly performed shoulder instability tests?**

TEST	SENSITIVITY (%)	SPECIFICITY (%)
Load-shift (under anesthesia)	83*	100
Sulcus sign	Not reported	Not reported
Apprehension	57	100
Relocation	30	50
Anterior release	92	89

*Hawkins suggests it may be overly sensitive.

17. **What type of grading scheme is used to assess increased glenohumeral translation?**
Anterior translation of 25% or less of the humeral head diameter is considered normal. Hawkins suggested a grading system that may be more appropriate for reporting the test results than distance or percentages:
    - Grade I—humeral head can be felt to ride up the face of the glenoid to the glenoid rim but cannot be felt to move over the rim edge. Grade I corresponds to approximately up to 50% of humeral head translation.
    - Grade II—humeral head can be felt to move over the glenoid rim but reduces with release of pressure, corresponding to clinical subluxation. For grade II the humeral head has more than 50% translation.
    - Grade III—head remains dislocated on release, corresponding to clinical dislocation.

18. **Describe the clinical tests for posterior shoulder instability.**
In addition to the load-shift test, posterior instability can be assessed with the jerk test. The arm is flexed to 90 degrees with internal rotation (IR), and an axial load is delivered to the shoulder in a posterior direction. The arm is brought into a horizontally adducted position, and posterior slippage is noted. The arm then is brought back into a horizontally abducted position. A jerk may be experienced when the humeral head relocates onto the glenoid fossa.

19. **What radiologic studies and views are best suited for confirming or evaluating shoulder instability?**
The recommended views in a trauma series include a true anteroposterior (AP) view, a true scapular lateral view, and an axillary view. The most commonly obtained views of the shoulder include the AP view of the shoulder with the humerus in both internal and ER, a true AP of the glenoid view, a scapulolateral (Y) view, an axillary view, a West Point projection, and a Stryker notch view.

20. **Describe the Hill-Sachs and reverse Hill-Sachs lesions.**
The Hill-Sachs lesion is a compression fracture of the posterolateral aspect of the humeral head. It results from impact to the anteroinferior rim of the glenoid during an anterior dislocation of the shoulder. A reverse Hill-Sachs lesion involves a compression fracture of the anteromedial humeral head as the result of a posterior dislocation.

21. **What is the suggested radiologic view to visualize a Hill-Sachs lesion?**
The Hill-Sachs lesion is demonstrated best by either the IR or the Stryker notch views; each has a sensitivity of 92%. The detection of a Hill-Sachs lesion is prognostically important because patients with a Hill-Sachs lesion may be prone to redislocation.

22. **What is a Bankart lesion? What is its significance?**
A Bankart lesion is an avulsion or detachment of the anterior portion of the inferior glenohumeral ligament complex and glenoid labrum off the anterior rim of the glenoid. Although a Bankart lesion can contribute to increased translation of the humeral head, complete dislocation requires associated capsular injury. Bankart lesions can contribute to recurrent instability.

23. **Describe the clinical presentation of a posterior shoulder dislocation.**
Observation is often difficult because most patients hold the shoulder in the traditional sling position of adduction and IR. ER usually is limited, and it is not uncommon to find the posteriorly dislocated shoulder locked into IR secondary to a fracture of the lesser tuberosity. Observation usually reveals a prominent coracoid process and a flattening of the anterior aspect of the shoulder.

24. **What is the suggested initial medical treatment for anterior shoulder dislocation? Why is early relocation important?**
Initial treatment includes application of ice and use of a sling. Acute glenohumeral dislocations should be reduced as quickly and gently as possible because early relocation quickly reduces stretch and compression of neurovascular structures, minimizes the degree of muscle spasm that must be overcome to reduce the joint, and prevents progressive enlargement of the humeral head defect in the locked dislocation.

25. **Following reduction for an anterior dislocation, should the arm be immobilized in IR or ER?**
Postreduction management after traumatic anterior shoulder dislocation is controversial. A 10-year prospective study by Hovelius comparing immobilization with no immobilization found no difference in recurrence rates. The position of immobilization is also controversial. Itoi et al. investigated immobilizing the arm in IR or ER after initial traumatic anterior dislocation. The recurrence rate was approximately 30% in the IR group and 0% in the ER group at a mean follow-up time of 15.5 months, suggesting ER as the position of immobilization. However, it is still more customary to immobilize the arm in IR at this time.

26. **What is the most common complication in managing a traumatic anterior dislocation?**
Recurrence is the most common complication. Other complications include fractures of the humerus, vascular injuries, neural injuries, and rotator cuff tears (more common in patients >40 years).

27. **What accounts for the high incidence of recurrent dislocation?**
Several factors have been identified as contributing to recurrence and instability. Age at the time of onset correlates most closely to recurrence. Patients under the age of 20 years may have a recurrence rate up to 80%, whereas after the age of 40 the rate drops to under 10%. Males have a higher recurrence rate than females, and most recurrences are seen within 2 years of the initial traumatic dislocation. The recurrence rate varies inversely with the severity of the initial trauma. If dislocation occurs a second time in younger patients, the chance of frequent recurrence is almost 100%.

28. **What is the normal shoulder ER/IR strength ratio and why is it important?**
Muscle weakness, specifically of the rotator cuff musculature, has been proposed as a possible risk factor for developing shoulder injury. Because of the critical functional role of the rotator cuff muscles, objective evaluation of shoulder IR and ER strength is important during rehabilitation and in preparticipation evaluation. Ideally, this ratio should be 1:1; however, in unilateral dominant sports such as baseball and tennis, the recommended muscle strength between shoulder internal rotators and external rotators is 65% to 75%. These data are important for clinicians to use when interpreting strength performance in athletes who are attempting to return to play after an injury and when individualizing training enhancement programs. Additionally, assessing preseason muscle strength might be an effective strategy for identifying athletes at risk for injury and might provide the opportunity to prescribe training programs for injury prevention.

29. **What is the incidence of associated rotator cuff tears in patients older than 40 years? Why is the rate increased?**
The incidence of rotator cuff tears after acute dislocation in patients older than 40 years ranges from 35% to 86%. The reason for the variability in numbers is the unknown amount of rotator cuff pathology before the initial dislocation. With dislocation of the humeral head anteriorly, the anterior and/or posterior structures are disrupted. With dislocations in younger patients, the anterior capsuloligamentous complex tends to disrupt because it is less strong than other tissues of the shoulder. In older patients, the posterior structures (rotator cuff and greater tuberosity complex) are weaker by attrition and tend to disrupt, leaving the anterior capsuloligamentous complex intact.

30. **What nonoperative management is appropriate after anterior shoulder dislocation?**
After an initial period of immobilization, a regimen of shoulder rehabilitation should be implemented. Initially, range of motion exercises are instituted to help prevent stiffness. Positions of abduction and ER should be avoided to prevent excessive stress on the anterior capsule. Strengthening of the shoulder musculature is of paramount importance to improve dynamic stability. Because the capsular stabilizing structures are compromised, the shoulder has a greater dependence on dynamic stabilizing mechanisms. Early focus is placed on the stabilizers of the scapula. The scapula must provide a stable base on which the humerus can rotate and maintain the glenoid in a position that provides maximal congruence with the humeral head. The core scapular exercises are scaption, protraction, retraction, and seated press-up.

Once scapular stability is addressed, emphasis is placed on reestablishing the strength of the rotator cuff musculature, which is the main dynamic stabilizer of the glenohumeral joint. Exercises should be performed in the scapular plane, which provides the greatest congruence between the humeral head and glenoid and minimizes the stress placed on the anterior capsule. The supraspinatus can be isolated with prone horizontal abduction and ER. Activation of the teres minor and infraspinatus draws the humeral head posteriorly and thus unloads the stress on the damaged anterior structures. These two muscles are best isolated with prone ER with the arm positioned in 90-degree abduction. In addition to strengthening exercises, proprioception exercises should be used to enhance the patient's sense of position.

31. **What nonoperative management is appropriate after posterior shoulder dislocation?**
Reduction is accomplished by longitudinal forward traction on the arm with the elbow bent, accompanied by anterior pressure on the humeral head. The arm then is brought into an adducted, externally rotated, and internally rotated position to reduce the humeral head back into the glenoid fossa. Principles of nonoperative treatment include pain management, activity modification, and a shoulder strengthening program involving the scapular and rotator cuff musculature. Nonoperative treatment produces superior results in posterior instability compared with anterior instability. The joint is immobilized for only 2 to 3 weeks in a handshake cast. Integral to the strengthening program is the periscapular and rotator cuff musculature. ER and posterior deltoid strengthening is emphasized during rehabilitation. Push-ups and bench press activities should be avoided. The patient must be instructed to avoid activities that place the shoulder at the limits of flexion, IR, or horizontal adduction. Otherwise the shoulder may redislocate.

32. **What nonoperative management is appropriate for multidirectional instability?**
Overall, patients tend to respond well to rehabilitation. Aggressive physical therapy with strengthening of the scapular stabilizers and rotator cuff musculature frequently provides sufficient dynamic stability. If the patient does not respond to conservative treatment, an inferior capsular shift should be included as part of the surgical procedure.

33. **Describe the modern surgical management of patients for whom operative treatment is advisable.**
Several different surgical procedures are used to control shoulder instability. The success and/or failure rate for each is quite variable and highly dependent on the skill of the surgeon. Currently, the gold standard is some variation of capsulorrhaphy, which directly affects the size and/or orientation of the glenohumeral capsule:
    - Bankart repair—suturing of the anterior capsule and labrum to the anterior glenoid rim
    - Capsular shift—tightening of the joint capsule, depending on the precise amount and location of laxity
    - Staple capsulorrhaphy—securing the detached anterior capsule and labrum onto the glenoid
    - Thermal capsulorrhaphy—thermal shrinkage of the capsular collagen tissue to restore normal stability
    - Putti-Platt procedure—subscapularis and capsular shortening

34. **Describe the Latarjet procedure for shoulder instability.**
The Latarjet operation, also known as the Latarjet-Bristow procedure, is a surgical procedure used to treat recurrent shoulder dislocations, typically caused by bone loss or a fracture of the glenoid. The procedure was first described by French surgeon Dr. Michel Latarjet in 1954. The Latarjet procedure involves the removal and transfer of a section of the coracoid process and its attached muscles to the front of the glenoid. This placement of the coracoid acts as a bone block that, combined with the transferred muscles acting as a strut, prevents further dislocation of the joint. While the Latarjet procedure can be used for surgical treatment of most cases of shoulder dislocations or subluxation, it is particularly indicated in cases with bone defects. The failure rate following arthroscopic Bankart repair has been shown to dramatically increase from 4% to 67% in patients with significant bone loss.

35. **How does the outcome of immediate surgical stabilization compare to the nonoperative management of shoulder instability in the young, healthy adult?**
Kirkley conducted a prospective randomized clinical trial comparing the effectiveness of immediate arthroscopic stabilization versus immobilization and rehabilitation in first-time, traumatic anterior shoulder dislocations. At an average of 32 months' follow-up, a significant reduction in redislocation and an improvement in disease-specific quality of life were afforded by early arthroscopic stabilization in patients less than 30 years of age with a first-time, traumatic anterior dislocation of the shoulder.
The Bankart lesion was noted in a very high percentage of traumatic first-time dislocations—97% in one series of patients who underwent arthroscopic evaluation soon after their injury. The standard of care in the overhead athlete is early repair of the capsular structures. With the Bankart lesion, the capsulolabral complex avulses from the glenoid. If the anteroinferior labrum and capsule do not heal in their anatomic position, the depth of the concavity will be lost in that isolated area, thereby contributing to an increased recurrence rate, especially when the arm is placed in a position of abduction and ER. Early stabilization in athletic high-risk patients should diminish progressive soft tissue and bony damage.

36. **What are superior labrum anterior and posterior (SLAP) lesions?**
SLAP lesions most often result from a sudden downward force on a supinated outstretched upper extremity or from a fall on the lateral shoulder. Patients complain of popping and sliding of the shoulder, especially with overhead activities. The average time to diagnosis from onset of symptoms is about 2.5 years.

37. **What are the types of SLAP lesions?**
In 1990 Stephen Snyder coined the name SLAP lesion to describe a more extensive injury pattern involving the superior labrum. Snyder further classified superior labrum disorders into four types:
- Type I—degenerative fraying of the labrum
- Type II—avulsion of the superior labrum and biceps tendon
- Type III—bucket-handle tears of the superior labrum
- Type IV—same as grade II or III with extension into the biceps tendon
- Maffet and co-workers described three additional types of SLAP lesions:
- Type V—an anterior-inferior Bankart lesion that propagates superiorly to the biceps tendon
- Type VI—an unstable flap tear of the labrum with separation of the biceps anchor
- Type VII—a superior biceps-labral detachment that extends anteriorly beneath the middle glenohumeral ligament

Bibliography

Anderson, M. J., Mack, C. D., Herzog, M. M., & Levine, W. N. (2021). Epidemiology of shoulder instability in the National Football League. *Orthopedic Journal of Sports Medicine, 9*(5), 23259671211007743.

Bahr, R., Craig, E. V., & Engebretson, L. (1995). The clinical presentation of shoulder instability including on field management. *Clinics in Sports Medicine, 14*, 761–776.

Barnes, L. F., Parsons, B. O., Lippitt, S. B., Flatow, E. L., & Matsen, F. A. (1998). Glenohumeral instability. In Rockwood, M. A., & Matsen, F. A. (Eds.), The shoulder Philadelphia, PA: Elsevier.

Bigliani, L. U. (Ed.). (1996). *The unstable shoulder.* Chicago: American Academy of Orthopedic Surgeons.

Bottoni, C. R., Wilckens, J. H., DeBerardino, T. M., et al. (2002). A prospective, randomized evaluation of arthroscopic stabilization versus nonoperative treatment in patients with acute, traumatic, first-time shoulder dislocations. *American Journal of Sports Medicine, 30*, 576–580.

Burkhead, W. Z., & Rockwood, C. A. (1992). Treatment of instability of the shoulder with an exercise program. *Journal of Bone and Joint Surgery, 74*(6), 890–896.

Cleeman, E., & Flatow, E. L. (2000). Shoulder dislocations in the young patient. *Orthopedic Clinics of North America, 31*, 217–229.

DiMaria, S., Bokshan, S. L., Nacca, C., & Owens, B. (2019). History of surgical stabilization for posterior shoulder instability. *Journal of Shoulder and Elbow Surgery, 3*(4), 350–356.

Dines, D. M., & Levinson, M. (1995). The conservative management of the unstable shoulder including rehabilitation. *Clinics in Sports Medicine, 14*, 797–816.

Eshoj, H. R., Rasmussen, S., Frich, L. H., et al. (2020). Neuromuscular exercises improve shoulder function more than standard care exercises in patients with a traumatic anterior shoulder dislocation: a randomized controlled trial. *Orthopedic Journal of Sports Medicine, 8*(1), 2325967119896102.

Galvin, J. W., Ernat, J. J., Waterman, B. R., Stadecker, M. J., & Parad, S. A. (2017). The epidemiology and natural history of anterior shoulder dislocation. *Current Review of Musculoskeletal Medicine, 10*(4), 411–424.

Hawkins, R. J., & Misamore, G. W. (1996). *Shoulder injuries in the athlete.* New York, NY: Churchill Livingstone.

Hovelius, L. (1996). Primary anterior dislocation of the shoulder in young patients: a ten year prospective study. *Journal of Bone and Joint Surgery, 78*(11), 1677–1684.

Itoi, E., Hatakeyama, Y., Kido, T., et al. (2003). A new method of immobilization after traumatic anterior dislocation of the shoulder: a preliminary study. *Journal of Shoulder and Elbow Surgery, 12*, 413–415.

Kavaja, L., Lähdeoja, T., Malmivaara, A., & Paavola, M. (2018). Treatment after traumatic shoulder dislocation: a systematic review with a network meta-analysis. *British Journal of Sports Medicine, 52*(23), 1498–1506.

Kirkley, A., Griffin, S., Richards, C., Miniaci, A., & Mohtadi, N. (1999). Prospective randomized clinical trial comparing the effectiveness of immediate arthroscopic stabilization versus immobilization and rehabilitation in first traumatic anterior dislocations of the shoulder. *Arthroscopy, 15*, 507–514.

Maffet, M. W., Gartsman, G. M., & Moseley, B. (1995). Superior labrum-biceps tendon complex lesions of the shoulder. *American Journal of Sports Medicine, 23*, 93–98.

Minkus, M., Königshausen, M., Pauly, S., et al. (2021). Immobilization in external rotation and abduction versus arthroscopic stabilization after first-time anterior shoulder dislocation: a multicenter randomized controlled trial. *American Journal of Sports Medicine, 49*, 857–865.

Moseley, J. B., Jr., Jobe, F. W., Pink, M., Perry, J., & Tibone, J. (1992). EMG analysis of the scapular muscles during a shoulder rehabilitation program. *American Journal of Sports Medicine, 20*, 128–134.

Neer, C. S. (1985). Involuntary inferior and multidirectional instability of the shoulder: etiology, recognition, and treatment. *Instructional Course Lectures, 34*, 232–238.

Nord, K. D., Masterson, J. P., & Mauck, B. M. (2004). Superior labrum anterior posterior (SLAP) repair using the Neviaser portal. *Arthroscopy, 20*(Suppl 2), 129–133.

Petersen, S. A. (2000). Posterior shoulder instability. *Orthopedic Clinics of North America, 31*, 263–274.

Pötzl, W., Thorwesten, L., Götze, C., Garmann, S., & Steinbeck, J. (2004). Proprioception of the shoulder joint after surgical repair for instability: a long-term follow-up study. *American Journal of Sports Medicine, 32*, 425–430.

Rhee, S. M., Nashikkar, P. S., Park, J. H., Jeon, Y. D., & Oh, J. H. (2021). Changes in shoulder rotator cuff strength after arthroscopic capsulolabral reconstruction in patients with anterior shoulder instability. *Orthopedic Journal of Sports Medicine, 9*(1), 2325967120972052.

Saha, A. K. (1971). Dynamic stability of the glenohumeral joint. *Acta Orthopaedica Scandinavica, 42*, 491–505.
Saha, A. K. (1983). Mechanism of shoulder movements and a plea for the recognition of the "zero" position of the glenohumeral joint. *Clinical Orthopaedics and Related Research, 173*, 3–10.
Snyder, S. J., Karzel, R. P., Del Pizzo, W., Ferkel, R. D., & Friedman, M. J. (1990). SLAP lesions of the shoulder. *Arthroscopy, 6*, 274–279.
Speer, K. P. (1995). Anatomy and pathomechanics of shoulder instability. *Clinics in Sports Medicine, 14*, 751–760.
Stayner, L. R., Cummings, J., Andersen, J., & Jobe, C. M. (2000). Shoulder dislocations in patients older than 40 years of age. *Orthopedic Clinics of North America, 31*, 231–239.
Taylor, D., & Arciero, R. (1997). Pathologic changes associated with shoulder dislocations. *American Journal of Sports Medicine, 25*, 306–311.
Tzannes, A., Paxinos, A., Callanan, M., & Murrell, G. A. C. (2004). An assessment of the interrater reliability of tests for shoulder instability. *Journal of Shoulder and Elbow Surgery, 13*, 18–23.
Vopat, M. L., Coda, R. G., Giusti, N. E., et al. (2021). Differences in outcomes between anterior and posterior shoulder instability after arthroscopic Bankart repair: a systematic review and meta-analysis. *Orthopedic Journal of Sports Medicine, 9*(5), 23259671211006437.
Yuehuei, H., & Friedman, R. J. (2000). Multidirectional instability of the glenohumeral joint. *Orthopedic Clinics of North America, 31*, 275–283.

CHAPTER 38 QUESTIONS

1. **With the arm positioned in 45 degrees of abduction, which of the glenohumeral ligaments is the primary restraint to ER?**
   a. Inferior glenohumeral ligament
   b. Middle glenohumeral ligament
   c. Posterior glenohumeral ligament
   d. Superior glenohumeral ligament

2. **Which of the following surgical procedures is performed for recurrent anterior instability or dislocation of the glenohumeral joint and involves reattachment and repair of the capsulolabral complex to the anterior rim of the glenoid?**
   a. Bankart repair
   b. Anterior capsular shift
   c. Hill-Sachs repair
   d. Repair of a SLAP lesion

3. **This lesion is seen in recurrent anterior glenohumeral dislocation as an indentation or compression fracture of the articular surface of the humeral head as created by the sharp edge of the anterior glenoid as the humeral head dislocates up and over it:**
   a. Hill-Sachs lesion
   b. Bankart lesion
   c. Reverse Hill-Sachs lesion
   d. Reverse Hills-Sachs is a real condition

4. **Which of the following does NOT contribute to the passive stability of the glenohumeral joint?**
   a. Negative intraarticular pressure
   b. Glenoid labrum
   c. Osseous geometry
   d. Supraspinatus

5. **A bicyclist falls off of a bike onto his outstretched arm, with the arm adducted and internally rotated. He has symptoms of severe pain, inability to move his shoulder, and an apparent prominence in the infraspinatus region. The most likely diagnosis is:**
   a. Anterior shoulder dislocation
   b. Brachial plexus injury
   c. Posterior shoulder dislocation
   d. Rotator cuff tear

6. **In the glenohumeral joint with the arm at the side, the presence of a sulcus sign is a reflection of laxity of what structure?**
   a. Inferior capsular ligament
   b. Coracoacromial ligament
   c. Supraspinatus tendon
   d. Superior glenohumeral ligament
   e. Biceps tendon

7. A 17-year-old high school quarterback experiences recurrent anterior shoulder pain in his throwing arm. Instability testing demonstrates a multidirectional instability with secondary impingement. Which of the following tests will not be positive?
   a. Hawkins test
   b. Sulcus test/sign
   c. Anterior/posterior load and shift test
   d. Adson's test

CHAPTER 39

ADHESIVE CAPSULITIS

J. Placzek, MD, PT, L. Placzek, and B. Ring, RN

1. **Describe the epidemiology of adhesive capsulitis.**
   Adhesive capsulitis, or "frozen shoulder," is more common in females than males and occurs most often in the age range of 40 to 60 years. Bilateral involvement is seen in about 12% of patients. The incidence is 2% in the general population and 10% to 35% in diabetic patients.

2. **What are the predominant cell types in adhesive capsulitis? What growth factors are present?**
   Fibroblasts and myofibroblasts are the predominant cell types. The presence of type III collagen in those with adhesive capsulitis indicates new deposition of collagen within the capsule. The frequency of staining for transforming growth factor-β, platelet-derived growth factor, and hepatocyte growth factor is greater in adhesive capsulitis tissue than in tissue from patients with nonspecific synovitis. Intercellular adhesion molecule-1 is present in the capsule of patients with frozen shoulder. Increased chondrogenesis is also seen along with fibrosis in the capsule of those with frozen shoulder.

3. **Define primary and secondary adhesive capsulitis.**
   Lundberg described stiff shoulder with insidious onset as primary adhesive capsulitis. Frozen shoulder after some type of trauma or inciting event is classified as secondary adhesive capsulitis.

4. **Are plain x-ray films beneficial in diagnosing adhesive capsulitis?**
   A disruption of the scapulohumeral arch is present in 80% of patients with adhesive capsulitis. Patients with scapulohumeral arch disruption had 16-fold increased odds of having adhesive capsulitis. Plain films are also useful in excluding other pathology.

5. **What imaging technique was previously used for the diagnosis of adhesive capsulitis?**
   Arthrography was the gold standard for diagnosis. The normal capsular volume decreases from 25 ml to about 6 ml with obliteration of the biceps sheath, axillary fold, and subscapular bursa.

6. **What MRI findings are associated with adhesive capsulitis?**
   Thickening of the coracohumeral ligament (CHL) to >4 mm is 95% specific and 59% sensitive for the diagnosis of adhesive capsulitis. Thickening of the capsule in the rotator interval to >7 mm has a specificity of 86% and sensitivity of 64%. Obliteration of the fat triangle between the CHL and the coracoid process was 100% specific but 32% sensitive. Enhancement of the axillary recess after intravenous contrast administration increases the sensitivity and specificity to 98% for the diagnoses of adhesive capsulitis.

7. **Describe ultrasound features of adhesive capsulitis.**
   Thickening of the axillary pouch of greater than 4 mm (93%), effusion of the bicep sheath (71%), thickening of the coracohumeral ligament (greater than 2.2 mm), or superior glenohumeral ligament (88%). The coracohumeral ligament is significantly thicker in stage 2 than in stage 1.

8. **What factors have been proposed in the pathogenesis of adhesive capsulitis?**
   Cervical spine disorders, autoimmune disorders, tendinitis, hypothyroidism, diabetes, hormonal disorders, and poor posture have been postulated as predisposing factors for capsulitis. Hypercholesterolemia is an independent risk factor for adhesive capsulitis.

9. **Describe the natural resolution of adhesive capsulitis.**
   Reeves described the three classic stages of adhesive capsulitis:
   - Early painful stage (freezing)—lasts 2 to 9 months; patients have diffuse pain and difficulty sleeping on the affected side; patients begin to have restricted movement secondary to pain
   - Stiffening stage (freezing)—lasts 4 to 12 months; progressive loss of ROM and decreased function are noted
   - Recovery stage (thawing)—lasts 5 to 24 months, with gradual increases in ROM and decreased pain

10. **What outcomes are associated with the natural resolution of adhesive capsulitis?**
    The time to resolution is quite variable, averaging 12 to 36 months. Approximately 20% to 60% of patients have some limitation in ROM and residual pain for up to 10 years.

11. **What are the outcomes associated with a home stretching program for adhesive capsulitis?**
Griggs et al. found that 90% of patients reported a satisfactory outcome. However, after 22 months, patients still had restricted range of motion compared with the contralateral side. Abduction was 145 degrees, flexion was 155 degrees, passive internal rotation at 90 degrees of abduction was 29 degrees, and external rotation was 60 degrees.

12. **What is the role of physical therapy for the treatment of capsulitis?**
Exercise is more effective than modalities, nonsteroidal antiinflammatory drugs, or steroid injections. Nicholson found that mobilization significantly improved ROM into abduction. However, mobilization offered no significant advantage over exercise alone in other motions. One study found mobilization to be more effective than manipulation for increasing ROM. Numerous case studies have found mobilization to be effective in treating adhesive capsulitis, especially when combined with a home stretching program.

13. **Do end range mobilization techniques improve range of motion in patients with adhesive capsulitis?**
Vermeulen et al. found that passive abduction increased from 96 to 159 degrees, flexion increased from 122 to 154 degrees, external rotation increased from 21 to 41 degrees, and the mean glenohumeral capsular volume increased from 10 to 15 ml.

14. **What outcomes are associated with steroid injections for capsulitis?**
Although steroid injections may provide transient relief of pain, no studies show conclusive evidence that they increase ROM or function. Pain relief is more effective when steroid injections are given in early in the disease process. Steroid injections appear to improve motion both in the short and long term, particularly when combined with a home exercise program.

15. **How does translational manipulation differ from traditional long lever manipulation?**
Translational manipulation uses linear forces applied at the humeral head to restore normal kinematic gliding associated with glenohumeral movements. By avoiding long lever forces, translational manipulation minimizes the stress applied to the brachial plexus and the glenohumeral, acromioclavicular, scapuloclavicular, and scapulothoracic joints.

16. **What outcomes are associated with traditional long lever manipulation under anesthesia for capsulitis?**
Despite reported complications of dislocation, fracture, brachial plexus injury, rotator cuff tearing, and failure to regain ROM secondary to pain, manipulation under anesthesia remains a proven treatment technique with a low incidence of the previously mentioned complications. Hill and Bogumill reported significant increases in ROM immediately and in the long term (flexion = 139 degrees, abduction = 143 degrees, external rotation = 54 degrees, and internal rotation = 63 degrees) after manipulation.

17. **Does manipulation tear the rotator cuff?**
Although the inferior capsule is torn, it is unusual for any tear of the rotator cuff to occur.

18. **What outcomes are associated with translational manipulation under anesthesia for capsulitis?**
Placzek et al. reported significant increases in ROM immediately and in the long term (flexion = 163 degrees, abduction = 163 degrees, external rotation = 84 degrees, and internal rotation = 69 degrees) after manipulation. Furthermore, pain was significantly reduced (7.6/10 down to 1.5/10), and function was significantly increased (Wolfgang score of 5.5/16 increased to 14.1/16).

19. **What outcomes are associated with the brisement technique (arthrographic distention)?**
Distention arthrography in general provides minimal immediate increases in ROM. However, it speeds improvement in ROM over the next several weeks to months. The steroids and local anesthetics used usually provide some pain relief.

20. **What outcomes are associated with arthroscopic release for capsulitis?**
In general, ROM gains have been somewhat less than with manipulation under anesthesia. The best results have been published by Jerosch et al., where abduction improved from 75 to 165 degrees, external rotation improved from 3 to 75 degrees, external rotation and abduction improved from 4 to 81 degrees, and internal rotation improved from 17 to 59 degrees. Arthroscopic capsular release may be particularly helpful in recalcitrant cases in which therapy and manipulation have failed.

21. **Is traditional long lever manipulation under anesthesia associated with intraarticular lesions?**
    Loew et al. found that in a group of 30 patients 22 had localized synovitis in the rotator interval and 8 had disseminated synovitis. After manipulation, the capsule was ruptured superiorly in 11 patients, anteriorly in 24, and posteriorly in 16. In four patients an iatrogenic SLAP lesion was found, three had partial tearing of the subscapularis, and four had anterior labral detachments. Two patients had tears of the middle glenohumeral ligament. Although manipulation is effective for increasing range of motion, certain iatrogenic intraarticular damage can occur.

Bibliography

Atoun, E., Funk, L., Copland, S. A., Even, T., Levy, O., & Rath, E. (2013). The effect of shoulder manipulation on rotator cuff integrity. *Acta Orthopaedica Belgica, 79*(3), 255–259.

Challoumas, D., Biddle, M., Mclean, M., & Millar, N. L. (2020). Comparison of treatments for frozen shoulder: A systematic review and meta-analysis. *JAMA Network Open, 3*(12), e2029581.

Dimitriou, D., Mazel, P., Hochreiter, B., et al. (2021). Superior humeral head migration might be a radiological aid in diagnosing patients with adhesive capsulitis of the shoulder. *JSES International, 5*(6), 1086–1090.

Do, J. G., Hwang, J. T., Yoon, K. J., & Lee, Y. T. (2021). Correlation of ultrasound findings with clinical stages and impairment in adhesive capsulitis of the shoulder. *Orthopaedic Journal of Sports Medicine, 9*(5), 23259671211003675.

Duenas, L., Bernat, M. B., Rodriguez, M. A., et al. (2019). A manual therapy and home stretching program in patients with primary frozen shoulder contracture syndrome: A case series. *Journal of Orthopaedic & Sports Physical Therapy, 49*(3), 192–201.

Griggs, S. M., Ahn, A., & Green, A. (2000). Idiopathic adhesive capsulitis. A prospective functional outcome study of nonoperative treatment. *Journal of Bone and Joint Surgery, 82*(10), 1398–1407.

Hagiwara, Y., Ando, A., Onoda, Y., et al. (2012). Coexistence of fibrotic and chondrogenic process in the capsule of idiopathic frozen shoulders. *Osteoarthritis and Cartilage, 20*(3), 241–249.

Harryman, D. T., Lazarus, M. D., & Rozencwaig, R. (1998). The stiff shoulder. In C. A. Rockwood & F. A. Matsen (Eds.), *The shoulder* (2nd ed., pp. 1064–1112). Philadelphia: WB Saunders.

Hill, J. J., Jr., & Bogumill, H. (1988). Manipulation in the treatment of frozen shoulder. *Orthopedics, 11*, 1255–1260.

Jerosch, J. (2001). 360 degree arthroscopic capsular release in patients with adhesive capsulitis of the glenohumeral joint—indication, surgical technique, results. *Knee Surgery, Sports Traumatology, Arthroscopy, 9*, 178–186.

Kim, Y. S., Kim, J. M., Lee, Y. G., Hong, O. K., Kwon, H. S., & Ji, J. H. (2013). Intercellular adhesion molecule-1 (ICAM-1, CD54) is increased in adhesive capsulitis. *Journal of Bone and Joint Surgery (American), 95*(4), 181–188.

Lo, S. F., Chu, S. W., Muo, C. H., et al. (2014). Diabetes mellitus and accompanying hyperlipidemia are independent risk factors for adhesive capsulitis: A nationwide population-based cohort study (version 2). *Rheumatology International, 34*(1), 67–74.

Loew, M., Heichel, T. O., & Lehner, B. (2005). Intra-articular lesions in primary frozen shoulder after manipulation under general anesthesia. *Journal of Shoulder and Elbow Surgery, 14*, 16–21.

Mengiardi, B., Pfirrmann, C. W., Gerber, C., Hodler, J., & Zanetti, M. (2004). Frozen shoulder: MR arthrographic findings. *Radiology, 233*, 486–492.

Michelin, P., Delarue, Y., Duparc, F., & Dacher, J. N. (2013). Thickening of the inferior glenohumeral capsule: An ultrasound sign for shoulder capsular contracture. *European Radiology, 23*(10), 2802–2806.

Pessis, E., Mihoubi, F., Feydy, A., et al. (2020). Usefulness of intravenous contrast-enhanced MRI for diagnosis of adhesive capsulitis. *European Radiology, 11*, 5981–5991.

Placzek, J. D., & Kulig, K. (1998). Translational manipulation under anesthesia: New concepts in adhesive capsulitis management. *Orthopaedic Physical Therapy Clinics of North America, 7*, 1–23.

Placzek, J. D., Roubal, P. J., Freeman, D. C., Kulig, K., Nasser, S., & Pagett, B. T. (1998). Long term effects of translational manipulation for adhesive capsulitis. *Clinical Orthopaedics and Related Research, 356*, 181–191.

Placzek, J. D., Roubel, P. J., Kulig, K., Pagett, B. T., & Wiater, J. M. (2004). Theory and technique of translational manipulation for adhesive capsulitis. *American Journal of Orthopedics, 33*(4), 173–179.

Stella, S. M., Gualtierotti, R., Ciampi, B., et al. (2021). Ultrasound of adhesive capsulitis. *Rheumatology and Therapy, 9*(2), 481–495.

Sung, C. M., Jung, T. S., & Park, H. B. (2014). Are serum lipids involved in primary frozen shoulder? A case-control study. *Journal of Bone and Joint Surgery (American), 96*(21), 1828–1833.

Vermeulen, H. M., Obermann, W. R., Burger, B. J., Kok, G. J., Pozing, P. M., & van Den Ende, C. H. (2000). End range mobilization techniques and adhesive capsulitis of the shoulder joint: A multiple subject case report. *Physical Therapy, 80*, 1204–1213.

Wang, W., Shi, M., Zhou, C., et al. (2017). Effectiveness of corticosteroid injections in adhesive capsulitis of shoulder: A meta-analysis. *Medicine (Baltimore), 96*(28), e7529.

CHAPTER 39 QUESTIONS

1. Adhesive capsulitis
   a. Is self-limiting within 6 months of onset
   b. Resolves with short-term NSAID use
   c. Is usually precipitated by a rotator cuff tear
   d. Lasts 15 to 18 months, often with some ongoing limitations

2. Which of the following is the least sensitive for diagnosing adhesive capsulitis?
   a. Ultrasound
   b. MRI
   c. X-ray
   d. Arthrogram

3. **Which of the following does not play a role in the pathogenesis of adhesive capsulitis?**
   a. Hypercholesterolemia
   b. Thyroid disorders
   c. Diabetes mellitus
   d. Hypogonadism

4. **Adhesive capsulitis is most common in____.**
   a. Men 60 to 80 years old
   b. Men 40 to 60 years old
   c. Women 60 to 80 years old
   d. Women 40 to 60 years old

5. **What ultrasound findings are diagnostic for adhesive capsulitis?**
   a. Articular-sided tearing of the bursal cuff
   b. Thickening of glenoid labrum
   c. Thickening of the axillary pouch of 2 mm
   d. Thickening of coracohumeral ligament of 3 mm

6. **Which is true regarding steroid injections for adhesive capsulitis?**
   a. Steroid injections are most effective when given in the recovery (thawing) phase and when coupled with an exercise program.
   b. Steroid injections provide no pain relief.
   c. Steroid injections are best given early in the disease process and when coupled with an exercise program.
   d. Steroid injections provide immediate normalization of ROM.

CHAPTER 40

TOTAL SHOULDER ARTHROPLASTY

O. Oshikoya, MD, PharmD and J.M. Wiater, MD

1. **Who is the typical patient who might undergo total shoulder arthroplasty (TSA)?**
Traditionally the age of the patient who undergoes TSA is 50 to 75 years. Patients with avascular necrosis or posttraumatic arthritis may be as young as 40. Total shoulder arthroplasty includes anatomic and reverse total shoulder arthroplasty. The typical patient who will undergo anatomic total shoulder arthroplasty has glenohumeral arthritis, avascular necrosis, or fracture in the setting of adequate glenoid bone stock and functioning rotator cuff. The typical patient who will undergo reverse total shoulder arthroplasty has rotator cuff tear arthropathy, irreparable rotator cuff tear without osteoarthritis, acute or malunited/nonunited proximal humeral fracture, glenohumeral arthritis, inflammatory arthritis, chronic locked glenohumeral joint dislocation, and revision arthroplasty.

2. **How many anatomic TSAs, reverse TSAs, and hemiarthroplasties are performed each year?**
Recent review using data from the National Inpatient Sample (NIS) of the Healthcare Cost and Utilization Project, Agency for Healthcare Research and Quality demonstrates an overall increase in total shoulder arthroplasties performed annually. Anatomic total shoulders in 2017 totaled 40,665, compared to 29,685 in 2012. Reverse total shoulders increased to 62,705 cases in 2017, up from 22,835 in 2012. The number of shoulder hemiarthroplasty decreased to 4930 in 2017 compared to 11,695 in 2012.

3. **What are the typical indications for TSA?**
Medical indications for TSA include severe proximal humerus fractures, primary osteoarthritis, posttraumatic arthritis, cuff tear arthropathy, inflammatory arthritis, shoulder girdle tumors, osteonecrosis of the humeral head, pseudoparesis caused by rotator cuff deficiency, and failed shoulder arthroplasty. Patients often present with shoulder pain, functional limitations in motion, and radiographic deterioration of the glenohumeral joint. Primary glenohumeral degenerative joint disease presents with central wearing of the humeral head, known as the "Friar Tuck" pattern of central baldness. The glenoid surface wears out primarily on the posterior margin, predisposing the joint to posterior subluxation.

4. **What are the typical contraindications for TSA?**
   - Anatomic Total Shoulder Arthroplasty
     - Active infection
     - Neurologic compromise of either deltoid or rotator cuff musculature
     - Brachial plexus palsy
     - Neurotrophic shoulder
     - Unrealistic expectation of shoulder function after surgery
     - Lack of appropriate motivation to perform rehabilitation program after surgery
   - Reverse Total Shoulder Arthroplasty
     - All of the above including
     - Acromion deficiency
     - Glenoid osteoporosis and insufficiency

5. **What is the difference between hemiarthroplasty, anatomic TSA, and reverse TSA?**
Hemiarthroplasty is the replacement of only the humeral component. This replacement can be stemmed or stemless. A hemiarthroplasty is indicated when the humeral head is deteriorated or fractured but the glenoid surface is intact. Hemiarthroplasty is the surgery of choice if the patient has insufficient glenoid bone to support a glenoid component. When the physical demands are heavy after surgery, such as weight-lifting or manual laborers, a hemiarthroplasty is indicated. Hemiarthroplasty is indicated when arthritis and rotator cuff deficiencies coexist. A badly eroded glenoid cannot stabilize a glenoid component securely, and a nonfunctional rotator cuff produces unbalanced muscular forces on the glenoid, leading to loosening.
Anatomic TSA is the anatomic replacement of both humeral head and glenoid. The humeral component can be stemmed or stemless. The glenoid component is typically minimally constrained and consists of a polyethylene glenoid component. This procedure is undertaken when both joint surfaces are damaged and both are reconstructible. TSA is recommended in patients with osteoarthritis with sufficient glenoid bone stock and intact, well-functioning rotator cuff. Additionally, patients with inflammatory arthritis, osteonecrosis with glenoid involvement, and posttraumatic degenerative joint disease with proximal humerus malunion can be considered for anatomic total shoulder arthroplasty.

Reverse TSA is the nonanatomic replacement of both humeral and glenoid component. The construct uses a convex glenoid hemispheric ball and a concave humeral articulating cup with polyethylene liner. This procedure medializes and distalizes the center of rotation of the joint while increasing the moment arm of the deltoid to power motion. The reverse TSA is preferred in patients with severe rotator cuff deficiency due to concerns for glenoid component loosening when anatomic TSA is used in this patient cohort.

6. **How does a reverse TSA allow a patient with severe rotator cuff deficiency to elevate the arm?**
There are four key principles described by Dr. Paul Grammont and his original reverse prosthesis introduced in 1985. (1) The center of rotation must be fixed, distalized, and medialized to the level of the glenoid surface; (2) the prosthesis must be inherently stable; (3) the lever arm of the deltoid must be effective from the start of movement; and (4) the glenosphere must be large and the humeral cup small to create a semi-constrained articulation. In rotator cuff deficiency, there is a loss of the force couple and the compressive effect on the proximal humerus that is required to initiate forward elevation. As a result of long-standing rotator cuff insufficiency, the proximal humerus migrates cranially decreasing the mechanical advantage of the deltoid muscle. Inferior placement of the center of rotation leads to tensioning of the deltoid and facilitates recruitment of the deltoid to achieve flexion and abduction. Internal and external rotation are initially compromised; however, rotational motion can be improved through tendon transfers and lateralization of the glenosphere. Scapulothoracic motion is significantly increased compared to the native shoulder, where the glenohumeral to scapulothoracic joint motions are 2:1, respectively.

7. **What is the difference between stemmed and stemless shoulder arthroplasty?**
Stemmed arthroplasty involves the implantation of a stemmed humeral component with extensive bone ingrowth or use of a cemented fixation. Long-stem implants typically achieve fixation within the diaphysis of the humerus. Removal of fixed, long-stem prostheses can be difficult in the setting of revision shoulder arthroplasty. Complications of stemmed implants include bone resorption around the proximal portion of the humerus due to stress shielding, osteolysis due to polyethylene microparticles and periprosthetic fracture. Short-stem implants typically achieve fixation within the metaphysis of the humerus. These were designed to reduce the risk of complications caused by long-stem implants. Stemless arthroplasty involves implantation of a stemless humeral component that achieves fixation on the metaphysis of the humeral neck. Stemless designs were pursued to allow for easier revision surgery and to take advantage of the preserved proximal humeral bone to further support the prosthesis. Limitations to stemless prostheses include inability to use in the setting of poor bone quality such as the elderly, where a stemmed prosthesis would be preferred.

8. **Is there a benefit for choosing hemiarthroplasty versus TSA?**
It appears that the TSA is the best option for the treatment of patients with glenohumeral arthritis. Consistent relief of pain and improved function in multiple studies support this statement. There are times when the bone stock of the glenoid cannot support the prosthesis or the deficiency of the rotator cuff requires the use of hemiarthroplasty. Additionally, hemiarthroplasty is preferred in younger patients who are highly active due to concerns regarding early glenoid component loosening. Hemiarthroplasty also is completed quicker and reportedly with less intraoperative blood loss.

9. **What factors and conditions should be present for a person to consider undergoing a TSA or hemiarthroplasty?**
Patients who have failed conservative management should have a functioning deltoid and rotator cuff musculature, demonstrate appropriate motivation toward rehabilitation, and be in sufficient health to undergo major surgical intervention. Patients without erosion of the glenoid have been found to have improved function after a hemiarthroplasty, although anatomic TSA patients have been found to have less pain, better motion, and better strength when compared to hemiarthroplasty. Patients suffering from osteoarthritis or osteonecrosis tend to have higher levels of function after surgery than patients with rheumatoid arthritis and cuff tear arthropathy.

10. **Can a hemiarthroplasty be converted to a TSA if the hemiarthroplasty fails?**
Yes, hemiarthroplasty can be converted to either anatomic or reverse TSA. Usual conversion is to reverse TSA due to violation of the rotator cuff during implantation of the hemiarthroplasty. Reasons for conversion include stiffness, tuberosity malunion or nonunion, rotator cuff tear, instability, progression of glenoid arthritis, infection, and component malpositioning. Patients typically manifest with severe pain and loss of function of the shoulder.

11. **What postoperative complications are associated with anatomic TSA and reverse TSA?**
The incidence of complications after a TSA is approximately 10%. According to Sperling, common complications are due to fractures, infection, anterior and posterior instability with an anatomic prosthesis, rotator cuff tear, and glenoid component loosening. A study published in 2006 found 53 surgical complications on 431 total shoulder arthroplasties (12%). In this study tearing of the rotator cuff accounted for approximately 32% of postoperative complications, fractures for approximately 24%, brachial plexopathy for approximately 15%,

subluxation for approximately 9%, and dislocation for approximately 7%. Humeral loosening, humeral and glenoid loosening, infection, hematoma, and long head of biceps rupture individually accounted for approximately 1% of postoperative complications.

The incidence of complications after a reverse TSA ranges from 15% to 50%. According to Zumstein, common complications are due to scapular notching, instability, infection, glenoid loosening, and scapular fractures. A systematic review in 2011 reviewed 782 cases and identified these most common complications: Scapular notching accounted for 35% of the complications; instability accounted for 5% of the complications; infection and glenoid loosening each accounted for 4% of the complications; and acromion and scapular spine fractures both accounted for 2% of the reverse TSA complications.

12. **What causes components to loosen?**

Symptomatic loosening of glenoid and humerus components occurs in 3.5% of patients with TSA. The many contributing factors include glenoid preparation, soft tissue balancing, wear debris, bone reabsorption, prosthetic design, component geometry, and biomaterials. One major concern is the eccentric load placed on the glenoid component by the humeral component, particularly if the humerus has migrated superiorly. The humerus can migrate superiorly because of rotator cuff tear, poor humeral fixation, and soft tissue imbalance. During arm elevation the eccentric load of a proximal migrated humeral component can produce a “rocking horse” effect on the glenoid component that loosens the glenoid component.

13. **What are the postoperative goals after TSA?**

The primary goal is to relieve pain while implanting a stable construct to motion. Approximately 90% of patients report no or slight pain after hemiarthroplasty or TSA. The secondary goal is to restore normal function, specifically shoulder range of motion, upper extremity strength, smooth motion between prosthetic components, prosthesis and bone interface, and smooth motion between proximal humerus, rotator cuff, and rotator cuff outlet.

14. **How long does a TSA last?**

Failure of prosthesis was defined as need for reoperation or patient dissatisfaction in a multicenter study of 470 cases of TSA. This study reported that, at 5-year follow-up, 3% of the procedures had failed. A smaller study of 53 operations, using similar criteria, reported that, at 11-year follow-up, 27% had failed. A study of 29 patients who had surgery at the age of 50 or younger revealed that 84% of the TSA prostheses were still intact 20 years postoperatively, with approximately 50% of these patients reporting satisfactory or better results.

Flurin et al. published their survivorship results in 2020. There were 778 procedures performed, including anatomic and reverse TSA. Both constructs demonstrated similar survivorship at 8 years. Anatomic TSA survivorship was 98.5% and 96% at 2 and 8 years, respectively. Reverse TSA survivorship was 98.7% and 96% at 2 and 8 years, respectively.

15. **How much pain, function, and motion improvement is expected after hemiarthroplasty, TSA, or reverse TSA?**

Recent publications have demonstrated that all of these procedures can produce improvements in function, decrease pain, and improve range of motion. For total shoulder arthroplasties at an average of 31.4 months' follow-up, 73 patients were found to have an average pain reduction on the numerical pain rating scale (NPRS) of 6 points out of a 10-point scale. Several different functional scales are used to assess patients undergoing a TSA, but, overall, the typical patient reports approximately 40% of normal function before surgery and improves to approximately 80% to 90% of normal function after surgery and rehabilitation. Active elevation improved approximately 42 degrees and external rotation 36 degrees.

Hemiarthroplasties at an average of 24 months' follow-up were found to have an average pain reduction on the McGill pain visual analog scale of 51 points out of 100 points. Several different functional scales are used to assess patients undergoing a hemiarthroplasty, but, overall, the typical patient reports approximately 30% to 40% of normal function before surgery and improves to approximately 70% to 80% of normal function after surgery and rehabilitation. Forward elevation has been seen to improve up to 50 degrees and external rotation 20 degrees after hemiarthroplasty.

In a study by Jobin, patients after primary reverse TSA at an average of 16 months' follow-up were found to have an average improvement in their American Shoulder and Elbow Surgeons pain and function score, which improved by 44% from 24 to 69 on a 100-point scale. Active forward elevation improved from 38 degrees to 144 degrees while active external rotation at side improved from 11 degrees to 23 degrees. Active external rotation with arm abducted improved on average from 18 degrees to 44 degrees.

16. **Can a patient participate in sports after TSA?**

Yes, most patients are able to return to sports after shoulder arthroplasty. Anatomic TSA has the highest rate of return. A systematic review and meta-analysis by Liu et al. looked at 944 patients (506 athletes) treated with shoulder arthroplasty. Average follow-up was 5.1 years. The most common sports were swimming, golf, fitness sports, and tennis. Overall rate of return to sport was 85.1%, including 72.3% returning to an equivalent or improved level of play after 1 to 36 months. Patients with anatomic TSA returned at a significantly higher rate (92.6%) compared to reverse TSA (74.9%) and hemiarthroplasty (71.1%).

The patient should be counseled by the physician and therapist that activities that expose the patient to high-impact events are not recommended because of the potential trauma to the prosthesis. However, sports such as swimming, bowling, dancing, and bicycling should be resumed when appropriate healing has occurred.

17. What is meant by limited-goal rehabilitation? To what type of patient is it applied?

Limited-goal rehabilitation is meant for patients who have deficient rotator cuff and deltoid musculature and significant bone deficiency that does not tolerate the typical rehabilitation program. Patients having long-standing rheumatoid arthritis; rotator cuff arthropathy and some revision arthroplasties may fall into this category. The focuses of limited-goal rehabilitation are pain relief and stability. The shoulder functions primarily at the side with elevation restricted at or below 100 degrees and external rotation of 20 degrees.

18. What are typical rehabilitation protocols for anatomic total shoulder arthroplasty?

Reverse total shoulder arthroplasty?

The main tenet of shoulder rehabilitation involves early joint protection with progressive functional mobilization and strengthening. For anatomic total shoulder arthroplasty, much of the focus with respect to rehabilitation is directed toward the balance of subscapularis protection and shoulder mobilization. There is no consensus on type and duration of sling immobilization. Options include simple sling, shoulder immobilizer, or abduction sling. Duration ranges from <24 hours to 6 weeks. Baumgarten et al. looked at neutral rotation sling versus internal rotation sling for 6 weeks after subscapularis tenotomy and found that the neutral rotation cohort had significantly better range of motion over time. The neutral rotation group had better active and passive external rotation and passive horizontal adduction long term, as well as significantly less night pain at 2 weeks. No long-term differences in pain were found. Biomechanical data suggest that having restrictions to external rotation and abduction following shoulder arthroplasty may be beneficial for decreasing strains on the repaired subscapularis. Limited evidence suggests that early motion may adversely influence healing rates after lesser tuberosity osteotomy. Strengthening is important to reestablish muscular balance through periscapular and rotator cuff strengthening. This becomes essential for the longevity of the prosthesis; however, strengthening is often delayed to allow for adequate healing of the subscapularis.

For reverse total shoulder arthroplasty, the biomechanics are altered and rely more heavily on deltoid and periscapular function than the anatomic total shoulder arthroplasty. There is similarly no consensus on the type and duration of sling use. Early instability is a more substantial concern after reverse than after anatomic total shoulder arthroplasty. Regarding initiation and progression of passive or active motion, there is no consensus. Important factors to consider include whether the subscapularis was repaired, risk of instability, and concern for early acromial stress reaction. Strengthening focusing on scapulothoracic and deltoid rehabilitation is critical for function. Most studies indicate waiting until at least 8 weeks postoperatively to start a strengthening regimen.

19. Describe the technique of early passive motion (EPM).

EPM, as described by Neer, begins on the second day postoperatively. The patient takes an appropriate pain medication 45 minutes before EPM and applies dry or moist heat to relax the muscles. The patient performs pendulum exercises forward, backward, and in circles with the muscle relaxed like a rag doll. The patient sits or lies in a recumbent position while the surgeon or therapist slowly elevates the relaxed arm in the scapular plane, applying slight traction. Observation of patient's face and constant communication with the patient are mandatory to assess pain during the exercise. Patients are reminded frequently to relax as the arm is elevated to maximal levels. This maneuver is repeated three to five times twice daily. The point of maximal elevation, based on the surgical procedure, should be determined by the surgeon and communicated to the therapist. Typically, passive external rotation is also started with the arm at the side. Because of the recent changes in health care, exercises often are started on day 1 postoperatively and must be taught to a family member because of early discharge.

20. Is all passive elevation the same?

No. Passive elevation in the supine position produces less electromyographic (EMG) activity in shoulder musculature than passive elevation in the upright position. Minimal EMG activity has been recorded in the supraspinatus, infraspinatus, and anterior deltoid during supine self-assisted and helper-assisted elevation. However, more EMG activity is noted in the supraspinatus, infraspinatus, and anterior deltoid during passive elevation in an upright position using a pulley or a stick.

21. What is the Neer-phased rehabilitation program?

Charles Neer popularized three phases of shoulder rehabilitation for TSA, hemiarthroplasty, and rotator cuff repairs. **Phase I** consists primarily of passive motion exercises, including passive movement of the involved arm by a therapist or family member. Phase I also incorporates the use of assist devices such as rope and pulley, stick, or tabletop to aid the patient in performing passive and active assisted exercises independently.

Phase II consists primarily of active motion exercises. The patient progresses from active assisted to active exercises without assistive devices. The treating clinician must respect healing time frames and incorporate creative techniques to regain coordinated active range of motion.

Phase III consists of resistive exercises. Use of resistive devices, such as light weights and rubber tubing, is incorporated to regain shoulder strength.

22. **Why do some patients need abduction pillows and others do not?**
The surgical repair and status of the rotator cuff musculature dictate the necessity of an abduction pillow or splint postoperatively. The surgeon examines the quality of the soft tissues during the operation and at closure decides whether excessive tension is placed on the rotator cuff tendons with the arm at the side. Patients with undue tension with the arm at the side or poor tissue may be placed in an abduction splint to reduce stress on the compromised structures and allow for healing.

23. **What are the standard precautions after TSA and reverse TSA?**
Each surgery is different, and communication with the surgeon is critical. Events during surgery must be communicated to the therapist to ensure postoperative rehabilitation that enhances rather than damages the repair. However, some standard precautions are recommended. Self-transfers and ambulation with crutches should be avoided until adequate strength is regained (often about 6 months). If the patient is suffering from osteoarthritis, therapists are urged to avoid cardinal plane flexion activities because posterior glenoid wear is common and may predispose the patient to posterior subluxation. Patients undergoing TSA because of arthritis from previous dislocations may have weak deltoid and/or unstable joints, which may delay the resistive exercise phase. Patients with rheumatoid arthritis often have weak or torn rotator cuff tissues and proceed slowly through rehabilitation; they need frequent verbal reinforcement. Patients undergoing TSA because of rotator cuff tear arthropathy, congenital defects, neoplasm, and Erb's palsy deformity most commonly fall into the limited-goal rehabilitation program.
Reverse TSA carries specific precautions. Most important, the reverse TSA is at great risk for dislocation; therefore, the patient must be made aware of positions of potential dislocation to avoid overstretching the anterior tissue of the subscapularis and anterior capsule. Instruct the patient to avoid internal rotation or hyperextension of the involved shoulder. The patient should not use the involved arm to assist in transfers from bed or chair.

24. **What are typical outcomes for reverse total shoulder prosthesis?**
Pain improves although it may not be completely eliminated because several studies have shown pain to decrease by 3 to 8 points. Active forward arm elevation usually improves to between 100 and 150 degrees. Function improves by a range between 30% and 50% on the American Shoulder and Elbow Surgeons Score (ASES) and Simple Shoulder Test (SST) scores. Complication rates are quite variable from 7% to 75% because of surgeon inexperience, prosthetic design, surgical technique, and case complexity. These include dislocation, infection, nerve palsy, glenoid loosening, humeral loosening, failure of the glenosphere to properly seat, glenoid fracture, polyethylene wear, and humeral osteolysis

Bibliography

Bacle, G., Nové-Josserand, L., Garaud, P., & Walch, G. (2017). Long-term outcomes of reverse total shoulder arthroplasty: A follow-up of a previous study. *Journal of Bone and Joint Surgery, 99*(6), 454–461.

Berliner, J. L., Regalado-Magdos, A., Ma, C. B., & Feeley, B. T. (2015). Biomechanics of reverse total shoulder arthroplasty. *Journal of Shoulder and Elbow Surgery, 24*(1), 150–160.

Best, M. J., Aziz, K. T., Wilckens, J. H., McFarland, E. G., & Srikumaran, U. (2021). Increasing incidence of primary reverse and anatomic total shoulder arthroplasty in the United States. *Journal of Shoulder and Elbow Surgery, 30*(5), 1159–1166.

Bishop, J. Y., & Flatow, E. L. (2005). Humeral head replacement versus total shoulder arthroplasty: Clinical outcomes—a review. *Journal of Shoulder and Elbow Surgery, 14*(1 Suppl), s141–s146.

Boileau, P., Watkinson, D. J., Harzidakis, A. M., & Balg, F. (2005). Grammont reverse prosthesis: Design, rationale, and biomechanics. *Journal of Shoulder and Elbow Surgery, 14*(1 Suppl), s147–s161.

Brems, J. J. (1994). Rehabilitation following total shoulder arthroplasty. *Clinical Orthopaedics, 307*, 70–85.

Carroll, R. M., Izquierdo, R., Vazques, M., Blaine, T. A., Levine, W. N., & Bigliani, L. U. (2004). Conversion of painful hemiarthroplasty to total shoulder arthroplasty: Long- term results. *Journal of Shoulder and Elbow Surgery, 13*(6), 599–603.

Chin, P. Y., Sperling, J. W., Cofield, R. H., & Schleck, C. (2006). Complications of total shoulder arthroplasty: Are they fewer or different? *Journal of Shoulder and Elbow Surgery, 15*(1), 19–22.

Cuff, D., Pupello, D., Virani, N., Levy, J., & Frankle, M. (2008). Reverse shoulder arthroplasty for the treatment of rotator cuff deficiency. *Journal of Bone and Joint Surgery, 90*(6), 1244–1251.

Cuomo, F., & Checroun, A. (1998). Avoiding pitfalls and complications in total shoulder arthroplasty. *Orthopedic Clinics of North America, 29*, 507–518.

Day, J., Paxton, E. S., Lau, E., Abboud, J., Gordon, V., & Williams, G. R. (2015). Utilization of reverse total shoulder arthroplasties in the Medicare population (abstract). *Orthopedic Research Society Annual Meeting, 24*(5), 766–772.

Familiari, F., Rojas, J., Doral, M. N., Huri, G., & McFarland, E. G. (2018). Reverse total shoulder arthroplasty. *EFORT Open Reviews, 3*, 58–69.

Flurin, P. -H., Marczuk, Y., Janout, M., Wright, T. W., Zuckerman, J., & Roche, C. P. (2013). Comparison of outcomes using anatomic and reverse total shoulder. *Bulletin of the Hospital for Joint Disease, 71*(2 Suppl), 101–107.

Flurin, P. H., Tams, C., Simovitch, R. W., et al. (2020). Comparison of survivorship and performance of a platform shoulder system in anatomic and reverse total shoulder arthroplasty. *JSES International*, *4*(4), 923–928.

Frankle, M., Siegal, S., Pupello, D., Saleem, A., Mighell, M., & Vasey, M. (2005). The reverse shoulder prosthesis for glenohumeral arthritis associated with severe rotator cuff deficiency: A minimum two-year follow-up study of sixty patients. *Journal of Bone and Joint Surgery*, *87*(8), 1697–1705.

Goetti, P., Denard, P. J., Collin, P., Ibrahim, M., Mazzolari, A., & Lädermann, A. (2021). Biomechanics of anatomic and reverse shoulder arthroplasty. *EFORT Open Reviews*, *6*(10), 918–931.

Healy, W. L., Iorio, R., & Lemos, M. J. (2001). Athletic activity after joint replacement. *American Journal of Sports Medicine*, *29*(3), 377–388.

Hettrich, C. M., Weldon, E., Boorman, R. S., Parsons, I. M., & Matsen, F. A. (2004). Preoperative factors associated with improvements in shoulder function after humeral hemiarthroplasty. *Journal of Bone and Joint Surgery*, *86*(7), 1446–1451.

Jobin, C. M., Brown, G. D., Bahu, M. J., Gardner, T. R., Bigliani, L. U., Levine, W. N., & Ahmad, C. S. (2012). Reverse total shoulder arthroplasty for cuff tear arthropathy; the clinical effect of deltoid lengthening and center of rotation medicalization. *Journal of Shoulder and Elbow Surgery*, *21*(10), 1269–1277.

Kelley, M. J., & Ramsey, M. J. (2000). Osteoarthritis and traumatic arthritis of the shoulder. *Journal of Hand Therapy*, *13*(2), 148–162.

Kim, S. H., Wise, B. L., Zhang, Y., & Szabo, R. M. (2011). Increasing incidence of shoulder arthroplasty in the United States. *Journal of Bone and Joint Surgery*, *93*(24), 2249–2254.

Kirsch, J. M., & Namdari, S. (2020). Rehabilitation after anatomic and reverse total shoulder arthroplasty: A critical analysis review. *JBJS Reviews*, *8*(2), e0129.

Liu, J. N., Steinhaus, M. E., Garcia, G. H., et al. (2018). Return to sport after shoulder arthroplasty: A systematic review and meta-analysis. *Knee Surgery, Sports Traumatology, Arthroscopy*, *26*, 100–112.

Lo, I. K., Litchfield, R. B., Griffin, S., Faber, K., Patterson, S. D., & Kirkley, A. (2005). Quality-of-life outcome following hemiarthroplasty or total shoulder arthroplasty in patients with osteoarthritis. A prospective, randomized trial. *Journal of Bone and Joint Surgery*, *87*(10), 2178–2185.

Matsen, F. A., Rockwood, C. A., Wirth, M. A., & Lippitt, S. B. (1998). Glenohumeral arthritis and its management. In C. A. Rockwood & F. A. Matsen (Eds.), *The shoulder* (2nd ed., pp. 840–964). Philadelphia, PA: W.B. Saunders.

McCann, P. D., Wootten, M. E., Kadaba, M. P., & Bigliani, L. U. (1993). A kinematic and electromyographic study of shoulder rehabilitation exercises. *Clinical Orthopaedics and Related Research*, *288*, 179–188.

Mehlko, M. J., & Fink, M. L. (2012). Reverse total shoulder arthroplasty versus shoulder hemiarthroplasty in patients with rotator cuff arthropathy: A literature review. *Orthopaedic Physical Therapy Practice*, *24*(3), 138–141.

Neer, C. S. (1990). *Shoulder reconstruction*. Philadelphia, PA: W.B. Saunders.

Orfaly, R. M., Rockwood, C. A., Esenyel, C. Z., & Wirth, M. A. (2003). A prospective functional outcome study of shoulder arthroplasty for osteoarthritis with an intact rotator cuff. *Journal of Shoulder and Elbow Surgery*, *12*(3), 214–221.

Shin, Y.-S., Lee, W.-S., & Won, J.-S. (2021). Comparison of stemless and conventional stemmed shoulder arthroplasties in shoulder arthropathy. *Medicine*, *100*(6), e23989.

Singh, J. A., Sperling, J., Buchbinder, R., & McMaken, K. (2011). Surgery for shoulder osteoarthritis: A Cochrane systematic review. *Journal of Rheumatology*, *38*(4), 598–605.

Smith, K. L., & Matsen, F. A., III. (1998). Total shoulder arthroplasty versus hemiarthroplasty: Current trends. *Orthopedic Clinics of North America*, *29*, 491–506.

Sperling, J. W., Cofield, R. H., & Rowland, C. M. (2004). Minimum fifteen-year follow- up of Neer hemiarthroplasty and total shoulder arthroplasty in patients aged fifty years or younger. *Journal of Shoulder and Elbow Surgery*, *13*(6), 604–613.

Sperling, J. W., Hawkins, R. J., Walch, G., & Zuckerman, J. D. (2013). Complications in total shoulder arthroplasty. *Journal of Bone and Joint Surgery*, *95*(6), 563–569.

Walker, M., Willis, M. P., Brooks, J. P., Pupello, D., Mulieri, P. J., & Frankle, M. A. (2012). The use of the reverse shoulder arthroplasty for treatment of failed total shoulder arthroplasty. *Journal of Shoulder and Elbow Surgery/American Shoulder and Elbow Surgeons*, *21*(4), 514–522.

Wiater, M. J., & Fabing, M. H. (2009). Shoulder arthroplasty: Prosthetic options and indications. *JAAOS-Journal of the American Academy of Orthopaedic Surgeons*, *17*(7), 415–425.

Wierks, C., Skolasky, R. L., Ji, J. H., & McFarland, E. G. (2009). Reverse total shoulder replacement: Intraoperative and early postoperative complications. *Clinical Orthopaedics and Related Research*, *467*(1), 225–234.

Zumstein, M. A., Pinedo, M., Old, J., & Boileau, P. (2011). Problems, complications, reoperations, and revisions in reverse total shoulder arthroplasties; a systematic review. *Journal of Shoulder and Elbow Surgery*, *20*(4), 146–157.

CHAPTER 40 QUESTIONS

1. **Which arthroplasty is associated with the highest return to sporting activities?**
   a. Resection arthroplasty
   b. Hemiarthroplasty
   c. Anatomic total shoulder arthroplasty
   d. Reverse total shoulder arthroplasty

2. **The center of rotation of a reverse total shoulder arthroplasty is ________ compared to the native shoulder?**
   a. Medialized
   b. Lateralized
   c. Superior
   d. Unchanged

3. **Phase III of the Neer-phased rehabilitation program consists of which of the following?**
   a. Primarily active range of motion exercises
   b. Primarily passive range of motion exercises
   c. Primarily resistive exercises
   d. Primarily active assistive range of motion exercises

4. **Tearing of the rotator cuff accounts for approximately _______ % of total shoulder complications.**
   a. 32
   b. 42
   c. 66
   d. 50

5. **Complications following reverse total shoulder arthroplasty range from 7% to 75%. Which of the following helps explain this large variation?**
   a. Surgeon inexperience
   b. Prosthetic design
   c. Case complexity
   d. All of the above

6. **Phase II of the Neer-phased rehabilitation program consists of which of the following?**
   a. Primarily active range of motion exercises
   b. Primarily passive range of motion exercises
   c. Primarily resistive exercises
   d. Primarily active assistive range of motion exercises

ACROMIOCLAVICULAR AND STERNOCLAVICULAR INJURIES: EVALUATION AND TREATMENT

T.R. Malone, EdD, MS, BS and A.L. Pfeifle, EdD, PT

ACROMIOCLAVICULAR (AC)

1. **What is the typical mechanism of injury?**
   The most common mechanism of acromioclavicular (AC) injury is a direct force as seen when an individual is driven into the ground with their arm adducted against the body. This occurs very often in athletic events involving a tackling or catching activity. In these situations, the acromion is driven "downward or inferiorly," with resultant ligament disruption. The location and number of ligaments affected are directly related to the level of force, with both the acromioclavicular and the coracoclavicular complexes at risk.
   A secondary mechanism of acromioclavicular injury can occur with an indirect force, as seen when an individual falls on an outstretched hand, generating an impact load at the acromion through the humeral head. This injury is typically to the acromioclavicular capsule/ligaments alone.
   Acromioclavicular injury occurs far more commonly in men than women and in the relatively young as opposed to the elder population. Acromioclavicular injuries are approximately four or five times more prevalent than SC injuries.

2. **What is the common descriptor for acromioclavicular joint injury?**
   The common name for this injury is "shoulder separation." Athletes often will refer to the joint as being "separated."

3. **What does this joint look like and what do these shapes allow?**
   The acromioclavicular joint is diarthrodial, with fibrocartilage surfaces. The facet (surface) shapes include a convex clavicle and a concave acromion. An interesting addition to the joint is the intraarticular fibrocartilaginous disc that is interposed between the surfaces and can be viewed as being meniscus like. This disc commonly degenerates during the third and fourth decades of life. Some patients are able to displace their disc into a superior "dislocated" position and voluntarily reduce the structure. Patients must be instructed not to do this as over time the disc can become resistant to reduction, even to the point of not reducing at all!
   The acromioclavicular joint, in concert with the sternoclavicular joint, allows the clavicle to serve as a crankshaft, keeping the arm in a functional position in relation to the body. The clavicle rotates early and late during abduction and elevation actions of the humerus.

4. **What are the ligaments supporting/controlling the acromioclavicular joint?**
   The acromioclavicular ligaments (superior and inferior) reinforce the joint capsule proper. The primary role of these structures is to control horizontal movements of the clavicle. The superior portion is likewise reinforced by the insertional fibers of the deltoid and trapezius muscles. When very large energy injury occurs, damage may include rupture of these insertions and make reduction of the clavicle impossible—these injuries are the 4 to 6 level of involvement.
   Vertical stability of the clavicle (acromioclavicular joint) is controlled by the coracoclavicular ligaments (conoid and trapezoid). The conoid lies medially, runs posteriorly, and is triangular in shape while the trapezoid is lateral, of the sagittal plane, and is quadrilateral in shape.
   The orientation of these coracoclavicular ligaments is critical to controlling the rotation of the clavicle to enable full elevation of the arm.
   In review: horizontal stability is controlled by the acromioclavicular structures (by contrast, coracoclavicular structures control vertical stability).

5. **What is the acute presentation of the patient with an acromioclavicular injury?**
   The individual will often "cradle" the involved arm by grasping and supporting the elbow with the uninvolved hand. This reduces the pull of the weight of the arm inferiorly and also somewhat stabilizes the arm to the trunk.

6. **What radiographs are taken to diagnose acromioclavicular injuries?**
   These patients are sometimes radiographed in loaded (weighted) and unloaded patterns to outline the level of clavicle displacement. The key to this is that the weight must be suspended from the arm not allowing muscular

actions. A second key to obtaining appropriate views of the acromioclavicular joint is for the intensity of the exposure to be decreased since overexposure will occur with normal intensities. (Bone is dense–joint space and muscle are not!)

Special angles have been used to better delineate the joint space as the normal AP view provides a superimposition of the joint onto the spine of the scapula. Zanca recommends a 10 to 15 degree superior angulation view while other modifications include a scapulolateral view (Alexander). The visualization of the coracoid is best provided by a supine notch view (Stryker).

The need for most imaging studies is somewhat in question. The primary question that the surgeon must ask is: "Will the results of this study change the treatment for this patient?" If the answer is no … probably shouldn't be getting the imaging! In special circumstances and severe injuries, the radiographs may be very useful to delineate care.

7. **How are acromioclavicular injuries classified?**
Since acromioclavicular injury may include two ligament complexes, the classification scheme is somewhat complex. Rather than the normal first-, second-, and third-degree pattern with specific ligamentous implications, the acromioclavicular scheme incorporates this but with modifications reflecting the horizontal and vertical motions. It also adds the rare extreme vertical displacement injuries as types IV–VI. Table 41.1 contains a summary of this scheme.

8. **What is the treatment for type I acromioclavicular injuries?**
These patients have no instability as they have less than third-degree injury to the acromioclavicular ligament complex. Thus the first key to treatment is not to require immobilization. The patient will complain of local tenderness at the acromioclavicular joint proper. We recommend the use of ice for pain modulation and return to activity as comfortably tolerated. If their activity exposes them to contact/impact forces, we use a pad placed over the shoulder made in a "donut format." The pad is designed to allow impact to be distributed around the

Table 41.1 Acromioclavicular Injury Classification

TYPE	CLINICAL FINDINGS	INSTABILITY	X-RAY FINDINGS
Type I: first-degree sprain of acromioclavicular ligaments	Mild to moderate pain at acromioclavicular joint, general movement is pain free; tender to palpation	None; minimal ligament damage	
Type II: second- and third-degree sprain of acromioclavicular ligaments; first- and second-degree sprain of coracoclavicular ligaments	Moderate to severe pain at both acromioclavicular joint and coracoclavicular interspace; limited function	Definite horizontal instability; possible slight change in vertical stability	Slight elevation of clavicle
Type III: third-degree sprain of acromioclavicular and coracoclavicular ligaments	High-riding clavicle; exquisite pain; unable to use UE, often cradling affected arm with unaffected extremity	Acromioclavicular (horizontal) and coracoclavicular (vertical) instability;	25%–100% increase in coracoclavicular space
Type IV, V, and VI (variations of type III—clavicle may be prevented from freely being positioned—it is caught or blocked into a position)	Severe pain and limited function; extreme "drooping" of the involved upper extremity	Horizontal and vertical (surgical intervention is directed to restoration of ligamentous complexes and muscular insertions)	Severe displacement of the clavicle as follows: Type IV: superior and posterior displacement of the clavicle Type V: superior displacement Type VI: clavicle is displaced inferior to the coracoid (subcoracoid dislocation)

acromioclavicular joint rather than onto it. We often use an oblong dense foam base with the center removed (area of the AC) and covered by thermoplastic material (taped in place). If used in athletic event, we then cover the thermoplastic surface with temper foam to protect others. If the activity has a shoulder pad, you should make a set of these pads and place a protective donut under the pads bilaterally to not enable the possible concentration of loading to one side of the athlete.

9. **What is the treatment for type II acromioclavicular injuries?**
Type II injured patients are quite uncomfortable on acute presentation. If the acromioclavicular ligament complex is disrupted (third degree) the patient will have horizontal instability. The coracoclavicular ligaments are intact (with first- or second-degree ligament injury), thus vertical stability is present, but the joint is painful if stressed. Left to their own devices, we see these folks placing their involved hand in a pocket or pants top/belt to support the weight of the arm. A sling can be used for comfort but does not require the use of special "AC immobilizing units," as there is no vertical component in these patients and the more limited treatment approach results in the same outcome.

Patients typically use a sling as desired and apply ice as a pain modulator. ROM exercises are initiated on an as-tolerated basis often beginning in a passive form to minimize muscle activation of the trapezius and deltoid groups. An exercise program that is designed to fit the individual patient's needs includes functional progression. If the patient's activity is such that the shoulder will be exposed to impact forces, the aforementioned donut pad should be used as they return to function. Specific strengthening exercises may be required dependent on patient activities. The deltoid and trapezius fibers do reinforce the acromioclavicular joint capsule and are thus often a part of the long-term rehabilitation program. Usually, the athlete can return to full function within 2 to 3 weeks of the injury.

10. **What is the treatment of type III acromioclavicular injuries?**
Controversy: To operate or not–That is the question!

There has been some controversy as to the most appropriate treatment for these patients. Surgical techniques have been used to address the disrupted ligament complexes. (Both the acromioclavicular and coracoclavicular complexes have sustained third-degree injury–horizontal and vertical instability.) The surgery is made more difficult since the more simplistic solutions do not recognize the three-dimensional aspects of the ligaments and their relationships to the clavicle. Surgeons have attempted to pull or stabilize the clavicle downward often to the coracoid via metal plates/screws, Dacron tape, suture/suture anchors, wire, or pins. These procedures were often described as "nonanatomic" and the results have been mixed. Complications of these procedures have included infection, pin breakage, pin/wire migration, and resection of the clavicle or coracoid as the wire cut through the bone. These factors led orthopaedists to create more anatomic surgical procedures designed to recreate the original dual ligament nature of the coracoclavicular complex. These surgeries require a precise placement into the clavicle and are challenging in the attempt to duplicate the conoid and trapezoid ligaments orientation and structure. Even after surgery, residual acromioclavicular joint deformity or discomfort can occur with either nonanatomic or anatomic procedures. Early postoperative management often includes 4 to 6 weeks of immobilization postsurgical intervention and a rehabilitation program thereafter. Functional outcomes for patients following these procedures appear to be quite similar to those obtained through nonsurgical management. Hence the treatment today continues to be more often directed toward nonsurgical patterns but with anatomic reconstruction becoming the surgery of choice particularly as it can be done long term rather than requiring it be acute.

Conservative management is very much like that for the second-degree acromioclavicular injury, but with a greater reliance on an immobilizing support device as there is vertical instability. Because there is associated vertical instability, a residual step deformity will remain at the distal clavicle, even after "healing" is complete. Fortunately, it is rare that this deformity becomes a disability and function is typically nearly equal in the patient managed without surgery compared to the operatively managed patient. Since disability is most likely a problem in those individuals exposing the arm to high-intensity demands, surgeons will consider surgical treatment under those conditions. However, it is becoming relatively rare for surgical intervention to be used acutely. The surgical treatment is more often used in type IV, V, and VI injuries, as the displacement is severe with significant muscle tissue disruption and the clavicle is not able to freely be positioned.

11. **What is the initial treatment for significant (type III or greater) acromioclavicular injuries?**
Reduction and maintenance for comfort is the rule. Because the type IV, V, and VI injuries may be surgically corrected, physician follow-up is important. Although the stated treatment is reduction, the reality is for the arm to be immobilized or supported in a sling, but true reduction is not maintained. Devices have been designed that pull the humerus superiorly and the clavicle inferiorly, but their success is minimal related to lack of patient compliance. (Let's be honest: Would you wear it 24/7? They don't either!) The most commonly used device was the Kenny Howard harness, which incorporates this combination. Reality: The outcome of treatment with a harness as opposed to benign neglect is very similar, but more importantly equal to or better than surgical long-term results.

12. **What can be done to minimize or prevent acromioclavicular injuries?**
As mentioned previously, the donut pad can be used to distribute loads around the acromioclavicular joint rather than on it. This can be accomplished through wearing "pads" or some type of device over the shoulders. In sports where tackling is the rule, shoulder pads are frequently worn. As described previously, one of the key rules is that if you place a donut pad under one side, it is important to also "pad" the uninjured side so as not to alter shoulder pad alignment. Athletes wear a shell under their shoulder pads, which can be seen as donut padding each acromioclavicular joint prophylactically. It should be noted that shoulder pads work via a cantilever design that enables forces to be placed onto the anterior and posterior thorax rather than the underlying area. This requires the pads to be fit properly and stabilized to the thorax. (This is precisely what often does not happen in high school athletes!)

13. **What are the long-term consequences of acromioclavicular injury?**
Patients will often develop a step deformity at the acromioclavicular joint where the clavicle appears to sit higher on the affected than on the normal side. In addition, the patient may experience some pain with high demand activity. (Personal note: Cross-country skiing with the "high poles" is a great way to irritate these unhappy joints!) Interestingly, it is relatively rare to experience significant disability even with an obvious deformity. Patients will see long-term arthritis of the joint but again with limited symptoms. In fact, postsurgical patients have similar long-term outcomes.

14. **What can be done for the patient who has pain associated with weight lifting?**
Pain with weight lifting is a common complaint in the athlete with a previous acromioclavicular injury. The wide grip bench press is the primary culprit for this pain. Another exercise that should be avoided is the anterior fly type maneuver, which replicates the cross-arm adduction test for acromioclavicular pain/provocation.
It is accepted that athletes hesitate to go to a more narrow grip during weight lifting as it decreases the maximal load that can be used during bench press. This is not particularly desirable, even though it often does provide significant pain relief. Antiinflammatories, local ice applications pre/postexercise, and exercise modification can be used successfully in some select patients. In other patients, there will not be a successful outcome of treatment, due to an established osteolysis of the distal clavicle. The continued wide grip bench press literally enables them to delete their distal clavicles but creates chronic acromioclavicular dysfunction.

15. **What other athletes are prone to acromioclavicular problems?**
Racquet and throwing athletes may develop acromioclavicular symptoms related to their activities. They may exhibit symptoms on follow-through (cross-arm motions) as well as during weight training involving wide grip bench press, dips, or cross-arm fly maneuvers. Partial ROM (restricted ranges) during weight training and decreased maximal effort and repetitions of throwing can also be helpful.

16. **What options are there for the patient who continues to complain of acromioclavicular pain during rehabilitation?**
First, the patient should be evaluated to determine if the pain is linked to specific exercise, posture, or activity. If it is either due to exercise or position linked, modifications can be made, much like the grip alteration described in Question 14. If little improvement occurs with exercise modification or positional change, an arthritic acromioclavicular joint is suspected. In those cases that respond poorly to rehabilitation, joint injection may be the best approach. This has been associated with significant success when it facilitates the advancement of rehabilitation, such as when the patient needs assistance to "get past a tough point" in management.

17. **What type of strengthening program is used with acromioclavicular injuries?**
The muscular training sequence has limited impact on these patients unless a significant level of disuse or immobility has been imposed. The program includes trapezius and deltoid exercise with both concentric and eccentric patterns. One major caveat is that the exercises must be executed pain free and cross-arm adduction should be minimized. The general balanced shoulder approach of rotations and functional patterns is the rule.

18. **What is the surgical procedure of choice for arthritic acromioclavicular disability?**
Physicians will often perform an excision of the distal clavicle for the patient with recalcitrant pain and disability of the acromioclavicular joint. The Mumford procedure is designed to remove approximately 0.5 to 2 cm (1/4–3/4 of an inch) of the distal clavicle, which prevents "impingement" of this structure with crossed arm movements. Rehabilitation after following the procedure is directed toward pain modulation and support for the first 10 to 14 days, followed by a functional progression related to the specific needs of the patient. Patients should not push too hard in the immediate postoperative period as it has a tendency to maintain the "inflamed state" resulting in greater pain and prolonged recovery. This is particularly true when attempting to do early aggressive abduction/elevation tasks at or above 90 degrees. It is generally best to wait until 10 to 14 days postoperatively to begin aggressive rehabilitation.

19. **Is there a role for acromioclavicular joint mobilizations?**
Acromioclavicular mobilization can be successfully used with patients presenting with decreased "elevation" and limited crossed arm motion (horizontal adduction). These are usually performed from behind, using the horizontally placed thumb to move the clavicle forward. In this mobilization, the therapist should maintain as much contact with the distal clavicle as possible so as to minimize the "point" of pressure. The arm is supported on a plinth or tabletop as the mobilization is performed. Significant improvements in range of motion may occur following this procedure.

STERNOCLAVICULAR (SC)

1. **What is the typical mechanism of sternoclavicular injury?**
Sternoclavicular (SC) injury is relatively rare but does occur through direct trauma, as seen when an athlete falls or sustains an impact with direct force to the clavicle via impact collision with another participant or hard surface such as a goalpost or equipment. The more common method of SC injury is an indirect force seen as when someone lying on their side loads (gets piled onto!) the upper shoulder, causing a loading force as it is "rolled or pushed" and resulting in compression with either anterior or posterior movement. Anterior injuries are more common than posterior, with posterior dislocation being very rare but possibly having serious implications.
These injuries occur relatively infrequently but are far more common in men than women and more common in the relatively young than the older population. Acromioclavicular injuries occur four or five times more frequently than sternoclavicular injuries.

2. **What does the sternoclavicular joint look like and what movements does it allow?**
The sternoclavicular joint is similar to the acromioclavicular joint, as it also contains a meniscus-like disc. The articulating surfaces of the sternum and clavicle are typically incongruent, such that the disc becomes the contact surface of the joint. The actual joint surfaces are saddle shaped and utilize the disc independently to enable unique actions of the clavicle in relation to the sternum (ie, the disc works/stays with either the sternum or clavicle during specific actions).
Both the acromioclavicular and sternoclavicular joints allow the clavicle to serve as a crankshaft that keeps the arm in a functional position in relation to the body. The clavicle rotates early and late during abduction and elevation actions of the humerus.

3. **What are the ligaments supporting/controlling the sternoclavicular joint?**
The sternoclavicular ligament complex includes the capsule itself, which is directly reinforced by the named anterior and posterior sternoclavicular ligaments. The costoclavicular ligament is quite strong and assists with the pivoting action of the clavicle in relation to the anchored/underlying first rib. The interclavicular ligament supports the superior aspect reinforcing the position of the clavicle so as to minimize inferior displacement, which would endanger the underlying brachial plexus and subclavian artery.

4. **What radiographic views are used to assess sternoclavicular injuries?**
Special radiographic views can be utilized to assess the sternoclavicular joint. These views provide the benefit of minimizing superimposed structures. Hobbs recommends that patients be radiographed while in a sitting position, leaning forward with elbows supported on the x-ray table. In this position a vertical (superior) x-ray is taken.
Rockwood uses a "serendipity" view in which the patient is positioned supine with the x-ray tube angled approximately 40 degrees from the vertical and directed toward the clavicle.

5. **How are sternoclavicular injuries classified?**
Sternoclavicular injuries resemble the "classic" ligamentous disruption sequence. Table 41.2 includes a classification scheme for these injuries.

6. **What is the treatment for type I sternoclavicular injuries?**
Type I injury is a first-degree sprain and as such no instability is present. For these patients, ice can be used for pain modulation, in addition to protection from additional trauma via a sling for 2 to 4 days, or until pain free. A gradual return to activities should follow as tolerated through a functional progression.

7. **What is the treatment for type II sternoclavicular injuries?**
Type II injuries involve third-degree sprain of the sternoclavicular ligaments and requires immobilization and protection. Most patients will wear a clavicle strap to keep proper clavicular orientation and a sling to support the weight of the arm. These are used for 2 to 4 weeks followed by a rehabilitation progression dictated by need and symptoms.
A couple of clinical pearls: while immobilized, showering can be a challenge. Instruct the patient on "cradling of the arm" and the use of liquid soap. A second idea is to do rehabilitation in midportions of the ROM. These

Table 41.2 Sternoclavicular Injury Classification

TYPE	DESCRIPTION
I	First/second-degree sprain of sternoclavicular and costoclavicular ligaments
II	Third-degree sprain of sternoclavicular and first/second-degree sprain of costoclavicular ligaments
III	Third-degree sprain of sternoclavicular and costoclavicular ligaments (true instability)

portions seem to be better tolerated and place minimal loads onto the sternoclavicular ligaments recognizing maximal rotation occurs at end range.

8. **What is the initial treatment for significant (type III) sternoclavicular injuries?**
   The first approach to treating a sternoclavicular injury is to ensure that reduction is present and maintained. The vast majority of sternoclavicular dislocations (type III) occur anteriorly and can be reduced through firm digital pressure. In some instances muscle relaxants or anesthesia is required for this procedure. To reduce the dislocation, the patient is positioned supine and a pad placed posteriorly allowing shoulder extension and a posterior force applied to the proximal (displaced) clavicle completes the reduction.
   The rare posterior dislocation requires shoulder extension while the trunk position is maintained, thus permitting a fulcrum/lever sequence. In these cases, reduction may occur in the operating room (as above), particularly because a closed technique may not be successful, necessitating an open procedure utilizing forceps to pull the clavicle into correct position. The patient with a posterior sternoclavicular dislocation may present as a medical emergency as significant injury to underlying organs/structures may accompany this insult.
   Following reduction, a sling is often worn (3–6 weeks) for the anterior patient while a figure-of-eight harness is similarly used for the posterior patient. Some physicians combine the clavicle harness with the arm sling. The use of ice, followed by gentle controlled movements after immobilization, then leads into a functional exercise progression for rehabilitation.

9. **What are the long-term consequences of sternoclavicular injuries?**
   After reduction of a sternoclavicular injury, the majority of patients will not have significant disability. If chronic instability does develop, surgical intervention can be performed. Surgical outcomes have improved in these chronic situations, but some complications may occur. Importantly, SC reconstructions have become relatively consistent in positive outcomes. Long-term outcomes may include a level of arthritis and pain, particularly in high-demand patients.

10. **What type of surgery is done for patients with sternoclavicular instability/disability?**
    Although relatively rare, some patients will experience recurrent dislocations and demonstrate instability leading to disability/pain. Surgical intervention is typically not performed acutely unless the joint remains unstable after reduction. Most procedures use some type of graft material (subclavius tendon, palmaris longus, gracilis, or toe extensor) to redevelop proximal stability of the SC pivot point. The postsurgical results are not easily predicted since the number of these procedures is small. Recent literature shows improving consistency of positive outcomes for these patients.

Bibliography

Classic Texts Related to the Shoulder – Specific AC/SC Chapters

Andrews, J. R., & Wilk, K. E. (Eds.). (1994). *The athlete's shoulder.* New York, NY: Churchill Livingstone.

Chan, K. M. (Ed.), (1995). *Sports injuries of the hand and upper extremity.* New York, NY: Churchill Livingstone.

Donatelli, R. A. (Ed.), (1997). *Physical therapy of the shoulder* (3rd ed.). New York, NY: Churchill Livingstone.

Hawkins, R. J., Bell, R. H., & Lippitt, S. B. (1996). *Atlas of shoulder surgery.* St. Louis, MO: CV Mosby.

Kelley, M. J., & Clark, W. A. (Eds.). (1995). *Orthopedic therapy of the shoulder.* Philadelphia, PA: J. B. Lippincott.

Nicholas, J. A., Hershman, E. B., & Posner, M. A. (Eds.), (1990). *The upper extremity in sports medicine.* St. Louis, MO: CV Mosby.

Rockwood, C. A., & Matsen, F. A. (Eds.). (1998). *The shoulder* (2nd ed.). Philadelphia, PA: W. B. Saunders.

Classic Specific AC/SC Articles

Boesmueller, S., Wech, M., Tiefenboeck, T. M., et al. (2016). Incidence, characteristics, and long-term follow-up of sternoclavicular injuries: An epidemiologic analysis of 92 cases. *Journal of Trauma and Acute Care Surgery, 80*(2), 289–295.

Bosworth, B. M. (1941). Acromioclavicular separation: New method of repair. *Surgery, Gynecology & Obstetrics, 73,* 866–871.

Branch, T. P., Burdette, H. L., Shahriari, A. S., et al. (1996). The role of the acromioclavicular ligaments and the effect of distal clavicle resection. *American Journal of Sports Medicine, 24,* 293–297.

Chaudhury, S., Bavan, L., Rupani, N., et al. (2018). Managing acromio-clavicular joint pain: A scoping review. *Shoulder & Elbow, 10*(1), 4–14.

Cheema, S. G., Hermanns, C., Coda, R. G., et al. (2021). Publicly accessible rehabilitation protocols for acromioclavicular joint reconstruction are widely variable. *Arthroscopy, Sports Medicine, and Rehabilitation, 3*(2), e427–e433.
Cook, F. F., & Tibone, J. E. (1988). The Mumford procedure in athletes: An objective analysis of function. *American Journal of Sports Medicine, 16*, 97–100.
Cox, J. S. (1981). The fate of the acromioclavicular joint in athletic injuries. *American Journal of Sports Medicine, 9*, 50–53.
Frank, R. M., Cotter, E. J., Leroux, T. S., et al. (2019). Acromioclavicular joint injuries: Evidenced based treatment. *Journal of the American Academy of Orthopaedic Surgeons, 27*, e775–e788.
Galpin, R. D., Hawkins, R. J., & Grainger, R. W. (1985). A comparative analysis of operative versus nonoperative treatment of grade III acromioclavicular separations. *Clinical Orthopaedics and Related Research, 193*, 150–155.
Inman, V. T., Saunders, J. B., & Abbott, L. C. (1944). Observations on the function of the shoulder joint. *Journal of Bone and Joint Surgery, 26*, 1–30.
Kirby, J. C., Edwards, E., & Moaveni, A. K. (2015). Management and functional outcomes following sternoclavicular dislocation. *Injury, 46*(10), 1906–1913.
Lemos, M. J. (1998). Current concepts: The evaluation and treatment of the injured acromioclavicular joint in athletes. *American Journal of Sports Medicine, 26*, 137–144.
Liu, T., Bao, F., Jiang, T., et al. (2020). Acromioclavicular joint separation: Repair through suture anchors for coracoclavicular ligament and nonabsorbable suture fixation for acromioclavicular joint. *Orthopaedic Surgery, 12*, 1362–1371.
Moatshe, G., Kruckeberg, B. M., Chahla, J., et al. (2018). Acromioclavicular and coracoclavicular ligament reconstruction for acromioclavicular joint instability: A systematic review of clinical and radiographic outcomes. *Arthroscopy, 34*(6), 1979–1995.
Morrison, D. S., & Lemos, M. J. (1995). Acromioclavicular separation: Reconstruction using synthetic loop augmentation. *American Journal of Sports Medicine, 23*, 105–110.
Snyder, S. J., Banas, M. P., & Karzel, R. P. (1995). The arthroscopic Mumford procedure: An analysis of results. *Arthroscopy, 11*, 157–164.
Soler, F., Mocini, F., Djemeto, D. T., et al. (2021). No differences between conservative and surgical management of acromioclavicular joint arthritis: A scoping review. *Knee Surgery, Sports Traumatology, Arthroscopy, 29*, 2194–2201.
Walsh, W. M., Peterson, D. A., Shelton, G., et al. (1985). Shoulder strength following acromioclavicular injury. *American Journal of Sports Medicine, 13*, 153–158.
Weaver, J. K., & Dunn, H. K. (1972). Treatment of acromioclavicular injuries: Especially complete acromioclavicular separation. *Journal of Bone and Joint Surgery, 54*(6), 1187–1194.
Wojtys, E. M., & Nelson, G. (1991). Conservative treatment of grade III acromioclavicular dislocations. *Clinical Orthopaedics and Related Research, 268*, 112–119.
Wylie, J. D., Johnson, J. D., DiVenere, J., et al. (2018). Shoulder acromioclavicular and coracoclavicular ligament injuries: Common problems and solutions. *Clinical Journal of Sports Medicine, 37*(2), 197–207.
Xara-Leite, F., Andrade, R., Moreira, P. S., et al. (2019). Anatomic and non-anatomic reconstruction improves post-operative outcomes in chronic acromioclavicular instability: A systematic review. *Knee Arthroscopy Surgery, Sports Traumatology, 27*, 3779–3796.
Yap, J. J. L., Curl, L. A., Kvitne, R. S., & McFarland, E. G. (1999). The value of weighted views of the acromioclavicular joint: Results of a survey. *American Journal of Sports Medicine, 27*, 806–809.

CHAPTER 41 QUESTIONS

A 23-year-old college student was seen 2 hours after he had been in a bicycle accident on campus–using a rental bicycle. (Today–it could be electric rental scooter!) He had "stuck his right shoulder" into the turf as he was thrown from the bicycle. On examination he had exquisite tenderness over the right acromioclavicular joint but a full but painful range of shoulder motions. The clavicle appeared consistent in general appearance with the left and did have some increased anterior to posterior displacement when assessed. There was no significant tenderness below the clavicle.

1. **What additional information would indicate the need for immediate referral to an orthopaedic surgeon?**
   a) Continued pain with palpation of the acromioclavicular joint after the third hour
   b) Continued pain at the extremes of ROM after icing
   c) Tenderness to palpation of the clavicle not related to soft tissue insertion
   d) Pain associated with scapular retraction

2. **The described injury with the presentation of acromioclavicular tenderness with palpation and increased A-P motion most likely reflects:**
   a) A first-degree sprain of the acromioclavicular ligaments.
   b) A second-degree injury of the acromioclavicular ligaments
   c) A third-degree injury to the acromioclavicular ligaments
   d) A third-degree injury to the coracoclavicular ligaments

3. **The most likely treatment for this bicyclist would be:**
   a) A sling for comfort and instruction in icing–slow exercise progression
   b) A sling for 3 weeks and slow exercise progression after the initial immobilization
   c) A sling for 3 weeks and early strengthening emphasizing maximal elevation
   d) A sling for 6 weeks to enable protected ligament healing and then aggressive strengthening

CHAPTER 42

SCAPULOTHORACIC DYSFUNCTION AND IMPAIRMENTS

C.A. Thigpen, PhD, PT, ATC and K. Shaughnessy, PT, DPT, OCS, CSCS

1. **What is the role of the scapula in glenohumeral movement?**
   The scapula provides a mobile base for humeral motions in all directions; assists in providing an appropriate muscle length-to-tension ratio for rotator cuff and deltoid musculature throughout arm elevation; and serves as a bony attachment for most of the upper quarter proximal musculature. The scapula and surrounding musculature are critical in force transmission from the lower extremities and trunk to the arm in overhead activities. While very mobile due to its single articulation with the clavicle, it most often functions in a static position to optimize force transmission.

2. **What is the 3-D kinematics of the scapula with respect to the humerus and trunk in arm elevation?**
   Scapular motion occurs in three cardinal planes during arm elevation: upward rotation, external rotation, and posterior tilt. In a healthy person, as the arm is elevated in the scapular plane, the scapula rotates upwardly $\approx 50° \pm 4.8°$, externally rotates about a vertical axis $\approx 24° \pm 12.8°$, and tilts posteriorly about a horizontal axis $\approx 30° \pm 13.0°$.

3. **What muscular force couples act on the scapula during arm elevation?**
   A force couple is two or more lines of force acting on different points of the same structure to produce rotation. The upper trapezius, lower trapezius, and serratus anterior are involved in scapular upward rotation and resist downward rotation. The posterior tilting and external rotation of the scapula are thought to result from action of the lower serratus anterior musculature and lower trapezius. Maintenance of relative scapular external rotation and posterior tilting is most critical from 90° to 120° to allow the greater tuberosity to clear the acromion during overhead activities.

4. **Does the scapular musculature activation pattern change when the glenohumeral joint is injured?**
   Yes. Several different studies have demonstrated that motor activity level or onset of motor activity is altered in patients with impingement or glenohumeral instability. Diminished serratus anterior activity has been documented in throwers with unstable shoulders and swimmers with impingement. Delayed onset of serratus anterior activity in overhead reaching has been demonstrated in swimmers with impingement.

5. **Can abnormal scapular movement be associated with rotator cuff impingement?**
   Yes, previous research suggests that patients with subacromial impingement syndrome will present with impaired scapular posterior tilt, upward rotation, and external rotation. Patients with internal impingement, on the other hand, have been found to have increased sternoclavicular elevation and scapular posterior tilt. Thus, relating the clinical examination and area of impingement with scapular movements is important.

6. **Define scapular dyskinesia.**
   Scapular dyskinesia describes abnormal or atypical movement of the scapular during normal active motion tasks, such as reaching overhead. Similar terms used in the literature include abnormal scapulohumeral rhythm, scapular winging, and scapular dysrhythmia.

7. **How common is scapular dyskinesia?**
   It is very common and may or may not be an associated impairment driving shoulder dysfunction. Based on the current literature, it can occur in 75% of the healthy asymptomatic population. In healthy overhead athletes it is typical to see asymmetry, primarily with more anterior tilt and internal rotation on the dominant side compared with the nondominant side. Warner found 64% of patients diagnosed with an unstable glenohumeral joint present with some form of scapula dyskinesia, while all patients with impingement demonstrated some degree of scapular dyskinesia. Similarly, Tate and Uhl have shown similar rates of dyskinesia without a clear link to symptoms and disease state. Most recently Plummer et al. have shown no greater incidence of scapular dyskinesia in patients with shoulder pain compared to health controls. Thus, the presence of scapular dyskinesia alone, without corollary pain and disability, should not be considered "pathologic."

8. **What populations need to be watched for scapular adaptations/impairments that require special focus?**
Scapular adaptations that are impairments related to shoulder pain should be evaluated in the context of the patients' presentation of shoulder pain. There are no clear links in the presence or resolution of scapular dyskinesis and shoulder pain. Thus, clinical examination techniques such as the active elevation test and scapular relocation test should be used to identify scapular dyskinesis and impairments that are most associated with shoulder pain and disability.

9. **What causes scapular dyskinesis?**
It is not clear whether the scapula dyskinesis is primary or secondary to shoulder pathology. The general consensus is that deficiency of the scapular musculature, particularly the serratus anterior and trapezius, is often involved. The deficiency may be simple weakness, tightness, or a compensatory motor pattern developed in response to pain. Congenital deformities, such as scoliosis or Sprengel's deformity, may contribute to scapular dyskinesis.

10. **What is Sprengel's deformity?**
Also called Eulenburg's deformity, Sprengel's deformity is failure of the scapula to descend during normal development. Typically, it is seen in infancy or early childhood as a prominent lump in the web of the neck. The scapula often is hypoplastic, abnormally shaped, and malrotated so that the superomedial angle is curved anteriorly into the supraclavicular region and the inferior angle abuts the thoracic spine. Arm abduction may be limited. Associated musculoskeletal deformities, such as scoliosis, rib abnormalities, Klippel-Feil syndrome, and spina bifida are common.

11. **How do you assess abnormal scapular movement?**
Static Assessment:
Scapular movement initiates from the scapula's resting posture. Therefore, assessment of scapular movement begins with observation of static scapular positioning on the thoracic spine. The clinician can assess prominence and tipping of the medial and inferior borders of the scapula as well as thoracic spine posture, since conditions such as thoracic scoliosis can have a profound impact on scapular positioning and movement. Recent studies suggest that abnormalities should be apparent and that subtle differences likely have little impact on overall scapular performance.
Dynamic Assessment:
Several observational clinical methods exist, with the most supported incorporating the two-type scapular observational method of "yes," scapular dyskinesis is observed, or "no," scapular dyskinesis is not observed. These approaches were found to have moderate to good (kappa = 0.4 to 0.6) reliability and to be less restrictive than a previous four-category approach. The patient elevates the arm through a full range of motion in either flexion, scapular plane abduction, or pure abduction multiple times. Hand weights during shoulder flexion and frontal-plane abduction can be used to help load the scapular muscles to enhance the observational analysis. The use of multiple repetitions or weight suggests that, to observe scapular dyskinesis, the musculature needs to be challenged.

12. **How do you treat an impairment of scapular dyskinesis?**
The first step is to do a complete neuromuscular examination of the shoulder girdle and cervical region. Based on your findings, tight structures need to be lengthened, often levator scapulae and pectoralis minor, while muscle that display altered timing and force production should be isolated to improve their function. For example, a winging scapula during arm elevation noted by inferior medial border prominence should focus on increasing the ability of the pectoralis minor to lengthen through soft tissue and stretching techniques. Then protraction and depression exercises (serratus/lower trap) should begin below chest level then progress to overhead as scapular control improves.
Recent studies suggest that including the entire kinetic chain can improve how the scapula functions to transfer energy from the patient's contralateral hip, core, and spine to the patient's glenohumeral joint. Underlying mobility, strength, and coordination deficits in these three areas decrease the efficiency of movements and increase the overall stress on the shoulder joint. Therefore, incorporating exercises aimed to improve muscle performance of the gluteus medius, maximus, and deep core in functional positions that replicate the demands of daily activities should be considered. Often biofeedback techniques, such as mirrors, verbal cueing, tactile cueing, and video monitoring during exercises, help the patient visualize the trunk and scapula. The patient benefits by observing the entire kinetic chain working with their scapula during exercises to learn how to voluntarily control each segment in functional overhead tasks.

13. **Which scapular muscles should be targeted for rehabilitation?**
There are approximately 20 muscles attached to the scapula; however, those most involved in stabilization of the scapula against the thoracic wall are the rhomboids, major and minor; upper, middle, and lower trapezius muscles; the rotator cuff musculature; and the serratus anterior.

14. **Which exercises target the scapular muscles?**
Current electromyographic (EMG) research on scapular rehabilitation suggests the following exercises most effectively target the scapular stabilizers. The push-up plus elicits 80% maximum voluntary isometric contraction (MVIC) of serratus anterior activity, prone flexion over head for lower trap elicits 95%, and rows elicit 112% MVIC for upper trap and middle trap muscles. Side-lying external rotation, side-lying forward flexion, prone horizontal abduction with external rotation, and prone extension stimulate lower and middle trapezius muscle activity while diminishing upper trapezius activity. Although it is a scapular stabilizer, excessive activation of the upper trapezius is a contributing factor to abnormal scapular motion.
The lower fibers of the serratus anterior are best activated with exercises that require the arm to be elevated to at least 120 degrees. Strengthening and stabilization of these muscles will help reestablish neuromuscular pathways and aid in prevention of instability and secondary impingement, labral pathology, and certain overuse pathologies by maintaining glenohumeral joint congruency. In addition, scapular rehabilitation should include a strong lower extremity and core strengthening program.

15. **How does dyskinesis differ from scapular winging?**
Scapular winging typically is associated with long thoracic nerve palsy. There are two ways to assess for scapular winging. In the first test, have the patient lean into a wall, supporting his or her weight with their arms. In the second test, apply resistance to a patient's outstretched arm as he or she attempts to forward flex. A positive test for either assessment is lifting of the entire medial and inferior border of the scapula off of the thoracic wall, indicating a serratus anterior deficiency.

16. **What is the standard treatment for long thoracic nerve palsy?**
The palsy usually resolves gradually over time. An electromyographic (EMG) study confirms the diagnosis and can be used to track progress. Strengthening exercises for the weak serratus anterior should be delayed until EMG indicates regeneration. The patient should restrict heavy pushing and overhead lifting activities. Some patients have benefited from a shoulder orthotic that keeps the scapula pressed against the thoracic wall to relieve pain. Long-term outcomes (6 years; range 2–11 years) of iatrogenic long thoracic palsy reported residual symptoms in 25 of 26 patients. Eighty-one percent could not lift or pull heavy objects, 54% could not work with hands above shoulder level, and 58% could not participate in sports such as tennis and golf.

17. **What are alternative treatments for long thoracic nerve palsy?**
Muscle transfer of the pectoralis major is a procedure that has shown (at a 2-year follow-up) improvement in function (58%) and pain reduction (50%) with a 40-degree increase in active arm elevation. Surgical release of the scalene muscles to relieve compression on the long thoracic nerve has been reported with good success. Case reports of nerve transfer of the thoracodorsal for the long thoracic have been reported. Outcomes demonstrated full shoulder flexion with no scapular winging and reported no functional limitations within his daily activities of living (at a 16-year follow-up). A case report describing a two-level motor nerve transfer of the pectoral fascicle of the middle trunk and part of the thoracodorsal nerve was conducted to reinnervate the serratus anterior muscle. Postsurgery, the patient's pain diminished from a 4 out of 10 to a 1 out of 10, and after 13 months of physical therapy, the patient was able to return to all normal activities, with mild difficulty with overhead activities.

18. **A patient presents with severe shoulder and neck pain and a drooped shoulder after cervical lymph node resection. What do you suspect is the cause?**
One complication of a lymph node or benign tumor removal is iatrogenic injury to spinal accessory nerve. The injury typically involves the trapezius but often spares the sternocleidomastoid muscle. Trapezius weakness is often noted with the inability to lift the arm above horizontal, and the involved side presents with drooped posture. Patients describe significant shoulder pain, with a sensation of heaviness or the feeling that the shoulder is being pulled out of the socket on the involved side.

19. **What is scapulothoracic dissociation?**
Scapulothoracic dissociation results from severe trauma involving lateral displacement of the scapula. It has been described as a closed, traumatic forequarter amputation. This injury typically is associated with motorcycle, motor vehicle, or farm implement accidents. The lateral displacement of the scapula ruptures surrounding soft tissue. Typical associated injuries are clavicle fracture, significant neurovascular damage, and major trauma.

20. **Define snapping scapula.**
Snapping scapula is attributed to friction between the mobile scapula and its attached soft tissues and the thoracic wall. The noise or grating sound may be audible or sensed by the patient. The incidence of grating in the general population has been reported to be as high as 70%. A general friction sound is typically nonpathologic. Grating, loud snap, or pop sounds associated with pain are thought to be pathologic. Anatomic explanations for snapping scapula include thickened bursa, bone spurs on scapula or a rib, Luschka's tubercle (an exostosis at the superomedial angle of the scapula), and osteochondroma (a common scapular tumor). A tangential scapulolateral

view or computed tomographic scan is more helpful in identifying anatomic anomalies associated with snapping scapula than standard anteroposterior scapular radiographs.

21. **What is the differential diagnosis of snapping scapula?**
Pain may be referred from the glenohumeral joint, cervical nerve root compression, or cervical joint disease. Thoracic disc disease should be ruled out, along with thoracic outlet syndrome. Tumors also must be considered and evaluated with appropriate imaging studies.

22. **How is snapping scapula treated?**
Conservative management with antiinflammatory medication, physical therapy modalities, and exercise to strengthen the lower trapezius and serratus anterior musculature often are prescribed. Supportive strapping or bracing may be beneficial. Injection of marcaine may be helpful. Surgical treatment is rare and should be considered only if diagnostic imaging demonstrates the presence of an exostosis or a space-occupying lesion in the scapulothoracic space. Recent studies from Provencher and Warth have shown releasing a recalcitrant pectoralis minor with and without removing bony overgrowth under the spine of the scapula can be effective when >6 months of conservative therapies have failed.

Bibliography

Burkhart, S. S., Morgan, C. D., & Kibler, W. B. (2003). The disabled throwing shoulder: Spectrum of pathology part III: The SICK scapula, scapular dyskinesis, the kinetic chain, and rehabilitation. *Arthroscopy, 19*, 641–661.

Butters, K. P. (1998). The scapula. In C. A. Rockwood & F. A. Matsen (Eds.), *The shoulder* (2nd ed., pp. 391–427). Philadelphia, PA: W.B. Saunders.

Cools, A. M., Dewitte, V., Lanszweert, F., et al. (2007). Rehabilitation of scapular muscle balance: Which exercises to prescribe? *American Journal of Sports Medicine, 35*(10), 1744–1751.

Donner, T. R., & Kline, D. G. (1993). Extracranial spinal accessory nerve injury. *Neurosurgery, 32*, 907–910.

Ekstrom, R. A., Donatelli, R. A., & Soderberg, G. L. (2003). Surface electromyographic analysis of exercises for the trapezius and serratus anterior muscles. *Journal of Orthopaedic and Sports Physical Therapy, 33*(5), 247–258.

Endo, K., Ikata, T., Katoh, S., & Takeda, Y. (2001). Radiographic assessment of scapular rotational tilt in chronic shoulder impingement syndrome. *Journal of Orthopaedic Science, 6*(1), 3–10.

Glousman, R., Jobe, F. W., Tibone, J. E., et al. (1988). Dynamic electromyographic analysis of the throwing shoulder with glenohumeral instability. *Journal of Bone and Joint Surgery, 70*(2), 220–226.

Hawkins, R. J., & Bokor, D. J. (1998). Clinical evaluation of shoulder problems. In C. A. Rockwood & F. A. Matsen (Eds.), *The shoulder* (2nd ed., pp. 164–197). Philadelphia, PA: W.B. Saunders.

Inman, V. T., Saunders, J. B., & Abbott, L. C. (1996). Observations of the function of the shoulder joint. 1944. *Clinical Orthopaedics and Related Research*, (*330*), 3–12.

Kauppila, L. I., & Vastamaki, M. (1996). Iatrogenic serratus anterior paralysis: Long-term outcome in 26 patients. *Chest, 109*, 31–34.

Kendall, F. P., McCreary, E. K., Provance, P. G., et al. (2005). *Muscles: Testing and function with posture and pain* (5th ed.). Baltimore, MD: Williams & Wilkins.

Kibler, W. B. (1998). The role of the scapula in athletic shoulder function. *American Journal of Sports Medicine, 26*, 325–337.

Kibler, W. B., & Livingston, B. (2001). Closed-chain rehabilitation for upper and lower extremities. *Journal of the American Academy of Orthopaedic Surgeons, 9*, 412–421.

Kibler, W. B., & Sciascia, A. (2006). The role of core stability in athletic function. *Sports Medicine, 36*, 189–198.

Laudner, K., Lynall, R., Williams, J. G., et al. (2013). Thoracolumbar range of motion in baseball pitchers and position players. *International Journal of Sports Physical Therapy, 8*, 777–783.

Laudner, K. G., Myers, J. B., Pasquale, M. R., Bradley, J. P., & Lephart, S. M. (2006). Scapular dysfunction in throwers with pathologic internal impingement. *Journal of Orthopaedic and Sports Physical Therapy, 36*(7), 485–494.

Ludewig, P. M., Cook, T. M., & Nawoczenski, D. A. (1996). Three-dimensional scapular orientation and muscle activity at selected positions of humeral elevation. *Journal of Orthopaedic and Sports Physical Therapy, 24*, 57–65.

Lukasiewicz, A. C., McClure, P., Michener, L., et al. (1999). Comparison of 3- dimensional scapular position and orientation between subjects with and without shoulder impingement. *Journal of Orthopaedic and Sports Physical Therapy, 29*, 574–586.

Manske, R. C., Reiman, M. P., & Stovak, M. L. (2004). Nonoperative and operative management of snapping scapula. *American Journal of Sports Medicine, 32*, 1554–1565.

Marin, R. (1998). Scapular winger's brace: A case series on the management of long thoracic nerve palsy. *Archives of Physical Medicine and Rehabilitation, 79*, 1226–1230.

McClure, P. W., Michener, L. A., Sennett, B. J., et al. (2001). Direct 3-dimensional measurement of scapular kinematics during dynamic movements in vivo. *Journal of Shoulder and Elbow Surgery, 10*, 269–277.

McClure, P. W., Tate, A. R., Kareha, S., Irwin, D., & Zlupko, E. (2009). A clinical method for identifying scapular dyskinesis, part 1: Reliability. *Journal of Athletic Training, 44*, 160–164.

Mourtacos, S. L., Sauers, E. L., & Downar, J. M. (2003). Adolescent baseball players exhibit differences in shoulder mobility between the throwing and nonthrowing shoulder and between divisions of play [abstract]. *Journal of Athletic Training, 38*, S72.

Myers, J. B., Laudner, K. G., Pasquale, M. R., et al. (2005). Scapular position and orientation in throwing athletes. *American Journal of Sports Medicine, 33*, 263–271.

Nath, R. K., Lyons, A. B., & Bietz, G. (2007). Microneurolysis and decompression of long thoracic nerve injury are effective in reversing scapular winging: Long-term results in 50 cases. *BMC Musculoskeletal Disorders, 8*, 25.

Novak, C. B., & Mackinnon, S. E. (2002). Surgical treatment of a long thoracic nerve palsy. *Annals of Thoracic Surgery, 73*(5), 1643–1645.

Oliver, G., Plummer, H., & Weimar, W. (2014). Gluteus medius and scapula muscle activations in youth baseball players. *Strength and Conditioning, 29*(6), 1494–1499.

Oyama, S., Myers, J. B., Wassinger, C. A., Ricci, R. D., & Lephart, S. M. (2008). Asymmetric resting scapular posture in healthy overhead athletes. *Journal of Athletic Training, 43*(6), 565–570.
Park, S. Y., Yoo, W. G., Kim, M. H., Oh, J. S., & An, D. H. (2013). Differences in EMG activity during exercises targeting the scapulothoracic region: A preliminary study. *Manual Therapy, 18*(6), 512–518.
Plafcan, D. M., Turczany, P. J., Guenin, B. A., et al. (1997). An objective measurement technique for posterior scapular displacement. *Journal of Orthopaedic and Sports Physical Therapy, 25*, 336–341.
Plummer, H. A., Sum, J. C., Pozzi, F., Varghese, R., & Michener, L. A. (2017). Observational scapular dyskinesis: Know-groups validity in patients with and without shoulder pain. *Journal of Orthopaedic & Sports Physical Therapy, 47*(8), 530–537.
Provencher, M. T., Kirby, H., McDonald, L. S., et al. (2017). Surgical release of the pectoralis minor tendon for scapular dyskinesia and shoulder pain. *American Journal of Sports Medicine, 45*(1), 173–178.
Ray, W. Z., Pet, M. A., Nicoson, M. C., Yee, A., Kahn, L. C., & Mackinnon, S. E. (2011). Two-level motor nerve transfer for the treatment of long thoracic nerve palsy. *Journal of Neurosurgery, 115*(4), 858–864.
Scovazzo, M. L., Browne, A., Pink, M., et al. (1991). The painful shoulder during freestyle swimming: An electromyographic cinematographic analysis of twelve muscles. *American Journal of Sports Medicine, 19*, 577–582.
Streit, J. J., Lenarz, C. J., Shishani, Y., et al. (2012). Pectoralis major tendon transfer for the treatment of scapular winging due to long thoracic nerve palsy. *Journal of Shoulder and Elbow Surgery/American Shoulder and Elbow Surgeons, 21*(5), 685–690.
Tate, A. R., McClure, P., Kareha, S., Irwin, D., & Barbe, M. F. (2009). A clinical method for identifying scapular dyskinesis, part 2: Validity. *Journal of Athletic Training, 44*(2), 165–173.
Tsuruike, M., & Ellenbecker, T. S. (2015). Serratus anterior and lower trapezius muscle activities during multi-joint isotonic scapular exercises and isometric contractions. *Journal of Athletic Training, 50*(2), 199–210.
Uhl, T. L., Kibler, W. B., Gecewich, B., & Tripp, B. L. (2009). Evaluation of clinical assessment methods for scapular dyskinesis. *Arthroscopy, 25*(11), 1240–1248.
Wadsworth, D. J., & Bullock-Saxton, J. E. (1997). Recruitment patterns of the scapular rotator muscles in freestyle swimmers with subacromial impingement. *International Journal of Sports Medicine, 18*, 618–624.
Warner, J. J. P., Micheli, L. J., Arslanian, L. E., et al. (1992). Scapulothoracic motion in normal shoulders and shoulders with glenohumeral instability and impingement syndrome. *Clinical Orthopaedics, 285*, 199.
Warth, R. J., Spiegl, U. J., & Millett, P. J. (2015). Scapulothoracic bursitis and snapping scapula syndrome: A critical review of current evidence. *American Journal of Sports Medicine, 43*(1), 236–245.
Woo, V. E., & Marchinksi, L. (1998). Congenital anomalies of the shoulder. In C. A. Rockwood & F. A. Matsen (Eds.), *The shoulder* (2nd ed., pp. 99–163). Philadelphia, PA: W.B. Saunders.
Zaremski, J. L., Wasser, J. G., & Vincent, H. K. (2017). Mechanisms and treatments for shoulder injuries in overhead throwing athletes. *Current Sports Medicine Reports, 16*(3), 179–188.

CHAPTER 42 QUESTIONS

1. **The push-up plus elicits ___________ % maximum voluntary contraction (MVC) of serratus anterior activity, while the prone flexion overhead elicits ________ % MVC of lower trapezius activity.**
   a. 90, 80
   b. 90, 115
   c. 80, 95
   d. 70, 95

2. **Which of the following is an exercise that best elicits muscle activity within the lower trapezius?**
   a. Push-up plus
   b. Prone horizontal abduction at 90 degrees with full external rotation
   c. Prone shoulder extension
   d. Prone 120-degree abduction with palms facing floor

3. **Which of the following is a common cause of long thoracic nerve palsy?**
   a. Viral illnesses
   b. Pithing the nerve during dry needling
   c. Obstetrical complications
   d. Shortening of the nerve

FRACTURES OF THE CLAVICLE, PROXIMAL HUMERUS, AND HUMERAL SHAFT

J.D. Keener, MD, PT

CHAPTER 43

1. **How are clavicle fractures classified?**
   Clavicle fractures are most commonly classified according to their location (Allman classification). Middle-third fractures are the most prevalent, occurring in about 80% to 85% of clavicle fractures. Proximal-third and distal-third fractures occur in 3% to 5% and 12% to 15%, respectively, of clavicle fractures.

2. **Describe the subclassification of distal-third clavicle fractures.**
   Distal-third fractures of the clavicle are subclassified by Neer into three groups. The classification is based upon location of the fracture line and integrity of the coracoclavicular ligaments. Type I fractures are minimally displaced or nondisplaced because the coracoclavicular ligaments remain attached to the medial fragment. Type II fractures result in detachment of the coracoclavicular ligaments from the medial fragment and displacement of the medial fracture fragment upward. Type IIa injuries are more medial where both the conoid and trapezoid ligaments are attached to the lateral fragment, and type IIb injuries occur between the conoid and trapezoid and the more medial conoid ligament is torn from the medial fragment. This is analogous to a clavicle fracture with a shoulder separation resulting in a high rate of fracture nonunion. Type III fractures involve the articular surface of the acromioclavicular joint without detachment of the coracoclavicular ligaments.

3. **What nerve is the most frequently injured nerve with a fracture of the clavicle?**
   The most frequently injured nerve is the ulnar nerve, as it passes between the first rib and the fractured clavicle.

4. **How are middle-third clavicle fractures usually treated?**
   Surgical indications are controversial. Closed treatment is used for middle-third clavicle fractures without displacement and shortening. The most common methods of closed immobilization include casting, sling and swathe, or figure-of-eight dressings. No closed method can maintain a reduction; therefore a sling and swathe is most commonly used to maintain patient comfort while the fracture heals. Operative treatment is recommended when there is complete displacement combined with either shortening and/or comminution of the fracture fragments.

5. **What are the indications for operative treatment of acute clavicle fractures?**
   - Open fractures
   - Midshaft fracture with >100% displacement with shortening of >10–15 mm and/or comminution
   - Nerve or vascular injury requiring repair
   - Displaced type II distal clavicle fractures
   - Multitrauma victim where upper extremity assist for weight bearing is needed

6. **What are the risks of fracture nonunion for displaced midshaft clavicle fractures treated conservatively?**
   While the healing rate of nondisplaced fractures of the clavicle is excellent, the rate of nonunion for displaced and shortened midshaft clavicle fractures is between 10% and 15%. Additionally, there is some evidence that fractures that heal in a shortened position can develop a painful malunion with loss of shoulder function.

7. **What are the results of operative treatment of displaced midshaft clavicle fractures?**
   Randomized trials of surgical and conservative treatment of displaced midshaft clavicle fractures show a lower risk of nonunion and better functional outcomes with surgical treatment. Healing can be successfully obtained with plating and intramedullary pinning (Figure). Most patients will regain normal shoulder motion and function after operative intervention. Approximately 20% to 25% of patients will elect for later implant removal due to local soft tissue irritation from plates and pins.

8. **When should shoulder motion be initiated with nonoperative treatment of clavicle fractures?**
   Most middle-third clavicle fractures require 6 to 8 weeks for union to occur. Gentle shoulder active motion is initiated once early swelling and pain are improved, usually around 2 to 3 weeks following injury. The sling is removed

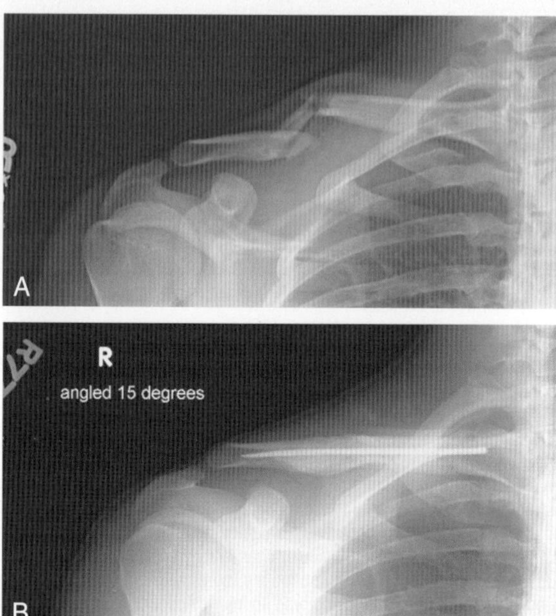

Clavicle fracture. (A) X-ray of comminuted right midshaft clavicle fracture. (B) Healed, well-aligned fracture following intramedullary nailing.

soon thereafter based on comfort. Active motion and stretching can be advanced as tolerated based on comfort but weight bearing and strengthening are generally avoided until 6 weeks following injury if healing is noted on x-ray. The elbow, wrist, and forearm should be used immediately after the fracture to prevent local stiffness and deconditioning.

9. **What is the incidence of proximal humerus fractures?**
   Proximal humerus fractures are common injuries, representing 4% to 5% of all extremity fractures. The majority of proximal humerus fractures occur in patients over 65 to 70 years of age. The majority of fractures result from ground-level falls, similar to distal radius and hip fractures. Several studies have shown that the incidence of proximal humerus fractures is increasing and felt to be related to the high prevalence of osteoporosis in the aging population.

10. **Describe the Neer classification of proximal humerus fractures.**
    Fractures of the proximal humerus can occur in several patterns. Fractures typically propagate through the greater tuberosity, lesser tuberosity, surgical neck, and/or anatomic neck. Fractures are classified according to the number of displaced fracture fragments and dislocation of the humeral head. The number of fragments can vary from one to four. Fracture fragments are considered to be present only when displaced 1 cm or more or angulated a minimum of 45 degrees. The interobserver agreement for the Neer classification is moderate at best. Furthermore, the Neer system does not account for other variables that influence treatment, such as bone quality, head split injuries, deforming muscle forces (fracture stability), and patient age and activity level.

11. **What are the deforming muscular forces responsible for the pattern of fracture displacement encountered with proximal humerus fractures?**
    The greater tuberosity is displaced in a posterior and superior direction from the pull of the supraspinatus and infraspinatus muscles. Displaced greater tuberosity fractures also create a tear in the rotator cuff in the region of the rotator interval. The subscapularis will pull displaced lesser tuberosity fractures medially. The humerus displaces medially and internally rotates from the pull of the pectoralis major with displaced surgical neck fractures. In addition, varus angulation and shortening are common because of the pull of the deltoid muscle on the humeral shaft. Often the humeral head will abduct because of the unopposed force of the rotator cuff, further contributing to the varus alignment of the humeral head. The biceps tendon frequently will become trapped within the fracture fragments with displaced surgical neck fractures.

12. **How often do nerve injuries accompany proximal humerus fractures?**
Nerve injury following proximal humerus fractures is common, especially with displaced fractures. Clinically detectable nerve injuries following proximal humerus fractures have been reported in up to 45% of cases. The axillary and suprascapular nerves are most commonly involved. Often these injuries are incomplete and may manifest as temporary weakness that recovers along the same course of time as fracture healing. One author reported a 6.1% incidence of brachial plexus injuries following displaced proximal humerus fractures. Electromyography (EMG) studies have revealed a very high incidence of occult (not clinically detectable) nerve injury following both nondisplaced (52%) and displaced (82%) fractures. The risk of neurovascular injury following fractures of the proximal humerus is greater with high-energy injuries, fracture-dislocations, and penetrating trauma.

13. **What percentage of proximal humerus fractures can be treated nonoperatively?**
The majority of proximal humerus fractures can be managed conservatively. Most fractures are minimally displaced (considered one-part fractures) and can be treated successfully with conservative measures. In addition, some displaced fractures, particularly valgus-impacted injuries, can be managed conservatively. Approximately 80% of proximal humerus fractures meet the criteria for conservative treatment. Fractures of the surgical neck are often accompanied by a moderate degree of displacement and angulation. Because of the high degree of mobility available at the glenohumeral joint, angulation of 30 to 45 degrees and translation of up to 75% of the width of the humeral shaft can be tolerated as long as there is good apposition of the fracture fragments.

14. **When is the treatment of conservatively managed proximal humerus fractures initiated?**
Numerous authors have noted that early range of motion is critical for successful outcomes following proximal humerus fractures. The shoulder is immobilized in a sling or cuff and collar for comfort and to facilitate fracture reduction afforded by the weight of the arm. Elbow, wrist, and hand range of motion exercises are initiated immediately. Pendulum exercises are initiated as soon as tolerable for most stable one-part fractures. The shoulder is evaluated clinically at 1-week intervals to assess for clinical signs of early union. Once the humerus and the proximal fragments move as one unit with gentle shoulder range of motion exercises, formal range of motion exercises are initiated. Early fracture stability is usually noted at 2 to 3 weeks from the time of injury at which time formal physical therapy is initiated starting with active range of motion rather than aggressive passive stretching.

15. **What are the outcomes of conservatively treated proximal humerus fractures?**
The outcomes of conservatively treated proximal humerus fractures are generally good. Fracture union rates are greater than 90% in those patients with minimally displaced fractures. Early range of motion of the shoulder has been shown to improve the functional outcome following proximal humerus fractures. Most patients will regain near normal function of the shoulder following these injuries and experience minimal residual pain. A patient can expect 130- to 150-degree elevation, near symmetric external rotation range of motion, and only mild weakness and functional limitations compared with the opposite shoulder. For displaced fractures managed nonoperatively the functional range of motion and strength may be more limited due to displacement of the tuberosities, which can lead to secondary cuff dysfunction. However, pain relief is generally good assuming fracture healing occurs.

16. **What are the indications for surgical management of proximal humerus fractures?**
The decision to operatively stabilize proximal humerus fractures is related to the severity of the fracture displacement, the age of the patient, bone quality, and coexisting humeral head dislocations. Surgical indications are controversial. For two-part fractures, there is some debate about the degree of deformity that is tolerable at the surgical neck. Fracture angulation at the surgical neck greater than 45 degrees or translation of the humeral shaft leading to minimal contact of the bony fragments is best treated surgically. Displacement of the greater tuberosity is not tolerated well because of the risk of fragment impingement within the subacromial space. Therefore, greater tuberosity displacement greater than 5 mm is another indication for surgery. Most three- and four-part fractures require surgery except in low-demand elderly patients but this is debatable. Some randomized trials have shown comparable clinical results between conservative treatment and surgical stabilization for displaced fractures with a higher complication rate with surgical treatment. This has prompted the use of more stringent selection criteria for surgical treatment. Anatomic neck and head split fractures generally require operative treatment in the form of shoulder arthroplasty. Fractures associated with humeral head dislocations require open reduction followed by fracture stabilization or arthroplasty.

17. **What are the general outcomes of open reduction and internal fixation of proximal humerus fractures?**
The outcomes of surgically managed proximal humerus fractures are good with proper indications and appropriate rehabilitation. Factors related to outcome include the type of fracture, the preoperative shoulder function, bone quality, and the development of a complication related to the injury or surgery itself. Both percutaneous pinning and open reduction and internal fixation provide reliable results as long as bony union occurs and avascular necrosis of the humeral head does not develop. Most patients will regain functional range of

motion of the shoulder. Most will attain active shoulder elevation to 120 to 150 degrees, external rotation to 30 to 45 degrees, and internal rotation to the lumbar spine. Studies using validated outcome scales note mild residual functional problems such as occasional pain, slight weakness, and limited function following two- and three-part fractures of the proximal humerus. These studies also note poor function or a significant complication, such as avascular necrosis, in 10% to 40% of patients with displaced three- and four-part fractures. Full recovery can take 6 months following surgery. There is a 20% to 30% risk of need for reoperation mostly due to hardware-related complications such as prominent screws.

18. **What are the potential complications of surgical fixation of proximal humerus fractures?**
Complications are relatively common following fixation of proximal humerus fractures ranging from 15% to 30% in most series. The rates of complications are more common in more severe fracture patterns and in fractures with poor bone quality. The use of fixed angle locking plates has decreased the risk of loss of fracture reduction, particularly when poor bone quality is present. The most frequent complications remain: loss of fracture reduction, avascular necrosis of the humeral head, glenohumeral joint screw penetration, poor return of function, and need for hardware removal.

19. **When is shoulder arthroplasty preferred over fracture fixation for the management of proximal humerus fractures?**
The decision to replace the proximal humerus in order to provide fracture stabilization is based on several factors including the risk of avascular necrosis of the humeral head, the quality of bone, and the age and functional demands of the patient. Some moderately displaced three- and four-part fractures can be treated conservatively in lower demand patients. Severely displaced four-part fractures, head split fractures, anatomic neck fractures, and three- and four-part fracture dislocations are best treated with arthroplasty. Severely displaced three-part fractures in older patients or those with poor bone quality is another indication for shoulder arthroplasty. Several studies have shown a higher complication and reoperation rates with open reduction and internal fixation of proximal humerus fractures compared to shoulder arthroplasty, particularly when bone quality is poor, which has resulted in the recent increase in popularity of reverse shoulder arthroplasty.

20. **For proximal humerus fractures that require arthroplasty, who should have a hemiarthroplasty as opposed to a reverse shoulder arthroplasty?**
Hemiarthroplasty has become less popular recently than reverse arthroplasty for managing severe proximal humerus fracture. Therefore, hemiarthroplasty is indicated generally only in younger patients (<55–60 years) with injuries that are not amenable to open reduction and internal fixation. Reverse arthroplasty produces more reliable results with a lower reoperation rate than hemiarthroplasty. However, due to concerns regarding the unknown longevity of reverse arthroplasty, hemiarthroplasty still plays a role in younger patients.

21. **What are the outcomes of hemiarthroplasty for the treatment of proximal humerus fractures?**
Most studies of displaced proximal humerus fractures report inferior results from hemiarthroplasty as compared to fracture fixation or reverse arthroplasty. Complications such as malunion and nonunion of the tuberosity fragments and humeral component malposition are thought to be related to poor outcomes. Most patients experience reliable pain relief following hemiarthroplasty for proximal humerus fractures; however, functional outcomes can be quite variable. The majority of patients can use the involved extremity well for activities of daily living below shoulder height, but overhead function is variable. A good outcome following hemiarthroplasty for humerus fracture is elevation to 110 to 130 degrees, external rotation to 45 to 60 degrees, minimal to no pain, and only a modest functional limit. These goals are generally achieved in between 60% and 70% of patients. Full recovery may take up to 12 months following surgery.

22. **What are the indications for reverse shoulder arthroplasty in patients with displaced proximal humerus fractures?**
Given the inconsistent clinical results with hemiarthroplasty for proximal humerus fracture, reverse total shoulder arthroplasty is more popular for displaced fractures not amenable to repair. Reverse total shoulder arthroplasty is generally indicated in older patients (60 years of age or older); however, the minimum age threshold is debated. Reverse arthroplasty is also preferred in cases with a concomitant glenoid fracture or rotator cuff tear. Reverse shoulder arthroplasty provides reliable return of shoulder function with a lower complication and reoperation rate than open reduction and internal fixation or hemiarthroplasty, which explains the rise in popularity of this procedure (Figure). Reverse shoulder arthroplasty requires an intact deltoid for function; therefore, careful assessment of the axillary nerve should be performed prior to surgery.

23. **How are humeral shaft fractures classified?**
Humeral shaft fractures are generally classified by the morphology of the fracture itself. The Orthopedic Trauma Association has subclassified these fractures as simple, wedge, and complex fractures. Simple fractures can

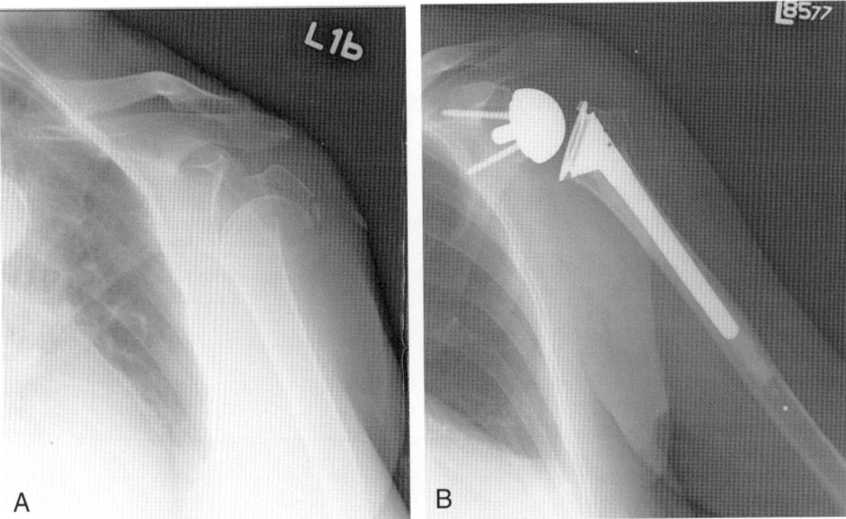

Proximal humerus fracture. (A) X-ray of four-part left proximal humerus fracture. (B) Reverse shoulder arthroplasty placement with fixation of greater tuberosity (GT).

either be spiral, oblique, or transverse. Wedge fractures have an intermediate bone fragment and are further subclassified as spiral, bending, and fragmented. Complex fractures include long spiral, segmental, and irregular (highly comminuted) fractures. Humeral shaft fracture classification is primarily descriptive and does not generally predict preferred treatment.

24. **How often do nerve injuries accompany humeral shaft fractures?**
Radial nerve injuries complicate between 6% and 18% of humeral shaft fractures. Other nerve injuries are rare, although brachial plexus injuries have been reported in higher energy trauma. Risk factors for radial nerve injuries include high-energy fractures, open fractures, and distal-third humeral shaft fractures. Over 90% of radial nerve injuries will recover spontaneously over a 4-month period. If there is no clinical or electrodiagnostic evidence of nerve recovery after 3 to 4 months, surgical exploration and nerve repair and/or grafting is often recommended.

25. **What is the recommended treatment for radial nerve palsies associated with humeral shaft fractures?**
The majority of radial nerve palsies represent neurapraxic injuries and will improve with observation alone (>90%). Splinting and range of motion exercises of the hand are encouraged to prevent contracture formation. Electromyography and nerve conduction tests are performed after 3 months if failure of improvement of the palsy is noted clinically. Exploration and neurolysis or repair of the nerve is performed if no signs of recovery are seen after 3 to 4 months. Indications for acute nerve exploration include penetrating open fractures, high-grade soft tissue injuries, or secondary nerve palsies (in some cases).

26. **What is the most common treatment for fracture of the humeral shaft?**
The majority of humeral fractures can be treated conservatively. The humeral shaft will heal well with good functional outcomes even with significant angular deformity (20–30 degrees) and displacement of the fracture. Most fractures are treated for a short period of time in a plaster or fiberglass coaptation splint. Within 1 to 2 weeks, the arm is placed in a prefabricated functional brace. The soft tissue compression and effects of gravity will often improve the alignment of the fracture over time as it heals.

27. **What are the outcomes of conservative management of humeral shaft fractures?**
Most patients with humeral shaft fractures do well with conservative treatment. Fracture union rates are between 90% and 95% for those injuries that meet the criteria for nonoperative treatment. Fracture union is usually obtained between 8 and 12 weeks. Between 80% and 98% of patients will obtain full range of motion and function of the shoulder and elbow joints.

28. **What are the indications for surgical management of humeral shaft fractures?**
There are several well-recognized indications for surgical management of humeral shaft fractures. These include pathologic fractures, associated brachial plexus injuries, associated forearm fractures (floating elbow), open fractures with high-grade soft tissue injury, vascular repair, bilateral humerus fractures, multiple trauma, and inability to maintain adequate alignment (varus angulation of 20 degrees, sagittal plane angulation of 30 degrees, or shortening of 3 cm).

29. **What are the outcomes of surgical management of humeral shaft fractures?**
Both open reduction and internal fixation (ORIF, Figure) and intramedullary fixation (IMF) produce reliable clinical results. The rate of fracture union following ORIF generally ranges from 94% to 98% whereas union rates following IMF range from 87% to 94%. Both types of surgery are associated with low but significant rates of complications. Residual elbow pain is more common following ORIF. Shoulder pain and the need for repeat surgery are more common following IMF. Direct comparisons between the two surgical techniques show trends toward slightly better outcomes following ORIF.

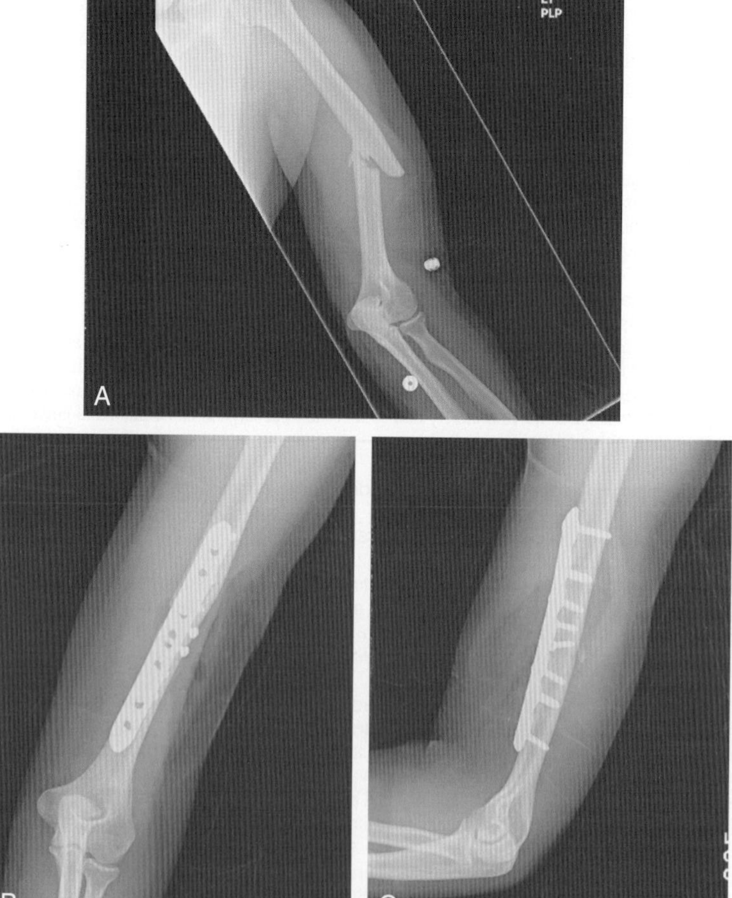

Humeral shaft fracture. (A) X-ray of angulated left humeral shaft fracture. (B) Anteroposterior x-ray following open reduction and internal fixation of humerus fracture. (C) Lateral view of left humerus.

Bibliography

Anakwenze, O. A., Zoller, S., Ahmad, C. S., & Levine, W. N. (2014). Reverse shoulder arthroplasty for acute proximal humerus fractures: A systematic review. *Journal of Shoulder and Elbow Surgery, 23*, e73–80.

Bigliani, L. U., Flatow, E. L., & Pollock, R. G. (1996). Fractures of the proximal humerus. In C. A. Rockwood et al. (Ed.), *Fractures in adults* (pp. 1055–1107). Philadelphia, PA: Lippincott-Raven.

Boileau, P., Alta, T. D., Decroocq, L., et al. (2019). Reverse shoulder arthroplasty for fractures in the elderly: Is it worth reattaching the tuberosities? *Journal of Shoulder and Elbow Surgery, 28*(3), 437–444.

Boileau, P., Trojani, C., Walch, G., Krishnan, S. G., Romeo, A., & Sinnerton, R. (2001). Shoulder arthroplasty for the treatment of the sequelae of fractures of the proximal humerus. *Journal of Shoulder and Elbow Surgery, 10*(4), 299–308.

Chapman, J. R., Henley, M. B., Agel, J., & Benca, P. J. (2000). Randomized prospective study of humeral shaft fracture fixation: Intramedullary nails versus plates. *Journal of Orthopaedic Trauma, 14*(3), 162–166.

Clavert, P., Adam, P., Bevort, A., Bonnomet, F., & Kempf, J.-F. (2010). Pitfalls and complications with locking plate for proximal humerus fracture. *Journal of Shoulder and Elbow Surgery, 19*(4), 489–494.

de Laat, E. A., Visser, C. P., Coene, L. N., Pahlplatz, P. V., & Tavy, D. L. (1994). Nerve lesions in primary shoulder dislocations and humeral neck fractures. A prospective clinical and EMG study. *Journal of Bone and Joint Surgery, 76*(3), 381–383.

Fraser, A. N., Bjørdal, J., Wagle, T. M., et al. (2020). Reverse shoulder arthroplasty is superior to plate fixation at 2 years for displaced proximal humerus fractures in the elderly: A multicenter randomized controlled trial. *Journal of Bone and Joint Surgery, 102*(6), 477–485.

Hawkins, R. J., & Switlyk, P. (1993). Acute prosthetic replacement for severe fractures of the proximal humerus. *Clinical Orthopaedics and Related Research, 289*, 156–160.

Hintermann, B., Trouillier, H. H., & Schafer, D. (2000). Rigid internal fixation of fractures of the proximal humerus in older patients. *Journal of Bone and Joint Surgery, 82*(8), 1107–1112.

Jakob, R. P., Miniaci, A., Anson, P. S., Jaberg, H., Osterwalder, A., & Ganz, R. (1991). Four-part valgus impacted fractures of the proximal humerus. *Journal of Bone and Joint Surgery, 73*(2), 295–298.

Jobin, C. M., Galdi, B., Anakwenze, O. A., Ahmad, C. S., & Levine, W. N. (2015). Reverse shoulder arthroplasty for the management of proximal humerus fractures. *Journal of the American Academy of Orthopaedic Surgeons, 23*(3), 190–201.

Jung, S.-W., Shim, S.-B., Kim, H.-M., Lee, J.-H., & Lim, H.-S. (2015). Factors that influence reduction loss in proximal humerus fracture surgery. *Journal of Orthopaedic Trauma, 29*(6), 276–282.

Kralinger, F., Blauth, M., Goldhahn, J., et al. (2014). The influence of local bone density on the outcome of 150 proximal humerus fractures treated with locking plates. *Journal of Bone and Joint Surgery, 96*(12), 1026–1032.

Lind, T., Kroner, K., & Jensen, J. (1989). The epidemiology of fractures of the proximal humerus. *Archives of Orthopaedic and Trauma Surgery, 108*(5), 285–287.

McCormack, R. G., Brien, D., Buckley, R. E., McKee, M. D., Powell, J., & Schemitsch, E. H. (2000). Fixation of fractures of the shaft of the humerus by dynamic compression plate or intramedullary nail. A prospective randomized trial. *Journal of Bone and Joint Surgery, 82*(3), 336–339.

McKee, R. C., Whelan, D. B., Schemitsch, E. H., & McKee, M. D. (2012). Operative versus nonoperative care of displaced midshaft clavicular fractures: A meta-analysis of randomized clinical trials. *Journal of Bone and Joint Surgery, 94*(8), 675–684.

Pollock, F. H., Drake, D., Bovill, E. G., Day, L., & Trafton, P. G. (1981). Treatment of radial nerve palsy associated with fractures of the humerus. *Journal of Bone and Joint Surgery, 63*(2), 239–243.

Rangan, A., Handoll, H., Brealey, S., et al. (2015). Surgical vs. nonsurgical treatment of adults with displaced fractures of the proximal humerus: the PROFHER randomized clinical trial. *JAMA, 313*(10), 1037–1047.

Robinson, C. M., Goudie, E. B., Murray, I. R., et al. (2013). Open reduction and plate fixation fixations versus nonoperative treatment for displaced midshaft clavicle fractures: A multicenter, randomized, controlled trial. *Journal of Bone and Joint Surgery, 95*(17), 1576–1584.

Rose, S. H., Melton, L. J., 3rd, Morrey, B. F., Ilstrup, D. M., & Riggs, B. L. (1982). Epidemiologic features of humeral fractures. *Clinical Orthopaedics and Related Research, 168*, 24–30.

Sarmiento, A., Zagorski, J. B., Zych, G. A., Latta, L. L., & Capps, C. A. (2000). Functional bracing for the treatment of fractures of the humerus humeral diaphysis. *Journal of Bone and Joint Surgery, 82*(4), 478–486.

Shao, Y. C., Harwood, P., Grotz, M. R. W., Limb, D., & Giannoudis, P. V. (2005). Radial nerve palsy associated with fractures of the shaft of the humerus: A systematic review. *Journal of Bone and Joint Surgery, 87*(12), 1647–1652.

Smekal, V., Irenberger, A., Struve, P., Wambacher, M., Krappinger, D., & Kralinger, F. S. (2009). Elastic stable intramedullary nailing versus nonoperative treatment of displaced midshaft clavicle fractures: A randomized, controlled, clinical trial. *Journal of Orthopaedic Trauma, 23*(2), 106–112.

Stableforth, P. G. (1984). Four-part fractures of the neck of the humerus. *Journal of Bone and Joint Surgery, 66*(1), 104–108.

Visser, C. P., Coene, L. N., Brand, R., & Tavy, D. L. (2001). Nerve lesions in proximal humeral fractures. *Journal of Shoulder and Elbow Surgery, 10*(5), 421–427.

Wijgman, A. J., Roolker, W., Patt, T. W., Raaymakers, E. L. F. B., & Marti, R. K. (2002). Open reduction and internal fixation of three- and four-part fractures of the proximal part of the humerus. *Journal of Bone and Joint Surgery, 84*(11), 1919–1925.

Yahuaca, B. I., Simon, P., Christmas, K. N., et al. (2020). Acute surgical management of proximal humerus fractures: ORIF vs. hemiarthroplasty vs. reverse shoulder arthroplasty. *Journal of Shoulder and Elbow Surgery, 29*(7S), S32–40.

Zagorski, J. B., Latta, L. L., Zych, G. A., & Finnieston, A. R. (1988). Diaphyseal fractures of the humerus. Treatment with prefabricated braces. *Journal of Bone and Joint Surgery, 70*(4), 607–610.

CHAPTER 43 QUESTIONS

1. Operative treatment of displaced midshaft clavicle fractures results in:
   a. More pain and disability
   b. Poorer return of function
   c. A greater chance of bony healing
   d. A higher risk of shoulder stiffness
   e. All of the above

2. A four-part displaced proximal humerus fracture in a 70-year-old, active, healthy female with osteoporosis should be treated with:
   a. Sling immobilization for 3 weeks, then therapy
   b. Open reduction and internal fixation with a plate
   c. Hemiarthroplasty
   d. Reverse shoulder arthroplasty
   e. Sling and bone stimulator

3. Which of the following is true regarding minimally displaced proximal humerus fractures?
   a. They are more common in the elderly.
   b. They have a relatively high rate of occult nerve injury.
   c. They can be treated nonsurgically in most cases.
   d. They typically result in only mild residual loss of shoulder function.
   e. All of the above.

4. What nerve is most commonly injured with a fracture of the clavicle?
   a. Median
   b. Ulnar
   c. Radial
   d. Nerve to subclavius

5. With proximal humerus fractures, the
   a. Humerus rotates externally due to pull of latissimus dorsi
   b. Varus angulation may occur from the pull of the deltoid
   c. Lesser tuberosity is pulled posteriorly from the subscapularis
   d. Greater tuberosity is pulled anteriorly from the supraspinatus

6. ORIF of the humeral shaft is indicated with
   a. Pathologic fractures
   b. Open fractures
   c. Floating elbow
   d. All of the above

NERVE ENTRAPMENTS OF THE SHOULDER REGION

E. Schrank, DSc, MPT and R.A. Sellin, PT, DSc, ECS

1. **How is the spinal accessory nerve usually injured?**
   The spinal accessory nerve (cranial nerve XI) is a purely motor nerve and supplies motor fibers to the upper, middle, and lower trapezius muscles as well as the sternocleidomastoid. Mechanisms of injury include tumor, surgical procedures to the posterior triangle, and stretch and whiplash injuries. The most common mechanism of injury to the accessory nerve is iatrogenic during lymph node biopsy in the posterior triangle of the neck. There is a single case report of injury after cervical manipulation.

2. **Describe the typical presentation of a patient with a spinal accessory nerve injury.**
   The patient's symptoms may include a drooping shoulder girdle and/or flat upper trapezius muscle on the involved side. Shoulder pain is a major disabling factor, often attributed to traction at the brachial plexus. Winging of the scapula caused by trapezius weakness increases with abduction, whereas winging caused by serratus anterior weakness increases with forward elevation. If there is wasting of the trapezius, the underlying bony scapula is easily visualized and often results in the mistaken impression of atrophy of the infra and supraspinatus. If the level of injury is above the innervation of the sternocleidomastoid, the patient also may demonstrate weakness in rotating the head toward the opposite shoulder. Symptoms may seem to mimic shoulder dysfunction, with pseudo-weakness of the rotator cuff secondary to decreased stability of the scapula, which, in turn, can contribute to rotator cuff pathology.

3. **How is the diagnosis of spinal accessory nerve injury made?**
   Delayed diagnosis of a spinal accessory nerve injury as the cause of shoulder pain remains a common problem, particularly in iatrogenic injuries. An electrophysiologic evaluation is required to precisely identify the level of the lesion and assess for the potential for regeneration. Electrophysiologic testing will also reveal the degree of damage and, in particular, whether or not the nerve is still intact or completely severed. Imaging procedures, such as MRI and neurosonography, can also deliver important information for planning interventions.

4. **What are the expected outcomes after a spinal accessory nerve injury?**
   If the injury was from a stretch or whiplash, recovery is typically spontaneous over the course of several months, with an excellent outcome. If the nerve suffered surgical trauma, the most important prognostic factor that can influence the outcome is the timing of the corrective operation. It should be performed within 3 to 4 months after the injury and, at the latest, before 6 months. Outcomes after spinal accessory nerve surgery are typically good although delays in diagnosis are common and may necessitate muscle transfer procedures, such as a modified Eden-Lange to help restore balance to the shoulder girdle.

5. **What are the common sites of entrapment of the suprascapular nerve?**
   The suprascapular nerve courses from nerve roots C5 and C6 and runs posterolaterally to the suprascapular notch beneath the transverse scapular ligament. The nerve is commonly injured at the suprascapular notch by ganglia or tumor. Injury at the suprascapular notch affects both the supraspinatus and the infraspinatus muscles and mimics rotator cuff pathology. The presenting symptoms include shoulder joint pain, weakness in external rotation, and, to a lesser degree, weakness in abduction.

   The suprascapular nerve is also susceptible to traction and compression injuries because it travels around the spine of the scapula through the fibro-osseous tunnel formed by the spinoglenoid ligament and the spine of the scapula. Injury at this level results in strength changes in the infraspinatus muscle and shoulder pain, with sparing of the supraspinatus muscle. There may be wasting in the infraspinatus fossa.

6. **What are common causes of injury to the suprascapular nerve?**
   A common cause of injury is traction on the nerve produced by a retracted superior or posterior rotator cuff tear. Electrodiagnostic findings of suprascapular neuropathy have been reported in patients with massive rotator cuff tears. There are also published reports that suggest that neuropathy associated with retracted rotator cuff tear may partially or completely resolve with repair of the rotator cuff. The suprascapular nerve may also be injured during surgery for rotator cuff repair because the cuff is pulled laterally to reattach, and tension is placed on the neurovascular bundle. Certain procedures for massive rotator cuff repair (double interval slide technique) place the suprascapular nerve close to the operative field, and iatrogenic injuries have been reported. Repetitive overhead athletes have been reported to experience neuropathy secondary to traction and microtrauma. Compression of

the nerve can also occur because of a bone tumor or cyst secondary to a labral or capsular injury. Other causes include brachial neuritis, shoulder dislocation, fracture in the shoulder girdle, and penetrating injury.

Prevalence ranges from 12% to 33% in athletic populations and 8% to 100% in patients with massive rotator cuff tears.

7. **What diagnostic tests are available to help confirm suprascapular nerve injury?**
Electromyography and nerve conduction studies are usually considered the criterion standard for diagnostic testing for suprascapular nerve injury, although when each test is used alone, it is not directly diagnostic. In patients with weakness, electrodiagnostic testing has shown a diagnostic accuracy of 91%, leading to a single, correct diagnosis. Diagnostic nerve blocks of the suprascapular nerve at the suprascapular notch have been used with a positive result—defined as temporary relief of the pain being experienced by the patient. Sensitivity and specificity studies are lacking with regard to the value of diagnostic nerve blocks for this problem. Magnetic resonance imaging has been shown to have a sensitivity and specificity of 94.5% and 100%, respectively, in detecting muscular edema associated with nerve injury, using electromyography and nerve conduction studies as the reference standard. Diagnostic ultrasound shows some promise in evaluation of this type of injury and is considered an advanced technique.

8. **What is the "Unhappy or Terrible Triad" in regard to the shoulder?**
The "Terrible Triad," or sometimes called the "Unhappy Triad," describes an anterior shoulder dislocation along with rotator cuff tear and peripheral nerve injury. Dislocations should be considered as a clinical spectrum that includes (1) isolated dislocations, (2) injuries producing either detachment of the rotator cuff or neurologic deficit alone, and (3) combined injuries.

9. **What nerve is most commonly injured after anterior shoulder dislocation?**
The most common neurologic deficit after anterior shoulder dislocation is isolated axillary nerve palsy, although any component of the brachial plexus may be injured. Neurologic injury occurs mostly in the young, predominantly male population during sports activities. The axillary nerve is most vulnerable to injury in anterior shoulder dislocations because it travels from the quadrilateral space, passing anteriorly and lying against the surgical neck of the humerus. The incidence of axillary nerve injury has been reported to be between 19% and 55% after anterior shoulder dislocations and up to 58% of proximal humeral fractures. Full recovery of axillary nerve injury, resulting from dislocation or fracture, occurs 85% to 100% of the time with nonoperative management within 6 to 12 months from the time of injury.

10. **Describe the motor and sensory distributions of the musculocutaneous nerve.**
The musculocutaneous nerve, which arises from the roots of C5, C6, and sometimes C7, is the terminal branch of the lateral cord of the brachial plexus. It innervates and penetrates the coracobrachialis muscle and travels between and innervates the biceps brachii and brachialis muscles. The musculocutaneous nerve emerges laterally to the biceps tendon as the lateral antebrachial cutaneous nerve, providing sensory innervation to the lateral forearm. Damage to this nerve causes weakness in elbow flexion and supination and numbness or paresthesias in the lateral forearm.

11. **What are the common mechanisms of injury to the musculocutaneous nerve?**
Isolated musculocutaneous nerve injury is very rare and is usually described in association with other nerve injuries, such as brachial plexus injury. Many of the reported cases have been sports related and include weight lifting, resistive exercise, rowing, football and baseball throwing, swimming, tennis, racquetball, and windsurfing. Traumatic causes include fractures or dislocations of the humerus, fracture of the clavicle, gunshot or stab wounds, entrapment by the coracobrachialis muscle, heavy exercise, and complications from anterior shoulder surgery.

12. **What are common causes for long thoracic nerve injuries?**
Isolated injury to the long thoracic nerve is rare. Traumatic causes of injury result from overuse and strenuous exercise of the shoulder, blunt trauma, or sudden depression of the shoulder. Iatrogenic nerve injury may occur after axilla or chest surgery or after incorrect positioning of the arm during general anesthesia. Long thoracic mononeuropathy is sometimes associated with infectious diseases, natural delivery, cervical manipulation, electric burn, C7 radiculopathy, or use of a single axillary crutch.

13. **What are expected outcomes for someone with a long thoracic nerve palsy?**
Overall, outcomes are generally favorable, even with no surgical intervention. If the cause of injury was inflammatory or idiopathic, the probability of a full recovery is increased. Electromyography (EMG) is an invaluable tool to confirm the clinical diagnosis of long thoracic mononeuropathy, but EMG findings do not seem to be a good predictor of the final outcome.

14. What are the common causes of brachial plexus injuries?
Motorcycle/snowmobile accidents, gunshot wounds, traction to arm or neck, fractures of the humerus, dislocations of the shoulder, primary nerve tumors, metastatic breast cancer, and radiation therapy can cause brachial plexus injuries. Closed injuries account for the majority of brachial plexus injuries, and 75% of injuries occur at the root level. Idiopathic brachial neuritis (Parsonage-Turner syndrome or neuralgic amyotrophy) is a postinfectious inflammatory condition that initially presents with acute onset of painful upper limb weakness. It is thought to be immune mediated. This initial phase is followed by a painless paresis that typically recovers over a 6- to 18-month time span.

15. What are the clinical signs and symptoms of typical brachial plexus injuries?

- Upper trunk lesions affect the suprascapular, musculocutaneous, and axillary nerves as well as parts of the median and radial nerves. Patients' symptoms include weakness in shoulder flexion, abduction, and extension as well as marked weakness in elbow flexion, supination, and pronation and in wrist flexion. Areas of numbness and paresthesia may include the lateral forearm and hands as well as the thumb and index fingers.
- The middle trunk is rarely injured in isolation. Lesions produce weakness in the general distribution of the radial nerve, partially involving the triceps and sparing the brachioradialis.
- Lower trunk lesions cause motor weakness in muscles innervated by the ulnar nerve, the C8 components of the radial nerve, and muscles innervated by the distal median nerve, including the thenar muscles and the lumbricals. Patients have profound weakness of hand intrinsic muscles and sensory changes in the medial forearm (medial antebrachial cutaneous nerve), the medial hand, and the entire ring and little fingers.
- Lesions of either the posterior or anterior division are rare in isolation, although a posterior division lesion has been reported.
- Lateral cord lesions are similar to upper trunk lesions with sparing of the suprascapular nerve and upper trunk contributions to the axillary and radial nerves. Normal shoulder strength in flexion, extension, abduction, and external rotation; weakness in elbow flexion, supination, and pronation and wrist flexion; and numbness in the lateral forearm implicate the lateral cord.
- Medial cord lesions are similar to lower trunk lesions with sparing of C8 contributions to the radial nerve. Finger extension has normal strength.
- Posterior cord lesions are rare in isolation.

16. What key muscle tests help differentiate a C5–C6 root injury from a lateral cord lesion?
A C5–C6 root lesion affects all C5–C6 muscles, whereas an upper trunk lesion typically spares the dorsal scapular nerve to the rhomboids and the long thoracic nerve to the serratus anterior. A lateral cord lesion spares the suprascapular nerve (shoulder external rotation and abduction) as well as contributions to the posterior cord.

17. What is thoracic outlet syndrome (TOS)?
Thoracic outlet syndrome (TOS) refers to the compression of the neurovascular structures (roots or trunks of the brachial plexus and axillary or subclavian arteries) between the neck and axilla. TOS can be subdivided into vascular or neural compression symptoms, or both, depending on which specific structures within the cervicoaxillary canal are compromised. Klaassen reports the majority of cases (nearly 95%) are neurogenic in nature. True neurologic TOS manifests as a chronic lower trunk brachial plexopathy, caused by anatomic anomalies. The anomalies include a taut band extending from near the tubercle of the first thoracic rib to the tip of either the C7 transverse process or a rudimentary cervical rib. The C8 and T1 anterior primary rami can be stretched around this band either before or after, forming the lower trunk. Electromyography may show evidence of denervation in the intrinsic hand muscles, but this is not common. Neural compression symptoms occur more commonly than vascular symptoms. The cause of TOS also can be traumatic. A midshaft fracture of the clavicle occasionally results in injury to the blood vessels or brachial plexus, which are situated between the clavicle and first thoracic rib. With this type of injury, the terminal portion of the subclavian artery, the initial portion of the subclavian vein, and the proximal aspects of the cords of the brachial plexus may be damaged. Urschel and Razzuk performed a 50-year analysis of 2210 patients treated surgically for TOS, describing 250 with upper plexus compression, 1508 with lower plexus compression, and 452 symptomatic for both.

18. What diagnostic tests are helpful in diagnosing TOS?
Klaassen describes one of the issues with TOS as a lack of a gold standard for definitive diagnosis. Radiographs, CT scans, and MRIs provide for detection of cervical ribs and fibrous bands for identification of potential factors causing TOS. Confirmation of a vascular abnormality is aided by the use of duplex ultrasound, which has been found to be 92% sensitive and 95% specific. In addition, electrophysiologic testing is valuable for differential diagnosis and determining the presence of additional abnormalities such as cervical nerve root or distal peripheral nerve pathology.

19. **Describe the clinical findings of a patient with Pancoast tumor.**
A Pancoast tumor (also known as a superior sulcus tumor) can compromise the C8–T1 roots of the brachial plexus via compression from the apex of the lung. The presenting symptoms of the patient are sensory changes in the medial forearm and hand, including the fourth and fifth digits. Other signs may include intrinsic muscle wasting, Horner syndrome, and a history of night pain. Clinicians should be especially suspicious of a Pancoast tumor in smokers who have these symptoms and no history of trauma or neurologic disease.

20. **What is a "burner" or "stinger"?**
"Burner" or "stinger" are commonly used terms to describe a transient upper trunk brachial plexus neuropraxia that usually occurs during a contact sport. The athlete often describes a "burning" or "stinging" sensation down the arm when injured. The disorder usually produces transient pain, numbness, and paresthesia. Chronic burner syndrome may result from nerve root compression in the intervertebral foramina secondary to disc disease in older collegiate and professional athletes. Several mechanisms of injury have been proposed, including traction of the plexus due to rapid lateral flexion of the neck as well as compression of the fixed brachial plexus between the shoulder pad and the superior medial scapula when the pad is pushed into the area of Erb's point, where the brachial plexus is most superficial. The disorder usually produces transient pain, numbness, and paresthesia. Researchers have identified high rates of structural abnormalities in the cervical spine in athletes with recurrent stingers, particularly spinal canal or neural foraminal stenosis.

Bibliography

Albritton, M. J., Graham, R. D., Richards, R. S., II, & Basamania, C. J. (2003). An anatomic study of the effects on the suprascapular nerve due to retraction of the supraspinatus muscle after a rotator cuff tear. *Journal of Shoulder and Elbow Surgery, 12*(5), 497–500.

Antoniadis, G., Kretschmer, T., Pedro, M. T., Konig, R. W., Heinen, C. P. G., & Richter, H.-P. (2014). Iatrogenic nerve injuries. *Deutsches Ärzteblatt International, 111*(16), 273–279.

Arzillo, S., Gishen, K., & Askari, M. (2014). Brachial plexus injury: treatment options and outcomes. *Journal of Craniofacial Surgery, 25*(4), 1200–1206.

Besleaga, D., Castellano, V., Lutz, C., & Feinberg, J. H. (2010). Musculocutaneous neuropathy: case report and discussion. *HSS Journal, 6*(1), 112–116.

Carofino, B. C., Brogan, D. M., Kircher, M. F., et al. (2013). Iatrogenic nerve injuries during shoulder surgery. *Journal of Bone and Joint Surgery, 95*(18), 1667–1674.

Chandra, V., Little, C., & Lee, J. T. (2014). Thoracic outlet syndrome in high performance athletes. *Journal of Vascular Surgery, 60*(4), P1012–1018.

Charbonneau, R. M., McVeigh, S. A., & Thompson, K. (2012). Brachial neuropraxia in Canadian Atlantic University sport football players: what is the incidence of "stingers"? *Clinical Journal of Sport Medicine, 22*(6), 472–477. https://doi.org/10.1097/JSM.0b013e3182699ed5

Collin, P., Treseder, T., Lädermann, A., et al. (2014). Neuropathy of the suprascapular nerve and massive rotator cuff tears: a prospective electromyographic study. *Journal of Shoulder and Elbow Surgery, 23*(1), 28–34.

Cordova, C. B., & Owens, B. D. (2014). Infraspinatus muscle atrophy from suprascapular nerve compression. *Journal of the American Academy of Physician Assistants, 27*(2), 33–35.

Costouros, J. G., Porramatikul, M., Lie, D. T., & Warner, J. J. P. (2007). Reversal of suprascapular neuropathy following arthroscopic repair of massive supraspinatus and infraspinatus rotator cuff tears. *Arthroscopy: The Journal of Arthroscopic & Related Surgery, 23*(11), 1152–1161.

Dramis, A., & Pimpalnerkar, A. (2005). Suprascapular neuropathy in volleyball players. *Acta Orthopaedica Belgica, 71*(3), 269–272.

Feinberg, J. H. (2000). Burners and stingers. *Physical Medicine and Rehabilitation Clinics of North America, 11*(4), 771–784.

Freehill, M. T., Shi, L. L., Tompson, J. D., & Warner, J. J. P. (2012). Suprascapular neuropathy: diagnosis and management. *The Physician and Sportsmedicine, 40*(1), 72–83.

Friedenberg, S. M., Zimprich, T., & Michel Harper, C. (2002). The natural history of long thoracic and spinal accessory neuropathies. *Muscle & Nerve, 25*(4), 535–539.

Glassman, L., & Hyman, K. (2013). Pancoast tumor: a modern perspective on an old problem. [Miscellaneous Article]. *Current Opinion in Pulmonary Medicine, 19*(4), 340–343.

Gustin, M., Olszewski, N., Parisien, R. L., & Li, X. (2020). The modified Eden-Lange tendon transfer for lateral scapular winging secondary to spinal accessory nerve injury. *Arthroscopy Techniques, 9*(10), e1581–e1589.

Henry, D., & Bonthius, D. J. (2011). Isolated musculocutaneous neuropathy in an adolescent baseball pitcher. *Journal of Child Neurology, 26*(12), 1567–1570.

Holzgraefe, M., Kukowski, B., & Eggert, S. (1994). Prevalence of latent and manifest suprascapular neuropathy in high-performance volleyball players. *British Journal of Sports Medicine, 28*(3), 177–179.

Jezierski, H., Podgórski, M., Wysiadecki, G., et al. (2018). Morphological aspects in ultrasound visualisation of the suprascapular notch region: a study based on a new four-step protocol. *Journal of Clinical Medicine, 7*(12), E491.

Jones, M. R., Prabhakar, A., Viswanath, O., et al. (2019). Thoracic outlet syndrome: a comprehensive review of pathophysiology, diagnosis, and treatment. *Pain and Therapy, 8*(1), 5–18.

Kim, D. H., Cho, Y. -J., Tiel, R. L., & Kline, D. G. (2003). Surgical outcomes of 111 spinal accessory nerve injuries. *Neurosurgery, 53*(5), 1106–1113.

Klaassen, Z., Sorenson, E., Tubbs, R. S., et al. (2014). Thoracic outlet syndrome: a neurological and vascular disorder. *Clinical Anatomy, 27*(5), 724–732.

Lajtai, G., Wieser, K., Ofner, M., Raimann, G., Aitzetmüller, G., & Jost, B. (2012). Electromyography and nerve conduction velocity for the evaluation of the infraspinatus muscle and the suprascapular nerve in professional beach volleyball players. *American Journal of Sports Medicine, 40*(10), 2303–2308.

Mallon, W. J., Wilson, R. J., & Basamania, C. J. (2006). The association of suprascapular neuropathy with massive rotator cuff tears: a preliminary report. *Journal of Shoulder and Elbow Surgery, 15*(4), 395–398.

Mautner, K., & Keel, J. C. (2007). Musculocutaneous nerve injury after simulated freefall in a vertical wind-tunnel: a case report. *Archives of Physical Medicine and Rehabilitation, 88*(3), 391–393.

Mondelli, M., Aretini, A., & Ginanneschi, F. (2013). Predictive factors of recovery in long thoracic mononeuropathy. *Orthopedics, 36*(6), e707–e714.

Peck, E., & Strakowski, J. A. (2015). Ultrasound evaluation of focal neuropathies in athletes: a clinically-focused review. *British Journal of Sports Medicine, 49*(3), 166–175.

Robinson, C. M., Shur, N., Sharpe, T., Ray, A., & Murray, I. R. (2012). Injuries associated with traumatic anterior glenohumeral dislocations. *Journal of Bone and Joint Surgery. American Volume, 94*(1), 18–26.

Shi, L. L., Freehill, M. T., Yannopoulos, P., & Warner, J. J. P. (2012). Suprascapular nerve: is it important in cuff pathology? *Advances in Orthopedics, 2012*, 516985.

Simonich, S. D., & Wright, T. W. (2003). Terrible triad of the shoulder. *Journal of Shoulder and Elbow Surgery/American Shoulder and Elbow Surgeons, 12*(6), 566–568.

Standaert, C. J., & Herring, S. A. (2009). Expert opinion and controversies in musculoskeletal and sports medicine: stingers. *Archives of Physical Medicine and Rehabilitation, 90*(3), 402–406.

Stephens, L., Kinderknecht, J. J., & Wen, D. Y. (2014). Musculocutaneous nerve injury in a high school pitcher. *Clinical Journal of Sport Medicine, 24*(6).

Takase, F., Inui, A., Mifune, Y., et al. (2014). Concurrent rotator cuff tear and axillary nerve palsy associated with anterior dislocation of the shoulder and large glenoid rim fracture: a "terrible tetrad." *Case Reports in Orthopedics, 2014*, 1–4.

Tom, J. A., Mesfin, A., Shah, M. P., et al. (2014). Anatomical considerations of the suprascapular nerve in rotator cuff repairs. *Anatomy Research International, 2014*, 674179.

Twaij, H., Rolls, A., Sinisi, M., & Weiler, R. (2013). Thoracic outlet syndromes in sport: a practical review in the face of limited evidence—unusual pain presentation in an athlete. *British Journal of Sports Medicine, 47*(17), 1080–1084.

Witvrouw, E., Cools, A., Lysens, R., et al. (2000). Suprascapular neuropathy in volleyball players. *British Journal of Sports Medicine, 34*(3), 174–180.

Yeap, J. S., Lee, D. J. K., Fazir, M., Kareem, B. A., & Yeap, J. K. (2004). Nerve injuries in anterior shoulder dislocations. *Medical Journal of Malaysia, 59*(4), 450–454.

Yoon, J. R., Kim, Y. K., Ko, Y. D., Yun, S. I., Song, D. H., & Chung, M. E. (2018). Spinal accessory nerve injury induced by manipulation therapy: a case report. *Annals of Rehabilitation Medicine, 42*(5), 773–776.

CHAPTER 44 QUESTIONS

1. **John is a 36-year-old male who complains of left shoulder pain and weakness in his shoulder. On examination he has full ROM of his shoulder but has 3/5 weakness in external rotation and 4+/5 shoulder abduction. His sensory exam was normal, and he does not have increased pain with resisted shoulder motions. John most likely has a lesion involving the:**
   a. Axillary nerve
   b. Spinal accessory nerve
   c. Suprascapular nerve
   d. Upper trunk of the brachial plexus

2. **The "Unhappy or Terrible Triad" related to the shoulder refers to a/an:**
   a. Acromioclavicular arthritis, rotator cuff tear, and peripheral nerve injury
   b. Anterior shoulder dislocation, rotator cuff tear, and peripheral nerve injury
   c. Glenohumeral arthritis, rotator cuff tear, and peripheral nerve injury
   d. Rotator cuff tear, labral lesion, and peripheral nerve injury

3. **Mary is a 23-year-old, right-hand-dominant volleyball player who has developed right shoulder pain and winging of her right scapula. She has full cervical and upper extremity ROM. She appears to have near normal strength in her shoulder, and resisted motions of the shoulder are painless. However, she has marked right scapular winging with wall push-ups. This is most likely a lesion of the:**
   a. Dorsal scapular nerve
   b. Long thoracic nerve
   c. Spinal accessory nerve
   d. Suprascapular nerve

CHAPTER 45

FUNCTIONAL ANATOMY OF THE ELBOW

J. Placzek, MD, PT and A. Placzek

1. **Describe the joints of the elbow.**
The elbow consists of three joints: the ulnohumeral, radiocapitellar, and proximal radioulnar joints. The olecranon forms the greater sigmoid notch of the ulna, which articulates with the trochlea to form a uniaxial ginglymoid joint. The radiocapitellar and proximal radioulnar joints form a trochoid or pivoted joint. The thin elbow capsule and synovial membrane define the confines of the joint, beginning proximal to the coronoid and olecranon fossae and ending beyond the tips of the coronoid and olecranon processes. Because the maximal volume of the capsule is 15 to 30 ml at 80-degree flexion, the elbow often is held in this position to minimize pain from capsular distention secondary to acute hemarthrosis.

2. **What is the normal carrying angle of the elbow?**
The carrying angle of the elbow varies with flexion and extension, ranging from 6 degrees of varus with full flexion to 11 degrees of valgus in full extension. In men the mean value is between 11 and 14 degrees (full extension). Some studies show that women tend to have larger carrying angles than men, with an average value between 13 and 16 degrees.

3. **Describe the articular geometry of the distal humerus.**
The articular surface has a 30-degree anterior angulation, 5 to 7 degrees of internal rotation, and 6 to 8 degrees of valgus tilt.

4. **Describe the interosseous membrane (IOM) of the forearm.**
The interosseous membrane is composed of the central band, the proximal band, several accessory bands, and the membranous portion. The most important structure is the central band, which originates from the radius and is angled distally to attach to the ulna at a 21-degree angle. The central band is 1.5 to 2 cm wide and is responsible for 71% of the IOM stiffness after excision of the radial head.

5. **What portion of the longitudinal growth of the upper arm does the elbow contribute?**
The elbow accounts for only 20% of the total longitudinal growth of the humerus. The proximal humerus accounts for the remaining 80%.

6. **What structures contribute to elbow stability?**
Elbow stability is maintained by a combination of bony and soft tissue components. Primary stabilizers include the coronoid (ulnohumeral joint), lateral ulnar collateral ligament, and anterior band of the medial collateral ligament. Secondary stabilizers include the radial head, extensor and flexor muscle masses, and joint capsule.

7. **Describe the medial ligamentous complex.**
The main constraint to elbow valgus instability is the medial collateral ligament (MCL). The MCL originates on the central two thirds of the anteroinferior medial condyle and inserts onto the anteromedial coronoid. It has three distinct bundles. The anterior bundle, which is the strongest, inserts on the anterior coronoid and greater sigmoid notch. The thin posterior bundle attaches to the posterior greater sigmoid notch. The oblique bundle is variable in its attachments. The anterior bundle is divided into anterior and posterior bands. The anterior band is the primary restraint to valgus stress from 30 to 90 degrees, while the posterior band tensions from 90 to 120 degrees.

8. **Describe the lateral ligamentous complex.**
The lateral collateral ligament (LCL) complex consists of the radial collateral ligament (lateral epicondyle to annular ligament), the annular ligament (anterior to posterior edge of sigmoid notch), the accessory collateral ligament (variable, posterior annular ligament to supinator crest), and the lateral ulnar collateral ligaments (LUCLs, lateral epicondyle to supinator crest), which blend intimately with the underlying joint capsule and more superficial extensor tendons. The LUCL insertion may be broad-based or bilobed and is the primary constraint to posterolateral rotatory instability.

9. **Describe the most important varus and valgus stabilizers of the elbow at 0 and 90 degrees of flexion.**
Varus stress at the elbow is resisted by the LCL, anconeus muscle, and joint capsule. With full extension, the LCL contributes 14% of the restraint to varus stress; 54% is provided by the joint surface and 32% by the capsule.

With 90 degrees of flexion, restraint to varus stress provided by the LCL, joint articulation, and capsule changes to 9%, 78%, and 13%, respectively.

Valgus stress is resisted mainly by the fan-shaped MCL complex, which consists of anterior, intermediate, and posterior fibers. The anterior oblique fibers are taut throughout flexion-extension and are the most important valgus stabilizers. The posterior oblique ligaments are taut only during flexion. At full extension, contributions from the MCL, joint surface, and anterior capsule to resisting valgus stress are equal. At 90 degrees of flexion, the MCL contributes 54% of the resistance, the radial head contributes 30%, and the remainder is supplied by articular congruity and the anterior capsule.

10. What provides the most dynamic stabilization of the medial elbow?

The flexor carpi ulnaris (FCU) provides the greatest stability followed by the flexor digitorum profundus (FDS) and pronator teres (PT).

11. Describe posterolateral rotatory instability.

Posterolateral rotatory instability (PLRI) is a common pattern of acute elbow instability, caused by a fall onto an outstretched arm. The humerus rotates internally on the elbow, which undergoes external rotation and valgus loading as the elbow flexes. Specifically, the ulnar rotates externally while the radiohumeral joint subluxes posterolaterally, allowing the coronoid to pass under the trochlea as the ulna swings into a valgus position.

12. What is the Morrey elbow instability scale?

Morrey described five elbow instability types based on damage to particular structures about the elbow:

- Type 0—elbow reduced and stable when stressed
- Type I—PLRI with a positive shift test; torn LUCL
- Type II—perched condyles, unstable elbow with varus stress; torn LUCL and anterior and posterior capsules
- Type IIIa—posterior dislocation of the elbow with valgus instability; torn LUCL, posterior MCL, and anterior and posterior capsules
- Type IIIb—posterior dislocation of the elbow with gross instability; torn LUCL, anterior MCL, posterior MCL, and anterior and posterior capsules

13. During closed-chain upper extremity exercise, how much weight is transmitted through the radiocapitellar and ulnohumeral joints?

Approximately 60% of the force is transferred through the radiocapitellar joint and 40% through the ulnohumeral joint. The greatest amount of force is transmitted between 0 and 30 degrees of flexion.

14. Describe normal arthrokinematics at the elbow.

Motion at the elbow is primarily gliding for both flexion and extension. Rolling occurs in the final 5 to 10 degrees of range of motion (ROM) for both flexion and extension. Minimal adduction may occur with flexion and minimal abduction with extension, although the magnitude of these movements is debated.

15. Differentiate "normal" from "functional" elbow ROM.

The normal average ROM of the elbow is from 0 degrees (full extension) to 150 degrees (full flexion) with 85 degrees of supination and 80 degrees of pronation. However, activities of daily living usually can be accomplished with a ROM of 30 to 130 degrees of flexion, 50 degrees of supination, and 50 degrees of pronation. If pronation and supination are normal with good motion of the wrist and shoulder, functional mobility may occur with as little as 75 to 120 degrees of motion.

16. Where is the axis of flexion and extension in the elbow? Where is the axis during pronation and supination?

The axis of flexion of the elbow is a line through the center of the capitellum and the center of curvature of the trochlear groove, colinear with the distal anterior humeral cortex. Motion resembles a "loose hinge," with 3 to 5 degrees of rotation and varus/valgus motion during the flexion arc. During pronation and supination, the radius rotates along an axis passing through the center of the radial head and the distal ulnar fovea. The radial head translates 1 to 2 mm proximally during pronation.

17. Which muscle is considered the "workhorse" of elbow flexion?

The brachialis muscle is the primary flexor of the elbow, inserting approximately 1 cm distal to the coronoid onto both the ulna and the capsule. The brachioradialis has the longest lever arm.

18. What is the primary function of the brachioradialis?

The brachioradialis is active during all aspects of elbow flexion regardless of forearm rotation, indicating its role as elbow stabilizer. It is also more active in pronation than supination, indicating it acts as a secondary pronator.

19. **Describe the effect of speed on muscle recruitment during supination.**
During slow, unresisted supination activity, the supinator may act independently. However, all rapid and resisted movements are assisted by the biceps. This holds true regardless of elbow position.

20. **Describe the effects of speed and joint angle on pronation activity.**
The pronator quadratus is the primary pronator of the forearm, regardless of elbow position. With increasing speeds or resistance, activity of the pronator teres increases.

21. **What is the effect of changing forearm position on muscle testing of elbow flexion strength?**
Resisting elbow flexion with the forearm in neutral position places maximal stress on the brachioradialis muscle. Testing the elbow with the forearm pronated minimizes bicep activity. Forearm position does not affect the activity of the brachialis.

22. **At what position are elbow flexion strength and supination strength maximal?**
Elbow flexion strength is maximal at 90 to 110 degrees of flexion. The biceps act most strongly as a supinator at 90 degrees of flexion. Pronation strength is 15% to 20% less than supination strength in the normal elbow.

23. **Describe the innervation of the various muscles controlling movement at the elbow.**

ACTION	MUSCLES	NERVE ROOT	NERVE
Flexion	Brachialis	C5, C6	Musculocutaneous
	Biceps brachii		—
	Brachioradialis		Radial
Extension	Triceps	C7	Radial
	Anconeus		
Pronation	Pronator teres	C6, C7	Median
	Pronator quadratus		
Supination	Biceps	C5, C6	Musculocutaneous
	Supinator	C5, C6, C7	Deep branch of radial

24. **Which arteries supply blood to the elbow?**
Three arcades surround the elbow joint. The medial arcade is formed by the superior and inferior ulnar collateral arteries and the posterior ulnar recurrent artery. The posterior arcade is formed by the medial and lateral arcades and the middle collateral artery. The lateral arcade is formed from the radial and middle collateral, radial recurrent, and interosseous recurrent arteries.

25. **What is the order (and approximate age) of ossification of structures around the elbow?**
Ossification follows the acronym CRMTOL: **c**apitellum (6 months to 2 years), which includes the lateral crista of the trochlea; **r**adial head (4 years); **m**edial epicondyle (6–7 years); **t**rochlea (8 years); **o**lecranon (8–10 years); and **l**ateral epicondyle (12 years).

26. **Describe the anatomy of the ulnar nerve at the elbow.**
The ligament of Osborne is present in all elbows, and two thirds of elbows will also display a discrete arcade of ligament of Struthers. An average of one capsular branch diverges from the ulnar nerve 7 mm proximally to the medial epicondyle. An average of three motor branches to the flexor carpi ulnaris (FCU) is typical. Approximately 45% of elbows will have an aponeurosis distal to Osborne's ligament, which runs between the FCU and medial epicondylar muscles.

27. **Does the ulnar nerve really innervate the medial triceps?**
Gross connection of the ulnar nerve to the medial triceps may be apparent; however, these fibers typically can be traced back as branches originally carried by the radial nerve that crossed over in the axillary region.

28. **The medial antebrachial cutaneous nerve is subject to painful neuromas if disrupted during surgery. Where do branches of this nerve typically cross the medial elbow?**
 In approximately 61% of the time, a branch is noted an average of 1.8 cm above the medial epicondyle; 100% of the time branches cross distally to the medial epicondyle at an average distance of 3.1 cm.

29. **What is the blood supply to the extensor carpi radialis brevis (ECRB) tendon?**
 The radial recurrent artery supplies the tendon through branches on its medial and lateral borders. Important contributions are given from the posterior branch of the radial collateral artery and more minor contributions from the interosseous recurrent artery. These arteries form a superficial network with the deep portion of the tendon being nearly avascular.

30. **Describe the anatomy of the lateral joint capsule.**
 The ECRB originates as a tendon with no muscular fibers, which are seen in other extensors. The anterior portion is thin under the ECRB, whereas the posterior portion was thicker and mingled with fibers from the supinator and annular ligament. This thin attachment can explain why patients with lateral epicondylitis often have pain with stressing of the lateral joint capsule, which may play a role in the development of lateral epicondylitis.

31. **What is the relationship of the posterior interosseous nerve (PIN) near the lateral elbow?**
 Pronation of the forearm increases the distance from the capitellum to the PIN to an average of 52 mm. Supination draws the nerve proximal with an average distance of 33 mm from the capitellum.

32. **What is the innervation pattern of the radial nerve in the forearm?**
 The most common innervation pattern in the forearm was brachioradialis, extensor carpi radialis longus, superficial sensory, extensor carpi radialis brevis, supinator, extensor digitorum/extensor carpi ulnaris, extensor digiti minimi, abductor pollicis longus, extensor pollicis brevis, extensor pollicis longus, and extensor indicis.

33. **What distal bicep tendon repair technique is at greatest risk for radioulnar impingement?**
 Repair with suture anchors carries greater risk than a bony trough or suture button technique.

34. **What are the differences in function regarding the long and short head of the biceps at the elbow?**
 The short and long heads of the biceps have separate insertions. The short head's insertion allows greater efficiency with the elbow flexed at 90 degrees. In the neutral and pronated forearm, the short head is a more efficient supinator. In the supinated forearm, the long head becomes more efficient at supination.

35. **What advantage does a two-incision technique have over a one-incision technique for distal biceps repairs?**
 A two-incision technique allows for a more anatomic repair to the tuberosity, likely allowing for increased strength, particularly into supination.

36. **How is elbow flexion strength affected after release of the brachioradialis tendon during repair of distal radius fractures?**
 Brachioradialis torque does not drop down to less than 80% of normal, and therefore, overall elbow flexion torque changes less than 5% because of the primary flexion effects of the biceps and brachialis.

37. **Describe the anatomy of the distal triceps tendon insertion.**
 The triceps inserts at 1.1 cm from the tip of the olecranon. The triceps width is approximately 2.6 cm. The tendon extends proximally at an average of 15.3 cm. Three distinct areas of insertion are present, the capsular insertion, the deep muscular portion, and the superficial tendinous portion.

38. **Describe kinematics at the elbow during throwing activities.**
 The elbow extends up to 2400 degrees per second when throwing while valgus torque at the elbow can reach 64 Nm.

39. **What throwing mechanics are correlated with loads of the medial collateral ligament?**
 Trunk rotation before front-foot contact increased elbow valgus torques. Side arm throwing increased elbow valgus torques compared to the overhand slot position. Increased elbow flexion is associated with decreased valgus torques.

Bibliography

Aguinaldo, A. L., & Chambers, H. (2009). Correlation of throwing mechanics with elbow valgus load in adult pitchers. *American Journal of Sports Medicine, 37*(10), 2043–2048.

Barco, R., Sánchez, P., Morrey, M. E., Morrey, B. F., & Sánchez-Sotelo, J. (2017). The distal triceps tendon insertional anatomy – implications for surgery. *JSES Open Access, 1*(2), 98–103.

Boland, M. R., Spigelman, T., & Uhl, T. L. (2008). The function of brachioradialis. *Journal of Hand Surgery, 33*(10), 1853–1859.

Branovacki, G., Hanson, M., Cash, R., & Gonzalez, M. (1998). The innervation pattern of the radial nerve at the elbow and in the forearm. *Journal of Hand Surgery (British), 23*(2), 167–169.

Degeorges, R., & Masquelet, A. C. (2002). The cubital tunnel: An anatomical part of its distal part. *Surgical and Radiologic Anatomy, 24*, 169–176.

Diliberti, T., Botte, M., & Abrams, R. (2000). Anatomical considerations regarding the posterior interosseous nerve during posterolateral approaches to the proximal part of the radius. *Journal of Bone and Joint Surgery, 82*(6), 809–813.

Gonzalez, M. H., Lofti, P., Bendre, A., Mandelbroyt, Y., & Lieska, N. (2001). The ulnar nerve at the elbow and its local branching: An anatomic study. *Journal of Hand Surgery (British), 26*, 142–144.

Hollinshead, W. H. (1969). *Anatomy for surgeons, vol. 3.* New York, NY: Harper & Row.

Jarrett, C. D., Weir, D. M., Stuffmann, E. S., Jain, S., Miller, M. C., & Schmidt, C. C. (2012). Anatomic and biomechanical analysis of the short and long head components of the distal biceps tendon. *Journal of Shoulder and Elbow Surgery, 21*(7), 942–948.

Krueger, C. A., Aden, J. K., Broughton, K., & Rispoli, D. M. (2014). Radioulnar space available at the level of the biceps tuberosity for repaired biceps tendon: A comparison of 4 techniques. *Journal of Shoulder and Elbow Surgery, 23*(11), 1717–1723.

Loftice, J., Fleisig, G. S., Zheng, N., & Andrews, J. R. (2004). Biomechanics of the elbow in sports. *Clinical Journal of Sports Medicine, 23*(4), 519–530.

Lowe, J. B., Maggi, S. P., & Mackinnon, S. E. (2004). The position of crossing branches of the medial antebrachial cutaneous nerve during cubital tunnel surgery in humans. *Plastic and Reconstructive Surgery, 114*, 692–696.

Mazzocca, A. D., Cohen, M., Berkson, E., et al. (2007). The anatomy of the bicipital tuberosity and distal biceps tendon. *Journal of Shoulder and Elbow Surgery, 16*(1), 122–127.

Nimura, A., Fujishiro, H., Wakabayashi, Y., Imatani, J., Sugaya, H., & Akita, K. (2014). Joint capsule attachment to the extensor carpi radialis brevis origin: An anatomical study with possible implications regarding the etiology of lateral epicondylitis. *Journal of Hand Surgery (American), 39*(2), 219–225.

O'Driscoll, S. W., Morrey, B. F., & Korinek, S. (1992). Elbow subluxation and dislocation: A spectrum of instability. *Clinical Orthopaedics and Related Research, 280*, 186–197.

Park, M. C., & Ahmad, C. S. (2004). Dynamic contributions of the flexor-pronator mass to elbow valgus stability. *Journal of Bone and Joint Surgery (American), 86*(10), 2268–2274.

Pascual-Font, A., Vazquez, T., Marco, F., Saæudo, J. R., & Rodriguez- Niedenführ, M. (2013). Ulnar nerve innervation of the triceps muscle: Real or apparent? An anatomic study. *Clinical Orthopaedics and Related Research, 471*(6), 1887–1893.

Schneeberger, A. G., & Masquelet, A. C. (2002). Arterial vascularization of the proximal extensor carpi radialis brevis tendon. *Clinical Orthopaedics, 398*, 239–244.

Simon, S. R. (Ed.), (1994). *Orthopaedic basic science.* Rosemont, IL: American Academy of Orthopaedic Surgeons.

Tirrell, T. F., Franko, O. I., Bhola, S., Hentzen, E. R., Abrams, R. A., & Lieber, R. L. (2013). Functional consequence of distal brachioradialis tendon release: A biomechanical study. *Journal of Hand Surgery, 38*(5), 920–926.

Yamaguchi, K., Sweet, F. A., Bindra, R., Morrey, B. F., & Gelberman, R. H. (1997). The extraosseous and intraosseous arterial anatomy of the adult elbow. *Journal of Bone and Joint Surgery, 79*(11), 1653–1662.

CHAPTER 45 QUESTIONS

1. **What is the last muscle in the forearm that is innervated by the radial nerve?**
   a. Extensor indicis
   b. Extensor digitorum
   c. Extensor digiti minimi
   d. Abductor pollicis longus

2. **The anterior lateral joint capsule of the elbow:**
   a. Is thick and stout
   b. Blends with the annular ligament
   c. Blends with the supinator
   d. Is thin under ECRB

3. **The last growth plate to ossify in the elbow is the:**
   a. Capitellum
   b. Lateral epicondyle
   c. Medial epicondyle
   d. Olecranon

4. **Which statement is false regarding the articular geometry of the distal humerus?**
   a. There is 30 degrees of anterior angulation.
   b. There is 5–7 degrees of internal rotation.
   c. There is 5–7 degrees of external rotation.
   d. There is 6–8 degrees of valgus tilt.

5. **Where is elbow flexion strength maximal?**
   a. 30 degrees of flexion
   b. 50 degrees of flexion
   c. 80 degrees of flexion
   d. 100 degrees of flexion

6. **What advantage does a two-incision distal bicep reconstruction have over a single incision technique?**
   a. Greater flexion ROM
   b. Greater extension ROM
   c. Greater supination strength
   d. Greater elbow flexion strength

CHAPTER 46

COMMON ORTHOPEDIC ELBOW DYSFUNCTION

T.K. Robinson, PT, DSc, OCS

1. **What are patient-reported outcome questionnaires, and which is best when working with patients with elbow pathologies?**
There are two basic types of outcome measures used in orthopedic practices, clinician-based outcome measures, and patient-reported outcome questionnaires. Clinician-based measures can be affected by observer bias. Patient-reported measures provide their perspective and have been associated with the prediction of return to work. Three of the most commonly used patient-reported outcome questionnaires are the Patient-Related Elbow Evaluation (PREE), the patient-reported form of the American Shoulder and Elbow Surgeons elbow Questionnaire (pASES-e), and the Disabilities of the Arm, Shoulder, and Hand Questionnaire (DASH). Vincent et al. (2014) compared the internal consistency, concurrent construct validity, longitudinal validity, and sensitivity to change features of these three commonly used questionnaires prospectively on 128 patients. They concluded that all three questionnaires have acceptable validity and sensitivity to change. However, the pASES-e function subscale was the least sensitive to change and is less correlated to the other measures.

2. **Describe an elbow with joint effusion.**
All three joints of the elbow complex are affected because they have a common joint capsule. The joint swelling is most evident in the triangular space between the radial head, tip of the olecranon, and lateral epicondyle. The elbow is held in the loosely packed position of about 70 degrees of flexion because, in this position, the joints have maximal volume.

3. **What is "little league elbow"?**
Little league elbow is a generic term referring to several overuse injuries in young throwers. Examples include osteochondritis dissecans of the capitellum with or without loose bodies, injury and premature closure of the proximal radial epiphysis, overgrowth of the radial head, and medially stressed valgus overuse. The repetitive valgus stress of throwing results in microtrauma of the medial anterior oblique ligament and compression of the radiocapitellar joint. Repeated traction on the olecranon at the site of the triceps brachii insertion may produce olecranon apophysitis or an olecranon stress fracture. Excessive repeated traction through the medial elbow may result in enlargement of the medial humeral epicondyle as well as inflammation of the medial humeral apophysis. Osteochondrosis dissecans of the radial head and/or capitellum or osteochondrosis of the capitellum (Panner's disease) may result from compressive forces through the lateral elbow during the throwing motion. These same forces can result in injury to the proximal radial epiphysis and early closure of its growth center.

4. **How is little league elbow treated?**
In general, little league elbow is treated with relative rest and absolutely no throwing for up to 1 year. If significant fragmentation or separation of the medial humeral apophysis is seen on plain radiographs, surgery may be indicated.

5. **Describe the recommended sequence of pitches for adolescent athletes.**
One of the main causes of elbow injury in adolescent athletes is throwing pitches that they are not physically prepared to perform. Baseball's Medical and Safety Advisory Committee has recommended when various pitches should be introduced. The first pitch introduced is the fastball at 8 years, followed by the change-up at 10 years, the curveball at 14 years, the knuckleball at 15 years, and the slider and forkball at 16 years.

6. **What functional tests help confirm the diagnosis of little league elbow?**
Flexing and extending the elbow with maintenance of valgus stress should elicit elbow pain. Valgus stress testing may reveal pain and increased range. Loss of passive elbow extension may result from early flexion contracture, which is common in professional pitchers and may represent serious damage in children or adolescents.

7. **What does the literature show as risk factors for elbow injuries in baseball?**
Risk factors for elbow injury differ among skill levels. Elbow varus and shoulder external rotation torque during maximal external rotation during pitching, passive shoulder rotational and flexion range of motion deficits, and high pitch velocity were risk factors for elbow injury among professional baseball players. For youth players, pitching >100 innings in 1 year, the player being 9 to 11 years of age, being a pitcher or catcher, and training >16 hours per week were significant risk factors for elbow injury.

8. **How effective are orthobiologics in the treatment of UCL injuries?**

Dugas et al. reported on 128 overhead athletes, mostly high school and collegiate level, who underwent UCL repair with type-1 bovine collagen-dipped Fibertape (Arthrex) augmentation. All study participants had MRI-confirmed partial or complete UCL tears. Of those with follow-up, 92% had returned to the same or higher level of competition at a mean time of 6.7 months.

There have been many clinical studies investigating the use of orthobiologics in the nonoperative treatment of UCL injuries. Three recent cases include:

1) Podesta et al. reported on 34 athletes with symptomatic partial-thickness UCL tears, 88% treated with one PRP injection, and a graded rehab program returned to competition at an average of 12 weeks.
2) Deal et al. reported on 25 high school and collegiate throwing athletes with symptomatic grade 2 tears. Each received two PRP injections and conservative measures. The results showed 22 athletes (88%) of the athletes returned to competition at an average of 12 weeks and 20 (80%) had full ligamentous restoration on follow-up MRI.
3) Kato et al. examined the effects of PRP injections after both partial and full-thickness UCL tears in 30 baseball players. Participants were amateur and professional-level players with MRI-confirmed UCL tears ranging from grades 1 to 3. The intervention included ultrasound-guided PRP injection followed by a graded rehab protocol. The results showed that 26 athletes returned to competition at an average of 12 weeks and four had persistent symptoms requiring reconstruction.

9. **What is lateral elbow tendinopathy?**

The term "tendinitis" has been used to describe a hypothetical chronic inflammatory process in the overused tendon. However, histologic examinations of excised pathologic tendons have consistently failed to display the presence of inflammatory cells. Instead, the tissue is characterized by the presence of dense populations of fibroblasts, vascular hyperplasia, and disorganized collagen, termed by Nirschl as angiofibroblastic hyperplasia. Angiofibroblastic hyperplasia appears to be the result of a failed healing response to microtears, combined with vascular deprivation in the tendon's origin, preventing healing from occurring.

10. **Which structure is most commonly involved in lateral elbow tendinopathy (tennis elbow)?**

The most commonly involved structure is the extensor carpi radialis brevis (ECRB) tendon, followed by the extensor digitorum communis (EDC) tendon. These tendons may be histologically indistinguishable at the common origin. The ECRB tendon has the greatest electromyography (EMG) activity of the forearm muscles, especially in the acceleration and early follow-through phases of the tennis swing. Tendon fibers attaching to the periosteum are relatively avascular and tend to heal very slowly. Immature granulation tissue is present at the injury repair site.

11. **What are the differential diagnoses for lateral elbow tendinopathy?**

- Entrapment of the radial nerve
- Degenerative changes of the radiocapitellar joint
- Posterolateral rotatory instability
- Occult fractures of the radial head or lateral humeral epicondyle
- Posterior tendinopathy of the triceps attachment to the olecranon
- Panner's disease
- Tumor of the capitellum or in the supinator muscle
- Rheumatoid arthritis
- Tendinitis of the long head of the biceps (caused by insertion on the radius)
- Cervical spinal problems

12. **Are forearm support bands (counterforce braces) an effective orthosis for lateral elbow tendinopathy?**

Counterforce braces consist of a flexible band that fits around the proximal forearm and applies pressure to the underlying tissues during activity. These braces may reduce acceleration forces by 46%. Although one study showed that they increase the rate of fatigue in unimpaired people, other studies have shown decreased pain threshold with no changes in isokinetic strength.

13. **Describe the incidence and demographics of lateral elbow tendinopathy.**

Lateral tendinopathy most commonly occurs in patients between 35 and 50 years of age. The incidence varies in different populations. In studies performed at industrial health clinics, tendinopathy was most commonly associated with work-related activities (35% to 64% of all reported cases). Tennis players also are at high risk: 10% to 50% will have symptoms at some time in their career. Risk increases with poor stroke mechanics, striking the ball off center, improper grip size, and harder court surfaces. Amateurs tend to have lateral tendinopathy secondary to the backhand, whereas professionals usually have medial tendinopathy because of forceful serving.

14. **What is the best treatment for lateral elbow tendinopathy?**

There is no universally effective treatment for all patients with later elbow tendinopathy (LET). However, in looking at the systematic reviews, the literature does show moderate evidence for manual therapy techniques to improve pain and grip strength. Two of these techniques include ulnar-humeral lateral glides and radial head posterior-anterior glides. Vicenzino et al. found that using these sustained mobilizations with the patient performing the pain-producing movement produced substantial immediate improvement in pain and impairment.

The entire patient has to be considered, as opposed to a patient just having an elbow complaint. Physical impairments have been demonstrated on manual exam of C4-7 segmental levels in patients with relatively localized symptoms of LET. There is moderate evidence that manual therapy techniques targeting the cervical and thoracic spines provide additional clinical benefits. This also serves as a reminder to the clinician to always perform a complete upper quarter screen with these patients so that these comorbidities are not missed.

15. **Is eccentric exercise an effective treatment for lateral elbow tendinopathy?**

Cullinane et al. conducted a systematic review of randomized and controlled clinical trials incorporating eccentric exercise to establish the effectiveness of eccentric exercise as a treatment intervention for lateral elbow tendinopathy. Twelve studies met the inclusion criteria. Eight of the studies were randomized trials investigating a total of 334 subjects. Following treatment, all groups inclusive of eccentric exercise reported decreased pain and improved function and grip strength from baseline. Seven studies reported improvements in pain, function, and/or grip strength for therapy treatments inclusive of eccentric exercise when compared with those excluding eccentric exercise. Additionally, Peterson et al. performed a randomized control trial comparing eccentric versus concentric graded exercise in chronic lateral elbow tendinopathy. Their results also showed that graded eccentric exercise reduced pain and increased muscle strength more effectively than concentric graded exercise.

16. **Are there biologic treatments available for lateral elbow tendinopathy?**

Mishra et al. examined PRP treatment in a multicenter randomized controlled trial of 230 patients with chronic lateral epicondylitis. Patients were evaluated at 12 and 24 weeks after injection and compared with active controls not receiving biologic therapy. At 12 weeks, there were no significant differences in outcome in either cohort, but at 24 weeks those who received leukocyte-rich PRP had significant decreases in VAS pain assessments when compared with controls. These studies, along with several other high-quality trials published in recent years, provide some of the strongest evidence of the use of PRP in musculoskeletal pathology.

Investigations of cellular-based treatments of lateral epicondylitis are more limited than those of PRP augmentation, but in general, also demonstrate favorable outcome improvement. In a case of 30 patients with previously untreated lateral epicondylitis, Singh et al. examined the efficacy of a single BMAC injection on functional outcomes. Short-term evaluations up to 12 weeks after injection were performed using the Patient-rated Tennis Elbow Evaluation score. At both 6 and 12 weeks, mean outcome scores were significantly improved when compared with the baseline. The efficacy of ADSC injections in lateral epicondylitis was examined by Lee et al. When considering VAS and modified Mayo Clinic performance index for the elbow outcomes, patients had significant improvements in outcome by 6 weeks after injection that were sustained for the entire 52-week study period. In addition, ultrasound assessments of the tendon were also performed and demonstrated a significant decrease in tendon defect size during the study period. While these early studies show safety and moderate efficacy of cellular-based biologic therapies, larger studies with a higher level of evidence are essential in determining clinical recommendations for their use.

17. **What is radial tunnel syndrome? Why is it confused with lateral elbow tendinopathy?**

The radial tunnel is about 2 inches in length, extending proximally from the capitellum of the humerus, between the brachioradialis and brachialis, and distally through the supinator muscle. The radial nerve may become entrapped in this tunnel, resulting in persistent pain around the lateral epicondyle and an aching sensation in the extensor and/or supinator muscle mass distal to the lateral epicondyle. The nerve is typically impinged at the arcade of Froshe. Tennis elbow straps may increase symptoms because of increased pressure compression over the radial tunnel.

18. **What is "nursemaid's elbow"?**

Nursemaid's elbow ("pulled elbow") is a subluxation of the radial head, usually in children younger than 5 years. It usually occurs when a child is forcefully pulled or jerked by the arm with the arm in extension. Radiographs are of little benefit, even with comparison views of the uninvolved elbow. The combination of patient history and limitation of motion, especially absence of supination of the elbow, usually makes the diagnosis. A sudden pull on the extended elbow while the forearm is pronated may produce a tear in the distal attachment of the annular ligament to the radial neck. The radial head penetrates partially through the tear as it is distracted from the capitellum. Then the proximal part of the annular ligament slips into the radiohumeral joint, where it becomes trapped between the joint surfaces once the pull is released. The source of pain is the trapped annular ligament. The entrapped ligament can be freed by suddenly supinating the forearm while the elbow is flexed.

19. **Describe medial elbow tendinopathy.**
Medial tendinopathy has been called golfer's elbow, medial tennis elbow, and even swimmer's elbow. It is an overuse injury that results from repetitive valgus stress on the medial elbow, combined with wrist flexion and pronation. The patient with medial tendinopathy usually presents with pain, inflammation, and point tenderness at the medial epicondyle where the flexor/pronator group originates.

20. **What are the differential diagnoses for medial elbow tendinopathy? How are they ruled out?**
The differential diagnoses for medial tendinopathy are medial collateral ligament (MCL) injuries, ulnar nerve injuries, and degenerative changes of the medial elbow joint. Both medial elbow tendinopathy and MCL injury can create pain on valgus stress testing. It is possible to differentiate the two injuries by applying valgus stress to a slightly flexed elbow while the wrist is flexed and the forearm is pronated. This arm position eliminates the symptoms attributed to medial elbow tendinopathy and results in a painless valgus stress test, provided that the ulnar collateral ligament (UCL) is uninjured. Passive wrist extension and active resisted wrist flexion and pronation can further distinguish medial elbow tendinopathy from UCL injury. A positive Tinel's sign, tenderness of the ulnar nerve to palpation, and paresthesia and numbness in the fourth and fifth fingers confirm ulnar nerve injuries. According to Nirschl, 60% of patients with medial elbow tendinopathy have ulnar nerve symptoms. Radiographic changes include bone spurs and degenerative disease.

21. **What is olecranon bursitis and how is it managed?**
The olecranon bursa is located between the skin and tip of the olecranon process. Bursitis is caused by trauma because of chronic overuse (eg, leaning on the elbow or "student's elbow") or by direct impact that results in inflammation or infection. The differential diagnoses include fracture of the olecranon process of the ulna, gout, rheumatoid arthritis, and synovial cyst of the elbow joint. Usually, the elbow joint is not involved because the bursa and joint do not communicate unless rheumatoid arthritis is present. If the joint is infected, all motion is resisted.
Traumatic bursitis is managed symptomatically with immobilization in a splint, compressive dressings, and contrast baths. Aspiration of the bursa usually does not prevent recurrence of swelling because of continued flexion and extension activities. If the bursa is painful and prevents activity, aspiration is indicated and may be both diagnostic and therapeutic.

22. **How common is a rupture of the distal biceps tendon, and what is the etiology of injury?**
Rupture of the distal biceps tendon is a relatively rare injury that can have a significant functional impact on the upper extremity. In a retrospective study performed by Safran and Graham, the incidence rate was found to be 1.2 per 100,000 patients with an average age of 47 years at the time of injury. The dominant arm was involved 86% of the time, and smokers were 7.5 times more likely to sustain the injury compared with nonsmokers.
The theories for rupture of the distal biceps tendon include hypovascular and mechanical mechanisms. Seiler et al. performed an anatomic study that included vascular injections of 27 cadavers. A consistent, hypovascular zone, measuring 2.14 cm in diameter, was found at the musculotendinous junction with light microscopy. Other studies used sequential computed tomography scans of patients with their forearms in positions of maximal pronation, neutral, and maximal supination. With the forearm in maximum pronation, the distance between the lateral border of the ulna and the radial tubercle was 48% less than the distance in full supination. Additionally, with the forearm in pronation, the biceps tendon consumed 85% of the radioulnar space at the level of the radial tubercle. Thus, mechanical impingement of the tendon is the other proposed theory for distal biceps tendon rupture.

23. **What is the clinical presentation for a patient with a distal biceps tendon rupture?**
Patients with a distal biceps tendon rupture frequently report sustaining an unexpected forced extension of the elbow, resulting in an eccentric contraction of the biceps and a tearing sensation in the antecubital fossa. The patient will also report weakness with elbow flexion and significant weakness with forearm supination.

24. **What clinical tests can be used to assess for a distal biceps tendon rupture?**
Despite the clinical presentation, distal biceps tendon ruptures can still be missed clinically, especially if the lacertus fibrosus remains intact. The two most common clinical tests are the biceps squeeze test and the hook test.
Ruland et al. developed the biceps squeeze test, which is similar to the Thompson test used to identify Achilles tendon ruptures. The biceps brachii is squeezed, which will result in forearm supination if the tendon is intact. In Ruland's study, 23 of 24 patients with a positive test had a complete distal biceps tendon rupture, which was confirmed surgically or by MRI.
O'Driscoll et al. developed the hook test to identify distal biceps tendon ruptures. The test is performed by placing the patient's elbow at 90 degrees of flexion and inserting a finger under the lateral edge of the biceps tendon and hooking the finger under the cord-like structure, crossing the antecubital fossa. The authors of this study reported 100% sensitivity and specificity for this test. One key with the hook test is to hook the lateral edge of the biceps tendon, not the medial edge, so that the lacertus fibrosus would not be mistaken for an intact biceps tendon.

25. **What are the outcomes for untreated, complete distal biceps tendon tears?**
    Flexion strength is decreased 20% to 30%, and supination strength is decreased 40% to 50%, compared with the uninvolved limb.

26. **What are the outcomes for surgically repaired acute distal biceps ruptures?**
    Typically, strength is 90% to 95% of the contralateral limb, and motion is normal or near normal. Slight decreases in extension, pronation, or supination may be present.

27. **What are potential complications of distal bicep tendon repairs?**
    Transient or permanent paresthesias, PIN palsy, re-rupture, tuberosity fracture, vascular injury, heterotopic bone formation, radial ulnar synostosis, infection, and hematoma.

28. **What is the clinical presentation of osteoarthritis of the elbow?**
    Primary osteoarthritis of the elbow is uncommon but usually presents on the dominant side in middle-aged males with a history of heavy use through sports or work. In the early stages, the typical presentation is pain at end-range extension and flexion. This has been associated with osteophytes at the tips of the coronoid process and the olecranon. As the disease progresses, there is pain throughout the range of motion. The osteophytes can enlarge and actually become space-occupying lesions, which will lead to capsular contracture.

Bibliography

Anz, A. W., Bushnell, B. D., Griffin, L. P., Noonan, T. J., Torry, M. R., & Hawkins, R. J. (2010). Correlation of torque and elbow injury in professional baseball pitchers. J Sports Med, 38(7), 1368–1374.

Agresta, Cristine E., et al. (2019). "Risk Factors for Baseball-Related Arm Injuries: a Systematic Review.". *Orthopaedic Journal of Sports Medicine*, *7*(2), 557–570..

Bennett, J. B., & Tullos, H. S. (1990). Acute injuries to the elbow In J. A. Nicholos & E. B. Hershman (Eds.), *Upper extremity in sports medicine* (pp. 319–334). St. Louis: Mosby.

Brody, L. T. (1999). The elbow, forearm, wrist and hand In C. M. Hall & L. T. Brody (Eds.), *Therapeutic exercise: moving toward function* (pp. 626–663). Philadelphia: Lippincott Williams & Wilkins.

Buettner, C. M., & Leaver-Dunn, D. (2000). *Prevention and treatment of elbow injuries in adolescent pitchers*. Champaign, Ill.: Athletic Therapy Today.

Bushnell, B. D., Anz, A. W., Noonan, T. J., Torry, M. R., & Hawkins, R. J. (2010). Association of maximum pitch velocity and elbow injury in professional baseball pitchers. *Am J Sports Med*, *38*(4), 728–732.

Cleland, A. J., Flynn, T. W., & Palmer, J. A. (2005). Incorporation of manual therapy directed at the cervicothoracic spine in patients with lateral epicondylalgia: a pilot clinical trial. *J Man Manip Ther*, *13*, 143–151.

Cullinane, F. L., Boocock, M. G., & Trevelyan, F. C. (2014 Jann). Is eccentric exercise an effective treatment for lateral tendinopathy? A systematic review. *Clin Rehabil*, *28*(1), 3–19. https://doi.org/10.1177/0269215513491974. Epub 2013 Jul 23. PMID: 23881334.

Deal, J. B., Smith, E., Heard, W., O'Brien, M. J., & Savoie, F. H., 3rd. (2017). Platelet-Rich Plasma for primary Treatment of Partial Ulnar Collateral Ligament Tears: MRI CorrelationWith Results. *Orthop J Sports Med*, *5* 2325967117738238. https://doi.org/10.1177/2325967117738238.

Dimberg, L. (1987). The prevalence and causation of tennis elbow (lateral humeral tendinopathy) in a population of workers in an engineering industry. *Ergonomics*, *30*, 573–580.

Dugas, J. R., Looze, C. A., Capogna, B., Walters, B. L., Jones, C. M., Rothermich, M. A., et al. (2019). Ulnar Collateral Ligament Repair With Collagen-Dipped FiberTape Augmenta-tion in Overhead-Throwing Athletes. *Am J Sports Med*, *47*, 1096–1102.

Fleisig, G. S., Andrews, J. R., Cutter, G. R., et al. (2011). Risk of serious injury for young baseball pitchers: a 10-year prospective study. *Am J SportsMed*, *39*(2), 253–257.

Hart, L. E. (2002). Corticosteroid injections, physiotherapy, or a wait-and-see policy for lateral tendinopathy? Clinical Journal of Sport Medicine: *Official Journal of the Canadian Academy of Sport Medicine*, *12*, 403–404.

Kato, Y., Yamada, S., & Chavez, J. (2019). Can platelet-rich plasma therapy save patients with ulnar collateral ligament tears from surgery? *Regen Ther*, *10*, 123–126. https://doi.org/10.1016/j.reth.2019.02.004.

Klaiman, M. D., et al. (1998). Phonophoresis versus ultrasound in the treatment of common musculoskeletal conditions. *Medicine & Science in Sports & Exercise*, *30*, 1349–1355.

Knebel, P. T., et al. (1999). Effects of the forearm support band on wrist extensor muscle fatigue. *Journal of Orthopaedic and Sports Physical Therapy*, *29*, 677–685.

L'Insalata, J. C., et al. (1997). A self-administered questionnaire for assessment of symptoms and function of the shoulder. *Journal of Bone and Joint Surgery (American)*, *79*, 738–748.

Lee, S. Y., Kim, W., Lim, C., & Chung, S. G. (2015). Treatment of Lateral Epicondylosis by Using Allogeneic Adipose-Derived Mesenchymal Stem Cells: a Pilot Study. *Stem Cells*, *33*, 2995–3005. https://doi.org/10.1002/stem.2110.

Mishra, A. K., Skrepnik, N. V., Edwards, S. G., Jones, G. L., Sampson, S., Vermillion, D. A., et al. (2013). Efficacy of Platelet-Rich Plasma for Chronic Tennis Elbow: A Double-Blind,Prospective, Multicenter, Randomized Controlled Trial of 230 Patients. *Am JSports Med*, *42*, 463–471. https://doi.org/10.1177/0363546513494359.

Matsuura, T., Iwame, T., Suzue, N., Arisawa, K., & Sairyo, K. (2017). Risk factors for shoulder and elbow pain in youth baseball players. *Phys Sportsmed*, *45*(2), 140–144.

Nirschl, R. P., & Pettrone, F. (1979). Tennis elbow. The surgical treatment of lateral tendinopathy. *Journal of Bone and Joint Surgery*, *61A*, 832–839.

Noteboom, T., et al. (1994). Tennis elbow: a review. *Journal of Orthopaedic and Sports Physical Therapy*, *25*, 357–366.

O'Driscoll, S. W., Goncalves, L. B., & Dietz, P. (2007). The hook test for distal biceps tendon avulsion. *American Journal of Sports Medicine*, *35*, 1865–1869.

Podesta, L., Crow, S. A., Volkmer, D., Bert, T., & Yocum, L. A. (2013). Treatment of partial ulnar collateral ligament tears in the elbow with platelet-rich plasma. *Am J SportsMed, 41*, 1689–1694. https://doi.org/10.1177/0363546513487979.
Peterson, M., Butler, S., Eriksson, M., & Svärdsudd, K. (2014 Sepp). A randomized controlled trial of eccentric vs. concentric graded exercise in chronic tennis elbow (lateral elbow tendinopathy). *Clin Rehabil, 28*(9), 862–872. https://doi.org/10.1177/0269215514527595. Epub 2014 Mar 14. PMID: 24634444.
Ruland, R. T., Dunbar, R. P., & Bowen, J. D. (2005). The biceps squeeze test for diagnosis of distal biceps tendon ruptures. *Clinical Orthopaedics and Related Research, 437*, 128–131.
Safran, M. R., & Graham, S. M. (2002). Distal biceps tendon ruptures: incidence, demographics, and the effect of smoking. *Clinical Orthopaedics and Related Research, 404*, 275–283.
Seiler, J. G., 3rd, Parker, L. M., Chamberland, P. D., Sherbourne, G. M., & Carpenter, W. A. (1995 May-Jun). The distal biceps tendon. Two potential mechanisms involved in its rupture: arterial supply and mechanical impingement. *J Shoulder Elbow Surg, 4*(3), 149–156. https://doi.org/10.1016/s1058-2746(05)80044-8. PMID: 7552670.
Singh, A., Gangwar, D. S., & Singh, S. (2014). Bone marrow injection: a novel treatment for tennis elbow. *J Nat Sci Biol Med, 5*(2), 389–391.
Spencer, G. E., & Herndon, C. H. (1953). Surgical treatment of tendinopathy. *Journal of Bone and Joint Surgery, 35A*, 421–424.
Vincent, J. I., et al. (2014). Validity and sensitivity to change of patient-reported pain and disability measures for elbow pathologies. *Journal of Orthopaedic and Sports Physical Therapy, 43*, 263–274.
Vicenzino, B., Paugmali, A., & Teys, P. (2007). Muligan's mobilization with movement, positional faults and pain relief: current concepts from a critical review of the literature. *Man Ther, 12*, 98–108.
Wilk, K. E., Macrina, L. C., Fleisig, G. S., et al. (2014). Deficits in glenohumeral passive range of motion increase risk of elbow injury in professional baseball pitchers: a prospective study. *Am J Sports Med, 42*(9), 2075–2081.
Wysocki, R. W., & Cohen, M. S. (2011). Primary osteoarthritis and posttraumatic arthritis of the elbow. *Hand Clinics, 27*, 131–137.

CHAPTER 46 QUESTIONS

1. What are common objective findings with cubital tunnel syndrome?
   a. Weak pinch grip from loss of thumb adduction
   b. Weakness of DIP flexion noted in the second finger
   c. Weakness of wrist flexion and radial deviation
   d. Positive "OK" sign (inability to flex the IP joint of the thumb and DIP joint of the second finger results in pulp to pulp versus tip to tip)

2. What are common objective findings with Anterior Interosseous Nerve (AIN) syndrome?
   a. Weakness of the pronator quadratus muscle (shown with weak resisted pronation with the elbow maximally flexed
   b. Weakness of the pronator teres muscle
   c. Weakness of flexion of the DIP joint of the 4th or 5th fingers
   d. Loss of sensation of the anterior medial aspect of the forearm

3. All of the following are true regarding Posterior Interosseous Nerve (PIN) syndrome except:
   a. Finger metacarpal extension weakness
   b. Common compression site for this nerve is the arcade of Frosch in the supinator muscle
   c. Wrist extension weakness. The wrist will extend with radial deviation due to weakness of the extensor carpi ulnaris
   d. Weakness of forearm supination

CHAPTER 47

ELBOW FRACTURES AND DISLOCATION: PATTERNS, CLASSIFICATIONS, AND MANAGEMENT

J. Placzek, MD, PT and Job A. Gallaher

1. **How are fractures of the distal humerus classified?**
Distal humeral fractures historically have been divided into extraarticular and intraarticular, with the following subdivisions: supracondylar, epicondylar, transcondylar, condylar, intercondylar, capitellar, and trochlear. In an attempt to develop a universal system, the AO/ASIF classification encompasses all periarticular distal humeral fractures.

AO/ASIF CLASS	DESCRIPTION	TREATMENT
Type A: extraarticular fractures		
A1	Avulsion fractures with no loss of column support to articular surface	Brief immobilization with early ROM
A2	Metaphyseal fractures with limited comminution	Nondisplaced: cast/brace <3 weeks
		Displaced: ORIF
A3	Significant metaphyseal comminution	ORIF
Type B: partial articular fractures		
B1	Lateral column disruption	ORIF with plates and/or screws
B2	Medial column disruption	ORIF with plates and/or screws
B3	Disruption of capitellum or trochlea	ORIF with or without primary fragment excision
Type C: entire articular fractures		
C1	Intercondylar split without comminution	ORIF
C2	C1 with metaphyseal comminution	ORIF with or without bone graft
C3	C2 with articular surface comminution	ORIF with or without excision and with or without bone graft

AO/ASIF, Arbeitsgemeinschaf fur Osteosynthesefragen/Association for the Study of Internal Fixation; ORIF, open reduction and internal fixation.

2. **Define Malgaigne (supracondylar) fractures.**
Most commonly seen in children, Malgaigne fractures occur above the olecranon fossa and are characterized by dissociation of the humeral diaphysis from the condyles of the distal humerus. Fracture lines may extend distally to involve the articular surface. In adults intercondylar fractures are much more common and must be suspected.

3. **Describe two classification systems for Malgaigne fractures.**
The simpler system, based on the mechanism of injury, includes either extension-type or flexion-type supracondylar fractures. Falls onto an outstretched hand can produce the more common extension-type supracondylar fracture (80%), in which the fracture line passes from anterodistal to posteroproximal on lateral radiographs. Flexion-type supracondylar fractures result from force directed against the posterior aspect of a flexed elbow. The fracture line passes obliquely from anteroproximal to posterodistal on lateral radiographs. When displaced, the sharp proximal bone fragment often pierces the triceps and overlying skin, creating an open fracture.

A more comprehensive classification system, based on the presence of intercondylar extension and fracture comminution, is used more commonly in adults. Four types of supracondylar fractures are recognized:

- Type I—fractures without intercondylar extension
- Type II—fractures with intercondylar extension but without comminution
- Type III—fractures with intercondylar extension and supracondylar comminution
- Type IV—fractures with intercondylar extension and intercondylar comminution

4. **How are supracondylar fractures managed in adults?**
Anatomic reduction with stable fixation in adults is best achieved with plate-and-screw fixation (see table). External fixators are used when rapid stabilization of the elbow is required (eg, vascular disruption), when an open wound is associated with significant soft tissue injury or loss, or when plate-and-screw fixation is precluded by extensive bone loss or comminution. External fixator pins are placed laterally into the distal humerus and dorsally into the ulna. Skin incisions that are followed by blunt dissection to bone under direct visualization help prevent injury to the radial nerve. Ulnar pins are inserted with the forearm in 30 degrees of supination to permit forearm rotation.

Treatment of Supracondylar Fractures in Adults

FRACTURE TYPE	OPERATIVE TREATMENT
Type I	Medial, lateral, or triceps, splitting with application of medial- and lateral-column plating
	Orthogonal configuration preferred over parallel placement
	Medial-column plate applied to medial ridge; lateral-column plate placed on posterior column surface
Types II and III	Transolecranon exposure, followed by reduction and lag-screw fixation of intercondylar fracture
	Reduce and stabilize supracondylar component with medial and lateral plates
	Use bone graft in regions of supracondylar comminution (autogenous graft)
Type IV	Same as type III, but do not use lag-screw construct to fix intercondylar component because mediolateral condylar distance will decrease, creating joint incongruity

5. **Describe the classification and management of supracondylar fractures in children.**
The Gartland classification of supracondylar humerus fractures in children is based on the degree of displacement. Treatment ranges from percutaneous pin placement to formal open reduction and internal fixation (ORIF). Short-term immobilization in a bivalved cast is common to all treatments.

Treatment of Supracondylar Fractures in Children

CLASS	DESCRIPTION	EXTENSION TYPE	FLEXION TYPE
Type I	Undisplaced fracture	Immobilization at 90 degrees of flexion	Immobilization in near-extension
Type II	Displaced with one intact cortex	Closed reduction and percutaneous pin placement (two lateral)	Closed reduction and percutaneous pin placement (two lateral)
Type III	Complete displacement	Closed reduction and crossed-pin placement (two lateral, one medial); ORIF if unstable	Closed reduction and crossed-pin placement (two lateral, one medial); ORIF if unstable

6. **How are Granger (epicondylar) fractures classified and managed?**
Lateral epicondylar fractures are extremely rare and usually are managed symptomatically with brief splinting, followed by early ROM exercises. The medial epicondyle—a traction apophysis for the wrist flexors and medial collateral ligament—is the last ossification center to fuse with the humeral metaphysis (age 15–20 years). Fractures are classified as undisplaced, minimally displaced, displaced >5 mm but proximal to the elbow joint, and entrapped (usually between the olecranon and trochlea). Acute fractures are differentiated from chronic

tension stress injuries (little league elbow). Treatment of nonincarcerated fragments involves closed manipulation with short-term immobilization (10–14 days) with the forearm pronated and the elbow and wrist flexed. ORIF is indicated for incarcerated fractures that cause ulnar neuropathy. Chronic stress fractures are treated conservatively with brief immobilization and activity modification.

7. **Which age group is most susceptible to transcondylar humerus fractures?**
Transcondylar fractures usually are seen in older adult patients as a consequence of osteoporotic bone. The fracture line passes between the articular surface and the old epiphyseal line, traversing the coronoid and olecranon fossae. Treatment ranges from closed reduction and splinting to percutaneous pinning or ORIF. Excessive callus formation in the coronoid or olecranon fossa may result in loss of motion.

8. **How are condylar fractures classified in adults?**
Condylar fractures are rare in adults, representing <5% of all distal humerus fractures. Lateral condylar fractures, which include the capitellum and lateral epicondyle, are more common than medial condylar fractures. In Rockwood's *Handbook of Fractures,* Milch describes two types of fractures based on the presence of the lateral trochlear ridge: type I fractures leave the lateral trochlear ridge intact, whereas type II fractures, which are less stable, include the lateral trochlear ridge as part of the fracture fragment. Jupiter describes Milch fractures as high or low, based on extension of the fracture line into the supracondylar region. Low Jupiter fractures are equivalent to Milch type I fractures and high Jupiter fractures to Milch type II fractures. Preferred treatment in adults is ORIF with early ROM exercises.

9. **How are condylar fractures classified in children?**
In children, both Milch and Jacob systems are used. The Jacob system accounts for fracture displacement:
   - Stage I fractures are undisplaced with an intact articular surface.
   - Stage II fractures have moderate displacement.
   - Stage III fractures are unstable elbow injuries with fragment displacement and rotation.

   Closed treatment of initially nondisplaced fractures in a long-arm cast is associated with a loss of reduction. Frequent serial radiographs are recommended to detect fracture displacement. ORIF is recommended for stage II fractures and for failed closed treatment.

10. **Define intercondylar fractures.**
Intercondylar fractures are the most common distal humerus fractures in adults. Usually they result from forces directed against the posterior aspect of a flexed elbow that cause the ulna to impact the trochlea. The resultant force splits the condyles, which are pulled apart by the flexor (medial) and extensor (lateral) muscle masses.

11. **Describe three classification systems for intercondylar fractures in adults.**
The universal AO/ASIF classification of intercondylar fractures includes subtypes C1, C2, and C3. The Jupiter classification describes the shape and direction of the fracture as high T, low T, Y, H, medial lambda, or lateral lambda. Riseborough and Radin describe four types: type I (undisplaced), type II (slight displacement with no condylar fragment rotation in the frontal plane), type III (displacement of the condylar fragments with rotation), and type IV (type III fracture with severe comminution of the articular surface).

12. **How are intercondylar fractures managed?**
Treatment of intercondylar fractures must be individualized according to the patient's age, medical status, bone quality, and fracture pattern. Older adult patients with osteoporotic bone and comminuted articular fractures may be managed with either closed treatment (cast/traction) or total elbow arthroplasty using a semiconstrained device. In general, ORIF with plates and screws is the preferred treatment for intercondylar fractures.

13. **What are typical functional outcomes after an intraarticular distal humerus fracture?**
Approximately 70% of patients have a good or excellent outcome; 25% have a fair outcome; and 5% have a poor outcome. Other typical outcomes are the following: mean flexion arc, ≈112 degrees; pronation and supination, ≈75 degrees each; grip strength, ≈80% of the contralateral side. About 75% of patients return to their previous occupation.

14. **Describe the three types of capitellar fractures.**
Capitellar fractures are rare, representing <1% of all elbow fractures. Shear stress in the coronal plane may produce three types of fracture patterns:
   - Type I fractures involve both osseous and cartilaginous portions of the capitellum, producing a Hahn-Steinthal fragment.
   - Type II fractures of the capitellum shear off the articular cartilage with little underlying subchondral bone. This "uncapped condyle" is called a Kocher-Lorenz fragment.
   - Type III fractures are markedly comminuted compression fractures of the capitellum.

15. **How are capitellar fractures managed?**
Treatment of nondisplaced fractures involves placing the elbow in maximal flexion and forearm pronation to allow for the radial head to act as an internal splint. However, extreme flexion in the face of soft tissue edema can cause vascular compromise and subsequent compartment syndrome. Immobilization at 90 degrees of flexion in a long-arm cast decreases the risk of compartment syndrome but is associated with loss of fracture reduction. Displaced fractures are treated with ORIF or fragment excision. Type I fractures are exposed through the anconeus surgical approach. Provisional fixation with Kirschner wires simplifies placement of small-fragment cancellous bone screws (directed posteriorly to anteriorly) or headless screws (placed anteriorly to posteriorly and buried below the articular surface). Excision of fracture fragments is indicated for most displaced type II fractures and for severely comminuted type III fractures.

16. **Define Laugier (trochlear) fractures.**
Trochlear fractures are rare injuries produced by coronal shear forces directed against the trochlea by the coronoid process. Often associated with capitellar fractures, trochlear fractures are distinguished by a double-arc sign on lateral distal humerus radiographs. One arc represents the lateral ridge of the trochlea, and the other arc represents capitellar subchondral bone.

17. **How are trochlear fractures managed?**
Trochlear fractures are managed much like capitellar fractures. Nondisplaced fractures are managed by splinting and casting with early ROM exercises. Displaced fractures with significant osseous fragments are exposed through an extended lateral Kocher approach and stabilized via cancellous or headless screws. Severely comminuted or extensive articular injuries are managed via excision followed by early ROM exercises.

18. **Describe the Colton classification of olecranon fractures.**
Colton modified the original Schatzker classification system of olecranon fractures to include the following classes: undisplaced, displaced, oblique, and transverse fractures; comminuted fractures; and fracture-dislocations.

19. **How are undisplaced olecranon fractures treated?**
Treatment of undisplaced fractures involves immobilization in a long-arm cast with the elbow in 45 to 90 degrees of flexion for approximately 3 weeks. Radiographic evaluation 5 to 7 days after cast application is needed to rule out fracture displacement. Protected ROM in a hinged brace with 90 degrees of maximal flexion is initiated at 3 weeks. Fracture union is not expected until 6 to 8 weeks after injury. Joint stiffness and loss of motion are common, particularly in older adult patients who undergo prolonged immobilization.

20. **How are displaced olecranon fractures treated?**
Displaced fractures or fractures associated with a loss of active elbow extension are commonly treated with tension band wiring, plate and screw fixation, or excision of up to 50% of the olecranon fragment and reattachment of the triceps. The coronoid must be intact.

21. **What outcomes are associated with olecranon fractures?**
Decreased ROM is noted in 50% of patients. Deficits usually are minimal, and patients maintain a functional ROM. Paresthesias, usually transient, are noted in 10% of patients. Nonunion occurs in about 5% of olecranon fractures. Approximately 85% of patients have no complaints at long-term follow-up; 50% will show arthritic changes compared with 11% in the uninjured extremity. Approximately 22% of plates used for fixation require removal, and up to 50% of tension band wires will need to be removed.

Treatment of Displaced Olecranon Fractures

MODIFIED COLTON TYPE	TREATMENT
Avulsion fracture	Tension band wiring or excision of small fragment
Oblique fracture	Bicortical screws/plates to prevent shortening
Transverse fracture	Tension band wiring
Comminuted fracture	
Coronoid intact	Excision (up to 50%) with triceps reattachment
Coronoid fracture	Plate/screw fixation
Fracture dislocation	Reduce dislocation; ORIF of radial head (no early excision); ORIF of olecranon as above

22. **What are the types of coronoid fractures?**
Regan and Morrey classified coronoid fractures as:
- Type I—tip avulsion fractures
- Type II—fractures of less than 50% of the coronoid height
- Type III—basal coronoid fractures
- The O'Driscoll classification recognizes subclassifications and anteromedial facet fractures because these often result in posterior medial instability.

23. **What is the treatment of coronoid fractures?**
Stable type I and type II fractures can be treated by early protected motion. If unstable, or associated with radial head fractures, these should undergo ORIF. Type III and anteromedial facet fractures usually undergo ORIF. Associated injuries should be treated as well, and, if ongoing instability is present, the use of an external fixator should be considered.

24. **What surgical approach gives the best view of anteromedial fractures?**
The flexor carpi ulnaris (FCU) splitting approach gives the most extensile exposure.

25. **What other structure is often injured with anteromedial coronoid fractures?**
Commonly tears of the lateral collateral ligament can allow for varus laxity and increased instability.

26. **Do type I fractures represent true avulsions of the coronoid?**
No. The brachialis inserts an average of 11 mm distal to the tip of the coronoid. Therefore, most type I fractures represent shear fractures of the tip of the coronoid.

27. **Summarize the mechanisms of injury and general management of radial head fractures.**
Radial head fractures result from indirect trauma (eg, fall onto an outstretched hand) when longitudinal forces drive the radial head into the capitellum. Because of the mechanism of injury, concomitant Essex-Lopresti injury to the distal radioulnar joint (DRUJ), capitellum, and medial collateral ligament must be ruled out. A mechanical block to motion or elbow instability is an indication for operative intervention. Aspiration of an elbow hemarthrosis with injection of lidocaine through a direct lateral approach can decrease pain and allow for evaluation of passive ROM. ORIF is accomplished by placing cortical screws, headless screws, or miniplates in the anterolateral quadrant of the radial head (nonarticulating surface).

28. **How are radial head fractures classified in adults?**
Mason's classification of radial head fractures in adults was modified by Johnston. Recommended treatment is listed in the following table.

FRACTURE	DESCRIPTION	MANAGEMENT
Type I	Undisplaced fracture involving <25% of head	Splint and ROM as pain subsides
Type II	Marginal fracture with displacement of head	Excision or ORIF if angulation >30°, more than one third of head is fractured, or displacement >3 mm
		Otherwise treat conservatively with splinting and early ROM
Type III	Entire head comminuted	Early vs late radial head excision; repair DRUJ; repair/reconstruct MCL
Type IV	Associated elbow dislocation or Monteggia fracture	Reduce elbow; assess Monteggia or Essex-Lopresti injury; repair DRUJ; reconstruct MCL

ROM, Range of motion; ORIF, open reduction and internal fixation; DRUJ, distal radioulnar joint; MCL, medial collateral ligament.

29. **How are radial head fractures classified in children?**
In children 90% of proximal radial fractures involve either the physis or the radial neck and are associated with fractures of the olecranon, coronoid, and medial epicondyle. The O'Brien classification is based on the degree of angulation of the radial neck. ORIF is indicated with angulation >60 degrees, failed closed reduction, complete displacement of the radial head, or >4 mm of radial head translocation. Radial head excision in children is associated with a high incidence of overgrowth and poor outcome.

O'BRIEN TYPE	ANGULATION	TREATMENT
Type I	<30°	Simple immobilization
Type II	30–60°	Closed reduction and immobilization
Type III	>60°	ORIF with Kirschner wires

30. **How are elbow dislocations classified?**

    Elbow dislocations are classified based on the position of the ulna and radius relative to the distal humerus. Several types of elbow dislocations are recognized: posterior, posterolateral, posteromedial, medial, lateral, anterior, and divergent.

31. **What are the most and least common types of elbow dislocations?**

    Posterolateral elbow dislocations account for 11% to 28% of injuries to the elbow and are more common than other types of elbow dislocations. The incidence of posterolateral dislocations is highest in the 10- to 20-year-old age group and frequently is associated with sports-related injuries.

    Divergent elbow dislocations are rare and consist of two types: anteroposterior and mediolateral (divergent).

32. **Which fractures are commonly associated with elbow dislocations?**

    Medial or lateral epicondyle fractures (12%–34%) can become entrapped in the joint, causing a mechanical block to motion. They are seen more commonly in children. ORIF is occasionally necessary.

    Coronoid process fractures (5%–10%) are seen most commonly with posterior dislocations. Fragments are graded as type I, II, or III as size increases. Type III fractures are associated with recurrent dislocations, and ORIF is recommended.

    Radial head fractures involving the proximal intraarticular portion of the radius are managed nonoperatively in the absence of a bony mechanical block to motion. ORIF is indicated with concomitant radial head dislocation.

33. **What complications are associated with elbow dislocations?**

    - Loss of motion (average of 10- to 15-degree loss of extension with simple dislocations)
    - Loss of strength (15% average)
    - Chronic instability
    - Redislocation
    - Posttraumatic arthritis
    - Neurologic or vascular injury
    - Compartment syndrome (Volkmann's ischemic contracture)
    - Ectopic calcification of the capsule or collateral ligaments (75% of cases)
    - Heterotopic ossification of the capsule (5%), collateral ligaments, or brachialis

34. **What are typical outcomes for triad injuries of the elbow (radial head fracture, coronoid fracture, and ligament instability)?**

    Typical outcomes include the following: flexion arc, ≈112 degrees; pronation/supination arc, ≈136 degrees; and complications resulting in reoperation, ≈20%. Approximately 78% of patients have a good to excellent result.

35. **What outcomes are associated with total elbow arthroplasty for comminuted distal humeral fractures?**

    Total elbow arthroplasty provides good pain relief and ROM. Survival rates at 10 years are lower for those with rheumatoid arthritis at the time of fracture. Deep infection, component loosening, and periprosthetic fractures are potential major complications (up to 36%).

Bibliography

Aslam, N., & Willett, K. (2004). Functional outcome following interim fixation of intra- articular fractures of the distal humerus (AO type C). *Acta Orthopaedica Belgica*, *70*, 118–122.

Bailey, C. S., MacDermid, J., Patterson, S. D., & King, G. J. (2001). Outcome of plate fixation of olecranon fractures. *Journal of Orthopaedic Trauma*, *15*, 542–548.

Barco, P., Streubel, P. N., Morrey, B. F., & Sanchez-Sotelo, J. (2017). Total elbow arthroplasty for distal humeral fractures: A ten year minimum follow-up study. *Journal of Bone and Joint. Surgery*, *18*, 1524–1531.

Bucholz, R. W. (1996). *Orthopedic decision making* (2nd ed.). St. Louis: Mosby.

Canale, S. T. (Ed.). (1998). *Operative orthopaedics* (9th ed.). St. Louis: Mosby.

Colton, C. L. (1973). Fractures of the olecranon in adults: Classification and management. *Injury*, *5*, 121–129.

Hotchkiss, R. N. (1997). Displaced fractures of the radial head: Internal fixation or excision? *Journal of the American Association of Orthopaedic Surgeons*, *5*, 1–10.

Ikeda, M., Sugiyama, K., Kang, C., Takagaki, T., & Oka, Y. (2005). Comminuted fractures of the radial head. Comparison of resection and internal fixation. *Journal of Bone and Joint Surgery, 87*, 76–84.

Jupiter, J. B., Neff, U., Holzach, P., & Allgöwer, M. (1985). Intercondylar fracture of the humerus. *Journal of Bone and Joint Surgery, 67*(2), 226–239.

Karlssson, M. K., Hasserius, R., Karlsson, C., Besjakov, J., & Josefsson, P. -O. (2002). Fractures of the olecranon: A 15 to 25 year follow-up of 73 patients. *Clinical Orthopaedics, 403*, 205–212.

Koval, K. J., & Zuckerman, J. D. (eds.). (2002). *Rockwood's handbook of fractures.* Philadelphia, PA: Lippincott Williams and Wilkins.

Levine, A.M. (ed.). (2015). Orthopaedic knowledge update: Trauma. Rosemont. American Academy of Orthopaedic Surgeons.

Park, S. M., Lee, J. S., Jung, J. Y., Kim, J. Y., & Song, K. S. (2015). How should anteromedial coronoid facet fracture be managed? A surgical strategy based on O'Driscoll classification and ligament injury. *Journal of Shoulder and Elbow Surgery, 24*(1), 74–82.

Pugh, D. M., Wild, L., Schemitsch, E. H., King, G. J., & McKee, M. D. (2004). Standard surgical protocol to treat elbow dislocations with radial head and coronoid fractures. *Journal of Bone and Joint Surgery, 86*(6), 1122–1130.

Regan, W., & Morrey, B. (1989). Fractures of the coronoid process of the ulna. *Journal of Bone and Joint Surgery, 71*(9), 1348–1354.

Riseborough, E. J., & Radin, E. L. (1969). Intercondylar T fractures of the humerus in the adult. A comparison of operative and non-operative treatment in twenty-nine cases. *Journal of Bone and Joint Surgery, 51*(1), 130–141.

Webb, L. X. (1996). Distal humerus fractures in adults. *Journal of the American Association of Orthopaedic Surgeons, 4*, 336–344.

CHAPTER 47 QUESTIONS

1. **Anteromedial coronoid fractures:**
   a. May result in posterolateral instability
   b. May result in posteromedial instability
   c. Are usually stable fractures
   d. Require surgery less often than type I fractures

2. **Radial head fractures that require ORIF include:**
   a. Type I fractures
   b. All type II fractures
   c. Fractures blocking full ROM
   d. Severely comminuted five-part fractures

3. **What is the most common elbow dislocation?**
   a. Medial
   b. Lateral
   c. Posterior
   d. Posterior lateral

4. **After ORIF, olecranon fractures**
   a. have normal ROM
   b. have few overall complaints
   c. have high rates of nonunion (20%)
   d. have low rates of long term arthritis (5%)

5. **What types of coronoid fractures typically require ORIF?**
   a. Type I
   b. Type II
   c. Type III
   d. Types II and III

6. **Surgical treatment of severe distal humeral fractures with total elbow arthroplasty result in**
   a. Severe ROM limitations
   b. Ongoing moderate pain
   c. Poor survivorship at 5 years
   d. High complication rates

NERVE ENTRAPMENTS OF THE ELBOW AND FOREARM

CHAPTER 48

*R.J. McKibben, PT, DSc, ECS, M.E. Brooks, DSc, PT, ECS, OCS, M. Skurja, Jr., DPT, ECS (Emeritus), and J.L. Echternach, PT, DPT, EDD, ECS, FAPTA**

1. **Describe the anatomic course of the ulnar nerve and compressive structures that commonly lead to ulnar neuropathy at the elbow.**

   The ulnar nerve traverses the distal medial intermuscular septum with the median nerve, then courses posterior to the medial epicondyle in the ulnar groove entering the cubital tunnel beneath the cubital tunnel retinaculum (CTR). The CTR is a fibrous band attaching from the medial epicondyle to the olecranon, then blends distally with the flexor aponeurosis, also called the humeroulnar arcade (HUA). The ulnar nerve exits the cubital tunnel beneath the two heads of the flexor carpi ulnaris. As the elbow is flexed, the fibrous structures of the cubital tunnel roof become taut and force the nerve against the bone. The nerve is more commonly compromised in the proximal cubital tunnel (retroepicondylar groove) but may also be compressed at the HUA.

2. **Can subluxation of the ulnar nerve cause ulnar neuropathy at the elbow?**

   Yes. The ulnar nerve can slip out of the ulnar groove when the elbow moves from extension to flexion in individuals lacking a cubital tunnel retinaculum (CTR). Repeated subluxation of the ulnar nerve at the elbow could result in neuritis. This phenomenon can be palpated or observed dynamically with neuromusculoskeletal ultrasound (NMSKUS)

3. **What are the sensitivity of provocation tests for ulnar neuropathy at the elbow?**

   Test results for ulnar neuropathy at the elbow (UNE) may include the following: Tinel's sign (0.62–0.70), elbow flexion (0.32), pressure provocation (0.55), combined pressure-flexion test (0.61–0.91)

4. **Describe typical electrodiagnostic findings in ulnar neuropathy at the elbow.**

   Electrodiagnostic studies (EMG/NCS) in suspected UNE should include standard NCS of the ulnar motor nerve across the elbow with NCV around 50 m/s. Demyelination could reduce motor nerve conduction velocity (NCV) across the elbow with normal speeds in the adjacent forearm and brachial segments. Advancing UNE severity may result in motor conduction block across the elbow, a decrement of distal ulnar sensory amplitude, and/or motor axon loss resulting in a decreased distal motor amplitude. Severe UNE may also demonstrate abnormal EMG activities consistent with motor axonopathy in ulnar innervated muscles below the lesion (flexor carpi ulnaris, ulnar ½ flexor digitorum profundus, and ulnar hand intrinsics).

5. **What are the clinical differences (sensory changes and muscle weakness) that would help distinguish a motor and sensory axonal loss lesion of the ulnar nerve (at the elbow or hand), from a brachial plexus injury?**

LESION SITE	SENSORY CHANGES	MOTOR CHANGES
Lower Trunk Plexopathy	Decreased sensation of the medial arm (medial cutaneous nerve of arm), medial forearm (medial cutaneous nerve of the forearm), medial hand (ulnar nerve), and digits IV–V (ulnar nerve)	Weakness in ulnar innervated muscles: flexor carpi ulnaris, ulnar ½ of the flexor digitorum profundus, and ulnar innervated hand intrinsicsWeakness in radial innervated muscles supplied by the C8 and T1 anterior rami, such as extensor indicis, extensor pollicis longus, and extensor digitorum longusWeakness in median innervated muscles supplied by the C8 and T1 anterior rami, such as flexor pollicis longus, pronator quadratus, abductor pollicis brevis, and opponens pollicisPotential weakness of the pectorals (medial pectoral nerve).

Continued

*Deceased.

LESION SITE	SENSORY CHANGES	MOTOR CHANGES
Medial Cord Plexopathy	Decreased sensation of the dorsum medial hand, digit V and medial ½ digit IV, medial arm (medial cutaneous nerve of arm) and medial forearm (medial cutaneous nerve of the forearm)	Weakness in ulnar innervated muscles: flexor carpi ulnaris, ulnar ½ flexor digitorum profundus, and ulnar intrinsic muscles of the handWeakness in median innervated muscles supplied by the C8 and T1 anterior rami, such as flexor pollicis longus, pronator quadratus, abductor pollicis brevis, and opponens pollicisPotential weakness of the pectorals (medial pectoral nerve).
Ulnar Neuropathy (Elbow)	Decreased sensation of the dorsum medial hand, digit V and medial ½ digit IV	Weakness in the flexor carpi ulnaris, ulnar ½ flexor digitorum profundus, and ulnar intrinsic muscles of the hand.
Ulnar Neuropathy (Wrist)	Decreased sensation of the dorsum medial hand, digit V and medial ½ digit IVMay also spare any decreased sensation if only involving the deep ulnar branch	Weakness in the ulnar intrinsic muscles of the handMay spare the abductor digit minimi if only involving the deep ulnar branch.

6. **What are the surgical options and outcomes for ulnar neuropathy at the elbow?**
   Surgical options include decompression, subcutaneous transposition, intramuscular transposition, submuscular transposition, medial epicondylectomy, and arthroscopic epicondylectomy. Positive surgical outcomes vary from 70% to 95%, with few differences between procedures other than minor benefits from submuscular transfer with advanced-stage ulnar nerve compression. Preoperative severity of neuropathy will also influence overall recovery.

7. **How frequently is there loss of ulnar nerve function after a total elbow joint arthroplasty?**
   The incidence of ulnar nerve complications after a total joint arthroplasty varies considerably. Some reports carry no information about ulnar neuropathy after this procedure. Others have reported an incidence of up to 26%. Most of the literature seems to indicate a 6% to 10% complication rate of ulnar nerve problems after a total joint arthroplasty, with most of these resolving over time. Many patients have subclinical nerve changes before surgery secondary to arthritis, synovitis, and swelling.

8. **At what sites above the elbow can the median and ulnar nerves be compressed?**
   - The ligament of Struthers runs from a bony projection on the supracondylar ridge of the humerus (avain spur) to the medial epicondyle. The median nerve, and in some instances the ulnar nerve, pass below this bony projection and may be a site of compression, but more typically only the median nerve is involved.
   - An epitrochleoanconeus muscle (prevalence up to 30%) attaches from the proximal medial epicondyle to the olecranon and impinge the ulnar nerve just proximal to the cubital tunnel. A thickening of the medial intermuscular septum may also compress the median or ulnar nerves in the arm.
   - Humeral fracture, elbow dislocation, or other space occupation in the arm could also involve the median or ulnar nerves.

9. **Why is the pronator teres spared in a pronator syndrome?**
   The pronator teres is innervated by a motor branch from the median nerve before the nerve passes between the two heads of the pronator teres. Therefore, the pronator teres would not demonstrate any weakness during a muscle test. Compression of the median nerve within the pronator teres could result in weakness of all or some of the muscles supplied by the median nerve distal to the pronator teres, such as the flexor carpi radialis, flexor digitorum superficialis, abductor pollicus brevis, opponens pollicus, and anterior interosseus nerve innervated muscles (flexor pollicis longus, flexor digitorum profundus [digits 2 and 3] and pronator quadratus).

10. **Would compromise of the anterior interosseus nerve result in a cutaneous sensory disturbance?**
    No. The anterior interosseus nerve (AIN) is a motor branch of the median nerve in the forearm. While it does provide sensory innervation to the capsules and periosteum of the volar carpal bones that could result in deep pain in the wrist, there is no cutaneous innervation to the skin of the forearm or hand. The AIN does provide motor innervation to the flexor pollicus longus, median ½ flexor digitorum profundus, and the pronator quadratus, and injury could result in weakness of these muscles.

11. **Compare the common signs, symptoms, and EMG/NCS changes noted in carpal tunnel syndrome, anterior interosseous syndrome, and pronator syndrome.**

SYNDROME	SYMPTOMS	SIGNS	EMG/NCS FINDINGS
Carpal tunnel syndrome	Nocturnal hand pain/ paresthesias improved with shaking the hands. Numbness and tingling in digits I–III and lateral ½ digit IV	Decreased sensation of digits I–III and lateral ½ digit IV Weakness of thenar muscles	Distal latency prolongation of median nerve (sensory and/or motor) across wrist Possible denervation of thenar muscles and lateral lumbricals
Anterior interosseous syndrome	Weak grip Volar forearm/wrist pain Weakness of pinch and lateral ½ FDP No paresthesias	Weakness of FPL, PQ, Normal sensation	Possible denervation of FPL, PQ, and lateral ½ FDP Normal median motor and sensory nerve, distal latencies at wrist, and normal forearm conduction velocity
Pronator syndrome	Numbness and tingling in digits I–III and lateral digit IV Deep anterior forearm pain Increased symptoms with forceful pronation activities (eg, twisting off lids) Hand weakness	Weakness of thenar muscles, wrist flexors (FCR/FDS) Questionable weakness of FPL, PQ, and FDP (lateral) Decreased sensation of digits 1–3½	Decreased forearm conduction velocity (may have conduction block across elbow) May have denervation in median and AIN muscles distal to pronator teres

12. **What is a Martin-Gruber anastomosis? Explain its clinical significance.**
A Martin-Gruber anastomosis (MGA) is a common communication anomaly of the median to ulnar nerve or ulnar to median nerve in the forearm. MGA can be confusing to the clinician if not fully understood. MGA has reported incidence of 8% to 54% in various studies. There are four types of MGA: type I (60%)—motor branches sent from the median to the ulnar nerve to innervate "median" muscles; type II (35%)—motor branches sent from the median to the ulnar nerve to innervate "ulnar" muscles; type III (3%)—motor fibers sent from the ulnar to the median nerve to innervate "median" muscles; type IV (1%)—motor fibers sent from the ulnar to the median nerve to innervate "ulnar" muscles.

13. **What is Wartenberg syndrome?**
Wartenberg syndrome is a superficial radial neuropathy. Occasionally, patients have symptoms of sensory loss in the distribution of the superficial radial nerve without other evident problems with the radial nerve. Compression may occur when the superficial radial nerve emerges from beneath the brachioradialis muscle and enters the fascia, investing the extensor muscles of the forearm or more distally where the nerve is superficial as it traverses along the radius. The nerve can also be irritated in de Quervain's tenosynovitis. Other names for this syndrome are cheiralgia paresthetica, handcuff palsy, or dog handler's syndrome.

14. **What is Saturday night palsy?**
The classic clinical presentation of a patient with Saturday night palsy is wrist drop of the involved upper limb. Saturday night palsy is a compression injury of the radial nerve in the arm anywhere along its course from the medial, posterior, or lateral humerus around the spiral groove. The typical patient is one who loses consciousness with the arm slung over the back of a chair causing compression of the radial nerve in the region of the posterior aspect of the humerus. However, the radial nerve is also susceptible to trauma from humeral fracture, lateral intermuscular septum compression, BP cuffs, fibrous arch of the lateral triceps, intramuscular injection, blunt trauma, or space-occupying lesions.

15. **Describe the symptoms and signs of radial neuropathy in the arm.**
Patients typically do not have weakness of the triceps because the injury usually occurs in the distal one-third of the humerus along the spiral groove and results in loss of radial function distally. This would include the brachioradialis, wrist extensors, finger, and thumb extensors. Sensory loss is common in the superficial radial distribution.

16. **How do you tell if a radial nerve palsy is likely to get better?**
Fortunately, radial neuropathies often result in transient conduction block and will recover within days to weeks. However, if symptoms persist, electrodiagnostic studies can assist in estimating the severity and prognosis by assessing the preservation of motor nerve function below the level of the lesion. Generally, the prognosis is good when there is a preservation of more than 20% of distal motor amplitude. When distal motor amplitudes are very low or absent, the prognosis is less favorable and likely to be protracted. It is worth noting that preservation of distal motor amplitude responses is applicable to most nerve lesions and can assist in patient management and education.

17. **Can you differentiate lateral epicondylitis from radial tunnel syndrome (RTS)?**
Yes, but it can be difficult as lateral epicondylitis can present 21% to 41% of the time with RTS. Conversely, RTS is only present about 5% of the time in patients with primary lateral epicondylitis. Lateral epicondylitis is the most common cause of lateral elbow pain. It is an overuse syndrome involving the common extensor insertion predominantly affecting the extensor carpi radialis brevis on the lateral epicondyle resulting in lateral elbow pain and palpable pain over the epicondyle. In RTS, it is postulated that the radial nerve is intermittently compressed at five potential sites from the distal radial head to the supinator, the most common being the Arcade of Froshe. Signs and symptoms include deep, aching pain in the upper dorsal forearm, worse at night, and arm fatigue without tenderness over the lateral epicondyle or radial head. Symptoms may be provoked with palpation, traction of the nerve, and contractile pain of the common extensor wad. The tenderness is located just below the radial head in the groove formed between the brachioradialis muscle and the extensor carpi radialis. Traction can be applied with combined wrist flexion, forearm pronation, and elbow extension. Patients also may have a positive long-finger sign (pain with resisted digit III extension) and painful resisted supination. Common extensor weakness is rare and is seemingly most limited by pain. Weakness of the posterior interosseous nerve may occur in advanced cases.

18. **What are special tests commonly used to aid in the clinical diagnosis of radial tunnel syndrome?**
    1. Compression over the radial tunnel
    2. Long-finger test
    3. Wrist extension
    4. Resisted supination
    5. Rule of Nine Test

19. **What are the five possible sites of compression in radial tunnel syndrome?**
From proximal to distal:
    1. Lateral elbow joint at the radial head (Osteoarthritis, fibrous bands, radiocapitellar joint arthrosis)
    2. Leash of Henry (Anastomosing branches of the recurrent radial artery at the radial neck)
    3. Fibrous edge of the extensor carpi radialis brevis
    4. The Arcade of Froshe (Proximal fibrous edge of the supinator)
    5. The distal radial tunnel (Distal edge of the supinator)

    Sites 1–3 may result in radial sensory symptoms, while 4 and 5 may only result in pain, tenderness to palpation, or weakness in the PIN distribution.

20. **Why are focal entrapments such as ulnar neuropathy at the elbow and carpal tunnel syndrome more easily identified with EMG/NCS and others not (such as radial tunnel syndrome, pronator syndrome, and anterior interosseus nerve syndrome)?**
Electrodiagnostic studies for focal neuropathies can be quite sensitive in detection of demyelinating and axonal loss nerve lesions. In carpal tunnel syndrome and ulnar neuropathy at the elbow, sites of stimulation can be performed immediately proximal and distal to the lesion allowing the examiner to observe conduction directly across the condition. However, in radial tunnel syndrome and pronator/anterior interosseus syndromes, there are no stimulation sites in proximity to the lesion to reliably detect changes in nerve conduction. In order to detect abnormal needle EMG, the lesion needs to be more advanced in severity to cause motor axonopathy, so mild to moderate conditions may test normally with both the EMG and NCS. It is important to trust the clinical examination recognizing that EMG/NCS is a useful tool in many but not all conditions.

Bibliography

Amoiridus, A., & Vladronikolis, I. G. (2003). Verification of the median-to-ulnar and ulnar-to-median nerve motor fiber anastomosis in the forearm: an electrophysiological study. *Clin Neurophysiol, 114*, 94–98.

Dawson, D. M., Hallett, M., & Welbourn, A. J. (1999). *Entrapment neuropathies* (3rd ed.). Philadelphia, PA: Lippincott-Raven.

Dimutru, D., Amato, A. A., & Zwarts, M. (2002). *Electrodiagnostic medicine* (2nd ed.). Philadelphia, PA: Hanley & Belfus, Inc.

Echternach, J. L. (2000). Loss of ulnar nerve function following a total elbow joint arthroplasty. *Clinical Electrophysiology Newsletter, 14*, 11–14.

Hildebrand, K. A., Patterson, S. D., Regan, W. D., MacDermid, J. C., & King, G. J. (2000). Functional outcome of semiconstrained total elbow arthroplasty. *J Bone Joint Surg Am, 82*(10), 1379–1386.

Kelly, E. W., Coghlan, J., & Bill, S. (2000). Five- to thirteen-year follow up of the GSB III total elbow arthroplasty. *J Shoulder Elbow Surg, 13*, 434–440.

Moradi, A., Ebrahimzadeh, M., & Jupiter, J. (2015). Radial tunnel syndrome, diagnostic and treatment dilemma. *Arch Bone Jt Surg, 3*(3), 156–162.

Omejec, G., & Podnar, S. (2016). What causes ulnar neuropathy at the elbow? *Clin Neurophysiol, 127*(1), 919–924.

CHAPTER 48 QUESTIONS

1. **A patient presents with paresthesias in the distal lateral brachium and antebrachium and weakness in shoulder external rotation, shoulder abduction, elbow flexion, and wrist flexion. Which of the following components of the brachial plexus is least likely to be involved?**
   a. C6 nerve root
   b. Upper trunk
   c. Lateral cord
   d. Medial cord

2. **What group of clinical special tests will best evaluate for an ulnar nerve entrapment at the elbow?**
   a. Tinel's, Wartenberg, and Froment's
   b. Phalen's, anterior compression, and Tinel's
   c. Finkelstein's, Hoffmans reflex, and reverse Phalen's
   d. Allen's test, Phalen's, and a square-shaped wrist

3. **Anterior interosseous nerve entrapment will most likely result in which of the following clinical presentations?**
   a. Weakness in the flexor pollicus longus with paresthesia in digits I-III and the lateral half of digit IV
   b. Deep aching in the forearm
   c. Weakness in the medial ½ of the flexor digitorum profundus
   d. Weakness in the pronator teres

CHAPTER 49

FUNCTIONAL ANATOMY OF THE WRIST AND HAND

D. Gustitus, OTR/L, CHT

DISTAL RADIOULNAR JOINT

1. **What is the triangular fibrocartilage complex (TFCC)?**
The triangular fibrocartilage complex (TFCC) is a structure of ligaments and cartilage located on the ulnar wrist. It includes the dorsal and volar radioulnar ligament, the central articular disc, the meniscus homologue, the ulnar collateral ligament (UCL) and the extensor carpi ulnaris (ECU) subsheath, and the origin of the ulnolunate and ulnotriquetral ligaments. The TFCC is responsible for stabilizing the joint, providing cushioning with movement and impact, and promoting smoothness of motion, especially during grip and forearm rotation.

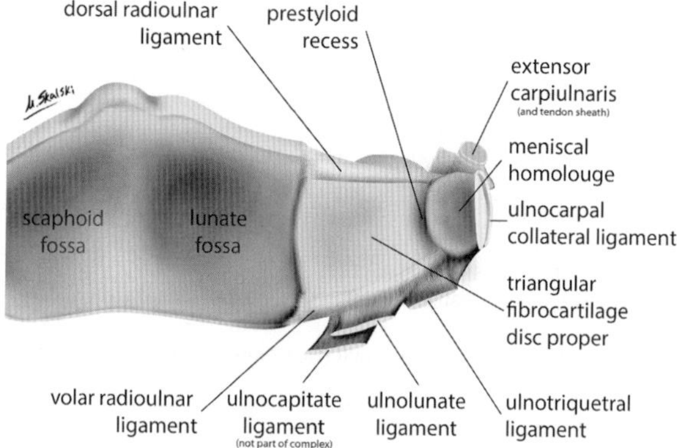

TFCC anatomy, thanks to Skalski, M. R., White, E. A., Patel, D. B., Schein, A. J., RiveraMelo, H., & Matcuk, G. R. (2016). The traumatized TFCC: An Illustrated Review of the anatomy and injury patterns of the triangular fibrocartilage complex. *Current Problems in Diagnostic Radiology, 45*(1), 39–50. https://doi.org/10.1067/j.cpradiol.2015.05.004

2. **What are the dynamic stabilizers of the distal radioulnar joint (DRUJ)?**
The pronator quadratus and ECU serve as dynamic stabilizers of the wrist. The ECU pulls the ulnocarpus dorsally and holds the ulnar head down during pronation. Since the ECU acts on the carpus, it is targeted during therapy to assist in the stabilization of lunotriquetral (LTq) tears. The pronator quadratus consists of a superficial and deep head. The deep head pulls the ulna into the sigmoid notch during pronation and passively holds it in place with supination. The superficial head acts as the primary pronator of the forearm.

3. **What is the function of the distal radius ulnar joint (DRUJ)? Forearm rotation. What kind of joint is the DRUJ?**
The DRUJ is a trochoid joint, meaning it consists of convex and concave components that rotate around a single axis. In the case of the DRUJ, the convex ulnar head fits into the concave sigmoid notch of the radius, allowing the radius to turn about the stationary ulna for pronation and supination. The palmar radioulnar and the dorsal radioulnar ligaments are the primary intrinsic stabilizers of this joint (Altman, E. 2016).

4. **Besides rotation of the radius around the ulna, what other accessory motions occur at the DRUJ?**
The distal ulna translates dorsally within the sigmoid notch with pronation and palmarly with supination restricted primarily by the aforementioned PRUL and DRUL. The radius translates proximally during forearm pronation and distally with forearm rotation that has an impact on ulnar variance.

5. **Describe the anatomy of the ECU and tears of the subsheath.**
The ECU resides within a groove on the dorsoulnar aspect of the distal ulna. Subsheath tears typically occur with forceful supination, wrist flexion, and ulnar deviation of the wrist and forearm. It is most common in athletes that grip and forcefully rotate items such as racquets, hockey sticks, and bats. When a tear has occurred in the tendon's subsheath, the ECU is unconstrained and subluxes volarly and ulnarly around the ulnar head with supination and ulnar deviation. The tendon returns to the groove with pronation.

WRIST

6. **Describe the structure of the carpal ligaments.**
The majority of the carpal ligaments are intracapsular. They can be categorized into two groups: intrinsic and extrinsic. The intrinsic ligaments begin and end on the carpal bones, and the extrinsic ligaments connect the radius and ulna to the carpus. The names of the carpal ligaments describe their origins and insertions. The volar ligaments are believed to be the strongest and most important. The major extrinsic ligaments are the radioscaphoid, radiocapitate, long radiolunate, ulnocapitate, short radiolunate, ulnotriquetral, and ulnolunate. Among the major intrinsic ligaments are the scapholunate interosseous, lunotriquetral, triquetral-hamate-capitate complex, and the numerous distal carpal row interosseous ligaments.

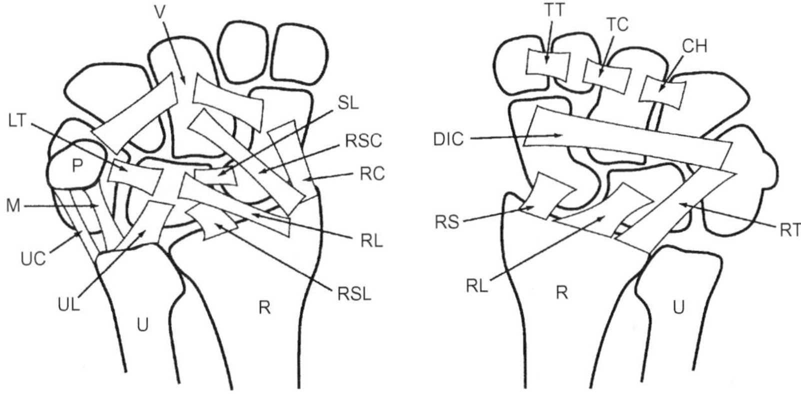

7. **Describe the blood supply of the scaphoid.**
The scaphoid receives its blood supply through its ligaments. The main arterial supply enters around the midpoint (waist) of the scaphoid; additional vessels enter distally. The more proximal portion of the scaphoid receives nutrients in a retrograde fashion. This precarious situation can be disrupted by fractures and explains the relatively high incidence of avascular necrosis.

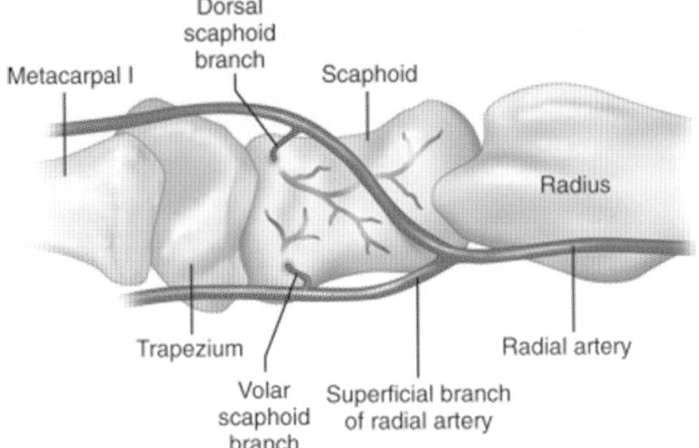

Illustration of retrograde blood supply to the scaphoid from Trumble TE, et al, editors: Core Knowledge in Orthopaedics: Hand, Elbow, and Shoulder. Philadelphia, Mosby, 2006, p 117.

8. **What wrist injury can be detected often with a clenched fist PA view of the wrist?**
A clenched fist view of the wrist can help detect a scapholunate ligament tear. When a scapholunate ligament tear is present, a gap will be present between the scaphoid and the lunate that is wider than with the nonclenched view of the wrist.

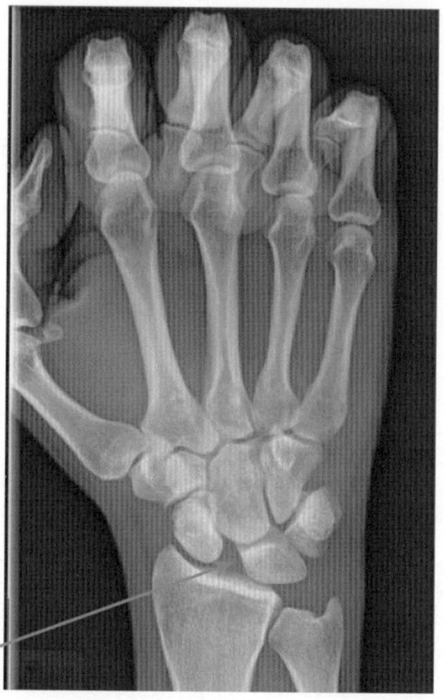

Clenched fist view eliciting an SL gap, courtesy of Michelotti, B., & Chung, K. C. (2018). Scapholunate ligament repair. Operative Techniques: Hand and Wrist Surgery, 180–191.

9. **What information can be obtained from a carpal tunnel view?**
Carpal fractures can be detected with this view as it shows the palmar surfaces of the carpus. Fractures of the triquetrum, hook of hamate, and the pisiform are especially detectable with this view.

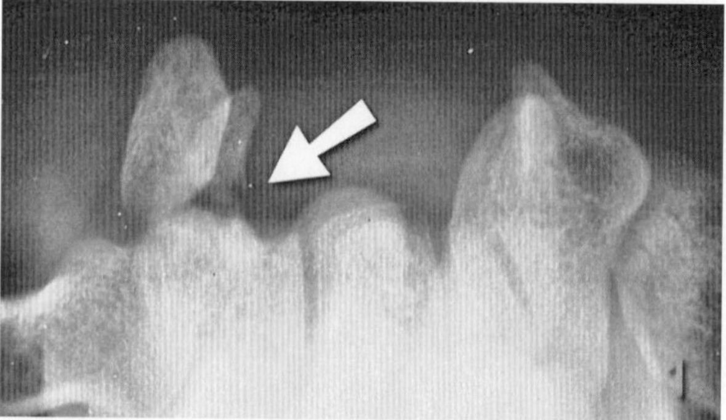

Carpal tunnel x-ray depicting a hamate fracture, courtesy of Weiss, S., Schwartz, D. A., & Anderson, S. C. (2007). Radiography: A review for the Rehabilitation Professional. *Journal of Hand Therapy*, *20*(2), 152–179. https://doi.org/10.1197/j.jht.2007.03.001

10. **Why is the dart thrower's motion being utilized in the rehabilitation of SLIL injury?**
Anatomical studies show that the dart thrower's motion causes limited motion at the proximal row of the carpus, thus minimizing stress to the dorsal and palmar SLIL during rehabilitation. Most of the dart thrower's motion occurs at the midcarpal joint.

11. **Describe the kinematics of the wrist.**
The distal carpal row interosseous ligaments are multiple and strong. Hence, the distal row moves as a unit. Excluding the pisiform, the proximal row has no tendinous attachments. Thus the distal row moves first, and the proximal row follows its lead. With wrist flexion the distal row flexes and the ulnar deviates. Extension causes the distal row to extend and deviate radially. With radial deviation, the distal row deviates radially, extends, and supinates. The exact opposite occurs with ulnar deviation. The proximal carpal row extends with ulnar deviation and flexes with radial deviation. In a normal wrist the scaphoid flexes and pronates, and the lunate and triquetrum extend and supinate with axially loading. During axial loading, the scaphoid flexes and pronates, and the lunate and triquetrum extend and supinate.

12. **Why is the proximal row of the carpus referred to as an intercalated segment?**
While consisting of three distinct bones, the proximal row acts as a continuous unit or segment, while being intercalated or located within layers of tissue without having any tendinous attachment to it.

13. **Describe the force transmission across the radiocarpal joint with axial wrist loading.**
With the wrist in neutral position during axial carpal loading:
- 80% across distal radius (60% through scaphoid facet, 40% lunate facet)
- 20% across distal ulna

14. **What is volar intercalated segment instability (VISI)?**
The lunotriquetral interosseus ligament (LTIL) is the primary stabilizer contributing to the VISI deformity (lunate extended); however, injuries to the secondary stabilizers are typically necessary to result in this deformity. These secondary stabilizers include the ulnar half of the volar arcuate ligament on the volar side and the dorsal radiocarpal ligament and dorsal intercarpal ligament on the dorsal side of the wrist (Pulos and Bonzentka). **Describe the abnormal wrist kinematics that cause the presence of a VISI**. The malposition of the lunate determines whether a wrist has a dorsal or volar intercalated segment instability. In a normal wrist the scaphoid flexes and pronates, and the lunate and triquetrum extend and supinate with axially loading. When the LTIL and the aforementioned secondary stabilizers are incompetent, the triquetrum follows the capitate and hamate into flexion and supination, rather than the lunate into extension and supination with axially loading. The lunate then follows the scaphoid into flexion and pronation. This abnormal volar flexion of the lunate is termed VISI.

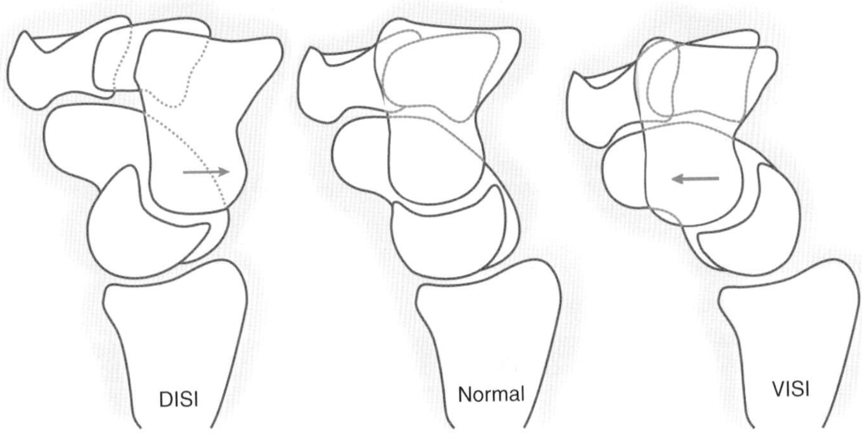

This abnormal volar flexion of the lunate is termed VISI. DISI (left) arrow shows abnormally extended lunate; VISI (right) arrow shows abnormally flexed lunate. (Courtesy of Wolfe, S. W., Pederson, W. C., Kozin, S. H., Cohen, M. S., & Kakar, S. (2022). Carpal Instability. In *Green's Operative Hand Surgery*. Elsevier.)

15. **What is dorsal intercalated segment instability DISI? What structures are injured to cause DISI deformity?**
The scapholunate interosseous ligament is a primary stabilizer of the wrist and the structure necessary to be torn to cause dynamic instability under loading of the wrist (eg, closed fist, ulnar deviation, axially loading). In order for a static deformity to occur (signet ring sign of the flexed scaphoid, and scapholunate disassociation on a standard

anteroposterior x-ray), the secondary stabilizers of the wrist need to also be injured, consisting of the distal scapho-trapezoid ligament complex, the dorsal intercarpal ligament (scaphoid to triquetrum), the palmar extrinsic ligaments (radioscaphocapitate ligament, long and short radiolunate), ulnolunate and lunotriquetral ligaments, and flexor carpi radialis. When the SLIL is torn and the aforementioned secondary stabilizers are incompetent, the scaphoid is no longer tethered to the lunate but is connected to the distal carpal row. Therefore, the scaphoid behaves like a distal row bone and further flexes and supinates with axially loading. The lunate and triquetrum continued to behave per normal. When the secondary stabilizers are torn, the lunate is allowed to extend dorsally out of the lunate fossa beyond normal. This dorsal displacement is termed DISI. If left untreated, it can progress into a SLAC wrist.

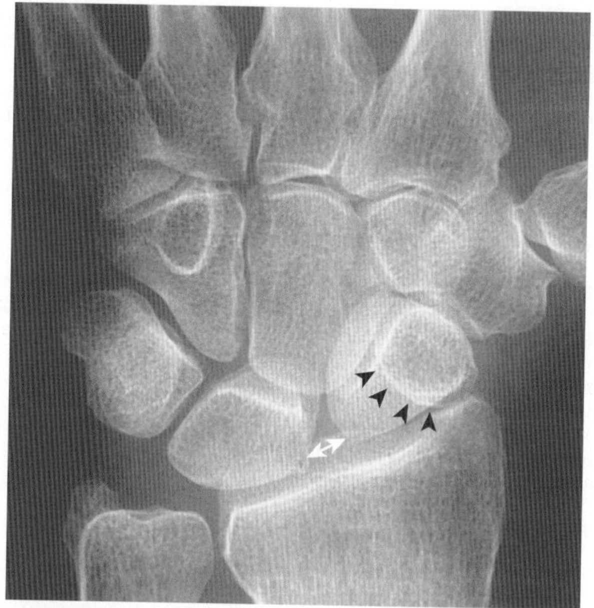

Cortical ring sign of the scaphoid, indicative of DISI, courtesy of Wolfe, S. W., Pederson, W. C., Kozin, S. H., Cohen, M. S., & Kakar, S. (2022). Carpal Instability. In *Green's Operative Hand Surgery*. essay, Elsevier.

16. **What position of the wrist allows maximal grip strength?**
    Maximal power grip is achieved with 35 degrees of extension and 7 degrees of ulnar deviation. In full flexion only 25% of grip strength can be achieved.

HANDS AND FINGERS

17. **Describe the musculature of the hand.**

Musculature of the Hand

MUSCLE	ORIGIN	INSERTION	ACTION	INNERVATION
Abductor pollicis brevis	Fr, Tm, Sc	Lateral base of proximal phalanx of thumb	Abduction of thumb	RBMN
Flexor pollicis brevis	Superficial head: Fr, Tm	Lateral base of proximal phalanx of thumb	Flexion of thumb	Superficial: RBMN
	Deep head: Ca, Td		MCP	Deep: deep ulnar

Musculature of the Hand

MUSCLE	ORIGIN	INSERTION	ACTION	INNERVATION
Opponens pollicis	Fr, Tm	Lateral/anterior shaft of 1st MC	Medial rotation during opposition	RBMN
Adductor pollicis	Oblique head: Ca, Td, base of 2nd MC	Medial base of proximal phalanx of thumb	Adduction of thumb	Deep ulnar
	Transverse head: shaft of 3rd MC			
Abductor digiti minimi	Pisiform	Medial base of 5th proximal phalanx	Abduction of 5th at MCP	Deep ulnar
Flexor digiti minimi	Hook of hamate	Medial base of 5th proximal phalanx	Flexion of 5th at MCP	Deep ulnar
Opponens digiti minimi	Hook of hamate	Anterior shaft of 5th MC	Opposition of 5th	Deep ulnar
Palmaris brevis	Medial palmar aponeurosis	Skin	Deepens palm	Superficial ulnar
Lumbricals	1 and 2: single heads from lateral FDP	Lateral sides of extensor expansions of 2–5	Flexion of MCPs and extension of PIPs and DIPs	1 and 2: median
	3 and 4: double heads from medial 3rd FDP			3 and 4: ulnar
Dorsal interossei	Double heads from adjacent MCs	Extensor expansions of fingers 2, 3, and 4 on side, allowing for abduction	Abduction of 2nd and 4th MCPs, medial/lateral deviation of 3rd MCP	Deep ulnar
Palmar interossei	Single heads from MCs 1, 2, 4, and 5	1 to medial thumb proximal phalanx 2, 4, and 5 to side of extensor expansions of 2, 4, and 5 for adduction	Adduction of fingers 1, 2, 4, and 5	Deep ulnar

Fr, flexor retinaculum; Tm, trapezium; Sc, scaphoid; Ca, capitate; Td, trapezoid; MC, metacarpal.

18. What is the total excursion of normal flexor and extensor tendons?

Extensor digitorum communis (EDC) ≈ 50 mm
Flexor digitorum profundus (FDP) ≈ 70 mm

19. What are the zones of injury of the extensor tendon?

1. Distal interphalangeal (DIP)
2. Middle phalanx
3. Proximal interphalangeal (PIP)
4. Proximal phalanx
5. Metacarpophalangeal (MCP)
6. Metacarpal
7. Dorsal retinaculum
8. Distal forearm

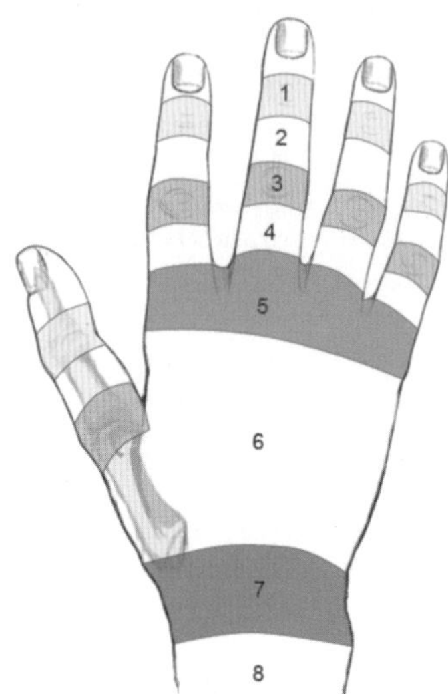

Extensor zone illustration courtesy of Sameem, Mojib, et al. "A Systematic Review of Rehabilitation Protocols after Surgical Repair of the Extensor Tendons in Zones V–VIII of the Hand." *Journal of Hand Therapy*, vol. 24, no. 4, Oct. 2011, pp. 365–373, 10.1016/j.jht.2011.06.005. Accessed 13 Apr. 2022.

20. Discuss the structure and function of the extensor mechanism.

Triangular Ligament: Prevents volar subluxation of the conjoined lateral bands during flexion of the IP joint.

Oblique Retinacular Ligament (Landsmeer Retinacular Ligament): The oblique retinacular ligament runs from the proximal volar aspect of the PIP to the dorsal terminal extensor tendon. This ligament links the movement of the DIP and PIP joints. PIP flexion allows for DIP flexion, whereas PIP extension promotes DIP extension. Tightness of the oblique retinacular ligament may limit DIP flexion.

Transverse Retinacular Ligament: The transverse retinacular ligaments attach from the flexor sheath to the conjoined lateral bands, thus stabilizing the lateral bands. Lateral displacement of the bands may lead to a boutonnière deformity, whereas contracture and dorsal displacement may lead to swan neck deformity. During PIP flexion, the TRL positions the lateral bands volarly and, during PIP extension, prevents dorsal displacement of the lateral bands.

Conjoined Tendons: The lateral slips of the extrinsic extensor merge with the lateral bands of the intrinsic muscles to form the conjoined lateral bands. The radial and ulnar conjoined tendons continue on to form the terminal tendon that goes on to insert on the base of the distal phalanx, allowing for extension of the DIP joint.

Central Slip: The central slip (CS) is formed by the central division of the extrinsic extensor tendon in combination with medial fibers from the intrinsic tendons. The CS continues distally to insert onto the base of middle phalanx, helping to initiate PIP extension.

Lateral Bands: The lateral bands are composed of tendons from the intrinsic interossei and lumbrical muscles. The lateral bands are located on each side of the proximal phalanx and travel distally toward the PIP joint, contributing and receiving fibers along the way. At the distal end of the proximal phalanx, the lateral bands join with the lateral slips of the extrinsic extensor and become the conjoined lateral bands. The lateral bands transmit tension force from the EDC, lumbricals, and interossei to assist with metaphalangeal (MP) flexion and interphalangeal (IP) joint extension.

Sagittal Bands: The sagittal bands and volar plate completely surround the MP joint and assist the juncturae tendinum with anchoring and maintaining the extensor tendon over the MP joint. It also assists with extension of the PIP joint by transmitting the pull of the extrinsic tendon.

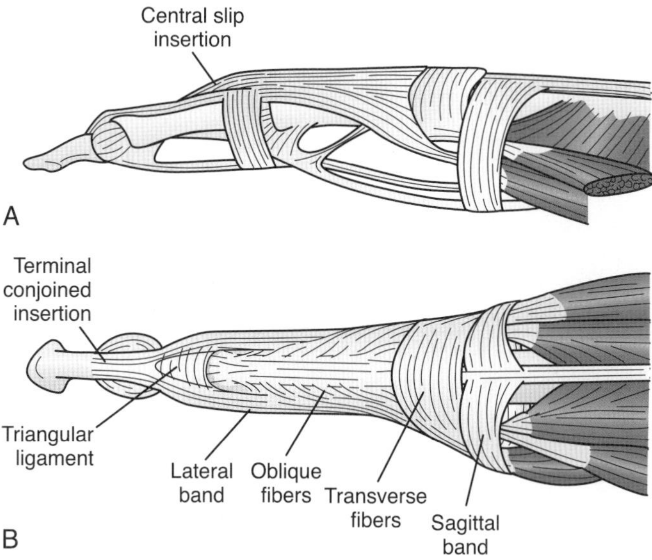

Twonsend, C. M. (2021). Hand Surgery In Sabiston Textbook of Surgery. The Biological Basis of Modern Surgical Practice.

21. Name the tendons in the six dorsal compartments of the hand.

The first compartment consists of the abductor pollicis longus and extensor pollicis brevis. The extensor carpi radialis brevis and extensor carpi radialis longus are in the second compartment. In the third compartment the extensor pollicis longus passes radially to Lister's tubercle to insert on the thumb. The fourth compartment contains the four tendons of the extensor digitorum and the "fellow traveler" extensor indicis proprius. In the fifth compartment is the tendon for the fifth digit—the extensor digiti minimi. Finally, the extensor carpi ulnaris passes through the sixth compartment.

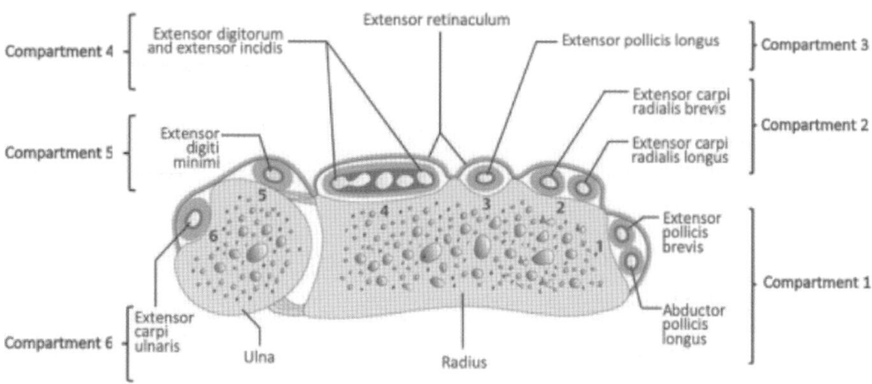

Ibrahim Engin Şimşek, Salih Angin. (2020). Kinesiology of the wrist and the hand. In Comparative Kinesiology of the Human Body: Normal and Pathological Conditions.

22. Where is Camper's chiasm and what is its function?

Camper's chiasm lies over the proximal phalanx. Just distal to the PIP joint, the flexor digitorum superficialis (FDS) tendon divides, allowing the deeper flexor digitorum profundus (FDP) to pass through to become the more superficial tendon. The two slips of the FDS wrap obliquely around the FDP and rejoin dorsally via the Camper's chiasm. The Camper's chiasm is not just one specific point but the "bed" for the FDP to glide upon, limiting hyperextension and increasing stability of the PIP joint.

23. What are the anatomic landmarks for the zones of flexor tendon injury in the hand?

- Zone 1—distal to the insertion of the FDS
- Zone 2—distal palmar crease, formerly called "no man's land"

- Zone 3—distal to the distal edge of the transverse carpal ligament
- Zone 4—carpal tunnel
- Zone 5—distal portion of the forearm

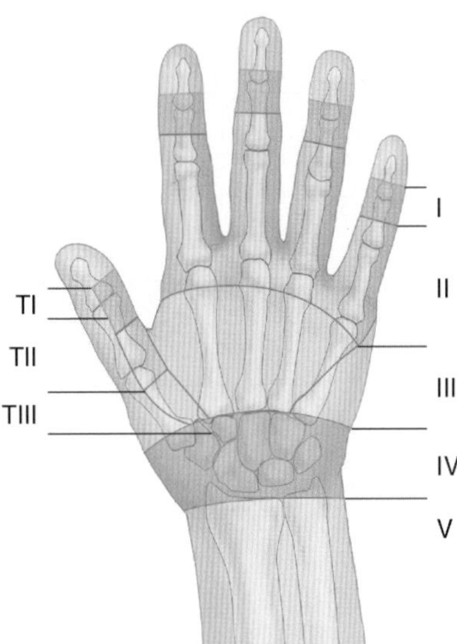

Flexor injury zones illustration From Chung KC. Operative Techniques: Hand and Wrist Surgery , 3rd ed. Elsevier; 2017 Fig. 64.3.

24. **Why are the lumbricals considered unique with regards to their attachment sites?**
    The lumbricals are the only muscle in the body to have its origin and insertion on a tendon. The origin of the lumbricals of the index and middle fingers is at the FDP tendon of each finger. The lumbrical to the ring finger originates on the FDP tendons of the middle and ring fingers, and the lumbrical to the small finger originates on the FDP tendons of the ring and small fingers. All of the lumbricals insert onto the radial aspect of the extensor hoods of the lateral bands.

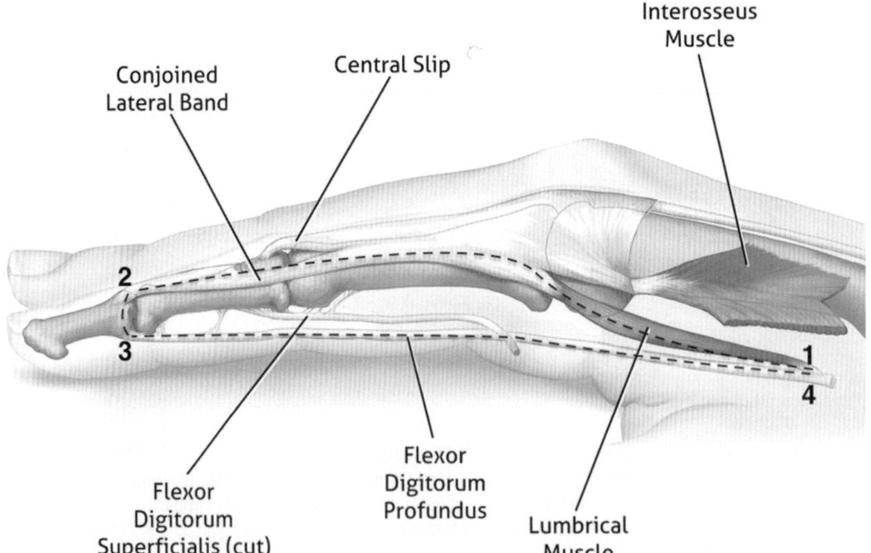

Relationship between the FDP and lumbrical muscle, courtesy of Crowley, J. S., Meunier, M., Lieber, R. L., & Abrams, R. A. (2021). The lumbricals are not the workhorse of digital extension and do not relax their own antagonist. *The Journal of Hand Surgery, 46*(3), 232–235. https://doi.org/10.1016/j.jhsa.2020.10.022

25. **Describe the nutrition and blood supply of the flexor tendon.**
Flexor tendons receive their nutrition intrinsically and extrinsically. Intrinsically flexor tendons receive their nutrition from the vincula in the digits and from blood vessels entering the tendon at the musculotendinous junction of the FDS and FDP. Extrinsically the flexor tendons receive nutrition from synovial fluid diffusion. Clinically it remains unclear which of these is most important. It is clear that the region of flexor tendon between the musculotendinous juncture and where the vincula begins is most reliant on synovial diffusion. The vincula are located on the dorsal half of the flexor superficialis and profundus tendons and begin proximally at the proximal phalanx. They are the longitudinal fibers visible when the FDS or FDP are lifted volarly during surgery.

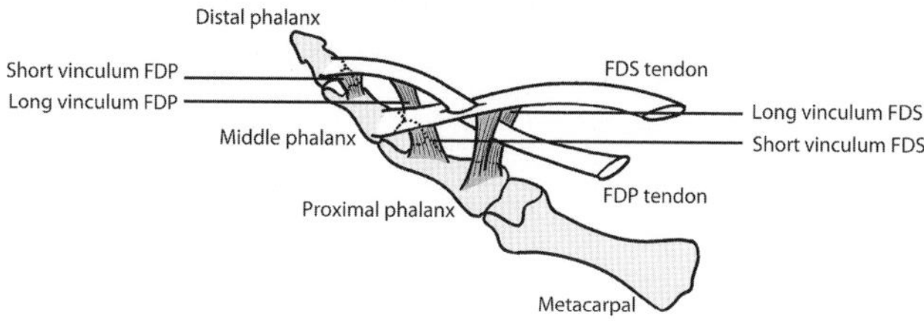

Flexor tendon nutrition illustration, courtesy of Newton, A. W., Tonge, X. N., Hawkes, D. H., & Bhalaik, V. (2019). Key aspects of anatomy, surgical approaches and clinical examination of the hand. *Orthopaedics and Trauma*, *33*(1), 1–13. https://doi.org/10.1016/j.mporth.2018.11.009

26. **Describe the anatomy of the flexor sheath.**
The pulleys are called annular (A) and cruciate (C), names derived from their respective configurations. They prevent the tendons from bowstringing when the fingers are flexed as well as improving the biomechanics of finger flexion.
- A1 pulley—on the volar plate of the metacarpal phalangeal joint
- A2 pulley—over the proximal portion of the proximal phalanx
- C1 pulley—over the midportion of the proximal phalanx
- A3 pulley—on the volar plate of the proximal interphalangeal (PIP) joint
- C2 pulley—over the proximal middle phalanx
- A4 pulley—at the midportion of the middle phalanx
- C3 pulley—on the distal aspect of the middle phalanx
- A5 pulley—attached to the volar plate of the distal interphalangeal (DIP) joint

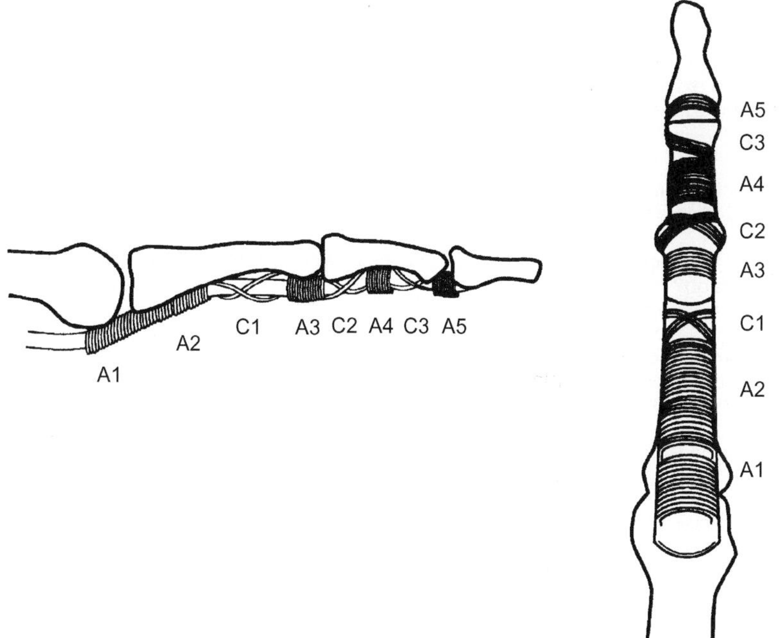

Flexor sheath illustration, courtesy of Wolfe, S. W., Pederson, W. C., Kozin, S. H., Cohen, M. S., & Wolf, J. M. (2022). Tendinopathy. In *Green's operative hand surgery*. Elsevier.

The odd-numbered annular pulleys (A1, A3, A5) are located at the joints, and even-numbered pulleys (A2 and A4) are located over bone. After the two initial annular pulleys, the cruciate and annular pulleys alternate. The A2 and A4 pulleys are considered the most crucial.

27. What are the pulleys of the thumb, and which thumb pulley is the most responsible for prevention of bowstringing of the FPL?

1. A1—annular pulley at the level of the volar plate at the thumb MP joint
2. A2—annular pulley at the level of the volar plate at the thumb IP joint
3. Oblique pulley—located between the annular pulleys at the diaphysis of the proximal phalanx

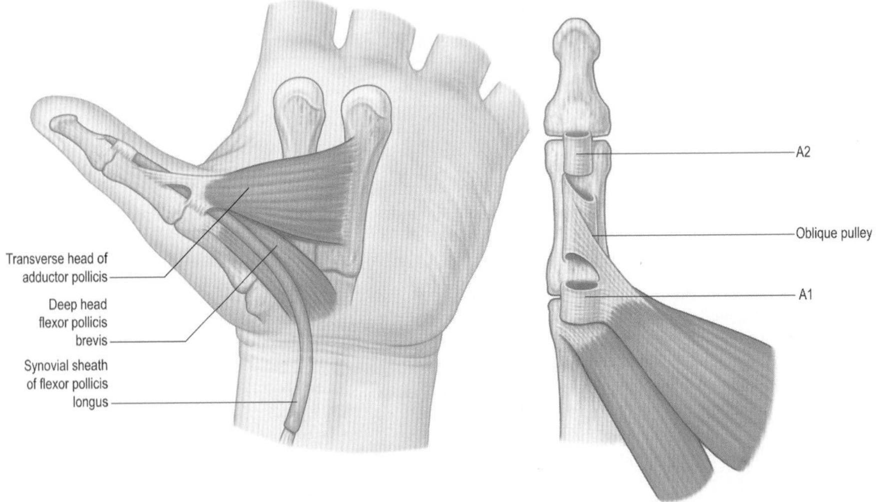

The oblique pulley is most responsible for preventing bowstringing of the FPL. Thumb pulley system, courtesy from Doyle, J. R., & Blythe, W. F. (1977). Anatomy of the flexor tendon sheath and pulleys of the thumb. *Journal of Hand Surgery (American), 2*, 149–151. With permission from the American Society for Surgery of the Hand.

28. How much extensor tendon excursion following an injury is thought to be needed to avoid significant adhesions?

3 to 5 mm

29. How much PIP motion is needed to achieve 3 to 5 mm of extensor excursion?

30 degrees of PIP flexion

30. How much tendon excursion is elicited in zone IV with DIP flexion while having the PIP in full extension?

3 to 4 mm

31. Besides increased risk of tendon adhesions from immobilization after injury, what other negative biomechanical impacts can occur to immobilized anatomical structures?

Increased stiffness and decreased strength of the tendon.

32. Describe the Boutonierre deformity. What causes this deformity to occur?

Boutonniere deformities occur either traumatically or via cumulative stress to the CS. The CS is formed by the central division of the extrinsic extensor tendon in combination with medial fibers from the intrinsic tendons. The CS continues distally to insert onto the base of middle phalanx, helping to initiate PIP extension. When it becomes inadequate (attenuated or lacerated/closed trauma), it can no longer transmit the force necessary to extend the PIP joint. The condyles of the P1 protrude through the tear in the central slip and triangular ligament (TL) becomes attenuated. The TL prevents volar subluxation of the conjoined lateral bands during flexion of the IP joint. When compromised, the conjoined lateral bands sublux volarly below the axis of the PIP joint. Due to this volar position, it now acts as a flexor of the PIP joint. The conjoined tendons continue to form the terminal tendon and due to altered mechanics, excessively pull the DIP into hyperextension (Dell, P. C., et al. 2005).

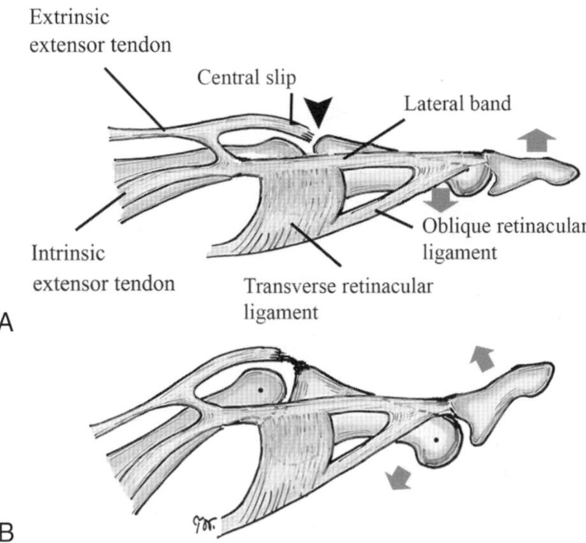

A. Central slip tear with lateral bands remaining dorsal to the PIP joint axis. B. Lateral bands have fallen volar to the PIP joint axis, eliciting PIP flexion, altered extensor mechanics cause the DIP to hyperextend. (Reprinted from Little KJ, Stern PJ. Rheumatoid arthritis—skeletal reconstruction. In: Trumble TE, Budoff JH, eds. Hand Surgery Update IV. Rosemont, Il: American Society for Surgery of the Hand, 2007:679. Courtesy of the American Society for Surgery of the Hand, https://www.assh.org)

33. **Describe the presentation of a swan neck deformity. What causes this deformity to occur?**
A swan neck deformity presents with hyperextension at the PIP joint and the DIP held in flexion. Swan neck deformities occur via a multitude of reasons, including altered mechanics due to a mallet deformity, laxity of the volar plate at the PIP joint, dorsal subluxation of the conjoined lateral band, FDS incompetence, intrinsic tightness, spasticity, and contractures of the intrinsics; chronic synovitis from rheumatoid arthritis (RA) at the PIPs can lead to UCL ligament instability, flexor tenosynovitis from RA can lead to MCP subluxation, and CMC osteoarthritis of the thumb in late phases can cause postures of the thumb that contribute to swan neck deformities. In fingers, laxity of the transverse retinacular ligament occurs due to the aforementioned causes allowing for dorsal displacement of the conjoined lateral bands. This causes shortening of the triangular ligament, further maintaining the dorsal displacement of the conjoined lateral bands, thus presenting with hyperextension at the PIP and flexion at the DIP.

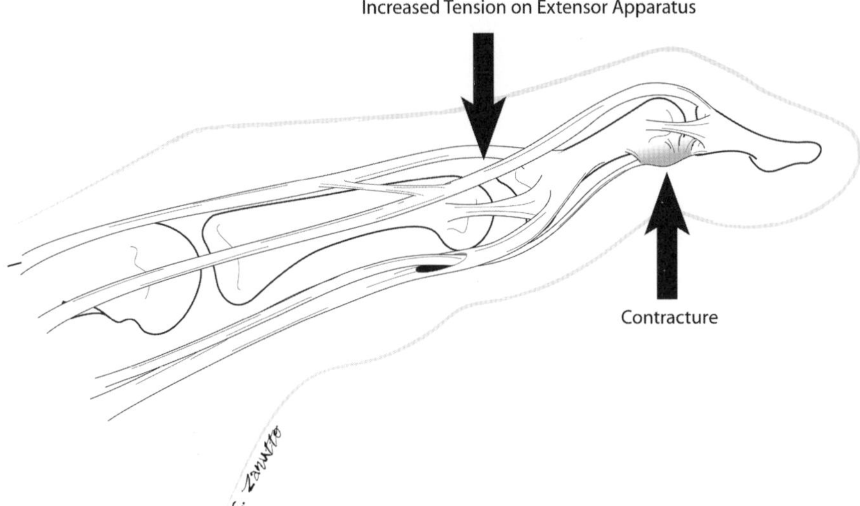

Swan neck deformity drawing courtesy of Shrikant J. Chinchalkar MThO, BScOT, OTR, CHT. Swan neck deformity after distal interphalangeal joint flexion contractures: A biomechanical analysis. *Journal of Hand Therapy*, *23*(4), 420–425. https://doi.org/10.1016/j.jht.2009.11.005

34. **Describe the tension in the collateral ligaments in relation to joint position at the MP and PIP joints.**
At the metacarpophalangeal joint, the ulnar and radial proper collateral ligaments are taut in flexion because they are stretched over the condyles of the metacarpal head, resisting radial and ulnar deviation. The MCP proper collateral ligaments are relaxed with MP extension. At the proximal interphalangeal joint, the collateral ligaments and volar plate are stretched when held in extension because of the shape of the phalangeal head. The IP collateral ligaments are relaxed with flexion.

35. **Do the A2 and A4 pulleys need to be salvaged at all costs with performance of flexor sheath–related injuries?**
Historically, surgeons have always tried to salvage the A2 and A4 pulleys with performance of surgeries in this region. It has been found that this is no longer the case. The A2 pulley can be released up to two-thirds of its length without significant bowstringing. The A4 pulley can be completely removed without concern, as long as the other pulleys are intact. Additionally, it has been found that up to 2 cm of pulley length can be removed without concern of diminished hand function (Tang and Lalonde).

NERVES

36. **Describe the anatomy of the carpal tunnel.**
TRANSVERSE CARPAL LIGAMENT
- Extends from proximal carpal row (pisiform and scaphoid tubercle) to distal row (hook of hamate and trapezial ridge) through proximal aspect of second through fifth metacarpals.
- Width = 22 mm
- Length = 26 mm
- Thickness:
  1. Proximal = 0.6 mm
  2. Midportion = 1.6 mm
  3. Distal = 0.6 mm

CARPAL CANAL
- Depth
  1. Entrance to canal = 12 mm
  2. Midportion = 10 mm
  3. Distal end = 13 mm
- Average cross-sectional area = 17 mm^2
- Smallest cross-sectional area = 16 mm^2 (at distal carpal row)
- Volume = 5.84 mL
- Carpal tunnel release increases canal volume by 25% and changes the shape from oval to round. This is associated with a concomitant change in the shape of Guyon's canal from triangular to a vertical oval.

37. **What is the average pressure (in mm Hg) in the carpal tunnel at different wrist positions?**

	NORMAL	WITH CARPAL TUNNEL SYNDROME
Neutral position	2	32
Full flexion	31	94
Full extension	35	110
After carpal tunnel release	5	—

38. **Describe the cross section of the median and ulnar nerves.**
- Median—6% motor, 94% sensory; motor branch may arise radial (60%), central (22%), or volar/radial (18%)
- Ulnar—45% motor, 55% sensory; motor branch arises dorsal ulnar

39. **What is the relationship between the digital nerves and arteries?**
The common digital arteries usually bifurcate 0.5 to 1.0 cm distally to the bifurcation of the common digital nerves in the palm. They are contiguous in the distal half of the fingers. The arteries are deep to the nerves. In general, if the artery is lacerated, so is the nerve. A simple mnemonic is "you hurt before you bleed."

40. **What are the two possible communications (anastomosis or interconnection) between the median and ulnar nerves?**
   - Martin-Gruber anastomosis: In this anomaly nerve fibers that were destined to be with the ulnar nerve when the median nerve was formed (by contributions from the lateral and medial cords of the brachial plexus) have stayed with the median nerve until the proximal forearm, where they finally join the ulnar nerve. This nerve interconnection explains why some patients with high ulnar nerve lesion have retained function in an area that typically is innervated by the ulnar nerve.
   - Riche-Cannieu interconnection: This less common anomaly occurs with a pattern similar to the Martin-Gruber anastomosis. In this case, however, motor nerves to intrinsic muscles have stayed with the median nerve rather than the ulnar nerve at the level of the brachial plexus and rejoin the ulnar nerve in the hand.

41. **Describe the anatomy of the superficial branch of the radial nerve (SBRN).**
   The superficial branch of the radial nerve (SBRN) exits between the brachioradialis (BR) and the extensor carpi radialis longus (ECRL) at approximately 9 cm proximal to the radial styloid. It bifurcates 5.1 cm proximally to the styloid and develops into five dorsal digital nerves

42. **What nerves are most vulnerable to injury with performance of surgeries at the wrist?**
   After the SBRN exits from between the BR and ECRL, it becomes more superficial within the thin subcutaneous tissue of the distal radius and dorsal hand. This superficial anatomical location makes it susceptible to compression, injury during surgery and injections, and entrapment following injury or surgery. It is also not uncommon for SBRN to be injured during fixation of distal radius fractures. Most commonly by traction to this nerve with volar plating, or irritation from K-wire fixation near the radial styloid.
   Additionally, during distal radius fracture treatment the palmar cutaneous branch of the median nerve is also at high risk of injury during the performance of open reduction and internal fixation of a distal radius fracture with performance of retraction with an anterior Henry approach to fixation. The dorsal ulnar sensory nerve (DUSN) is also commonly irritated during dorsal approaches to the distal ulna with repairs of ulnar-sided TFCC repairs.

NAIL

43. **What is the function of the eponychium?**
   The eponychium consists of the intermediate nail, ventral nail, and the dorsal nail. The intermediate nail produces the bulk of the nail plate, the ventral nail produces laminates that keep the nail plate attached to the nail bed, and the dorsal nail provides the hard, shiny coat of the nail.

Bibliography

Altman, E. (2016). The ulnar side of the wrist: Clinically relevant anatomy and biomechanics. *Journal of Hand Therapy, 29*(2), 111–122.

Amin, R. M., & John. (2019). Anatomy and biomechanics of the hand and wrist: *DeLee & Drez's Orthopaedic Sports Medicine*. Elsevier.

Chinchalkar, S. J., Lanting, B. A., & Ross, D. (2010). Swan neck deformity after distal interphalangeal joint flexion contractures: A biomechanical analysis. *Journal of Hand Therapy, 23*(4), 420–425.

Clavero, J. A., Golanó, P., Fariæas, O., Alomar, X., Monill, J. M., & Esplugas, M. (2003). Extensor mechanism of the fingers: MR imaging-anatomic correlation. *Radiographics, 23*(3), 593–611.

Colditz, J. C., OTR/L, CHT, & FAOTA. (2012). The intrinsic muscles of the hand: An overview: *2012 Philadelphia meeting: Surgery and rehabilitation of the hand*. Philadelphia: Lecture.

Crowley, J. S., Meunier, M., Lieber, R. L., & Abrams, R. A. (2021). The lumbricals are not the workhorse of digital extension and do not relax their own antagonist. *The Journal of Hand Surgery, 46*(3), 232–235.

Dell, P. C., & Sforzo, C. R. (2005). Ulnar intrinsic anatomy and dysfunction. *Journal of Hand Therapy, 18*(2), 198–207.

Erickson, M., Smith, H. F., Waggy, C., & Pratt, N. E. (2021). Anatomy and kinesiology of the hand In T. M. Skirven (Ed.), *Rehabilitation of the hand and upper extremity, seventh edition*. Elsevier.

Flowers, K. R., & LaStayo, P. C. (2007). A case of ulnar positive variance found on x-ray. *Journal of Hand Therapy, 20*(2), 148–151.

Gellman, H., Kauffman, D., Lenihan, M., Botte, M. J., & Sarmiento, A. (1988). An in vitro analysis of wrist motion: The effect of limited intercarpal arthrodesis and the contributions of the radiocarpal and midcarpal joints. *Journal of Hand Surgery, 13*(3), 378–383.

Johnson, C., Swanson, M., & Manolopoulos, K. (2021). Treatment of a zone III extensor tendon injury using a single relative motion with dorsal hood orthosis and a modified short arc motion protocol—A case report. *Journal of Hand Therapy, 34*(1), 135–141.

Ko, J. H., & Wiedrich, T. A. (2012). Triangular fibrocartilage complex injuries in the elite athlete. *Hand Clinics, 28*(3), 307–321.

Lane, L. B., Daher, R. J., & Leo, A. J. (2010). Scapholunate dissociation with radiolunate arthritis without radioscaphoid arthritis. *The Journal of Hand Surgery, 35*(7), 1075–1081.

Loisel, F., Orr, S., Ross, M., Couzens, G., Leo, A. J., & Wolfe, S. (2022). Traumatic nondissociative carpal instability: A case series. *The Journal of Hand Surgery, 47*(3), 285.e1–285.e11.

Mackin, & Evelyn. (2002). *Rehabilitation of the hand and upper extremity*. St. Louis: Mosby.

Micucci, C. J., & Schmidt, C. C. (2007). Arthroscopic repair of ulnar-sided triangular fibrocartilage complex tears. *Operative Techniques in Orthopaedics, 17*(2), 118–124.

Michelotti, B., & Chung, K. C. (2018). Scapholunate ligament repair. *Operative techniques: Hand and wrist surgery*, 180–191.

Miller, M. D., Thompson, S. R., Amin, R. M., & Ingari, J. V. (2019). Anatomy and biomechanics of the wrist and hand: *DeLee & Drez's Orthopaedic sports medicine* (pp. 785–792). Elsevier.

Miller, M. D., Hart, J., & MacKnight, J. M. (2020). *Essential orthopaedics.* Philadelphia, PA: Elsevier.
Moses, K. P. (2013). *Atlas of clinical gross anatomy.* Philadelphia, PA: Elsevier, Saunders.
Newton, A. W., Tonge, X. N., Hawkes, D. H., & Bhalaik, V. (2019). Key aspects of anatomy, surgical approaches and clinical examination of the hand. *Orthopaedics and Trauma, 33*(1), 1–13.
Poublon, A. R., Kraan, G., Lau, S. P., Kerver, A. L. A., & Kleinrensink, G. -J. (2016). Anatomical study of the dorsal cutaneous branch of the ulnar nerve (DCBUN) and its clinical relevance in TFCC repair. *Journal of Plastic, Reconstructive & Aesthetic Surgery, 69*(7), 983–987.
Pratt, N. (2005). Anatomy of nerve entrapment sites in the upper quarter. *Journal of Hand Therapy, 18*(2), 216–229.
Preston, D. C., & Shapiro, B. E. (2021). Radial neuropathy: *Electromyography and neuromuscular disorders.* Elsevier.
Pulos, N., & Bozentka, D. J. (2015). Carpal ligament anatomy and biomechanics. *Hand Clinics, 31*(3), 381–387.
Rhee, P. C., Dennison, D. G., & Kakr, S. (2012). Avoiding and treating perioperative complications of distal radius fractures. *Hand Clinics, 28*(2), 185–198.
Ross, P. R., & Chung, K. C. (2022). Acute repair of flexor tendon injuries in zones I to V In K. C. Chung (Ed.), *Operative techniques: Hand and wrist surgery* (pp. 2022). Elsevier.
Sarah, R. D. (2022). Wrist and hand: *Orthopaedics for physician assistants* (pp. 110–180). Elsevier.
Sameem, M., Wood, T., Ignacy, T., Thoma, A., & Strumas, N. (2011). A systematic review of rehabilitation protocols after surgical repair of the extensor tendons in zones V–VIII of the hand. *Journal of Hand Therapy, 24*(4), 365–373.
Skalski, M. R., White, E. A., Patel, D. B., Schein, A. J., RiveraMelo, H., & Matcuk, G. R. (2016). The traumatized TFCC: An illustrated review of the anatomy and injury patterns of the triangular fibrocartilage complex. *Current Problems in Diagnostic Radiology, 45*(1), 39–50.
Smith, J. L., & Ebraheim, N. A. (2019). Anatomy of the palmar cutaneous branch of the median nerve: A review. *Journal of Orthopaedics, 16*(6), 576–579.
Strickland, J. W. (2005). The scientific basis for advances in flexor tendon surgery. *Journal of Hand Therapy, 18*(2), 94–110.
Tägil, M. (2022). Distal radius fractures In S. W. Wolfe (Ed.), *Green's operative hand surgery.* Elsevier.
Tang, J. B., & Lalonde, D. (2021). Surgery management of flexor tendon injuries In T. M. Skirven (Ed.), *Rehabilitation of the hand and upper extremity.* Elsevier.
Trumble, T. E., Baratz, M. E., Budoff, J. E., & Ryan, G. M. (2010). *Principles of hand surgery and therapy (includes Dvd).* Saunders.
Tuffaha, S. H., & Lee, W. P. A. (2018). Treatment of proximal interphalangeal joint contracture. *Hand Clinics, 34*(2), 229–235.
Umay, E., Gurcay, E., Serce, A., Gundogdu, I., & Uz, C. (2021). Is superficial radial nerve affected in patients with hand osteoarthritis? *Journal of Hand Therapy, 35*(3), 461–467.
Williams, K., & Terrono, A. L. (2011). Treatment of boutonniere finger deformity in rheumatoid arthritis. *The Journal of Hand Surgery, 36*(8), 1388–1393.
Wolfe, S. W., Hotchkiss, R. N., Pederson, W. C., Kozin, S. H., & Cohen, M. S. (2017). *Green's operative hand surgery.* Elsevier.
Wolfe, S. W., Pederson, W. C., Kozin, S. H., & Cohen, M. S. (2022). The stiff finger: *Green's operative hand surgery.* Elsevier.
Wolfe, S. W., Pederson, W. C., Kozin, S. H., Cohen, M. S., & Kakar, S. (2022). Carpal instability: *Green's operative hand surgery.* Elsevier.
Wolfe, S. W., Pederson, W. C., Kozin, S. H., Cohen, M. S., & Leversedge, F. J. (2022). The distal radioulnar joint: *Green's operative hand surgery.* Elsevier.
Wolfe, S. W., Pederson, W. C., Kozin, S. H., Cohen, M. S., & Leversedge, F. J. (2022). The distal radius fracture: *Green's operative hand surgery.* Elsevier.
Wolfe, S. W., Pederson, W. C., Kozin, S. H., Cohen, M. S., & Wolf, J. M. (2022). Tendinopathy: *Green's operative hand surgery.* Elsevier.
Wolff, A. L., & Wolfe, S. W. (2016). Rehabilitation for scapholunate injury: Application of scientific and clinical evidence to practice. *Journal of Hand Therapy, 29*(2), 146–153.

CHAPTER 49 QUESTIONS

1. **What intrinsic muscles of the hand are innervated by the median nerve?**
   a. Dorsal interosseous
   b. Palmar interosseous
   c. 1st and 2nd lumbricals
   d. 3rd and 4th lumbricals

2. **What is the role of the lateral bands of the extensor mechanism?**
   a. Distributes force from the FDS, lumbricals, and interossei to the middle phalanx
   b. Distributes force from the FDP, lumbricals, and interossei to the distal phalanx
   c. Distributes force from the EDC, lumbricals, and interossei to the distal phalanx
   d. Distributes force from the EDC, lumbricals, and interossei to the middle phalanx

3. **What is the function of the dorsal interossei muscles?**
   a. Flexes IP joints
   b. Adducts digits and assists with MCP flexion and IP extension
   c. Flexes the thumb
   d. Abducts digits and assists with MCP flexion and IP extension

4. **Which of the following muscles uses the flexor retinaculum, scaphoid, and trapezium as their proximal attachment?**
   a. Adductor pollicis
   b. Opponens pollicis, flexor pollicis brevis, and abductor pollicis brevis
   c. Medial lumbricals
   d. Opponens digiti minimi, flexor digiti minimi, and abductor digiti minimi

5. **What tendon resides in the third dorsal compartment?**
   a. Extensor pollicis brevis
   b. Abductor pollicis longus
   c. Extensor pollicis longus
   d. Extensor carpi radialis longus

6. **Tearing of the scapholunate ligament and secondary stabilizers results in the development of what type instability?**
   a. Dorsal intercalated segment instability (DISI)
   b. Volar intercalated segment instability (VISI)
   c. Midcarpal instability
   d. DRUJ instability

7. **What sensory nerve is most at risk during a volar approach to the distal radius for fixation of a distal radius fracture?**
   a. Sensory branch of the radial nerve
   b. Palmar cutaneous branch of the median nerve
   c. Dorsal sensory branch of the ulnar nerve
   d. Terminal branch of the posterior interosseous nerve

CHAPTER 50

COMMON ORTHOPEDIC DYSFUNCTION OF THE WRIST AND HAND

J. Cronin, OTR/L, CHT

1. **What special test is used to evaluate scapholunate ligament disruption?**
   - Scaphoid shift test: test for scapholunate ligament.

   Pressure is applied to volar surface of the scaphoid with thumb while passively holding wrist in ulnar deviation. While maintaining pressure, passively move wrist into radial deviation and slight flexion. At this time the evaluator releases pressure from deviation of the wrist. If the scapholunate (S-L) ligament is disrupted, pressure from thumb on scaphoid will cause the scaphoid to glide on to the dorsal rim of the radius. Releasing thumb pressure causes scaphoid to fall back to volar flexion with a painful "clunk."

2. **How are scapholunate ligament injuries treated?**
   Primary repair is considered when the injury is acute. If this is not possible, a dorsal wrist capsulodesis (sometimes referred as Blatt capsulodesis) or tenodesis using the flexor carpi radialis are common techniques. Ligamentous repairs using tendon grafts are also utilized.

   Postoperative care of a scapholunate ligament repair focuses on achieving functional range of motion (ROM) in the wrist of 40 degrees of flexion and 40 degrees of extension. The stability of the joint is most important over trying to gain more ROM. Patients can be immobilized up to 12 weeks if the ligament is repaired. High stress to the wrist is avoided for 4 to 6 months. In chronic situations where arthritis is already present, partial wrist fusion may be necessary.

3. **What happens if S-L ligament is not repaired?**
   When left untreated the patient can develop arthritis in the midcarpal and radiocarpal joints that is apparent within 4 years and more severe by 15 years post injury. At this time the patient may require more salvage wrist procedures such as partial wrist fusion.

4. **Why is a "dart thrower's motion" and dart thrower's orthosis used in treating scapholunate interosseous ligament (SLIL) tears in conservative management for this injury?**
   Movement in this direction allows for less stress to the healing ligament while allowing for early active motion. This is due to very little movement of the scaphoid tuberosity during this motion, which allows decreased load on the ligament and radius.

5. **What is the function of the triangular fibrocartilage complex (TFCC)?**
   The function of the TFCC is to stabilize the distal radioulnar joint (DRUJ) and take compressive load with grip. The TFCC absorbs 20% of these forces and the radius 80%. The deep portion of the volar and dorsal radioulnar ligaments are the primary stabilizers with pronation and supination of the forearm.

6. **What are common causes of ulnar-sided wrist pain?**
   Fracture, instability of DRUJ/TFCC, lunotriquetral or midcarpal joint, TFCC tear, tendonitis (Extensor Carpi ulnaris [ECU] or Flexor Carpi ulnaris [FCU]), pisotriquetral arthritis, or ulnar nerve compression at the wrist.

7. **What are two provocative tests for ulnar-sided wrist pain?**
   - Ulnocarpal stress test:

   Wrist is placed in maximal ulnar deviation, axially loaded, while passively pronating and supinating the forearm. Pain with performance can indicate ulnocarpal impaction syndrome, L-T ligament tear, TFCC injury, or ulnocarpal arthritis.
   - Ulnar fovea sign:

   Tenderness with palpation of the soft region around the distal ulna (between the ulnar styloid and FCU and between the ulnar head and pisiform) could indicate foveal disruption of the distal radioulnar ligaments and/or ulnotriquetral ligament injury.

8. **How are TFCC injuries identified and treated?**
   Arthrography has a 27% false-positive rate, and false positives may be as high as 50% with MRI. The sensitivity of both modalities is about 85%. Treatment options for TFCC tears include debridement, which will decompress the tear but doesn't change the structural anatomy (usually for central or nonrepairable tears). For degenerative

tears, typically from ulnar impaction, arthroscopic debridement or ulnar shortening osteotomy can be performed. Following surgery for debridement, ROM is initiated early, progressing to strengthening at 6 weeks post op. When a peripheral tear is repaired, the wrist is immobilized for 6 weeks. AROM is then started, with strengthening beginning at 10 to 12 weeks. Start with strengthening in supination and progress to neutral and then pronation.

9. **What is the etiology of de Quervain's syndrome?**
   de Quervain's is stenosing tenosynovitis in the first dorsal compartment of the wrist. This compartment contains the abductor pollicis longus and extensor pollicis brevis. Symptoms include pain along the radial side of the wrist. The patient may report pain with palpation of the first dorsal compartment at the wrist, pain with resisted thumb abduction, and extension. Causes can include repetitive pinching with radial or ulnar deviation, opening jars, using scissors, new moms nursing their babies, knitting, and trauma.

10. **What are the provocative tests for de Quervain's and intersection syndrome?**
    For de Quervain's, a positive Finkelstein's test is noted when the thumb is flexed into palm and wrist is ulnarly deviated passively causes pain. For intersection syndrome, testing is the same as a Finkelstein's with added wrist flexion.

11. **What is the treatment for de Quervain's?**
    Conservative treatment can include splinting in a thumb spica orthosis and activity modification to eliminate the extreme wrist and thumb positions that aggravate the patient's symptoms along with stretching, heat, and massage. When resistant to conservative management many patients get complete relief after one or two steroid injections. For those persistent cases, surgical release of the first dorsal compartment is indicated. Success rates for various interventions are as follows:
    - Splinting (wrist in 20 degrees extension with thumb in metacarpal (MP) and IP extension)—30%
    - Splinting with injection—57%
    - Injection—69% (50%–90% success rate with 1–2 injections)
    - Operative management—91%

12. **What is intersection syndrome?**
    Intersection syndrome is tenosynovitis located mid-forearm where the thumb extensors and wrist extensors cross (1st and 2nd dorsal compartments). This can occur with repetitive forceful wrist extension with radial deviation. Also, activities with a tight fist and thumb abducted such as rowing can provoke symptoms. Treatment is similar to de Quervain's.

13. **What is a ganglion cyst?**
    Ganglion is a Greek word meaning "cystic tumor." Ganglions are mucus-filled cysts that account for 50% to 70% of all soft tissue tumors of the hand and wrist; they are more prevalent in women (female to male ratio of 3:1). There is no occupational proclivity, although the tendency to develop ganglions is seen with repetitive wrist activity. Dorsal wrist ganglions are the most common and account for 60% to 70% of all ganglions. The next most common site is the radial volar wrist (20%), followed by the flexor sheath of the fingers and the distal interphalangeal (DIP) joint. When ganglions become painful or noticeably enlarged, aspiration and cortisone injection may be indicated. Surgical removal of the cyst, in most cases, provides reliable definitive treatment with relatively low reoccurrence rates of 3% to 5%.

14. **What is a mallet finger and how is it treated?**
    Mallet finger is an injury to the tip of a finger, where the extensor tendon attached to the distal phalanx is torn or lacerated, causing the tip to droop. The patient usually cannot straighten the DIP joint on their own. A classification system of mallet fingers was developed by Doyle as follows: type I (closed injury, with or without small dorsal avulsion fracture), type II (open injury, with laceration of the tendon), type III (open injury, with loss of skin, subcutaneous cover, and tendon substance), and type IV (mallet fracture).
    - Type I mallet fingers are typically treated nonoperatively via 8 weeks of immobilization in a dorsal extension fixation device (Alum Foam, Stack finger splint, or custom-made orthotic), placing the DIP joint in slight hyperextension. The patient is encouraged to maintain PIP joint flexion during the immobilization.
    - Type II–III mallet fingers are typically treated operatively via an open repair of the tendon with K-wire fixation of the DIP in extension. The K wire is typically removed at 4 weeks postoperatively, followed by dorsal extension splinting full time for 2 weeks and slowly weaning from splint to prevent droop.
    - Type IV mallet fingers are often treated nonoperatively, but operative treatment with K-wire fixation may be appropriate when a large fracture with volar subluxation is present. Patients treated nonoperatively are splinted in extension 8 weeks.
    - Active ROM of the DIP joint post immobilization is encouraged; however, passive stretching of the DIP is not recommended because this could lead to an elongation of the extensor tendon with a subsequent increase in extensor lag.

- Maximum DIP ROM will take months to achieve, typically with a small residual extensor lag present. Treatment intensity should be adjusted according to the patient's progression and the amount of extensor lag present.

15. **What is swan neck deformity?**
Swan neck deformity is when the proximal interphalangeal (PIP) joint of the finger is positioned in hyperextension and DIP joint is flexed. This deformity is common with rheumatoid arthritis as a result of laxity of the ligaments and volar plate combined with muscle tendon imbalance. It can also be seen with chronic mallet injuries, flexor digitorum superficialis (FDS) weakness, intrinsic muscle contracture, and excessive traction by the extensor apparatus. This deformity usually does not respond to conservative splinting or an exercise program and requires operative management.

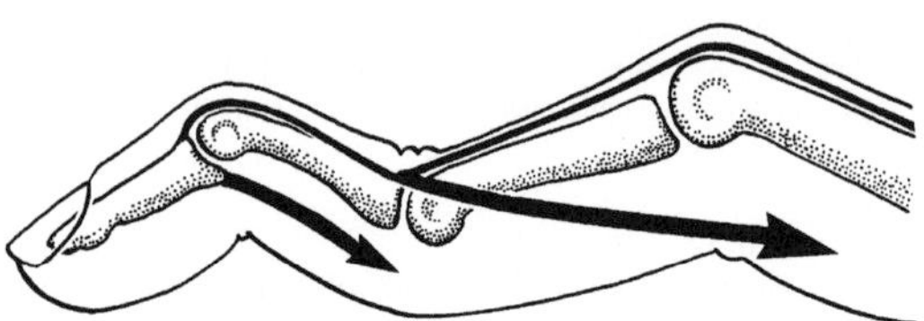

16. **What is a boutonnière deformity?**
A boutonnière deformity occurs when there is an injury to the PIP joint extensor mechanism, causing the PIP to form a flexion deformity and the DIP to pull into extension. This can be caused by trauma, the so-called "jammed finger," volar PIP dislocation, collateral ligament injury, central slip rupture, and rheumatoid arthritis.

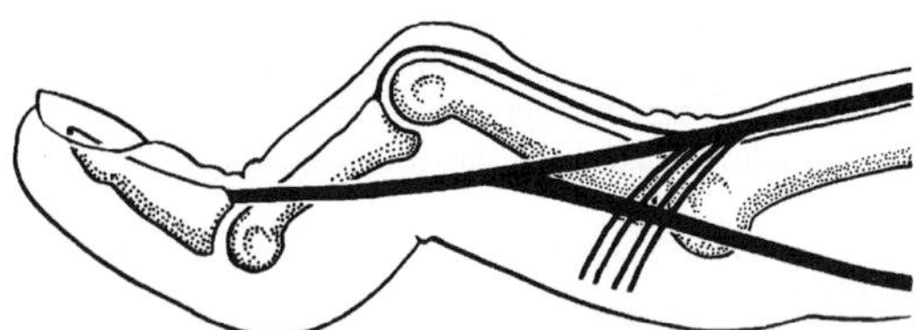

17. **Describe the treatment for boutonnière deformity.**
The traditional way to treat a boutonnière is to splint the PIP joint in extension and allow the DIP to be active into full flexion for a period of time. This allows for the active DIP flexion to stretch to oblique retinacular ligament at the DIP and help pull the lateral bands more dorsally. However, Judy Colditz OT/L, CHT, FAOTA points out that the DIP cannot do this unless the PIP is in full passive extension. When initially splinting or casting the PIP for the flexion contracture, the DIP can be included for better ability to achieve full PIP extension. Once PIP joint extension is achieved then a relative motion orthosis (RMO) can be used to provide "active redirection" of the tissues to regain motion at the PIP joint. In a boutonnière the DIP joint can be splinted in slight flexion to pull the lateral bands dorsally. The RMO is fabricated with the affected finger 15 to 20 degrees more flexed at the metacarpophalangeal (MCP) than the other digits; it is worn throughout the day to focus the tension to the affected joint and block normal joints. A night extension splint can be worn for preventing further contracture. This is beneficial if only one joint is involved. If multiple joints are affected, or the patient has developed chronic stiffness, then treatment with a nonremovable CMMS (casting motion to mobilize stiffness) cast may be an option. Here fingers can be casted to focus movement at specific joint to facilitate normal motion and are nonremovable for a period of time as motion improves.

18. **How do you assess if DIP loss of motion is due to oblique retinacular ligament tightness or joint contracture?**
DIP flexion is measured with PIP joint extended and with PIP flexed. If the DIP flexion is better with PIP flexion than when extended, the ORL ligament is shortened or tight. If DIP motion is limited equally with PIP motion, then it is joint contracture.

19. **How is the Bunnell-Littler test for intrinsic tightness performed?**
The patient's MP joint is held in extension while passively flexing the PIP joint, then again with the MP joint held in full flexion. If the PIP joint has more motion with the MP flexed and more limited with MP extended this is positive for intrinsic muscle tightness. Intrinsic muscles are at their shortest length when the MP joint is flexed and IP joints extended. They are at their longest length when MP joint is hyperextended and the IPs flexed.

20. **What options are available for splinting and casting of stiff joints?**
- Static progressive splinting: the splint holds the joint or shortened tissue to its maximum length, and as the tissue responds and elongates the splint can be adjusted to progress the ROM.
- Serial casting is often used for PIP contractures for a more prolonged stretch over 2 to 4 days, then recasting as tissue lengthens.
- CMMS (casting motion to mobilize stiffness) uses plaster of Paris to immobilize certain joints in order to redirect motion to other joints and facilitate more normal movement patterns.
- Relative motion splinting is used for finger motion to improve boutonnière deformity by redirecting motion and pulling the lateral bands dorsally.

21. **In general, what is the appropriate position of the MCP joints in splinting? Why?**
The MCP joints should be splinted in some degree of flexion and not in an extended position. In the extended position, the collateral ligaments are shortened, whereas in the flexed position they are stretched. Consequently, it is easier to regain full flexion when the MCP joints are splinted in the flexed position. Because of the cam effect of the metacarpal head, the collateral ligaments are lengthened and therefore stretched in flexion.

22. **List and briefly describe the three rehabilitative approaches to the treatment of flexor tendons.**
- Immobilization: a conservative treatment approach, immobilizing the patient for a duration of 3 to 4 weeks in a dorsal blocking splint with the wrist in 10 to 30 degrees of flexion, 40 to 60 degrees of MCP flexion, and full IP extension. This treatment approach is primarily used with children and other individuals who are unable to adhere to more complex protocols.
- Early passive mobilization: a treatment approach having various subprotocols including, but not limited to, Kleinert, modified Duran, and Washington. These protocols exist on the theory that passive mobilization of the tendon will result in increased tendon excursion with fewer adhesions and increased healing of the tendon. The modified Duran protocol uses a dorsal blocking splint (DBS) to protect the repair, and PROM is performed to the digits in flexion. The IP joints are actively extended while holding the MPs in full passive flexion. The Kleinert and Washington protocols also use a DBS; however, they use rubber band traction with a palmar pulley, providing passive flexion to the digit(s). The patient performs hourly active extension within the brace. The splints are worn for 3 to 6 weeks as appropriate with treatment, progressing according to the patient's progress.
- Early active mobilization: early active mobilization (EAM) protocols apply a controlled amount of stress to the repaired tendons, encouraging increased tendon glide with fewer adhesions.

23. **What factors come into play that may affect tendon healing and adhesions to form?**
Preoperative condition of tendon, multiple tendons repaired, and thickness of repair. Location of injury, amount of time hand is immobilized, gapping at repair site, postoperative infection, significant edema, or ischemia. Patient's age, health, and cooperation for following protocol will also come into play.

24. **What are the nutritional sources of flexor tendon healing?**
Vascular through the vincula, and by synovial fluid diffusion in the tendon sheath.

25. **How much does a flexor tendon repair have to glide to prevent adhesions during the healing phase?**
3 to 5 mm.

26. **How much gliding of flexor tendons does joint motion produce?**
Each 10 degrees of DIP motion produces 1 to 2 mm of FDP gliding, whereas each 10 degrees of PIP motion produces about 1.5 mm of FDP and FDS gliding.

27. **When is the flexor tendon repair the weakest and at risk for rupture?**
6 to 12 days postoperative.

28. **EAM protocols for flexor tendon repairs are becoming more common. When should they be started and what are the risks?**
EAM should start between days 4 to 7 post op; after 7 days adhesions start to form.
- A review of 34 articles that compared rehabilitation approaches and rupture rates indicated:

- Passive protocol—4% rupture rate (57/1598 patients).
- Early active protocol—5% rupture rate (75/1598).
- Of the 75 patients who ruptured with an early active protocol, 72 had a 2-strand core suture, 3 had a 4-strand core suture, and no patients ruptured with a 6-strand core suture.

29. **What position is the hand for a DBS when using the early motion protocols and what problem can occur if MPs are placed in high degrees of flexion?**
Wrist is positioned in 0 to 30 degrees flexion (this is most common position with all protocols) with the MPs in 15 to 30 degrees flexion and IPs extended. This position is good for repairs distal to zone 4. If MPs are placed in an intrinsic plus position, it is harder to flex the fingers with the extrinsic flexor muscles. There can also be adaptive shortening of the interosseous muscles and the patient learns to initiate finger flexion with MP joint first rather than the IP joints.

30. **What is wide awake hand surgery and what is the benefit for flexor tendon repairs?**
In this type of surgery, there is no general anesthesia given to the patient. They are injected with lidocaine and epinephrine (which decreases bleeding during the procedure without using a tourniquet). The patient is awake and can move the fingers after the surgeon repairs the tendon, allowing the physician to alter the repair to make sure it glides easily through the pulleys and tendon sheath. This allows for early motion to start with less chance of rupture postoperatively.

31. **Briefly describe the St. John Protocol for postop wide awake flexor repairs.**
Dorsal blocking splint (DBS) with wrist in 20 to 30 degrees of extension, MP's in 60 degrees flexion with IP joints extended. Passive motion is first in preparation for active. Active extension to splint, mid-range flexion starting at day 3 only if low edema and easy PROM. MP flexion to comfort and max 45 degrees at the PIP/DIP joints. Movement is frequent to prevent adhesions. Wean from splint 4 to 6 weeks.

32. **In general, what are the expected outcomes after flexor tendon repair?**
On average, patients regain 75% of grip strength, 77% of finger pressure, 75% of pinch strength, 76% of PIP motion, and 75% of DIP motion.

33. **Define the syndrome of the quadriga.**
If a surgical procedure or injury prevents the proximal excursion of a single flexor profundus tendon, the full flexion of the adjacent profundus tendon may be impaired. This phenomenon can occur only in the long, ring, and small fingers because of the anatomic arrangement of the flexor profundus tendons and their origin from a common muscle belly. If the excursion of one profundus tendon is limited, the muscle cannot move the other tendons to their full extent. Verdan coined the term quadriga from the Roman chariot in which the reins to four horses were controlled and operated by a single rider.

34. **How do you isolate FDS flexion and FDP flexion in the hand?**
FDS is isolated by holding all fingers in extension except the test finger and asking the patient to bend at the PIP joint. This will glide only the FDS of that finger. To isolate FDP the examiner holds MP and PIP of test finger in extension and asks patient to bend DIP. This blocking exercise is used frequently in therapy treatment for improving tendon gliding in the hand after injury.

35. **Describe the "lumbrical plus" finger. What causes it?**
A lumbrical plus finger results in paradoxical extension of the PIP joint during attempted flexion of the finger. It occurs when the FDP is ineffective because of laceration, scarring, or amputation. "Pull" of the FDP through the lumbrical attachment to the finger causes extension of the PIP joint, which may also occur when a flexor tendon graft is "too long."

36. **Briefly describe postoperative rehab for extensor tendon repairs in zone IV.**
    1. Delayed motion: hand is splinted with fingers in full extension, treatment focus on edema management and scar care. At 4 weeks post op, patient can begin AROM starting with short arc to mid arc flexion and full extension focus on minimizing any extensor lag. Full AROM at 5 weeks, discontinue splint at 6 weeks, and PROM can begin if extensor lag is less than 10 degrees.
    2. Early active motion: two splints are fabricated, with one finger in full extension, and a second one with fingers flexed to 30 degrees (IP joints). The second splint is used for short arc motion exercise program. This allows for gentle extension with 30 degrees of flexion to be performed 4 to 6 times per day. This exercise splint is progressed to 45 at 2 weeks, 60 at 3 weeks, and 75 at 4 weeks. This is dependent on each patient's response and if there is an extension lag. At 5 and 6 weeks, motion continues to progress and passive stretching can be added. The extension orthosis is gradually weaned to night only and discontinued at 10 weeks.

37. **What is the rehab for extensor tendon repairs in zone V and VII?**
    1. Custom orthosis with wrist in 30 to 40 degrees extension and outrigger holding IP joints and MP joints in full extension. Active flexion to about 30 to 35 degrees at the MP with passive extension. The amount of flexion is increased over time transitioning to AROM out of the splint at 4 to 6 weeks. Passive flexion can be initiated at 7 weeks with precautions to prevent extensor lag. Splint is weaned to night only and discontinued at 10 to 12 weeks.
    2. Relative motion extension splint: a relative motion splint is fabricated with the repaired digit maintaining 15 to 20 degrees more extension relative to the other MCP joints. A separate static extension splint can also be fabricated to allow patient to rest hand intermittently, and at night for comfort, and if extensor lag develops. This RME is worn for 4 to 6 weeks, cautioning patient to not flex wrist at the same time as the fingers. A complete and specific exercise plan is provided to the patient with education on precautions.

38. **Explain extrinsic tightness with respect to the extensor tendons.**
    If the extrinsic (long) extensor tendons are shortened or adherent after trauma-like metacarpal fracture, or healing tendon, excursion distal to this point is limited. If MP and PIP joints are passively normal individually but limited with composite fist (MPs and IPs fully flexed), this means the extrinsic muscle is shortened, or adhered.

39. **Describe splinting techniques for various upper extremity nerve injuries.**
    - Median nerve—must maintain thumb abduction.
    - Radial nerve—must maintain wrist extension; may use outrigger for passive finger extension.
    - Ulnar nerve—must attempt to avoid claw deformity; use a splint to keep MCP joints flexed and IP joint extended.

40. **What is Dupuytren's contracture? Which structures in the hand are typically involved?**
    Dupuytren's contracture is a familial disease characterized by the development of new fibrous tissue in the form of nodules and cords in the palmar and digital fascia of the hand. The fibrous tissue leads to flexion contractures of the digits. Dupuytren's contracture is more common in northern Europeans, diabetic patients, alcoholic patients, patients with liver disease, and patients who smoke. Men outnumber women by about 9 to 1. Dupuytren's contracture involves certain components of the palmar fascia, the pretendinous bands, and superficial transverse ligament, the spiral band, the natatory ligament, and lateral digital sheet, and Grayson's ligament. Treatment is usually surgical, followed with static and dynamic splinting, wound care and scar management, and ROM and strengthening.

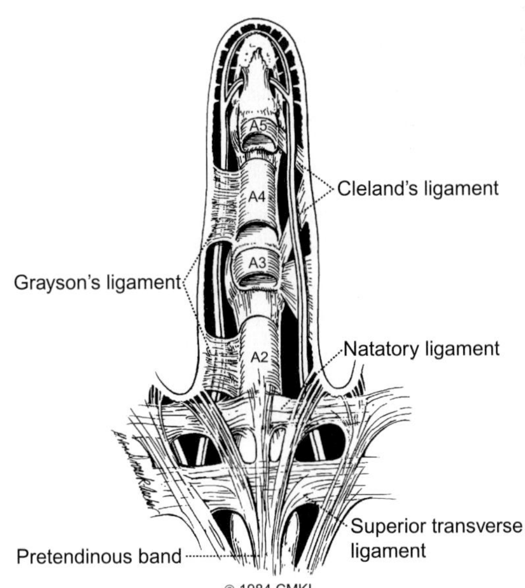

Structures involved in Dupuytren's contracture. (From the Christine M Kleinert Institute for Hand and Microsurgery, Inc., with permission, Figure from previous edition.)

41. **What are the three techniques commonly used to treat Dupuytren's contracture?**
Collagenase clostridium histolyticum (xiaflex) injection followed with a manipulation, fasciectomy (surgical removal of diseased tissue), and percutaneous needle fasciotomy. Recurrence rates vary for each procedure but are higher for collagenase injection and needle fasciotomy when compared to surgical excision (fasciectomy).

42. **What is trigger finger?**
Trigger finger is an inflammatory process involving the flexor tendon and A1 pulley. Most cases are idiopathic (no definitive cause) with increased occurrence in patients with diabetes, RA, and hypothyroidism. This may be due to changes to collagen or other components of the tendon or pulley. This affects 2% to 3% of the general population.
Trigger finger can also develop from direct trauma to the A1 pulley, excessive tool use, or from increased force to the flexor tendon with pinching activities using the tips of the fingers. This puts a lot of tension on the tendon at the proximal end of the tendon sheath and the A1 pulley. There may be swelling or thickening of the tendon. The patient will experience pain over the pulley, or catching and locking of the finger in a flexed position as the tendon tries to pass under the pulley. Conservative treatment with corticosteroid injection has a success rate in the literature between 50% to 94%. For patients with multiple trigger fingers, or failed conservative treatment, surgery to release the A1 pulley would be the next option.

43. **Is there conservative treatment available for CMC arthritis that can help with pain and create stability for the joint?**
Yes, there are three main exercises that can be taught to the patient: stretching the adductor pollicis muscle to open the first web space, isolating the muscles that stabilize the CMC joint with an isometric contraction (one being the first dorsal interosseous muscle), then adding others pertinent to the individual patient needs. Education in joint protection and adaptive equipment are also helpful to these patients to slow down wear and tear on their joints.

44. **What treatment technique can be used for digit malrotation due to soft tissue restrictions?**
Patients can develop digit overlap or malrotation due to muscle weakness, scarring, and edema in the intrinsics of the hand following a fracture. Although there is not a lot of evidence-based literature for using therapeutic taping methods for finger alignment many therapists are utilizing what they know from principles of taping to influence soft tissues of the digits to realign fingers during ROM. Kinesio Tape being the tape of choice is placed on the fingers to guide their motion into more normal movement patterns. Clinicians use their knowledge of k-tape and clinical judgment to assist their patients gain more normal function.

45. **What is graded motor imagery (GMI) and what diagnosis is it used for?**
GMI is a treatment that is used for people with complex chronic pain. It is a brain-based treatment stimulating different regions of the brain in a specific order and pace. It is divided into three stages that exercise your brain differently: left right discrimination, motor imagery, and mirror therapy. It is beneficial to use with patients who have pain after any UE trauma, but has been successful with CRPS, phantom limb pain, and brachial plexus injuries.

46. **Define Raynaud's phenomenon and discuss its etiology, clinical presentation, and treatment.**
Raynaud's phenomenon is a vasospastic disorder of unknown origin. It is often experienced by individuals with vascular disorders, including systemic lupus erythematosus and atherosclerosis, as well as with rheumatoid arthritis. It is also commonly seen in response to repeated digital trauma, vibration, and prolonged cold exposure. The presenting symptoms of Raynaud's phenomenon often include a "triple response" of vascular changes, although not all individuals experience three color changes, and the order of the color changes varies. Typically, the digit(s) will assume a blanched appearance (lack of blood flow because of vasospasm), then cyanosis (venous pooling), and then reddening of the digit(s) as arterial blood flow returns to the digit(s). Raynaud's phenomenon can also occur in the feet, nose, ears, and tongue. Treatment for this disorder consists of oral vasodilatory medications, patient education on the effects of smoking and caffeine, avoidance of cold and vibration and of vasoconstrictive medications, biofeedback, and rarely surgical sympathectomy.

Bibliography

Alter, S., Feldon, P., & Terrono, A. L. (2002). Pathomechanics of deformities in the arthritic hand and wrist (*5th ed.*) *Rehabilitation of the hand* (Vol. 2, pp. 1545–1554). St. Louis, MO: Mosby.

Anderson, H., & Hoy, G. (2016). Orthotic intervention incorporating the dart-thrower's motion as part of conservative management guidelines for treatment of scapholunate injury. *Journal of Hand Therapy*, *29*(2), 199–204.

Aulicino, P. L. (2002). Clinical examination of the hand (*5th ed.*) *Rehabilitation of the hand* (Vol. 1, pp. 120–142). St. Louis, MO: Mosby.

Brazzelli, M., Cruickshank, M., Tassie, E., et al. (2015). Collagenase clostridium histolyticum for the treatment of Dupuytren's contracture: Systematic review and economic evaluation. *Health Technology Assessment*, *19*(90), 1–202.

Cannon, N. M. (2001). *Diagnosis and treatment manual for physicians and therapists* (*4th ed*). Indianapolis, IN: Hand Rehabilitation Center of Indiana.

Colditz, J. (2017). *Clinical Pearls: Leaving the DIP joint free when treating a boutonniere injury.* Retrieved from Brace Lab: www.HandLab.com
Colditz, J. (2020). *Nuances of flexor tendon rehab: Video course.* Retrieved from Brace Lab: www.handlab.com
Duke Orthopaedics. (n.d.). *Wheeless' textbook of orthopaedics.* Retrieved from Wheelessonline.com.
Frykman, G., & Watkins, B. E. (2002). The distal radioulnar joint (*5th ed.*) *Rehabilitation of the hand and upper extremity* (Vol 2, pp. 1124–1135). St. Louis, MO: Mosby.
How the wide awake approach is changing hand surgery and hand therapy. (2012). *Inaugural AAHS sponsored lecture at the ASHT meeting* (pp. 175–178). San Diego, CA: Elsevier.
Kleinert, H. E., & Cash, S. L. (1985). Management of acute flexor tendon injuries in the hand. *Instructional Course Lectures, 34,* 361–372.
Kleinert, H. E., Kutz, J. E., Atasoy, E., & Stormo, A. (1973). Primary repair of flexor tendons. *Orthopedic Clinics of North America, 4,* 865–876.
Kleinert, H., & Meares, A. (1974). In quest of the solution to severed flexor tendons. *Clinical Orthopaedics, 104,* 23–29.
Lee, M. J., & LaStayo, P. C. (2002). Ulnar wrist pain and impairment: A therapist's algorithmic approach to the Triangular Fibrocartilage Complex (*5th ed.*) *Rehabilitation of the hand* (Vol. 2, pp. 1156–1170). St. Louis, MO: Mosby.
Masker, K. A. (2016). Therapeutic taping for soft tissue-based digit malrotation. *Journal of Hand Therapy, 29*(3), 334–338.
Miller, L. K., Jerosch-Herold, C., & Shepstone, L. (2017). Effectiveness of edema management techniques for subacute hand edema: A systematic review. *Journal of Hand Therapy, 30*(4), 432–446.
Moseley, G. L., Butler, D. S., & Beames, T. B. (2019). *The graded motor imagery handbook.* Adelaide: Noigroup Publications.
Petersen, L. , M., Nasser-Sharif, S., & Zelouf, D. S. (2002). Surgeon's and therapist's management of tendinopathies in the hand and wrist (*5th ed.*) *Rehabilitation of the hand and wrist* (Vol. 1, pp. 931–951). St. Louis, MO: Mosby.
Pettengill, K., & Van Strien, G. (2002). Postoperative management of flexor tendon injuries *Rehabilitation of the hand and upper extremity* (Vol. 2, pp. 439–452). St. Louis: Mosby.
Porretto-Loehrke, A., Schuh, C., & Szekeres, M. (2016). Clinical manual assessment of the wrist. *Journal of Hand Therapy, 29*(2), 123–135.
Rodner, C.M., & Peter, W.M. (2010). Ulnar wrist pain. *Plastic surgery secrets plus* (pp. 984–987). Mosby.
Schultz-Johnson, K. (2002). Static progressive splinting. *Journal of Hand Therapy, 15*(2), 163–178.
See how xiaflex demonstrates sustained results over time. (2022). Retrieved from xiaflex.com.
Werner, F., Sutton, L., Basu, N., W.H., S., Moritomo, H., & St-Amand, H. (2016). Scaphoid tuberosity excursion is minimized during a dart-throwing motion: A biomechanical study. *Journal of Hand Therapy, 29*(2), 175–182.
Wong, A. L., Wilson, M., Girnary, S., Nojoomi, M., Acharya, S., & Paul, S. M. (2017). The optimal orthosis and motion protocol for extensor tendon injury in zones IV-VIII: A systematic review. *Journal of Hand Therapy, 30*(4), 447–456.
Wright, T. W., & Michlovitz, S. L. (2002). Management of carpal instability (5th ed.) *Rehabilitation of the hand* (Vol. 2, pp. 1185–1193). St. Louis: Mosby.
Young, K. (2019). *Clinical Pearls: Exercise for a painful thumb CMC joint?* Retrieved from Brace Lab website: www.HandLab.com
Young, K. (2019). *Clinical Pearls: Living the supinated life: Solutions for ulnar sided wrist pain.* Retrieved from Brace Lab: www.HandLab.com
Young, L., Bartell, T., & Logan, S. (1988). Ganglions of the hand and wrist. *Southern Medical Journal, 81,* 751–760.

CHAPTER 50 QUESTIONS

1. **What is the position of immobilization of a mallet finger?**
   a. Neutral
   b. Slight hyperextension
   c. Flexion
   d. Maximal hyperextension

2. **Which joint is hyperextended in a swan neck deformity?**
   a. PIP joint
   b. MCP joint
   c. Wrist joint
   d. DIP joint

3. **What splints are commonly used now for treating extensor tendon repairs zone V–VII?**
   a. Relative motion splint
   b. Tenodesis splint
   c. Dynamic extension splint
   d. Both a and c

4. **What forearm/wrist position should you start strengthening in after TFCC repair?**
   a. Neutral
   b. Supination
   c. Pronation
   d. Wrist flexion

CHAPTER 51

FRACTURES AND DISLOCATIONS OF THE WRIST AND HAND

J.A. Hyland, PA-C

1. **Define boxer's fracture.**
   Typically, fractures of the metacarpal necks of the ring and small fingers are called boxer's fractures. The name is derived from the mechanism of injury. The fracture usually occurs when a person strikes or punches. The fracture usually angulates the apex dorsally because the volar cortex comminutes and the intrinsic muscles cause a flexed position secondary to crossing the metaphalangeal (MP) joints volar to their axis of motion. Usually boxer's fractures can be treated nonoperatively with closed reduction and casting. The acceptable degree of angulation is undecided, but most surgeons accept up to 10 to 15 degrees in the second and third digits, 30 to 35 degrees in the fourth, and 50 degrees in the fifth.

2. **What is a baseball finger?**
   Baseball finger, another name for mallet or drop finger, is typically a flexion deformity of the distal interphalangeal (DIP) joint resulting from injury of the extensor tendon to the base of the distal phalanx. This injury usually occurs during catching a ball (hence the name) or striking something with the finger extended and the tendon tight. The extensor tendon can pull directly off the dorsal distal phalanx or be associated with a dorsal articular fracture. The usual treatment is splinting of the DIP joint for 4 to 6 weeks. Average extensor lag after stack splinting is 8 degrees. Late management includes tenodermodesis, Fowler's tenotomy, or oblique retinacular ligament (ORL) reconstruction.

3. **What is a jersey finger?**
   A jersey finger is avulsion of the flexor digitorum profundus (FDP) tendon from the distal phalanx. The result is inability to flex the DIP. Treatment is surgical reattachment. Some loss of extension is common. Surgery should be performed soon after injury, especially if the tendon is completely retracted to the palm.

4. **Describe the usual angulation of proximal phalanx fractures.**
   The angulation of proximal phalanx fractures, like that of most fractures, depends on two factors: the mechanism of injury and the muscles acting as a deforming force on the fractured bone. Typically, proximal phalanx fractures present with apex volar angulation. The proximal fragment is flexed by the interossei, which insert into its base, and the distal fragment is pulled into hyperextension by the central slip, which inserts into the base of the middle phalanx.

5. **What is the usual or ideal position of immobilization of phalanx fractures?**
   Stable fractures often can be treated with buddy taping and early movement. If a fracture requires reduction and immobilization, the best position is the position of function, with the MP joints in almost full flexion and the interphalangeal (IP) joints in full extension. The MP joints rarely become stiff in full flexion because of the cam effect of the metacarpal hands on the collateral ligaments. The proximal interphalangeal (PIP) joints are least likely to become stiff in full extension.

6. **What are phalangeal condylar fractures?**
   Unicondylar and bicondylar fractures occur from axial loads. These fractures are usually very unstable and require intervention. Conservative treatment can be attempted in nondisplaced fractures, but a close eye with follow-up is required to avoid displacement. Closed reduction with pin fixation is acceptable if anatomical reduction can be achieved. Fractures that demonstrate any displacement require open reduction.

7. **Describe Bennett's fracture and Rolando's fracture.**
   Both are fractures of the base of the thumb metacarpal. Bennett's fracture typically results from an axial force directed against a partially flexed metacarpal (often in a fight). The smaller of the two fracture fragments stays in place, attached to the anterior oblique ligament. The rest of the digit is pulled dorsally and radially by the abductor pollicis longus, whereas the more distal attachment of the adductor pollicis contributes additional dorsal displacement. Rolando's fracture involves more comminution with the two fragments; usually a third large dorsal fragment in a Y- or T-shaped pattern is also present.

8. Describe the diagnosis and treatment of lateral collateral ligament injuries of the PIP joint.
Lateral dislocations are caused by an abduction or adduction force across the extended finger, usually in such sports as basketball, football, and wrestling. The radial collateral ligament (RCL) is injured more often than the ulnar collateral ligament (UCL). The PIP joint is stressed radially and ulnarly between 0 and 20 degrees. Angulation >20 degrees is an indication of collateral injury. The injury is treated with buddy taping and motion. The length of treatment depends on the degree of injury (complete or incomplete).

9. What are the differences between a dorsal and a volar PIP dislocation?
Dorsal dislocation is more common and results from hyperextension of the joint. The volar plate usually is injured at its attachment to the distal phalanx. Such injuries usually are treated with buddy taping for 3 to 6 weeks. Volar PIP dislocations are much less common. The injured tissue is the central slip. If the dislocation is treated with buddy taping, a boutonnière deformity probably will result. Hence, volar dislocation should be treated with immobilization of the PIP joint in full extension.

10. Define gamekeeper's thumb.
An injury to the UCL of the thumb MP joint is called a gamekeeper's thumb because British gamekeepers often developed UCL laxity, resulting from their method of putting down wounded rabbits. Today, however, it is seen most commonly in skiers. On examination the thumb is most tender over the ulnar aspect of the MP joint. The MP joint is stressed in both flexion and extension and in comparison with the other side. Often radiographic stress views confirm the diagnosis.

11. What is a Stener lesion?
With a complete tear of the UCL, the adductor aponeurosis often will be found under the torn UCL. This is called a Stener lesion and can prevent the ligament from healing. For this reason, most physicians recommend surgical treatment of complete UCL ruptures.

12. How is gamekeeper's thumb treated?
Acute partial ruptures can be treated with a thumb spica cast for 4 weeks. The treatment of complete ruptures is controversial. Most believe that it should be treated surgically. Tears in the middle of the ligament can be repaired directly. If the ligament is avulsed, it is reattached with a bone anchor or tied over a button.

13. How are metacarpophalangeal radial collateral ligament tears of the thumb treated?
These injuries occur by an impact on the radial thumb region. Partial tears are treated with 6 to 8 weeks of immobilization. Treatment of complete RCL tears remains controversial. The ligament rarely displaces, similar to a Stener lesion; therefore, immobilization can allow for complete ligament tears to heal. However, the EPL can pull the thumb MCP into ulnar deviation, causing the RCL ligament to heal in an attenuated position. Some are advocating surgical repair to avoid subjective instability and joint degenerative changes.

14. Describe the radiographic evaluation of the wrist.
1. Anteroposterior (AP): three smooth arcs should be visible on the normal AP radiograph—across the distal radius; across the distal scaphoid, lunate, and triquetral; and across the proximal capitate and hamate.
2. Lateral: the radiolunatocapitate should form a straight line with the third metacarpal joint.
   - Normal scapholunate (SL) angle—30 to 60 degrees
   - Normal capitolunate (CL) angle—0 to 30 degrees
3. Flexion, extension, radial deviation, and ulnar deviation views, along with the previously mentioned, are enough to diagnose 90% of wrist injuries.
4. Special views
   - Scaphoid-radial oblique (supinated posteroanterior view)—with the forearm pronated 45 degrees from neutral, a full profile view of the scaphoid is obtained.
   - AP with fist compression or passive longitudinal compression may accentuate scapholunate dissociation and widen the scapholunate interval.
   - Carpal tunnel view—for this view, the wrist is in maximal dorsiflexion with the beam directed 15 degrees toward the carpus.

15. Describe Colles', Barton's, and Smith's fractures.
The most common of the three is Colles' fracture, which is extraarticular with dorsal angulation, displacement, and shortening. Barton's fracture is an intraarticular shear fracture that may be dorsal or volar. A Smith's fracture is often called a reverse Colles' fracture. It is an extraarticular fracture with volar displacement and angulation.

16. What are chauffeur's and die-punch fractures?
A chauffeur's fracture is an intraarticular, triangular-shaped fracture involving the radial styloid. A die-punch fracture describes a depressed fracture of the lunate fossa.

17. **When is surgery indicated for distal radius fractures?**
An unstable fracture (one that cannot be held in position with a splint or cast) is an indication for surgery. Radial shortening >5 mm, dorsal angulation >20 degrees, and articular step-off >1 to 2 mm are also reasons to consider surgery.

18. **Name the five factors that may contribute to instability of a distal radius fracture after closed reduction.**
    - Initial angulation >20 degrees
    - Dorsal metaphyseal comminution >50% of the width of the radius
    - Intraarticular fracture
    - Age >60 years
    - Considerable osteoporosis

19. **What are the outcomes from volar plating of distal radius fractures?**
Flexion and extension average 55 to 60 degrees, pronation/supination averages 75 degrees, and grip is approximately 75% to 80% of the contralateral side.

20. **What is the second most common fracture of the wrist?**
Scaphoid fractures are the second most common wrist fracture after distal radius fractures. They usually result from a fall on a dorsiflexed wrist. The diagnosis is made from the patient's history and from examination findings of pain and swelling in the anatomic snuff box. Of course, radiographs are taken, but pain and tenderness justify initiation of treatment.

21. **Where is the scaphoid most commonly fractured?**
Around 65% of scaphoid fractures occur at the waist, while 10% occur at the distal body, 15% through the proximal pole, and 8% at the tuberosity. Because of differences in blood supply, fracture location can determine healing rates and times to union. The average time to union for waist fractures is 10 to 12 weeks, and 90% heal. It takes 12 to 20 weeks for proximal pole fractures to heal, and only 60% to 70% heal with cast treatment. Tuberosity and more distal fractures almost always heal in 4 to 6 weeks.

22. **What are the treatment guidelines for scaphoid fractures?**
    1. Nondisplaced fractures: long-arm thumb spica for 6 weeks, then short-arm cast until the fracture is radiographically healed
    2. Displaced fractures (ie, 1-mm step-off, >60-degree scapholunate angulation, or >15-degree lunatocapitate angulation):
        - With acceptable reduction (ie, <1-mm step-off, <25-degree lateral intrascaphoid angulation, or <35-degree anteroposterior angulation), use a long-arm spica cast.
        - With unacceptable reduction, use open reduction with Herbert or compression screw or staple fixation; cast for 2 to 3 weeks, then encourage early movement.

23. **When is surgery indicated for ulnar styloid fractures?**
Ulnar styloid fractures are relatively common fractures. They can present alone or in association with a distal radius fracture (seen in approximately 50% of distal radius fractures). Surgical treatment is only indicated if the fracture leads to distal radioulnar joint (DRUJ) instability. Fortunately, the most common pattern seen is an avulsion fracture of the tip of the styloid. These rarely lead to DRUJ instability and can be treated conservatively. Fractures involving the base of the styloid have a higher incidence of DRUJ instability and may need surgical fixation with a tension band or screw fixation.

24. **Define Kienböck's disease.**
Kienböck's disease is defined by the radiographic finding of avascular necrosis of the lunate. The exact etiology is uncertain, but the probable cause is some combination of a traumatic event, repeated microtrauma, and/or injury to the ligaments carrying blood supply to the lunate. It also has been associated with relative shortening of the ulna compared with the radius (ulnar negative variance).

25. **What are the four stages of Kienböck's disease?**
    - Stage 1—sclerosis
    - Stage 2—fragmentation
    - Stage 3—collapse
    - Stage 4—arthritis

26. **What are the treatment options for Kienböck's disease?**
Surgical treatment before lunate collapse (stage 1 and stage 2 disease) involves decreasing the load across the lunate and/or improving the vascular supply to the lunate. The load is decreased by a radial shortening osteotomy in ulnar negative variance or capitates shortening osteotomy in ulnar neutral or ulnar positive variant wrists. Revascularization is performed by inserting a vascularized bone graft or a blood vessel into the lunate to promote blood flow. Once significant collapse has occurred (stage 3 and stage 4 disease), salvage procedures are employed. If the articular surfaces of the capitate and lunate fossa of the radius are intact, a proximal row carpectomy can be performed. In the setting of significant degenerative changes, a heavy laborer, or failure of previous surgical procedures, a total wrist arthrodesis is recommended.

27. **Describe the classification of carpal instabilities.**
The loss of the normal carpal ligaments and/or normal bony anatomy can lead to wrist instability. Wrist instability is classified as dissociative (CID) or nondissociative (CIND).
- CID—Carpal instability dissociative results from loss of the intrinsic ligaments. There are two types of CID:
  1. Dorsal intercalated segment instability (DISI) results from disruption between the scaphoid and lunate, allowing the scaphoid to rotate into volar flexion. The remaining components of the proximal row, the lunate and triangular muscles, rotate into dorsiflexion because of loss of connection to the scaphoid. DISI is the most common clinical pattern of carpal instability. The SL angle is >60 degrees, and the CL angle is >30 degrees.
  2. Volar intercalated segment instability (VISI) results from disruption of the ligamentous support to the triangular and lunate and leads to volar rotation of the lunate and extension of the triangular. It is the second most common instability. The SL angle is <30 degrees, and the CL angle is >30 degrees.
- CIND—A tear of the extrinsic ligaments can cause midcarpal or radiocarpal instability and is called carpal instability nondissociative.
- CIC—Carpal instability combined is caused by disruption both within and between rows, as seen in a transscaphoid perilunate fracture dislocation.
- Axial carpal instability—This is usually caused by violent trauma that results in longitudinal disruption.

28. **What is scapholunate dissociation?**
A complete tear of the scapholunate ligaments may result from a hyperextension injury and can lead to scapholunate dissociation, which disrupts normal proximal row kinematics. The lunate and triquetrum extend abnormally, supinate, and deviate radially. The scaphoid tilts into flexion, pronation, and ulnar deviation. This abnormal positioning affects how the wrist bears loads and can lead to pain, weakness, and arthritis.

29. **What is the Terry Thomas sign?**
A posteroanterior radiograph of the wrist that shows a gap >3 to 5 mm between the scaphoid and lunate, especially in comparison with the other side, suggests scapholunate dissociation (SLD). It is named after the English comedian who had a space between his front teeth. A more familiar eponym might be the Alfred E. Newman sign.

30. **How is SLD treated?**
Acute SLD can be treated with closed reduction and percutaneous pinning or open reduction, internal fixation, and repair of the ligament. Less than acute injuries can be treated with repair or reconstruction of the ligament and reinforcement of the capsule. Chronic injuries can be treated with limited or complete fusion, proximal row carpectomy, styloidectomy, or total wrist arthroplasty.

31. **How are thumb UCL avulsion fractures best treated?**
Small avulsion fractures of the thumb ulnar collateral ligament with minimal (<2.0 mm) displacement are best treated with open reduction and internal fixation. Minimally displaced UCL avulsion fractures frequently have significant rotation, which prevents successful fracture healing even with prompt cast immobilization.

32. **Describe the Galeazzi fracture-dislocation.**
In the Galeazzi fracture-dislocation of the forearm, fracture of the radial shaft includes a distal ulna dislocation. This injury was termed a "fracture of necessity," stemming from the inherent instability of the fracture-dislocation and the need for surgical intervention. A key element of treatment is to stabilize the radius with internal fixation and restore the length of the radius. The stability of the DRUJ is assessed, and, if unstable, repair of the triangular fibrocartilage complex (TFCC) and/or the capsule of the DRUJ is recommended.

33. **Describe the Essex-Lopresti injury.**
Essex-Lopresti injuries are a variant of Galeazzi fractures, except that the radial head has an intraarticular fracture combined with a dislocation of the distal ulna, tearing the capsule of the DRUJ and/or the TFCC. Injuries that have less than 1 to 2 mm of articular step-off have less than 30% of the radial head joint surface involved, and those that are angled less than 30 degrees can be treated nonoperatively by immobilizing the forearm in supination to

help reduce the DRUJ for 3 weeks before starting range of motion exercises. Fractures not within these criteria are best treated with open reduction and internal fixation.

34. **Define Seymour fracture.**
Seymour fractures are Salter-Harris I or II of the distal interphalangeal joint with associated nailbed injury in the pediatric patient. The injury usually occurs as result of a direct trauma or crush injury. Most often, the patient will have a mallet finger–type appearance to the digit while at rest. The nail plate is often lying superficial to the eponychial fold. Diagnosis can be aided with a lateral view of the digit, which will show a widened distal phalangeal physis. Treatment includes oral antibiotics with open reduction of the fracture, pinning the joint, and repair of the nailbed. Failure to treat properly can cause physis arrest and chronic osteomyelitis.

35. **What is a fight bite infection?**
The fight bite infection, or clenched fist injury, occurs when a closed fist strikes an opposed tooth, exposing the soft tissue to the metacarpal head. This impregnates the soft tissue of the MCP joint with the bacteria of the oral flora. This can appear somewhat benign in nature, but can cause septic arthritis. In fight bite, the appropriate treatment is exploration of the wound with incision and debridement. Prophylactic antibiotic coverage is advised.

36. **What is an extra-octave fracture?**
Extra-octave fractures are the most common fracture of the proximal phalanx in the pediatric population. This fracture involves a Salter-Harris II of the proximal phalanx of the small finger with lateral deviation. The fracture was described due to the fact that without treatment, a piano player would be able to reach an extra octave with the displacement of the small finger. Nondisplaced variants can be splinted and buddy taped. Displaced fractures require closed reduction of the fracture to prevent permanent deformity.

37. **Define a triangular fibrocartilage complex tear (TFCC).**
Triangular fibrocartilage complex is an intricate set of tissue that spans the DRUJ and ulnocarpal joint. Tears of the complex can be defined as acute versus degenerative in nature. Degenerative tears of the TFCC are most often caused by chronic, excessive load between the ulna and the carpus. Treatment for degenerative tears includes activity modification, NSAIDs, splinting, and injection of the ulnocarpal joint. Surgery is only held for patients who fail conservative treatment. Acute tears can be put into different classes defined by Palmer as follows:
Class 1A Tear: A slit-like injury near the radial insertion of the disk that does not involve the radioulnar ligaments. These are common injuries that do not require open repair.
Class 1B Tear: A partial or complete avulsion of the TFCC from its ulnar attachments, which may or may not include an ulnar styloid fracture. Most times, this type of injury will respond to conservative treatment. Open or scope repairs are only needed with persistent symptoms or instability.
Class 1C Tear: A partial or complete tear of the ulnocarpal ligaments. Majority of these cases can be treated conservatively unless instability is present early.
Class 1D Tear: Is a partial or complete traumatic avulsion of the TFCC directly from the radius, with or without a bony avulsion, involving one of both radioulnar ligaments. These are frequently associated with displaced distal radius fractures and usually respond well with the reduction of the radius. With instability of the DRUJ, these can be repaired arthroscopic or open.

Bibliography

Allan, C. H., Joshi, A., & Lichtman, D. M. (2001). Kienbock's disease: Diagnosis and treatment. *Journal of the American Academy of Orthopaedic Surgeons, 9*, 128–136.
Cooney, W. P., Linscheid, R. L., & Dobyns, J. H. (1996). Fractures and dislocations of the wrist. In R. W. Bucholz et al. (Eds.), *Fractures in adults* (4th ed., pp. 745–867). New York: Lippincott-Raven.
Dinowitz, M., Trumble, T., Hanel, D., Vedder, N. B., & Gilbert, M. (1997). Failure of cast immobilization for thumb ulna collateral ligament avulsion fractures. *Journal of Hand Surgery, 22*, 1057–1063.
Fernandez, D. L., & Palmer, A. K. (1999). Fractures of the distal radius. In D. P. Green (Ed.), *Operative hand surgery* (4th ed., pp. 929–985). New York: Churchill Livingstone.
Glickel, S. Z., Malerich, M., Pearce, S. M., & Littler, J. W. (1993). Ligament replacement for chronic instability of the ulnar collateral ligament of the metacarpophalangeal joint of the thumb. *Journal of Hand Surgery, 18*(5), 930–941.
Green, D. P., & Butler, T. E. (1996). Fractures and dislocations in the hand. In R. W. Bucholz et al. (Eds.), *Fractures in adults* (4th ed., pp. 607–745). New York: Lippincott-Raven.
Heyman, P., Gelberman, R. H., Duncan, K., & Hipp, J. A. (1993). Injuries of the ulnar collateral ligament of the thumb metacarpophalangeal. Biomechanical and prospective clinical studies on the usefulness of valgus stress testing. *Clinical Orthopaedics and Related Research, 292*, 165–171.
Kozin, S. H., Thoder, J. J., & Lieberman, G. (2000). Operative treatment of metacarpal and phalangeal shaft fractures. *Journal of the American Academy of Orthopaedic Surgeons, 8*, 111–121.
Logan, A. J., & Lindau, T. R. (2008). The management of distal ulnar fractures in adults: A review of the literature and recommendations for treatment. *Strategies in Trauma and Limb Reconstruction, 3*, 49–56.
Orbay, J. L., & Fernandez, D. L. (2004). Volar fixed-angle plate fixation for unstable distal radius fractures in the elderly patient. *Journal of Hand Surgery, 29*, 96–102.

Ruby, L. (1992). Carpal fractures and dislocations. In B. D. Browner et al. (Eds.), *Skeletal trauma: Fractures, dislocations, and ligamentous injuries* (pp. 1025–1059). Philadelphia: WB Saunders.
Ruby, L. K. (1995). Carpal instability. *Journal of Bone and Joint Surgery, 77A*, 476–487.
Trumble, T., Rayan, G. M., Budoff, J. E., & Baratz, M. E. (2010). *Principles of hand surgery and therapy* (pp. 126–129) (2nd ed.). Philadelphia, PA: Saunders, an imprint of Elsevier Inc.
Wright, T. W., Horodyski, M., & Smith, D. W. (2005). Function outcome of unstable distal radius fractures: ORIF with a volar fixed-angle tine plate versus external fixation. *Journal of Hand Surgery, 30*, 289–299.

CHAPTER 51 QUESTIONS

1. **What form of carpal instability is seen with a chronic scapholunate ligament tear?**
   a. Volar intercalated segment instability (VISI)
   b. Dorsal intercalated segment instability (DISI)
   c. Carpal instability nondissociative (CIND)
   d. Carpal instability complex (CIC)

2. **In a Stener lesion, what structure traps the UCL in a displaced position?**
   a. Extensor pollicis longus
   b. Volar plate
   c. Abductor aponeurosis
   d. Adductor aponeurosis

3. **What position should you immobilize phalanx fractures?**
   a. MCP flexion and PIP flexion
   b. MCP flexion and PIP extension
   c. MCP extension and PIP flexion
   d. MCP extension and PIP extension

4. **What degree of angulation is acceptable to treat nonoperatively in a Boxer's fracture of the fifth metacarpal?**
   a. 20 degrees
   b. 30 degrees
   c. 50 degrees
   d. 60 degrees

5. **In a Mallet finger, what part of the tendon in ruptured in the injury?**
   a. Terminal extensor tendon
   b. The central slip
   c. The sagittal band
   d. The FDP tendon

6. **A Seymour fracture is**
   a. A fracture of the small finger proximal phalangeal physis
   b. A fracture of the ulnar styloid physis
   c. A Salter-Harris I or II of the proximal phalangeal physis
   d. A Salter Harris I or II of the distal phalangeal physis

CHAPTER 52

NERVE ENTRAPMENTS OF THE WRIST AND HAND

J.J. Palazzo, PT, DSc, ECS and K. Galloway, PT, DSc, ECS

1. Describe the difference between Wartenberg's disease and sign.

Wartenberg's disease is also known as superficial radial nerve entrapment or cheiralgia paresthetica. It occurs infrequently and can be confused with de Quervain's disease and intersection syndrome. The superficial radial nerve is easily compressed between the brachioradialis and extensor carpi radialis longus tendons along the distal radius with pronation and ulnar deviation. Superficial radial nerve entrapment creates a pattern of pain, numbness, and tingling over the dorsal lateral aspect of the hand in the web space between the thumb and index finger, with no motor loss.

In contrast, Wartenberg's sign is a classic neurological sign suggesting underlying ulnar motor nerve injury producing weakness in control of the small finger. This is mostly seen in more advanced stages of ulnar nerve injury presenting as the inability to adduct the small finger toward the ring finger. Clinically this imbalance occurs as a combination of abductor digiti minimi and palmar interosseous muscle weakness. This results in unopposed abduction action of the small finger from the radial innervated extensor digiti minimi muscle which inserts into the dorsal medial proximal phalanx of the small finger. The patient therefore cannot actively adduct or move the small finger toward the ring finger. This sign is, however, nonlocalizing as ulnar nerve lesions at the elbow, wrist, or higher level neuroaxis conditions like cervical myelopathy or upper motor neuron disease can cause this condition.

2. Describe the sensory loss in the hand with ulnar neuropathy at the wrist.

Typical sensory loss is in the palmar aspect of the entire small finger and the medial half of the ring finger, with sparing of the dorsal aspect of the small and ring fingers. The dorsal sensory sparing occurs because the dorsal ulnar cutaneous branch leaves the ulnar nerve proper proximal to the wrist. The palmar sensory loss may extend to the lateral half of the ring finger and into the middle finger in cases of a connection between the median and ulnar palmar sensory branches. This connection is called a Berettini branch and has been reported in cadaver studies in 60% to 94% of hands.

3. How often does carpal tunnel syndrome coexist with cervical nerve root pathology?

Carpal tunnel syndrome may occur in isolation, or may be a component of a multiple crush syndrome. This concept proposes that a proximal nerve compromise makes the nerve more susceptible at more distal entrapment sites possibly due to reduced axoplasmic flow. Upton and McComas (1973) identified a higher rate of distal nerve compression in patients with cervical nerve root pathology. Others have extended this concept to multiple compressions that can happen in those who have underlying pathology such as a diabetic polyneuropathy. The exact rate of a multiple compression is difficult to identify; however, a full evaluation of entrapment sites to include the cervical spine and common nerve entrapment sites in the arm would be recommended in evaluation of entrapment neuropathy in the hand.

4. Describe how an ulnar claw hand develops and the differences between a low and high ulnar palsy.

The extensor digitorum and the ulnar innervated lumbricals and palmar/dorsal interossei work together to fully extend the digits at the PIP and DIP joints. The extensor digitorum attaches to the dorsal proximal phalanx to extend the metacarpophalangeal (MCP) joint. The interossei and lumbrical muscles also attach in part to the dorsal extensor mechanism distal to the MCP joint and provide a counterforce for the extensor digitorum in order for the fingers of the hand to fully extend at the DIP and PIP joints. An ulnar claw hand develops because the interossei and medial two lumbrical muscles become weak after an ulnar nerve injury. The radial innervated extensor digitorum is able to extend the MCP joint but is ineffective at extending the PIP and DIP joints fully without the counterforce provided by the lumbricals and interossei.

A low ulnar palsy occurs with an ulnar nerve injury distal to the midpoint of the forearm, while a high ulnar palsy would be proximal to midpoint of the forearm. Both lesions would result in weakness of the ulnar intrinsic muscles of the hand to include the palmar and dorsal interossei as well as the medial two lumbricals. The high ulnar nerve injury would also produce weakness in the flexor digitorum profundus to the small and ring fingers as well as possible weakness of the flexor carpi ulnaris. The low ulnar palsy produces a more significant clawing of the hand since the medial half of the flexor digitorum profundus muscles are spared and the weak lumbrical and interosseous muscles cannot counter the intact long finger flexors. The clawing is milder in a higher ulnar lesion.

5. **Is there a surgical intervention for loss of median recurrent motor nerve function?**
Both tendon transfers and nerve transfers have been used to treat median recurrent branch injury and to improve thumb function/opposition. An anterior interosseous nerve (from pronator quadratus) to median recurrent branch transfer is one option to improve thenar muscle function.

6. **What is the significance of a positive Froment's sign?**
Ulnar nerve lesions result in a significant loss in hand grip strength. Weakness of the adductor pollicis, flexor pollicis brevis, and first dorsal interosseous muscles sharply impairs the pinching power of the thumb against the index finger. A simple test is to ask the patient to pinch a piece of stiff paper between the thumb and index finger while the examiner attempts to pull it away. The patient with an ulnar-deficient hand substitutes the AIN supplied flexor pollicis longus, causing hyperflexion of the thumb DIP joint to hold the thumb opposed to the radial side of the index finger. As the patient tries harder, the thumb flexes more and the pinch becomes weaker and fails.

7. **Describe the tunnel of Guyon and a related nerve entrapment.**
The lateral border of the tunnel of Guyon is the hook of the hamate, and the medial border is the pisiform bone. The floor is the joining of the ulnar extension of the transverse carpal ligament and pisohamate ligament. The overlying palmar fascia and palmaris brevis form the roof. The principal contents of the tunnel include the ulnar nerve and ulnar artery. The flexor carpi ulnaris inserts on the pisiform, but no tendons are contained within the tunnel of Guyon. Ganglions, fracture of the hamate hook, displacement of the pisiform bone, anomalous muscles, repetitive trauma, hypothenar hammer syndrome, arthritis, ulnar artery thrombosis, or aneurysm can cause various patterns of ulnar nerve involvement, ranging from complete motor and sensory to partial motor or sensory-only symptoms. The ulnar nerve bifurcates into a deep motor and sensory branch within or near Guyon's canal. Varying patterns of clinical presentation may be related to the particular area of entrapment within Guyon's canal, which is typically divided into four zones. Zone 1 is the proximal portion of Guyon's canal before the bifurcation of the ulnar nerve into the terminal motor and sensory branches. Zone 1 compression produces mixed sensory and motor symptoms with weakness in all ulnar innervated intrinsic muscles and sensory loss in the medial palm and into the palmar aspects of the small finger and medial half of the ring finger. A Zone 2 injury involves the deep motor branch just distal to the sensory and motor bifurcation. Zone 2 injury results in weakness in all ulnar intrinsic muscles. Zone 3 level involvement refers to a more distal motor nerve injury within the deep palmar arch so that the hypothenar muscles are spared while the palmar and dorsal interossei and the medial 2 lumbricals are weak. Zone 4 compression at Guyon's canal refers to compression of the superficial sensory branch resulting in sensory loss in the palmar medial ring finger and medial and lateral palmar small finger with no weakness.

8. **Describe the clinical signs and symptoms and describe clinical tests for median nerve compression at the wrist.**
Median nerve compression at the wrist results in numbness or pain in the radial three and one-half digits. Numbness is often aggravated while sleeping. Patients report an increased frequency of dropping items and difficulty with fine motor tasks. Two-point discrimination may be reduced along the second and third digits and the radial aspect of the fourth digit. Positive results on both the median nerve compression test and Phalen test have an 80% sensitivity and 92% specificity for identifying carpal tunnel syndrome (CTS). The flick sign or maneuver is described as shaking the wrist to relieve numbness associated with CTS and has a 93% sensitivity and 96% specificity for identifying CTS. The Scratch collapse test (SCT) is performed with the examiner scratching the skin over the carpal tunnel while the patient performs bilateral resisted shoulder external rotation. The test is positive if there is a loss of shoulder external rotator resistance for a short period of time. Initial studies described the accuracy rate for the SCT at 82% with a positive predictive value of 99% and a negative predictive value of 73% for CTS. However, other authors have not consistently replicated these results.

9. **Are clinical exam tests valid for evaluating carpal tunnel syndrome?**
   - Phalen's test is described as a wrist flexion test when a patient is asked to flex the wrist with the dorsum of each hand pressed together. It was originally described as having a sensitivity of 74%, however a 60 second timed Phalen's test was reported to have a sensitivity of 85%.
   - The combined wrist flexion/median nerve pressure test is accomplished by placing the wrist in full flexion while placing manual or digital pressure on the median nerve just proximal to the distal wrist crease. When this test was completed at 30 seconds the sensitivity was reported at 82% and the specificity at 99%
   - The combined wrist extension/median nerve pressure test is accomplished by placing the wrist in full extension and placing manual pressure on the median nerve just proximal to the distal wrist crease. This test had a sensitivity of 89% at 60 seconds duration and a specificity of 83% at 30 seconds duration

10. What are the most sensitive electromyographic indicators for carpal tunnel syndrome when reading an EMG report?

Median sensory studies typically show the earliest abnormalities in carpal tunnel syndrome. The most sensitive nerve conduction finding is a prolonged latency or slow nerve conduction velocity in the palmar segment reflecting focal demyelination within the wrist to palm segment.

11. What is the clinical difference between a proximal median nerve injury at pronator teres and median nerve injury at the wrist?

The anterior interosseous nerve (AIN), which innervates the flexor pollicis longus, pronator quadratus, and flexor digitorum profundus to the index and long fingers, may be involved in pronator teres muscle entrapment of the median nerve, depending on the location of the AIN branch from the median nerve proper. In addition, the pronator teres and wrist flexor muscles would also be involved with median nerve compromise at the pronator teres. These forearm and AIN innervated muscles would be spared in CTS. Sensory loss in a proximal median nerve injury would include the digits 1–3 and the radial half of digit 4 as well as the thenar palm. The median palmar sensory component is not usually involved in CTS as the palmar cutaneous branch of the median nerve typically leaves the median nerve proper proximal to the anatomic carpal tunnel.

12. What are the normative EMG and nerve conduction values used to define pathology in carpal tunnel syndrome? How are they applied in a patient case setting?

The following are some commonly used criteria for nerve conduction values:

Median motor latency greater than 4.2 msec is considered abnormal

Sensory digital latency over a 14-cm distance greater than 3.6 msec is considered abnormal. Sensory palmar latency (orthodromic) greater than 2.2 msec over a 7- to 8-cm distance is considered abnormal. A difference greater than 10 m/sec in velocity or 0.5 msec in latency between median and ulnar sensory studies in the palm-to-wrist segment is considered abnormal.

A difference greater than 0.5 m/sec between radial and median sensory studies (stimulate at wrist and record from thumb) over a 10-cm distance is considered abnormal.

For example, a 51-year-old female patient has numbness and tingling in the hand worse at night and when driving and playing golf. She has a nerve conduction examination with findings of a median motor distal latency of 5.4 msec and an orthodromic palmar sensory latency of 3.2 msec. Her ulnar motor and sensory values are within normal limits. These findings may indicate that she has a focal carpal tunnel syndrome.

13. What are the common risk factors associated with carpal tunnel syndrome?

There are several anthropometric characteristics associated with carpal tunnel syndrome to include the following:

- Increased body mass index/obesity
- Deceased hand length–to–body height ratio
- Greater wrist width
- Wrist index greater than 0.69

The wrist index is measured using calipers at the distal wrist crease to measure wrist width in centimeters in the anteroposterior (AP) and mediolateral (ML) planes. The AP measurement is then divided by the ML measurement to calculate the wrist index. This index may be related to obesity as well.

Other risk factors have been identified as: smoking, alcohol use, kidney disease, liver disease, thyroid disease, pregnancy, menopause, lactation, diabetes, and chemotherapy.

14. What may produce carpal tunnel syndrome in children?

Several congenital genetic syndromes may increase the prevalence of CTS. The genetic syndromes such as Scheie and Hunter syndrome often have other associated features such as joint contracture. Other cases of CTS in children have been reported to be associated with thickening of the flexor retinaculum in familial cases and with scleroderma. Malformation of the palmaris longus, flexor digitorum superficialis, first lumbrical, and palmaris brevis muscles, or the presence of a vestigial or supernumerary muscle in the forearm or hand, has also been reported to have a link with childhood CTS.

15. Are there different classifications or degrees of carpal tunnel syndrome, and, if so, how would an electromyographer grade carpal tunnel syndrome?

There have been several proposed electrophysiologic classification systems for CTS that categorize motor and sensory nerve conduction findings into different levels of CTS. Some systems are using a numeric scale with 0 indicating a normal study, with higher numbers representing progressively more significant pathology. Other scales use a range of mild, moderate, severe to extremely severe classifications. Typically, sensory findings are earlier than motor findings and are categorized as mild or with a lower number. The progression into motor involvement tends to move the categorization into a moderate to severe level. An extremely severe CTS would indicate loss of sensory response and potentially a loss of motor response from the thenar muscles with needle EMG abnormalities in the abductor pollicis brevis.

16. **A patient complains of numbness and tingling in the small and ring fingers on only the palmar side of the hand with no complaints of numbness in the forearm or in the dorsal hand. What is your suspected location of injury and why?**
The injury is to the ulnar nerve distal to or at the level of the wrist. The ulnar nerve supplies sensation to the small and ring fingers and is a derivative of the C8 and T1 roots, the lower trunk and medial cord of the brachial plexus. A lesion in any one of these sections could produce tingling in the small and ring fingers; however, a proximal lesion at the level of the lower trunk or proximal medial cord would most likely produce numbness in the medial forearm via the medial cutaneous nerve of the forearm, which is a derivative of the medial cord. In addition, tingling would be present on the dorsum of the small and ring fingers in a lesion at the level of the midforearm or proximal to this location because the supply to the dorsal aspect of the small and ring fingers is from the dorsal ulnar cutaneous sensory branch of the ulnar nerve proper that exits the ulnar nerve approximately 10 cm proximal to the wrist.

BIBLIOGRAPHY

Becker, J., Nora, D. B., Gomes, I., et al. (2002). An evaluation of gender, obesity, age and diabetes mellitus as risk factors for carpal tunnel syndrome. *Clinical Neurophysiology, 113*(9), 1429–1434.

Bland, J. D. (2000). A neurophysiological grading scale for carpal tunnel syndrome. *Muscle Nerve, 23*, 1280–1283.

Chang, C. W., Wang, Y. C., & Chang, K. F. (2008). A practical electrophysiological guide for non-surgical and surgical treatment of carpal tunnel syndrome. *Journal of Hand Surgery (European), 33*, 32.

Chatterjee, R., & Vyas, J. (2016). Diagnosis and management of intersection syndrome as a cause of overuse wrist pain. *BMJ Case Reports, 2016*, bcr2016216988.

Dellon, A. L., & Mackinnon, S. E. (1986). Radial sensory nerve entrapment in the forearm. *Journal of Hand Surgery, 11*(2), 199–205.

Dias, J. J., Burke, F. D., Wildin, C. J., Heras-Palou, C., & Bradley, M. J. (2004). Carpal tunnel syndrome and work. *Journal of Hand Surgery (British), 29*(4), 329–333.

Don Griot, J. P., Zuidam, J. M., van Kooten, E. O., Prosé, L. P., & Hage, J. J. (2000). Anatomic study of the ramus communicans between the ulnar and median nerves. *Journal of Hand Surgery (American), 25*(5), 948–954.

Durkan, J. (1991). A new diagnostic test for carpal tunnel syndrome. *Journal of Bone and Joint Surgery, 73*(4), 535–538.

Finkelstein, H. (1930). Stenosing tendovaginitis at the radial styloid process. *Journal of Bone and Joint Surgery, 12A*, 509–539.

Hirani, S. (2020). An update to the present carpal tunnel syndrome (CTS) nerve conduction grading tool. *International Archives of Clinical Physiology, 2*, 006.

Hlebs, S., Majhenic, K., & Vidmar, G. (2014). Body mass index and anthropometric characteristics of the hand as risk factors for carpal tunnel syndrome. *Collegium Antropologicum, 38*(1), 219–226.

Kane, P. M., Daniels, A. H., & Akelman, E. (2015). Double crush syndrome. *Journal of the American Academy of Orthopaedic Surgeons, 23*(9), 58–62.

Kouyoumdjian, J. A., Zanetta, D. M., & Morita, M. P. (2002). Evaluation of age, body mass index, and wrist index as risk factors for carpal tunnel syndrome severity. *Muscle and Nerve, 25*(1), 93–97.

Kwon, J. -Y., Ko, K., Sohn, Y. B., et al. (2011). High prevalence of carpal tunnel syndrome in children with mucopolysaccharidosis type II (Hunter syndrome). *American Journal of Medical Genetics Part A, 155*, 1329–1335.

Lew, H. L., Date, E. S., Pan, S. S., Wu, P., Ware, P. F., & Kingery, W. S. (2005). Sensitivity, specificity, and variability of nerve conduction velocity measurements in carpal tunnel syndrome. *Archives of Physical Medicine and Rehabilitation, 86*, 12–16.

Michaud, L. J., Hays, R. M., Dudgeon, B. J., & Kropp, R. J. (1990). Congenital carpal tunnel syndrome: case report of autosomal dominant inheritance and review of the literature. *Archives of Physical Medicine and Rehabilitation, 71*(6), 430–432.

Nora, D. B., Becker, J., Ehlers, J. A., & Gomes, I. (2005). What symptoms are truly caused by median nerve compression in carpal tunnel syndrome? *Clinical Neurophysiology, 116*, 275–283.

Novak, C. B., & Mackinnon, S. E. (2005). Evaluation of nerve injury and nerve compression in the upper quadrant. *Journal of Hand Therapy, 18*, 230–240.

Padua, R., & Tonali, P. (2009). Neurophysiological classification and sensitivity in 500 carpal tunnel syndrome hands. *Acta Neurologica Scandinavica, 96*, 211–217.

Sasaki, T., Koyama, T., Kuroiwa, T., et al. (2022). Evaluation of the existing electrophysiological severity classifications in carpal tunnel syndrome. *Journal of Clinical Medicine, 11*, 1685.

Senel, S., Ceylaner, G., Yuksel, D., Erkek, N., & Karacan, C. (2010). Familial primary carpal tunnel syndrome with possible skipped generation. *European Journal of Pediatrics, 169*(4), 453–455.

Seror, P. (1987). Tinel's sign in the diagnosis of carpal tunnel syndrome. *Journal of Hand Surgery (British), 12*(3), 364–365.

Simon, J., Lutsky, K., Maltenfort, M., & Beredjiklian, P. K. (2017). The accuracy of the scratch collapse test performed by blinded examiners on patients with suspected carpal tunnel syndrome assessed by electrodiagnostic studies. *Journal of Hand Surgery (American), 42*(5), e1–e5. 386.

Szabo, R. M. (1989). Superficial radial nerve compression syndrome. In R. M. Szabo (Ed.), *Nerve compression syndromes diagnosis and treatment* (pp. 194–195). Thorofare, NJ: Slack.

Thoma, A., Veltri, K., Haines, T., & Duku, E. (2004). A systematic review of reviews comparing the effectiveness of endoscopic and open carpal tunnel decompression. *Plastic and Reconstructive Surgery, 113*, 1184–1191.

Tseng, C. H., Liao, C. C., Kuo, C. M., Sung, F. C., Hsieh, D. P., & Tsai, C. H. (2012). Medical and non-medical correlates of carpal tunnel syndrome in a Taiwan cohort of one million. *European Journal of Neurology, 19*(1), 91–97.

Wiesman IM, Novak, CB, Mackinnon SE, Winograd JM. Sensitivity and specificity of clinical testing for carpal tunnel syndrome. Can J Plast Surg. 2003 Summer; 11(2): 70–72. doi: 10.1177/229255030301100205

Wilbourn, A. J. (1985). Ulnar neuropathy. *Rochester, MN: American Association of Electromyography and Electrodiagnosis.* p. 27.

CHAPTER 52 QUESTIONS

1. **Which of the following nerve conduction studies indicate CTS?**
   a. Motor latency of 4.1
   b. Sensory latency of 4.1
   c. Digital sensory latency of 3.2
   d. 0.4 msec difference in latencies between median and ulnar nerve

2. **Which of the following is not associated with CTS?**
   a. Obesity
   b. Parathyroid disease
   c. Diabetes
   d. Thyroid disease

3. **What is not weak with a high median palsy?**
   a. APB
   b. Pronator quadratus
   c. FPL
   d. Adductor pollicus

FUNCTIONAL ANATOMY OF THE SPINE

B. Vibert, MD and H.N. Herkowitz, MD*

1. **Describe the blood supply to the spinal cord.**

   The spinal cord is supplied by three arteries. The anterior spinal artery supplies 80% of the spinal cord, and paired dorsal arteries supply the remainder. The anterior spinal artery is often mistaken as one contiguous artery. It actually is three separate anterior arteries, with the superiormost artery supplying C1-T3, the middle supplying approximately T3-T8, and the inferiormost anterior spinal artery supplying the area from T8 to the conus. The superior anterior spinal artery is fed by branches of the vertebral artery. The middle and inferior sections are fed by direct radicular branches from the aorta.

2. **Describe the cross-sectional location and function of the lateral corticospinal tracts, the spinothalamic tracts, and the dorsal column tracts of the spinal cord.**
   - The lateral corticospinal tracts are located laterally and slightly posteriorly. Within the column, arm function is located medially, truncate function in the middle, and leg function most laterally. This controls ipsilateral motor function.
   - The spinothalamic tracts are anterior and lateral. They transmit pain and temperature sensation from the contralateral side of the body.
   - The dorsal column tracts are located dorso medially. Within the dorsal column, arm function is most centrally located and leg function is most peripheral. These columns transmit light touch, proprioception, and vibration.

3. **Describe the six major incomplete spinal cord injury syndromes and their characteristics.**
   - Anterior cord syndrome: Injury to the anterior two thirds of the spinal cord either due to direct compression or disruption of the anterior spinal artery supply. Usually results in complete paralysis and spasticity (lateral corticospinal tracts are nonfunctional) but maintains proprioception and deep pressure (dorsal columns).
   - Central cord syndrome: This is the most common and results in motor injury in the upper extremities more than the lower extremities. Usually the result of a hyperextension injury in the cervical spine. This has the best prognosis.
   - Posterior cord syndrome: Injury to the dorsal columns, resulting in loss of proprioception.
   - Brown-Séquard syndrome: Injury to one half of the spinal column, resulting in loss of ipsilateral motor function and proprioception, with contralateral loss of pain and temperature.
   - Conus medullaris syndrome: Can result in urinary incontinence because of spastic bladder (high conus lesion) or flaccid bladder (low conus lesion). Usually results in asymmetric weakness and loss of sensation. May have a mix of upper and lower motor neuron syndromes.
   - Cauda equina syndrome: Results from compression of the nerves of the cauda equina (disc herniation, space occupying lesion, etc). Classic symptoms include saddle paresthesia, urinary retention and lower extremity weakness. Urgent surgery is required for decompression of the nerve roots.

4. **Describe Fryette's laws of spinal biomechanics.**
   - In the cervical spine, side-bending and rotation occur to the same side.
   - When the lumbar and thoracic areas of the spine are in neutral position, side-bending, and rotation occur to the opposite side.
   - When the lumbar and thoracic areas of the spine are in extreme flexion, side-bending, and rotation occur to the same side.
   - In actuality, spinal movement is highly variable among different people and even in the same person in different regions of the thoracolumbar spine.

5. **Describe the normal ranges of motion of each section of the spine.**
   - C0-C1—10 to 15 degrees of flexion/extension, 8 degrees of lateral flexion, minimal rotation
   - C1-C2—10 degrees of flexion/extension, 45 degrees of rotation, little or no lateral flexion
   - C3-C7—64 degrees of flexion, 24 degrees of extension, 40 degrees of lateral flexion, 40 degrees of rotation
   - T1-S1—80 degrees of flexion, 25 degrees of extension, 45 degrees of rotation, 35 degrees of lateral flexion

   In general, flexion/extension and lateral flexion increase from cranial to caudal. Rotation decreases from cranial to caudal.

---

*Deceased.

6. **List the important ligaments of the cervical and lumbar spine. Specify their origin, insertion, attachment, and function.**

NAME	ORIGIN	INSERTION	ATTACHMENT	FUNCTION	UPPER CERVICAL NAME CHANGE
Anterior longitudinal ligament	Skull	Sacrum	Anterior surface of vertebral bodies	Limits extension	Atlantoaxial and anterior atlanto-occipital membrane
Posterior longitudinal ligament	Skull	Sacrum	Posterior surface of vertebral bodies	Resists hyperflexion, posterior disc protrusion	Tectoral ligament
Ligamentum flavum	Anterior surface of lamina above	Superior margin of lamina below		Prestresses disc Helps extend membrane	Posterior atlanto-occipital membrane
Interspinous ligament	Posterior aspect of superior spinous process	Anterior/inferior aspect of interior spinous process		Limits flexion	
Supraspinous ligament	Occipital protuberance to upper lumbar spine	Across tips of spinous processes		Limits flexion	Ligamentum nuchae
Transverse ligament	Body of C1	Body of C1	Across posterior dens	Retains odontoid process of C2 in place against anterior arch of atlas	
Alar ligament	Bilateral extension from sides of dens	Occipital condyles		Secondary stabilizer C1-C2	
Apical ligament	Tip of dens	Foramen magnum		Secondary stabilizer C1-C2	

7. **Describe the anatomy of the intervertebral disc.**

Each motion segment has one disc, with the exception of C1-C2. The disc is an avascular structure composed of an outer annulus fibrosus, an inner nucleus pulposus, and a cartilaginous end plate interface superior and inferior to the vertebral body. The jellylike nucleus pulposus acts as a shock absorber, and the annulus helps stabilize and transmit the loads transmitted to the nucleus pulposus by axial loading. The biomechanical vertical compression forces to which the nucleus is exposed are converted into horizontally directed forces that the tough outer annulus helps absorb and distribute to the motion segment. The fibers of the annulus are arranged in alternating perpendicular lamellar fibers, arranged at a 45-degree angle to the vertebral endplates. Disc height is larger anteriorly in the cervical and lumbar spine and shorter anteriorly in the thoracic spine, which accounts for the cervical and lumbar lordosis and thoracic kyphosis.

8. **How does the disc obtain its nutrition?**
Because the disc is avascular, the disc cells must obtain their nutrition through local diffusion. Diffusion of uncharged solutes, such as glucose, occurs primarily through the endplates. Negatively charged solutes diffuse through the annulus.

9. **What is the effect of exercise on disc nutrition?**
Exercise provides nutrition through pumping of the disc, which aids in solute transport and possibly promotes nutrition through increasing external local vascularity.

10. **What changes occur in the disc with aging?**
As the spine ages, degenerative changes occur, and the chemical composition of the nucleus pulposus changes. In the nucleus pulposus of a youth, type II collagen, proteoglycans, and water are abundant. Over time, the nucleus decreases proteoglycan production, loses water, and produces less type II collagen. It begins to resemble the annulus, which consists mostly of type I collagen. Whereas young discs maintain height, aging discs lose height with degeneration and water loss.

11. **Describe the facet articulations of the spine.**
   - Occiput anterior (OA)—At the atlanto-occipital joint is an articulation between the condyles of the occipital bone and superior facets of the atlas (C1). The anterior and posterior occipital membranes and joint capsule support this articulation.
   - Atlanto-axial (AA)—Great mobility is needed at C1-C2, where 50% of cervical rotation occurs. As a result of the strong coupling pattern at this joint, axial rotation is associated with vertical translation and contralateral side-bending. The facets of C1-C2 are horizontally aligned but biconvex in design. As a result, C1 is vertically at its highest position in neutral rotation and in its lowest position in full left or right lateral rotation.
   - Cervical—The facet joints are angulated at 45 degrees to the vertical in the sagittal plane at C2-C7. This orientation allows increased mobility compared with the thoracic and lumbar portions of the spine, including the coupled axial rotation observed with lateral bending.
   - Thoracic—In the thoracic spine, the facet joints are oriented at 60 degrees to the vertical in the sagittal plane. This orientation leads to increased rigidity in the thoracic spine, with decreased axial rotation in the lower thoracic spine compared with the upper thoracic spine. This decrease is secondary to transitioning of the facets to a more lumbar-type facet.
   - Lumbar—In the lumbar spine, the facet joints are vertically oriented, and their configuration allows little rotation and flexion. The superior facets are oriented dorsomedially, almost facing each other. The inferior facet processes face ventrolaterally. This configuration allows for a locking-in of each articulation of the superior facets from the lower vertebrae with the inferior processes of the upper vertebrae.

12. **How does the spine receive loads in different postures? What is the effect of a backrest or lumbar support?**
Nachemson measured intradiscal pressure with pressure transducers placed at L3-L4 in normal patients at different postures. His research showed that the least loaded condition is lying supine. In vivo, loads increase sequentially with lying on the side, standing, sitting in a chair, standing with flexed spine, sitting in a chair with flexed spine, standing with flexed spine carrying a weight, and sitting in a chair with flexed spine carrying a weight. The relative loads are as follows:
   - Lying on the side—25%
   - Standing—100%
   - Seated—145%
   - Standing with forward bend—150%
   - Seated with forward bend—180%

   The loads on the lumbar spine are lower during supported sitting than during unsupported sitting because part of the weight of the upper body is supported by the backrest. Backward inclination and use of a lumbar support further reduce the loads.

13. **What are the dimensions of the spinal canal? How does the canal size change in different areas of the spine?**
The space available for the cord (SAC) is defined as the area posterior to the posterior longitudinal ligament and anterior to the ligamentum flavum. The normal canal opening is about 17 to 20 mm in the cervical spine. Stenotic symptoms often occur when this space decreases to <14 mm. The SAC is narrowest at T5. The spinal cord is approximately 42 cm long in women, 45 cm long in men, and 10 mm in diameter. Two levels of enlargement correlate with the levels of upper and lower extremity innervation: the C4-T1 level and the L2-S3 level. The end of the cord, the conus medullaris, starts at the T10-T11 disc level. The L1-L2 disc level marks the end of the conus medullaris and the start of the cauda equina.

14. **How are the facet joints innervated?**
The spinal nerve divides into ventral and dorsal rami. The dorsal primary ramus gives medial, lateral, and intermediate branches to the facet joints and paraspinal muscles. The medial branches are especially important in facet joint innervation. Two branches—superior and inferior—innervate the facet joint above and below the level of the nerve root. For example, the descending medial branch of L1 and the ascending medial branch of L3 innervate the L2-L3 facet.

15. **Where is the nerve root in relation to the pedicle and disc in the cervical and lumbar portions of the spine?**
In the cervical spine, the spinal nerve roots exit directly lateral from the spinal canal adjacent to the corresponding disc and superior to the inferior pedicle. The nerve roots are numbered for the cervical vertebra above which they pass. For example, the C4 nerve root exits beneath the C3 pedicle and above C4. Because there are eight cervical nerve roots but only seven cervical vertebrae, the numbering changes at C7-T1. Here the eighth cervical root passes. Thus the nerve root passing under the pedicle of T1 is the T1 nerve root.
In the lumbar spine, the nerve root passes directly under the pedicle for which it is named. For example, the L4 nerve root passes beneath the pedicle of L4 at the L4-L5 intervertebral level. The nerve root is usually superior to the disc at that level, whereas the cervical nerve roots exit at the level of the disc.

16. **How does spinal movement affect the size of the intervertebral foramen?**
Cadaver studies indicate that foramen size increases in flexion by 24% and decreases in extension by 20%. Changes caused by lateral bending and axial rotation are not as impressive.

17. **Where do compressive loads have the greatest effect in the vertebra?**
Compressive loading of the spine is a common occurrence leading to injury. The most common site of failure of the vertebra is at the endplates. Furthermore, the superior endplate is more likely to fail than the inferior endplate. This is especially common in the osteoporotic population resulting in compression fractures.

18. **Describe the function of the facet joints and their role in load bearing.**
The facets are thought to protect the lumbar spine against torsional disc damage. They decrease the allowable rotation to which an intervertebral disc is exposed and share spinal load with the disc. Investigators debate the exact amount of load that the facets bear, but estimates range from 9% to 25%, depending on whether the spine is flexed or extended. If the spine is arthritic, the facets may bear almost 50% of the load.

19. **Describe the form and function of the uncinate processes.**
The uncinate processes, which are fully developed by age 18, are thought to prevent posterior translation as well as some degree of lateral bending. They are also thought to be a guiding mechanism for flexion and extension in the cervical spine.

20. **What happens during the straight-leg raise test?**
Investigators have shown that the L4, L5, S2, and S3 nerve roots run in a sigmoid course through the foramina, with slack that can be taken up. The S1 nerve root runs a relatively straight course through the foramen. During a straight-leg raise (SLR) test, the sciatic nerve trunk is drawn downward through the greater sciatic notch, pressing tightly against the anterior bony structures. From 0 to 30 degrees, at 5 cm above the horizontal position, movement of the nerve at the greater sciatic notch already has begun. After a bit more elevation, the lumbosacral plexus is moving against the sacral ala, without root movement. From 35 to 70 degrees, the nerve roots begin moving. At 70 to 90 degrees, the nerve roots no longer move, but more tension is placed on all of the neural structures. The seated SLR has been shown in some studies to be more sensitive than the supine SLR.

21. **Which muscles are recruited to initiate and complete lumbar flexion and extension?**
Flexion is initiated by the abdominal muscles and the vertebral portion of the psoas. With further flexion, the erector spinae muscles are recruited as the forward moment acting on the spine increases. As the spine is further flexed, the posterior hip muscles are activated. At full flexion, the erector spinae muscles become inactive and are at full stretch. These muscles and the posterior ligaments supply passive restriction to further forward flexion. To extend from this position, the pelvis tilts backward and the spine extends backward, using the above muscles in reverse sequence.

22. **How effective are lumbosacral corsets for relief of spinal disc pressure?**
Maximal disc load reduction with tight corsets is approximately 20% to 30%. The use of an abdominal corset with a chair back brace also may be helpful in diminishing loads applied to the lumbar spine.

23. What is sagittal balance of the spine? What is normal and what are the effects of an abnormal sagittal balance?

Sagittal balance, also referred to as the sagittal vertical axis, is the relative position of the mid portion of the C7 vertebra with respect to the sacrum. In normal sagittal balance, a plum line drawn from the midportion of the C7 vertebral body should land in the posterior corner of the superior endplate of the S1 segment. A positive sagittal balance describes a forward flexed position of the trunk over the pelvis and has been shown to be a common cause of back pain.

24. List the ratios of disc height to vertebral body height in the cervical, lumbar, and thoracic areas of the spine.

- Cervical—1:4
- Thoracic—1:7
- Lumbar—1:3

25. What active range of motion in the cervical spine is required to perform activities of daily living?

In order to perform activities of daily living, 65 to 70 degrees of both rotation and flexion and extension is needed. In a recent study, shoe-tying required the greatest amount of flexion and extension (66.7 degrees), while driving a car in reverse (67.6 degrees) and crossing the street (≈85 degrees) necessitated the greatest rotation.

26. Describe the effect on spinal loading of the double SLR, supine sit-up, trunk curl, and reverse curl.

- A double SLR involves mostly the psoas muscle; little abdominal muscle function can be measured.
- A supine sit-up with the knees and hips bent eliminates psoas recruitment and actively strengthens the abdominal muscles; however, because of greatly increased disc pressure, these exercises should be avoided.
- A trunk curl or half sit-up, in which only the shoulder blades clear the floor, lessens lumbar motion, recruits abdominal muscle function, and lessens the load on the discs.
- A reverse curl, in which the knees are brought to the chest and the buttocks are raised from the floor, activates the internal and external obliques as well as the rectus abdominus but with less disc pressure than sit-ups.

27. What lumbar pressures are involved in commonly used exercises and postures?

Standing—100%	Sit-up—210%
Fowler's position—35%	Reverse curl—140%
Bilateral SLR—150%	Prone extension—130%

28. What are the differences in lumbar spine muscle kinematics between patients with chronic low back pain and normal subjects?

Chronic low back pain patients have been found to have earlier activation and significantly longer activation of their erector spinae musculature compared with normal controls during a lifting exercise. Longer contraction may suggest that chronic low back pain patients have changed their motor program from an open to a closed loop system.

29. What is the effect of age on cervical spine range of motion?

Average adolescent flexion-extension measures approximately 130 degrees whereas adult men (average age 37) have only 117 degrees of flexion-extension. Similarly, rotation decreased from 160 to 153 degrees for these same age groups. This exemplifies the importance of cervical spine range of motion exercises beginning in young adulthood.

30. What are the effects of lumbar discectomy on trunk musculature?

At 2 months after surgery, patients undergoing lumbar spine discectomy were found to have 44% decreased trunk flexion strength and 36% decreased trunk extension strength compared with controls. This may indicate a need for formal trunk strengthening after lumbar spine surgery.

31. What is the effect of leg length discrepancy on spinal motion during gait?

There is a significant asymmetric lateral bending motion in the lumbar spine during gait in patients with leg length discrepancies of 3 cm. This may lead to accelerated degenerative changes in the lumbar spine.

32. **How much nerve root movement occurs in the lumbar spine with SLR?**
    - L4—1.5 mm
    - L5—3.0 mm
    - S1—4.0 mm
    - Sacral ala—4.5 mm
    - Sciatic notch—6.5 mm

33. **How much nerve root movement occurs in the lumbar spine with forward flexion while standing?**
    - L1-L2—2 to 5 mm
    - L3—2.0 mm
    - L4—0 mm

34. **How much dural movement occurs in the cervical spine with flexion and extension?**
    - C5—Approximately 3 mm
    - C8—Approximately 9 mm
    - T1—Approximately 13 mm
    - T5—Approximately 7 mm
    - T10—Approximately 2 mm

35. **Describe key vertebral landmarks.**
    - L5—Smallest lumbar spinous process
    - L3—Largest lumbar transverse process
    - C7—Most prominent cervical spinous process
    - C6—Most inferior bifid cervical spinous process

36. **Discuss the 3-column model of the spine.**
    - The anterior column consists of the anterior longitudinal ligament to the mid-vertebral body.
    - This middle column includes the posterior vertebral body of the posterior longitudinal ligament.
    - The posterior column includes the pedicles, facets, laminal transverse processes, spinous processes, and interspinous ligament.

37. **What are the most common levels for cervical and lumbar disc herniations and what are the most common findings for each of these?**

    In the cervical spine, the most common levels for disc herniations occur at the C5–6 and C6–7 levels. At the C5–6 level, the C6 nerve is most commonly affected which results in any combination of pain, numbness, and tingling in the radial forearm and into the thumb and index finger. C6 weakness manifests as decreased wrist extension strength. At the C6–7 level, the C7 nerve root is affected, resulting in similar symptoms in the mid dorsum of the forearm into the middle finger as well as triceps weakness.

    In the lumbar spine, the L4–5 herniated disc results in L5 radiculopathy in the anterolateral leg and weakness in great toe dorsiflexion. At L5-S1, the S1 nerve is affected with radicular symptoms into the calf and lateral foot, and weakness of the gastroc-soleus complex.

38. **Describe the sacroiliac joint.**

    The sacroiliac joint is an irregularly shaped articulation between the lateral-facing facet of the sacrum and the medial-facing facet of the ilium. The joint is supported by three very strong ligaments, including the posterior sacroiliac ligaments (strongest), the interosseous ligaments, and the anterior sacroiliac ligaments. The curvature of the joint and the strong ligaments allow for very little motion of the sacroiliac joint.

Bibliography

Alderink, G. J. (2002). Three-dimensional analysis of active head and cervical spine range of motion: effect of age in healthy male subjects. *Clinical Biomechanics, 17*, 611–614.

Bennett, S. E., Schenk, R. J., & Simmons, E. D. (2002). Active range of motion utilized in the cervical spine to perform daily functional tasks. *Journal of Spinal Disorders & Techniques, 15*, 307–311.

Denis, F. (1983). The three-column spine and its significance in the classification of acute thoracolumbar spinal injuries. *Spine, 8*, 817–831.

Ferguson, S. A., Marras, W. S., Burr, D. L., Davis, K. G., & Gupta, P. (2004). Differences in motor recruitment and resulting kinematics between low back pain patients and asymptomatic participants during lifting exertions. *Clinical Biomechanics, 19*, 992–999.

Glassman, S. D., Bridwell, K., Dimar, J. R., et al. (2005). The impact of sagittal balance in adult spinal deformity. *Spine, 30*(18), 2024–2029.

Grieve, G. P. (1988). *Common vertebral joint problems* (2nd ed.). New York, NY: Churchill Livingstone.

Hakkinen, A., Kuukkanen, T., Tarvainen, U., & Ylinen, J. (2004). Trunk muscle strength in flexion, extension, and axial rotation in patients managed with lumbar disc herniation surgery and in healthy control subjects. *Spine, 28*, 1068–1073.

Huang, R. C., Girardi, F. P., Cammisa, F. P., Jr., Tropiano, P., & Marnay, T. (2003). Long-term flexion-extension range of motion of the prodisc: Total disc replacement. *Journal of Spinal Disorders & Techniques, 16*, 435–440.

Lazorthes, G., Gouaze, A., Zadeh, J. O., et al. (1971). Arterial vascularization of the spinal cord. *Journal of Neurosurgery, 35*, 253–262.

Mitchell, F. L., Moran, P. S., & Pruzzo, M. A. (1979). *An evaluation and treatment manual of osteopathic muscle energy procedures* (pp. 23). Valley Park, MO: ICEOP.

Mototaka, K., Kei, M., & Katsuji, S. (2003). The effect of leg length discrepancy on spinal motion during gait. *Spine, 28*, 2472–2476.

Nachemson, A. (1975). Towards a better understanding of back pain: a review of the lumbar disc. *Rheumatology and Rehabilitation, 14*, 129.

Panjabi, M. M., Takata, K., & Goel, V. K. (1983). Kinematics of lumbar intervertebral foramen. *Spine, 8*, 348.

White, A. A., III, & Panjabi, M. M. (1990). *Clinical biomechanics of the spine* (2nd ed.). Philadelphia, PA: JB Lippincott.

Zehra, U., Robson-Brown, K., Adams, M. A., et al. (2015). Porosity and thickness of the vertebral endplate depend on local mechanical loading. *Spine, 40*(15), 1173–1180.

CHAPTER 53 QUESTIONS

1. **Where does the greatest amount of nerve root movement occur with SLR?**
   a. L4
   b. L5
   c. S1
   d. Sciatic notch

2. **Lumbar pressures are greatest:**
   a. Standing
   b. Laying on side
   c. Standing with forward bend
   d. Seated with forward bend

3. **Cervical rotation is greatest at:**
   a. C0-C1
   b. C6-C7
   c. C7-T1
   d. C1-C2

4. **What are the most likely findings of an L5-S1 herniated disc?**
   a. Groin pain
   b. Numbness in the thigh
   c. Pain and numbness in the calf and lateral foot
   d. Anterolateral shin pain that travels into the great toe

5. **Signs and symptoms of a positive sagittal balance include which of the following?**
   a. The head and neck anterior to the pelvis and low back pain with prolonged standing
   b. The head and neck lateral to the pelvis and low back pain with prolonged standing
   c. The head and neck in a neutral position over the pelvis and no pain with prolonged standing
   d. The head and neck posterior to the pelvis and low back pain with prolonged standing

6. **The most common site of injury to the vertebra during compression is the**
   a. Spinous process
   b. Facets
   c. Anterior longitudinal ligament
   d. Endplate

CHAPTER 54

CERVICAL SPINE

L.L. Devaney, PT, ATC, PhD, OCS, FAAOMPT and B.T. Swanson, PT, DSc, OCS, FAAOMPT

1. **Is neck pain a common problem?**

   Neck pain is a common problem. Lifetime prevalence has been reported to be high, with the results of a systematic review with meta-analysis estimating that 48.5% of the global adult population will experience neck pain. Prevalence estimates for the adult population suggest neck pain will be experienced by 37.2% in 1 year, 23.3% each month, 12.5% each week, and by 4.9% to 7.6% of the population at any point in time. Neck pain is more common in women, and prevalence appears to peak in middle age. On a global perspective, neck pain is most common in North America followed by Western Europe.

2. **What is the economic burden of neck pain?**

   The economic burden due to disorders of the neck is high. Low back and neck pain represent the third-largest health care expenditure by condition at $87.6 billion. Additional impact includes lost wages and compensation expenditures, with neck pain second to only low back pain for workers' compensation expenses in the United States. These costs continue to increase, as annual spending on low back and neck pain increased more than any health condition except diabetes between 1996 and 2013.

3. **What are risk factors for developing neck pain?**

   Demographic, physical, and psychosocial factors are associated with the development of *new onset* neck pain. Although there is some conflict the most consistently observed predisposing factors for new onset (atraumatic) neck pain include female sex and prior history of neck pain. Additionally, occupational factors such as high job demands, low social or work support, prior history of low back pain, and being an ex-smoker are associated with incidence of neck pain. "Leisure activity" and neck extensor endurance were associated with reduced risk of neck pain in workers. New research on *first episode* neck pain reported the strongest overall risk factors include high perceived muscular tension, depressed mood, role conflict, and high job demand. This most recent review highlights the importance of psychosocial factors and suggests that many predisposing factors for new onset neck pain are modifiable.

4. **What findings have meaningful prognostic value for individuals with neck pain?**

   Schellingerhout et al. (2010) predicted recovery based on age, pain intensity (0–10), concurrent headache, radiation to elbow/shoulder, previous neck complaints, concurrent low back pain, employment status, and quality of life. Consistent with previous work, higher pain intensity and a history of previous neck pain, older age (≥40), concurrent low back pain and headaches were associated with a worse prognosis. When a patient presents with age >40 years and "concomitant back pain" these factors were prognostic for higher pain intensity, while "a previous period of neck pain" and "accompanying headache" were associated with perceived nonrecovery. Interestingly, Schellingerhout (2010) and Borghouts (1998) both reported that radiation to the arm was not associated with a worse prognosis, while Borghouts (1998) further concluded that radiologic findings (degenerative disc/joints) are not associated with a worse prognosis.

5. **What are the most common structural changes associated with neck pain?**

   Based on innervation, the cervical spine facet joints, discs, ligaments, musculature, and vasculature are all potential sources of neck pain. The challenge is identifying which structures are symptomatic in individuals with neck pain. Nakashima et al. (2015) assessed the MR images of 1211 healthy volunteers between the ages of 20 and 70. Their study found disc bulging in over 87% of participants, including individuals in their 20s (73%–78%). The prevalence of disc bulges progressed through age 50, after which the severity rather than frequency of disc bulging progressed. Manchikanti et al. (2002), using diagnostic blocks, found a prevalence rate of facet joint pain in chronic neck pain of 60%. Alterations in the physical structure and function of the cervical musculature are also frequently observed in individuals with mechanical neck pain. These changes include atrophy and fatty replacement of the cervical extensor muscles as well as weakness/inhibition of the deep cranio-cervical flexors. Excessive superficial muscle activity is frequently observed, likely in response to inhibition of the deep stabilizers. While current recommendations are nearly universal in their support of retraining altered muscular firing patterns, recommendations regarding pathoanatomic findings generally focus on treatment of the clinical presentation and subgrouping rather than pathoanatomy.

6. **What are the possible pain generators in the cervical spine?**
Potential pain generators in the spine include the zygapophyseal (facet) joints, vertebral bodies, surrounding musculature and ligaments, intervertebral discs, and exiting nerve roots. Cervical facet joints are well recognized as a source of local neck pain. The characteristics of lower cervical facet involvement include parasagittal pain that does not cross midline and does not extend down the arm, although the lower cervical facets may refer into the ipsilateral scapular region, while the upper cervical facets are most commonly associated with ipsilateral headache. The disc itself can cause local and referred pain into the scapular region.

7. **Is poor posture related to neck pain?**
Research results are conflicting, and the relationship between neck pain and posture appears to vary with age. Despite common assumptions, there are no studies indicating a causal effect of forward head posture on neck pain. However, a recent meta-analysis found that adults aged 18 to 50 with neck pain had greater craniovertebral angle than age-matched asymptomatic controls. There was no difference in adolescents (under 18 years) nor in adults older than 50 years. Additionally, there is weak to moderate evidence of a moderate correlation between neck pain and forward head posture in adults that increases with age. Increased thoracic kyphosis is also associated with limited neck range of motion, a common impairment in patients with neck pain. Despite lack of definitive evidence indicating that poor posture "causes" neck pain, postural assessment and interventions may be indicated to address limited neck mobility and neck pain particularly if symptoms are modified with reduced craniovertebral angle.

8. **Why is screening for red flags important in evaluating patients with neck pain?**
As stated in the Clinical Practice Guidelines Neck Pain: Revision 2017, medical screening is the first component of the physical therapy evaluation for a patient with neck pain. Early identification and timely management of nonmusculoskeletal conditions and serious spinal pathology presenting as neck pain are vital to safe and optimal outcomes for patients. The physical therapist incorporates findings including red flags from the history and physical exam to determine whether the patient is appropriate for physical therapy examination/intervention or referral to another healthcare provider. The IFOMPT Cervical Framework and International Framework for Red Flags for Potential Serious Spinal Pathologies are clinical reasoning pathways that guide this decision-making process. Examples of systemic conditions that may present as neck pain include but are not limited to primary or metastatic cancer (lung, thyroid, etc.), infection, cardiac disease, and cervical artery dissection. Examples of serious spinal pathology include but are not limited to fracture, myelopathy, and craniocervical instability.

9. **What are the red flags for serious spinal pathology in patients with neck pain?**
See Table 54.1.

10. **How is neck pain classified?**
Neck pain has historically been classified in a variety of ways including etiology, severity, treatment approach, and duration. A mechanism-based classification categorizes neck pain as systemic, neuropathic, and mechanical. Examples of systemic neck pain are those attributed to vascular pathology or rheumatoid arthritis. Neuropathic neck pain typically refers to radiculopathy with associated radiating pain, while mechanical neck pain originates from musculoskeletal structures in the cervical spine. A more global classification defines neck pain as specific versus nonspecific neck pain. Specific neck pain has an identifiable pathoanatomic source (ie, myelopathy), while nonspecific neck pain cannot be attributed to an identified tissue pathology. A secondary consideration in classification schemes is duration of neck pain that is traditionally defined as acute <6 weeks, subacute 6 to 12 weeks, and chronic or "persistent" >3 months.

Neck pain may be further divided into traumatic and nontraumatic neck pain, and the Quebec Task Force (QTF) model defines five categories of whiplash-associated disorder based on presence and severity of physical and psychological impairments. With the exception of the modified QTF classifications, a limitation of current classification models is the reliance on physical findings versus acknowledgment of the psychosocial and behavioral factors that inform management of patients with neck pain.

11. **What are the four categories of neck pain described in the Neck Pain: Revision 2017 Clinical Practice Guidelines?**
The International Classification of Functioning, Disability and Health classification for neck pain provides a framework for an impairment and treatment-based approach to managing patients with neck pain. Physical therapists assess for movement limitations, associated headache, traumatic injury history, sensory and motor impairments, and pain that radiates to the arm or scapular region in order to classify patients into one of the following categories:
    1. Neck pain with mobility deficits
    2. Neck pain with headache
    3. Neck pain with radiating pain
    4. Neck pain with movement coordination impairment

Table 54.1 Primary Risk Factors and Red Flags for Nonmusculoskeletal and Serious Spinal Pathology in Patients with Neck Pain

	RISK FACTORS	SYMPTOMS	SIGNS
Fracture (Stiell 2001) (Finucane 2020)	Age >65 Female Decreased bone density Trauma Corticosteroid use	Immediate onset pain Unrelenting pain Paresthesias	Decreased AROM (hesitancy) Midline tenderness Proximal muscle weakness
Myelopathy (Cohen 2015) (Vijiaratnam 2018)	Age Trauma	Bowel/bladder dysfunction Fine motor fatigue Gait impairment	Upper motor neuron signs Nonmyotomal weakness Ataxia/balance impairment Lhermitte's sign Micrographia
Craniocervical Instability (Rushton 2014)	Trauma Systemic disease Connective tissue disorder	Headache Difficulty holding head up/ unwillingness to move Extrasegmental paresthesias Nausea Dizziness	Sharp's Purser test Alar ligament test Worsening symptoms with neck flexion and/or end range rotation
Cervical Artery Dissection (Rushton 2014)	High blood pressure Hypercholesterolemia Recent trauma	Sudden onset Headache Dizziness Nausea Double vision	Elevated BP Unilateral weakness Cranial nerve signs
Neoplasm (Finucane 2020) (Vijiaratnam 2018)	Age Personal history of cancer	Unrelenting night pain Unexplained weight loss Progressive, worsening pain	Palpable mass Neurological signs

These classifications take into account patient history and subjective reporting combined with physical exam features to guide the physical therapist in selecting evidence-based interventions. Treatment-based categories are further stratified into acute, subacute, and chronic classification to better reflect the increased complexity in managing patients with delayed recovery.

12. **What are the clinical presentations of a patient with neck pain?**
With respect to the Clinical Practice Guidelines, the classifications of neck pain present with different patterns of symptoms and physical findings. Patients with neck pain with mobility deficits generally present with recent onset unilateral neck pain, no symptoms distal to the shoulder, restricted neck AROM, and no signs of nerve root compression. Patients with neck pain with headache present with unilateral-dominant headache with neck pain, headache associated with neck movements, limited neck motion and upper cervical segmental mobility, and tenderness in upper three cervical facet joints. Patients with neck pain with radiating pain (cervical radiculopathy) report unilateral neck and arm/periscapular pain and peripheralization/centralization of symptoms with active and/or repeated movements, and they show signs of nerve root compression, and positive distraction, Spurling's, or upper limb tension testing. Patients in the neck pain with movement coordination impairment have a history of trauma (ie, whiplash mechanism), pain with mid-to-end range neck movements, impaired cervical muscle strength and movement control, and sensorimotor impairment. Additionally, they may report symptoms consistent with concussion (headache, dizziness, concentration difficulty). Patients with subacute and chronic neck pain in these categories present with longer symptom duration, regional strength and endurance deficits, reduced pain pressure thresholds, and more complex management needs.

13. **What clinical tests and measures are useful in the management of patients with neck pain?**
The physical exam includes provocation/alleviation tests to identify patients with cervical radiculopathy and tests/measures that quantify physical impairments (joint mobility, muscle performance, and movement patterns) and sensory impairments (sensorimotor and sensory processing). Spurling's test, the distraction test, and the upper limb tension test are useful in conjunction with myotome/dermatome/reflex exam to aid in identifying patients

with neck pain with radiating pain. Range of motion, passive accessory motion testing, the cervical flexion rotation test (CFRT), and visual inspection of movement patterns detect joint mobility and muscle length limitations that may contribute to pain and functional loss. The craniocervical flexion test, neck flexion endurance test, and joint position sense assess movement control and muscle performance that is most likely to be impaired in patients with neck pain with delayed recovery. Emerging evidence points to the use of sensory testing (pressure pain threshold and quantitative sensory testing) to assess sensory and pain processing function in patients with subacute and chronic neck pain.

14. What are the most common impairments and activity limitations in patients with neck pain?

The most common physical impairments in patients with neck pain are limited neck mobility, decreased strength of neck and upper quarter muscles, and decreased proprioception. Patients with neck pain have less active range of motion in all directions when compared with those without neck pain, and patients with traumatic neck pain (WAD) demonstrate less motion than those with atraumatic neck pain. Impaired muscle performance of the neck and shoulder girdle muscles is a common characteristic of patients with mechanical neck pain. Patients with mechanical neck pain demonstrate decreased muscle force production and decreased endurance to moderate loads particularly in the neck flexors and extensors, which influences the ability to maintain sustained postures. Impaired spatial acuity/proprioception coupled with deficits in mobility and muscle performance subsequently results in altered movement strategies. The most common activity limitations associated with the above impairments include difficulty with driving, maintaining sustained postures for work, lying in bed/sleeping, sport-specific tasks, and lifting/carrying.

15. How is cervical radiculopathy differentiated from other sources of upper limb pain?

Neck pain that radiates into the arm or scapular region accompanied by pain, weakness, and/or sensory changes in an accepted dermatomal and/or myotomal distribution is suggestive of cervical radiculopathy. Cervical radiculopathy results from compression of the exiting spinal nerve roots, generally caused by either disc herniation or hypertrophy of the facet and uncovertebral joints. Cervical radicular symptoms are most likely to originate from the C6-7 segment (C7 root) followed by the C5-6 and C4-5 segments.

While there have been many tests proposed to diagnose cervical radiculopathy, a test cluster developed by Wainner et al. (2003) is generally the most widely accepted in physical therapy practice. The four tests in the cluster include Spurling's test, upper limb tension test 1, the distraction test, and ipsilateral cervical rotation AROM of 60 degrees or less. When all four tests are positive, the posttest probability is 90%, although this decreases to 65% if only three tests are positive. Within the cluster, the Spurling test has been proposed to be the most specific (spec. 0.93), while the ULTT 1 has been proposed to be the most sensitive (sens 0.97). Among other tests that may help differentiate cervical radiculopathy from other sources of UE pain are the Valsalva maneuver (sens 0.22, spec 0.94), the shoulder abduction test (sens 0.17–0.78, spec 0.75-0.92), and the arm squeeze test (sens 0.96, spec 0.91–1.00). The combination of the test cluster and neurological screening guide the physical therapist in clinical recognition of cervical radiculopathy.

16. When is radiography indicated for patients with neck pain?

For new or progressive nontraumatic neck pain with no red flags as well as chronic neck pain, cervical radiography is the most appropriate test. However, imaging is generally not required at the time of initial presentation. Abnormal imaging findings are common in patients >30 years of age, and abnormal imaging findings have been shown to be poorly correlated with the presence of neck pain. The American College of Radiology (ACR) has presented an extensive set of guidelines regarding the appropriateness of imaging. The determination of appropriate imaging is based on the context of the patient presentation and mechanism of injury.

17. When is imaging indicated for patients with neck pain following traumatic injury?

In the presence of trauma, the first determination is based on the indications of either the NEXUS or Canadian C-spine Rules (CCR) clinical criteria. The NEXUS criteria identify five factors that indicate if a patient is at risk for significant cervical injury; no imaging is required if 0/5 factors are present. These factors include focal neurologic deficit, midline spinal tenderness, altered level of consciousness, intoxication, and distracting injury. In a validation study of over 34,000 cases, these five simple factors have been demonstrated to have 99.6% sensitivity and 99.9% negative predictive value for the detection of significant cervical injury. The CCR consists of a slightly more complex decision-making matrix but may have 100% sensitivity to detect serious cervical spine injuries. Imaging is automatically indicated for individuals with high-risk injuries. These factors include age >65 years, paresthesia in extremities, or a dangerous mechanism: falls from ≥3 feet/five stairs; axial load to head; motor vehicle crash with high speed, rollover, or ejection; bicycle collision; or motorized recreational vehicle accident. If no high-risk factors are present, the patient is assessed for low-risk factors: simple rear-end motor vehicle crash; patient in sitting position in emergency center; patient ambulatory at any time after trauma; delayed onset of neck pain; and absence of midline cervical spine tenderness. If the low-risk criterion is met, the patient is asked to rotate the head to the left and right. The ability to rotate 45 degrees to each side clears the individual, while an inability to rotate 45 degrees to either side indicates the need for imaging. For individuals over 16 years of age, in cases where the NEXUS and CCR are negative, imaging is usually not required.

18. When is advanced imaging suggested for patients with neck pain following traumatic injury?
In cases where the CCR or NEXUS indicate imaging is appropriate, CT scan of the cervical spine is usually appropriate, despite the higher levels of radiation exposure. CT scan is considered the gold standard for identifying cervical spine fractures, while having the added benefit of identifying the majority of cervical spine instabilities. In cases when spinal cord or nerve root injury is suspected, MRI without contrast is usually appropriate; however, in cases with contraindications such as pacemaker or severe claustrophobia CT myelography provides an acceptable alternative.

19. When is MRI indicated for individuals with neck pain?
For individuals with nontraumatic neck pain and/or radiculopathy, the ACR suggests that for new or progressive nontraumatic radiculopathy, MRI without contrast is usually appropriate, while CT scan without contrast may be appropriate in some instances. However, in the absence of red flag symptoms, imaging is not generally required at the initial examination. A recent meta-analysis concluded that the correlation between MRI findings of nerve root compression and physical examination findings was limited, perhaps due to high levels of both false-positive and false-negative findings on MRI in this patient population. One notable exception is the patient who presents with signs of myelopathy, who requires imaging studies to assess for extrinsic compression of the spinal cord.

20. What treatments should physical therapists use for patients with neck pain?
Current guidelines recommend specific treatments for individuals with neck pain and mobility deficits, movement coordination impairments, radiating pain, and headaches. While the recommendations are based on a compilation of current best evidence, they do not replace the need for a thorough examination and application of techniques based on individual patient presentation, including irritability, and thoughtful clinical reasoning. With that caveat, the following treatment categories are supported by the evidence and practice guidelines:

For individuals with acute neck pain with mobility deficits, mobilization/manipulation of the cervical and thoracic spine are primary recommendations supported by ROM and stretching exercises. The role of exercise, particularly endurance-based activities, is emphasized for the treatment of individuals with subacute neck pain, in addition to mobilization/manipulation. A similar approach is supported for chronic neck pain with mobility deficits with a progressive emphasis on mixed exercises including endurance, stretching, strengthening, and proprioception. The clinician should also emphasize the importance of physical activity and addressing affective considerations.

For individuals with neck pain and headache (generally including cervicogenic headaches), the majority of recommendations include mobility focused interventions with special attention to C1-2. In the acute phase, supervised active mobility exercises and self-SNAGs to C1-2 are recommended. This conservative approach considers the known prodromal symptoms of neck pain and headache that accompany acute vertebral artery dissection. Once symptoms are more stable (subacute), manual therapies such as manipulation/mobilization are generally recommended and can be augmented with the addition of mobility exercises such as the C1-2 self-SNAG. In the chronic stage, mobilization/manipulation remains the treatment of choice, accompanied by a multimodal exercise program including stretching, strengthening, and endurance activities targeting the neck and shoulder girdle.

For individuals with acute neck pain with radiating pain, treatments may include mobilizing and stabilizing exercises. Short-term use of a cervical collar may allow symptomatic relief, but should be reserved for individuals who do not gain relief with other interventions. Unlike the lumbar spine, repeated motion activities have not been shown to be consistently beneficial in the cervical spine, and based on updated evidence neural mobilizations also do not appear to offer significant benefits in this population. In the presence of more chronic symptoms, in addition to advice to remain active, treatment may include intermittent cervical traction. In the authors' opinion, the clearest indication for traction is relief of peripheral symptoms during a distraction test as performed during a radiculopathy testing cluster. Cervical and/or thoracic mobilization/manipulation may also be appropriate, both to improve mobility or for neuromodulatory purposes. This should most likely be combined with exercise interventions (stretching and strengthening).

The treatment recommendations change when considering individuals with acute neck pain with movement coordination impairments. Of primary interest is minimizing the likelihood of transition to chronicity. Reassurance that recovery occurs for the majority of individuals within 2 to 3 months is a hallmark of this phase of treatment. Early return to familiar activities, particularly if they do not provoke symptoms, is encouraged. Collar use is minimized, and postural and mobility exercises are utilized. For individuals with persistent symptoms and impairments, a multimodal exercise program including strength, endurance, and coordination activities is the most appropriate intervention. For individuals with significant delays in recovery, the addition of pain education is recommended.

21. Should traction be used in the treatment of patients with neck pain?
Intermittent mechanical traction is supported in the literature for the treatment of individuals with cervical radiculopathy. Current clinical practice guidelines recommend its use in patients within the chronic neck pain with radiating pain category based on moderate evidence. Systematic reviews have identified favorable studies supporting intermittent application, but not continuous cervical traction while also finding moderate evidence to support the use of both manual and mechanical traction in the treatment of cervical radiculopathy. A clinical prediction rule identified individuals likely to respond to traction if a patient had four or more of the following factors: patient reported peripheralization with lower cervical spine mobility testing, a positive shoulder abduction

test, age 55 or greater, a positive ULTT A, and a positive neck distraction test. Of these, the authors believe the distraction test may be the most useful, as it serves as an immediate test of mechanical forces similar to those proposed to be beneficial, and may help to improve patient acceptance and understanding of the treatment.

22. **Should patients with neck pain wear a collar or brace?**
There is limited evidence to support collar use. The 2017 clinical practice guidelines provide recommendations based on moderate strength of evidence to minimize collar use for individuals in the acute stage of the neck pain with movement coordination impairments category. In an extensive systematic review of interventions following acute WAD, Teasell et al. (2010) concluded that immobilization with a soft collar appears to be generally less effective than active mobilization while there are no significant differences in outcome between collar use and advice to act as usual. There is weak evidence to support use in the acute neck pain with radiating pain category. In a systematic review by Gross et al. (2013), a semi-rigid collar was identified as having a short-term effect on pain and global perceived function compared to a waitlist comparison, although there were no significant difference when compared to active therapy. Aksoy et al. (2017) found that both soft and semi-rigid collars improved pain and NDI scores at 2 and 6 weeks in patients in radiculopathy compared to a control group, with the soft collar demonstrating greater pain relief. Thoomes et al. (2013), based on low-quality evidence, concluded that a collar was no more effective than physical therapy for cervical radiculopathy, but that both appear to be promising interventions at short-term follow-up. The authors suggest that collars may be appropriate in the short-term management in the presence of high irritability, such as instances of nerve root edema, or where traction or other physical interventions may not be tolerated by the patient.

23. **When is surgery indicated for a patient with neck pain?**
The indications for anterior cervical spine surgery remain controversial, and studies have shown that pragmatic physical therapy and surgery have equivalent outcomes in the treatment of radiculopathy. However, when symptoms do not subside despite appropriate conservative intervention, radiculopathy is accompanied by progressive neurologic deficit, or in cases of spinal cord compression (see question on myelopathy), surgery may be the most appropriate course of action. In cases of radiculopathy where surgery is required, arm pain has been shown to improve more if surgery is performed within the first 6 months, although neck pain may not differ significantly.

24. **Is treatment by a physical therapist helpful for cervical myelopathy?**
There is conflicting evidence regarding physical therapist intervention for cervical myelopathy. In a systematic review of nonoperative therapies for cervical myelopathy, Rhee et al. (2013) suggested that physical therapy might be appropriate for individuals with mild myelopathy, particularly those with concurrent neck and/or radicular pain. Outcomes of patients with mild CSM were similar to surgical treatment at 1, 2, and 3 years after treatment. Conversely, in patients with moderate to severe myelopathy surgery resulted in superior results. Browder et al. (2004) published a case series, detailing the use of intermittent cervical traction and thoracic manipulation to treat seven patients with grade I myelopathy with decreased pain and improved functional scores. While there may be symptomatic improvements in patients with early myelopathy, it is suggested that they be monitored carefully for signs of neurologic deterioration.

25. **Is surgery recommended for patients with cervical myelopathy?**
Surgery is generally recommended for patients with cervical myelopathy. The natural history of spondylotic myelopathy is that of a progressive disorder, with neurologic deterioration occurring in up to 60% of patients. While the natural history is not absolute, surgical intervention eliminates the chances of the neurological deterioration, halts the progression of existing neurologic symptoms, and may improve neurological outcomes.

26. **How should the outcomes of treatment for patients with neck pain be measured?**
Outcomes should be considered from multiple perspectives. From a more traditional view of change, baseline measures of pain, ROM, endurance, and provocative tests can be reassessed to track progress. Pain is most commonly tracked using either a numeric pain rating scale (NPRS) or a visual analog scale (VAS). To capture additional domains, it is important to also include validated, objective measures of self-reported function. For the cervical spine, the most commonly used patient reported outcome is the neck disability index (NDI), a tool that measures self-reported disability and the impact of neck pain on an individual's daily life. Reported minimal clinically important difference (MCID) for the NDI range from 3.5/50 for nonspecific neck pain to 8.5/50 for radiculopathy. Additional tools supported by clinical guidelines include the SF-36 (a generic measure of multiple health domains) and the SF-12 (a measure of health-related quality of life). Particularly useful in clinical practice is the patient-specific functional scale (PSFS), which has been shown to be reliable, valid, and responsive in individuals with neck pain. The PSFS offers a patient-centered approach to outcomes assessment that may be more responsive than the NDI for individuals with neck pain. While data regarding the MCID for the PSFS in individuals with neck pain remains limited, Abbott and Schmitt (2014) reported that differences of 1.3 (small change) to 2.7 (large change) were relatively stable across multiple body regions.

BIBLIOGRAPHY

Abbott, J. H., & Schmitt, J. (2014). Minimum important differences for the patient-specific functional scale, 4 region-specific outcome measures, and the numeric pain rating scale. *Journal of Orthopaedic & Sports Physical Therapy, 44*(8), 560–564.

Agarwal, V., Shah, L.M., Parsons, M.S., et al. (2020). Myelopathy. Available at: https://acsearch.acr.org/docs/69484/Narrative/. American College of Radiology. Accessed August 31, 2021.

Aksoy, M. K., Altan, L., & Güner, A. (2017). The effectiveness of soft and semi-rigid cervical collars on acute cervical radiculopathy. *The European Research Journal, 4*(1), 16–25.

Beckmann, N. M., West, O. C., Nunez Jr, D., et al. (2018). Suspected spine trauma. Available at: https://acsearch.acr.org/docs/69359/Narrative/. American College of Radiology. Accessed August 31, 2021.

Bier, J. D., Scholten-Peeters, W. G. M., Staal, J. B., et al. (2018). Clinical practice guideline for physical therapy assessment and treatment in patients with nonspecific neck pain. *Physical Therapy, 98*(3), 162–171.

Blanpied, P. R., Gross, A. R., Elliott, J. M., et al. (2017). Neck pain: revision 2017. *Journal of Orthopaedic & Sports Physical Therapy, 47*(7), A1–A83.

Bogduk, N. (2003). The anatomy and pathophysiology of neck pain. *Physical Medicine and Rehabilitation. Clinics, 14*(3), 455–472.

Borghouts, J. A., Koes, B. W., & Bouter, L. M. (1998). The clinical course and prognostic factors of non-specific neck pain: a systematic review. *Pain, 77*, 1–13.

Borghouts, J. A., Koes, B. W., Vondeling, H., & Bouter, L. M. (1999). Cost-of-illness of neck pain in The Netherlands in 1996. *Pain, 80*, 629–636.

Brinjikji, W., Luetmer, P. H., Comstock, B., et al. (2015). Systematic literature review of imaging features of spinal degeneration in asymptomatic populations. *American Journal of Neuroradiology, 36*, 811–816.

Browder, D. A., Erhard, R. E., & Piva, S. R. (2004). Intermittent cervical traction and thoracic manipulation for management of mild cervical compressive myelopathy attributed to cervical herniated disc: a case series. *Journal of Orthopaedic & Sports Physical Therapy, 34*(11), 701–712.

Burneikiene, S., Nelson, E. L., Mason, A., Rajpal, S., & Villavicencio, A. T. (2015). The duration of symptoms and clinical outcomes in patients undergoing anterior cervical discectomy and fusion for degenerative disc disease and radiculopathy. *The Spine Journal, 15*(3), 427–432.

Cassidy, J. D., Boyle, E., Côté, P., et al. (2009). Risk of vertebrobasilar stroke and chiropractic care: results of a population-based case-control and case-crossover study. *Journal of Manipulative and Physiological Therapeutics, 32*(2), S201–208.

Childs, J. D., Flynn, T. W., Fritz, J. M., et al. (2005). Screening for vertebrobasilar insufficiency in patients with neck pain: manual therapy decision-making in the presence of uncertainty. *Journal of Orthopaedic & Sports Physical Therapy, 35*(5), 300–306.

Cloward, R. B. (1959). Cervical diskography: a contribution to the etiology and mechanism of neck, shoulder and arm pain. *Annals of Surgery, 150*(6), 1052.

Cloward, R. B. (1960). The clinical significance of the sinu-vertebral nerve of the cervical spine in relation to the cervical disk syndrome. *Journal of Neurology, Neurosurgery, and Psychiatry, 23*(4), 321.

Cohen, S. P. (2015). Epidemiology, diagnosis, and treatment of neck pain. *Mayo Clinic Proceedings, 90*(2), 284–299.

De-la-Llave-Rincón, A. I., Fernández-de-las-Peñas, C., Palacios-Ceña, D., & Cleland, J. A. (2009). Increased forward head posture and restricted cervical range of motion in patients with carpal tunnel syndrome. *Journal of Orthopaedic & Sports Physical Therapy, 39*(9), 658–664.

Dieleman, J. L., Baral, R., Birger, M., et al. (2016). US spending on personal health care and public health, 1996–2013. *JAMA, 316*(24), 2627–2646.

Dwyer, A., Aprill, C., & Bogduk, N. (1990). Cervical zygapophyseal joint pain patterns. I: a study in normal volunteers. *Spine (Phila Pa 1976), 15*(6), 453–457.

Engquist, M., Löfgren, H., Öberg, B., et al. (2015). Factors affecting the outcome of surgical versus nonsurgical treatment of cervical radiculopathy. *Spine, 40*(20), 1553–1563.

Engquist, M., Löfgren, H., Öberg, B., et al. (2017). A 5-to 8-year randomized study on the treatment of cervical radiculopathy: anterior cervical decompression and fusion plus physiotherapy versus physiotherapy alone. *Journal of Neurosurgery: Spine, 26*(1), 19–27.

Fejer, R., Kyvik, K. O., & Hartvigsen, J. (2006). The prevalence of neck pain in the world population: a systematic critical review of the literature. *European Spine Journal, 15*(6), 834–848.

Finucane, L. M., Downie, A., Mercer, C., et al. (2020). International framework for red flags for potential serious spinal pathologies. *Journal of Orthopaedic & Sports Physical Therapy, 50*(7), 350–372.

Godek, P., Murawski, P., Ruciński, W., & Guzek, M. (2020). Biological, mechanical or physical? Conservative treatment of cervical radiculopathy. *Ortopedia, Traumatologia, Rehabilitacja, 22*(6), 409–419.

Graham, N., Gross, A. R., Carlesso, L. C., et al. (2013). Suppl 4: an ICON overview on physical modalities for neck pain and associated disorders. *The Open Orthopaedics Journal, 7*, 440.

Gross, A. R., Kaplan, F., Huang, S., et al. (2013). Suppl 4: psychological care, patient education, orthotics, ergonomics and prevention strategies for neck pain: a systematic overview update as part of the ICON project. *The Open Orthopaedics Journal, 7*, 530.

Hill, J., Lewis, M., Papageorgiou, A. C., Dziedzic, K., & Croft, P. (2004). Predicting persistent neck pain: a 1-year follow-up of a population cohort. *Spine, 29*, 1648–1654.

Hoffman, J. R., Mower, W. R., Wolfson, A. B., Todd, K. H., & Zucker, M. I. (2000). Validity of a set of clinical criteria to rule out injury to the cervical spine in patients with blunt trauma. National Emergency X-Radiography Utilization Study Group. *New England Journal of Medicine, 343*, 94–99.

Horn, M. E., Brennan, G. P., George, S. Z., Harman, J. S., & Bishop, M. D. (2015). Description of common clinical presentations and associated short-term physical therapy clinical outcomes in patients with neck pain. *Archives of Physical Medicine and Rehabilitation, 96*(10), 1756–1762.

Hoving, J. L., de Vet, H. C., Twisk, J. W., et al. (2004). Prognostic factors for neck pain in general practice. *Pain, 110*, 639–645.

Hoy, D., March, L., Woolf, A., et al. (2014). The global burden of neck pain: estimates from the global burden of disease 2010 study. *Annals of the Rheumatic Diseases, 73*(7), 1309–1315.

Jain, N. K., Dao, K., & Ortiz, A. O. (2014). Radiologic evaluation and management of postoperative spine paraspinal fluid collections. *Neuroimaging Clinics of North America, 24*, 375–389.

Jull, G., Amiri, M., Bullock-Saxton, J., Darnell, R., & Lander, C. (2007). Cervical musculoskeletal impairment in frequent intermittent headache. Part 1: subjects with single headaches. *Cephalalgia*, *27*(7), 793–802.

Karadimas, S. K., Erwin, W. M., Ely, C. G., Dettori, J. R., & Fehlings, M. G. (2013). Pathophysiology and natural history of cervical spondylotic myelopathy. *Spine*, *38*(22S), S21–36.

Kelly, J., Ritchie, C., & Sterling, M. (2017). Clinical prediction rules for prognosis and treatment prescription in neck pain: a systematic review. *Musculoskeletal Science & Practice*, *27*, 155–164.

Kim, R., Wiest, C., Clark, K., Cook, C., & Horn, M. (2018). Identifying risk factors for first-episode neck pain: a systematic review. *Musculoskeletal Science & Practice*, *33*, 77–83.

Kjellman, G., Skargren, E., & Oberg, B. (2002). Prognostic factors for perceived pain and function at one-year follow-up in primary care patients with neck pain. *Disability and Rehabilitation*, *24*, 364–370.

Kuijper, B., Tans, J. T., van der Kallen, B. F., Nollet, F., Nijeholt, G. J. L. A., & de Visser, M. (2011). Root compression on MRI compared with clinical findings in patients with recent onset cervical radiculopathy. *Journal of Neurology, Neurosurgery and Psychiatry*, *82*, 561–563.

Mahmoud, N. F., Hassan, K. A., Abdelmajeed, S. F., Moustafa, I. M., & Silva, A. G. (2019). The relationship between forward head posture and neck pain: a systematic review and meta-analysis. *Current Reviews in Musculoskeletal. Medicine*, *12*(4), 562–577.

Manchikanti, L., Singh, V., Rivera, J., & Pampati, V. (2002). Prevalence of cervical facet joint pain in chronic neck pain. *Pain Physician*, *5*(3), 243–249.

March, L., Smith, E. U., Hoy, D. G., et al. (2014). Burden of disability due to musculoskeletal (MSK) disorders. *Best Practice & Research: Clinical Rheumatology*, *28*, 353–366.

Matsumoto, M., Fujimura, Y., Suzuki, N., et al. (1998). MRI of cervical intervertebral discs in asymptomatic subjects. *Journal of Bone and Joint Surgery (British)*, *80*, 19–24.

McDonald, M. A., Kirsch, C. F. E., Amin, B. Y., et al. (2018). Cervical neck pain or cervical radiculopathy. Available at: https://acsearch.acr.org/docs/69426/Narrative/. American College of Radiology. Accessed August 31, 2021.

McLean, S. M., May, S., Klaber-Moffett, J., Sharp, D. M., & Gardiner, E. (2010). Risk factors for the onset of non-specific neck pain: a systematic review. *Journal of Epidemiology and Community Health*, *64*(7), 565–572.

Moeri, M., Rothenfluh, D. A., Laux, C. J., & Dominguez, D. E. (2020). Cervical spine clearance after blunt trauma: current state of the art. *EFORT Open Reviews*, *5*(4), 253–259.

Nakashima, H., Yukawa, Y., Suda, K., Yamagata, M., Ueta, T., & Kato, F. (2015). Abnormal findings on magnetic resonance images of the cervical spines in 1211 asymptomatic subjects. *Spine (Phila Pa 1976)*, *40*(6), 392–398.

Nordin, M., Carragee, E. J., Hogg-Johnson, S., et al. (2008). Assessment of neck pain and its associated disorders: results of the bone and joint decade 2000–2010 Task Force on Neck Pain and Its Associated Disorders. *Spine (Phila Pa 1976)*, *33*, S101–122.

Ogince, M., Hall, T., Robinson, K., & Blackmore, A. M. (2007). The diagnostic validity of the cervical flexion-rotation test in C1/2-related cervicogenic headache. *Manual Therapy*, *12*(3), 256–262.

O'Leary, S., Falla, D., Elliott, J. M., & Jull, G. (2009). Muscle dysfunction in cervical spine pain: implications for assessment and management. *Journal of Orthopaedic & Sports Physical Therapy*, *39*(5), 324–333.

Persson, L. C., Carlsson, C. A., & Carlsson, J. Y. (1997). Long-lasting cervical radicular pain managed with surgery, physiotherapy, or a cervical collar: a prospective, randomized study. *Spine*, *22*(7), 751–758.

Pool, J. J., Ostelo, R. W., Hoving, J. L., Bouter, L. M., & de Vet, H. C. (2007). Minimal clinically important change of the Neck Disability Index and the Numerical Rating Scale for patients with neck pain. *Spine (Phila Pa 1976)*, *32*(26), 3047–3051.

Quek, J., Pua, Y. -H., Clark, R. A., & Bryant, A. L. (2013). Effects of thoracic kyphosis and forward head posture on cervical range of motion in older adults. *Manual Therapy*, *18*(1), 65–71.

Raney, N. H., Petersen, E. J., Smith, T. A., et al. (2009). Development of a clinical prediction rule to identify patients with neck pain likely to benefit from cervical traction and exercise. *European Spine Journal*, *18*(3), 382–391.

Rempel, D. M., Harrison, R. J., & Barnhart, S. (1992). Work-related cumulative trauma disorders of the upper extremity. *JAMA*, *267*, 838–842.

Rhee, J. M., Shamji, M. F., Erwin, W. M., et al. (2013). Nonoperative management of cervical myelopathy: a systematic review. *Spine*, *38*(22S), S55–67.

Ritchie, C., & Sterling, M. (2016). Recovery pathways and prognosis after whiplash injury. *Journal of Orthopaedic & Sports Physical Therapy*, *46*(10), 851–861.

Romeo, A., Vanti, C., Boldrini, V., et al. (2018). Cervical radiculopathy: effectiveness of adding traction to physical therapy—a systematic review and meta-analysis of randomized controlled trials. *Physical Therapy*, *98*(4), 231–242.

Rushton, A., Rivett, D., Carlesso, L., Flynn, T., Hing, W., & Kerry, R. (2014). International framework for examination of the cervical region for potential of cervical arterial dysfunction prior to orthopaedic manual therapy intervention. *Manual Therapy*, *19*(3), 222–228.

Saifi, C., Fein, A. W., Cazzulino, A., et al. (2018). Trends in resource utilization and rate of cervical disc arthroplasty and anterior cervical discectomy and fusion throughout the United States from 2006 to 2013. *The Spine Journal*, *18*(6), 1022–1029.

Schellhas, K. P., Smith, M. D., Gundry, C. R., & Pollei, S. R. (1996). Cervical discogenic pain: prospective correlation of magnetic resonance imaging and discography in asymptomatic subjects and pain sufferers. *Spine*, *21*(3), 300–311.

Schellingerhout, J.M., Heymans, M.W., & Verhagen, A.P., et al. (2010). Prognosis of patients with nonspecific neck pain: development and external validation of a prediction rule for persistence of complaints. Spine, 35, E827–E835.

Shedid, D., & Benzel, E. C. (2007). Cervical spondylosis anatomy: pathophysiology and biomechanics. *Neurosurgery*, *60*(suppl_1), S1–7.

Slipman, C. W., Plastaras, C., Patel, R., et al. (2005). Provocative cervical discography symptom mapping. *The Spine Journal*, *5*(4), 381–388.

Sterling, M. (2004). A proposed new classification system for whiplash associated disorders—implications for assessment and management. *Manual Therapy*, *9*(2), 60–70.

Sterling, M. (2007). Patient specific functional scale. *Australian Journal of Physiotherapy*, *53*(1), 65–66.

Stiell, I. G., Wells, G. A., Vandemheen, K. L., et al. (2001). The Canadian C-spine rule for radiography in alert and stable trauma patients. *JAMA*, *286*, 1841–1848.

Sugawara, T. (2015). Anterior cervical spine surgery for degenerative disease: a review. *Neurologia medico-chirurgica*, *55*(7), 540–546.

Teasell, R. W., McClure, J. A., Walton, D., et al. (2010). A research synthesis of therapeutic interventions for whiplash-associated disorder (WAD): part 2–interventions for acute WAD. *Pain Research and Management*, *15*(5), 295–304.

Thoomes, E. J., Scholten-Peeters, W., Koes, B., Falla, D., & Verhagen, A. P. (2013). The effectiveness of conservative treatment for patients with cervical radiculopathy: a systematic review. *The Clinical Journal of Pain*, *29*(12), 1073–1086.

Thoomes, E. J., van Geest, S., van der Windt, D. A., et al. (2018). Value of physical tests in diagnosing cervical radiculopathy: a systematic review. *Spine Journal*, *18*, 179–189.
Thoomes-de Graaf, M., Fernández-De-Las-Peñas, C., & Cleland, J. A. (2020). The content and construct validity of the modified patient specific functional scale (PSFS 2.0) in individuals with neck pain. *Journal of Manual & Manipulative Therapy*, *28*(1), 49–59.
Vernon, H. (2008). The Neck Disability Index: state-of-the-art, 1991-2008. *Journal of Manipulative and Physiological Therapeutics*, *31*(7), 491–502.
Verwoerd, M., Wittink, H., Maissan, F., de Raaij, E., & Smeets, R. J. (2019). Prognostic factors for persistent pain after a first episode of nonspecific idiopathic, non-traumatic neck pain: a systematic review. *Musculoskeletal Science and Practice*, *42*, 13–37.
Vincent, M. B., & Luna, R. A. (1999). Cervicogenic headache: a comparison with migraine and tension- type headache. *Cephalalgia*, *19*(S25), 11–16.
Wainner, R. S., Fritz, J. M., Irrgang, J. J., et al. (2003). Reliability and diagnostic accuracy of the clinical examination and patient self-report measures for cervical radiculopathy. Spine, 28(1), 52–62.
Walton, D. M., & Elliott, J. M. (2017). An integrated model of chronic whiplash-associated disorder. *Journal of Orthopaedic & Sports Physical Therapy*, *47*(7), 462–471.
Westaway, M. D., Stratford, P. W., & Binkley, J. M. (1998). The patient-specific functional scale: validation of its use in persons with neck dysfunction. *Journal of Orthopaedic & Sports Physical Therapy*, *27*(5), 331–338.
Wingbermühle, R. W., van Trijffel, E., Nelissen, P. M., Koes, B., & Verhagen, A. P. (2018). Few promising multivariable prognostic models exist for recovery of people with non-specific neck pain in musculoskeletal primary care: a systematic review. *Journal of Physiotherapy*, *64*(1), 16–23.
Wright, A., Mayer, T. G., & Gatchel, R. J. (1999). Outcomes of disabling cervical spine disorders in compensation injuries. A prospective comparison to tertiary rehabilitation response for chronic lumbar spinal disorders. *Spine (Phila Pa 1976)*, *24*, 178–183.
Young, B. A., Walker, M. J., Strunce, J. B., Boyles, R. E., Whitman, J. M., & Childs, J. D. (2009). Responsiveness of the Neck Disability Index in patients with mechanical neck disorders. *Spine Journal*, *9*(10), 802–808.
Zito, G., Jull, G., & Story, I. (2006). Clinical tests of musculoskeletal dysfunction in the diagnosis of cervicogenic headache. *Manual Therapy*, *11*(2), 118–129.

CHAPTER 54 QUESTIONS

1. **How is red flag screening utilized in the assessment of patients with neck pain?**
   a. During the physical examination only
   b. in the history and physical examination
   c. in response to the intervention
   d. when reviewing diagnostic imaging

2. **What are common impairments for patients with neck pain in each of the 4 categories identified in the CPGs?**
   a. Limited neck mobility, pain at rest, and reduced strength of muscles within a single myotome.
   b. Pain, increased fear avoidance behaviors, difficulty lifting, limited ADLs.
   c. Limited neck mobility, decreased strength of neck and upper quarter muscles, and decreased proprioception.
   d. Increased fear avoidance behaviors, limited mobility, decreased sensation, decreased reflexes.

3. **When is traction indicated for a patient with neck pain?**
   a. With acute or subacute neck pain with pain relief after repeated axial extension.
   b. With subacute neck pain with irritability and pain with movement and limited cervical flexion.
   c. With acute neck pain only, less than ten days in duration and negative neurological signs and no radiating pain into the extremity.
   d. With chronic neck pain and when relief of peripheral symptoms occur during a distraction test as performed during a radiculopathy testing cluster.

4. **How do physical therapists determine an appropriate intervention strategy/plan of care for patients with neck pain?**
   a. Physical therapists can use the International Classification of Functioning, Disability and Health classification for neck pain which provides a framework for an impairment and treatment-based approach to managing patients with neck pain. These classifications consider patient history and subjective reporting combined with physical exam features to guide the physical therapist in selecting evidence-based interventions.
   b. Physical therapists can use the International Classification of Functioning, Disability and Health classification for diagnostic purposes to guide the referral of patients to other practitioners. The classification system is of limited use for guiding intervention choices.
   c. Physical therapists can use the International Classification of Functioning, Disability and Health classification for screening radiculopathy but it is of little value with other conditions.
   d. Physical therapists can use the International Classification of Functioning, Disability and Health classification for research purposes to quantify and classify subjects into specific categories. It is of little value guiding the physical therapist in selecting evidence-based interventions.

TEMPOROMANDIBULAR JOINT

S. Ho, PT, DPT, MS, OCS

CHAPTER 55

1. **What are the unique features of the temporomandibular joint (TMJ)?**
   The TMJ is divided by a disk into an upper and a lower joint cavity. During mouth opening, rotation of the condylar head takes place in the inferior cavity and translation occurs in the superior cavity. The TMJ and the disk are both covered with fibrocartilage that has a superior reparative property to wear and tear. The TMJ, functioning as one of a pair, must perform coordinated movements.

2. **How does temporomandibular dysfunction (TMD) manifest clinically?**
   Clinical symptoms of TMD include pain in the masseter, temporalis, head, face and neck area; headaches; dizziness; vertigo; earache or fullness; tinnitus; TMJ noises; toothache; myofascial pain; swallowing difficulty; speech disturbance; etc.

3. **What are the causes of TMD?**
   Macrotrauma: a blow to the face (by a direct force as in a fist fight or from a fall), auto accident resulting in neck and jaw injury, prolonged opening of the mouth during oral/dental procedure, etc.
   Microtrauma: parafunction, eg, clenching and bruxing, or playing with tongue and lips; strain of masticatory and cervical muscles due to poor posture or daily stress, etc.

4. **What is the anatomic attachment and the function of the disk?**
   Anteriorly, the disk is attached to the superior belly of the lateral pterygoid muscle. The posterosuperior portion of the disk is attached to the superior stratum, and the posteroinferior portion is attached to the inferior stratum. Medially and laterally, the disk is attached to the medial/lateral poles of the condylar head, respectively, through the medial and lateral collateral ligaments. The disk protects and lubricates the articulating surfaces. It also accepts force that is exerted upon the TMJ.

5. **Describe the innervation of the TMJ.**
   The anterior and medial regions of the TMJ are innervated by the deep temporal and masseteric nerves. The posterior and lateral regions of the TMJ are innervated by the auriculotemporal nerve. These three nerves arise from the mandibular division of the trigeminal nerve.

6. **What are the kinematic movements of mouth opening?**
   During the early phase of mouth opening (11–25 mm), anterior rotation of the condylar head is the primary movement. During the late phase (25 mm to end range) of mouth opening, anterior translation of the condylar head is the primary movement. Currently, the predominant opinion of researchers is that rotation and translation occurs simultaneously, with varying dominance during different phases.

7. **Describe the functional range and normal range of mouth opening.**
   The functional range of mouth opening (approximately 35 mm) is measured by three fingers' width (or two knuckles' width) of the nondominant hand; the normal range is measured by four fingers' width (or three knuckles' width) of the nondominant hand. For men, the normal range of opening is between 40 and 45 mm; for women, the normal range of opening is between 45 and 50 mm.

8. **What is the normal range of motion for lateral excursion, protrusion, and retrusion?**
   The normal range of lateral excursion is usually one fourth of the normal opening. For example, if a person has a 48 mm opening, then the lateral excursion is expected to be 12 mm. The normal range of protrusion is approximately 6 to 9 mm, and the retrusion range is approximately 3 mm.

9. **What are the elevators of the mandible?**
   The masseter, temporalis, and medial pterygoid muscles are the three major elevators of the mandible. The superior belly of the lateral pterygoid muscle is active during the closing phase of the mouth, but its function is primarily for stabilization of the disk in relationship to the condylar head.

10. What are the depressors of the mandible?

The depressors of the mandible are the inferior belly of the lateral pterygoid, digastric, mylohyoid, geniohyoid, and stylohyoid muscles.

11. Describe the muscle function and kinematics of lateral deviation.

When the mandible deviates to one side, the muscles involved are the ipsilateral temporalis, the contralateral medial pterygoid, and the contralateral lateral pterygoid. Arthrokinematically, the ipsilateral condyle rotates and spins forward, downward, and medially, while the contralateral condyle translates horizontally toward the ipsilateral side.

12. What is the role of the masseter muscle in oral function?

Superficial masseter fibers: mandible elevation and protrusion.

Deep masseter fibers: mandible elevation and retrusion.

Unilateral contraction of the masseter muscle causes slight ipsilateral excursion.

13. What is the role of the temporalis in oral function?

Mandible elevation, ipsilateral deviation, retrusion.

14. What is the role of the lateral pterygoid in oral function?

Approximately 30% of the superior belly of the lateral pterygoid muscle attaches to the anteromedial portion of the articular disk. This superior belly is active during mandibular elevation, especially in the last phase of forceful chewing between molars. It helps to stabilize the disk and the condyle in a functional position. Spasm of the superior belly of the lateral pterygoid muscle can result in anterior displacement of the disk because of its anteromedial pull on the disk during contraction.

The inferior belly of the lateral pterygoid muscle inserts on the anterior surface of the condylar neck. When it contracts, the lateral pterygoid depresses, protrudes, and deviates the mandible to the contralateral side.

Unilateral contraction of both bellies of the lateral pterygoid muscle produces effective contralateral deviation. Bilateral contraction of the lateral pterygoid muscles produces strong protrusion of the mandible.

15. How is pain arising from the disk differentiated from pain arising from muscular contraction?

Using a cotton roll, the patient bites down with the back molars. If pain increases, muscular or ligamentous involvement is indicated. If pain decreases (because of decreased pressure on the disk caused by gapping the TMJ), the disk is involved. This finding can be further confirmed by asking the patient to bite down on the cotton roll with the contralateral molars. If pain increases on the ipsilateral side (due to compression on the TMJ), then the disk is affected.

16. Define parafunctional habits.

Clenching, bruxing, biting nails, sucking on cheeks, chewing gum, and biting lips are examples of parafunctional habits. These nonfunctioning, repetitive movements can cause microtrauma to the soft tissue and the hard structure. Microtrauma may result in pain, spasm, altered mandibular dynamics, abnormal development, osteoarthritis, and TMJ dysfunction.

17. How does an anteriorly displaced disk present clinically?

There are two categories of anteriorly displaced disk. In the case of anteriorly displaced disk with reduction (ADDwR), a louder opening click, and a milder closing click (reciprocal clicks), may be heard. The mouth opening pattern is usually demonstrated by a "C" curve or "S" curve, with pain during the pathway.

In the case of anteriorly displaced disk without reduction (ADDwoR), the patient usually has pain and limited opening with deflection to the involved side. Mouth opening is limited to less than 40 mm and the joint noise is absent.

When the ADDwR is not properly treated, it very often will progress to the ADDwoR condition. At this time, patient will report a history of reciprocal clicks before the occurrence of the absent joint noise with limited opening.

18. What is the cluster of clinical tests recommended by Julsvoll et al. to be used in diagnosing ADDwoR when 5/7 tests are positive?

1. The joint provocation test (mouth opening with pain)
2. The deviation test (deflection to the ipsilateral side at end of opening
3. The laterotrusion test (limited lateral excursion, less than 9 mm to the contralateral test)
4. The joint mobility test (reduced anterior translation of the condylar head upon palpation)
5. The joint sound test (absent joint noise)

6. The dental stick test (pain elicited either in the ipsilateral or contralateral joint when the patient is being asked to bite down on a tongue depressor placed between the back molars)
7. The isometric test (pain is elicited when manual isometric resistance is given to lateral excursion contralaterally)

19. **What is an open lock?**
An open lock is the inability to close the mouth when the condyle is locked in an open position. This usually happens after wide opening from yawning or a prolonged dental procedure. The most likely cause is a posteriorly displaced disk.
Patient with an open lock will demonstrate an open mouth occlusion and may report closing click in the case of reduction.

20. **Explain the significance of opening with a C curve or S curve.**
Altered TMJ kinematics is often presented by mouth opening with deviation. A "C" curve usually indicates a capsular pattern, or in the case of ADDwR, when the jaw returning to the center after the disk is relocated. An "S" curve during opening usually indicates muscle imbalance or incoordination. This can also occur in the case of ADDwR. (Reciprocal clicks is another symptom that can confirm the condition of ADDwR.) In the case of ADDwoR, the mandible will deflect to the ipsilateral side with limited range, and without joint noise.

21. **What is the ideal resting position of the tongue?**
With the head and neck in neutral position, the tip of the tongue is placed lightly against the roof of the mouth (the palate), not touching the back of the upper front teeth. Upper and lower lips are kept together, and back molars are kept apart. This position is especially important for patient who clenches or grinds at night.

22. **Describe the connection between TMD and forward-headed posture.**
Patients with TMD demonstrate a more forward-headed posture than patients without TMD. Generally, it is believed that approximately 85% of patients with TMD hold a forward-headed posture.
The tight suboccipital muscles caused by the habitual forward-headed posture rotate the cranium posteriorly and may pressure the greater occipital nerve, which may result in symptoms in the head, neck, and facial area.
A forward-headed posture stretches infrahyoid and suprahyoid muscles, which in turn pulls the mandible in a direction of retrusion and depression. The change of the condyle position within the fossa will set off a vicious cycle of muscle spasm and disk displacement.

23. **How can TMJ problems cause dizziness, headache, and ear symptoms?**
The TMJ is innervated by the trigeminal nerve. The neurons from the trigeminal nerve (cranial nerve V) share the same neuron pool as the upper cervical nerves (cervical nerves 1, 2, and 3) and cranial nerves VII, IX, X, and XI. Consequently, all the afferent nerves converge and may affect each other's innervation. This area, the so-called trigeminocervical nucleus, is considered the principal nociceptive center for the entire head, face, and upper neck. Any pain in the TMJ area can be transmitted through the trigeminocervical nucleus to the head and neck area and can be perceived as symptoms arising from the head and neck.
Patients with TMJ problems usually demonstrate forward-headed posture and suffer from cervical dysfunction. Tightness of the cervical musculature may compromise vertebrobasilar blood flow, which is one of the causes of dizziness. On the other hand, disturbances in the cervical column, whether they originate from muscles, ligaments, or joints, can interfere with tonic neck reflexes and also affect the function of the vestibular nuclei.
The auriculotemporal nerve (a branch of the trigeminal nerve that is both efferent and afferent of the TMJ) innervates the posterolateral region of the TMJ. This nerve also sends a few branches to innervate the tympanic membrane, the external auditory meatus, and the lateral surface of the superior auricle. Therefore, any symptom that affects the auriculotemporal nerve may cause earache, ear fullness, or tinnitus.

24. **Can PT be helpful for patients suffering from nonotological ear symptoms?**
Yes. The nonotological ear symptoms are often caused by poor posture, cervical dysfunction, and TMJ disorder. PT intervention is effective in managing these areas and therefore can be helpful in relieving ear symptoms.

25. **Describe current evidence-informed PT management for patients with TMD.**
- Patient education: posture, body mechanics, tongue resting position, soft diet.
- Modalities: heat/cold, ultrasound, electrical stimulation, light therapy.
- Manual therapy: myofascial release (intra-oral and extra-oral), joint mobilization, manipulation.
- Home exercise program: TMJ exercise, cervical spine exercise, postural exercise, diaphragmatic breathing, progressive relaxation, aerobic reconditioning, sleep hygiene.
- Stress management, chronic pain management.

26. **Discuss the roles of splints.**

The repositioning splint is generally used to recapture the anteriorly dislocated disk and/or manage the disk-condyle discoordination. It should be worn continuously throughout the day and night except during oral cleaning or eating. The duration may last from a few weeks to several months, depending on the progress in joint stability. The goal of the repositioning splint is to achieve the centric occlusion position of the mandible to relax the masticatory muscles and to stabilize the disk-condyle complex.

The resting splint is preferred when relaxation or balancing of soft tissue is desired. This type of splint can be worn during the day or only at night to offset the soft tissue reaction from nocturnal clenching and/or bruxing.

27. **What imaging modalities are used to diagnose TMD?**

Plain radiography of the TMJ includes lateral transcranial, transpharyngeal, and transorbital projections. The lateral transcranial projection is used most often; it images the lateral one third to one half of the condyle and fossa but does not include the condylar neck. The transpharyngeal projection images the lateral and medial portions of the condyle; in combination with the transorbital projection, it images the condylar neck.

Panoramic radiography is a modified tomogram used to provide a comprehensive view of the dental and bony structure.

Arthrograms are used to identify soft tissue abnormalities (eg, disk displacement, disk perforation, or retrodiskal inflammation). This technique involves the injection of a contrast medium into the joint space followed by static or dynamic imaging. Arthrography is the most sensitive technique for detecting soft tissue perforation; however, it is invasive and involves high levels of radiation exposure.

Magnetic resonance imaging (MRI) provides the most accurate information about the soft tissues of the TMJ. Disk position and disk condition can be identified with MRI. The use of dynamic MRI can reveal functional information of the joint studied (ie, ADD wR or ADDwoR).

Ultrasonic imaging has gained increasing popularity in recent years for the study of TMD. It is noninvasive, nonradioactive, cost effective, and easy to operate. The bony structures and the soft tissues of the TMJ can be clearly visualized with ultrasound. However, the disk material is difficult to detect due to its location.

28. **What evidence exists in the literature regarding the efficacy of physical therapy for TMD?**

Calixtre conducted a systematic review of RTCs on manual therapy for patients with TMD. They concluded that manual therapy techniques (myofascial release and massage) can improve pain and maximal mouth opening in patients with TMD.

Armijo-Olivo et al. conducted a systematic review and meta-analysis to study the effectiveness of manual therapy and therapeutic exercises for TMDs. They concluded that the combination of these two treatments produced superior outcome in pain reduction and mouth opening.

Gil-Martinez recommended using a biobehavioral model (medical, physiotherapeutic, psychological, and dental) to manage patients with TMD, especially in the case of chronic condition.

Porto De Toledo et al., through their systematic review and meta-analysis, reported that a high prevalence of fullness (74.8%), otalgia (ear pain, 55.1%), tinnitus (52.1%), vertigo (40.8%), and hearing loss (38.9%) is present in patients with TMD. Marciel et al. reported that the number of ontological symptoms was considerably higher in patients with moderate and severe TMD.

Michiels et al. reported the positive effect of PT treatment to CS and TMJ in patients with nonotological tinnitus.

Durham et al. reported the definition of self-management (through an international Delphi process) included: education, self-exercise, self-massage, thermal therapy, dietary advice and nutrition, parafunctional behavior identification, monitoring, and avoidance.

29. **What is the evidence of dry needling in TMD management?**

According to the systemic review and meta-analysis conducted by Machado et al. and Vier et al. the evidence is weak in favor of dry needling for myofascial pain connected to TMD.

Gonzalez-Perez et al. reported positive dry needling effect in the lateral pterygoid muscles than the oral medication in the management of chronic myofascial pain.

Blasco-Bonora and Martin-Pintado-Zugasti reported positive effect of dry needling for myofascial trigger points in patients with sleep bruxism and TMD.

Butts et al. in their literature review of the conservative management of TMD reported that dry needling to the lateral pterygoid muscle and posterior peri-articular connective tissues is the most evidence-based method for reducing pain and disability in patients with TMD.

30. **How does one palpate the pterygoid place intraorally?**

With the small finger of the therapist's hand, follow the patient's maxillary arch all the way to behind the back molar; there is a small indentation that can be palpated that is the so-called "pterygoid place." This is usually a very sensitive area when the patient is suffering from TMD.

31. **What is the "condylar remodeling exercise"?**
Also known as the "tubing" exercise, the patient is instructed to place a 1 cm plastic tubing between the maxillary and mandibular incisors. Movement in the direction of lateral excursion, protrusion, and retrusion is then recommended. At the end of each range, if no pain is reported, then the patient is instructed to bite down on the tubing to stabilize the joint and return to the neutral position. Attempt to distract the plastic tube while patient bites down on the tube in the neutral position is another way to provide the condyle-disk congruency. This exercise can recruit the muscles of mastication to stabilize the disk and provide remodeling of the condyle.

Bibliography

Armijo-Olivo, S., Pitance, L., Singh, V., Neto, F., Thie, N., & Michelotti, A. (2016). Effectiveness of manual therapy and therapeutic exercise for temporomandibular disorders: systematic review and meta-analysis. *Physical Therapy, 96*(1), 9–25.

Blasco-Bonora, P. M., & Martin-Pintado-Zugasti, A. (2017). Effects of myofascial trigger point dry needling in patients with sleep bruxism and temporomandibular disorders: a prospective case series. *Acupuncture in Medicine, 35*(1), 69–74.

Butts, R., Dunning, J., Pavkovich, R., Mettille, J., & Mourad, F. (2017). Conservative management of temporomandibular dysfunction: a literature review with implications for clinical practice guidelines (Narrative review part 2). *Journal of Bodywork and Movement Therapies, 21*(3), 541–548.

Calixtre, L. B., Moreira, R. F., Franchini, G. H., Alburquerque-Sendin, F., & Oliveira, A. B. (2015). Manual therapy for the management of pain and limited range of motion in subjects with signs and symptoms of temporomandibular disorder: a systematic review of randomized controlled trials. *Journal of Oral Rehabilitation, 42*(11), 847–861.

Durham, J., Al-Baghdadi, M., Baad-Hansen, L., et al. (2016). Self-management programs in temporomandibular disorders: results from an international Delphi process. *Journal of Oral Rehabilitation, 43*(12), 929–936.

Gil-Martinez, A., Paris-Alemany, A., Lopez-de-Uralde-Villanueva, I., & La Touche, R. (2018). Management of pain in patients with temporomandibular disorder (TMD): challenges and solutions. *Journal of Pain Research, 11*, 571–587.

Gonzalez-Perez, L. M., Infante-Cossio, P., Granados-Nunez, M., Urresti-Lopez, F. J., Lopez-Martos, R., & Ruiz-Canela-Mendez, P. (2015). Deep dry needling of trigger points located in the lateral pterygoid muscle: efficacy and safety of treatment for management of myofascial pain and temporomandibular dysfunction. *Medicina Oral, Patologia Oral, Cirugia Bucal, 20*(3), e326–e333.

Julsvoll, E. H., Vøllestad, N. K., & Robinson, H. S. (2016). Validation of clinical tests for patients with long-lasting painful temporomandibular disorders with anterior disc displacement without reduction. *Manual Therapy, 21*, 109–119.

Machado, E., Machado, P., Wandscher, V. F., Marchionatti, A. M. E., Zanatta, F. B., & Kaizer, O. B. (2018). A systematic review of different substance injection and dry needling for treatment of temporomandibular myofascial pain. *International Journal of Oral and Maxillofacial Surgery, 47*(11), 1420–1432.

Maciel, L. F. O., Landim, F. S., & Vasconcelos, B. C. (2018). Otological findings and other symptoms related to temporomandibular disorders in young people. *British Journal of Oral and Maxillofacial Surgery, 56*(8), 739–743.

Michiels, S., De Hertogh, W., Truijen, S., & Van de Heyning, P. (2014). Physical therapy treatment in patients suffering from cervicogenic somatic tinnitus: study protocol for a randomized controlled trial. *Trials, 15*, 297.

Porto De Toledo, I., Stefani, F. M., Porporatti, A. L., et al. (2017). Prevalence of otologic signs and symptoms in adult patients with temporomandibular disorders: a systematic review and meta-analysis. *Clinical Oral Investigations, 21*(2), 597–605.

Vier, C., Almeida, M. B., Neves, M. L., Santos, A., & Bracht, M. A. (2019). The effectiveness of dry needling for patients with orofacial pain associated with temporomandibular dysfunction: a systematic review and meta-analysis. *Brazilian Journal of Physical Therapy, 23*(1), 3–11.

CHAPTER 55 QUESTIONS

JM is a 24-year-old female who was involved in a rear-end automobile accident 6 months prior to her first visit to your clinic.

Patient reports that she only noticed pain in her cervical spine area with intermittent headache initially. The physical therapy intervention she received after the accident was primarily focused on her cervical spine complaint. After 2 months, she noticed increasing pain in her right TMJ area, with limited opening. She also reports that she used to hear a loud clicking noise when she opened her mouth, followed by a milder click when she closed her mouth, and now the joint noise has disappeared.

Upon objective assessment, you found that the patient had a limited mouth opening to 35 mm, with her jaw deflected to the right side. Her lateral excursion was 7 mm to the left and 10 mm to the right. There is no audible joint noise on either side during auscultation.

1. **What will be your working hypothesis at this time?**
   a. OA of the TMJ.
   b. ADDwR of the Left TMJ.
   c. ADDwoR of the Left TMJ.
   d. ADDwR of the Right TMJ.
   e. ADDwoR of the Right TMJ.

2. **Which of the following statements is accurate?**
   a. There is no connection between CS symptoms and TMJ disorder.
   b. Posture only affects the symptoms of CS, not TMJ.
   c. Education regarding proper posture and relaxation can relieve this patient's TMJ symptoms.
   d. Sleep hygiene should be addressed by OTR only.

3. What would be a most desirable outcome of PT for this patient?

a. Opening to 45 mm.
b. Return to the stage of reciprocal joint noises.
c. Normalize opening pattern.
d. Opening to 40 mm, with lateral excursion to 10 mm bilaterally.

4. Which of the following is the best combination of PT intervention for patients with TMD?

a. Heat, ultrasound, soft tissue release, stretching, home exercise program.
b. Postural correction, stress management, home exercise program.
c. Patient education regarding TMJ care, soft tissue release, joint mobilization, home exercise program.
d. Dry needling, postural correction, body mechanics instruction, home exercise program.

THORACIC SPINE AND RIB CAGE DYSFUNCTION

M.W. Reynolds, PT, DPT, EdD and T.W. Flynn, PT, PhD, OCS, FAAOMPT, FAPTA

1. **What is the prevalence of thoracic spine pain and pathologies?**
   Prevalence estimates for thoracic spine pain vary widely. The point prevalence in adolescent 13- to 20-year-olds ranged from 4.0% to 41.0% and in children from 4.0% up to 72.0%, seemingly making children more likely to experience thoracic spine pain. Thoracic disc herniations are prevalent in individuals 20 to 59 years of age, depending on the literature source. Of all disc herniations, the thoracic region was the least likely region for these to occur. Thoracic disc herniations were most common at T7-8. The T8-9 segment was the second most common followed by the T11-12 segment. Those with a thoracic disc herniation were likely to have more than one disc herniation in the thoracic spine. Schmorl's nodes are degenerative impairments that could present in the thoracic spine. Individuals 40 years and older were more prone to Schmorl's nodes than those in the first three decades of life.

2. **Describe the normal range of motion (ROM) of the thoracic spine.**
   The rib cage and sternum attachments limit ROM of the thoracic spine. Inclinometry of T1–T12 indicates that the total range of sagittal plane motion is approximately 36 degrees (16 degrees of flexion and 20 degrees of extension from neutral posture). Frontal plane motion is approximately 44 degrees (24 degrees of right-side bending and 20 degrees of left-side bending from neutral posture).

3. **Describe the preferred side-bending and rotation-coupling pattern of the thoracic spin.**
   Systematic review of the literature to date shows variability in the coupling patterns of the thoracic spine. Study design and methodology variations may be to blame for some of the differences in findings. No consistent coupling pattern has been recognized whether the thoracic spine is flexed, extended, or in neutral position or whether axial rotation, side-bending, or upper extremity movement was initiated first. Even with recent advances in the accuracy of three-dimensional computed tomography assessments, consistency could only be found in the upper thoracic spine (T1–6), where axial rotation was coupled with side bending to the same side. The middle and lower thoracic spine (T6–L1) side bending occurred to the same and opposite direction as the axial rotation.

   Past premise has been that when the spine is neither flexed nor extended, side bending and rotation were coupled in opposite directions (right-side bending with left rotation). It had also been suggested that the coupling pattern was sensitive to which plane of movement was introduced first; Lee suggested that rotation and side bending couple to the same side in the thoracic spine when rotation is introduced first.

4. **How accurate can a physical therapist be with manual examination of the thoracic spine?**
   Similar to the lumbar and cervical mobility assessment, intrarater-reliability findings are often variable but can reach substantial agreement in some studies while interrater reliability rarely exceeds fair. Passive physiologic intervertebral motion examination has shown agreement between 63.4% and 82.5%. Palpation for tenderness or pain typically increases the reliability measures. However, we should be cautious of false positives when relying heavily on the subjective report of pain provocation, especially in those patients with chronic widespread pain presentations.

5. **What effects has thoracic spine manipulation been found to have?**
   There is a growing body of evidence emerging on the study of treatment directed at the thoracic spine. A systematic review by Walser et al. in 2009 screened 242 articles pertaining to thoracic spine or cervicothoracic manipulation. Quality research is showing that thoracic spine manipulation has a positive effect on patients with shoulder or neck pain and disability. The exact mechanism by which these effects occur has not been determined, but accepted theories include a regional interdependence model that may also include neurophysiologic and other nonspecific effects. In patients with mechanical neck pain, thoracic thrust manipulation at thoracic level(s) with limited mobility can provide immediate improvement in a patient's Visual Analog Scale (VAS) rating and the Neck Disability Index (NDI).

6. **How many articulations are present on the typical thoracic vertebra?**
   A typical thoracic vertebra has 12 separate articulations: 4 zygapophyseal articulations, 2 costotransverse articulations, 4 costovertebral articulations, and 2 body-IV disc-body articulations. At present, individual passive assessment of these components is likely to be fraught with difficulty and poor reliability.

7. **Describe the typical pattern of rib cage motion.**
The typical upper rib motion during respiration is termed pump handle (sagittal plane elevation), whereas lower rib motion is termed bucket handle (frontal plane flaring). Lee's model suggests that during spinal flexion, the rib rotates anteriorly; posterior elements move superiorly and anterior elements move inferiorly. This pattern is termed internal torsional movement. During spinal extension, the opposite movement is proposed, with the rib rotating posteriorly; posterior elements move inferiorly and anterior elements move superiorly. This pattern is termed external torsional movement. This model has not been validated with in vivo motion studies. Various authors and one case report have outlined the potential clinical presentation and significant loss of this movement.

8. **Describe the cervical rotation lateral flexion (CRLF) test.**
The CRLF determines the presence of first rib hypomobility in patients with brachialgia. The test is performed with the patient in a sitting position. The cervical spine is rotated passively and maximally away from the side being tested (ie, rotation to the left to test the right side). In this position, the spine is gently flexed as far as possible, moving the ear toward the chest. A test is considered positive when lateral flexion movement is blocked. Lindgren and colleagues reported excellent interrater reliability (K = 1.0) and good agreement with cineradiographic findings (K = 0.84).

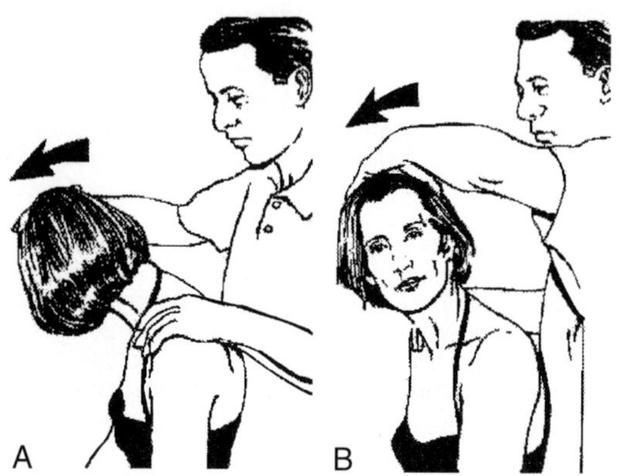

Cervical rotation lateral flexion (CRLF) test: A, negative; B, positive.

9. **Define thoracic outlet syndrom.**
Thoracic outlet syndrome (TOS) is perhaps the most controversial symptom complex in surgery. Even the use of established operation criteria before surgery results in the relief of symptoms in only 28% of patients undergoing first-rib resection. Diagnoses using the traditional positional provocation tests of the upper extremity are unreliable and result in a large number of false positives. Conservative therapy aimed at restoring function to the upper thoracic aperture in patients with TOS decreased symptoms and returned patients to work after intervention and at a 2-year follow-up. Therefore conservative management is advocated. Lower-level evidence (case series) describes treating a "subluxation" of the first rib with manual therapy techniques with subsequent reduction of symptoms attributed to TOS.

10. **Describe the typical pattern of movement and positional dysfunction of the thoracic spine and rib cage.**
In general, the upper two segments of the thoracic spine often have restricted ability to extend fully, resulting in a flexed (kyphotic) posture in this region. The T3–T7 segments often have restricted ability to flex and concurrent external rib torsional dysfunction, resulting in an extended (flat) posture in this region. The T8–T12 segments often have restricted ability to extend, resulting in a flexed (kyphotic) posture in this region.

11. **Describe a classification system for thoracic spine and rib cage dysfunction.**
Patients in whom specific mobilization is indicated have primary single segmental restriction of either flexion or extension, torsional rib cage dysfunction, and/or first-rib restriction. The immobilization category includes patients who require motion restriction. The rib subluxations are the primary candidates for this treatment, which is geared at using the patient's muscle activity to restore normal symmetry and to avoid movement stresses in directions that promote asymmetry. Segmental thoracic hypermobility or instability also is placed in this category.

The nonspecific mobilization category does not imply gross mobilization but rather the treatment of multiple segments in the neutral (neither flexed nor extended) spine. Rib cage restrictions in either inhalation or exhalation also fall into this category.

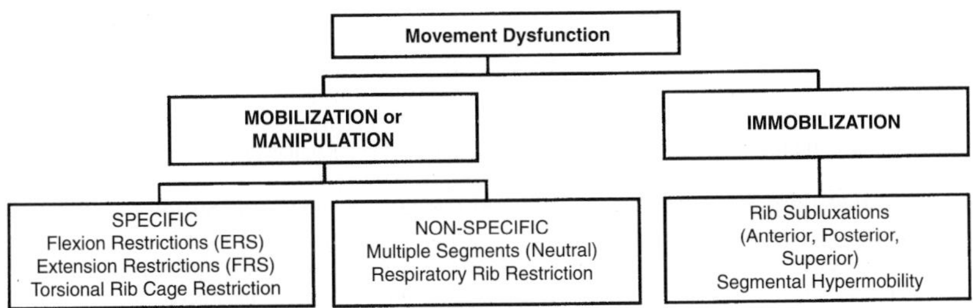

Classification and treatment scheme for thoracic spine and rib dysfunction.

12. Does osteoporosis frequently involve the thoracic spine?

Osteoporosis is associated with loss of bone mass per unit of volume. Loss of bone mass in the axial skeleton predisposes vertebral bodies to fracture, which results in back pain and deformity. An anterior wedge compression fracture is manifested by a decrease in anterior height, usually 4 mm or greater, compared with the vertical height of the posterior body.

13. What are the symptoms of thoracic osteoporosis? How are they treated?

Symptomatic osteoporosis presents as midline back pain localized over the thoracic or lumbar spine, the most common location for fractures. The treatment of osteoporosis is often complex and, in severely affected patients, should be coordinated with an endocrinologist. Treatment should include exercise, which has been shown to increase or slow the decline of skeletal mass. Weight-bearing activities should be emphasized.

14. What systemic pathologies could present to as a potential thoracic musculoskeletal dysfunction?

Pain in the thoracic region should be carefully screened due to visceral structure pain referral patterns. The organs from the cardiovascular, pulmonary, urinary, and gastrointestinal systems have innervation from the thoracic nerves. Musculoskeletal chest wall syndromes have been reported in as many as 28% of patients admitted to the ED with acute chest pain but without acute myocardial infarction. In a 2021 published case report, a spontaneous spleen rupture mimicked nonspecific thoracic pain that warranted immediate medical attention. Correlating findings from the subjective and objective assessments would aid in the clinical reasoning process for proper intervention or a referral for additional medical screening.

15. A 35-year-old man presents with pain and stiffness in the thoracic region, which is worse in the morning. On physical examination you note limited chest expansion. What should your differential diagnosis include?

Ankylosing spondylitis (AS) is a chronic inflammatory disease characterized by a variable symptomatic course. Back pain and stiffness are the initial symptoms in 81% of patients. In the thoracic spine, AS causes decreased motion at the costovertebral joints, reduced chest expansion, and impaired pulmonary function. Chest expansion is measured at the fourth intercostal space in men and below the breasts in women. The patient raises both hands over the head and is asked to take a deep inspiration. Normal expansion is ≥2.5 cm.

16. A 44-year-old man presents with pain in the right T7–T9 region just below the inferior lateral angle of the scapula. Further questioning reveals that the symptoms are worse 2 to 3 hours after a meal. What should your differential diagnosis include?

Pain from cholecystitis (inflamed gallbladder) typically occurs 1 to 2 hours after ingestion of a heavy meal with severe pain peaking at 2 to 3 hours. Pain from gallbladder disease is generally transmitted along T8 and T9 nerve segments. Right upper quadrant or epigastric pain is characteristic, but pain often is referred to the angle of the scapulae on the right side.

17. Can thoracic spine and rib cage musculoskeletal dysfunction mimic anginal pain?

The T4–T7 thoracic segments frequently have been implicated as the source for initiation of pseudoanginal pain. The primary evidence is in the form of case reports and case series. Hamburg and Lindahl reported six cases of "anginal" pain relieved by manipulation of the midthoracic segments. In many cases, the primary symptoms of diabetic thoracic radiculopathy are severe abdominal and anterior chest pain with minimal back pain.

18. **What is Scheuermann's disease? Is it safe to use manual therapy in affected patients?**
Scheuermann first described the radiographic changes of anterior wedging and vertebral end-plate irregularity in the thoracic spine associated with kyphosis. The disease also is known as juvenile kyphosis, vertebral osteochondritis, and osteochondritis deformans juvenilis dorsi. Disc material herniated into the vertebral bodies (Schmorl's nodes) is a common associated finding. Patients benefit from even slight increases in motion of the posterior elements at the involved segments. Despite the fact that the basic deformity is not "corrected," maintenance and improvement in range of motion and function may be achieved.

19. **Do postural abnormalities of the cervical and thoracic spine contribute to pain?**
Poor upper quadrant posture has been implicated as a source of neck and shoulder pain. Patients with more severe postural abnormalities of the thoracic, cervical, and shoulder regions have a significantly increased incidence of pain. In particular, patients with thoracic kyphosis and rounded shoulders reportedly have an increased incidence of cervical, interscapular, and headache pain.

20. **Define T4 syndrome.**
T4 syndrome describes a group of patients with dysfunction within the T2–T7 segments. The clinical presentation includes various combinations of pain in the upper limbs and in the neck, upper thoracic, and scapular regions with cranial headaches. However, the T4 segment is nearly always involved. In addition, patients may report glove-like paresthesias and numbness in one or both hands, often nocturnal in nature. Differential diagnoses include systemic illness, polyneuritis, and nerve root compression. Typical examination findings include tenderness, asymmetry, and limited segmental range of motion and tissue thickening. Furthermore, posteroanterior pressure over the involved thoracic segment reproduces the symptoms. McGuckin (not peer-reviewed) reported 90 cases in which the syndrome occurred more frequently in women (4:1) than in men, with a typical presentation between 30 and 50 years. DeFranco and Levine reported two cases of apparent T4 syndrome of 6 to 12 months' duration that were treated successfully by two sessions of T3–T4 manipulation. Treatment includes localized segmental mobilization and/or manipulation.

21. **What role can the thoracic spine play in headaches?**
Dysfunction of the thoracic spine, in particular the upper five segments, has been implicated as the primary generator of headaches. Examination of the upper thorax in patients with headaches is warranted. Treatment using segmental mobilization and/or manipulation has been advocated. The mechanism for the referred pain to the head is unknown.

22. **What symptoms may arise from or at least be affected by treatment directed at the thoracolumbar region?**
Dysfunction at the thoracolumbar spine has been described as thoracolumbar junction syndrome as early as 1974 by Maigne. There may often be clinical manifestations of lower lumbar pain, pseudovisceral pain, and pseudopain on the posterior iliac crest, as well as irritable bowel symptoms. The lateral branches of the dorsal rami of lower thoracic and upper lumbar segments become cutaneous over the buttocks, iliac crest, and greater trochanter. Symptoms may also be perceived in the area of the inguinal ligament, groin, and testicles. Symptoms in any of these regions can be referred from the lower thoracic and upper lumbar spine, and the thoracolumbar junction should be examined thoroughly in their presence.

23. **During the history portion of the examination of patients over 50 years of age with thoracic spine pain that is not associated with trauma, why is it important to identify red flags associated with cancer?**
Metastatic lesions in the skeleton are much more common than primary tumors of bone (overall ratio = 25:1). The presence of metastases increases with age. Patients who are 50 years old or older are at greatest risk of developing metastatic disease. Metastases occur more commonly in the axial skeleton than in the appendicular skeleton. The thoracic spine is the area of the spine most frequently affected by metastases. Breast cancer is the most common site of tumor origin. In addition, skeletal metastases from tumors of prostate, lung, thyroid, kidney, rectum, and uterine cervix are quite common.

24. **Describe the clinical presentation of postherpetic neuralgia.**
Postherpetic neuralgia is pain that persists for longer than 1 month after the rash of acute herpes zoster (reactivated chickenpox virus) resolves. The pain can be lancinating or manifest as a steady burning or ache along a thoracic dermatomal pattern. The involved skin area is often hypersensitive to light touch. Postherpetic neuralgia can mimic thoracic radiculopathy or referred pain of thoracic spine origin.

25. Define costochondritis. What can the physical therapist do about it?

Costochondritis is an inflammation or irritation of the costochondral junction. Frequently it is referred pain from thoracic or rib dysfunction, probably in the corresponding vertebral level. Examination of the thoracic spine and posterior chest wall is warranted. Treatment using segmental mobilization and/or manipulation has been advocated.

26. If the patient demonstrates inhibition or difficulty in activating the lower trapezius muscle, what arthrokinematics should the physical therapist consider?

The physical therapist should screen the T8–T12 segments for extension restrictions. Segmental mobilization or manipulation to improve extension often results in immediate improvement of lower trapezius muscle activation.

27. If a patient demonstrates inhibition of the serratus anterior muscle or has difficulty in stabilizing the scapula during arm movements, what should the physical therapist consider?

In the absence of long thoracic neuropathy, the physical therapist should screen the T3–T7 vertebral segments for flexion restrictions. Segmental mobilization or manipulation to improve flexion often results in immediate improvement of serratus anterior muscle activation. The mechanism is unclear; it may be secondary to localized pain that inhibits maximal muscle firing.

28. What areas of the cervical spine typically refer pain to the thoracic region?

C4–C5—nape of the neck to the upper trapezius region

C5–C6—nape of neck, over entire upper trapezius region, and upper medial border of the scapula

C6–C7—over entire upper trapezius region, extending inferiorly over the entire scapula

29. When performing dry needling techniques in the thoracic region, what anatomical considerations are needed for patient safety?

Thoracic musculature can benefit from dry needling techniques. The anatomy of the thoracic region should be carefully considered prior to using this intervention. Careful palpation is needed along with solid anatomy knowledge to avoid puncturing the lung cavity, peripheral nerves, spinal cord or blood vessels. Sterile technique for dry needling should also utilized to avoid potential infections.

Bibliography

Briggs, A. M., Smith, A. J., Straker, L. M., & Bragge, P. (2009). Thoracic spine pain in the general population: prevalence, incidence and associated factors in children, adolescents and adults. A systematic review. *BMC Musculoskeletal Disorders, 10*(1), 77.

Brismee, J. M., Gipson, D., Ivie, D., et al. (2006). Interrater reliability of a passive physiological intervertebral motion test in the mid-thoracic spine. *Journal of Manipulative and Physiological Therapeutics, 29*(5), 368–373.

Cleland, J. A., Childs, M. J. D., McRae, M., Palmer, J. A., & Stowell, T. (2005). Immediate effects of thoracic manipulation in patients with neck pain: a randomized clinical trial. *Manual Therapy, 10*(2), 127–135.

Fernández-de-Las-Peñas, C., Layton, M., & Dommerholt, J. (2015). Dry needling for the management of thoracic spine pain. *Journal of Manual & Manipulative Therapy, 23*(3), 147–153.

Flynn, T. (1999). An evidence-based description of clinical practice: thoracic spine and ribs. *Orthopaedic Physical Therapy Clinics of North America, 8*, 1–20.

Flynn, T. W., & Hall, R. C. (1998). An evidence-based description of clinical practice: thoracic spine and ribs. *Journal of Manual and Manipulative Therapy, 6*, 202–203.

Fruergaard, P., Launbjerg, J., Hesse, B., et al. (1996). The diagnoses of patients admitted with acute chest pain but without myocardial infarction. *European Heart Journal, 17*, 1028–1034.

Greigel-Morris, P., Larson, K., Mueller-Klaus, K., & Oatis, C. A. (1992). Incidence of common postural abnormalities in the cervical, shoulder, and thoracic regions and their association with pain in two age groups of healthy subjects. *Physical Therapy, 72*, 425–431.

Grieve, G. P. (1994). Thoracic musculoskeletal problems. In J. D. Boyling & N. Palastanga (Eds.), *Grieve's modern manual therapy* (2nd ed., pp. 401–428). New York, NY: Churchill Livingstone.

Hamberg, J., & Lindahl, O. (1981). Angina pectoris symptoms caused by thoracic spine disorders: clinical examination and treatment. *Acta Medica Scandinavica Supplementum, 644*, 84–86.

Huijbregts, P. A. (2002). Spinal motion palpation: a review of reliability studies. *Journal of Manual and Manipulative Therapy, 10*(1), 24–39.

Kikta, D., Breder, A., & Wilbourn, A. (1982). Thoracic root pain in diabetes: the spectrum of clinical and electromyographical findings. *Annals of Neurology, 11*, 80–85.

Lee, D. (1993). Biomechanics of the thorax: a clinical model of in vivo function. *Journal of Manual and Manipulative Therapy, 1*, 13–21.

Lillegard, W. (1996). The thoracic spine and ribcage: musculoskeletal evaluation and treatment. In T. Flynn (Ed.), *The thoracic spine and ribcage: musculoskeletal evaluation and treatment* (pp. 107–120). Newton, MA: Butterworth-Heinemann.

Lindgren, K. -A. (1997). Conservative treatment of thoracic outlet syndrome: a 2-year follow-up. *Archives of Physical Medicine and Rehabilitation, 78*, 373–378.

Lindgren, K. -A., Leino, E., Hakola, M., & Hamberg, J. (1990). Cervical spine rotation and lateral flexion combined motion in the examination of the thoracic outlet. *Archives of Physical Medicine and Rehabilitation, 71*, 343–344.

Lindgren, K. -A., Leino, E., & Manninen, H. (1989). Cervical rotation lateral flexion test in brachialgia. *Archives of Physical Medicine and Rehabilitation, 73*, 735–737.

Maigne, R. (1974). Thoracolumbar origin of some low back pain: role of facet joints and posterior branches of spinal nerves. *Revue du Rhumatisme, 41*, 781–789.
Martin, G. T. (1993). First rib resection for the thoracic outlet syndrome. *British Journal of Neurosurgery, 7*, 35–38.
McDevitt, A. W., Cleland, J. A., Rhon, D. I., Altic, R. A., Courtney, D. J., Glynn, P. E., & McGuckin, N. (1986). The T4 syndrome. In G. Grieve (Ed.), *Modern manual therapy of the vertebral column* (pp. 370–376). New York, NY: Churchill Livingstone.
McInerney, J., & Ball, P. A. (2000). The pathophysiology of thoracic disc disease. *Neurosurgical Focus, 9*(4), 1–8.
Mintken, P. E. (2022). Thoracic spine thrust manipulation for individuals with cervicogenic headache: a crossover randomized clinical trial. *Journal of Manual & Manipulative Therapy, 30*(2), 78–95.
Sarsılmaz, A., Yencilek, E., Özelçi, Ü., Güzelbey, T., & Apaydın, M. (2018). The incidence and most common levels of thoracic degenerative disc pathologies. *Turkish Journal of Physical Medicine and Rehabilitation, 64*(2), 155.
Sforza, C., Margelli, M., Mourad, F., Brindisino, F., Heick, J. D., & Maselli, F. (2021). Spontaneous spleen rupture mimicking non-specific thoracic pain: a rare case in physiotherapy practice. *Physiotherapy Theory and Practice, 39*(3), 641–649.
Sizer, P. S., Jr, Brismee, J. -M., & Cook, C. (2007). Coupling behavior of the thoracic spine: a systematic review of the literature. *Journal of Manipulative and Physiological Therapeutics, 30*(5), 390–399.
Walser, R. F., Meserve, B. B., & Boucher, T. R. (2009). The effectiveness of thoracic spine manipulation for the management of musculoskeletal conditions: a systematic review and meta-analysis of randomized clinical trials. *Journal of Manual and Manipulative Therapy, 17*(4), 237–246.
Willems, J. M., Jull, G. A., & Ng, J. K. -F. (1996). An in vivo study of the primary and coupled rotations of the thoracic spine. *Clinical Biomechanics, 11*, 311–316.
Wood, K. B., Garvey, T. A., Gundry, C., & Heithoff, K. B. (1995). Magnetic resonance imaging of the thoracic spine. Evaluation of asymptomatic individuals. *Journal of Bone and Joint Surgery, 77*(11), 1631–1638.

CHAPTER 56 QUESTIONS

1. **When dry needling the multifidi muscle of the thoracic region, the physical therapist needles over which anatomical structure?**
   a. Lamina
   b. Pedicle
   c. Spinous process
   d. Transverse process

2. **Which segment of the thoracic spine would be most prone to a disc herniation due to the surrounding anatomical structures?**
   a. T2/3
   b. T4/5
   c. T7/8
   d. T11/12

3. **A patient is being evaluated by a physical therapist after being hospitalized for 29 days due to complications from COVID-19. Which of the following would improve respiratory inhalation?**
   a. Thoracic flexion
   b. Thoracic extension
   c. Thoracic rotation
   d. Thoracic sidebending

SCOLIOSIS

P.J. Roubal, PhD, DPT, OCS

1. **What are the major types of scoliosis?**
   - Functional scoliosis—This may be caused by muscle spasm (secondary to lumbar or thoracic injuries) or leg length discrepancy (which causes a lateral shift in the spine). Functional scoliosis resolves with healing of the lumbar or thoracic injuries or correction of a leg length discrepancy.
   - Structural scoliosis—This type of scoliosis is usually idiopathic.
   - Congenital scoliosis—This type is caused by vertebral anomalies and is much less common than the other two types of scoliosis.

2. **What is the incidence of idiopathic structural scoliosis?**
   Idiopathic scoliosis affects one to four people per thousand. Curves >20 degrees are seven times more common in females than in males, and curves >30 degrees have a 10:1 female-to-male ratio. Idiopathic scoliosis usually occurs in adolescents between 11 and 14 years of age.

3. **What are the possible causes of idiopathic scoliosis?**
   The role of genetics has been debated. Family history is not helpful in determining curve magnitude. Some form of multifactorial or autosomal dominant inheritance seems to be involved, although most recent research suggests a polygenic inheritance pattern. The proprioceptive system and equilibrium imbalances, possibly related to asymmetry in the brainstem, also may be implicated.

4. **Describe the clinical presentation of idiopathic scoliosis.**
   Curves do not strengthen when the trunk is flexed forward (Adam's test). Structural curves exhibit rotatory components during forward flexion, and the patient's symptoms usually include rib hump or asymmetry in the trunk, referred to as the angle of trunk rotation (ATR). The ATR is easily measured with the scoliometer.

5. **What screening methods are most effective for detection of scoliosis?**
   The Scoliosis Research Society, American Academy of Orthopedic Surgeons, as well as the Pediatric Orthopedic Surgeons of North America suggest early screening for scoliosis has great benefits. Adam's testing as well as scoliometer testing are the best and most cost-effective early screening methods.

6. **When is further evaluation of idiopathic scoliosis advisable?**
   In general, patients with curves >15 to 20 degrees and a 5- to 7-degree ATR usually are referred for further follow-up by an orthopedist. Current data, however, recommend at least a 20-degree curve and 7-degree ATR.

7. **Describe the Risser classification.**
   The Risser classification uses ossification of the iliac epiphysis to grade remaining skeletal growth. Ossification starts laterally and runs medially. Ossification of the lateral 25% indicated Risser type 1; of 50%, Risser type 2; of 75%, Risser type 3; complete excursion, Risser type 4; and fusion to the ilium, Risser type 5. Growth in females is usually complete in Risser type 4. It is best to treat patients at Risser 0–1 if able for the best results of bracing.

8. **Describe classification systems for scoliosis.**
   The King classification system describes curve types in idiopathic scoliosis, and the system helps determine surgical treatment.
   - Type I—primary lumbar and secondary thoracic curves
   - Type II—primary thoracic and secondary lumbar curves
   - Type III—thoracic curves only
   - Type IV—large thoracic curves extending into the lumbar spine
   - Type V—double thoracic curves

   Recent studies have demonstrated some reliability problems with the King classification system. A newer system, the Lenke classification of adolescent idiopathic scoliosis, uses three components: curve type, lumbar spine modifiers, and sagittal thoracic modifiers. All of the classification systems have limited inter-observer reliability, and thus it is possible that all classification systems will be obsolete and instead detailed descriptions derived from 3D radiography may be utilized instead.

9. **What are the recommendations for screening of adolescent idiopathic scoliosis?**
   Adolescent idiopathic scoliosis generally starts in immature patients older than 10 years of age. Approximately 2% to 4% of patients 10 to 16 years of age have some degree of spinal curvature. Recommendations now are that females are screened twice at ages 10 and 12 years old and males once at approximately age 13. Evaluation of curvature combined with level of skeletal maturity (Risser 0–5) will then help guide treatment.

10. **Will physical therapy work in correction of idiopathic scoliosis?**
    No recent literature reports physical therapy alone will help in the correction of idiopathic scoliosis. Exercises based on individual evaluation with the use of bracing may be more effective than bracing alone. More research must be done on this combination of therapies.

11. **When should bracing be considered?**
    Curves <20 degrees generally do not require bracing, particularly when patients are more mature (Risser type 3–5). Curves <30 degrees that progress 5 degrees or more over 12 months should be braced. For curves >30 degrees, bracing should be initiated immediately. Bracing is not indicated in skeletally mature patients. All braces are custom-fit, worn 23 hours/day, and need to be changed every 12 to 18 months. The primary corrective forces in bracing is lateral correction.

12. **Describe the bracing used for scoliosis. How long should the brace be worn?**
    The first brace, developed immediately after World War II by Blount was named the Milwaukee brace. It was fairly cumbersome, made with stainless steel bars, and fitted with side straps to reduce lateral deflection and rotation of the spine at the specific points of apexes of curves. Newer, more comfortable braces include the Boston brace (thoracolumbosacral orthosis [TLSO]), which appears to be the most effective; it is made of molded plastic and fitted to the patient. Boston braces enhance adherence to treatment protocols because of ease of use. Braces are usually changed once every 12 to 18 months, depending on the patient's growth and body changes. Braces are most effective when worn 23 hours per day until skeletal maturity is achieved. The effectiveness of bracing is time dependent: the more the brace is worn, the better the outcome.

13. **What forces in braces reduce progression of scoliotic curves?**
    Computer evaluation of braces determined that the primary correction forces in braces are lateral. Muscle forces and longitudinal traction play minimal roles, if any. Reduction in hyperlordosis also is needed to reduce the curve.

14. **What are the outcomes of major brace types in treating idiopathic scoliosis?**
    For most curves, the Boston brace appears more effective at preventing curves from progressing, as defined by a lower rate of surgery. Boston braces are most appropriate for curves with the apex below T8. Recent strides have been made in developing strap tension systems with strap transducers instrumented to the Boston brace. These tension systems allow for optimal prescribed levels of tensioning, so the patient may achieve the best curve correction along with a reduction in curve progression.

15. **What curves respond best to bracing?**
    Curves without severe lumbar hyperlordosis, thoracic lordosis, or hyperkyphosis respond best to bracing. Risser type 0 curves respond best, whereas Risser type 4 or 5 curves rarely respond well. Double major curves respond less favorably to bracing than other curves.

16. **How effective is bracing?**
    Over the years, the efficacy of bracing has been one of the most intensely debated subjects in the treatment of idiopathic scoliosis. Recent reports, however, indicate that the efficacy may be as high as 74% to 81% in halting the progression of idiopathic structural scoliosis. In contrast, only 33% of patients do not progress without the use of bracing. Recent studies also show that wearing braces did not affect the quality of life in adolescents compared with the observed counterparts. Other recent studies show that brace compliance and a high initial correction are strong indicators for bracing success.

17. **What are the indications for surgical intervention?**
    - Curves >50 degrees in skeletally mature patients.
    - Curves progressed beyond 40 degrees in skeletally mature patients
    - Curves >30 degrees with marked rotation
    - Double major curves >30 degrees

18. **What can occur with untreated adolescent idiopathic scoliosis?**
    Generally the patients can function well as adults. The major problems of nontreatment may lead to increased back pain, pulmonary and cardiac symptoms, and substantial deformity. The cosmetic aspect cannot be disregarded.

19. **What is the most common form of surgical intervention in idiopathic scoliosis?**
Posterior segmental instrumentation utilizing hooks, screws, wires, and rods is the most common approach. For more advanced and rigid curves, both anterior and posterior fusions may be incorporated. Patients should be evaluated on an individual basis.

20. **What type of correction can be expected with surgical intervention?**
Surgery in idiopathic scoliosis generally reduces the major coronal curve by approximately 50%, vertebral rotation by approximately 10%, and apical translation by an average of approximately 60%.

21. **Define "crankshaft phenomenon."**
In a patient with an immature spine, correction of scoliosis with successful posterior fusion may be complicated by continued anterior vertebral body growth, which can increase the curve and vertebral rotation. This problem may be corrected with combined anterior and posterior fusion procedures if a skeletally immature patient must undergo surgery.

22. **List potential complications of surgical intervention for idiopathic scoliosis.**
- Migration of rods
- Neurologic damage
- Pseudarthrosis
- Renal failure
- Psychological stress
- Blood loss
- Failure of fixation
- Infection
- Respiratory distress

23. **Compare the costs of bracing and surgery.**
Most research shows that the costs of bracing and surgery are somewhat comparable. At the start of the new millennium, total surgical costs, which include preoperative and postsurgical care and bracing as well as other medical care, average approximately $50,000. These costs do not include screening. Overall costs would be decreased if screening were used with bracing. Cost estimates do not include loss of income, welfare, social programs, or other direct or indirect medical costs associated with surgical intervention.

24. **What are the long-term curve progressions for surgical-treated versus brace-treated curves?**
After 22 years, brace-treated curves progressed 7.9 degrees versus 3.5 degrees for surgically treated curves.

25. **What are the long-term (20 years or more) quality-of-life outcomes for surgery versus bracing treatment?**
No correlation exists between curve size after treatment, curve type, total treatment time, or age at completion of treatment. Approximately 49% of those undergoing surgery, 34% of those treated with braces, and 15% of controls will have some limitation of social activities, mostly because of physical participation in activities or self-consciousness about appearance. Patients treated for scoliosis have about the same health-related quality of life as the general population.

26. **What is the natural history of patients with untreated idiopathic scoliosis?**
Untreated people with scoliosis are productive and function at a high level at 50-year follow-up. Back pain occurs in 61% compared with 35% of controls. However, of those with pain, 68% describe it as minor or moderate.

Bibliography

Burton, M. S. (2013). Diagnosis and treatment of adolescent idiopathic scoliosis. *Pediatr Ann, 42*(11), 224–228.

Climent, J. M., & Sanchez, J. (1999). Impact of the type of brace on the quality of life in adolescents with spine deformities. *Spine, 24*, 1903–1908.

Comité Nacional de Adolescencia SAP., (2016). Adolescent idiopathic scoliosis. *Archivos Argentinos De Pediatria, 114*(6), 585–594.

Danielsson, A. J., & Nachemson, A. L. (2001). Radiologic findings and curve progression 22 years after treatment for adolescent idiopathic scoliosis: comparison of brace and surgical treatment with matching control group of straight individuals. *Spine, 26*, 516–525.

Danielsson, A. J., Wiklund, I., Pehrsson, K., & Nachemson, A. L. (2001). Health related quality of life in patients with adolescent idiopathic scoliosis: a matched follow-up at least 20 years after treatment with brace or surgery. *Eur Spine J, 10*, 278–288.

Dubousset, J., Herring, J. A., & Shufflebarger, H. (1989). The crankshaft phenomenon. *J Pediatr Orthop, 9*, 541–550.

Hawasli, A. H., Hullar, T. E., & Dorward, I. G. (2015). Idiopathic scoliosis and the vestibular system. *Eur Spine J, 24*(2), 227–233.

Horne, J. P., Flannery, R., & Usman, S. (2014). Adolescent idiopathic scoliosis: diagnosis and management. *Am Fam Physician, 89*(3), 193–198.

Howard, A., Wright, J. G., & Hedden, D. (1998). A comparative study of TLSO, Charleston, and Milwaukee braces for idiopathic scoliosis. *Spine, 23*, 2404–2411.
Katz, D. E., & Durrani, A. A. (2001). Factors that influence outcome in bracing large curves in patients with adolescent idiopathic scoliosis. *Spine, 26*, 2354–2361.
King, H. A., Moe, J. H., Bradford, D. S., & Winter, R. B. (1983). The selection of fusion levels in thoracic idiopathic scoliosis. *J Bone Joint Surg, 65A*, 1302–1313.
Korbel, K., Kozinoga, M., Stoliński, Ł., & Kotwicki, T. (2014). Scoliosis Research Society (SRS) criteria and Society of Scoliosis Orthopaedic and Rehabilitation Treatment (SOSORT) 2008 guidelines in non-operative treatment of idiopathic scoliosis. *Pol Orthop Traumatol, 79*, 118–122.
Kuznia, A. L., Hernandez, A. K., & Lee, L. U. (2020). Adolescent idiopathic scoliosis: common questions and answers. *Am Fam Physician, 101*(1), 19–23.
Landauer, F., Wimmer, C., & Behensky, H. (2003). Estimating the final outcome of brace treatment for idiopathic thoracic scoliosis at 6-month follow-up. *Pediatr Rehabil, 6*, 201–207.
Lenke, L. G., Betz, R. R., Harms, J., et al. (2001). Adolescent idiopathic scoliosis: a new classification to determine extent of spinal arthrodesis. *J Bone Joint Surg, 83*(8), 1169–1181.
Lenke, L. G., Edwards, C. C., 2nd, & Bridwell, K. H. (2003). The Lenke classification of adolescent idiopathic scoliosis: how it organizes curve patterns as a template to perform selective fusions of the spine. *Spine, 28*, S199–207.
Lonstein, J. E., & Winter, R. B. (1994). The Milwaukee Brace for the treatment of adolescent idiopathic scoliosis. *J Bone Joint Surg, 76*(8), 1207–1221.
Lou, E., Benfield, D., Raso, J., Hill, D., & Durdle, N. (2002). Intelligent brace system for the treatment of scoliosis. *Stud Health Technol Inform, 91*, 397–400.
Nachemson, A. L., & Petersen, L. E. (1995). Effectiveness of treatment with a brace in girls who have adolescent idiopathic scoliosis. *J Bone Joint Surg, 77*(6), 815–822.
Peng, Y., Wang, S. -R., Qiu, G. -X., Zhang, J. -G., & Zhuang, Q. -Y. (2020). Research progress on the etiology and pathogenesis of adolescent idiopathic scoliosis. *Chin Med J, 133*(4), 483–493.
Rigo, M., Reiter, Ch, & Weiss, H. R. (2003). Effect of conservative management on the prevalence of surgery in patients with adolescent idiopathic scoliosis. *Pediatr Rehabil, 6*, 209–214.
Roubal, P. J., Freeman, D. C., & Placzek, J. D. (1999). Costs and effectiveness of scoliosis screening. *Physiotherapy, 85*, 259–268.
Steffan, K. (2015). Physical therapy for idiopathic scoliosis. *Orthopade, 44*(11), 852–858.
Tolo, V. T., & Herring, J. A. (2020). Scoliosis-specific exercises: a state of the Art Review. *Spine Deform, 8*(2), 149–155.
Ugwonali, O. F., Lomas, G., Choe, J. C., et al. (2004). Effect of bracing on the quality of life of adolescents with idiopathic scoliosis. *Spine J, 4*, 254–260.
Weinstein, S. L., Dolan, L. A., Spratt, K. F., Peterson, K. K., Spoonamore, M. J., & Ponseti, I. V. (2003). Health and function of patients with untreated idiopathic scoliosis: a 50 year natural history study. *JAMA, 5*, 559–567.
Weinstein, S. L. (2019). The natural history of adolescent idiopathic scoliosis. *J Pediatr Orthop, 39*(Issue 6, Supplement 1 Suppl 1), S44–S46.
Weiss, H. R., Weiss, G., & Schaar, H. J. (2003). Incidence of surgery in conservatively treated patients with scoliosis. *Pediatr Rehabil, 6*, 111–118.
Yaman, O., & Dalbayrak, S. (2014). Idiopathic scoliosis. *Turk Neurosurg, 24*(5), 646–657.

CHAPTER 57 QUESTIONS

1. **Costs of evaluation and bracing versus surgery?**
   a. Approximately the same
   b. Bracing with multiple changes in braces costs most
   c. Surgery is more expensive
   d. Surgery is less expensive

2. **What appears to be the best brace to use in treating idiopathic scoliosis?**
   a. Milwaukee brace
   b. TLSO-Boston
   c. Charleston brace
   d. Depends on the type curve

3. **When is it the best time to start bracing?**
   a. When the curve is greater than 30 degrees
   b. Risser at 0-1, curve approximately 20 degrees
   c. Patient at age of 15
   d. Once vertebral endplates are closed

4. **Risser type 3 indicates:**
   a. Complete fusion to the ilium
   b. Ossification of lateral 50% of iliac crest
   c. Ossification of lateral 75% of iliac crest
   d. Complete excursion of ossification

CLASSIFICATIONS OF LOW BACK PAIN

N.W. Ayotte III, PT, MPT, DSc, FAAOMPT and J. Magel, PT, PhD, DSc

LOW BACK PAIN: CLINICAL PRACTICE GUIDELINES LINKED TO THE ICF MODEL

1. **What is the International Classification of Functioning, Disability, and Health (ICF) Model as it relates to low back pain (LBP)?**

   The ICF utilizes a biopsychosocial model to acknowledge the relationship between biological, social, and personal factors and how they impact an individual's functioning and disability. Additionally, the ICF provides a common language and conceptual framework for measuring health and disability.

2. **What is the difference between the ICF model and International Statistical Classification of Diseases and Related Health Problems (ICD 10) classification?**

   The ICF model recognizes that function and disability are multidimensional and attempts to describe how the four domains of body function/structure, activities, participation, and environmental factors interact. The ICD 10 classification system is a standardized code set that provides a common language for reporting and monitoring diseases.

3. **According to the LBP: Clinical Practice Guidelines, when treating a patient with low back pain, the clinician should place the highest priority on which of the following?**
   a. Return to optimal function
   b. Prevention of recurrence and transition to chronic low back pain
   c. Identification and treatment of all impairments
   d. Determining the optimal course of care within the biopsychosocial model

   Answer: Given the high prevalence of recurrent and chronic LBP, special emphasis should be placed on the interventions that prevent the recurrence or movement of low back pain to a chronic state. This is based on theoretical and foundational evidence.

4. **What are the most common ICD-10 categories used to classify patients with LBP?**

   Low back pain, lumbago, lumbosacral segmental/somatic dysfunction, low back strain, spinal instabilities, flatback syndrome, lumbago due to displacement of intervertebral disc, and lumbago with sciatica.

5. **Using the ICF model, what are the most common impairment-based categories for LBP?**

   b28013 Pain in back
   b28018 Pain in body part, specified as pain in buttock, groin, and thigh

6. **When using the ICF model, a. why is it important to utilize both function and disability when providing diagnostic codes and b. what are some examples commonly utilized in low back pain patients?**
   a. The use of both function and disability reflects the unique interaction the person has with their environment at biological, individual, and social levels. Most often physical therapists describe impairments or limitations an individual has but fall short in describing their capabilities; the ICF model allows for both.
   b. Some examples include:
      I. Acute or subacute low back pain with mobility deficits (b7101 Mobility of several joints)
      II. Acute, subacute, or chronic low back pain with movement coordination impairments (b7601 Control of complex voluntary movements)
      III. Acute low back pain with related (referred) lower extremity pain (b28015 Pain in lower limb)
      IV. Acute, subacute, or chronic low back pain with radiating pain (b2804 Radiating pain in a segment or region)
      V. Acute or subacute low back pain with related cognitive or affective tendencies

7. **According to the APTA's 2012 low back pain clinical practice guidelines, briefly describe the symptoms and impairments of body function for each of the eight interventional categories?**

ICF-Based Category – Symptoms and Impairments of Body Functions		
ICF-BASED CATEGORY (*WITH ICD-10 ASSOCIATIONS*)	**SYMPTOMS**	**IMPAIRMENTS OF BODY FUNCTION**
Acute Low Back Pain With Mobility Deficits *Lumbosacral segmental/ somatic dysfunction*	• Acute low back, buttock, or thigh pain (duration 1 month or less • Unilateral pain • Onset of symptoms is often linked to a recent unguarded/awkward movement or position	• Lumbar range of motion limitations • Restricted lower thoracic and lumbar segmental mobility • Low back and low back–related lower symptoms are reproduced with provocation of the involved lower thoracic, lumbar, or sacroiliac segments

Subacute Low Back Pain With Mobility Deficits
Lumbosacral segmental/ somatic dysfunction
	• Subacute, unilateral, low back, buttock, or thigh pain
	• May report sensation of back stiffness
		• Symptoms reproduced with end-range spinal motions
		• Symptoms reproduced with provocation of the involved lower thoracic, lumbar, or sacroiliac segments
		• Presence of one or more of the following:
		  • Restricted thoracic range of motion and associated segmental mobility
		  • Restricted lumbar range of motion and associated segmental mobility
		  • Restricted lumbopelvic or hip range of motion and associated accessory mobility

Acute Low Back Pain With Movement Coordination Impairments *Spinal instabilities*	• Acute exacerbation of recurring low back pain that is commonly associated with referred lower extremity pain • Symptoms often include numerous episodes of low back and/or low back–related lower extremity pain in recent years	• Low back and/or low back–related lower extremity pain at rest or produced with initial to mid-range spinal movements • Low back and/or low back–related lower extremity pain reproduced with provocation of the involved lumbar segment(s) • Movement coordination impairments of the lumbopelvic region with low back flexion and extension movements
Subacute Low Back Pain With Movement Coordination Impairments *Spinal instabilities*	• Subacute, recurring low back pain that is commonly associated with referred lower extremity pain • Symptoms often include numerous episodes of low back and/or low back–related lower extremity pain in recent years	• Lumbosacral pain with mid-range motions that worsen with end-range movements or positions Low back and low back–related lower extremity pain reproduced with provocation of the involved lumbar segment(s) • Lumbar hypermobility with segmental mobility assessment may be present • Mobility deficits of the thorax and/or lumbopelvic/ hip regions • Diminished trunk or pelvic region muscle strength and endurance • Movement coordination impairments while performing self-care/home management activities

ICF-Based Category – Symptoms and Impairments of Body Functions		
ICF-BASED CATEGORY (*WITH ICD-10 ASSOCIATIONS*)	**SYMPTOMS**	**IMPAIRMENTS OF BODY FUNCTION**
Chronic Low Back Pain With Movement Coordination Impairments *Spinal instabilities*	• Chronic, recurring low back pain and associated (referred) lower extremity pain	• Presence of one or more of the following: • Low back and/or low back–related lower extremity pain that worsens with sustained end-range movements or positions • Lumbar hypermobility with segmental motion assessment • Mobility deficits of the thorax and lumbopelvic/hip regions • Diminished trunk or pelvic region muscle strength and endurance • Movement coordination impairments while performing community/work-related recreational or occupational activities
Acute Low Back Pain With Related (Referred) Lower Extremity Pain *Flatback syndrome* *Lumbago due to displacement of intervertebral disc*	• Acute low back pain that is commonly associated with referred buttock, thigh, or leg pain • Symptoms are often worsened with flexion activities and sitting	• Low back and lower extremity pain that can be centralized and diminished with specific postures and/or repeated movements • Reduced lumbar lordosis • Limited lumbar extension mobility • Lateral trunk shift may be present • Clinical findings consistent with subacute or chronic low back pain with movement coordination impairments classification criteria
Acute Low Back Pain With Radiating Pain *Lumbago with sciatica*	• Acute low back pain with associated radiating (narrow band of lancinating) pain in the involved lower extremity • Lower extremity paresthesias, numbness, and weakness may be reported	• Lower extremity radicular symptoms that are present at rest or produced with initial to mid-range spinal mobility, lower-limb tension tests/straight leg raising, and/or slump tests • Signs of nerve root involvement may be present It is common for the symptoms and impairments of body function in patients who have acute low back pain with radiating pain to also be present in patients who have acute low back pain with related (referred) lower extremity pain
Subacute Low Back Pain With Radiating Pain *Lumbago with sciatica*	• Subacute, recurring, mid-back and/or low back pain with associated radiating pain in the involved lower extremity • Lower extremity paresthesias, numbness, and weakness may be reported	• Mid-back, low back, and back-related radiating pain or paresthesia that are reproduced with mid-range and worsen with end range: 1. Lower limb tension testing/straight leg raising tests, and/or ... 2. Slump tests • May have lower extremity sensory, strength, or reflex deficits associated with the involved nerve(s)
Chronic Low Back Pain With Radiating Pain *Lumbago with sciatica*	• Chronic, recurring, mid- and/or low back pain with associated radiating pain in the involved lower extremity • Lower extremity paresthesias, numbness, and weakness may be reported	• Mid-back, low back, or lower extremity pain or paresthesias that are reproduced with sustained end-range lower-limb tension tests and/or slump tests • Signs of nerve root involvement may be present

Continued

ICF-Based Category – Symptoms and Impairments of Body Functions—cont'd		
ICF-BASED CATEGORY (*WITH ICD-10 ASSOCIATIONS*)	**SYMPTOMS**	**IMPAIRMENTS OF BODY FUNCTION**
Acute of Subacute Low Back Pain With Related Cognitive of Affective Tendencies *Low back pain* *Disorder of central nervous system, specified as central nervous system sensitivity to pain*	• Acute or subacute low back and/ or low back–related lower extremity pain	One or more of the following: • Two positive responses to Primary Care Evaluation of Mental Disorders screen and affect consistent with an individual who is depressed • High scores on the Fear-Avoidance Beliefs Questionnaire and behavioral processes consistent with an individual who has excessive anxiety or fear • High scores on the Pain Catastrophizing Scale and cognitive process consistent with rumination, pessimism, or helplessness
Chronic Low Back Pain With Related Generalized Pain *Low back pain* *Disorder of central nervous system* *Persistent somatoform pain disorder*	• Low back and/or low back–related lower extremity pain with symptom duration for longer than 3 months • Generalized pain not consistent with other impairment-based classification criteria presented in these clinical guidelines	One or more of the following: • Two positive responses to Primary Care Evaluation of Mental Disorders screen and affect consistent with an individual who is depressed • High scores on the Fear-Avoidance Beliefs Questionnaire and behavioral processes consistent with an individual who has excessive anxiety and fear • High scores on the Pain Catastrophizing Scale and cognitive process consistent with rumination, pessimism, or helplessness

8. **With respect to the ICF model what are the three types of codes used to define low back pain?**
   a. Body function
   b. Body structure
   c. Activity and participation

9. **What are some of the relevant pathoanatomical structures present in patients with low back pain?**
   Potential structures include: muscles, ligaments, dura mater and nerve roots, zygapophyseal joints, annulus fibrosis, thoracolumbar fascia, and vertebrae.

   Note: Any innervated structure in the region of the low back is a potential source of pain and, therefore, the rate of false positive findings is high with advanced imaging and therefore reliance on MRI findings to guide physical therapy treatment should be considered cautiously.

10. **According to the APTA's 2012 low back pain clinical practice guidelines, what are the prognostic factors associated with the development of recurrent low back pain?**
    a. History of previous episodes
    b. Excessive spine mobility
    c. Excessive mobility in other joints

11. **According to the APTA's 2012 low back pain clinical practice guidelines, what are the prognostic factors associated with the development of chronic low back pain?**
    a. Presence of symptoms below the knee
    b. Psychological stress or depression
    c. Fear of pain, movement, and reinjury or low expectation of recovery
    d. Pain of high intensity
    e. A passive coping style

12. **What are the four subgroups of the treatment-based classification system by Fritz et al., 2007?**
    a. Mobilization
    b. Specific exercise
    c. Stabilization
    d. Traction

13. **What are some differences between the treatment-based classification system by Fritz et al., 2007 and the ICF linked clinical practice guidelines published by the APTA in 2012?**
    a. The ICF linked CPG incorporates ICF impairments of body function such as low back pain with mobility deficits, low back pain with movement coordination impairments
    b. The ICF linked CPG adds low back pain with "related cognitive or affective tendencies" and "generalized pain" categories to provide a classification for patients with mental and/or sensory function impairments, and acute low back pain with radiating pain.
    c. The ICF linked CPG adds the patient level of acuity as defined by time since onset of symptoms and movement/pain relations.

14. **According to the ICF model what are three clinical findings that are consistent with the category of acute low back pain with movement coordination impairments?**
    a. Acute exacerbation of recurring low back pain that is commonly associated with referred lower extremity pain
    b. Symptoms produced with initial to mid-range spinal movements and provocation of the involved lumbar segment(s)
    c. Movement coordination impairments of the lumbopelvic region with low back flexion and extension movements

15. **The following is a patient scenario regarding chronic LBP with movement impairments:**
    A 30-year-old male presents to a physical therapy clinic for evaluation and treatment of chronic low back pain with radiating leg pain. The patient developed low back pain 4 weeks ago and then recently developed shooting leg pain that extends down the left posterior thigh but does not extend below the knee. He denies any numbness or tingling sensations. During the physical examination he is noted to have limits in his mobility forward and backward bending. He has difficulty with static positions of sitting or standing and is not able to lift more than 25 pounds from the ground.
    a. According to the Low Back Pain CPG ICD-10 coding guidelines, which code should be used to classify this patient (choose 1)?
        I. M54.5 Low back pain
        II. M54.5 Lumbago with sciatica
        III. M54.1 Lumbar radiculopathy
        IV. M51.2 Other specified intervertebral disc displacement
        V. G96.8 Disorder of central nervous system, specified as central nervous system sensitivity to pain
    b. **According to the ICF codes, which of the following codes would be most appropriate for this patient? (choose all that apply)**
        VI. Body functions b28013 Pain in back
            b28018 Pain in body part, specified as pain in buttock, groin, and thigh
            b7101 Mobility of several joints
            b7108 Mobility of joint functions, specified as mobility in a vertebral segment
        VII. Body structure s76002 Lumbar vertebral column
            s7401 Joints of pelvic region
            s7402 Muscles of pelvic region
            s75001 Hip joint
            s75002 Muscles of thigh
            s75003 Ligaments and fascia of thigh
        VIII. Activities and participation
            d4108 Bending
            d4153 Maintaining a sitting position
            d4154 Maintaining a standing position
            d4158 Maintaining a body position as maintaining the lumbar spine in an extended or neutral position with lifting, carrying, or putting down objects

    Answer: a. Based on the patient's presentation with symptoms extending from the back to the posterior thigh but not below the knee, the best ICD 10 code is M51.2 Other specified intervertebral disc displacement. b. Based on the patient's with pain starting in the low back and extending into his hip and posterior thigh, all of the body function and structure codes listed would be appropriate. Lastly, all of the activity and participation codes would be appropriate based on the patient's limitations in bending, static positions of standing and sitting, and lifting.

16. **In 2021, the APTA published a revision to their low back pain clinical practice guidelines. In general, what changes were made in this revision?**
    a. They provided recommendations on interventions delivered specifically by physical therapists or in health care setting that included physical therapists.
    b. They eliminated the subacute classification for the purpose of treatment.
    c. Interventions reviewed fell into four categories:
        I. Exercise
        II. Manual and other directed therapies
        III. Classification systems
        IV. Patient education
    d. Subgrouping for patient populations included:
        V. Acute or chronic LBP
        VI. LBP with leg pain
        VII. LBP in older adults
        VIII. Postoperative LBP
    e. To make the update applicable to physical therapist practicing globally, the literature search was not limited to the research conducted in the United States.

17. **The 2021 low back pain clinical practice guidelines provide Grades of Recommendation (A, B, C, D) for treatment options. These grades of recommendations provide the reader with a level of confidence based on the strength of the evidence. What is the difference between receiving a letter grade of A versus B?**
    A letter grade of A would suggest a strong level of evidence with a preponderance of level I and II studies that support use of the intervention, whereas a grade of B suggests a moderate level of evidence with only one level I study or a preponderance of level 2 studies which support the intervention. The letter grades have a level of obligation in their verbiage where a grade of A utilizes the word *should* and level B utilizes the word *may*.

18. **Have the ICD-10 classification codes changed with the 2021 update?**
    No, there has been no significant change in ICD-10 coding, therefore there was no revision to this section. However, ICD-11 codes were released in January of 2022 that include codes for chronic pain, so the reader should expect a revision with the next CPG update.

19. **According to the 2021 low back pain clinical practice guidelines, what are the recommendations for exercise interventions for acute and chronic low back pain?**
    a. Exercise training interventions, including trunk strengthening and endurance, multimodal exercise interventions, specific trunk muscle activation exercise, aerobic exercise, aquatic exercise, and general exercise for patients with chronic LBP should be used
    b. Exercise training interventions, including trunk muscle strengthening and endurance and specific trunk muscle activation to reduce pain and disability in patients with acute LBP with leg pain may be used
    c. Movement control exercise or trunk mobility exercise for patients with chronic LBP may be used

20. **According to the 2021 low back pain clinical practice guidelines, what are the recommended treatment options for acute low back pain?**
    a. Thrust and nonthrust joint mobilizations should be used
    b. Soft tissue mobilization, massage, treatment-based classifications (TBC), and patient education involving active education, BPS contributors to pain, self-management, and favorable natural history
    c. General exercise and mechanical diagnosis and therapy (MDT) can be used

21. **According to the 2021 low back pain clinical practice guidelines, what are the recommended treatment options for acute low back pain with leg pain?**
    Muscle strengthening and endurance training and specific trunk activation may be used.

22. **According to the 2021 low back pain clinical practice guidelines, what are the recommended treatment options for chronic low back pain?**
    a. General exercise, muscle strengthening and endurance, specific trunk activation, aerobic, aquatic exercise, thrust and nonthrust joint mobilization, and patient education involving pain neuroscience and active treatment should be used
    b. Trunk control, trunk mobility, soft tissue mobilization, massage, MDT, prognostic risk stratification, pathoanatomic-based classification, and patient education involving active education not as a stand-alone treatment may be used
    c. Dry needling, TBC, movement system impairment, and cognitive functional therapy can be used

23. **According to the 2021 low back pain clinical practice guidelines, what are the recommended treatment options for chronic low back pain with movement control impairment?**
Chronic LBP in the presence of movement control impairment, specific trunk activation, and movement control exercises should be used.

24. **According to the 2021 low back pain clinical practice guidelines, what are the recommended treatment options for chronic low back pain in older adults?**
General exercise should be used.

25. **According to the 2021 low back pain clinical practice guidelines, what are the recommended treatment options for chronic low back pain with leg pain?**
Specific trunk activation and movement control exercises, thrust and nonthrust joint mobilization, and neural tissue mobilization may be used.

26. **According to the 2021 low back pain clinical practice guidelines, what are the recommended treatment options for postoperative chronic low back pain?**
General education may be used and general exercise training can be used.

BIBLIOGRAPHY

Delitto, A., George, S. Z., Van Dillen, L., et al. (2012). Low back pain: clinical practice guidelines linked to the International Classification of Functioning, Disability, and Health from the Orthopaedic Section of the American Physical Therapy Association. *Journal of Orthopaedic & Sports Physical Therapy*, *42*(4), A1–A57.

Fritz, J. M., Cleland, J. A., & Childs, J. D. (2007). Subgrouping patients with low back pain: evolution of a classification approach to physical therapy. *Journal of Orthopaedic & Sports Physical Therapy*, *37*(6), 290–302.

George, S. Z., Fritz, J. M., Silfies, S. P., et al. (2021). Interventions for the management of acute and chronic low back pain: revision 2021: clinical practice guidelines linked to the international classification of functioning, disability and health from the academy of orthopaedic physical therapy of the American Physical Therapy Association. *Journal of Orthopaedic & Sports Physical Therapy*, *51*(11), CPG1–CPG60.

CHAPTER 58 QUESTIONS

1. **The 2012 APTA Low Back Pain Clinical Practice Guidelines introduced eight interventional categories. Which of those categories had the following characteristics: Symptoms often with numerous episodes of low back pain with or without a history of related lower extremity pain; Subacute low back pain that is commonly associated with referred lower extremity pain; Pain with mid-range motions that worsen with end-range movements or positions.**
   a. Subacute low back pain with mobility deficits
   b. Subacute low back pain with movement coordination impairments
   c. Subacute low back pain with radiating pain
   d. Subacute low back pain with related generalized pain

2. **According to the 2021 Low Back Pain Clinical Practice Guidelines, what are the best treatment strategies for a patient with chronic low back with leg pain?**
   a. General education and general exercise training
   b. General exercise only
   c. Specific trunk activation and movement control exercises
   d. Specific trunk activation and movement control exercises, thrust and nonthrust joint mobilization and neural tissue mobilization

3. **In the 2021 Low Back Pain Clinical Practice Guidelines, the authors describe grades of recommendation based on the level of evidence with respect to treatment options. They also use the term level of obligation using the terms should, may, can, and should not. Which is the most accurate description of these levels of obligation?**
   a. Should—strong evidence, may—moderate evidence, can—weak evidence, should not—conflicting evidence or no evidence
   b. May—strong evidence, should—moderate evidence, can—weak evidence, should not—conflicting evidence or no evidence
   c. Should—strong evidence, can—moderate evidence, may—weak evidence, should not—conflicting evidence or no evidence
   d. Can—strong evidence, may—moderate evidence, should—weak evidence, should not—conflicting evidence or no evidence

CHAPTER 59

MECHANICAL AND DISCOGENIC BACK PAIN

S. Paris, PhD PT, FAPTA, Hon LLD (Otago) and M.E. Lonnemann, PT, DPT, OCS, FAAOMPT

1. **What is the role of bed rest in acute back pain?**
   Bed rest has a very limited role; evidence-based treatment guidelines for acute LBP and a review of 13 national guidelines by Koes (2010) recommend early and gradual activation of patients and discourage bed rest. "Rest from activity but not from function" is a good adage to follow in this situation.

2. **Describe the structure of the intervertebral disc.**
   Moving centrally from the outer neurovascular capsule are fibrous annular plates, often erroneously called rings (they do not circle the disc). Because the number of anterior and lateral plates is greater than the number of posterior plates, the nucleus in the lumbar spine is positioned slightly posteriorly within the disc. Between the fibrous outer annulus and the inner fluid nucleus is a transition zone consisting of a loosely arranged collection of fibrous tissue that is highly deformable and acts as a buffer between the nucleus and annulus. The nucleus pulposus is a mucoid protein that binds approximately three times its weight in water and allows for distribution of forces.

3. **Describe the functions of the intervertebral disc.**
   Rather surprisingly, because of its extensive water content, the disc is not a shock absorber. Instead, the muscles of the spine are responsible for shock absorption. The functions of the intervertebral disc include the following: (1) It provides space and position for the segment to allow for the nerve root to pass through the foramen without compromise. (2) It permits, guides, and restrains motion in all directions, with the nucleus acting as an incompressible ball while the ligamentous annulus (90% type I collagen) restrains the nucleus and prevents excessive motion within the segment.

4. **What position facilitates disc nutrition?**
   Side lying or lying on the back with the knees bent and the back flat facilitates nutritional pressure changes. Approximately 80% of the nutrition absorbed within a night's rest occurs within the first hour of rest. Therefore, by resting during the lunch hour and again at the end of the workday as well as at night, it is possible to more than double the nutrition to the disc.

   Side lying is of value if the knees are drawn up so as to flatten or slightly round the back. However, the moment the back assumes lordosis, it loads the posterior disc, restricting its ability to imbibe nutrient fluids through the cartilaginous end plate. Likewise, prone lying is not recommended unless there is a large, firm pillow beneath the abdomen to prevent the formation of lordosis.

5. **Describe the innervation of the disc.**
   The recurrent sinu-vertebral nerve and a gray ramus communicans from the sympathetic chain innervate the disc. They penetrate the outer capsule and may extend as far as the second or third annular lamella.

6. **What is the source of discogenic low back pain?**
   Peng et al. (2009) studied the histologic characteristics of the painful disc. They noted the formation of a zone of vascularized granulation tissue from the nucleus pulposus to the outer part of the annulus fibrosus. Nerve growth was found deep into the annulus fibrosis and nucleus pulposus following the zone of granulation tissue in painful discs. Immunoreactive nerve fibers (such as substance P, neurofilament 2000, and vasoactive intestinal peptide) were more extensive in painful discs than in control discs. Annular tears noted at the periphery of discs were associated with this increased vascular granulation tissue, and these fibers may be the source of discogenic low back pain.

7. **Describe the articular receptor distribution in the spine.**
   - Type I—Postural receptors such as Ruffini's corpuscles (greatest in the cervical spine) sense joint position; they have a low threshold and are slow to adapt.
   - Type II—Dynamic receptors such as Golgi-Mazzoni fat pads (deep seated in synovium) sense movement; they have a low threshold but adapt rapidly.
   - Type III—Inhibitory receptors are found in the outer layers of the facet capsules, in associated ligaments, and in the deep layer of the multifidus.
   - Type IV—Nociceptive receptors have a high threshold; they are nonadapting and chemosensitive.

8. **Which structure is most commonly involved in the patient with low back pain?**
Regardless of the primary source of pain—disc, facet, or sacroiliac—the muscles will always be involved, whether voluntarily in a protective manner or involuntarily to guard against low back pain. However, they may also be the primary source of pain after unaccustomed overuse (eg, the first day of spring gardening). The most common cause of initial low back pain would be injury of the facet joints, followed by ligamentous weakness, sacroiliac strain, and ligamentous pain from the outer annulus. Pain may also develop from ligamentous laxity in a segment that is often adjacent to a stiff segment.

9. **Describe the outcomes of physical therapy for acute low back dysfunction.**
Only in the area of acute low back pain (with no specific diagnosis) have satisfactory outcomes been established. The treatments determined to be effective were, in descending order, manipulation, patient instruction, and exercise. Cook et al. (2013) compared the effectiveness of early use of thrust and nonthrust manipulation during the first two visits of physical therapy in patients with mechanical low back pain. Both groups improved with either thrust or nonthrust manipulation. Based on a systematic review of the evidence, spinal manipulation performed by physical therapists is safe and resulted in improved clinical outcomes for patients with low back pain.

10. **How does a therapist determine when manipulation of the spine for mechanical low back pain is indicated?**
Clinical research studies that have demonstrated the effectiveness of thrust and nonthrust manipulation for treatment of LBP used a clinical decision-making framework that incorporates an impairment-based approach. A framework to consider would be the following:
- Rule out red flags and assess for yellow flags
- Assess pain location and behavior
- Assess patient expectations

Assess impairments—Mobility deficits with active spinal mobility and passive intervertebral motion testing and pain provocation with passive accessory intervertebral motion testing guide the therapist to determine the location of focus for the manipulation, direction, intensity, and speed of force application.
- Classify patient—Hypomobility with concurrent pain in the low back and/or buttock with or without symptoms in the thigh

11. **Discuss the potential sources of pain associated with dysfunction of the disc.**
Several researchers have found nerve endings in the outer two to three layers of the disc. Furthermore when the disc degenerates to the degree that it becomes engorged with blood vessels in an effort to repair the disc, sympathetic nerves accompany the blood vessels. Substance P, a pain facilitator, has also been found in degenerative discs.

Early back pain, particularly that associated with developing instability, is mostly from the disc, is usually felt in the back and buttocks, and is of a deep and vague nature, often poorly localized.

When the disc herniates, one source of pain may be from the mechanical strain on the outer fibers of the annulus. If the prolapse places pressure on a nerve root, a sharper radicular radiating pain may pass from the back into the leg from compression of the dorsal root ganglia. With initial nerve root pressure, there is little pain because it appears that the nerves first have to become engorged and sensitized. Thus nearly 30 minutes may pass from the initial, sharp low back pain (tearing of the annulus) to the onset of radicular leg pain (pressure on the nerve root). Chemical irritation from inflammatory agents of the nociceptive fibers of the outer annulus may also cause pain. Other anatomic structures associated with the disc that are innervated and may cause nociception include the posterior longitudinal ligament (PLL), dural root sleeve, and dural sheath. Discogenic pain is mediated by the sinu-vertebral nerves; it reaches the rami communicans through the L2 spinal ganglion. The pain may also take another route through the sympathetic nervous system.

12. **Does disc herniation result from weakness and damage to the annulus (outside in) or from pressure pushing the disc outward (inside out)?**
The first change noted with discography is that the nucleus deforms and starts to "leak" or move laterally. The inner annulus has few fibers, like the loose-knit weave of a woolen sweater. It can be stretched considerably without tearing. The fibrous annulus, however, has many fibers. It is more like a cotton shirt, having little elasticity before tearing. Although the inner annulus may degenerate, tears begin at the outer annulus and spread inwardly, eventually allowing the nucleus to deform. The outer annulus is approximately three times as vascular as the capsule of the knee and thus can heal, as postmortem specimens have shown. Therefore, determining which patients have an outer annulus injury can aid in selection of the appropriate therapy to promote healing and prevent herniation. Glycosaminoglycan turnover within the annulus requires approximately 500 days; collagen turnover is even slower. Healing, if possible, is still remarkably slow.

13. **At what levels do cervical spondylosis most typically occur?**
The prevalence of cervical spondylosis is as follows: C5/C6 > C6/C7 > C3/C5 > C7/T1. These changes affect 70% of the population by age 70.

14. **At what levels do lumbar disc prolapse most commonly occur?**
The prevalence of lumbar disc prolapse usually occurs in the following order: L4/L5 > L5/S1 > L3/L4 > L2/L3 > L1/L2.

15. **In the thoracic spine, what are the most common levels of dysfunction that present with clinical symptoms?**
The junctional sites T1/2, T12/L1, and T4/5 are the most common levels of dysfunction.

16. **Describe a classification of disc herniations.**
DISC PROTRUSION (ANNULAR FIBERS INTACT)
- Localized annular bulge (usually laterally)
- Diffuse annular bulge (usually posteriorly and bilaterally)

DISC HERNIATIONS (ANNULAR FIBERS DISRUPTED)
- Prolapsed (nucleus has migrated through the inner layers but is still contained)
- Extruded (nucleus has broken through the outermost layer)
- Sequestered (nucleus has broken from the disc and is in the spinal or intervertebral canals)

17. **Does spontaneous disc resorption occur? What are the proposed mechanisms?**
Results reported by Kawaguchi et al. (2001) maintain that regression of herniated discs is a process of general tissue repair and remodeling observable in a range of disc herniations rather than a specific autoimmune response.

18. **What is the effect of facet angle on disc herniation?**
A study by Karacan et al. (2004) showed a positive correlation in patients with lumbar disc herniation and asymmetry to sagittalization of facet joints. They noted these alterations were more prominent in the taller patients. Park et al. (2001) found that the degree of facet tropism and disc degeneration might be considered a key factor when distinguishing the development of far lateral lumbar disc herniation from posterolateral lumbar disc herniation. A direct relationship between the extent of the degree of facet tropism and the extent of disc herniation was not seen. Other studies by Hagg and Farfan (1990) found an unclear relationship between facet tropism and disc degeneration.

19. **What is the incidence of disc herniation?**
The incidence of disc herniations cannot be answered for the simple reason that it is now believed that most disc herniations do not hurt. Computed tomography (CT) scans of the lumbar spine in asymptomatic subjects with no history other than minor back discomfort indicate that the rate of disc herniation is 39%. A similar study by Weisel (1984) showed 50% of abnormalities on CT scans in asymptomatic hospital workers. Disc protrusions are seen in 24% of asymptomatic patients.

20. **What are the common causes of radiculopathy?**
Neurologic signs arising from the lumbar spine most commonly occur in middle age, are more prevalent in men, and are typically a result of disc herniations, whereas neurologic signs arising from the cervical spine occur later in life, are more prevalent in women, and result from lateral foraminal stenosis caused by osteophytes from the lateral interbody, osteoarthrosis of the facet joints, and perhaps some disc material along with shortening and thickening of the ligamentum flavum.

21. **Describe the classic presentation of disc herniations at various spinal levels.**

LEVEL	NERVE ROOT	DERMATOME	MYOTOME	REFLEX
C2/C3	C3	Anterior neck and posterior neck	Lateral neck press	None
C3/C4	C4	Nape and anterior shoulder	Shoulder shrug	None
C4/C5	C5	Deltoid anterior arm to base of thumb	Biceps	Biceps
C5/C6	C6	Lateral arm thenar eminence, thumb and index finger	Wrist extensors	Brachioradialis

LEVEL	NERVE ROOT	DERMATOME	MYOTOME	REFLEX
C6/C7	C7	Posterior arm to index, long, and ring fingers	Triceps	Triceps
C7/C8	C8	Inner aspect of forearm and hand, lateral three fingers	None	
T12/L1	L1	Iliac crest and groin	Psoas	None
L1/L2	L2	Anterior thigh	Psoas	None
L2/L3	L3	Anterior lower thigh and shin	Quadriceps	Knee jerk
L3/L4	L4	Medial calf and big toe	Tibialis anterior	Knee jerk
L4/L5	L5	Lateral leg and anterior foot	Extensor hallucis longus	Extensor digitorum brevis
L5/S1	S1	Lower half of posterior calf, sole of foot, and lateral two toes	Flexor hallucis longus; gastrocnemius	Achilles
L5/S1	S2	Posterior thigh, sole, and plantar aspect of heel	Hamstrings	Lateral hamstrings

22. Describe the natural history of disc disease.

In 90% to 95% of patients, spinal pain (which often is disc related) resolves in 3 to 4 months. Lumbar disc herniations are quite common, and most cases have a favorable prognosis. Approximately 45% of patients demonstrate resorption of the herniation over time. In Norway, Weber (1997) randomly denied surgery to half of the patients selected for surgery by good and fair criteria (not as liberal as in the United States). At the end of the first year, those who had surgery scored twice as well on assessment as those who did not. By 3 years, however, there was no significant difference between the two groups. Five-year follow-up examination also found no difference.

23. Which is more successful for acute disc herniation—surgery or conservative care?

Evidence-based treatment guidelines (2012, 2017) for acute LBP and a review of 13 national guidelines by Koes (2010) recommend early and gradual activation of patients, the discouragement of prescribed bed rest, spinal manipulation, and screening for psychosocial factors that would be risk factors for chronicity. Surgery has not been determined to be more successful than conservative care, as indicated by guideline recommendations and published literature.

24. Is disc degeneration associated with low back pain?

In the past, studies of asymptomatic individuals have demonstrated that there is little or no correlation between low back pain and disc pathology. More recently, several large population studies have demonstrated that disc degeneration is associated with LBP. Cheung et al. (2013) demonstrated by visualization on MRI that the risk of back pain increased directly with increasing disc degeneration. De Schepper et al. (2010) showed a similar association with annulus collapse from disc narrowing visualized on x-rays. Other degenerative changes, such as radial fissures, end plate damage, and disc extrusions, have been linked with pain. The variations in the literature may be based on the variety of structural changes that can occur with degeneration such as annular tears, herniation, annular collapse, Schmorl's nodes, dehydration, and annular bulging.

25. Describe the Impairment-Based Classification System (IBCS) and International Classification of Functioning (ICF) and associated findings in a patient likely to present with discogenic pain.

1. IBCS: Lumbar and related leg pain that centralizes with repeated movements (specific exercise)
   ICF: Low back pain with related (referred) lower extremity pain
   Findings:

- Low back and leg pain that moves below the knee
- Extension syndrome
  Symptoms centralize with lumbar backward bending
  Symptoms peripheralize with lumbar forward bending
- Lateral shift

Visible frontal plane deviation of the shoulders relative to the pelvis
Symptoms centralize with side glide and backward bending

- IBCS: Lumbar radiculopathy that does not centralize with repeated movements
  ICF: Classification: Acute, subacute, or chronic low back pain with radiating pain
  Findings:
- Low back with associated radiating leg pain that tends to travel beyond the knee
- Poor tolerance to weight-bearing postures (ie, sitting or standing)
- Symptoms alleviated with traction
- Lower extremity paresthesias, numbness, and weakness may be reported
- No lumbar movements centralize symptoms
- No directional preference noted with history or clinical examination to alleviate lower leg pain
- Peripheralization of leg pain with lumbar backward bending
- Positive SLR for lower leg pain
- Positive crossed SLR test
- Lower extremity neurologic signs (weakness, numbness, DTR)

26. Discuss the role of manipulation and manual therapy in the treatment of disc herniation.

Manual therapy has no direct role in the reduction of disc herniations because neither traction nor manipulation has been shown to reduce the disc. However, manual therapy has been demonstrated to be effective by relaxing the muscles and allowing for movement in the segment.

Manipulation has not been shown to reduce disc herniation. However, Maitland grade I and II oscillations may help reduce discomfort and pain, thereby promoting return to active function. More physical techniques involving stretching and thrust may be of value at the neighboring stiff segments to increase motion and thus improve overall function of the spine, lessening the strain on the level with the disc herniation.

27. What is the effect of rehabilitation after disc surgery?

A 2011 systematic review of the literature by Wilco et al. provided the following conclusions:

- Exercise programs starting 4 to 6 weeks post surgery seem to lead to a faster decrease in pain and functional disability compared with no treatment, and high-intensity programs lead to a faster decrease in pain and functional disability than low-intensity programs.
- There is no evidence that these active programs increase the reoperation rate or that patients need to have their activities restricted after first-time lumbar surgery.
- It is still unclear the exact components that should be included in rehabilitation programs.
- High-intensity programs seem to be more effective, but they could also be more expensive.
- Therefore, cost-effectiveness analysis should be performed to assess whether intensive rehabilitation programs, if started early after surgery, lead to a reduction in costs in terms of less health care utilization or earlier return to work.
- Future research should also focus on the implementation of rehabilitation programs in daily practice.
- The effect of active rehabilitation on the main outcome of functional status is clinically significant in the short term and over the long term.

28. How does exercise relieve back pain?

1. Repetitive motion gates pain. For example, repetitive motion (eg, pendulum exercises) centralizes the pain to the shoulder, relaxes spasm, enables more motion, and hastens recovery.
2. If the pain is from an intradiscal source, repetitive motion may alter the chemical balance. T2-weighted MR studies showed a definite increase in disc water content after repetitive backward bending but no reduction in the size of the protrusion.
3. Extension places a higher stretch on the facet joint capsules than forward bending. Placing the hands in the small of the back and using them as a fulcrum mobilize the facet joints.
4. Repetitive motion enables a patient to get over "fear of movement" and undoubtedly relaxes muscle splinting, thus improving function, decreasing load on the disc, and allowing for earlier return to function.
5. Motion performed repetitively may reduce swelling around the nerve and thus the pressure that may cause ischemia.

29. What is the definition of spinal instability?

According to Panjabi (1992), spinal range of motion can be divided into neutral- and elastic-zone components. Instability is thought to occur when neutral-zone motion increases beyond normal (thus decreasing the elastic zone). Stabilization of the spine is thought to revolve around three subsystems: passive, active, and neutral. When either of these subsystems is impaired, aberrant movement can occur and lead to pain or disability. Rehabilitation should be directed at all three of these systems to increase function and decrease spine pain.

30. **Describe the innervation of the facet joints and types of afferent nerve fibers.**
The innervation of the facet joints is a branch of the posterior primary ramus, which supplies the skin and muscles to the back. A deep branch arises near the facet joint and innervates that joint, with a larger branch supplying the joint below and another branch traveling to the level above (perhaps only in the lumbar spine). Thus, the facet joints on their larger posterior surface have in common with most other joints a triple level of innervation. The anterior innervation is by the recurrent branch of the sinu-vertebral nerve that arches over the intervertebral foramen to supply the ligamentum flavum and the anterior facet joint capsule.

31. **What muscles increase abdominal tone and pressure for stabilization of the lumbar spine?**
The oblique and transverse abdominal muscles are important contributors to abdominal tone, while the multifidus muscle provides stabilization for the posterior spinal structures.

32. **Discuss the significance of the multifidus muscle.**
The multifidus arises from the mamillary process just lateral to the facet joint and then passes upward and medially, attaching to the adjacent facet joint capsule and to the capsule above before inserting into the spinous process one and two levels above. Acting unilaterally, it tends to bend the spine to the same side and rotate it to the opposite side. Acting bilaterally, it extends the spine. Because the multifidus inserts into the capsules of the facet joints, it tends to pull the capsule out of the way, helping to prevent capsular impingement. As one of the deepest muscles in the back, it is considered to be a primary stabilizer. The multifidus may be damaged during laminectomy or fusion. Even at 5 years after surgery, extensive damage may still be present. It is important that clinicians are able to target the multifidus when prescribing motor control exercises because it plays a significant role in lumbar stability. Decreased lumbar multifidus muscle activation is associated with the presence of factors predictive of clinical success with a stabilization exercise program. Hebert et al. (2010) studied the degree of transversus abdominis and lumbar multifidus activation by ultrasound imaging while looking at the prognostic factors associated with a successful stabilization exercise program. The factors included a positive prone instability test, age <40 years, aberrant movements, straight leg raise >91 degrees, and presence of lumbar hypermobility. Significant relationships were identified between decreased LM muscle activation and the number of prognostic factors present. A positive prone instability test and segmental hypermobility were associated with decreased LM muscle activation. These findings provide evidence for the clinical importance of targeting the lumbar multifidus muscle for motor control exercises.

33. **What are the effects of dynamic lumbar stabilization exercise programs after discectomy?**
One study demonstrated that after a microdiscectomy, a 4-week postoperative exercise program can improve pain relief, disability, and spinal function. The exercise program, designed by a physical therapist, concentrated on improving the strength and endurance of the back and abdominal muscles and the mobility of the spine and hips. The program included aerobic exercise and strengthening exercises, such as curl-ups and leg lifts, to strengthen the erector spinae musculature. A prospective randomized clinical trial by Yilmaz et al. (2003) demonstrated with controls that dynamic lumbar stabilization exercises are an efficient and useful technique in the rehabilitation of patients who have undergone microdiscectomy. Outcomes were good for relief of pain and for functional parameters such as strength of the trunk, abdominal, and lumbar spine muscles.

34. **What are the effects of disc herniation and surgery on proprioception and postural control?**
Leinonen (2003) studied proprioception and postural control in patients before and after discectomy. These variables were found to be diminished when comparing postoperative patients with chronic low back pain caused by disc herniation versus healthy controls.

35. **What are the functional results and risk factors for reoperation after disc surgery?**
It has been documented that factors including sedentary occupations, exposure to considerable vibration (such as from driving a motor vehicle), cigarette smoking, previous full-term pregnancies, physical inactivity, increased body mass index (BMI), and a tall stature are associated with symptomatic disc herniations. Increased fitness levels and strength have been noted to reduce the risk of disc rupture. Lack of regular physical exercise was a significant predictor for reoperation, while gender, age, BMI, occupation, or smoking did not hold as much significance as regular exercise. The reoperation rate within 5 years for patients having disc surgery has varied in studies from 7% to 35.3%.

36. **What are the effects of surgery on pain, spine mobility, and disability?**
In a prospective cohort study from the Maine Lumbar Spine Study (Atlas et al., 2005), 400 patients with sciatica caused by lumbar disc herniation were treated either surgically or nonsurgically, and then assessed in 10-year follow-up visits. Changes in the modified Roland back-specific functional status scale favored surgical treatment throughout the follow-up period. However, work and disability status at 10 years did not demonstrate a difference between those treated surgically from those treated nonsurgically. A cross-sectional survey by Hakkinen et al. (2007) reviewed the results of patients' status post lumbar disc herniation surgery. They found that 2 months after

the operation median leg pain had decreased by 87% and back pain by 81%. However, moderate or severe leg pain was still reported in 25% and back pain in 20% of the patients. Hakkinen noted that pain, decreased trunk muscle strength, and decreased mobility were still present in a considerable proportion of patients 2 months after surgery.

37. What are the effects of low back pain, disc herniation, and surgery on the lumbar multifidus?

Functional instability with motor coordination impairments of the core musculature, including the multifidus, has been the clinical assumption after an episode of low back pain because of disc herniation or other impairments as well as surgery. In patients with first-episode low back pain, ultrasound measurements indicate that multifidus muscle recovery does not occur spontaneously when the low back pain resolves. Disc herniation has been associated with selective atrophy of type I fibers while the atrophy of type II fibers was more frequent and severe. Findings such as decreased size of type 2 muscle fibers and core/targetoid and/or moth-eaten changes in the type 1 muscle fibers have been noted. Selective type 2 muscle fiber atrophy has been found during intraoperative muscle biopsies. Pathologic changes were present in 88% of patients before surgery. Rantanen et al. (1993) reviewed the intraoperative biopsies of patients with disc herniation and 5-year follow-up biopsies. Results showed that patients who have a positive outcome have positive changes in the structure of the multifidus. After a posterior surgical approach, biopsies of the multifidus showed significantly more signs of denervation in the tissue than before surgery. Clinicians should progress patients with a spinal stabilization and conditioning program with emphasis on retraining the motor control of the deep abdominal and multifidus muscles.

Bibliography

Atlas, S. J., Keller, R. B., Wu, Y. A., Deyo, R. A., & Singer, D. E. (2005). Long-term outcomes of surgical and nonsurgical management of sciatica secondary to a lumbar disk herniation: 10 year results from the Maine lumbar spine study. *Spine, 30*, 927–935.

Boden, S. D., Davis, D. O., Dina, T. S., Patronas, N. J., & Wiesel, S. W. (1990). Abnormal magnetic-resonance scans of the lumbar spine in asymptomatic subjects. A prospective investigation. *Journal of Bone and Joint Surgery (American), 72*(3), 403–408.

Boos, N., Rieder, R., Schade, V., Spratt, K. F., Semmer, N., & Aebi, M. (1995). 1995 Volvo Award in clinical sciences. The diagnostic accuracy of magnetic resonance imaging, work perception, and psychosocial factors in identifying symptomatic disk herniations. *Spine, 20*(24), 2613–2625.

Botsford, D. J., Esses, S. I., & Ogilvie-Harris, D. J. (1994). In vivo diurnal variation in intervertebral disk volume and morphology. *Spine, 19*, 935–940.

Cheng, J., Wang, H., Zheng, W., et al. (2013). Reoperation after lumbar disk surgery in two hundred and seven patients. *International Orthopaedics, 37*(8), 1511–1517.

Cook, C., Learman, K., Showalter, C., Kabbaz, V., & O'Halloran, B. (2013). Early use of thrust manipulation versus non-thrust manipulation: A randomized clinical trial. *Manual Therapy, 13*, 191–198.

Creighton, D. S. (1993). Positional distraction: A radiological confirmation. *Journal of Manual and Manipulative Therapy, 1*, 83–86.

de Schepper, E. I., Damen, J., van Meurs, J. B., et al. (2010). The association between lumbar disk degeneration and low back pain: The influence of age, gender, and individual radiographic features. *Spine, 35*(5), 531–536.

Delitto, A., George, S. Z., Van Dillen, L., et al. (2012). Low back pain: Clinical practice guidelines linked to the international classification of functioning, disability, health from the orthopaedic section of the American Physical Therapy Association. *Journal of Orthopaedic & Sports Physical Therapy, 42*(4), A1–A57.

Desmoulin, G. T., Pradhan, V., & Milner, T. E. (2020). Mechanical aspects of intervertebral disc injury and implications on biomechanics. *Spine, 45*(8), E457–E464.

Dolan, P., Greenfield, K., Nelson, R. J., & Nelson, I. W. (2000). Can exercise therapy improve the outcome of microdiskectomy? *Spine, 25*, 1523–1532.

Farfan, H., Huberdeau, R., & Dubow, H. (1972). Lumbar intervertebral disk degeneration: The influence of geometric features on the pattern of disk degeneration: A post mortem study. *Journal of Bone and Joint Surgery (American), 54*, 492–510.

Hagen, K., Jamtvedt, G., Hilde, G., & Winnem, M. F. (2005). The updated Cochrane Review of bed rest for low back pain and sciatica. *Spine, 30*, 542–546.

Hagg, O., & Wallner, A. (1990). Facet joint asymmetry and protrusion of the intervertebral disk. *Spine, 15*, 356–359.

Häkkinen, A., Kiviranta, I., Neva, M. H., Kautiainen, H., & Ylinen, J. (2007). Reoperations after first lumbar disk herniation surgery; A special interest on residives during a 5-year follow-up. *BMC Musculoskeletal Disorders, 8*(1), 2.

Häkkinen, A., Ylinen, J., Kautiainen, H., et al. (2003). Pain, trunk muscle strength, spine mobility and disability following lumbar disk surgery. *Journal of Rehabilitation Medicine, 35*, 236–240.

Hebert, J. J., Koppenhaver, S. L., Magel, J. S., & Fritz, J. M. (2010). The relationship of transversus abdominis and lumbar multifidus activation and prognostic factors for clinical success with a stabilization exercise program: A cross-sectional study. *Archives of Physical Medicine and Rehabilitation, 91*, 78–85.

Hides, J. A., Stokes, M. J., Saide, M., Jull, G. A., & Cooper, D. H. (1994). Evidence of lumbar multifidus muscle wasting ipsilateral to symptoms in patients with acute subacute low back pain. *Spine, 19*, 165–172.

Jacobs, W. C. H., vanTulder, M., Arts, M., et al. (2011). Surgery versus conservative management of sciatica due to a lumbar herniated disk: A systematic review. *European Spine Journal, 20*(4), 513–522.

Jensen, M. C., Brant-Zawadzki, M. N., Obuchowski, N., Modic, M. T., Malkasian, D., & Ross, J. S. (1994). Magnetic resonance imaging of the lumbar spine in people without back pain. *New England Journal of Medicine, 331*(2), 69–73.

Kara, B., Tulum, Z., & Acar, U. (2005). Functional results and the risk factors of reoperations after lumbar disk surgery. *European Spine Journal, 14*, 43–48.

Karacan, I., Aydin, T., Sahin, Z., et al. (2004). Facet angles in lumbar disk herniation: Their relation to anthropometric features. *Spine, 29*, 1132–1136.

Kawaguchi, S., Yamashita, T., Yokogushi, K., Murakami, T., Ohwada, O., & Sato, N. (2001). Immunophenotypic analysis of the inflammatory infiltrates in herniated intervertebral disks. *Spine, 26*, 1209–1214.

Koes, B. W., van Tulder, M., Lin, C. W. C., Macedo, L. G., McAuley, J., & Maher, C. (2010). An updated overview of clinical guidelines for the management of non-specific low back pain in primary care. *European Spine Journal, 19*, 2075–2094.

Kuczynski, J. J., Schwieterman, B., Columber, K., Knupp, D., Shaub, L., & Cook, C. E. (2012). Effectiveness of physical therapist administered spinal manipulation treatment of low back pain: A systematic review of the literature. *International Journal of Sports Physical Therapy, 7*(6), 647–662.

Leinonen, V., Kankaanpää, M., Luukkonen, M., et al. (2003). Lumbar paraspinal muscle function, perception of lumbar position and postural control in disk herniation-related back pain. *Spine, 28*, 842–848.

Moneta, G. B., Videman, T., Kaivanto, K., et al. (1994). Reported pain during lumbar diskography as a function of anular ruptures and disk degeneration. A re-analysis of 833 diskograms. *Spine, 19*(17), 1968–1974.

Olson, K. A. (2009). *Manual physical therapy of the spine*. St. Louis: W.B. Saunders Company.

Ostelo, R. W., Costa, L. O. P., Maher, C. G., de Vet, H. C. W., van Tuler, M. W., & Ostelo, R. W. J. G. (2006). Rehabilitation after lumbar disk surgery. *Cochrane Database of Systematic Reviews, 3*, CD003007.

Paris, S. V. (1983). Anatomy as related to function and pain. *Orthopedic Clinics of North America, 14*, 3.

Paris, S.V., & Nyberg, R. (1989). Healing of the lumbar intervertebral disk. Presented at the International Society for the Study of the Lumbar Spine, Kyoto, Japan, May.

Park, J., Chang, H., Kim, K. W., & Park, S. J. (2001). Facet tropism: A comparison between far lateral and posterolateral lumbar disk herniations. *Spine, 26*, 677–679.

Peng, B., Chen, J., Kuang, Z., Li, D., Pang, X., & Zhang, X. (2009). Diagnosis and surgical treatment of back pain originating from endplate. *European Spine Journal, 18*(7), 1035–1040.

Peng, B., Hou, S., Wu, W., Zhang, C., & Yang, Y. (2006). The pathogenesis and clinical significance of a high-intensity zone (HIZ) of lumbar intervertebral disk on MR imaging in the patient with diskogenic low back pain. *European Spine Journal, 15*(5), 583–587.

Peng, B., Wu, W., Hou, S., Li, P., Zhang, C., & Yang, Y. (2005). The pathogenesis of diskogenic low back pain. *Journal of Bone and Joint. Surgery (British), 87*(1), 62.

Quaseem, A., Wilt, T. J., & McLean, R. M. (2017). Noninvasive treatments for acute, subacute, and chronic low back pain: A clinical practice guideline from the American College of Physicians. *Annals of Internal Medicine, 166*(7), 514–530.

Rantanen, J., Hurme, M., Falck, B., et al. (1993). The lumbar multifidus muscle five years after surgery for a lumbar intervertebral disk herniation. *Spine, 18*, 568–574.

Raoul, S., Faure, A., Robert, R., et al. (2003). Role of the sinu-vertebral nerve in low back pain and anatomical basis of therapeutic implications. *Surgical and Radiologic Anatomy, 24*, 366–371.

Saal, J. A. (1996). Natural history and nonoperative treatment of lumbar disk herniation. *Spine, 21*(Suppl), 2S–9S.

Videman, T., Battie, M. C., Gibbons, L. E., Maravilla, K., Manninen, H., & Kaprio, J. (2003). Associations between back pain history and lumbar MRI findings. *Spine, 28*(6), 582–588.

Weber, B. R., Grob, D., Dvorák, J., & Müntener, M. (1997). Posterior surgical approach to the lumbar spine and its effect on the multifidus muscle. *Spine, 22*, 1765–1772.

Weisel, S. W., Tsourmas, N., Feffer, H. L., Citrin, C. M., & Patronas, N. (1984). A study of computer-assisted tomography. I: The incidence of positive CAT scans in an asymptomatic group of patients. *Spine, 9*, 549–551.

Yílmaz, F., Yílmaz, A., Merdol, F., Parlar, D., Sahin, F., & Kuran, B. (2003). Efficacy of dynamic lumbar stabilization exercise in lumbar microdiscectomy. *Journal of Rehabilitation Medicine, 35*, 163–167.

Zhao, W. P., Kawaguchi, Y., Matsui, H., Kanamori, M., & Kimura, T. (2000). Histochemistry and morphology of the multifidus muscle in lumbar disk herniation: Comparative study between diseased and normal sides. *Spine, 25*, 2191–2199.

Zoidl, G., Grifka, J., Boluki, D., et al. (2003). Molecular evidence for local denervation of paraspinal muscles in failed-back surgery/postdiscotomy syndrome. *Clinical Neuropathology, 22*, 71–77.

CHAPTER 59 QUESTIONS

1. **Which of the following is associated with impairment-based classifications in patients with discogenic low back pain?**
   a. Poor sitting tolerance
   b. Poor standing tolerance
   c. LBP and buttock pain that does not move below the knee
   d. Symptoms centralize with forward bending

2. **What finding that will predict clinical success of a stabilization program is associated with the following prognostic factors: positive prone instability test, age <40 years, aberrant movements, straight leg raise >91 degrees, and presence of lumbar hypermobility?**
   a. Decreased transversus abdominus function
   b. Normal transversus abdominus activation
   c. Decreased multifidus function
   d. Normal multifidus activation

3. **Which of the following statements is true regarding rehabilitation after lumbar disc surgery?**
   a. Exercise programs starting 4 to 6 weeks post surgery lead to faster pain reduction and less functional disability compared with no treatment.
   b. Low-intensity programs lead to a faster decrease in pain and functional disability than high-intensity programs.
   c. Specific components of exercise, such as stabilization, have been shown to be more effective than general aerobic conditioning.
   d. There is significant evidence that active exercise programs increase the reoperation rate after first-time lumbar surgery.

LUMBAR SPINAL STENOSIS

R.E. DuVall, PT, DHSc, MMSc, OCS, SCS, ATC, FAAOMPT, J.M. Whitman, PT, DScPT, OCS, FAAOMPT, and J.M. Fritz, PhD, PT, ATC

1. **What is lumbar spinal stenosis (LSS)?**
   LSS can be defined as any narrowing of the lumbar spinal canal, nerve root canals, and/or intervertebral foramina that may encroach on the nerve roots of the lumbar spine. LSS can become a painful and potentially disabling condition in affected individuals.

2. **How is LSS classified?**
   There are two means of classification commonly used to describe patients with LSS; one is based on the anatomic location of the narrowing, and the other on the etiology of the narrowing.

ANATOMIC CLASSIFICATION

- Lateral stenosis—narrowing that occurs within the lumbar intervertebral foramina and/or the nerve root canal, causing encroachment around the spinal nerve as it exits
- Central stenosis—narrowing that occurs within the spinal canal, causing encroachment around the nerve roots of the cauda equina housed within the dural sac

ETIOLOGIC CLASSIFICATION

- Primary stenosis—narrowing caused by a congenital malformation or defect in postnatal development. Only about 10% of cases of lumbar stenosis can be considered to be primary stenosis.
- Secondary stenosis—narrowing resulting from acquired conditions such as degenerative changes, spondylolisthesis, fractures, and postsurgical scarring. The most common cause of secondary stenosis is degenerative changes. Secondary stenosis may occur in individuals who already have a degree of primary stenosis.

3. **What are the most common structural changes associated with LSS?**
   The majority of cases of LSS occur secondary to degenerative changes. Facet joint arthrosis and hypertrophy, bulging and thickening of the ligamentum flavum, loss of disc height and posterior/lateral bulging of the intervertebral disc, and degenerative spondylolisthesis are the most common changes contributing to LSS. Other, less common causes of secondary stenosis include fractures, postoperative fibrosis, tumors, and systemic diseases of the bone, such as Paget's disease.

4. **Is lumbar stenosis a common problem?**
   Yes; LSS is a common cause of low back pain, particularly in older adults. It is the most common reason for undergoing spinal surgery in individuals over the age of 65. Because of increases in life expectancy and improved diagnostic technology, rates of diagnosis of LSS and rates of surgery have increased substantially in the past several decades. Even Egyptian burial grounds for the workers who helped build the great pyramids of the 18th to early 20th Dynasties have shown radiographic evidence of significant LSS. These heavy laborers were studied and found to have LSS degenerative changes with the most common lesions of their spines affecting the articular facets more than the vertebral bodies.

5. **How will the typical patient with lumbar stenosis present clinically?**
   In general, because degenerative changes are the predominant cause leading to LSS, affected individuals are typically older than age 50 with a long history of low back pain. Patients who have a history of performing heavy labor are at greatest risk. Most patients will have symptoms of pain and/or numbness in one or both legs. Chronic nerve compression may lead to diminished lower extremity reflexes and strength or sensation deficits. Lumbar range of motion, particularly in extension, will be limited and painful, often reproducing lower extremity symptoms. Symptoms tend to be posture dependent, worsening with spinal extension and improving with flexion. Because of this, patients will generally feel better in a sitting position and worse when standing or walking.

   Several authors have provided information that helps quantify the impact of these various clinical indicators on the ultimate diagnosis of LSS. Katz et al. and Fritz et al. identified several clinical findings with associated sensitivity (Sn) and/or specificity (Sp) values for establishing the diagnosis of LSS. These findings are as follows: age over 65 – Sn = 0.77; pain below buttocks – Sn = 0.88; no pain when seated – Sp = 0.93; pain with flexion – Sn = 0.88; sitting is the best position – Sn = 0.89; standing/walking are worst positions – Sn = 0.89.

Sugioka et al. sought to develop a score-based prediction rule to assist with diagnosis of LSS from self-report items only. The final predictors of LSS and associated risk scores are shown in Table 60.1. Scores of 7 or more yielded positive likelihood ratios of 1.90 to 3.91.

Last, Konno et al. also developed a score-based prediction rule for diagnosing LSS. In this analysis, the researchers also included items from the physical examination. Their final predictors for LSS and associated risk scores are shown in Table 60.2. For this prediction rule, total risk scores of 7 or higher yield the following diagnostic indices: sensitivity = 0.93, specificity = 0.72, positive likelihood ratio = 3.31.

6. **Why do patients with LSS feel worse when standing than when sitting?**
Standing places the lumbar spine in a position close to full extension. While standing, many patients will fail to activate their core musculature, whereby they passively position themselves in a relaxed lumbar extended position. Lumbar extended compressive loads fall upon the posterior aspects of their vertebral bodies and facet joints. Tonic axial compression results in osteophytic facet hypertrophy, which causes narrowing of the spinal foramen. In individuals without stenosis, this narrowing is tolerated without difficulty; however, patients with stenotic narrowing tend to have worse symptoms when standing or when standing and walking. Sitting facilitates lumbar flexion in the spine with decompressive widdening of the lumbar foramen which generally reduce the symptoms of individuals with LSS.

Table 60.1

PREDICTIVE VARIABLE	ASSIGNED RISK SCORE
Age: 60–70 >70	2 3
Onset of symptoms >6 months	1
Symptoms: Improve with bending forward Improve with bending backward Exacerbate while standing up	2 −2 2
Intermittent claudication present	1
Urinary incontinence present	1

Table 60.2

PREDICTIVE VARIABLE	ASSIGNED RISK SCORE
Age: 60–70 >70	1 2
Absence of diabetes	1
Symptoms: Improve with bending forward Exacerbate while standing up	3 2
Intermittent claudication present	3
Examination: Symptoms induced by having patients bend forward Symptoms induced by having patients bend backward	−1 1
Good peripheral artery circulation	3
Abnormal Achilles tendon reflex	1
SLR test positive	−2

7. **Are there other factors that exacerbate symptoms for patients with LSS?**
Axial compression, as is experienced during weight-bearing and high impact bipedal activities, also creates increased narrowing of both the spinal canal and intravertebral foramen which may exacerbate the symptoms of LSS. Because intravertebral discs are 80% composed of water, they can compress and decompress with different loads and movements. When these intravertebral discs are vertically loaded with axial compression they lose their vertical height and the facet joints now become more compressed. It is not uncommon for patients suffering with LSS to experience exacerbated symptoms toward the end of the day as their intravertebral discs have lost some of their water volume due to axial compression of being upright. Upright postures are further exacerbated by additional compressive forces associated with lifting, carrying, walking and even worse with running. Research has demonstrated that the narrowing effects of axial compression are similar in magnitude to those of spinal extension. This helps explain why walking can be difficult for patients with lumbar stenosis. Walking involves extension of the lumbar spine which creates increased compressive forces upon the posterior aspects of the intervertebral joints; whereby, narrowing the neural foramen.

8. **What is neurogenic claudication?**
Neurogenic claudication is defined as poorly localized pain, paresthesias, and cramping of one or both lower extremities of a neurologic origin; symptoms are often worsened by walking and relieved by sitting. Again, the lumbar spine is extended beyond a neutral position in the walking position that narrows the central canal and neural foramen, whereby inducing mechanical compression upon the respective cauda equina and/or exiting nerve roots. These mechanical compressors can result in altered sensibility, pain or motor weakness. The pathoanatomy and pathophysiology of this neurologic compression has to do with altered microcirculation leading to ischemic dysfunction of the encroached nervous tissues. There can be many causes of claudication; therefore the key distinguishing feature of neurogenic claudication is its neurologic origin enduced by mechanical compression of the cauda equina and/or exiting nerve roots. The symptoms of neurogenic claudication are often the reason that an individual with LSS is prompted to seek medical treatment.

9. **Are there other conditions that might be confused with lumbar stenosis?**
Other conditions that have been confused with LSS include osteoarthritis of the hip, vascular claudication (with peripheral arterial disease), unstable spondylolisthesis, and lumbar intervertebral disc herniation. Other frequent concomitant problems that may mandate additional differential diagnosis for those with lumbar stenosis may include diabetic neuropathy, other peripheral neuropathies, other local musculoskeletal abnormalities, lower extremity (LE) disorders, iliacus arterial involvement, abdominal aortic aneurysm and spinal tumors. It is important to recognize other comorbid conditions that can mimic symptoms associated with lumbar stenosis, especially conditions associated with mortality. These life-threatening comorbid conditions can include abdominal aortic aneurysms and infrarenal aortic pseudoaneurysms. Differential medical screening is necessary to rule out pathological conditions with similar symptoms to neurogenic claudication.

10. **How can LSS be differentiated from other conditions with a similar presentation in the clinic?**
The postural-dependency of symptoms (ie, better with flexion or sitting; worse with extension, standing, and walking) is a unique characteristic of patients with LSS. A thorough history, including exacerbating and relieving positions or activities, will often reveal this posture-dependent nature of symptoms.

Clinical tests have also attempted to capitalize on the posture-dependency of stenosis symptoms to differentiate spinal stenosis from other conditions with similar symptoms. A "bicycle test" has been described in which the patient first pedals in an upright, seated position with the lumbar spine in extension and then with the spine in a flexed position. If the individual pedals farther in the spine-flexed position, the test is considered positive for LSS. Walking tests have also been described for use in differential diagnosis. The patient walks on a level surface in an upright posture and also in a slumped or flexed posture. If the patient can walk farther with the spine flexed, the test is considered positive for LSS. A variation on this test, called the Two Stage Treadmill Test (TSTT), compares walking on a level treadmill versus an inclined treadmill (15% incline). The incline of the treadmill causes the patient to flex the spine while walking and usually will improve walking capacity in patients with LSS. Earlier onset of symptoms and prolonged recovery with level treadmill walking yields a specificity (Sp) of 0.95 and a positive likelihood ratio (+LR) of 14.5. A longer total walking time on the inclined treadmill versus the level treadmill yields an Sp of 0.92 and a + LR of 6.5.

Additionally, a thorough abdominal, illial and lower extremity neurovascular assessment should be performed, often including assessment of lower extremity muscle strength, reflexes, sensation, and pulses. The clinician should also look for trophic changes of the skin and nails and may opt to perform an ankle-brachial index test. This neurovascular assessment will help with differentiation from other neuropathic or vascular conditions.

11. **Are diagnostic imaging studies or electrodiagnostic studies helpful in confirming a diagnosis of LSS?**
Diagnostic imaging modalities are generally used to confirm the diagnosis of LSS. The most commonly used tests are the following:
- Magnetic resonance imaging—MRI is one of the most commonly used imaging studies to confirm a diagnosis of LSS. The anterior-posterior diameter of the spinal canal or the cross-sectional area of the dural sac can be measured to determine the extent of narrowing.
- CT scan—The CT scan is also commonly used to assess the diameter or cross-sectional area in the same manner as described for the MRI.

It is important to remember that the presence of stenosis with imaging is prevalent in the asymptomatic aging population; therefore correlation of imaging findings with clinical presentation is essential. Hence, imaging cannot be considered the gold standard in the diagnosis of LSS. It must only be considered as an adjunctive to a thorough physical examination.

Examination with electrodiagnostics is occasionally used to assist in the diagnosis of LSS. According to Haig et al., the following factors can help with this diagnosis:
- Miniparaspinal mapping with a one side score >4: sensitivity = 0.3; specificity = 1.0
- Fibrillation potential in limb muscles: sensitivity = 0.33; specificity = 0.88
- Absence of tibial H-wave: sensitivity = 0.36; specificity = 0.92
- Composite limb and paraspinal fibrillation score: sensitivity = 0.48; specificity = 0.88

12. **Are plain film x-rays helpful in the diagnosis of LSS?**
Plain film x-rays can show the degenerative changes such as osteophytes and disc degeneration that are often the cause of LSS. Lateral views can demonstrate the angle of lordotic curvature, diameter of the intervertebral foramina. However, plain film x-rays are limited in their usefulness by their inability to image the central spinal canal and the soft tissue changes that may contribute to LSS.

13. **What are the most common impairments and functional limitations found in patients with LSS?**
The most common impairments found during the examination of the patient are restrictions in spinal range of motion. Lumbar passive intervertebral mobility testing reveals facet joint hypomobility. Side-bending is often limited bilaterally; lumbar extension may be quite limited and reproduce or intensify the patient's symptoms. Lumbar flexion is also frequently limited in range but will often somewhat relieve the symptoms. Deficits in vibratory or pinprick sensation in one or both lower extremities can occur, along with strength or reflex deficits. Many patients will have a positive straight leg raise test. Another common area of impairment is the hip joint. Restricted range of motion, particularly in extension, and weakness of the hip extensors and abductors are common findings. The most widespread functional limitation in patients with LSS is diminished walking tolerance because of leg symptoms that are relieved by sitting, as well as limitation in prolonged standing postures.

14. **Describe the surgical procedure for a patient with LSS.**
Surgical treatment of LSS is performed to relieve compression on the contents of the central and lateral spinal canals. The most common surgical procedure for patients with LSS is a decompression laminectomy in which portions of the vertebral arch are removed to reduce compression of the lumbar spinal nerves. Sometimes a fusion, with or without instrumentation, will also be performed, although this is usually only done if there is evidence of spondylolisthesis along with the spinal stenosis.

15. **Should a patient with LSS have surgery?**
The decision to pursue surgery should be determined based on careful and shared decision making between providers and patients, with heavy emphasis on patient preferences.

Clinical outcomes are generally good for surgical treatment, with high percentages of patients expressing satisfaction and reporting improvement early postoperatively. However, these outcomes tend to deteriorate with time, with only about 60% to 70% of patients satisfied after 4 to 7 years and between-group clinical outcomes for those treated with surgery versus conservative care diminishing within 2 to 8 years after surgery.

Sufficient literature describing positive clinical outcomes from various nonsurgical approaches to care is available and often with no reported adverse outcomes. These nonsurgical approaches typically include treatments such as aerobic exercise, stretching, strengthening, mobilization/manipulation, and patient education.

Based on the known risks of surgical complications and the stable nature of spinal stenosis, current recommendations are that patients should be offered a rigorous trial of physical therapy care before pursuing surgery. Patients who do not improve should be well informed of the potential risks and benefits of surgery, including the fact that benefits from surgery will most likely diminish over time.

16. **Will the symptoms of lumbar stenosis continue to worsen over time?**
Research to date shows that LSS is a generally stable condition. Although some patients will deteriorate over time, this is not inevitable, and large percentages of patients can maintain or improve their condition with time.

17. **Will epidural steroid injections help patients with lumbar stenosis?**
Epidural steroid injections have been frequently recommended as a nonsurgical option for patients with LSS. Some patients will receive short-duration benefits from epidural steroid injections. The effectiveness of injections in reducing symptoms beyond a couple of weeks, however, is less likely.

18. **What is the best physical therapy treatment for patients with lumbar stenosis?**
Numerous treatment options have been proposed for use by physical therapists in the treatment of patients with LSS. Flexion-oriented exercises are advocated to capitalize on the postural dependency of symptoms of spinal stenosis. General conditioning activities are useful and may include stationary cycling, aquatic exercise, and walking as tolerated by the patient. Any strength or flexibility deficits identified during the physical examination should be addressed. Manual therapy (including mobilization, manipulation, and stretching) targeting the thoracic and lumbopelvic spine regions and hips may also be helpful. LSS is caused by mechanical compressive forces, so the best physical therapy treatments must include intgerventions directed toward revieving the mechanical compressive forces.

19. **Should traction be used in the treatment of patients with LSS?**
Lumbopelvic traction has been recommended for the treatment of LSS in an attempt to relieve compression that results from the pathology. Although traction may be helpful for pain reduction in some patients, it should be combined with patient education and more active forms of therapy to restore optimal postures, lessen symptoms and improve function.

20. **Can deweighted treadmill ambulation help patients with LSS?**
Deweighted treadmill ambulation uses a harness-and-traction device to provide a vertical traction force during ambulation on a treadmill. The traction force reduces the axial compression associated with weight bearing and may permit some individuals with LSS to walk with reduced symptoms of neurogenic claudication. This treatment technique may hold promise for selected patients with stenosis because it provides the benefit of traction while keeping the patient active and exercising. However, in a randomized trial by Pua et al. that compares exercise plus cycling versus exercise plus deweighted treadmill walking, both groups achieved similar pain and disability outcomes at 6 weeks. Therefore the use of deweighting should be considered as a potential rehabilitation tool on a case-by-case basis, based on clinical response, and, in general, should not be viewed as superior to cycling as a part of a comprehensive treatment program.

21. **Is it possible to identify patient-centered factors that predict better versus worse outcomes from surgery for lumbar stenosis?**
Although many researchers have investigated this question, there is some conflicting information in the literature. Some identified predictors of worse surgical outcomes to date include depression, worse emotional health, smoking, Workers' Compensation, anxiety, life dissatisfaction, higher BMI, longer duration of leg pain/symptoms, cardiovascular comorbidity, scoliosis, other disorders influencing walking ability, predominant back pain (>leg pain), prior lumbar surgery, history of psychiatric disease, female gender, and low baseline disability.
In addition to not having these identified predictive factors for worse outcomes, the following factors have been identified as predicting better surgical outcomes: greater central canal stenosis, good or above average self-rated health, younger age, lower duration use of analgesics preoperatively, greater preoperative disability, more ambitious preoperative expectations related to pain and functional improvements, and no lifting required at work.

22. **Are there published studies documenting patient outcomes with defined physical therapy treatment approaches?**
Many studies are now available demonstrating positive clinical outcomes of care for patients treated with interventions often provided by physical therapists, including aerobic exercise, stretching, strengthening, aerobic exercise, and mobilization/manipulation. Some studies also include traction, physical modalities, or lumbopelvic orthoses. Selected studies are described as follows:
- Simotas et al. reported on the results of 49 patients treated with a program of physical therapy (flexion-oriented exercises) and epidural steroids. After 3 years, 9 patients (18%) had undergone surgery, 12 patients (24%) reported no change in symptoms, 23 patients (47%) had some amount of improvement, and 5 patients (10%) experienced worsening of symptoms.
- Murphy et al. reported clinically meaningful long-term improvements in disability and pain for 57 patients treated with manipulation, neural mobilization, flexion exercises, and lumbar stabilization training in a prospective observational cohort.
- Pua et al. conducted a trial that included 68 patients. Both treatment groups received lumbar flexion exercises, lumbar traction, and thermal modalities. One group also performed deweighted treadmill walking, and the other performed stationary cycling. Although there were no between-group differences, both groups improved from baseline to 6 weeks.
- Ammendolia and Chow reported on clinically meaningful improvements in pain and disability for a cohort of 49 patients after a 6-week program, including manual therapy (soft tissue and neural mobilization, manipulation, lumbar flexion-distraction, and muscle stretching), home exercises, and self-management strategies.
- Cambron et al. included 60 patients in a pilot RCT that investigated optimal dosages of spinal manipulation. The treatment groups receiving a total of 12 and 18 manipulations over 6 weeks demonstrated significant

within-group improvements up through 6 months in symptom severity, and the group receiving 18 manipulations had significant within-group improvements in physical function.

- Whitman et al. conducted an RCT with 58 patients that compared an individualized approach (impairment-based manual therapy interventions to the thoracic spine, lumbopelvic spine, and lower extremities; deweighted treadmill walking; and abdominal retraining exercises) to walking, a standardized flexion exercise, and a subtherapeutic ultrasound program. A greater proportion of patients in the pragmatic, individualized program reported recovery at 6 weeks versus the flexion exercise/walking group. Although both groups demonstrated positive outcomes over the 24-month follow-up, improvements in disability, satisfaction, and treadmill walking tests favored the individualized treatment group at all follow-up points.
- Delitto et al. conducted a multisite, randomized controlled trial that included 169 surgical candidates with lumbar stenosis. Patients were treated with either surgical decompression or a 6-week, well-defined, twice weekly physical therapy (PT) intervention program, including lumbar flexion exercises, patient education, general conditioning (cycling or treadmill walking), and individualized lower extremity strengthening and flexibility exercises. Those patients undergoing physical therapy intervention had similar outcomes to those treated with surgical decompression at the 2-year follow-up.

23. Should patients with lumbar stenosis wear a brace or corset?

The use of a rigid corset to limit spinal extension or a soft corset for general support has been recommended. A soft corset may provide a measure of relief for patients. A more rigid brace, although effective in limiting or preventing extension, is often cumbersome and restrictive for the patient and should likely be reserved for those individuals not responding to other forms of nonoperative treatment. Additionally, proprioceptive taping may be utilized to cue patient to maintain their optimal decompressive postures.

24. How should the outcomes of treatment for patients with lumbar stenosis be measured?

Measuring the effectiveness of any treatment for LSS is an important consideration. Patient-reported measures, such as the Oswestry or Roland Morris disability scales, as well as the condition-specific Swiss Spinal Stenosis Questionnaire, are useful for documenting functional limitations and disability. The measurement of walking tolerance, usually conducted on a treadmill or with a 6-minute walking test, is an important assessment and monitoring tool because it measures the most common and troublesome functional limitation in these patients.

25. Does stenosis occur in the cervical spine as well?

Yes; stenotic narrowing can and does occur in the cervical spine. Similar to the lumbar spine, the narrowing may occur laterally, in the intervertebral foramen, or centrally, in the spinal canal. The etiology may be primary (ie, congenital), secondary to degenerative conditions, or a combination of these two factors. The presence of congenital stenosis of the central canal in the cervical spine is a particular concern for participants of collision sports, such as football. The normal sagittal plane diameter of the spinal canal in the cervical region is 17 to 18 mm. The diameter of the spinal cord is about 10 mm. If the sagittal plane diameter of the canal is diminished with osteophytic changes, the safety margin within the canal is compromised, and symptoms of compression of the spinal cord may result. As with lumbar stenosis, the presence of cervical stenosis on imaging may be present in absence of clinical symptoms, therefore mandating corroboration of clinical and imaging findings.

26. What symptoms will a patient with cervical stenosis exhibit?

The symptoms of lateral and central cervical stenosis differ substantially. Lateral cervical stenosis typically results in compression of the cervical nerve root and produces symptoms of radiculopathy. Central cervical stenosis may compress the spinal cord, resulting in a condition termed cervical myelopathy. Symptoms of radiculopathy include neck and upper extremity pain and paresthesia in a dermatomal pattern. There may also be complaints of upper extremity muscle weakness in the affected arm. Symptoms of cervical myelopathy are often subtler, particularly in the early stages. Neck pain is not always present. Impaired bipedal coordination, unsteadiness in gait, clumsiness or ataxia are often early symptoms. Wasting of the intrinsic hand muscles is common. An extrasegmental distribution of paresthesia in one or both hands and feet may be present, followed by a perception of weakness. Gait disturbances can become severe, significantly interfering with functional activities and safety.

27. What is the typical clinical presentation for patients with central cervical stenosis?

The signs of central cervical stenosis (myelopathy) are those of upper motor neuron, or long tract, disorders. Clinical signs may include weakness with spasticity, hypertonic deep tendon reflexes, clonus, present Hoffmann and Babinski signs, hand withdrawal reflex, and an inverted supinator sign. Vibratory sensation is typically diminished in the lower extremities, and both upper and lower extremity reflexes may become hyperactive. Cervical range of motion is typically restricted in all planes. Lhermitte's sign (spinal pain and/or radiating extremity pain and paresthesias with forced cervical flexion or extension) may be present. Spurling's sign is expected to be negative, and manual cervical traction will not have any effect on symptoms. According to Cook et al., at least three of the following five clinical tests help rule in cervical myelopathy: (1) gait deviation, (2) present Hoffmann's test, (3) + inverted supinator sign, (4) present Babinski test, (5) age >45 years (specificity = 0.99; CI = 0.97–0.99); + LR = 30.9; 95% CI = 5.5–181.8).

28. **Is treatment by a physical therapist helpful for cervical myelopathy?**
Nonsurgical care is often recommended for patients with mild myelopathy, although scant evidence exists investigating the impact of treatment by a physical therapist for this disorder. Intermittent cervical traction is often recommended as a potentially helpful intervention. In a small case series, Browder et al. reported improvements in pain and disability for seven patients with cervical myelopathy who were all treated with intermittent cervical traction and thrust manipulation targeting the thoracic spine. It is plausible that manual therapy directed to rectifying the upper thoracic spine would provide optimal functioning of the cervical spine by increasing the axial dimensions of the central spinal canal space. No adverse events or outcomes were reported.

29. **Is surgery recommended for patients with cervical myelopathy?**
The disorder is considered to be progressive in nature and potentially disabling, but those with cervical myelopathy (CM) often experience long periods of stable neurologic status between episodes of exacerbation. Conservative nonsurgical treatment is often recommended for patients with mild cervical myelopathy. In contrast, surgical management is typically considered for those with moderate to severe CM. Although one prospective RCT demonstrated no significant differences between groups (surgery versus no surgery) at 10 years, several other studies conclude that those with moderate to severe CM who undergo surgery experience improved outcomes over those who do not. Performing surgery early in the course of the condition is believed to lead to a better long-term outcome. Laminotomy or laminoplasty is typically performed to increase the dimensions of the central spinal canal and may be accompanied by cervical fusion.

Bibliography

Ammendolia, C., & Chow, N. (2015). Clinical outcomes for neurogenic claudication using a multimodal program for lumbar spinal stenosis: A retrospective study. *Journal of Manipulative and Physiological Therapeutics*, *38*(3), 188–194.

Atlas, S. J., Deyo, R. A., Keller, R. B., et al. (1996). The Maine lumbar spine outcome study, part III. 1-year outcomes for surgical and non-surgical management of lumbar spinal stenosis. *Spine*, *21*, 1787–1795.

Backstrom, K. M., Whitman, J. M., & Flynn, T. W. (2011). Lumbar spinal stenosis— diagnosis and management of the aging spine. *Manual Therapy*, *16*, 308–317.

Bridwell, K. H. (1994). Lumbar spinal stenosis. Diagnosis, management, and treatment. *Clinics in Geriatric Medicine*, *10*, 677–701.

Browder, D. A., Erhard, R. E., & Piva, S. R. (2004). Intermittent cervical traction and thoracic manipulation for management of mild cervical compressive myelopathy attributed to cervical herniated disc: a case series. *Journal of Orthopaedic and Sports Physical Therapy*, *34*(11), 701–712.

Cambron, J. A., Schneider, M., Dexheimer, J. M., et al. (2014). A pilot randomized controlled trial of flexion-distraction dosage for chiropractic treatment of lumbar spinal stenosis. *Journal of Manipulative and Physiological Therapeutics*, *37*(6), 396–406.

Chang, Y., Singer, D. E., Wu, Y. A., Keller, R. B., & Atlas, S. J. (2005). The effect of surgical and nonsurgical treatment on longitudinal outcomes of lumbar spinal stenosis over 10 years. *Journal of the American Geriatrics Society*, *53*, 785–792.

Cook, C., Brown, C., Isaacs, R., Roman, M., Davis, S., & Richardson, W. (2010). Clustered clinical findings for diagnosis of cervical spine myelopathy. *Journal of Manual & Manipulative Therapy*, *18*(4), 175–180.

Delitto, A., Piva, S. R., Moore, C. G., et al. (2015). Surgery versus nonsurgical treatment of lumbar spinal stenosis: a randomized trial. *Annals of Internal Medicine*, *162*, 465–473.

Deyo, R. A., Cherkin, D. C., & Loeser, J. D. (1992). Morbidity and mortality in association with operations on the lumbar spine. The influence of age, diagnosis, and procedure. *Journal of Bone and Joint. Surgery*, *74*(4), 536–543.

Dvorak, J. (1998). Epidemiology, physical examination and neurodiagnostics. *Spine*, *23*, 2663–2673.

Fritz, J., Erhard, R., Delitto, A., Welch, W., & Nowakowski, P. (1997a). Preliminary results of the use of a two-stage treadmill test as a clinical diagnostic tool in the differential diagnosis of lumbar spinal stenosis. *Journal of Spinal Disorders*, *10*(5), 410–416.

Fritz, J. M., Erhard, R. E., & Vignovic, M. (1997b). A nonsurgical approach for patients with lumbar spinal stenosis. *Physical Therapy*, *77*, 962–973.

Fritz, J. M., Delitto, A., Welch, W. C., & Erhard, R. E. (1998). Lumbar spinal stenosis: a review of current concepts in evaluation, management, and outcome measurements. *Archives of Physical Medicine and Rehabilitation*, *79*, 700–708.

Fuchs, C., Niemeier, T. E., Neway, W. E., & Manoharan, S. R. R. (2016). Concomitant lumbar stenosis and aortic pseudoaneurysm: a case report. *Cureus*, *8*(10), e822.

Haig, A. J., Tong, H. C., Yamakawa, K. S. J., et al. (2005). The sensitivity and specificity of electrodiagnostic testing for the clinical syndrome of lumbar spinal stenosis. *Spine*, *30*, 2667–2676.

Hurri, H., Slätis, P., Tallroth, K., et al. (1998). Lumbar spinal stenosis: assessment of long-term outcome 12 years after operative and conservative care. *Journal of Spinal Disorders*, *11*, 110–115.

Johnsson, K. E., Rosen, I., & Uden, A. (1992). The natural course of lumbar spinal stenosis. *Clinical Orthopaedics*, *279*, 82–86.

Katz, J. N., Dalgas, M., Stucki, G., et al. (1995). Degenerative lumbar spinal stenosis: diagnostic value of the history and physical examination. *Arthritis and Rheumatism*, *38*, 1236–1241.

Katz, J. N., Lipson, S. J., Chang, L. C., Levine, S. A., Fossel, A. H., & Liang, M. H. (1996). Seven- to 10-year outcome of decompressive surgery for degenerative lumbar spinal stenosis. *Spine*, *21*, 92–98.

Konno, S., Hayashino, Y., Kukuhara, S., Kikuchi, S., Kaneda, K., & Seichi, A. (2007). Development of a clinical diagnosis support tool to identify patients with lumbar spinal stenosis. *European Spine Journal*, *16*, 1951–1957.

Murphy, D. R., Hurwitz, E. L., Gregory, A. A., & Clary, R. (2006). A non-surgical approach to the management of lumbar spinal stenosis: a prospective observational cohort study. *BMC Musculoskeletal Disorders*, *7*, 16.

Penning, L. (1992). Functional pathology of lumbar spinal stenosis. *Clinical Biomechanics*, *7*, 3–17.

Porter, R. W. (1996). Spinal stenosis and neurogenic claudication. *Spine*, *21*, 2046–2052.

Pua, Y. H., Cai, C. C., & Lim, K. C. (2007). Treadmill walking with body weight support is no more effective than cycling when added to an exercise program for lumbar spinal stenosis: a randomised controlled trial. *Australian Journal of Physiotherapy*, *53*(2), 83–89.

Saleem, S. N., & Hawass, Z. (2014). Ankylosing spondylitis or diffuse idiopathic skeletal hyperostosis (DISH) in Royal Egyptian mummies of 18th–20th Dynasties? CT and archaeology studies. *Arthritis & Rheumatology*, *66*(12), 3311–3316.

Schonstrom, N., Lindahl, S., Willén, J., & Hansson, T. (1989). Dynamic changes in the dimensions of the lumbar spinal canal: an experimental study in vitro. *Journal of Orthopaedic Research*, *7*, 115–121.
Simotas, A. C., Dorey, F. J., Hansraj, K. K., & Cammisa, F., Jr. (2000). Nonoperative treatment for lumbar spinal stenosis: clinical outcome results and a 3-year survivorship analysis. *Spine*, *25*, 197–203.
Sugioka, T., Hayashino, Y., Konno, S., Kikuchi, S., & Fukuhara, S. (2008). Predictive value of self-reported patient information for the identification of lumbar spinal stenosis. *Family Practice*, *25*(4), 237–244.
Whitman, J. M., Flynn, T. W., Childs, J. D., et al. (2006). A comparison between two physical therapy treatment programs for patients with lumbar spinal stenosis: a randomized clinical trial. *Spine*, *31*(22), 2541–2549.
Willen, J., Danielson, B., Gaulitz, A., Niklason, T., Schönström, N., & Hansson, T. (1997). Dynamic effects on the lumbar spinal canal: axially loaded CT-myelography and MRI in patients with sciatica and/or neurogenic claudication. *Spine*, *22*, 2968–2976.
Zdeblick, T. A. (1995). The treatment of degenerative lumbar disorders: a critical review of the literature. *Spine*, *20*(Suppl), 126s–137s.

CHAPTER 60 QUESTIONS

1. **Current best evidence leads us to include the following in our physical therapy–related care for patients with lumbar spinal stenosis:**
   a. Double and single knee to chest exercises, quadruped "cat and camel" (flexion and extension) exercises, hot packs, and electrical stimulation
   b. Repeated flexion exercises, double and single knee to chest exercises, and abdominal ("core") retraining
   c. Aerobic exercise (cycling and/or walking), manual therapy to the lower quarter, lower quarter and abdominal muscle stretching and strengthening, and lumbo-pelvic flexion exercises
   d. Traction, electrical stimulation, cycling, and thermal modalities
   e. None of the above

2. **Which findings are most helpful in making a clinical diagnosis of lumbar spinal stenosis?**
   a. Standing and walking aggravate symptoms, and sitting eases symptoms; younger age; low back pain only (none in the lower extremities)
   b. Standing and walking aggravate symptoms, and sitting eases symptoms; older age; presence of pain, paresthesia, and/or cramping into one or both lower extremities below the buttocks
   c. Sitting aggravates symptoms and standing and walking ease symptoms; older age; low back pain only (none in the lower extremities)
   d. Sitting aggravates symptoms and standing and walking ease symptoms; younger age; presence of pain, paresthesia, and/or cramping into one or both lower extremities below the buttocks

3. **Which answer below includes disorders that may present similarly to lumbar spinal stenosis in the clinical exam? Pick the best answer.**
   a. Deep vein thrombosis, spondylitis of the lumbar spine, post-polio syndrome
   b. Femoral neck fracture, mechanical low back pain, hip and knee osteoarthritis
   c. Iliacus arterial disorder, fibular nerve adverse neural dynamics, mechanical low back pain
   d. Hip osteoarthritis, peripheral arterial disease, lumbar radiculopathy, peripheral neuropathy, spinal tumors

4. **What are common symptoms for a patient with cervical stenosis?**
   a. Neck pain and headache, referral of symptoms into the thoracic region, absence of symptoms below the acromioclavicular joint
   b. Unsteadiness and clumsiness in gait, lower motor neuron changes in the upper and lower extremities, and an absence of neck pain
   c. Neck and upper extremity pain and paresthesia, intrinsic muscle wasting of the hands, upper extremity weakness, absence of symptoms beyond the upper quarter
   d. Neck and upper extremity pain and paresthesia, upper extremity muscle weakness, unsteadiness in gait, wasting of the intrinsic muscles of the hands

5. **Which answer below includes a list of clinical signs that are most helpful in identifying the presence of central cervical stenosis?**
   a. Gait deviation, present Hoffmann's test, positive inverted supinator sign, present Babinski test, age >45 years, hand withdrawal reflex
   b. Age range of 20–40, present Hoffman's test, absent Babinski test, positive inverted pronator sign, hand withdrawal reflex, relief with manual cervical traction
   c. Gait deviation, present Babinski test, absent Hoffman's test, abnormal lower extremity neural dynamics tests, positive inverted pronator sign
   d. Age >45 years, neck pain and headache, referred symptoms to the medial scapular border, lower motor neuron findings in both the upper and lower extremities

SPONDYLOLYSIS AND SPONDYLOLISTHESIS

M. Schmidt, PT, DPT, MHA and M.G. Roman, PT, MHA, MMCi

1. **How is spondylolisthesis measured and graded?**
   Anterior slippage of one vertebral body on an adjacent body is graded I, II, III, and IV, according to the percentage of slippage of the posterior margin of one vertebral body relative to the next inferior body (25%, 50%, 75%, and 100%, respectively). For example, a grade II spondylolisthesis indicates a 25% to 50% subluxation of the vertebral body, a grade III indicates a 50% to 75% translation, etc. Grade V spondylolisthesis indicates the superior vertebral body slips entirely forward on and anterior to the subjacent body, known as spondyloptosis. These measurements are made on a standing lateral radiograph. Subsequently, Taillard has described a method that expresses the slippage in terms of percentage of the anteroposterior diameter of the distal segment (measurement of forward displacement of the anterior aspect of one vertebral body on the one below, divided by the anteroposterior dimension of the distal vertebral body). This method is considered to be more accurate and more reproducible than the Meyerding method. Both methods, however, continue to be commonly used.

2. **What is sacral inclination?**
   Sacral inclination, also known as sacral tilt, is the angle of displacement of the sacrum from the vertical. It is the measurement of the angle between a line drawn along the posterior margin of the first sacral vertebra and its bisection with the true vertical. This angle is measured on a standing lateral radiograph. The sacrum is angled anteriorly in normal upright standing postures, but the angle tends to decrease as the listhesis increases. The sacrum becomes more vertical with progressive listhesis.

3. **What is the slip angle?**
   Also known as sagittal roll, sagittal rotation, and angle of kyphosis, the slip angle is considered to be the most sensitive indication of potential segmental instability. This angle is measured between a line drawn perpendicular to the S1 and S2 vertebral bodies (through the disc space) and a line drawn along the superior end plate of the L5 body. The inferior end plate can also be used; however, the inferior end plate is more commonly deformed with degenerative changes and is more difficult to consistently identify than the superior end plate. This measurement is critical because it is felt to be the most sensitive measurement to predict progression of the listhesis.

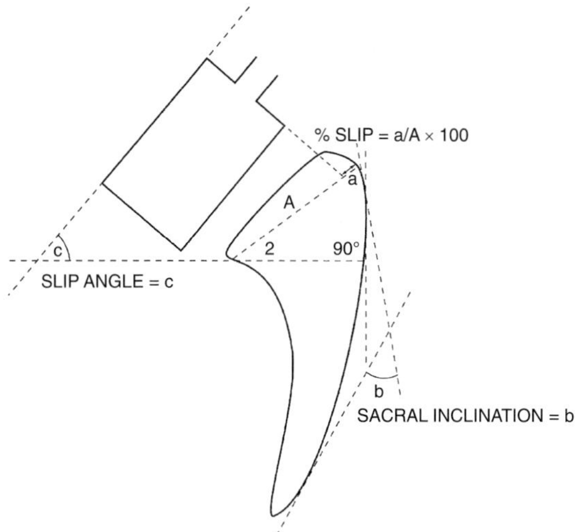

Measurement of sacral inclination, slip angle, and percent slip.

4. **What are the types (classifications) of spondylolistheses and the etiologies of each?**

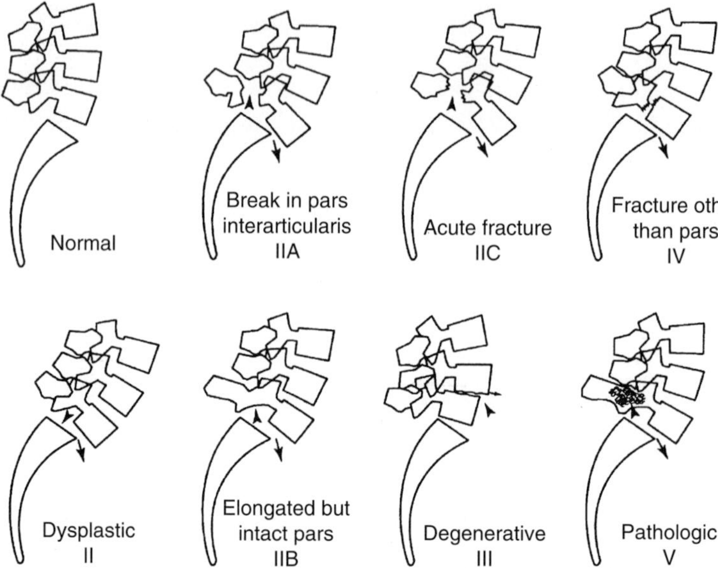

Types of spondylolistheses. Also see Table 61.1.

5. **What is the rate of occurrence of isthmic spondylolisthesis?**
The incidence of spondylolysis or spondylolisthesis was found to be 4.4% at age 6 with approximately 90% of spondylolysis occurring at the L5 level. These children were followed into adulthood, where the incidence increased to 6%. The degree of slip was seldom found to progress after adolescence because listhesis generally occurs concurrently with fatigue fracture. Interestingly, the spondylolysis was never found to be symptomatic in the population studied by Fredrickson et al. yet was reported by Micheli to be the most common cause of low back pain in adolescents.

6. **Does spondylolysis always progress to spondylolisthesis?**
No; nearly 50% of patients who present with isthmic spondylolysis do not progress to spondylolisthesis. Generally speaking, listhesis occurs at the time of fatigue fracture. If the anterior translation has not occurred during childhood or adolescence, it seldom occurs in adulthood. In the longitudinal study by Fredrickson et al., progression of listhesis was found to be unusual after it was initially appreciated in childhood or adolescence. Degenerative spondylolisthesis can occur without isthmic defect because of long-standing segmental instability and/or intervertebral disc degeneration. In a similar fashion, dysplastic spondylolisthesis can occur without a disrupted pars interarticularis. Some cases of dysplastic spondylolisthesis occur with intact, but attenuated posterior elements.

7. **Should neurologic compromise be anticipated with spondylolisthesis?**
Lower extremity radicular pain in the child is said to be more representative of dysplastic spondylolisthesis, suggesting irritation of the L5 or S1 nerve root, although isthmic spondylolisthesis can present similarly. Isthmic defects are often filled with fibrocartilaginous tissue that is formed in response to the stress fracture and resultant listhesis. The exiting nerve root then is stretched across this fibrous defect, causing nerve root irritation and associated lower extremity radicular symptoms. Neurologic signs can occur in the form of lower extremity weakness, paresthesia, and occasional bowel or bladder incontinence. Cauda equina symptoms are most commonly associated with dysplastic spondylolisthesis as the nerve roots are stretched across the defect as they exit the sacral foramina. Degenerative spondylolisthesis often results in neurogenic claudication signs consistent with associated spinal stenosis.

8. **Does the isthmic pars defect heal when treated?**
If diagnosed early and treated with rigid bracing for up to 6 months, the results have been favorable according to radiographic evaluation, clinical improvement in symptoms, and bone scan criteria. Bone scan evaluation is typically used to determine whether the fatigue fracture is sufficiently acute to warrant immobilization. Steiner and Micheli describe 78% clinical results as good or excellent with the use of a modified Boston brace in grade I

Table 61.1 Subtypes of Spondylolisthesis

	CONGENITAL	ISTHMIC	DEGENERATIVE	TRAUMATIC	PATHOLOGIC	IATROGENIC
Gender	Females > males, 2:1	Males > females, 2:1	Females > males, 5:1	Seldom seen	Data unavailable	Data unavailable
Age at onset	Congenital	Adolescents	Generally after 40 years	Seldom seen	Data unavailable	Data unavailable
Comorbidities	Questionable accelerated degenerative disc disease; spina bifida occulta	Questionable accelerated degenerative disc disease; spina bifida occulta		Seldom seen	Local or systemic bone disease	Lumbar stenosis
Most common level	L5–S1	L4–5	L4–5	Seldom seen	Data unavailable	Data unavailable
Progressive or not?	Yes, often caused by attenuation of posterior elements	Uncommon after stress fracture occurs	Gradually, occasionally will autofuse, related to degenerative changes		Data unavailable	Data unavailable
Associated symptoms	Radicular pain is common, associated with nerve root stretch and irritation	LBP, may present with radiculopathy in adulthood; "crisis" LBP at onset possible	Neurogenic claudication associated with stenosis		Data unavailable	Data unavailable
Cause	Dysplastic pars interarticularis, dysplastic sacral facets may have sagittal or axial orientation, attenuates with weight bearing	Stress fracture of pars interarticularis, more common in young gymnasts and football linemen	Degenerative lumbar spine and intervertebral disc changes	Traumatic, producing fracture other than at pars interarticularis that follows listhesis	Tumor, infection, osteoporosis	Excessive decompression of facets at time of surgery

LBP, Low back pain.

spondylolisthesis. The brace was used for 6 months full time, while allowing for a flexion exercise program and sports participation within limits of pain complaints. Other reports indicate that the pars defect rarely heals, but clinical results tend to be favorable in response to bracing for the acute spondylolytic crisis. Early in the immobilization period, aggressive abdominal strengthening and stabilization exercises are begun, with return to activity, including sports, as tolerated. It should be noted that literature indicates that clinical results and return-to-activity orders are not significantly different in patients who demonstrate solid bony healing compared with those whose stress fractures go to fibrous healing. Clinical results are similar. Although bracing has been shown to be helpful in these acute time periods, many adolescents have difficulty following protocols that require the patient to spend 23 hours a day in a brace and may not limit the spinal motion as much as once thought.

9. **What associated morbidity is seen with spondylolisthesis?**
When isthmic spondylolisthesis occurs at the L5–S1 level, local instability is rarely seen. However, when it occurs at L4–L5, instability is more common because of the absence of the contribution of the iliolumbar ligament to segmental stability. The fiber direction of this ligament allows for it to offer strong support against anterior translation of the L5 vertebra, but it has no insertion to L4, leaving the L4 body without this strong passive support. This level has been shown to be hypermobile or unstable into the third or fourth decade of life. Degenerative changes occurring over the next several years tend to stabilize the progressive isthmic spondylolisthesis but may lead to degenerative spondylolisthesis later in life.

There is some belief that intervertebral disc degeneration occurs more rapidly in the presence of isthmic spondylolisthesis than in a population without spondylolisthesis. Studies indicate a more rapid rate of degenerative processes after age 25 in patients with isthmic spondylolisthesis than in those without the disorder. Evidence of spina bifida occulta is seen four times more often in patients with isthmic and dysplastic spondylolisthesis compared with uninvolved control populations. Reported incidence of spina bifida occulta in dysplastic spondylolisthesis is 40%, with the normal incidence in adults without dysplastic spondylolisthesis being 6%. Spina bifida contributes to the predisposition to isthmic defects in involved patients by the dysplastic posterior elements not forming completely, leaving the posterior ring inherently weak. Transitional anatomy (sacralization of the L5 segment or lumbarization of the S1 segment) is four times more likely in those with degenerative spondylolisthesis than in age-matched controls.

10. **How is spondylolisthesis diagnosed radiologically?**
Standard x-rays are adequate in diagnosing a spondylolisthesis. A lateral lumbar spine film will demonstrate the listhesis of one segment on the next distal segment. Studies have confirmed that the anterior translation is greater in standing, weight-bearing films than in supine, nonweight-bearing films. Therefore some authors suggest both views be taken to demonstrate intersegmental motion. Lumbar spine oblique views are used to evaluate the integrity of the pars interarticularis. The well-described "Scotty dog" sign shows the presence of the fatigue fracture by a radiolucent area across the "neck" of the Scotty dog. Bone scan technology is used to diagnose an acute fatigue fracture of the pars or to differentiate local tumor or infection as the cause of symptoms. Neuroimaging studies (MRI or CT scan) are used to confirm suspicion of nerve root impingement associated with disc degeneration or the listhesis itself. Serial radiographs can be taken to assess for progression of listhesis. Repeat films are taken at 6- to 12-month intervals when spondylolisthesis is initially diagnosed and then after a greater interval if no progression is identified. Spondylosis, however, can be more difficult to diagnose before a stress fracture occurs. The single-photon-emission computed tomography (SPECT) scan is considered to be the most sensitive in detecting early metabolic changes that may preclude stress fracture. An uptake noted on this study indicates bone turnover, a response to stress reaction.

11. **What are the basic principles of conservative management of spondylolisthesis?**
Isthmic spondylolisthesis often presents with a "spondylolytic crisis"—acute low back pain—in a child or adolescent. When confirmed radiographically, bracing is recommended in the acute case, defined by active findings on CT or SPECT bone scan. When worn continuously for 3 to 6 months, the brace provides the pars defect an opportunity to heal. While still in the brace, specific trunk stabilization exercises are performed. The purpose of the exercises is to aggressively and functionally facilitate abdominal muscle contraction without causing segmental lumbar spine movement, which is undesirable during the healing stage because it may disrupt the healing pars. Attempts to restore "normal" lordosis through aggressive repeated extension activities, either standing or prone, are not indicated in treatment as this would cause increased pressure on the pars and bony structure of the spinal column. A patient with spondylolisthesis may demonstrate a compensatory reduction in lumbar lordosis as a mechanism to limit the anterior translation stress involved with upright postures. Repeated lumbar extension exercises increase this stress and have been shown to increase pain complaints in spondylolisthesis patients. As with many sources of mechanical low back pain, balance of flexibility of lower extremity muscles should be assessed and addressed. Patients with spondylolisthesis often demonstrate inadequate hamstring flexibility, resulting in increased shearing forces through the lumbar spine with movement. These shearing forces across an inherently weaker pars intraarticularis may contribute to low back pain symptoms.

12. **What is the role of flexibility exercises in conservative treatment of spondylolisthesis?**
Lower extremity flexibility exercises are an integral part of any complete low back rehabilitation program along with a primary focus on strengthening of the core. Hamstring flexibility is often limited in patients with symptomatic spondylolisthesis. Hamstrings become tight reactively to produce and maintain a posterior pelvic tilt and subsequent reduction in lumbar lordosis, thereby reducing the anterior shear force of the lumbar spine vertebral body. An anterior pelvic tilt may be adopted, allowing the iliopsoas and rectus femoris to adaptively shorten. These opposing forces of reactively shortening lower extremity musculature increase the overall stress and tension within the muscular system of the lumbosacral spine and pelvis, resulting in potentially increased symptoms of pain and dysfunction. Hamstring spasm that is unresponsive to conservative measures is often relieved by decompression of the L5 or S1 nerve roots at the time of surgery.

13. **What are the surgical indications in the child or adolescent with spondylolisthesis?**
Surgical indications for children and adolescents with spondylolisthesis are fairly well established. According to Amundson et al., surgical indications include:
- Persistence or recurrence of major symptoms in spite of aggressive conservative management for at least 1 year
- Tight hamstrings, persistently abnormal gait, or postural deformities that are unrelieved by physical therapy
- Sciatic scoliosis, or lateral shift
- Progressive neurologic deficit
- Progressive slip beyond grade II spondylolisthesis, even when asymptomatic
- A high slip angle (greater than 40–50 degrees), because high slip angles are considered to be the most sensitive indicator for progressive listhesis and instability
- Psychological problems associated with postural deformity, or gait deviations associated with a high-grade listhesis

Outcomes from in situ fusion in adolescents with spondylolisthesis have been well documented with very favorable results. Children and adolescents generally fare well after posterolateral fusion procedures, usually returning to unrestricted activity. It is interesting to note that most symptoms associated with spondylolisthesis in the child and adolescent are associated with segmental instability; therefore in situ fusion can adequately control the symptoms without requiring nerve root decompression. Current recommendations are that decompression without fusion should not be performed "in patients under age 40, and is rarely needed in the child and adolescent years."

14. **List the surgical indications for adults with spondylolisthesis.**
- Isthmic spondylolisthesis that becomes symptomatic as an adult
- Segmental instability or neurologic compromise post trauma
- Associated with progressive degenerative changes
- Degenerative spondylolisthesis associated with progressive symptoms
- Persistent symptoms lasting more than 4 months, interfering with patient's quality of life
- Progressive neurologic deficits
- Progressive weakness
- Bowel/bladder dysfunction
- Sensory loss
- Reflex loss
- Limited walking tolerance (because of neurologic claudication)
- Associated segmental instability
- Pathologic fracture

15. **What types of surgical interventions are available for treatment of spondylolisthesis?**
In situ fusion has long been the procedure of choice for symptomatic spondylolisthesis, both in adolescent and adult populations. Commonly, reduction procedures have been complicated by nerve root symptoms, radiculopathy, and occasional motor deficits from disrupting the nerve root during surgery. There is further controversy regarding the need for nerve root decompression accompanying posterolateral fusion in the adult with isthmic spondylolisthesis. Some authors claim decompression is necessary in the presence of any neurologic deficit, while others claim that decompression is effectively accomplished by a successful fusion. Wiltse and Winter claim that the fibrocartilage mass decreases in size with successful posterolateral fusion, effectively decompressing the nerve root. All authors, however, agree that the presence of bowel or bladder dysfunction and a motor deficit that is significant enough to cause loss of normal ambulation are reasons to decompress the offending nerve root during surgery. Decompression without fusion is often proposed in the treatment of degenerative spondylolisthesis as well. However, wide laminectomy and involvement of the facet joints with decompression without fusion may result in an increased prevalence of associated instability and could lead to iatrogenic spondylolisthesis. As a result, substantial debate continues regarding the efficacy of decompression alone versus decompression with fusion in degenerative spondylolisthesis.

16. **Are athletes more prone to spondylosis than others?**
Generally speaking, the prevalence of spondylosis is not greater in athletes than in nonathletic populations; however, there are some sports in which there appears to be a higher incidence. Various reports have suggested a higher incidence of spondylosis in sports such as gymnastics, diving, wrestling, weight lifting, throwing sports, and volleyball. Note all of these sports include frequent, loaded, or extreme ranges of motion of the lumbar spine (flexion or extension). These end range, externally loaded, and repeated ranges of motion are felt to contribute to the higher incidence in these athletes than in other populations.

17. **By what criteria can an athlete or nonathlete return to activity after being diagnosed with spondylolisthesis?**
There is no absolute agreement on criteria for return to sport or other activity with diagnosis of spondylolisthesis. Various authors have suggested functional or time-based criteria (see Hopkins and White). Others determine activity on the basis of clinical signs and symptoms. Presence of increasing or peripheralizing pain with activity and persistent or increasing weakness are indications to limit or reduce activity. Most literature suggests that bracing in the presence of an acute injury (metabolically active scan) is indicated, generally allowing activity within the brace. A Boston or other brace is felt to be unnecessary in absence of positive findings on bone scan but may be used if helpful in controlling symptoms associated with activity. Postoperatively, these patients are managed as other postlumbar fusion patients are, following the same physiologic guidelines as any patient status post instrumented lumbar spine fusion.

Bibliography

Amundson, G., Edwards, C., & Garfin, S. (1992). In Rothman, R. H., & Simone, F. A. (Eds.), *The spine: 1* (3rd ed., pp. 913–969). Philadelphia, PA: WB Saunders.

Bono, C. M. (2004). Low back pain in athletes. *Journal of Bone and Joint Surgery, 86*(2), 382–396.

Farfan, H. F. (1980). The pathological anatomy of degenerative spondylolisthesis: a cadaver study. *Spine, 5*, 412–418.

Fredrickson, B. E., Baker, D., McHolick, W. J., Yuan, H. A., & Lubicky, J. P. (1984). The natural history of spondylolysis and spondylolisthesis. *Journal of Bone and Joint Surgery, 66*(5), 699–707.

Gaines, R. W., & Nichols, W. K. (1985). Treatment of spondyloptosis of two-stage L5 and reduction of L4 onto S1. *Spine, 10*, 680–686.

Garet, M., Reiman, M., Mathers, J., & Sylvain, J. (2013). Nonoperative treatment in lumbar spondylolisthesis: a systematic review. *Sports Health: A Multidisciplinary Approach, 5*, 225–232.

Grobler, L. J., & Wiltse, L. J. (1991). Classification, non-operative, and operative treatment of spondylolisthesis. In J. W. (1991). Frymoyer (Ed.), *The adult spine: principles and practice*, Vol. 2. New York, NY: Raven Press.

Grobler, L. J., Robertson, P. A., Novotny, J. E., & Pope, M. H. (1993). Etiology of spondylolisthesis. Assessment of the role played by lumber facet joint morphology. *Spine, 18*, 80–91.

Hensinger, R. N. (1983). Spondylolysis and spondylolisthesis in children. *Instructional Course Lectures, 32*, 132–151.

Hodges, S. D., Shuster, J., Asher, M. A., & McClarty, S. J. (1999). Traumatic L5-S1 spondylolisthesis. *Southern Medical Journal, 92*, 316–320.

Hopkins, T. J. (1993). White AA 2nd. Rehabilitation of athletes following spine injury. *Clinics in Sports Medicine, 12*, 603–619.

Ishida, Y., Ohmori, K., Inoue, H., & Suzuki, K. (1999). Delayed vertebral slip and adjacent disc degeneration with an isthmic defect of the fifth lumbar vertebra. *Journal of Bone and Joint. Surgery, 81*(2), 240–244.

Klein, G., Mehlman, C. T., & McCarty, M. (2009). Nonoperative treatment of spondylolysis and grade I spondylolisthesis in children and young adults: a meta-analysis of observational studies. *Journal of Pediatric Orthopedics, 29*(2), 146–156.

Kurd, M. F., Patel, D., Norton, R., Picetti, G., Friel, B., & Vaccaro, A. (2007). Nonoperative treatment of symptomatic spondylolysis. *Journal of Spinal Disorders and Techniques, 20*(8), 560–564.

Love, T. W., Fagan, A. B., & Fraser, R. D. (1999). Degenerative spondylolisthesis: developmental or acquired? *Journal of Bone and Joint Surgery, 81*(4), 670–674.

Meyerding, H. W. (1932). Spondylolisthesis. *Surgery, Gynecology & Obstetrics, 54*, 371–377.

Micheli, L. J., & Wood, R. (1995). Back pain in young athletes: significant differences from adults in causes and patterns. *Archives of Pediatrics and Adolescent Medicine, 149*, 15–18.

Miller, R., Hardcastle, P., & Renwick, S. (1992). Lower spinal mobility and external immobilization in the normal and pathologic condition. *Orthopedic Review, 21*(6), 753–757.

Nance, D. K., & Hickey, M. (1999). Spondylolisthesis in children and adolescents. *Orthopedic Nursing, 18*, 21–27.

Ralston, S., & Weir, M. (1998). Suspecting lumbar spondylolysis in adolescent low back pain. *Clinical Pediatrics, 37*, 287–293.

Rubery, P., & Bradford, D. (2002). Athletic activity after spine surgery in children and adolescents. *Spine, 27*(4), 423–424.

Sakai, T., Sairyo, K., Takao, S., Nishitani, H., & Yasui, N. (1976). Incidence of lumbar spondylolysis in the general population in Japan based on multidetector computed tomography scans from two thousand subjects. *Spine, 34*(21), 2346.

Sanderson, P. L., & Fraser, R. D. (1996). The influence of pregnancy on the development of degenerative spondylolisthesis. *Journal of Bone and Joint Surgery, 78*(6), 951–954.

Shaffer, B., Wiesel, S., & Lauerman, W. (1997). Spondylolisthesis in the elite football player: an epidemiologic study in the NCAA and NFL. *Journal of Spinal Disorders, 10*, 365–370.

Steiner, M. E., & Micheli, L. J. (1985). Treatment of symptomatic spondylolysis and spondylolisthesis with the modified Boston brace. *Spine, 10*, 937–943.

Sys, J., Michielsen, J., Bracke, P., Martens, M., & Verstreken, J. (2001). Nonoperative treatment of active spondylolysis in elite athletes with normal X-ray findings: literature review and results of conservative treatment. *European Spine Journal, 10*, 498–504.

Taillard, W. (1954). Le spondylolisthesis chez l'enfant et l'adolescent. *Acta Orthopaedica Scandinavica, 24*, 115–144.

Tuong, N., Dansereau, J., Maurais, G., & Herrera, R. (1998). Three-dimensional evaluation of lumbar orthosis effects on spinal behavior. *Journal of Rehabilitation Research & Development, 35*(1), 34–42.

Wiltse, L. L., & Winter, R. B. (1983). Terminology and measurement of spondylolisthesis. *Journal of Bone and Joint Surgery, 65*(6), 768–772.

CHAPTER 61 QUESTIONS

1. An 18-year-old college cheerleader comes to your clinic 1 week after suffering a fall onto her buttocks in a tuck position when her teammates failed to catch her landing from a throw. She reports significant pain throughout her lower back that is not tender to touch but causes constant pain that is aggravated with any upright or loaded activities. She has been unable to go to class, as sitting is too painful. Standing feels better, but she can only tolerate this for short periods. She is most comfortable lying down, where she notes her pain to decrease from 8 to 4/10. She denies any past medical history or any neurologic signs. Her motion is limited by pain, but strength, sensation, reflexes, and neural tension signs are normal. She had an x-ray completed at an urgent care visit immediately following the fall that she asks you to help interpret. The imaging report indicates presence of a unilateral pars fracture with anterior slip Grade II slip of L4 vertebrae on L5. A Grade II slip indicates:
   a. 1%–25% translation
   b. Up to 50% translation
   c. Up to 75% translation
   d. 76%–100% translation

2. What of the following would be the most appropriate treatment for this patient at this stage?
   a. Recommend continued rest and avoidance of sports until next season
   b. Initiate core stabilization, avoiding brace because the patient will become dependent on it
   c. Initiate core stabilization, use brace if needed to tolerate return to sports
   d. Order flexion-biased brace and avoid exercise for the next 6–8 weeks

3. The patient expresses concern about her spinal translation and the likely prognosis. Which of the following is the most appropriate expectation?
   a. The slip will likely progress because she is so young and it will likely progress over time.
   b. The slip will likely not progress because she is active and strong and this will help to stabilize her spine.
   c. The slip will likely not progress because it has occurred at L4-L5 as opposed to L5-S1.
   d. The slip will likely not progress because her fracture is unilateral.

CHAPTER 62

SPINE FRACTURES AND DISLOCATIONS: PATTERNS, CLASSIFICATIONS, AND MANAGEMENT

E. Truumees, MD and R. Shah, MD

1. **How common is trauma to the spinal column?**
   There are over 1 million spine injuries per year in the United States alone; 50,000 of these injuries include fractures to the bony spinal column. Males outnumber females 4 to 1 for spinal trauma. Injury is most common at the cervicothoracic and thoracolumbar junctions. The improvement in automobile restraint systems has increased survival rates from major spinal column injuries.

2. **How many spinal cord injuries occur per year in the United States?**
   An estimated 17,700 people sustain survivable spinal cord injuries each year. Overall, 10% to 25% of spinal column injuries are associated with at least some neurologic changes. These changes are more common with injuries at the cervical level (40%) than at the lumbar level (20%).

3. **What are the most common modes of spinal column injury?**
   Almost half (45%) are related to motor vehicle accidents (MVAs). Falls account for another 20%. In children falls account for only 9% of significant spine injuries, whereas in older patients, they account for 60%. Sports injuries account for another 15%. Of these, diving injuries are the most common. Trampoline, ice hockey, and wrestling are other frequent culprits. Organized football accounts for 42 cervical fractures and 5 cases of quadriplegia per year. This statistic has decreased from 110 and 34, respectively, from 1976 (before the spear tackling rules were enacted). Another 15% of spinal column injuries are related to acts of violence.

4. **In what scenarios are spinal column injuries most likely to be missed?**
   Worsening neurologic deficits occur in only 1.5% of patients diagnosed early but in 10% of patients with missed injuries. Injuries are most commonly missed in patients with a decreased level of consciousness, intoxication, head trauma, or polytrauma. Two separate, noncontiguous spinal injuries occur in as many as 20% of cases. The presence of one obvious spinal injury increases the chance of missing another, subtler injury. Red flags to alert the practitioner to subtle spine injury are facial trauma, calcaneus fracture, hypotension, and localized tenderness or spasm. Significant injury is also more likely in patients with osteopenia or neuromuscular disease, and missed injuries often occur in conditions that make the spine "rigid" such as ankylosing spondylitis.

5. **What is the long-term prognosis of a spinal cord–injured patient?**
   The average 10-year survival rate in all patients with spinal cord injury is 86%. In patients over 29 years of age, this number drops to 50%. Cervical spine injuries and patients with decreased function have higher rates of mortality. Pneumonia, cancer, heart disease, and suicide are the chief causes of death.

6. **What are incomplete cord syndromes, and how do they affect rehabilitation?**
   Incomplete cord syndromes reflect injuries in which only part of the cord matter is damaged. Although severe, some function below the level of injury is preserved.

SYNDROME	MOI/PATHOLOGY	CHARACTERISTICS	PROGNOSIS
Central	Age >50 y, extension	UE > LE, M + S loss	Fair
Anterior	Flexion-comp (vert art)	Incomplete motor, some sensory	Poor
Brown-Séquard	Penetrating trauma	Ipsilateral motor, contralateral pain/temp	Best
Root	Foraminal comp/disc	Based on level, weakness	Good
Complete	Burst, canal comp	No function below level	Poor

comp, compression; *LE*, lower extremity; *M + S*, motor and sensory; *MOI*, Method of injury; *UE*, upper extremity; *vert art*, vertebral artery injury.

7. **How is the pediatric spine differently susceptible to trauma?**
For children older than 8 to 10 years, the spine behaves biomechanically like an adult's. Younger children have more elastic soft tissues that make multiple, contiguous fractures much more common than in adults. The large size of the child's head, relative to the body, places the fulcrum for spinal flexion at C2–C3 in children. For children older than 8 years, the fulcrum is at C5–C6. Younger children are therefore far more likely to have upper cervical spine injuries (occiput to C3).

8. **What is SCIWORA?**
The marked elasticity of the pediatric spinal column is greater than the elastic limit of the cord. Therefore in rare cases, the Spinal Cord can be Injured Without Obvious Radiographic Abnormality (SCIWORA). More than half of these children will have delayed onset of neurologic symptoms, and therefore close and repeated examinations are needed. In recent years, the concept of SCIWORA has been challenged. In any case, the ready availability of MRI makes the concept less critical than in years past.

9. **How are gunshot wounds to the spine treated?**
Because there is little ligamentous injury associated with civilian weapons, most can be treated nonoperatively with external immobilization. As bullet removal often worsens neurologic deficits, surgery is recommended only if the neurologic deficit is progressive, a CSF fistula ensues, or lead poisoning occurs. Surgical indications after colonic perforation are controversial.

10. **Describe appropriate steps in the early evaluation of spinal column injury.**
In trauma patients, the spine is assumed to be unstable until a secondary survey and radiographs have been performed. Directly examine the back by log-rolling the patient while maintaining in-line traction on the neck. Ecchymosis, lacerations, or abrasions on the skull, spine, thorax, and abdomen suggest that force was imparted to underlying spinal elements. Deformity, localized tenderness, step-off, or interspinous widening warrant further evaluation.

11. **Describe appropriate steps in the early management of spinal column injury.**
First, immobilize the spine on a backboard with sandbags and a hard collar. In a sports sidelines setting, do not attempt to remove helmets or pads. Remove any faceguards. In a hospital setting, after radiographs and a secondary survey have excluded major instability, transfer the patient to a regular bed. Maintain a hard cervical collar until the cervical spine has been formally cleared. When definitive stabilization must be delayed, patients with significant thoracolumbar injury should be transferred to a rotating frame or other protective bed. For unstable cervical trauma, traction may be required. High-dose steroid protocols are no longer considered the standard of care in the acute management of spinal cord injury. Operative stabilization, when indicated, should be undertaken as soon as possible.

12. **How is the level determined in spinal cord injury?**
Because the cord usually ends at the L1–L2 disc space, the level of injury to the spinal column may not match the level of cord injury. The cord level is defined as the lowest functional motor level, that is, the lowest level with useful motor function (grade 3 of 5, or antigravity strength). In some cases, a given cord injury will be described as "T8 motor and T12 sensory."

13. **Are there any radiographic clues that an injury might be unstable?**
The most common spine injuries lead to compression of the spinal column. These injuries are more likely to be stable. Any distraction or translation of the spine means the spine is unstable. Ligamentous injuries less predictably heal than bone injuries. Significant injury to the facet capsules, posterior longitudinal ligament, and interspinous ligaments (the posterior ligament complex) tend to predict for instability as well. Other radiographic parameters have also been defined but vary by spinal level and remain controversial. Clues include significant loss of vertebral height (perhaps >50%), marked or progressive spinal angulation (in some studies, segmental kyphosis >20 degrees), or more than 3 to 4 mm of spondylolisthesis, defined by the translation of one vertebra in relation to the one below it. Significant neurological injury also renders the injury unstable, for treatment purposes (sometimes called neurological instability).

14. **Why is the level of injury important?**
The room available for the cord and the native stability of the spinal column varies significantly from the occiput to the sacrum. In the upper cervical spine, the bony elements are highly mobile, and stability comes from the ligaments. Also, the ratio of the size of the canal to that of the cord is large. This extra room allows for more displacement before cord injury. In the lower cervical spine, the narrow canal leaves little room for translation before cord compression.

The rib cage and sternum render the thoracic spine inherently more stable than the rest of the spine. Yet here the canal is narrowest versus cord size. The transition zone between the fixed thoracic and mobile lumbar spine subjects the thoracolumbar junction at higher risk for injury. The mobile lower lumbar spine has a large canal with ample room for the nerve roots. Nerve roots are more resilient than the spinal cord, so injuries at this level tend to be less neurologically devastating.

15. How are spinal column injuries classified?

There are dozens of classification systems for spinal trauma in general and injuries to certain vertebrae in particular. There is no widespread consensus as to which system to use. Mechanistic classifications divide injuries into groups based on the force that caused them. The groups are divided into grades to signal increasing severity. More recently, anatomic classifications of cervical and thoracolumbar trauma have focused on the status of the posterior ligamentous complex (Figures).

16. What common force vectors cause spinal column injury?

When a car hits a tree, the seat belt holds the passenger back but inertia keeps the skull moving. An accident of this type imparts force to the cervical spine. A distraction vector, for example, lengthens the spinal column by tearing its ligaments. If the patient's head then hits the windshield, a compression vector shortens the vertebral column by fracturing its bones. Flexion (forward and lateral), extension, and rotation are the other major vectors. In reality, most injuries result from multiple simultaneous forces with one vector predominating.

17. What types of injuries are caused by compression-flexion moments?

MVAs or diving accidents often impart compression and flexion vectors to the spinal column. Early, the anterior column fails in compression. Later, the posterior and middle column ligaments fail in distraction. When the ligaments fail, the fractured level slides posteriorly over the underlying intact vertebra. These injuries are most common in the midcervical spine (C4–C5 and C5–C6). There are many classification systems to describe these fractures. One named the Ferguson-Allen classification of cervical spine trauma defines spinal injury subtypes by the vector of force that caused the injury (Figure).

Compression fractures represent early-stage injuries with no significant ligamentous failure and heal within 8 to 12 weeks of immobilization. When ligaments and their secondary restraints are torn (complete ligamentous disruption), healing is unlikely without surgery. Therefore higher energy compression-flexion injuries require operative stabilization.

18. What is a flexion teardrop fracture?

The most severe flexion-compression injury—the flexion teardrop fracture—is the most devastating of all cervical spine injuries compatible with life. Most patients will have either anterior cord syndrome or a complete cord injury. The lateral radiograph demonstrates a large triangular fragment of anteroinferior vertebral body with marked kyphosis at the injured level, leading to subluxation or dislocation of the facets. Complete disruption of the disc

Morphology		**Points**
	No Abnormality	0
	Compression	1
	Burst	2
	Translation/Rotation	3
	Distraction	4
Integrity of PLC		
	Intact	0
	Suspected to be injured	2
	Injured	3
Neurological Injury		
	Intact	0
	Nerve root injury	2
	Complete cord injury	2
	Incomplete cord injury	3
	Cauda equina	3

Surgical Decision Making		
		Indication
Total Points:	0-3	Nonsurgical treatment
	4	Surgeon's Choice
	>4	Surgical treatment

The TLIC classification of thoracolumbar spine trauma. Injuries are graded in terms of three major criteria the morphology of the fracture itself (which is determined by x-ray or CT scan), the integrity of the posterolateral ligamentous complex (which is often determined by MRI), and the presence of neurologic injury (which is determined by physical exam). If the total points (which is determined by adding the number of points you have in each criterion) is greater than 4, then surgical intervention may be indicated.

Morphology		**Points**			
	No Abnormality	0			
	Compression	1			
	Burst	2			
	Distraction	3			
	Translation/Rotation	4			
Injury of Discoliagmentous Complex					
			Surgical Decision Making		
	Intact	0			
	Undetermined	1			Indication
			Total Points:	0-3	Nonsurgical treatment
	Torn	2			
				4	Surgeon's Choice
Neurological Injury				>4	Surgical treatment
	Intact	0			
	Nerve root injury	1			
	Complete cord injury	2			
	Incomplete cord injury	3			
	Incomplete cord injury with ongoing cord compression	4			

The SLIC classification of cervical spine trauma. Injuries are graded in terms of three major criteria the morphology of the fracture itself (which is determined by x-ray or CT scan), the integrity of the discoligamentous complex (which is often determined by MRI), and the presence of neurologic injury (which is determined by physical exam). If the total points (which is determined by adding the number of points you have in each criterion) is greater than 4, then surgical intervention may be indicated.

and all the ligaments at the level of injury leads to translation and rotation of the involved vertebrae. Surgical stabilization is usually required.

19. **How are vertical compression injuries differentiated from compression-flexion injuries?**
If an MVA or diving accident leads to a blow to the top of the head rather than flexion, both the anterior and middle columns fail in compression (ie, a burst fracture). With increasing force, vertebral arch fractures become more common. In cervical spine trauma, this is the only mechanism wherein the bony injury is more important than the ligamentous injury. The absence of ligamentous disruption allows for some of these injuries to heal in a halo. A halo is an external rigid brace that is connected to the skull and immobilizes the cervical spine. In higher level injuries or those with neurologic injury, anterior decompression and fusion are recommended.

20. **What is the most common type of cervical spine injury?**
Distractive flexion injuries account for 61% of all subaxial spine injuries. In early stages, only the posterior ligaments fail (ie, a flexion sprain). Later, the middle and, finally, the anterior columns fail. As the spine displaces, the superior end plate of the subjacent vertebra may compress, but this should not be confused with flexion-compression injuries. The key differences are marked kyphosis with mild bony collapse and displacement between the fractured vertebra and its cranial neighbor.

21. **How are distractive flexion injuries treated?**
Low-energy injuries disrupt only the posterior column, resulting in facet subluxation only. Collar immobilization allows for complete healing. Increasing trauma leads to facet dislocation that merits reduction with skull tongs (Gardner-Wells tongs) followed by a posterior fusion to prevent late deformity, chronic pain, or worsening neurologic injury.

22. **What are the characteristics of compressive extension injuries?**
Accounting for almost 40% of cervical spine trauma, these injuries may result from a downward blow to the forehead. They may occur anywhere but are concentrated at C6–C7. Most are stable. At higher energy levels, tension shear failure through the middle and anterior columns allows the superior vertebra to move forward on the subjacent vertebra, leaving the posterior elements behind. In injuries without displacement, halo immobilization yields acceptable healing rates. Injuries with translation are best treated with operative stabilization.

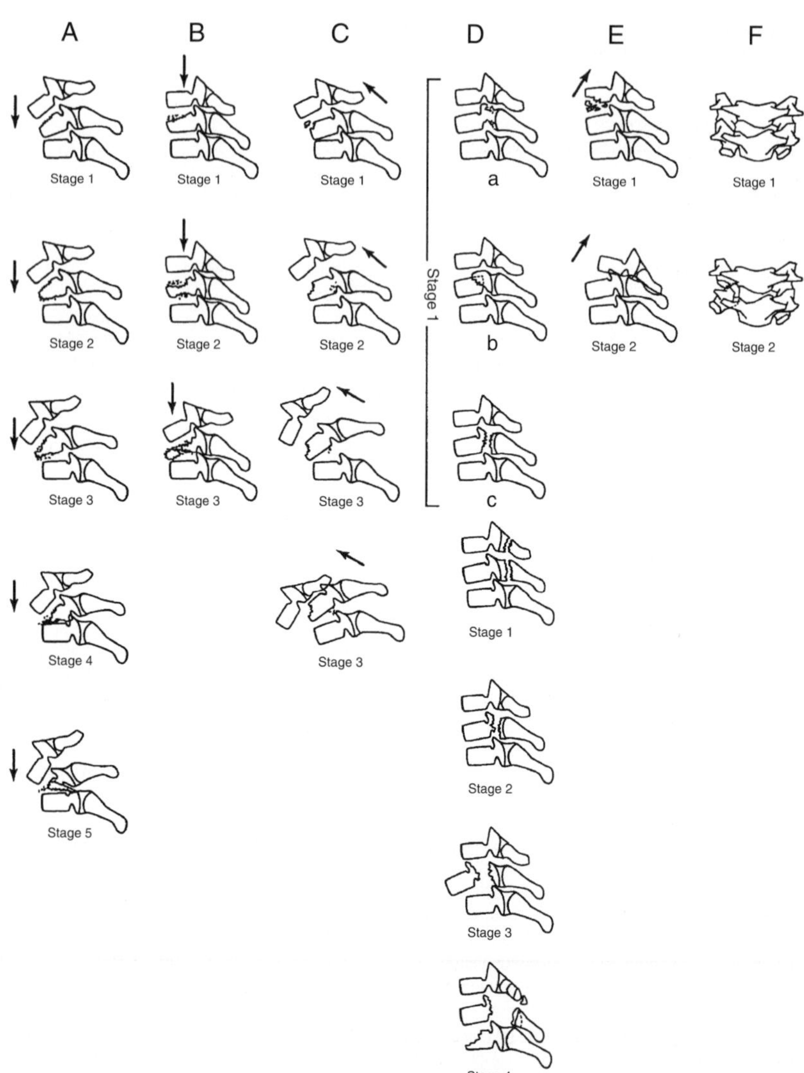

The Ferguson-Allen classification of cervical spine trauma. Spinal injuries are divided into subtypes based on the vector of force that produced them. Group A represents compressive flexion injuries of increasing severity. Group B includes types of vertical compression injuries. Distractive flexion injuries are part of group C. Group D represents compression-extension patterns. The distractive extension patterns are found in group E, whereas lateral flexion injuries are shown in group F.

23. What is an odontoid fracture?

Also called the dens, the odontoid is a peg of bone extending from the body of C2 into the arch of C1. This unique geometry maintains stability while allowing for rotation of the skull on C2 with the circular C1 acting like a passive washer. In younger patients, odontoid fractures are associated with high-energy trauma. Patients report pain and a sense of instability; occasionally, the patient's presenting symptoms include holding the head with the hands. In children under age 7, the fracture passes through the growth plate and is treated with reduction and a halo or Minerva cast for 6 to 12 weeks.

In adults, dens fracture subtypes associated with poor healing and late instability have been identified. For example, the injuries through the cortical waist of the dens (type II fractures) have poor blood supply and a higher nonunion rate. Type III fractures pass through the cancellous bone of the C2 body and are more likely to heal. A trial of halo immobilization is attempted. However, in severely displaced injuries, early stabilization is recommended. Recently, halo use has been associated with significant cardiopulmonary morbidity in the elderly;

therefore, an emphasis on rigid, operative stabilization of dens fractures in these otherwise frail patients is recommended.

24. **What is a hangman's fracture?**
Also known as traumatic spondylolisthesis of the axis, a hangman's fracture represents a bilateral fracture of the C2 pars interarticularis. Because bilateral pars fractures enlarge the canal, neurologic injuries are rare. Minimally displaced injuries are immobilized in a Philadelphia collar. Displaced injuries benefit from reduction and halo immobilization. If significant subluxation of C2 on C3 is noted, a posterior stabilization procedure is required.

25. **What is a Jefferson fracture?**
A Jefferson bursting fracture (of the atlas) is a relatively uncommon injury, usually seen in the context of another spine injury, particularly an odontoid fracture or hangman's fracture. Classically, this injury encompasses bilateral fractures in both the anterior and posterior arches of the C1 ring. Most isolated Jefferson fractures heal in an orthosis. Minimally displaced or isolated single or double fractures through the C1 ring may be treated with a Philadelphia collar. With increased loading, the fragments displace more widely. Beyond 5–8 mm lateral displacement, the transverse atlantal ligament (TAL) ruptures or avulses, rendering the C1–C2 motion segment unstable. The TAL acts as a sling keeping the dens in contact with the atlas. If the CT scan suggests bone avulsion of the ligament, traction for reduction followed by halo immobilization may allow for adequate healing. Rupture of the midsubstance of the ligament necessitates C1–C2 fusion.

26. **What is whiplash?**
Whiplash is a poorly understood clinical syndrome in which seemingly inconsequential trauma leads to chronic neck pain. This injury complex, also called acceleration injury, cervical sprain syndrome, or soft tissue neck injury, usually follows a rear-end collision. Patients treated for whiplash are commonly involved in accident-related litigation. For some of these patients, economic incentives interfere with clinical improvement.

27. **How is whiplash different from other cervical spine trauma?**
Most cervical spine trauma results from contact force (eg, striking the head on the dashboard, leading to an extension injury). Whiplash, on the other hand, results from inertial forces applied to the head. Anatomic structures including the sternocleidomastoid and longissimus colli muscles, intervertebral disc, facet capsule, and anterior longitudinal ligament have been implicated as pain generators.

28. **Who tends to be susceptible to whiplash?**
Although there are 4 million rear-end collisions per year, only 1 million result in reported whiplash injuries. Of those involved in these injuries, 70% are women, usually between 30 and 50 years of age. The injury is more common in those with low physical activity jobs.

29. **What are the typical symptoms of whiplash?**
Most patients report neck pain and/or occipital headaches. These headaches can be dull, sharp, or aching and are usually worse with movement. The pain is associated with stiffness and often radiates to the head, arm, or between the scapulae. Some patients report vertigo, auditory or visual disturbances, hoarseness, temperature changes, fatigue, depression, and sleep disturbances. These symptoms are often provoked or exacerbated by emotion, temperature, humidity, or noise and variably have been attributed to cranial nerve and sympathetic chain disruption.

30. **Describe the physical examination and radiologic signs of whiplash.**
On examination, decreased range of motion and spasm are noted; however, other objective findings are absent. Similarly, various radiologic modalities have a poor correlation with symptoms. Often a loss of normal cervical lordosis is noted. Preexisting degenerative disease of the spine is associated with a worse prognosis in whiplash. An MRI scan usually appears normal and is rarely indicated.

31. **What is the natural history of whiplash?**
Symptom onset usually occurs within 2 days. Of patients diagnosed with whiplash, 57% recover completely in 3 months, and 8% remain so severely affected that they are unable to work. For the remaining 35% of patients, a partial recovery occurs. Maximum improvement is usually reached by 1 year.

32. **How is whiplash treated?**
The goal of treatment is to reengage patients in their normal activities as soon as possible. In mild cases, an immediate return to work is warranted. Otherwise, a 3-week respite to allow for pain control may be advised. Nonsteroidal antiinflammatory medications are usually recommended. Muscle relaxants and narcotics are not recommended. A collar should be used only for the first few days after the injury. The critical element in treatment is active early mobilization. Short-arc active motion is used for pain and spasm. Gentle passive range of motion

can be employed to counteract stiffness. After 48 hours, progression to active motion is suggested. After the acute pain subsides, proceed with isometric strengthening to tolerance. Other modalities are commonly employed, including traction, biofeedback, ultrasound, manipulation, massage, heat, and ice. Combinations of treatment measures in addition to early mobilization have often been the most successful. If significant pain continues after 3 months, a multidisciplinary pain clinic approach has been found to be useful. In addition, symptoms of anxiety, depression, and posttraumatic stress often accompany chronic pain associated with whiplash and can increase the morbidity of this condition. Understanding who is at risk and who would benefit from screening and management can improve outcomes.

33. **How are injuries to the thoracolumbar spine classified?**
A number of classification schemes have been devised for the thoracolumbar spine. Some are descriptive; some are mechanistic. In general, however, the same principles apply as for the cervical spine (see table). Many divide injuries into major and minor types.

34. **What might be considered a minor injury of the thoracolumbar spine?**
Minor injuries account for 15% of thoracolumbar fractures. They include isolated fractures of the spinous and transverse processes, pars, and facets. They may be caused by direct trauma or violent muscular contraction in response to injury.

35. **How are these minor injuries evaluated?**
Obtain radiographs of the remainder of the spine to exclude other injuries. Then further assess the affected level for subtle injury with axial CT slices. If the CT is negative, flexion-extension views are important to exclude dynamic instability. For example, a pars fracture may be the only plain film evidence of a flexion-distraction injury. Assuming these tests are negative, the patient can be mobilized without braces or restrictions, except as needed for the relief of symptoms.

36. **What are the broad types of major injuries of the thoracolumbar spine?**
Major injuries include axial loading injuries such as compression and burst fractures. When additional, directional force is applied to the spine, flexion-distraction injuries and fracture dislocations may occur.

37. **What are compression fractures, and how are they treated?**
Compression fractures represent almost half of all major thoracolumbar spinal injuries. They result from a compression failure of the anterior column with the middle and posterior columns left intact. Traditionally, these fractures were treated with orthosis. In younger patients with higher energy levels imparted to the spine, a full contact orthosis (such as a thoracolumbosacral orthosis [TLSO]) was recommended and for osteoporotic patients with lower energy trauma, a limited contact orthosis (such as a Cash or Jewett brace) was appropriate. Braces, however, are criticized for being uncomfortable and for possibly causing delays in rehabilitation and muscle atrophy. In addition, more recent research shows that the treatment of these fractures without a brace can lead to the same recovery timeline and pain relief as treatment with a brace. For patients with low energy compression fractures and osteoporotic bone, percutaneous injection of bone cement (polymethyl methacrylate [PMMA]) either with (kyphoplasty) or without (vertebroplasty) balloon reduction of the deformity can be considered if nonoperative treatment has been ineffective.

38. **Are vertebral body augmentation (VBA) procedures (kyphoplasty and vertebroplasty) always indicated in spine fractures?**
While opinions vary, VBAs are not typically indicated in high energy trauma, especially in young patients with good bone quality. Additionally, these procedures cannot offer stabilization outside of the PMMA's role as a grout. That is, the bone cement is not a glue, so it only works to resist axial loads (compression). These procedures are most typically indicated in low-energy trauma (eg, falls from standing) in patients with osteoporosis. Even in these patients, if ambulatory, a trial of nonoperative management should be attempted before recommended VBA.

39. **How is a burst fracture different from a compression fracture?**
A burst fracture includes compression failure of the middle and posterior columns as well. This injury is associated with greater height loss of the anterior column, often with retropulsion of the middle column bone into the canal. A great deal of attention and controversy have been directed to what defines a stable and an unstable burst fracture. Therefore recommendations for treatment of given injuries are often variable. However, the angulation (kyphosis), loss of vertebral height, and canal encroachment as well as the presence or absence of neurologic deficits are evaluated. In general, a neurologically intact patient with little deformity is managed nonoperatively by use of an extension cast or TLSO. Unstable injuries, including those with posterior ligamentous disruption, neurologic deficit, or unacceptable deformities, are treated by surgical decompression and stabilization. This type of surgical procedure may be performed either with a direct anterior decompression and strut graft fusion or with a posterior approach using indirect reduction techniques and screw stabilization.

40. What is a seat-belt injury?

Historically seen in belted passengers in an MVA without a shoulder harness, a seat-belt injury results in a flexion-distraction injury of the spine. The anterior longitudinal ligament is intact, but there may be compression failure of the vertebral body and distraction through the posterior elements. This injury may occur through bone or soft tissue. If it occurs through bone, it is termed a Chance fracture. Such bony injuries are treated nonoperatively with an extension cast or thoracolumbar spinal orthosis. Close follow-up is required to exclude progressive deformity. If significant soft tissue or ligamentous injury is involved, less predictable healing occurs with closed means, and a posterior stabilization procedure is recommended.

41. How are fracture dislocations different from other types of thoracolumbar traumas?

In these injuries, the entire segment, anterior to posterior, fails and vertebral translation occurs. Translation may cause canal occlusion and cord compression. Therefore fracture-dislocations are associated with a high incidence of neurologic deficits. These injuries may be divided into subtypes based on the direction of translation: flexion-rotation, shear, and flexion-distraction. Almost all of these injuries require operative stabilization.

42. What are some complications associated with the surgical treatment of spinal trauma?

Implant displacement, which is most common after posterior instrumentation, is an important consideration in any patient describing increased pain or deformity. Such displacement is often related to poor bone quality, implant placement error, and noncompliance with brace/activity recommendations. Another common problem is postoperative wound infection. Increased drainage, redness, fever, and pain are signs of such an infection.

43. When may a spinal trauma patient be safely mobilized?

Mobilization is a critical issue in trauma patients and must be individualized. The benefits of immobilization in shielding the healing spine from excessive external loads are counterbalanced with the drawbacks, including increased muscular stiffness and weakness. In patients with polytrauma or neurologic injury, external bracing is burdensome and interferes with optimal rehabilitation.

Stable injuries are mobilized immediately with gentle, passive ROM. In these patients, modalities such as ice, heat, ultrasound, and massage appear helpful in symptomatic relief. A stretching and strengthening program is gradually added as pain levels decrease and motion increases. Unstable spinal column injuries will not tolerate early motion. In general terms, however, an injury with significant instability should be converted to a stable configuration by way of external bracing, surgery, or both.

A rigidly stabilized spine is often mobilized within 2 weeks. In injuries treated with less than rigid fixation or in those patients with poor bone quality or other factors compromising their fixation, 6 to 12 weeks of external orthosis wear is followed by the initiation of gentle, active ROM. Strengthening is instituted upon attainment of full and painless motion in patients for whom x-rays demonstrate no change in position of hardware or vertebral elements.

In patients with unstable injuries treated with nonoperative means, mobilization is started at times predicted by tissue healing. Therefore compression fractures through cancellous bone may tolerate mobilization at 4 weeks. On the other hand, cortical bone injuries (such as dens fractures) and injuries with a significant ligamentous component (burst fractures with severe collapse) will require 12 to 16 weeks of immobilization. Dynamic radiographs (flexion-extension views) are often useful to evaluate healing before aggressive rehabilitation.

44. Name other common postoperative medical problems to which spinal trauma patients are prone.

Deep venous thrombosis (DVT), pulmonary embolism, and pressure sores are very serious potential consequences of the immobilization required after major spinal injury. Pneumonia, pneumothorax, and other pulmonary problems are common as well. Autonomic dysreflexia is seen in patients with cervical and upper thoracic spinal cord injuries. In this disorder, bladder overdistention or fecal impaction causes an autonomic nervous system reaction, which leads to severe hypertension. The patient's presenting symptoms often include a pounding headache, anxiety, profuse head and neck sweating, nasal obstruction, and blurred vision. Treatment begins with immediate placement of a Foley catheter and rectal disimpaction. If the symptoms do not quickly resolve, medications are required.

45. What is the role of physical therapy in the status of osteoporotic patients after a vertebral compression fracture?

Osteoporotic patients are at risk for additional fractures. In particular, lifting while flexing, lifting overhead, and falls increases the risk of fracture. A rehabilitation program, including gait and balance training and extensor muscle strengthening, is being recommended in conjunction with a therapist-centered educational program about appropriate lifting techniques and back protection. Therapy to help improve technique and conditioning can prevent circumstances that increase the risk for injury.

46. How can therapy help prevent osteoporotic fractures?
A combination of strength training and weight-bearing exercise can increase bone density in postmenopausal women. In the absence of weight-bearing exercise, bone density will continue to deteriorate. Aerobic training has been shown to limit the reduction of bone mineral density loss, while strength training can increase specific site bone density especially in the lumbar spine. Consistent exercise (at least 3×/week for a year) is necessary for any meaningful improvement in bone density. A multimodal therapy program—including improving conditioning and technique through gait training and teaching on lifting techniques in combination with exercises to augment bone density—can help patients avoid further fragility fractures. The physical therapist should also support efforts to test the patient's bone mineralization (DEXA scans) and placement on appropriate anti-osteoporotic or bone building medications. Absent this approach, a high rate of subsequent fracture and mortality has been reported.

BIBLIOGRAPHY

An, H. S., & Simpson, J. M. (1994). *Surgery of the cervical spine*. London: Martin Dunitz Ltd.

Copley, P. C. C., Aimun, A. B., & Jamjoom, S. K. (2020). The management of traumatic spinal cord injuries in adults: a review. *Orthopaedics and Trauma, 34*(5), 255–265.

d'Amato, C. (2005). Pediatric spinal trauma: injuries in very young children. *Clinical Orthopaedics, 432*, 34–40.

Delamarter, R. B., & Coyle, J. (1999). Acute management of spinal cord injury. *Journal of the American Academy of Orthopaedic Surgeons, 7*, 166–175.

Denis, F. (1983). The three column spine and its significance in the classification of acute thoracolumbar spinal injuries. *Spine, 8*, 8.

DeVine, J. G., Agochukwu, U. F., & Jackson, K. L. (2021). Thoracolumbar and lumbosacral trauma. In E. Truumees & H. Prather H (Eds.), *Orthopaedic knowledge update* (6th ed.). Lippincott Williams and Wilkins.

Gu, C. N., Brinjikji, W., Murad, M. H., & Kallmes, D. F. (2016). Outcomes of vertebroplasty compared with kyphoplasty: a systematic review and meta-analysis. *Journal of NeuroInterventional Surgery, 8*, 636–642.

Joaquim, A. F., Patel, A. A., & Vaccaro, A. R. (2014). Cervical injuries scored according to the Subaxial Injury Classification system: An analysis of the literature. *Journal of Craniovertebral Junction & Spine, 5*(2), 65–70.

Karnes, J., Anderson, P., & Hah, R. (2021). Subaxial cervical trauma. In E. Truumees & H. Prather (Eds.), *Orthopaedic knowledge update* (6th ed.). Lippincott Williams and Wilkins.

Lee, J. Y., Vaccaro, A. R., Lim, M. R., et al. (2005). Thoracolumbar injury classification and severity score: a new paradigm for the treatment of thoracolumbar spine trauma. *Journal of Orthopaedic Science, 10*(6), 671–675.

Levine, A. M., Eismont, F.J., Garfin, S.R., & Zigler, J.E. (eds.). (1998). *Spine trauma*. Philadelphia: Saunders.

Müller, E. J., Wick, M., Russe, O., & Muhr, G. (1999). Management of odontoid fractures in the elderly. *European Spine Journal, 8*, 360–365.

Sliker, C. W., Mirvis, S. E., & Shanmuganathan, K. (2005). Assessing cervical spine stability in obtunded blunt trauma patients: review of medical literature. *Radiology, 234*, 733–739.

Spivak, J. M., Vaccaro, A. R., & Cotler, J. M. (1995). Thoracolumbar spine trauma I and II. *Journal of the American Academy of Orthopaedic Surgeons, 3*, 345–360.

Truumees, E. (2004). Osteoporosis of the spine. In C. M. Bono & S. R. Garfin (Eds.), *Orthopaedic surgery essentials: Spine*. Philadelphia: Lippincott.

Truumees, E., Hilibrand, A. S., & Vaccaro, A. R. (2004). Percutaneous vertebral augmentation. *The Spine Journal, 4*, 218–229.

Vaccaro, A. R. (Ed.), (2005). *Orthopaedic knowledge update* (8th ed.). Rosemont, Ill: AAOS.

White, A. A., 3rd, Panjabi, M. M., Posner, I., Edwards, W. T., & Hayes, W. C. (1981). Spinal stability: evaluation and treatment. *Instructional Course Lectures, 30*, 457–483.

Wood, K., Buttermann, G., Mehbod, A., Garvey, T., Jhanjee, R., & Sechriest, V. (2003). Operative compared with nonoperative treatment of a thoracolumbar burst fracture without neurological deficit: a prospective, randomized study. *Journal of Bone and Joint Surgery (American), 85*, 773–781.

Zhao, R. 1, Zhao, M., & Xu, Z. (2015). The effects of differing resistance training modes on the preservation of bone mineral density in postmenopausal women: a meta-analysis. *Osteoporosis International, 26*(5), 1605–1618.

CHAPTER 62 QUESTIONS

1. Which incomplete cord syndrome has the best prognosis for recovery?
   a. Central
   b. Anterior
   c. Brown-Séquard
   d. Lateral

2. Which of the following regarding whiplash is false?
   a. It is due to inertial forces on the head.
   b. Men are more commonly involved.
   c. More common in 30- to 50-year-olds.
   d. Eight percent never return to work.

3. How can therapy help prevent osteoporotic fractures?
   a. Electric stim can increase bone density.
   b. Aerobic exercise can increase bone density.

c. Weight-bearing and resistance exercises can increase bone density.
d. Aquatic exercise can increase bone density.

4. **Which of the following is true of the incidence and management of compression fractures?**
   a. These are commonly high-volume injuries in the elderly population.
   b. Treatment principles and options are the same in younger and elder populations.
   c. Bracing has shown to have an unequivocal benefit that improves the recovery timeline and pain relief.
   d. The majority of these injuries require surgical intervention.
   e. Kyphoplasty, the insertion of cement into the deformity caused by the fracture, can help pain control and function in certain patients.

5. **Which of the following is not a red flag to alert a practitioner to a possible spine injury?**
   a. Facial trauma
   b. Calcaneus fracture
   c. Hypotension
   d. Myocardial infarction
   e. Intoxication
   f. Worsening neurologic deficit

6. **Which of the following principles are important rehabilitation principles in spinal cord injury?**
   a. Tilt tables are an effective tool in physical rehabilitation to prevent syncope in patients with orthostatic hypotension.
   b. A bowel/bladder program is important to develop to help patients live with neurogenic bowel/bladder and prevent urinary tract infections.
   c. Mobilization and splinting can help reduce the risk of DVT, contractures, pressure ulcers, and osteoporosis.
   d. Autonomic dysreflexia is a temporary disorder that is self-resolving in the first few weeks after injury.
   e. Consultation with mental health professionals and working with occupational therapy to find a patient's role in society may be needed to help patients deal with symptoms of depression.

CHAPTER 63

FUNCTIONAL ANATOMY OF THE SACROILIAC JOINT

M.E. Lonnemann, PT, DPT, OCS, FAAOMPT and A. Grant, PT, DPT, MTC, CLT

1. **Name the osseous structures of the pelvic ring.**
   The ilia, sacrum, coccyx, femora, and pubis are the osseous structures of the pelvic ring.

2. **How is the sacroiliac joint (SIJ) classified?**
   The SIJ has been classified in several ways. Vleeming (2012) has classified the joint as an amphiarthrosis (synarthrodial cartilaginous) joint. However, Gray (2013) has classified the joint as a modified synovial joint (diarthrosis). The variation in classification is most likely because there are two aspects of the joint. The main portion of the joint is auricular and is surrounded by a complex capsule lined with cartilage (diarthrosis). There is a second dorsally located fibrous articulation that is extracapsular and is considered a synarthrosis stabilized by the interosseous ligaments. To simplify the classification, the SIJ can be considered to consist of two parts: a synovial joint (intraarticular) and a syndesmosis (extraarticular).

3. **Within which sacral segments does the SIJ form?**
   S1, S2, and S3.

4. **Is the sacrum fully fused at birth?**
   No, fusion of the sacral vertebrae begins early in the second decade of life.

5. **Which surface of the SIJ is concave?**
   The sacral surface is for the most part concave; however, often an intraarticular bony tubercle is present in the anterior and middle aspect of the surface of the sacrum. The iliac part is predominantly convex. Variations do exist.

6. **Describe the composition of the articular surfaces of the sacroiliac joint.**
   The sacral articular cartilage resembles typical hyaline cartilage, and its thickness ranges from 1 to 3 mm. The iliac cartilage resembles fibrocartilage and is usually <1 mm in thickness.

7. **What is the function of the sacroiliac joint?**
   The SIJ is the link between the axial skeleton and the lower appendicular skeleton, and thus its main function is to transmit forces from the axial skeleton to the lower limbs and vice versa.

8. **How does the orientation of the SIJ make it difficult to establish a specific axis of motion using conventional planes?**
   In general, the axes of motion lie in a transverse plane at the level of S2. However, motion and rotational axes at the SIJ have been found to vary considerably because of contour variations in the joint surfaces of both the frontal and the sagittal planes. Motion variations also may result from individual differences in ligamentous laxity.

9. **Are clinical exam tests valid for evaluating carpal tunnel syndrome?**
   - Phalen's test is described as a wrist flexion test when a patient is asked to flex the wrist with the dorsum of each hand pressed together. It was originally described as having a sensitivity of 74%, however a 60 second timed Phalen's test was reported to have a sensitivity of 85%.
   - The combined wrist flexion/median nerve pressure test is accomplished by placing the wrist in full flexion while placing manual or digital pressure on the median nerve just proximal to the distal wrist crease. When this test was completed at 30 seconds the sensitivity was reported at 82% and the specificity at 99%
   - The combined wrist extension/median nerve pressure test is accomplished by placing the wrist in full extension and placing manual pressure on the median nerve just proximal to the distal wrist crease. This test had a sensitivity of 89% at 60 seconds duration and a specificity of 83% at 30 seconds duration.

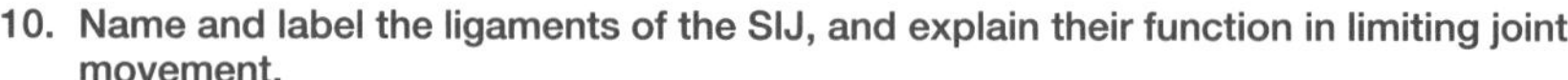

10. Name and label the ligaments of the SIJ, and explain their function in limiting joint movement.

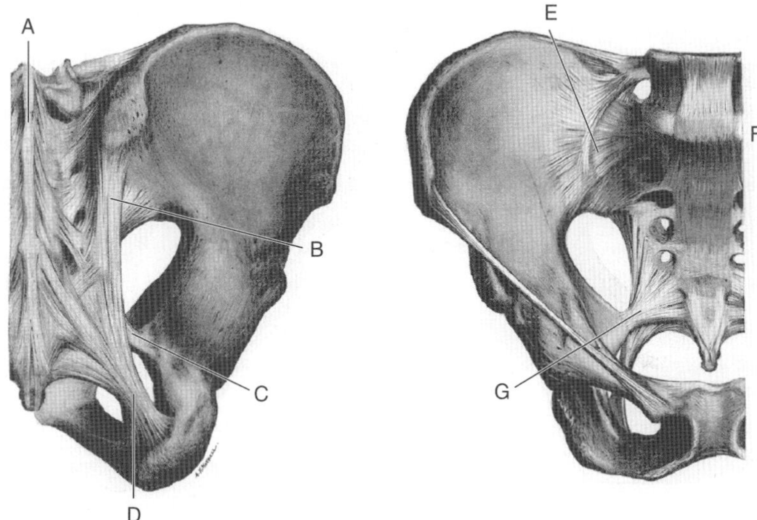

Interosseous sacroiliac ligament binds the ilium to the sacrum (not pictured). Long and short posterior sacroiliac ligaments: the long ligaments prevent counterrotation of the ilium (B) whereas the short ligament (A) binds the ilium to the sacrum. Anterior sacroiliac ligament prevents anterior displacement and diastasis of the joint (F). Sacrospinous (C and G) and sacrotuberous (D) ligaments prevent nutation of the sacrum by anchoring it to the ischium. Iliolumbar ligament prevents downward and anterior displacement of the ilium (E). (From Gray H. (1918). *Anatomy of the human body* (20th ed.). Philadelphia, PA: Lea & Febiger.)

11. Describe the attachments of the anterior sacroiliac and sacrospinous and sacrotuberous ligaments.

The anterior sacroiliac ligament covers the ventral aspect of the joint and extends from the sacral ala and anterior sacral surface to the anterior surface of the ilium beyond the margins of the joint. It is larger in males than in females. The sacrospinous ligament originates from the inferior lateral angle of the sacrum to the ischial spine of the ilium. The sacrotuberous ligament arises from the posterior superior iliac spine (PSIS), merges with the long posterior sacroiliac ligaments and the lateral margin of the sacrum (where it combines with the sacrospinous ligament), and attaches to the ischial tuberosity.

12. Describe the attachments and function of the interosseous sacroiliac ligaments.

The interosseous sacroiliac ligament is one of the strongest ligaments in the SIJ, with the most extensive volume and bony attachment compared with other SIJ ligaments regardless of gender. It fills the joint spaces of the axial joint/ventral auricular joint, as well as the dorsal, cephalic portion of the synovial joint. It provides multidirectional stability and binds the joint together.

13. Which muscles contribute to the stability of the SIJ?

The muscles that cross the SIJ are designed to create movement of the lumbar spine or hip, as well as contribute to the stability of the SIJ. They are not prime movers of the SIJ. The adjacent muscles, including the quadratus lumborum, multifidus, erector spinae, gluteus minimus, piriformis, iliacus, and latissimus dorsi, contribute to the strength of the joint capsule and ligaments. Other muscles attaching to the pelvic girdle and contributing to the function of the SIJ include the abdominal muscles: internal and external obliques, rectus abdominis, and transversus abdominis. Several studies have demonstrated that, among other muscles, contraction of the internal oblique and transversus abdominus creates force closure of the pelvis, and the superficial layer of the thoracolumbar fascia attaches to the latissimus dorsi and gluteus maximus, thereby contributing to compression of the SIJ through its contraction.

14. Describe the innervation of the SIJ.

The SIJ innervation is best described when comparing the intraarticular part of the SIJ and compared to the extraarticular portion. The intraarticular part of the joint is innervated primarily by the anterior rami of L4 and/or L5 or the lumbosacral trunk along with innervation from the posterior sacral network. The extraarticular part of the

SIJ is innervated by the posterior sacral network or the plexus formed by the lateral branches of the posterior rami of S1–S3 and L5–S4.

15. **What neurologic structures emerging from the sacrum innervate the pelvic region and lower limbs?**

NERVE	STRUCTURES INNERVATED
Tibial (L4–S3)	Medial hamstrings, adductor magnus, posterior compartment of leg, intrinsics of foot
Fibular (L4–S2)	Lateral hamstrings, lateral compartment of leg, EDB of foot
Pudendal (S2–S4)	External urethral and anal sphincters, levator ani, and skin of perineum, penis, clitoris
Superior gluteal (L4–S1)	Gluteus medius, gluteus minimus, tensor fasciae latae
Inferior gluteal (L5–S2)	Gluteus maximus
Nerve to obturator internus and superior gemellus (L5–S2)	Obturator internus, superior gemellus
Nerve to quadratus femoris and inferior gemellus (L4–S1)	Quadratus femoris and inferior gemellus
Posterior femoral cutaneous (S1–S3)	Skin on posterior thigh
Nerve to piriformis (S1–S2)	Piriformis muscle
Nerves to levator ani, coccygeus, external anal sphincter (S4)	Levator ani, coccygeus, and external anal sphincter; skin between anus and coccyx
Anococcygeal nerves (S4–CO)	Perianal skin

16. **What are the anatomic differences between the male and female pelvis?**
The male pelvis is larger with regard to overall pelvic dimensions (measured from crest to crest). In males the iliac crests also extend higher than the female pelvis. The male pelvis is heavy and thick with larger joint surfaces. The female pelvis is light and thin with small joint surfaces. The muscle attachments in the male pelvis are well defined, whereas the female muscle attachments are rather indistinct. The male sacrum is longer, narrower, and more curved, whereas the female sacrum is short and wide. The pelvic cavity is longer and cone shaped in males, whereas the female pelvic cavity is shorter and cylinder shaped.

17. **What are the functional differences between the male and female pelvis? How do they affect the SIJ?**
In males the weight of the body is situated in a direct vertical position above the axis of support of the legs. The body weight in females falls behind the axis of support (upward through the acetabulum) so that the gravity vector tends to create a posterior rotation force on the pelvis. Morphologic changes in the joint surface appear earlier in men and are more extensive with regard to joint surface irregularities. Such changes may be a normal response to greater forces on the SIJs of men compared with women. The primary function of the SIJ in women is to increase the pelvic diameter during labor for vaginal delivery.

18. **Describe the influence of hormones on the SIJ.**
Relaxin, a hormone secreted by the corpus luteum, is present throughout pregnancy. The role of relaxin is to remodel collagen, thus creating ligamentous laxity in target tissues, including the pubic symphysis, in preparation for delivery. Relaxin is produced during the luteal phase of menstruation, at which time the endometrium of the uterus prepares for pregnancy (between ovulation and menses). The increased levels of relaxin may provoke symptoms in patients with mobility dysfunctions of the SIJ. Changes in progesterone levels also may affect the laxity of the joint.

19. **Describe the amount of potential movement at the SIJ.**
Minimal range of motion of the SIJ has been reported in studies with good methodology and reproducibility. Sturesson et al. (1989) used roentgen stereophotogrammetry of metal balls inserted into the sacrum and ilium and found 1 to 3 degrees or 1 to 3 mm of motion at the sacroiliac joint. Walheim and Selvik (1984) used a similar method at the symphysis pubis and found rotation did not exceed 3 degrees and translation did not exceed 2 mm.

Recent data support that small movements or the normal range of movement are maintained in the SIJ through the sixth decade, with a slight reduction of movement in males after the sixth decade.

20. **Describe the possible movements of the sacrum and innominate/ilium.**
Research has demonstrated that with application of flexion, extension, lateral bending, and axial rotation loads, rotational and translational movements are seen in all three planes as depicted below.

PLANE OF MOTION	ILIAL/INNOMINATE MOVEMENT	SACRAL MOVEMENT
Sagittal	Anterior and posterior rotation	Flexion extension
Frontal	Superior and inferior translation	Side-bending
Transverse	External and internal rotation	Rotation

21. **Discuss the theoretic movements of the ilium and sacrum that may occur during trunk forward bending, backward bending, hip flexion, hip extension, and gait.**
After about the first 60 degrees of trunk forward bending, the pelvis rotates anteriorly around the hip joints. The sacrum follows the lumbar spine to the extreme of flexion in both standing and sitting positions, when counternutation or backward nodding of the sacrum occurs. During trunk hyperextension of the spine, nutation of the sacrum occurs. With hip flexion, rotation of the ilium occurs in a backward direction, and the opposite occurs with hip extension. Inman studied walking and describes posterior iliac rotation during hip flexion through the swing phase, which is accentuated by heel contact and initial loading. During the loading response, the ipsilateral ilium begins to rotate anteriorly. The sacrum seems to rotate forward about a diagonal axis, creating torsion on the side of loading at midstance.

22. **Describe the age-related changes in the SIJ.**
Over time the SIJ develops a coarse texture with ridges and depressions that enhance the stability of the joint. During the first 10 years of life, the joint surfaces remain flat, but in the second and third decades they begin to develop uneven articular surfaces. By the third decade, the iliac surface has developed a convex ridge through the center of the joint surface with a corresponding ridge on the sacrum. By the fourth and fifth decades, the joint surfaces become yellowed and roughened with plaque formation and peripheral joint erosions. In all specimens, marked degenerative arthrosis is the rule by the fourth decade. Sacral osteophytes begin to form in the fourth decade at the joint margins. By the sixth and seventh decades, the osteophytes enlarge and begin to interdigitate across the joint surface. The joint surfaces become irregular with deep erosions that sometimes expose the subchondral bone. By the eighth decade, osteophyte interdigitation increases to the extent that some specimens exhibit true bony ankylosis. The joint surfaces demonstrate marked degenerative changes with diminished articular cartilage on both surfaces.

23. **Why does the SIJ begin as a mobile joint and progress toward a stable joint?**
In the nonweight-bearing infant, the SIJ is not required to provide stability. As the child progresses to weight-bearing movements, the SIJ undergoes a transformation into a stable interlocking joint that serves as a force transmission center from the spine to the lower limbs and vice versa.

24. **Explain the standard views for radiographic evaluation of the SIJ, and discuss the anatomic structures that are best visualized in each image.**
Standard radiographic views of the SIJ include anteroposterior (AP), axial, and right and left posterior obliques (RPO and LPO, respectively). In the AP view, the articular surfaces present as two radiolucent lines because they are superimposed on each other. The joints are assessed for symmetry and joint margin contour. In the posterior oblique view, the entire margin of the joint space can be visualized. Assessment from this view includes extent of joint width, location of bony margins, and degenerative or fibrous changes within the joint.

25. **What is the incidence of sacralization in the United States, and how is the presence of a cervical rib associated with sacralization?**
Sacralization is when the transverse processes of the fifth lumbar vertebrae fuse to the sacrum or ilium (unilaterally or bilaterally). It occurs in 6% of adults. Studies tend to suggest a weak association between sacralization and low back pain. In a recent study of 1053 patients, 73% with cervical ribs had sacralization, and 64% with sacralization had cervical ribs. The value of this information is that if a patient is determined to have either a cervical rib or sacralization, the clinician should be aware of the association, which may help with the differential diagnosis of musculoskeletal complaints.

26. What is lumbarization?

Lumbarization is when the S1 vertebrae is separated from the sacrum and could be considered a sixth lumbar vertebrae. The incidence ratio of sacralization to lumbarization is 2:1.

Bibliography

Bakland, O., & Hansen, J. H. (1984). The "axial sacroiliac joint." *Anatomia Clinica, 6,* 29–36.

Beales, D. J., O'Sullivan, P. B., & Briffa, N. K. (2010). The effects of manual pelvic compression on trunk motor control during an active straight leg raise in chronic pelvic girdle pain subjects. *Manual Therapy, 15,* 190–199.

Bernard, T. N., & Cassidy, J. D. (1991). The sacroiliac joint syndrome: pathophysiology, diagnosis and management. In J. W. Frymoyer (Ed.), *The adult spine: principles and practice* (pp. 2107–2130). New York, NY: Raven Press.

Bogduk, N. (1997). *Clinical anatomy of the lumbar spine and sacrum* (3rd ed.). New York, NY: Churchill Livingstone.

Bowen, V., & Cassidy, J. D. (1981). Macroscopic and microscopic anatomy of the sacroiliac joint from embryonic life until the eighth decade. *Spine, 6,* 620–628.

Cox, M., Ng, G., Mashriqi, F., et al. (2017). Innervation of the anterior sacroiliac joint. *World Neurosurgery, 107,* 750–752.

Fast, A., Shapiro, D., & Ducommun, E. J. (1987). Low-back pain in pregnancy. *Spine, 12,* 368–371.

Goldthwait, J. E., & Osgood, R. B. (1905). A consideration of the pelvic articulations from an anatomical, pathological, and clinical standpoint. *New England Journal of Medicine, 152,* 593–601.

Gray, H. (2013). *Grays Anatomy.* London, England: Arcturus Publishing.

Greenman, P. (1996). *Principles of manual medicine* (2nd ed.). Philadelphia, PA: Williams & Wilkins.

Hayne, C. (1981). Manual transport of loads by women. *Physiotherapy, 67,* 226–231.

Hu, H., Meijer, O. G., van Dieen, J. H., et al. (2010). Muscle activity during the active straight leg raise (ASLR), and the effects of a pelvic belt on the ASLR and on treadmill walking. *Journal of Biomechanics, 43,* 532–539.

Inman, V. T., Ralston, J. H., & Todd, F. (1981). *Human walking.* Baltimore, MD: Williams & Wilkins.

Kapandji, I. A. (1947). Chapter 2. *The physiology of the joints*: Vol. 3 (pp. 54–71). New York, NY: Churchill Livingstone.

Lee, D. (1989). *The pelvic girdle: an approach to the examination and treatment of the lumbo-pelvic-hip region.* Edinburgh: Churchill Livingstone.

MacLennan, A. H. (1991). The role of the hormone relaxin in human reproduction and pelvic girdle relaxation. *Scandinavian Journal of Rheumatology, 20,* 7–15.

McKinnis, L. (1997). *Fundamentals of orthopedic radiology.* Philadelphia, PA: FA Davis.

Odeh, K., Wu, W., Taylor, B., Leasure, J., & Kondrashov, D. (2021). In-vitro 3D analysis of sacroiliac joint kinematics. *Spine, 46,* E467–E473.

Paquin, J. D., van der Rest, M., Marie, P. J., et al. (1983). Biochemical and morphologic studies of cartilage from the adult human sacroiliac joint. *Arthritis and Rheumatism, 26,* 887–895.

Paris, S. V. (1983). Anatomy as related to function and pain. *Orthopedic Clinics of North America, 14,* 475–489.

Pool-Goudzwaard, A. L., Vleeming, A., Stoeckart, R., Snijders, C. J., & Mens, J. M. A. (1998). Insufficient lumbopelvic stability: a clinical, anatomical and biomechanical approach to "a-specific" low back pain. *Manual Therapy, 3,* 12–20.

Sashin, D. (1930). A critical analysis of the anatomy and the pathological changes of the sacroiliac joints. *Journal of Bone and Joint Surgery, 12,* 891–910.

Scheuer, L., & Black, S. (2000). *Developmental juvenile osteology.* San Diego: Elsevier.

Solonen, K. A. (1957). The sacroiliac joint in the light of anatomical, roentgenological and clinical studies. *Acta Orthopaedica Scandinavica, Supplement, 27,* 1–127.

Standring, S. (2009). *Gray's anatomy: the anatomical basis of clinical practice* (40th ed.). St Louis, MO: Elsevier.

Steinke, H., Hammer, N., Slowik, V., et al. (2010). Novel insights into the sacroiliac joint ligaments. *Spine (Phila Pa 1976), 35,* 257–263.

Stevens, V. K., Vleeming, A., Bouche, K. G., et al. (2007). Electromyographic activity of trunk and hip muscles during stabilization exercises in four-point kneeling in healthy volunteers. *European Spine Journal, 16,* 711–718.

Stewart, T. D. (1984). Pathological changes in aging sacroiliac joints. *Clinical Orthopaedics and Related Research, 183,* 188–196.

Sturesson, B., Selvik, G., & Udén, A. (1989). Movements of the sacroiliac joints: a roentgen stereophotogrammetric analysis. *Spine, 14,* 162–165.

Tague, R. G. (2009). High assimilation of the sacrum in a sample of American skeletons: prevalence, pelvic size, and obstetrical and evolutionary implications. *American Journal of Physical Anthropology, 138,* 429–438.

Vleeming, A., Pool-Goudzwaard, A. L., Stoeckart, R., van Wingerden, J. P., & Snijders, C. J. (1995). The posterior layer of the thoracolumbar fascia: its function in load transfer from spine to legs. *Spine, 20,* 753–758.

Vleeming, A., Schuenke, D., Masi, A. T., Carreiro, J. E., Danneels, L., & Willard, F. H. (2012). The sacroiliac joint: an overview of its anatomy, function and potential clinical implications. *Journal of Anatomy, 221,* 537–567.

Vleeming, A., Stoeckart, R., Volkers, A. C., & Snijders, C. J. (1990). Relation between form and function in the sacroiliac joint. I: clinical anatomical aspects. *Spine, 13,* 133–135.

Walheim, G. G., & Selvik, G. (1984). Mobility of the pubic symphysis: in vivo measurements with an electromechanic method and a roentgen stereophotogrammetric method. *Clinical Orthopaedics, 191,* 129–135.

Walker, J. (1992). The sacroiliac joint: a critical review. *Physical Therapy, 72,* 903–916.

Weisl, H. (1954). The ligaments of the sacroiliac joint examined with particular reference to their function. *Acta Anatomica, 22,* 1–14.

Wiesman IM, Novak, CB, Mackinnon SE, Winograd JM. Sensitivity and specificity of clinical testing for carpal tunnel syndrome. Can J Plast Surg. 2003 Summer; 11(2): 70–72. doi: 10.1177/229255030301100205

Wilder, D. G., Pope, M. H., & Frymoyer, J. W. (1980). The functional topography of the sacroiliac joint. *Spine, 5,* 575–579.

CHAPTER 63 QUESTIONS

1. **Which of the following set of terms best describes the male pelvis compared with the female pelvis?**
   a. Larger in width and height, larger joint surfaces, narrow and curved sacrum, and a cone-shaped pelvic cavity
   b. Larger in width and height, smaller joint surfaces, narrow and curved sacrum, and a cone-shaped pelvic cavity
   c. Smaller in width and height, larger joint surfaces, narrow and curved sacrum, and a cylindrical-shaped pelvic cavity
   d. Smaller in width and height, small joint surfaces, short and wide sacrum, and a cone-shaped pelvic cavity

2. **The main portion of the SIJ is surrounded by a joint capsule and lined with cartilage. This portion of the joint is considered the _________ joint.**
   a. Diarthrodial
   b. Synarthrodial
   c. Synchondrosis
   d. Symphysis

3. **Contraction of which of the following muscles would best contribute to forced closure of the pelvic ring?**
   a. Hamstrings and gluteus maximus
   b. Gluteus medius and quadratus lumborum
   c. Rectus abdominus and multifidus
   d. Transversus abdominis and internal oblique

CHAPTER 64

SACROILIAC DYSFUNCTION

M.E. Lonnemann, PT, DPT, OCS, FAAOMPT and A.Grant, PT, DPT, MTC, CLT

1. **How are pelvic girdle disorders classified from an impairment-based model and the Impairment Classification of Functioning, Disability, and Health (ICF) model?**
   Lee (1989) distinguishes three types of impairment-based pelvic girdle disorders: 1) hypomobility with or without pain, 2) hypermobility with or without pain, and 3) normal mobility with pain.
   Clinton et al. (2017) defined the ICF codes as 1) acute, subacute, and chronic pelvic girdle pain with or without pregnancy low back pain; 2) acute, subacute, and chronic pelvic girdle pain with mobility deficits during pregnancy; 3) acute, subacute, and chronic pelvic girdle pain with movement coordination impairments during pregnancy; 4) chronic–recurrent pelvic girdle pain during pregnancy; 5) chronic pelvic girdle pain with related generalized pain during pregnancy.

2. **What are the typical mechanisms of injury of the sacroiliac joint (SIJ)?**
   Activities that produce posterior torsion stress on the SIJ include heavy lifting, falls on the ischial tuberosity, vertical thrusts on the extended leg (such as a sudden, unexpected step off a curb), and persistent postures (such as standing on one leg, bowling, and kicks that miss the ball or target).
   Activities that produce anterior torsion stress include golf swings and horizontal thrusts on the knee with the hip flexed (such as during a motor vehicle accident when the knee is suddenly thrust against the dashboard).
   Repetitive strain to the SIJ can result from decreased extensibility of muscles associated with the pelvic girdle. Decreased extensibility of the hip flexor musculature can create a repetitive anterior torsion strain during gait. Decreased extensibility of the hamstrings can produce a repetitive posterior torsion strain.
   Pregnancy-related strain to the SIJ due to ligamentous laxity secondary to hormonal changes (relaxin), mechanical changes due to fetus growth in utero and during childbirth, and postural changes postpartum.

3. **When a patient's symptoms include sacroiliac dysfunction, are there certain activities that either aggravate or relieve the pain as supported by a base of evidence in physical therapy practice?**
   Evidence indicates that no aggravating or relieving factors are of value for the diagnosis of SIJ-related pain. Anecdotal evidence has supported walking, unilateral standing, sexual intercourse, climbing or descending stairs, sit-to-stand movements, and getting in and out of a car as activities that aggravate the SIJ. Rolling over in bed also may cause pain by gapping or compressing the involved joint.

4. **Do age and gender play a role in the development of SIJ pathology?**
   Women tend to have smaller and flatter joint surfaces that increase joint mobility. Sacroiliac hypermobility and dysfunction associated with hypermobility are most common in females between the ages of 10 and 40. Joint hypermobility in females may be exacerbated by hormonal changes caused by relaxin not only while pregnant but also prior to menopause. The increase in mobility may lead to hypermobile conditions of the SIJ. The female patient usually presents when age-related changes in degenerative arthrosis are mild. Because the female's body weight (just anterior to S2) falls behind the axis of support (through the acetabulum), the gravity vector tends to create a posterior rotation force on the pelvis that causes strain on the posterior ligaments of the SIJ. In a recent retrospective review of patients who received dual anesthetic blocks of the SIJs, it was noted that the average age of patients diagnosed with SIJ pathology based on injection was in the mid-50s. This finding may be attributed to the degenerative process and potential for movement impairment in this population. There was no statistically significant difference in the propensity for SIJ pathology in males or females in this age group and population.

5. **Describe the pattern of pain referral from the SIJ, as mapped by injection.**
   The pain referral pattern from the SIJ has been described by Fortin and April (1994) as unilateral to the involved side in an area approximately 3 by 10 cm immediately inferior to the posterior superior iliac spine. Slipman (2000) found a similar pain pattern using intraarticular injection and reported the following pain patterns: 94% buttocks, 48% posterior thigh, 28% posterior lower leg, 13% foot/ankle, 14% groin, and 2% abdomen.

6. **Has limitation in lumbar range of motion been determined to be a predictor of SIJ dysfunction?**
   No; Schwarzer and Maigne (1995) both assessed range of motion in patients with SIJ dysfunction and found no statistical significance for the use of decreased lumbar range of motion as an indicator of SIJ dysfunction.

7. **Based on current literature, which appears to be more useful for evaluating the SIJ—assessment of anatomic symmetry or pain provocation?**
Assessment of pain provocation is more useful because many asymptomatic patients have minor structural asymmetry.

8. **Which provocation tests have been found to be the most useful in terms of reliability, sensitivity, specificity, and validity?**
   - Compression
   - Distraction
   - Thigh thrust
   - FABER (fixed abduction external rotation)
   - Gaenslen's
   - Resisted hip abduction
   - Sacral thrust
   - Active Straight Leg Raise The thigh thrust is the most sensitive test (0.88), the distraction test is most specific (0.81), and the compression test has the strongest positive likelihood ratio (2.20). Three or more positive pain provocation tests showed optimal sensitivity (0.85–0.94) and specificity (0.78–0.79) values with high positive likelihood ratios (4.02–4.29).

TEST NAME	TEST–RETEST RELIABILITY	SENSITIVITY	SPECIFICITY	POSITIVE LIKE-LIHOOD RATIO
Compression (ASIS)	0.84	0.04–0.59	0.5–1	—
Distraction (ASIS)	0.79	0.13–0.70	0.67–1	1.6
Thigh thrust	—	0.88	0.69	2.8
FABER	0.54	0.40–0.70	0.99	40–70
Gaenslen's	—	0.47	0.1	—
Resisted hip abduction	—	0.33	0.83	2.0
Sacral thrust	—	0.63	0.75	2.5
Active straight leg raise	0.82	0.44	0.83	2
Lunge	—	0.44	0.83	2.6
Mennell's test	0.87	0.54–0.70	1	—
Posterior pelvic pain provoking test	—	0.98	0.94	16.3

Data from *Orthopaedic Physical Examination Tests* (2013, Cook and Hegedus) as well as *CPGs for Women's Heath.*

9. **Why is the Patrick's/FABER test used to assess for SIJ dysfunction?**
Patrick's/FABER theoretically uses a long lever arm to apply a distraction (anterior separation) force to the SIJ. Pain reproduced below the lumbosacral junction overlying the SIJ would be considered a positive test.

10. **How could SIJ dysfunction cause acetabular retroversion? And why might this be important to the clinician?**
Individuals with SIJ dysfunction oftentimes develop functional asymmetry of the pelvis with resulting anterior or posterior innominate rotation/tilt, as well as internal or external innominate rotation/tilt. Acetabular retroversion is considered to be the result of a change in orientation of not just the acetabulum but also of the innominate. Acetabular retroversion is associated with rotation of the innominate, and this positioning may change the orientation of the acetabulum and increase the propensity for femoroacetabular impingement and hip osteoarthritis.

11. **Describe the posterior shear or thigh thrust test.**
This test is performed with the patient in a supine position. The therapist places one of their hands under the sacrum for stabilization. The therapist's other hand applies a gentle progressive posterior shearing stress to the SIJ through the femur by contracting the knee and pushing the thigh posterior while 90 degrees of hip flexion is maintained. Care must be taken to limit excessive hip adduction. This test assesses the ability of the ilium

to translate independently on the sacrum. A painful reaction may be attributed to strain placed on the posterior elements of the joint on the side of the loaded (thrust) side.

12. **Describe the right posterior rotation pelvic torsion provocation test.**
Posterior rotation of the right ilium on the sacrum is achieved by flexion of the right hip and knee and simultaneous left hip extension with the patient in the supine position. Overpressure is applied through both lower extremities force the right SIJ to its end range. This provocation is sometimes called Gaenslen's test. A painful reaction may be reproduced by strain on the posterior elements and by joint irritability caused by movement within the joint.

13. **Discuss the method and benefits of using injections to diagnose the SIJ as a cause of low back pain.**
Diagnostic injections with a local anesthetic and contrast medium can be introduced precisely into the joint via fluoroscopy or computed tomography to assess relief or provocation of pain. A control block eliminates placebo effects. Thus relief of pain gives compelling evidence that the intraarticular SIJ dysfunction is the source. However, it should be noted that pain that arises from the surrounding ligaments or muscles would not be affected by this type of injection. This may give us a reason to question the guided double SIJ injection as the gold standard for validity testing.

14. **According to the evidence in the current literature, why is it erroneous to consider hypomobility as a clinical syndrome or classification of dysfunction in the SIJ?**
The anatomic and biomechanical literature, based on stereophotogrammetric methods, suggests that the SIJ is an inherently stable joint with only approximately two to three degrees of motion. This amount of motion has made it difficult, if not impossible, for clinicians to establish reliable and valid motion assessment techniques in routine clinical examinations. Therefore, the diagnosis of hypomobility alone is not recommended. The evidence has suggested that excessive mobility—ie, hypermobility or instability—is more likely to contribute to pain associated with mechanical sacroiliac dysfunction. When the clinician finds asymmetry, a positive provocation test, and differences in passive mobility of the SIJ, the potential diagnosis may better be presented as a "fixated instability." Theoretically, the joint has become fixated in a nonneutral position, and a discernible difference in passive mobility indicates that it must be excessive to precipitation in the position of fixation. Therefore, the joint that appears to be hypomobile is actually an unstable joint that has become displaced or fixated.

15. **Describe the clinical signs and treatment of sacroiliac hypermobility.**
Increased passive or active mobility of either the innominate or the sacrum and concurrent loss of neuromuscular control presents with sacroiliac hypermobility dysfunction. Treatment may consist of therapeutic exercises for muscle imbalances, joint manipulation of neighboring hypomobilities in the lumbar spine or hips, patient education about reducing postural and functional stresses through positioning and normal movement for activities of daily and nightly living, and use of a sacroiliac binder. The use of a sacroiliac binder has been studied in cadavers and found to enhance pelvic stability.

16. **What special test is good for determining sacroiliac laxity in postpartum patients?**
    - Mens et al. in 1999 found that a positive active straight leg raise (ASLR) test is associated with increased SIJ mobility.
    - Damen et al. (2002) found that the ASLR test and the thigh thrust test are good for identifying postpartum patients who have SIJ laxity.

17. **What may cause sacroiliac pain when mobility of the SIJ is normal?**
    - Mild sprain or strain injury
    - Inflammatory disease
    - Overuse of the adjacent articular or myofascial tissues

18. **How can excellent diagnostic accuracy be achieved in the prediction of sacroiliac dysfunction?**
Use of a thorough evaluation to exclude pain of discogenic origin or red flags in combination with the use of three or more positive provocation tests has been shown to have excellent diagnostic accuracy for sacroiliac dysfunction.

19. **What percentage of patients will develop significant SIJ degeneration 5 years after a lumbar fusion?**
Up to 75% of postlumbar fusion patients will develop significant SIJ degeneration.

20. **What common medical conditions affect the SIJ?**
    - Ankylosing spondylitis (AS) begins as inflammation involving the synovium of SIJs. The ligaments are transformed to bone, beginning at the insertion point, which ends in bony fusion or ankylosis of the SIJ. The incidence varies with ethnic groups: AS is most common in Haida Indians (4.2 per 1000) and Caucasians (1 per 1000). It is more prevalent in males than females by a ratio of 3:1 and is most common in males under the age of 40. Symptoms usually begin in the lumbar spine. Radiologic changes vary from blurring to complete obliteration of the joint margins, resulting in bony fusion of the sacrum to the ilium. AS often appears first with abnormal narrowing of the upper half of the SIJs.
    - Reiter syndrome is precipitated by an infection in the genitourinary or gastrointestinal tract. Although the infection is not found within the joint, the organism causes reactive arthritis, which can cause sacroiliitis. Radiologic changes demonstrate erosions at the insertion points of ligaments.
    - About 15% of patients with inflammatory bowel disease (Crohn's disease or ulcerative colitis) have sacroiliitis clinically. The radiologic changes resemble those in AS.
    - Psoriatic spondylitis causes bone spur formation and partial bony ankylosis of the SIJs, often asymmetrically. Psoriasis affects 1.2% of the general population; 7% of patients with psoriasis may have arthritis.
    - Other conditions that may affect the SIJ include rheumatoid arthritis, pyogenic infection, tuberculosis, brucellosis, gout, hyperthyroidism, Paget's disease, diffuse idiopathic skeletal hyperostosis, and osteitis condensans ilii.

21. **What are the best imaging modalities for diagnosing the cause of SIJ pain?**
    No specific imaging studies provide precise findings that are helpful in the diagnosis of SIJ pain. Computed tomography and MRI provide an unobstructed view of the joint and the ability to view the joint margins superiorly and inferiorly for the presence of osteophytes. However, they are predominantly used to exclude other causes of sacroiliac pain (tumor, spondyloarthropathies). Bone scans are helpful in determining the presence of stress fractures, infection, inflammation, and tumor.

22. **What are the radiologic signs of pubic symphysis instability?**
    Instability of the pubic symphysis is suggested by radiographic findings of pubic symphysis separation >10 mm and vertical displacement >2 mm with the single leg stance.

23. **Do sacroiliac braces provide pain relief?**
    They may provide pain relief; however, randomized controlled trials do not show significant improvement in function and pain when worn. Proper application, duration of use, and underlying cause of SIJ pain all impact the effectiveness of an SIJ belt. Biomechanical studies of sacroiliac motion while wearing a sacroiliac belt directly superior to the greater trochanter showed an approximately 30% decrease in SIJ motion in cases of peripartum instability. This stabilizing effect could be linked to pain reduction in patients considered to have greater than normal SIJ motion, especially in the case of patients postpartum.

24. **Do osseous positional changes occur following a high-velocity manipulation to the SIJ?**
    No. Radiographic stereophotogrammetric analysis before and after manipulation does not demonstrate positional changes of the sacrum and ilium.

25. **What is prolotherapy, and is it effective in the treatment of SIJ pain?**
    Prolotherapy is a form of injection therapy. Sclerosing agents are injected into injured ligaments, which provokes a localized inflammatory reaction. Prolotherapy is proposed to stimulate regrowth of collagen, thus strengthening the ligaments and improving their elasticity and possibly function. Prolotherapy has been found to have superior results to sham injections for chronic nonspecific low back pain; however, its specific application to the SIJ has not been studied.

26. **What are some other forms of medical treatments for SIJ pain?**
    - Nerve stimulators (implanted)—partial pain relief has been reported with selective stimulation of sacral root 3
    - Viscosupplementation—partial pain relief has been reported with intraarticular injection of Hylan G-F 20
    - Radiofrequency neurotomy—64% of 14 patients with SIJ pain who underwent radiofrequency neurotomy demonstrated a >50% pain reduction at a 6-month follow-up visit
    - Arthrodesis—a very controversial treatment approach for idiopathic SIJ pain

27. **What motor control strategies should a physical therapist assess when considering force closure mechanisms of the SIJ and pelvis?**
    Alteration in the onset and timing of feed-forward muscular response of the transverse abdominis (TrA) has been identified in patients with SIJ pain.
    1. Activation of the transversus abdominus, pelvic floor musculature, gluteus maximum
    2. Assessment of diaphragmatic breathing

3. Balanced activation between abdominal muscles and trunk extensors
4. Assessment of aberrant movement of active motion of the SIJ/pelvis
5. Postural assessment

28. What is the prevalence and severity of pregnancy low back pain (PLBP) and pelvic girdle pain (PGP)?

According to Clinton et al., (2017) the prevalence of both impairment-based diagnoses is approximately 56% to 72% of the antepartum population.

WEEKS PREGNANT	% OF REPORTED PLBP/PGP
>20 weeks' gestation	33%–50%
20–30 weeks' gestation	20%
<30 weeks' gestation	60%–70%

29. Do three or more positive provocation tests indicate the type of SIJ dysfunction?

No, three or more positive provocation tests rule in SIJ involvement/irritation; however, they do not indicate the type or severity of the dysfunction.

30. What are the appropriate interventions for someone with an SIJ dysfunction?

a. SIJ belt, especially in the postpartum and antepartum populations
b. Exercise with consideration for patient (and fetus) safety per ACOG standards, including stabilization of the back, pelvis, and stretching hip musculature
c. Manual therapy including joint manipulation/mobilization to hypomobile joints surrounding the SIJ, soft tissue. and myofascial manipulation
d. Patient education including posture education and ergonomic instruction

Bibliography

Alderink, G. (1991). The sacroiliac joint: review of anatomy, mechanics, and function. *Journal of Orthopaedic and Sports Physical Therapy, 13*, 71–84.

Cibulka, M. T., & Koldenhoff, R. (1999). Clinical usefulness of a cluster of sacroiliac joint tests in patients with and without low back pain. *Journal of Orthopaedic and Sports Physical Therapy, 29*, 83–89.

Clinton, S. C., Newell, A., Downey, P. A., et al. (2017). Pelvic girdle pain in the antepartum population. *Journal of Women's Health Physical Therapy, 41*(2), 102–125.

Damen, L., Buyruk, H. M., Güler-Uysal, F., Lotgering, F. K., Snijders, C. J., & Stam, H. J. (2002). The prognostic value of asymmetric laxity of the sacroiliac joints in pregnancy-related pelvic pain. *Spine, 27*, 2820–2824.

Dehghan, F., Haerian, B.S., Muniandy, S., Yusof, A., Dragoo, J.L., & Salleh, N. (2014). The effect of relaxin on the musculoskeletal system. Scandinavian Journal of Medicine & Science in Sports, 24(4), e220–e229.

Delitto, A., George, S. Z., Van Dillen, L., et al. (2012). Low back pain. *Journal of Orthopaedic & Sports Physical Therapy, 42*(4), A1–A57.

DePalma, M., Ketchum, J., & Saullo, T. (2011). Etiology of chronic low back pain in patients having undergone lumbar fusion. *Pain Medicine, 12*(5), 732–739.

Dreyfuss, P., Michaelsen, M., Pauza, K., McLarty, J., & Bogduk, N. (1995). The value of medical history and physical examination in diagnosing sacroiliac joint pain. *Spine, 21*, 2594–2602.

Fortin, J. D., Dwyer, A. P., West, S., & Pier, J. (1994). Sacroiliac joint: pain referral maps upon applying a new injection/arthrography technique. *Spine, 19*, 1475–1482.

Freburger, J. K., & Riddle, D. L. (1999). Measurement of sacroiliac joint dysfunction: a multicenter intertester reliability study. *Physical Therapy, 79*, 1134–1141.

Goode, A., Heedus, E., Sizer, P., Brismeee, J. M., Linberg, A., & Cook, C. (2008). Three-dimensional movements of the sacroiliac joint: a systematic review of the literature and assessment of clinical utility. *Journal of Manual and Manipulative Therapy, 16*(1), 225–238.

Greenman, P. (1996). *Principles of manual medicine* (2nd ed.). Philadelphia, PA: Williams & Wilkins. 1996.

Ha, K. -Y., Lee, J. -S., & Kim, K. -W. (2008). Degeneration of sacroiliac joint after instrumented lumbar or lumbosacral fusion: a prospective cohort study over five-year follow-up. *Spine, 33*(11), 1192–1198.

Hayne, C. (1981). Manual transport of loads by women. *Physiotherapy, 67*, 226–231.

Hazle, C., & Nitz, A. (2008). Evidence-based assessment and diagnosis of pelvic girdle disorders: a proposal for an alternate diagnostic category. *Physical Therapy Reviews, 13*, 25–36.

Helms, C. (1995). *Fundamentals of skeletal radiology* (2nd ed.). Philadelphia, PA: WB Saunders.

Hodges, P. W., & Richardson, C. A. (1996). Inefficient muscular stabilization of the lumbar spine associated with low back pain. A motor control evaluation of transversus abdominis. *Spine, 21*, 2640–2650.

Huijbregts, P. A. (2004). Sacroiliac joint dysfunction: evidence-based diagnosis. *Orthopaedic Division Reviews. 18*(32), 41–44.

Hungerford, B., Gilleard, W., & Hodges, P. (2003). Evidence of altered lumbopelvic muscle recruitment in the presence of sacroiliac joint pain. *Spine, 28*, 1593–1600.

Irwin, R. W., Watson, T., Minick, R. P., & Ambrosius, W. T. (2007). Age, body mass index, and gender differences in sacroiliac joint pathology. *American Journal of Physical Medicine and Rehabilitation, 86*, 37–44.

Kakaty, D. K., Fischer, A. F., Hosalkar, H. S., Siebenrock, K. A., & Tannast, M. (2010). The ischial spine sign: does pelvic tilt and rotation matter? *Clinical Orthopaedics and Related Research*, *468*, 769–774.
Laslett, M. (1998). The value of the physical examination in diagnosis of painful sacroiliac joint pathologies: Comment. *Spine*, *23*, 962–964.
Laslett, M., & Williams, M. (1994). The value of the physical examination in diagnosis of painful sacroiliac joint pathologies: comment. *Spine*, *19*, 1243–1249.
Laslett, M., Young, S. B., Aprill, C. N., & McDonald, B. (2003). Diagnosing painful sacroiliac joints: a validity study of a McKenzie evaluation and sacroiliac provocation tests. *Australian Journal of Physiotherapy*, *49*, 89–97.
Lee, D. (1989). *The pelvic girdle: an approach to the examination and treatment of the lumbo-pelvic-hip region.* Edinburgh: Churchill Livingstone.
Maigne, J., Aivaliklis, A., & Pfefer, F. (1996). Results of sacroiliac joint double block and value of sacroiliac pain provocation tests in 54 patients with low back pain. *Spine*, *21*, 1889–1892.
Mens, J., Vleeming, A., Snijders, C. J., Koes, B. W., & Stam, H. J. (2002). Validity of the active straight leg raise test for measuring disease severity in patients with posterior pelvic pain after pregnancy. *Spine*, *27*, 196.
Mens, J., Vleeming, A., Snijders, C. J., Stam, H. J., & Ginai, A. Z. (1999). The active straight leg raise test and mobility of the pelvic joints. *European Spine Journal*, *8*, 468–473.
Potter, N., & Rothstein, J. (1985). Intertester reliability for selected clinical tests of the sacroiliac joint. *Physical Therapy*, *65*, 1671–1675.
Saueressig, T., Owen, P. J., Diemer, F., et al. (2021). Diagnostic accuracy of clusters of pain provocation tests for detecting sacroiliac joint pain: systemic review with meta-analysis. *Journal of Orthopaedic & Sports Physical Therapy*, *51*(9), 422–431.
Schwarzer, A. C., Aprill, C. N., & Bogduk, N. (1995). The sacroiliac joint in chronic low back pain. *Spine*, *20*, 31–37.
Sivayogam, A., & Banerjee, A. (2011). Diagnostic performance of clinical tests for sacroiliac joint pain. *Physical Therapy Reviews*, *16*(6), 472–476.
Slipman, C. W., Jackson, H. B., Lipetz, J. S., Chan, K. T., Lenrow, D., & Vresilovic, E. J. (2000). Sacroiliac joint pain referral zones. *Archives of Physical Medicine and Rehabilitation*, *81*, 334–338.
Tannast, M., Pfannebecker, P., Schwab, J. M., Albers, C. E., Siebenrock, K. A., & Buchler, L. (2012). Pelvic morphology differs in rotation and obliquity between developmental dysplasia of the hip and retroversion. *Clinical Orthopaedics and Related Research*, *470*, 3297–3305.
Vleeming, A., Buyruk, H. M., Stoeckart, R., Karamursel, S., & Snijders, C. J. (1992). An integrated therapy for peripartum pelvic instability: a study of the biomechanical effects of pelvic belts. *American Journal of Obstetrics and Gynecology*, *166*, 1243–1247.

CHAPTER 64 QUESTIONS

1. **Which of the following tests is most useful in the diagnosis of sacroiliac dysfunction based on its psychometric properties (reliability, sensitivity, specificity, and validity)?**
   a. FABER's, Stork or Gillette's test, and the standing flexion test
   b. Gaenslen's, resisted hip abduction, and the supine to sit leg length test
   c. Sacral thrust, sacral shear, and palpation of posterior SIJ ligaments
   d. Compression, distraction, and thigh thrust

2. **Which of the following diseases/disorders begins as inflammation involving the synovium of the SIJs and causes early onset of bilateral pain in the SIJ region?**
   a. Reiter's syndrome
   b. Ankylosing spondylitis
   c. Psoriatic arthritis
   d. Paget's disease

3. **Which is best test to determine SIJ hypermobility or instability?**
   a. Compression/distraction provocation test
   b. Active straight leg raise
   c. Transversus abdominus muscle activation test
   d. Thigh thrust

CHAPTER 65

FUNCTIONAL ANATOMY OF THE HIP AND PELVIS

T. Gibbons, MPT

1. **Describe a systematic layered classification of the anatomy of the hip and pelvis that helps to guide evaluation.**

   Lynch et al. describes a "layered approach" to understanding the hip and finding the source of pathology. The hip is divided into four layers:

   1. The osseous layer: the femur, pelvis, and acetabulum
   2. The intraarticular layer: the labrum, joint capsule, ligaments, and ligamentum teres
   3. The muscular layer: all the muscles around the hip, pelvis, lumbosacral region, and pelvic floor
   4. The neural layer: thoracolumbosacral plexus, lumbopelvic tissues and ilioinguinal, iliohypogastric, genitofemoral, and pudendal nerves

   Abnormality in layer one will impact joint surface contact that can lead to injury to tissues in layer two, altering muscular activity in layer three, which can lead to tendinopathies. Layer four then becomes impacted due to changes in the kinetic chain.

2. **Describe the articular surfaces of the hip joint.**

   The hip joint is created by the acetabulum of the pelvis and the head of the femur. The acetabulum is a cup-shaped structure located laterally on the pelvis and formed by the fusion of the ilium, ischium, and pubis. Only a horseshoe-shaped portion of the acetabulum is covered with articular cartilage and contacts the head of the femur. The acetabular notch lies inferior to this cartilage and is bridged by the acetabular labrum, which also covers the entire periphery of the acetabulum. The acetabular fossa is thus nonarticular and contains a fat pad covered with synovial fluid. The acetabulum faces laterally, anteriorly, and inferiorly.

   The head of the femur is covered completely by articular cartilage except for the fovea capitis, or central portion, which serves as the location for the ligamentum teres. Articular cartilage is thickest in the anterosuperior region and is thickest in the central portion around the ligamentum teres where weight-bearing forces are at a maximum. Articular cartilage is avascular and aneural. The femoral head is circular and attaches to the shaft of the femur by the femoral neck. The femoral head faces medially, superiorly, and anteriorly.

3. **How is the hip joint classified?**

   The hip joint is a diarthrodial, ball-and-socket joint with three degrees of movement: 1) flexion and extension occur in the sagittal plane around a coronal axis; 2) abduction and adduction occur in the frontal plane around an anteroposterior axis; and 3) internal and external rotation occur on the transverse plane around a longitudinal axis.

4. **What is the angle of inclination of the femur?**

   It is the angle between 1) the axis of the femoral head and neck and 2) the axis of the femoral shaft in the frontal plane. It begins at approximately 150 degrees in infants and decreases to 125 degrees in adults and 120 degrees in elderly people. The angle is slightly smaller in females than in males because of a female's increased pelvic width. Coxa valga (>150 degrees) is a pathologic increase in the angle of inclination, and coxa vara (<120 degrees) is a pathologic decrease.

5. **What is the angle of torsion of the femur?**

   It is the angle between the axis of the femoral condyles and the axis of the head and neck of the femur in the transverse plane. The plane of the head and neck is anterior to the plane of the condyles. It is approximately 40 degrees in infants and decreases to approximately 12 to 15 degrees in adults. An increase in the angle of torsion is called anteversion, and a decrease is called retroversion.

6. **How is the angle of torsion assessed clinically?**

   Femoral anteversion may be assessed using Craig's test (also called Ryder's method). The patient is prone with the knee flexed to 90 degrees. The leg is then rotated internally and externally until the greater trochanter is parallel to the table. The amount of anteversion is measured by the angle of the lower leg to the vertical.

7. **What gender differences exist in the anatomy of the hip?**

   Acetabula are shallower in females than in males. The female pelvis is broader with a greater pubic arch angle. The difference in pelvic geometry creates a reduced tolerance for hip fractures in front-end motor vehicle collisions. The female femur is shorter, lighter, and thinner than the male femur with a smaller femoral head diameter and shorter bicondylar width. This creates a shorter moment arm for the gluteus medius in females and an increase in femoral head pressure. These differences in pelvic and femoral geometry can create a reduced tolerance for hip fractures in female patients.

8. **Describe the joint capsule of the hip.**
The joint capsule is a strong and dense structure that figures prominently in hip joint stability. It attaches proximally to the entire rim of the acetabular labrum and distally to the base of the neck of the femur. The joint capsule covers the head of the femur like a sleeve. It is thickest anterosuperiorly, where the most protection is needed. The posteroinferior attachment is thinner and loose. Capsular innervation is from a variety of nerves from the lumbosacral plexus and muscular branches, but its primary nerve supply seems to be from the nerve to quadratus femoris and obturator nerve.

9. **Which ligaments contribute to the stability of the hip?**
Two ligaments reinforce the hip anteriorly: 1) the iliofemoral ligament (or Y-shaped ligament of Bigelow), which is the stronger and checks hip hyperextension; and 2) the pubofemoral ligament, which checks hip abduction and extension. The ischiofemoral ligament is located posteriorly; its fibers tighten with hip extension. All of these ligaments are major contributors to stability in an upright standing posture. The ligamentum teres, which passes from the acetabular notch under the transverse acetabular ligament or labrum and attaches to the head of the femur at the fovea, is important for delivering blood supply and added stability to the neonatal hip. In adulthood, it provides secondary stabilization and may help to prevent subluxation.

10. **Describe the arthrokinematics of the hip joint.**
The convex femoral head glides in a direction opposite to the movement on the concave acetabulum in an open-chain condition. In the more common closed-chain condition, the concave acetabulum moves in the same direction as the opposite side of the pelvis.

11. **Describe the osteokinematics of the hip joint.**
Movement of the femur is affected in most directions by the passive tension of two-joint muscles. Passive range of motion is as follows:
    - Flexion—120 to 135 degrees (90 degrees if the knee is extended because of tension in the hamstrings)
    - Extension—10 to 30 degrees (limited by the rectus femoris if combined with knee flexion)
    - Abduction—30 to 50 degrees
    - Adduction—10 to 30 degrees
    - External rotation—45 to 60 degrees
    - Internal rotation—30 to 45 degrees

    The normal end-feel for all directions of the hip is either tissue approximation or tissue stretch. The movements of the pelvis include anterior and posterior tilting, lateral pelvic tilt, and pelvic rotation.

12. **Name the muscles that cross the hip joint.**
    - Flexors—iliopsoas, rectus femoris, tensor fascia latae, sartorius, pectineus, adductor brevis, adductor longus, and oblique fibers of adductor magnus
    - Extensors—gluteus maximus, biceps femoris, semimembranosus, and semitendinosus
    - Abductors—gluteus medius, gluteus minimus, tensor fascia latae, and upper fibers of gluteus maximus
    - Adductors—adductor magnus, adductor longus, adductor brevis, pectineus, and gracilis
    - External rotators—obturator externus, obturator internus, quadratus femoris, piriformis, gemellus superior, gemellus inferior, gluteus maximus, sartorius, and biceps femoris
    - Internal rotators—gluteus minimus, tensor fascia latae, anterior fibers of gluteus medius, semitendinosus, and semimembranosus

13. **What is inversion of muscle action?**
Muscles that cross a joint with 3 degrees of freedom may have alternate or even opposite (inverted) actions than their classically described actions. The action of the muscle depends on joint position and has important implications for muscle stretching and resistive exercise.

14. **Describe inversion of the flexor component of the adductor muscles.**
All adductors of the hip are also flexors (except the adductor magnus) with the hip in neutral position. With flexion, the femur lies anterior to the origin of the muscle and the adductors become extensors. The adductor longus is a flexor to 70 degrees, the adductor brevis to 50 degrees, and the gracilis to 40 degrees, at which point they become extensors.

15. **Describe inversion of muscle action for the piriformis.**
With the hip in neutral position, the piriformis is primarily an external rotator and a weak flexor and abductor. At 60 degrees of flexion, the piriformis becomes primarily an abductor and medial rotator of the hip.

16. **What is the iliocapsularis muscle?**
- Origin—anteromedial hip capsule and the inferior border of the anterior inferior iliac spine
- Insertion—distal to the lesser trochanter

The iliocapsularis muscle may tighten the anterior hip capsule to increase stability of the femoral head. The muscle is a landmark during hip surgery to expose the anteromedial hip capsule and the psoas tendon interval. The muscle hypertrophies in dysplastic hips and atrophies in hips with acetabular overcoverage.

17. **Are there differences in the strength of hip musculature, with versus without, osteoarthritis (OA) of the hip?**
Arokoski et al. found a significant reduction in isometric hip abduction (31%) and adduction (25%) strength in males with OA versus without. Hip flexion strength was lower (18%–22%) in males with OA versus without. Hip extension strength was not significantly lower in men with OA versus without, but in those who had bilateral hip OA, the more deteriorated side was 13% to 22% weaker. The cross-sectional area of the hip and thigh musculature did not differ between groups. Weakness in the knee extensors and flexors has also been found on the arthritic side.

18. **Which muscles are active during two-legged erect stance?**
None. Stability is maintained by the capsule and ligamentous support.

19. **How much force is unloaded from the hip when a cane is used in the opposite hand?**
A cane can decrease force loads by 40%. A single contralateral crutch can decrease loads up to 50%.

20. **What structures pass through the sciatic notch?**
- Vessels—superior gluteal artery and vein, inferior gluteal artery and vein, internal pudendal artery and vein
- Nerves—sciatic, superior gluteal, inferior gluteal, posterior gluteal, nerve to quadratus femoris, nerve to obturator externus
- Muscle—piriformis

21. **Describe the blood supply to the femoral head.**
- Extracapsular arterial ring—formed posteriorly by a large branch of the medial femoral circumflex artery and anteriorly by the lateral circumflex femoral artery, which are branches of the femoral artery or the profunda femoris artery. The extracapsular ring supplies most of the head and neck of the femur. These arteries surround the neck of the femur and ascend along it, forming rings around the upper neck and subcapital sulcus. The medial circumflex artery branches into the lateral, superior, and inferior epiphyseal arteries, with the lateral epiphyseal artery supplying more than half of the femoral head.
- Ascending cervical branches—formed by the lateral circumflex artery, travel into the joint capsule, and run along the neck of the femur, deep to the synovial lining of the neck. They are at risk with any disruption of the capsule, as may occur in a femoral neck fracture.
- Artery of the ligamentum teres—contributes little, if any, significant supply to the adult femoral head.

22. **Describe the anatomy of the trochanteric bursa.**
A series of three bursae exist: 1) between the gluteus maximus and the gluteus medius tendon; 2) between the gluteus maximus and the greater trochanter; and 3) between the gluteus medius and the greater trochanter. Dunn et al. found that multiple bursae could exist and tended to be acquired with age because of excessive friction between the greater trochanter and the insertion of the gluteus maximus at the insertion into the fascia lata.

23. **What is the functional range of motion (ROM) of the hip?**
Hyodo et al. measured ROM with 22 ADLs. ROM required as follows:
- Hip flexion 101°
- Hip extension 8°
- Hip adduction 17°
- Hip abduction 31°
- Hip internal rotation 39°
- Hip external rotation 61°

24. **Describe the function of the acetabular labrum.**
The fibrocartilage labrum covers the entire border of the acetabulum and increases the coverage of the femoral head by 30%. It functions to improve joint stability by providing a vacuum effect. It also helps absorb shock and transmits stress that would be applied to the cartilage of the femur and acetabulum.
Maintenance of synovial fluid and its lubrication is another function of the labrum.

25. **What is the maximal loose or open-packed position of the hip?**
30 degrees flexion, 30 degrees abduction, and 15 degrees external rotation.

26. **What is the maximal close-packed position of the hip?**
Unlike other joints, a position does not exist that includes maximal capsuloligamentous tightness and maximal intraarticular pressure during maximal joint surface contact. Intraarticular pressure is greatest with extension combined with internal rotation or during upright standing. The greatest capsuloligamentous tension occurs during maximal extension combined with either maximal adduction and maximal internal rotation or with maximal abduction and maximal external rotation. Joint surface contact is greatest in maximal flexion combined with maximal abduction and maximal external rotation.

Bibliography

Arokoski, M.H., Arokoski, J.P., & Haara, M., et al. (2002). Hip muscle strength and muscle cross sectional area in men with and without hip osteoarthritis. *The Journal of Rheumatology*, 29(10), 2185–2195.

Babst, D., Steppacher, S. D., Ganz, R., Siebenrock, K. A., & Tannast, M. (2011). The iliocapsularis muscle: an important stabilizer in the dysplastic hip. *Clinical Orthopaedics and Related Research*, *469*(6), 1728–1734.

Dunn, T., Heller, C. A., & McCarthy, S. W. (2003). Anatomical study of the "trochanteric bursa." *Clinical Anatomy*, *16*, 233–240.

Enseki, K., Harris-Hayes, M., White, D. M., Orthopaedic Section of the American Physical Therapy Association (2014). Nonarthritic hip joint pain. *Journal of Orthopaedic & Sports Physical Therapy*, *44*(6), A1–32.

Hyodo, K., Masuda, T., Aizawa, J., Jinno, T., & Morita, S. (2017). Hip, knee, and ankle kinematics during activities of daily living: a cross-sectional study. *Brazilian Journal of Physical Therapy*, *21*(3), 159–166.

Loureiro, A., Mills, P. M., & Barrett, R. S. (2013). Muscle weakness in hip osteoarthritis: a systematic review. *Arthritis Care Res (Hoboken)*, *65*(3), 340–352.

Lynch, T. S., Terry, M. A., Bedi, A., & Kelly, B. T. (2013). Hip arthroscopic surgery: patient evaluation, current indications, and outcomes. *American Journal of Sports Medicine*, *41*(5), 1174–1189.

Lynch, T. S., Bedi, A., & Larson, C. M. (2017). Athletic hip injuries. *Journal of the American Academy of Orthopaedic Surgeons*, *25*(4), 269–279.

Murphy, N. J., Eyles, J. P., & Hunter, D. J. (2016). Hip osteoarthritis: etiopathogenesis and implications for management. *Advances in Therapy*, *33* (11), 1921–1946.

O'Donnell, J. M., Devitt, B. M., & Arora, M. (2018). The role of the ligamentum teres in the adult hip: redundant or relevant? A review. *Journal of Hip Preservation Surgery*, *5* (1), 15–22.

Robbins, C. E. (1998). Anatomy and biomechanics. In T. L. Fagerson (Ed.), *The hip handbook* (pp. 1–37). Boston: Butterworth Heinemann.

Tomlinson, J., Ondruschka, B., Prietzel, T., Zwirner, J., & Hammer, N. (2021). A systematic review and meta-analysis of the hip capsule innervation and its clinical implications. *Scientific Reports*, *11*(1), 5299.

CHAPTER 65 QUESTIONS

1. **You are assessing PROM of a patient's hip. Which of these are abnormal findings?**
   a. Extension 20 degrees with a capsular end feel
   b. Abduction 40 degrees with a firm end feel
   c. Flexion 100 degrees with a bony end feel
   d. External rotation 50 degrees with a capsular end feel

2. **Your patient has mild hip OA and you want to teach them the resting position of the hip to provide pain reduction. Which position do you teach them?**
   a. 30 degrees flexion, 30 degrees abduction, 15 degrees external rotation
   b. Neutral flexion/extension, 30 degrees abduction, 45 degrees external rotation
   c. 10 degrees flexion, 0 degrees abduction, neutral internal/external rotation
   d. 30 degrees flexion

3. **Postural assessment indicates possible femoral anteversion on the patient's right side. Which clinical special test would be the most helpful to estimate the angle of torsion?**
   a. Patrick's test
   b. Ober's test
   c. Q angle measurement
   d. Craig's test

CHAPTER 66

COMMON ORTHOPEDIC HIP DYSFUNCTION

T. Gibbons, MPT

1. **How are muscle strains classified?**
   - Grade I—little tissue disruption, low-grade inflammatory response; strength testing produces pain without loss of strength; no loss of range of motion (ROM)
   - Grade II—some disruption of muscle fibers, but not complete; strength and ROM decreased; pain significant
   - Grade III—complete rupture with complete loss of strength of involved muscle; palpable or visible defect may be present

2. **Describe the treatment for muscle strain.**
   The length of time for each stage will depend on the severity of the injury.
   - Stage 1 (acute phase, first 24–72 hours)—follow basic first-aid protocols of rest, ice, compression, and elevation (RICE). NSAIDs may be administered and crutches may be required for severe strains.
   - Stage 2 (reduction of acute symptoms, 2–7 days)—use gentle ROM and isometric exercise with modalities to reduce pain and swelling as needed. Modalities may include ultrasound, hydrotherapy, and muscle stimulation. Gentle friction massage may help avoid adhesion of scarred muscle tissue.
   - Stage 3 (pain-free isometrics)—continue with stage 2 treatment as needed for pain, but begin pain-free isotonic and isokinetic exercise. Include stretching and aerobic activity with proper warm-up. Stretching should include static stretches and proprioceptive neuromuscular facilitation (PNF) techniques, such as contract-relax, hold-relax, and contract-relax-contract. Sanders and Nemeth also suggest the use of ballistic stretching, which should follow static stretches and proper warm-up and involves only small movements in the last 10% of the available ROM.
   - Stage 4 (ROM 95% of normal, strength 75% of normal)—begin sport-specific exercise with emphasis on endurance and coordination activities. Jogging and running should be progressed gradually. Strength development should focus on eccentric training.
   - Stage 5 (strength 95% of normal)—return to sports with education for maintenance of proper warm-up, stretching, and strengthening program.

3. **How do adductor strains occur?**
   Strains of the hip adductors, most commonly the adductor longus, occur in sports that require quick acceleration or direction changes. In contact sports, ice hockey and soccer have the highest incidence of injury. Ice hockey players may be predisposed to groin pulls because of a lack of strengthening (specifically abduction to adduction strength ratio deficits) and stretching of the adductors, previous injury in that area, and lack of experience. During a stride in ice hockey, the adductors fire eccentrically to control push-off, but then quickly transition to concentric to bring the foot back under the body during recovery. Therefore, eccentric and concentric control is important. Most adductor strains in soccer occur from kicking with the adductor longus being under pressure as the leg transitions from eccentric in wind up to concentric as the leg begins to kick forward. Most injuries are grades I and II; complete ruptures are rare. Injuries occur at the musculotendinous junction or the adductor enthesis, which is the fibrocartilaginous insertion of the adductor tendon at the pubic bone. Examination reveals palpatory tenderness and pain and/or weakness with resisted hip adduction.

4. **What treatments are effective in treating adductor strains?**
   Passive physical therapy (massage, stretching, and modalities) is ineffective in treating groin pulls. However, an active strengthening program has proven effective in treating chronic groin strains and allows return to sport. The adductor muscles should be within 80% of the strength of the abductors to avoid reinjury. Tyler has developed a program emphasizing eccentric resistive exercise, balance training, core strengthening, and sport-specific movements, which has been supported throughout the literature. A review of the literature finds compressive clothing, manual therapy with strength training, and prolotherapy to be of the strongest (moderate) level of evidence as an effective treatment for adductor strains.

5. **Are there recommendations for adductor strain prevention?**
   Nunez describes a program for professional soccer players that maintains 10.37% dominant to nondominant strength ratio and 92% adductor to abductor ratio to reduce adductor injury. Similar ratios have been found to prevent injury in hockey players as well with assessment not only preseason, but throughout the playing season.

6. **When is surgery necessary to treat an adductor strain?**
   If symptoms persist after 6 months of appropriate physical therapy, and other pathology is ruled out, adductor tenotomy can be performed. Return to play (RTP) with this procedure is estimated at 75%.

7. **What is a "sports hernia"?**
   "Sports hernia" is a general term to describe deep groin or lower abdominal pain that is brought on by exertion and relieved by rest, with the presence of palpable tenderness over the pubic ramus, pain with resisted hip adduction and/or flexion, and pain with abdominal curl-up. No clinically palpable hernia is present, and the patient does not need to be an athlete to develop this injury.
   As understanding of this injury evolves, better terms to describe it are inguinal disruption and athletic pubalgia. The term inguinal disruption is used to describe injury of the inguinal canal soft tissues, ultimately causing the pain syndrome. Structures that may be at fault include the transverse fascia at the posterior inguinal wall, the rectus abdominis insertion, the conjoined tendon at its distal attachment to the anterior-superior pubis, and/or the external oblique aponeurosis. Athletic pubalgia is the disruption and/or separation of the more medial common aponeurosis from the pubis, usually with some degree of adductor tendon pathology.

8. **What is the treatment for athletic pubalgia?**
   Conservative care begins with rest and pain management. ROM and gentle stretching with hip and lumbar joint mobilization are used in early phases. The patient progresses to strength training to include the transverse abdominis, multifidus, and hip muscles of movement and stabilization. Weight-bearing exercises should progress from double to single limb challenges with less stable surfaces. PNF pattern challenges of the upper and lower extremities while maintaining a neutral spine are beneficial. Training should progress to sport-specific patterns with a gradual increase in speed, impact, and directional changes. If an athlete fails conservative care (6 months), then surgery is recommended. There is a high probability (80%–100%) for return to sport following surgical intervention for athletes, and return to play can occur in 6 to 8 weeks following surgery. The athletic population has a high probability of femoroacetabular impingement (FAI) being present with athletic pubalgia, and outcomes are greatly improved when both conditions are corrected.

9. **How do hamstring strains occur?**
   The hamstrings muscle group is the most frequently strained in the body. The mechanism of injury is a rapid, uncontrolled stretch or forceful contraction, usually eccentric. The biceps femoris is most frequently involved. An example of injury is forceful eccentric contraction in late swing/early heel strike during forceful running. Forceful overstretching can occur with maximal hip flexion with the knee extended such as hurdling or kicking. Sports with a high prevalence of hamstring strains include running, sprinting, soccer, football, and rugby. Most injuries are grade I or II. True grade III injuries are rare; an avulsion fracture of the ischial tuberosity is more common. Re-injury rates are high and athletes with a past strain are 3.6 times more likely to reinjure.

10. **How are hamstring strains treated?**
    Proper rehabilitation (improved muscle balance, stretching, proper education about warming up, endurance training, eccentric training, and coordination) is imperative to avoid reinjury. Croisier et al. trained 18 athletes with hamstring strains using specific isokinetic exercises to address their specific strength deficits (quadriceps/hamstring ratios, both concentrically and eccentrically). Of these 18 athletes, 17 improved their isokinetic profiles and returned to sport within 2 months. All 17 remained hamstring injury free at a 1-year follow-up. Although a reduction in strength in the injured hamstring is a predictor of reinjury, Sherry and Best found that a rehabilitation program needs to include progressive agility and trunk stabilization exercises to avoid reinjury. Proximal strains typically take longer to resolve than distal. Neural mobilization may be performed to reduce adhesion to surrounding tissue as the patient moves through the stages of healing.

11. **What are factors for determining RTP for hamstrings injuries?**
    History of recent (<8 weeks) hamstring injury should be taken into account. The presence of an appropriately progressed rehabilitation program that is impairment based reduces re-injury risk. RTP may be delayed if eccentric training was not included in the rehabilitation program. The decision for RTP should be dictated by clinical assessment including hamstring strength, pain level at the time of injury, number of days from injury to pain-free walking, and area of tenderness measured at initial evaluation. The Functional Assessment Scale for Acute Hamstring Injuries (FASH) may help measure improvement over time. Rudisill et al. found that proximal injuries were more successful in RTP with surgical intervention while distal/muscular injuries responded well to proper rehabilitation programs.

12. **What exercises should be components of a program to prevent a first-time hamstring injury?**
    The Nordic Hamstring Exercise should be included with a program of warm-up, stretching, stability training, strengthening, and functional movements (sport specific, agility, and high-speed running).

13. **How is hamstring length assessed?**
    - Active Knee Extension (AKE) test—patient is positioned supine with the hip flexed 90 degrees (either actively or passively). The knee is then actively extended from a starting position of 90-degree flexion toward full extension. The test is positive for hamstring tightness if the angle of knee flexion is >20 degrees. AKE test: individuals with a hamstring injury were categorized into grades based on the lack of full AKE compared to the uninjured side. Individuals with a grade I injury had less than a 15 degree deficit and required 25.9 days of rehabilitation. Those with a grade II injury exhibited a 16 degree to 25 degree deficit and required 30.7 days of rehabilitation. Athletes with a grade III injury demonstrated a 26 degree to 35 degree deficit and required 75 days of rehabilitation.
    - Tripod sign—patient sits with knees over the table in 90 degrees of flexion. The examiner passively extends the knee. The test is positive for hamstring tightness if the pelvis is forced into a posterior tilt.
    - Hamstring contracture test—patient sits with the tested leg extended while the untested leg is held toward the chest. The patient is instructed to reach the arm ipsilateral to the test leg toward the toes. The test is positive for hamstring tightness if the patient cannot reach the toes while maintaining knee extension.
    - Straight-leg raising—patient rests supine while the examiner passively raises the leg with the knee fully extended, and the angle of hip flexion is measured. This test has been found to be highly reliable but does not differentiate between elastic and inelastic posterior hip structures.

    The medial and lateral hamstrings can be differentiated with a manual muscle test. The semitendinosus and semimembranosus are isolated by positioning the patient in prone with the hip internally rotated and resisted knee flexion. The biceps femoris is isolated by positioning the patient prone with external rotation of the hip and resisted knee flexion. Hamstring tightness should be differentiated from radicular symptoms caused by the sciatic nerve or lumbar spine.

14. **Are quadriceps strains common?**
    No. However, when they occur, they are usually the result of rapid deceleration from a sprint. The rectus femoris is the most commonly affected of the quadriceps muscles because of its two-joint action, but the vastus medialis and vastus lateralis also can be injured. Most damage occurs either in the middle of the thigh or approximately 8 cm from the anterior superior iliac spine for grade I and II strains. Strains are seen in soccer, weight lifting, football, sprinting, and rugby. Tight quadriceps, muscle imbalance between the two extremities, leg length discrepancy, and improper warm-up may be contributing factors. Injury rates are also higher in female athletes.

15. **Describe greater trochanteric pain syndrome.**
    Greater trochanteric pain syndrome (GTPS) is a common cause of lateral hip pain that includes the diagnoses of trochanteric bursitis, abductor tendon pathology, and external coxa saltans. The bursae are rarely injured without the presence of tendinopathy or tears of the gluteus medius and/or minimus tendons. Proximal iliotibial band (ITB) tears may also be present. Onset can occur from microtrauma, blunt trauma, or idiopathic origin. External coxa saltans may be present with a palpable snapping of the ITB or gluteus maximus as it moves over the greater trochanter. Incidence is higher in females in the fourth to sixth decade. Risk factors include age, obesity, hip or knee OA, low back pain, and leg length discrepancy.

    Subjective complaints include pain lying on the affected side, sitting with legs crossed, single limb stance and climbing stairs. Onset is usually gradual except for blunt trauma. Palpatory tenderness is present over the greater trochanter, especially the posterior insertion of the gluteus medius. Resisted abduction may be painful and weak. Trendelenburg sign may be positive. External coxa saltans may be reproduced with palpable snapping with active flexion of the hip and may be ceased with the application of pressure to the ITB at the greater trochanter. Lateral hip pain with the FABER test indicates GTPS.

16. **What is the treatment for GTPS?**
    Conservative care includes activity modification, physical therapy, NSAIDs, and corticosteroid injections. Stretching of tightened structures including the tensor fascia latae, hip flexors, gluteals, and hamstrings is important. Strength training should correct muscle imbalances across the hip, focusing on the gluteals. Persistent pain may respond to extracorporeal shock wave therapy, with longer lasting improvement than corticosteroid injection. Platelet-rich plasma is not yet considered standard of care, but percutaneous ultrasonic tenotomy is an effective option for those who do not improve with less invasive treatment. Surgical treatment can include endoscopic bursectomy, ITB release, tendon repair, and augmentation in those who fail conservative care.

17. **Describe iliopectineal bursitis.**
    The iliopectineal bursa lies deep to the iliopsoas tendon anterior to the hip joint. Bursitis commonly results from osteoarthritis or rheumatoid arthritis. Other causes include overuse or direct trauma. Overuse can occur with sports such as weight lifting, rowing, uphill running, and competitive track and field. It occurs more commonly in women. An attachment of the bursae to the joint capsule is seen in 15% of cases. Hip joint pathology should be ruled out by checking for a capsular pattern of pain or restriction. Pain occurs at the anterior hip and groin with radiation in an L2 or L3 distribution. Passive hip flexion with adduction is painful, as is passive hip extension.

Strength testing of the hip flexors may be painful and external rotation may be weak when tested with the hip flexed. Palpation elicits tenderness just lateral to the femoral artery at the femoral triangle. The patient may have a palpable snapping at the anterior hip as the involved hip is passively moved from a flexed position into abduction/external rotation and then passively returned to neutral. Little information is available in the literature about conservative treatment.

18. **How does ischial tuberosity bursitis present? What is its treatment?**
The involved bursa lies between the ischial tuberosity and gluteus maximus. Bursitis usually occurs in people with sedentary occupations or results from a direct fall onto the ischial tuberosity. Pain worsens with sitting and may refer to the posterior thigh; therefore it is important to rule out lumbar pathology. Palpation over the ischial tuberosity is painful. Hamstring stretching is painful. Hip extension may be reduced in the late stance phase of gait with a shortened stride on the affected side.
NSAIDs and rest are usually successful. The patient should avoid sitting, or sit only on well-cushioned surfaces.

19. **How are contusions in athletes classified?**
- Grade I—produces minimal discomfort and should not limit participation in competition
- Grade II—more painful and limits ability to perform at extremes of ROM or strength
- Grade III—more pain, swelling, and bleeding

20. **What is a hip pointer?**
A hip pointer is a contusion of the lateral hip, which usually results from a blow to the iliac crest. In most cases, the TFL muscle belly is impacted and presents with hematoma; however, the injury may involve tearing of the external oblique at its iliac insertion, periostitis of the iliac crest, or contusion to the greater trochanter. Contact sports such as football, ice hockey, volleyball, soccer, wrestling, lacrosse, and rugby often produce hip pointers from impact with other players. Gymnasts may suffer this injury from impact with equipment. It can also result from a fall with any activity.

21. **Describe the clinical findings of a hip pointer.**
The injured athlete is immediately disabled by pain. The trunk is flexed forward and toward the side of injury because any side bending or rotation of the trunk is extremely painful. Abrasion or swelling may be present over the iliac crest. Bruising may be immediately present or may become apparent a few days after injury. Pain is caused by any movement involving the muscles that attach to the iliac crest, including the gluteus maximus, gluteus medius, TFL, sartorius, quadratus lumborum, and transverse abdominals. The abdominals may be in spasm.

22. **How are hip pointers treated?**
Initial treatment is RICE. Crutches may be needed if the patient has pain with ambulation. NSAIDs should not be used until 48 hours after injury because their blood-thinning properties may lead to hematoma. Ice massage is recommended as often as three to four times per day or as pain levels dictate. Gradual stretching keeps the injured area from healing in a contracted position. All exercises should be kept pain free, and pain-relieving modalities may be used. Strengthening programs should include trunk and leg muscles. The athlete must try to prevent hip pointers in the future by the maintenance of a flexibility program and wearing proper protective padding over the iliac crest. Return to sports is allowed in 1 week for grade I injuries; up to 6 weeks may be required for grade II and III injuries.

23. **What tests are useful in the diagnosis of hip pointers?**
No imaging is necessary, but radiographs help to rule out iliac crest fracture or displaced epiphyseal fracture in athletes who have not reached skeletal maturity.

24. **What is the mechanism for a quadriceps contusion? What are the clinical findings?**
Usually, a direct blow from another player is the cause. In football, contact may be made with a helmet, thigh, or padding. Quadriceps contusion also is seen in rugby, soccer, basketball, and ice hockey. The anterior thigh and lateral thigh are most commonly affected.
Pain occurs with ambulation. The patient is unable to flex and extend the knee fully and may not be able to perform an active straight-leg raise or isometric quadriceps contraction. A hematoma may be palpable.

25. **How does treatment for a quadriceps contusion progress?**
Initial RICE must be followed strictly for at least 48 hours. Crutches should be used for ambulation. For 48 hours the patient should be nonweight bearing and immobilized in knee flexion to maintain motion. Then weight bearing should progress once the patient has good quadriceps control and 90-degree pain-free range of motion. Patients should gradually begin passive ROM to avoid contracture. Ice, pulsed ultrasound, and high-voltage galvanic stimulation help to reduce pain and swelling. Patients should begin with isometric exercise and try to

progress to straight-leg raises without a quadriceps lag. Massage should be avoided because it may increase hematoma. As patients progress toward pain-free ambulation, crutch use is discontinued, and strengthening should progress gradually as pain allows. Return to sport can begin after full ROM and sport-specific training. There should be less than a 10% difference in strength between the injured and noninjured quadriceps before full return to sport.

26. **What causes myositis ossificans?**
Myositis ossificans can occur following trauma to a muscle. The injury can be sudden, as in blunt force trauma, or can be from repetitive minor trauma. Following initial edema, the patient may have a loss of ROM in the adjacent joints. A few weeks following injury, heterotropic bone forms in the muscle. The knee extensors are the most common muscle to develop this process, but it can happen throughout the body. Surgery or paraplegia also can cause myositis ossificans, or it may result from early treatment of a contusion with massage or heat, premature return to aggressive stretching or strengthening, or premature return to sport. About 7 to 10 days after injury, radiographs may show beginning ossification, which can progress to heterotopic bone in 2 to 3 weeks. Acute contusions should be monitored to watch for thigh and gluteal compartment syndromes.

27. **How is myositis ossificans treated?**
Early treatment consists only of rest. Weight bearing is reduced with crutches. Once pain and swelling decrease and rehabilitation can begin, initial treatment is geared at gently regaining ROM. Aggressive passive stretching should be avoided for 4 months after injury. Initially, no strengthening takes place, but once swelling subsides, gentle isometrics can begin. NSAIDs or corticosteroids may be required to reduce persistent swelling. Once radiographs show that bony growth has subsided, a gradual return to activity is progressed. One case study by Wieder showed possible resolution of the bony defect with iontophoresis with acetic acid followed by pulsed ultrasound.

28. **Is surgery indicated for myositis ossificans?**
Generally, no surgery is indicated. If the defect causes significant loss of function, surgery should be performed 9 to 12 months after injury when a bone scan shows no active calcification.

29. **What is "snapping hip" syndrome? How is it treated?**
Also known as coxa saltans, snapping hip can be internal, external, or intraarticular. The syndrome is characterized by reproduction of a snap or click at the hip with repetitive motion. Most commonly, the cause of external coxa saltans is snapping of the ITB or anterior fibers of gluteus maximus over the greater trochanter. Causes of internal coxa saltans include snapping of the iliofemoral ligaments over the femoral head, the suction phenomenon of the hip joint, and the movement of the iliopsoas tendon over the iliopectineal eminence or lesser trochanter. Intraarticular coxa saltans can be caused by the suction phenomenon of the hip joint, subluxation, a torn acetabular labrum, a loose body, synovial chondromatosis, and osteocartilaginous exostosis. The long head of the biceps tendon snapping over the ischial tuberosity can cause "snapping bottom." The syndrome is most common in female athletes, such as dancers, runners, gymnasts, and cheerleaders. The clicking in the hip is a greater complaint than pain.

Evaluation of which structure is causing the snap or click is made through palpation and while the causative movement is reproduced. Asymptomatic snapping hip doesn't require treatment. If needed, treatment should progress toward alleviating muscle tightness or weakness that may contribute to the disorder.

30. **What is osteitis pubis?**
Osteitis pubis is chronic inflammation of the symphysis pubis. It may occur after operations of the prostate or bladder or result from athletic activity such as soccer, race walking, running, fencing, weight lifting, hockey, swimming, and football. The mechanism of injury is repetitive stress of muscles with attachments at the symphysis pubis, such as the rectus abdominis, gracilis, and adductor longus. Injury to any of these muscles alters symphyseal biomechanics and can lead to a stress injury/reaction of the pubic bone. This can progress to degeneration of the cartilage of the pubic symphysis.

31. **How is osteitis pubis diagnosed and treated?**
Pain in the groin or medial thigh is reproduced with palpation over one side of the symphysis pubis and during a positive spring test on the pubic rami. Abdominal and adductor muscle spasm may accompany pain, and gait may be antalgic with movement adapted to reduce pain.

Radiographs show loss of definition of bony margins with widening of the symphysis pubis. In chronic cases, the area may appear "moth eaten." Bone scans are hot over the pubic symphysis. MRI shows subchondral bone marrow edema. Treatment consists of rest and administration of NSAIDs with possible use of corticosteroid injections, if possible, within 2 weeks of diagnosis to improve outcomes. Surgical treatment may be required in 5% to 10% of cases that do not resolve with conservative care.

32. **How does damage occur to the acetabular labrum?**

Tears to the labrum can be from acute trauma, repetitive injury, or can be insidious. Damage can occur in a dysplastic hip from changes in the congruence of the joint and abnormal joint stress. It can also occur in nondysplastic hips where labral microtearing, impingement, and cyst formation are precursors to arthritis. Dislocation can result in a labral tear. Anatomic variations in the proximal femur, such as a reduction in anteversion or head-neck offset, can lead to labral tears. Labral tears are commonly seen in conjunction with FAI. They are more common in males with cam impingement and in females with pincer-type impingement. In North Americans, damage is more common to the ant/sup labrum while in the Japanese population, damage to the posterior labrum is more common. Studies show a high incidence (48%–95%) of damage to the acetabular cartilage and early onset of osteoarthritis with labral tears.

33. **What clinical tests identify labral tears?**

- Fitzgerald's acetabular labral test—if passively moving the hip from flexion, adduction, and external rotation into extension, abduction, and internal rotation reproduces pain, with or without clicking, an anterior labral tear is suspected. If pain is reproduced by moving from extension, abduction, and internal rotation into flexion, adduction, and external rotation, a posterior labral tear is suspected. Fitzgerald found that 54 of 55 hips that tested positive also showed labral tears on MRI or arthrogram.
- Impingement provocation test—the patient is supine with the hip flexed to 90 degrees, adducted 25 degrees, and then maximally internally rotated. Pain indicates a possible torn labrum, acetabular rim, or snapping hip syndrome. This test is able to detect incomplete detaching tears of the posterosuperior portion of the acetabular labrum of dysplastic hips, but it does not correlate well with other arthroscopic findings of dysplastic hips.

34. **What imaging tests are used to detect labral tears?**

X-ray and CT scan are limited to indirect diagnosis by identifying dysplasia and FAI that may accompany tears. Ultrasonography can be useful but is limited by the technician's skill level and the habitus of the patient. MRI is less reliable than MRA (magnetic resonance arthrography) at detecting tears. MRA is considered the gold standard but is more invasive and has higher radiation exposure.

35. **How are acetabular labral tears treated?**

Acetabular tears are treated by reduced weight bearing using crutches and performing range of motion exercises for 4 weeks. Per Harris, due to the high prevalence of asymptomatic labral tear, the clinician must ensure that the patient's complaints match their imaging studies ("treat the patient, not the MRI"). Physical therapy should emphasize optimizing pelvic stability to minimize dynamic FAI, via gluteus maximus activation, abductor control, transversus abdominis and rectus abdominis activation, iliopsoas stretching, adductor stretching, rectus femoris stretching, core control, and pelvic floor control. Optimizing sagittal balance with the thoracolumbosacral spine and pelvis should be stressed, as improved strength and flexibility as part of a nonsurgical management program would significantly ease postoperative rehabilitation in the event of failure of nonoperative treatment. Fitzgerald found 13% of patients recovered when treated conservatively. Of those who underwent open arthrotomy or arthroscopic surgery, outcomes were improved if surgery was performed before damage occurred to the femoral head (which created unfavorable outcomes for approximately 12% of subjects). Labral tear resection with repair is the most promising arthroscopic treatment and is more successful with surgical treatment of FAI. Preserving as much healthy labral tissue as possible is important as the capsular side of the labrum has good vascularity and healing potential is maximal at the capsulolabral junction. Labral reconstruction may be necessary when repair is not possible.

36. **What are the three types of femoral acetabular impingements (FAI)?**

When there is reduced joint clearance between the femur and the acetabulum, FAI results are as follows:

1. Cam impingement is a deformity of the femoral head where an abnormally large radius causes abnormal joint contact, especially with hip flexion combined with adduction and internal rotation.
2. Pincer impingement occurs when the acetabulum covers the femoral head and causes premature abutment of the femoral head into the acetabulum.
3. Combined cam and pincer impingement

All types of FAIs can lead to labral and chondral damage. Imaging testing involves x-ray, MRI, and MRA (due to risk of labral tears). Per Palmer et al., symptomatic cases demonstrate better outcomes with surgical intervention than with physiotherapy and activity modification.

37. **How do you test for FAI clinically?**

A combination of these tests can be used:

1. FADIR (flexion–adduction–internal rotation) impingement test—hip is placed in 90 degrees of flexion with maximal adduction and internal rotation. This test is specific for pain provocation in patients with intraarticular, nonarthritic hip joint pain.

2. Patrick/FABER (flexion–abduction–external rotation) test—the patient is supine with the heel of the tested limb crossed above the opposite knee while the pelvis is stabilized at the contralateral iliac crest and overpressure is given into abduction and external rotation. A positive finding does not correlate well to a specific hip joint pathology.
3. Scour test—compression is applied to the hip through the femur, over a hip range of motion.
4. Internal rotation at 90 degrees—pain provocation has been associated with bony impingement as a result of FAI, especially if IR is less than 90°.

38. **What is the postoperative physical therapy progression following hip arthroscopy for FAI?**
Rehabilitation is a standard 3-month duration. Weight bearing is with flat foot immediately following surgery for the first week, with the use of crutches if labral repair is also performed. The phases of rehab are: 1) maximum protection and mobility, 2) controlled stability, 3) strengthening, 4) return to sport. Return to full activity is a minimum of 4 months postoperatively.

39. **How do you test for ligamentous laxity of the hip joint?**
    1. Log roll test—the patient is positioned supine and the leg is passively rolled into internal rotation and external rotation. Clicking may be indicative of a labral tear, and increased external rotation range of motion may indicate iliofemoral ligament laxity.
    2. Long axis distraction—clinician applies a longitudinal distraction force on 30 degrees' flexion, 30 degrees' abduction, and 10 to 15 degrees' external rotation. Excessive motion and apprehension are signs of laxity.

40. **Define piriformis syndrome.**
Piriformis syndrome is a pain in the buttock or posterior thigh and calf caused by inflammation or spasm of the piriformis muscle. Pain is referred in a sciatic distribution because of the proximity of the piriformis to the sciatic nerve, as the two exit the pelvis. Patients complain of pain with walking, ascending stairs, or trunk rotation.

41. **How is piriformis syndrome clinically assessed?**
    1. Frieberg test—the patient is positioned supine with the thigh resting against the table while the examiner applies passive internal rotation of the hip.
    2. Pace test—the patient is positioned in a sitting position while the examiner resists hip abduction.
    3. Piriformis test or FAIR test (flexion, adduction, and internal rotation)—the patient is positioned in side-lying position with the tested leg facing upward. The test hip is flexed to 60 degrees with the knee flexed. The examiner stabilizes the hip at the iliac crest and passively moves the hip into adduction. A variation of this test is performed in the supine position; with the hip and knee maximally flexed, the examiner moves the hip into full adduction. EMG studies performed in the FAIR position have been found to identify patients who will respond to physical therapy intervention. The FAIR test has been found to have a sensitivity of 0.881 and a specificity of 0.832.
    4. Beattie test—the patient is positioned side lying as for the piriformis test. With the hip and knee flexed and the knee resting on the examining table, the patient actively externally rotates the hip by lifting the knee off the table and then holding the position.
    5. Lee test—the patient is positioned in the supine hook-lying position (hip flexed 60 degrees with the foot flat on the table). The examiner resists hip abduction.

A positive result for any of these tests is the reproduction of pain symptoms either occurring in the buttock or radiating along the sciatic nerve. Restricted mobility is also a positive finding. Further examination should rule out the hip joint and lumbosacral pathology.

42. **How is piriformis syndrome treated?**
Modalities such as ultrasound or cold pack/ice massage can help to reduce pain and spasm. Fagerson suggests that massage or spray and stretch can help to reduce pain from trigger points in the muscle. Static stretching may be more beneficial than contract-relax if pain is caused by resisted external rotation of the hip. Modifications may be needed in the patient's base of support in the seated position. Crossing the legs should be avoided, and wallets should be removed from back pockets. Shock-attenuating insoles may help patients who spend a lot of time on their feet, especially on hard surfaces. Correction of leg length discrepancy with a heel lift reduces tension on the piriformis. NSAIDs may be necessary to reduce inflammation. Injection of botulinum toxin A in conjunction with physical therapy has also been found to be of benefit, but the duration of relief is limited. Trigger point injection combined with PT is beneficial.

43. **What outcome measures are validated for orthopedic hip conditions?**
The Western Ontario and McMaster Universities Osteoarthritis Index (WOMAC) physical function subscale, the Lower Extremity Functional Scale (LEFS), and Harris Hip Score (HHS).

Bibliography

Baker, C. L., Jr., & Mahoney, J. R. (2020). Ultrasound-guided percutaneous tenotomy for gluteal tendinopathy. *Orthopaedic Journal of Sports Medicine, 8*(3), 2325967120907868.

Bisciotti, G. N., Chamari, K., Cena, E., et al. (2021). The conservative treatment of longstanding adductor-related groin pain syndrome: a critical and systematic review. *Biology of Sport, 38*(1), 45–63.

Croisier, J. L., Ganteaume, S., Binet, J., Genty, M., & Ferret, J. M. (2008). Strength imbalances and prevention of hamstring injury in professional soccer players: a prospective study. *Am J Sports Med, 36*(8): 1469–1475. doi: 10.1177/0363546508316764. Epub 2008 Apr 30. PMID: 18448578.

Eckard, T. G., Kerr, Z. Y., Padua, D. A., Djoko, A., & Dompier, T. P. (2017). Epidemiology of quadriceps strains in national collegiate athletic association athletes, 2009–2010 through 2014–2015. *Journal of Athletic Training, 52*(5), 474–481.

Ellsworth, A. A., Zoland, M. P., & Tyler, T. F. (2014). Athletic pubalgia and associated rehabilitation. *International Journal of Sports Physical Therapy, 9*(6), 774–784.

Enseki, K., Harris-Hayes, M., White, D. M., et al. (2014). Nonarthritic hip joint pain: clinical practice guidelines linked to the international classification of functioning, disability and health from the orthopaedic section of the American Physical Therapy Association. *Journal of Orthopaedic and Sports Physical Therapy, 44*, A1–A32.

Fagerson, T. L. (1998). Diseases and disorders of the hip. In T. L. Fagerson (Ed.), *The hip handbook* (pp. 39–95). Boston: Butterworth Heinemann.

Harris, J. D. (2016). Hip labral repair: options and outcomes. *Current Reviews in Musculoskeletal Medicine, 9*(4), 361–367.

Hatem, M., Martin, R. L., & Bharam, S. (2021). Surgical outcomes of inguinal-, pubic-, and adductor-related chronic pain in athletes: a systematic review based on surgical technique. *Orthopaedic Journal of Sports Medicine, 9*(9), 23259671211023116.

Hicks, B. L., Lam, J. C., & Varacallo, M. (2022). Piriformis syndrome: In: StatPearls [Internet]. Treasure Island (FL): StatPearls Publishing.

Larson, C. M. (2014). Sports hernia/athletic pubalgia: evaluation and management. *Sports Health, 6*(2), 139–144.

Liu, Y., Lu, W., Ouyang, K., & Deng, Z. (2021). The imaging evaluation of acetabular labral lesions. *Journal of Orthopaedics and Traumatology, 22*(1), 34.

Lynch, T. S., Bedi, A., & Larson, C. M. (2017). Athletic hip injuries. *Journal of the American Academy of Orthopaedic Surgeons, 25*(4), 269–279.

Lynch, T. S., Minkara, A., Aoki, S., et al. (2020). Best practice guidelines for hip arthroscopy in femoroacetabular impingement: results of a Delphi process. *Journal of the American Academy of Orthopaedic Surgeons, 28*(2), 81–89.

Lynch, T. S., Terry, M. A., Bedi, A., & Kelly, B. T. (2013). Hip arthroscopic surgery: patient evaluation, current indications, and outcomes. *American Journal of Sports Medicine, 41*(5), 1174–1189.

Martin, R. L., Cibulka, M. T., Bolgla, L. A., et al. (2022). Hamstring strain injury in athletes. *Journal of Orthopaedic & Sports Physical Therapy, 52*(3), CPG1–CPG44.

Núñez, J. F., Fernandez, I., Torres, A., et al. (2020). Strength conditioning program to prevent adductor muscle strains in football: does it really help professional football players? *International Journal of Environmental Research and Public Health, 17*(17), 6408.

Palmer, A. J. R., Ayyar Gupta, V., Fernquest, S., et al. (2019). Arthroscopic hip surgery compared with physiotherapy and activity modification for the treatment of symptomatic femoroacetabular impingement: multicentre randomised controlled trial [published correction appears in BMJ. 2021 Jan 18;372:m3715]. *BMJ, 364*, I185.

Pianka, M. A., Serino, J., DeFroda, S. F., & Bodendorfer, B. M. (2021). Greater trochanteric pain syndrome: evaluation and management of a wide spectrum of pathology. *SAGE Open Medicine, 9*, 20503121211022582.

Rodriguez, R. (2020). Measuring the hip adductor to abductor strength ratio in ice hockey and soccer players: a critically appraised topic. *Journal of Sport Rehabilitation, 29*(1), 116–121.

Rudisill, S. S., Kucharik, M. P., Varady, N. H., & Martin, S. D. (2021). Evidence-based management and factors associated with return to play after acute hamstring injury in athletes: a systematic review. *Orthopaedic Journal of Sports Medicine, 9*(11), 23259671211053833.

Sherry, M. A., & Best, T. M. (2004). A comparison of 2 rehabilitation programs in the treatment of acute hamstring strains. *Journal of Orthopaedic and Sports Physical Therapy, 34*, 116–125.

Smirnova, L., Derinov, A., & Glazkova, I. (2020). Hamstring structural injury in futsal players: the effect of active range of motion (AROM) deficit on rehabilitation period. *Muscles, Ligaments and Tendons Journal, 10*, 645–650.

Varacallo, M., & Bordoni, B. (2022). Hip pointer injuries: In: StatPearls [Internet]. Treasure Island (FL): StatPearls Publishing.

Walczak, B. E., Johnson, C. N., & Howe, B. M. (2015). Myositis ossificans. *Journal of the American Academy of Orthopaedic Surgeons, 23*(10), 612–622.

Wieder, D. L. (1992). Treatment of traumatic myositis ossificans with acetic acid iontophoresis. *Physical Therapy, 72*, 133–137.

Yazbek, P. M., Ovanessian, V., Martin, R. L., & Fukuda, T. Y. (2011). Nonsurgical treatment of acetabular labrum tears: a case series. *Journal of Orthopaedic and Sports Physical Therapy, 41*, 346–363.

CHAPTER 66 QUESTIONS

1. **Your patient is a 16-year-old hockey player who wants to avoid "groin pulls." Which of these exercises is the best choice for injury prevention?**
   a. Bridging with resisted hip abduction
   b. Adductor strengthening
   c. Nordic hamstring exercise
   d. Adductor stretching

2. **A patient with a distal hamstring injury wants to return to play. Which of the following is NOT a factor in making the best decision for your patient?**
   a. History of a prior hamstring injury 6 weeks ago
   b. The patient was unable to walk pain free for 2 weeks following injury

c. Whether eccentric training of the hamstrings was included in the rehabilitation program
d. Active SLR is >75 degrees

3. **You suspect that a patient might have an acetabular tear. Which imaging test is considered the gold standard for this diagnosis?**
   a. X-ray
   b. MRI
   c. MRA
   d. Ultrasonography

FRACTURES AND DISLOCATIONS OF THE HIP AND PELVIS

T. Gibbons, MPT

1. **Describe the Garden classification of femoral neck fractures.**
   - Type I—incomplete and valgus impacted
   - Type II—complete, nondisplaced
   - Type III—complete, displaced <50%
   - Type IV—complete, displaced >50%

2. **Where is the pain from femoral neck fractures typically felt?**
   Pain from femoral neck fractures is usually deep in the anterior groin. Pain in the groin with log rolling, in the case of negative x-rays, should be explored with MRI.

3. **What are the treatment options for femoral neck fractures?**
   In older patients, Garden fractures type I and II may be treated with three percutaneously placed pins. Type III and IV are treated with hemiarthroplasty because of disruption of the femoral head blood supply and high rates of osteonecrosis and nonunion. Patients with preexisting degenerative joint disease may benefit from total hip arthroplasty, although morbidity and mortality are slightly higher. Younger patients (<65) should undergo open reduction and internal fixation (ORIF), if possible, in an attempt to save the femoral head.

4. **What is the difference between unipolar and bipolar hemiarthroplasties?**
   - Unipolar (Austin-Moore)—only the femoral head is replaced; the native acetabulum is retained. This noncemented prosthesis is used primarily for bedridden and low-demand patients.
   - Bipolar—femoral head is replaced and snaps into a rotating polyethylene shell, which sits in the acetabulum. Bipolar prostheses attempt to reduce acetabulum wear. The superiority of bipolar prostheses has not been proved, although the dislocation rate is lower than with unipolar prostheses.

5. **What preventive measures can elderly people take to avoid hip fractures?**
   Performing weight-bearing exercises, maintaining adequate calcium intake, maintaining adequate vitamin D intake, eliminating household and environmental hazards (eg, throw rugs), treating impaired vision and cataracts, medication withdrawal, gait stabilization devices, and hormonal implementation can decrease hip fracture risk.

6. **Describe the Evans classification of intertrochanteric (IT) hip fractures.**
   The Evans classification is based on 2D x-ray findings.
   - Type I—fracture line extends superiorly and laterally from the lesser trochanter
   - Type II—fracture line extends inferiorly and laterally from the lesser trochanter

   Evans further divides the two types into stable and unstable patterns.

7. **Describe the Tang classification of IT hip fractures.**
   The Tang classification is based on 3D CT imaging.
   - Type I: simple fracture with intact lateral femoral wall and greater trochanter fragment
   - Type II: simple fracture with intact lateral femoral wall with/without lesser trochanter detachment
   - Type III: fractures with intertrochanteric crest detachment involving the lesser trochanter and greater trochanter with an intact lateral femoral wall
   - Type IV: fractures with large intertrochanteric crest detachment and large lesser trochanter and greater trochanter detachment partially involving the lateral femoral wall and less medial cortical support
   - Type V: a combination of pertrochanteric and lateral fracture line involving the entire lateral femoral wall and lesser trochanter detachment

8. **What are the treatment options for IT fractures?**
   IT fractures can be treated with internal fixation either by intramedullary nail into the femoral bone marrow cavity (ie, intramedullary hip screw, gamma nail) or with extramedullary fixation applied outside the marrow cavity (lateral side plate with sliding head screw, ie, dynamic hip screw, sliding hip screw). Intramedullary fixation has been found to have lower rate of implant failure, deep infection, and reoperation than extramedullary fixation.

9. **How successful are MRI and bone scans in detecting nondisplaced hip fractures?**
Bone scans detect approximately 80% of fractures within 24 hours of injury. Sensitivity improves to nearly 100% at 3 days. MRI offers immediate, nearly 100% sensitivity in the detection of occult hip fractures.

10. **Describe the mortality rates associated with hip fractures.**
Mortality is 14% to 58% in the first year following hip fracture. Mortality rates decrease 2 years following fracture but never reach the same rate as controls. Risk of death is increased with lower level of prefracture activity, living in an institution before fracture, prior dementia diagnosis, advanced age, having three or more comorbidities, and male sex (although females more frequently suffer a fracture).

11. **What is the incidence of hip fracture?**
Incidence of hip fracture increases with age. For women, the risk at 35 years of age is 2/100,000 but at age 85+ is 3032/100,000. In men, the rates are 4/100,000 at 35 and 190/100,000 at 85 years.

12. **What functional losses occur after hip fracture?**
Hip fracture survivors experience worse mobility, independence in function, health, quality of life, and higher rates of living in an institution than age matched controls. Ten to twenty percent of hip fracture patients are institutionalized following fracture.

13. **What is the treatment for isolated avulsion fracture of the greater or lesser tuberosities?**
These rare fractures usually do well with limited bed rest and progression of weight bearing and ambulation as tolerated. ORIF may be indicated for widely displaced fragments.

14. **How are subtrochanteric femur fractures defined?**
Fractures that occur within 5 cm distal to the lesser trochanter are termed subtrochanteric (ST) femur fractures. Two thirds of these fractures occur in patients >50 years old and in women more than men. Risk factors include pharmacologic treatment of osteoporosis with bisphosphonates, low bone mineral density, and diabetes.

15. **What is the recommended treatment for femoral shaft and ST femur fractures?**
Intramedullary nails are the gold standard for surgical fixation. Extramedullary plates are a less frequently used option.

16. **Should THA be considered in patients with displaced femoral neck fractures?**
Hemiarthroplasty and total hip arthroplasty are both used to treat femoral neck fractures with hemiarthroplasty preferred with patients with more severe comorbidities. THA usually results in improved functional outcome and reduced pain than hemiarthroplasty. THA is becoming more common.

17. **What rehabilitation considerations are important after hip fracture?**
Because falls are the cause of 90% of hip fractures, fall risk assessment and management are important in rehabilitation of these patients. Knee extension strength, Verbal Rating Score for pain management, NMS score, Cumulated Ambulation Score, Timed Up and Go test, and gait speed are all valid tools for documenting function in hip fracture patients following surgery. Interdisciplinary care is essential to watch for delirium from medication, pressure ulcers, and to prevent repeat falls. Physical therapy programs need to include structured exercise, including progressive high-intensity resistive strength, balance, weight bearing, and functional mobility training, to older adults after hip fracture.

18. **What features distinguish a stable pelvis fracture from an unstable one?**
Several classification systems attempt to identify which fractures of the pelvis are stable and may be treated nonoperatively and which fractures are unstable and require operative stabilization. Essentially the pelvis is a ring structure. Therefore, a single break in the ring usually does not lead to pelvic instability, whereas double breaks (bony or ligamentous) may lead to vertical and/or rotatory instability. The posterior sacroiliac ligamentous complex is the single most important structure for pelvic stability. Fractures that lie entirely outside of the ring (ie, inferior pubic rami fractures) are stable.

19. **What is the usual mechanism of injury for pelvis fracture?**
Low-velocity injuries in older osteoporotic bones often result from lateral compression of the pelvis secondary to a fall. Patients often present with fracture to the superior and/or inferior pubic ramus. High-velocity trauma may result in fractures caused by lateral compression, anteroposterior compression, and vertical shear. These fractures tend to cause significant disruption of the pelvic ring and are therefore more likely to be unstable. Fractures that lie entirely outside of the ring (ie, inferior pubic rami fractures) are stable.

20. **Describe the usual mechanism of injury for acetabular fractures.**
    Fractures of the acetabulum often occur when a direct force is transmitted from the proximal femur. When the hip is flexed (as in an automobile accident), the posterior wall fails. When the hip is extended (as in falls from a height), the anterior wall fails.

21. **What are the long-term complications of unstable pelvic ring disruptions?**
    Chronic low back pain, sacroiliac pain, residual gait abnormalities, and leg length discrepancy are common complaints. Fewer than 30% of patients with >1-cm displacement of the pelvic ring are pain free at 5-year follow-up.

22. **How do avulsion fractures of the pelvis occur?**
    Avulsion fractures are most common in adolescents and occur at the unfused apophysis at the location of a tendon attachment. Violent muscle contraction during sporting activity is the most common mechanism of injury. Avulsion fractures can also occur in adults, but if they occur without trauma, pathologic lesion is suspected. Treatment is usually rest and avoiding use of the attached muscle. Surgical care is only needed for wide displacements.

23. **What is the post reduction treatment of traumatic hip dislocation?**
    After closed reduction, thorough neurovascular assessment continues for 24 hours. Patients may be placed in gentle traction for 24 to 48 hours. At that time gentle range of motion may begin. Weight-bearing restrictions continue to be a subject of debate, but in general patients without fracture may slowly begin progressive weight bearing.

24. **What complications are associated with hip dislocation?**
    - Osteonecrosis—1% to 17%; early reduction decreases the rate
    - Degenerative joint disease—33% to 50%
    - Sciatic nerve injury—8% to 19%; approximately 50% of patients recover spontaneously
    - Femoral head fracture—7% to 68%

Bibliography

Dhanwal, D. K., Dennison, E. M., Harvey, N. C., & Cooper, C. (2011). Epidemiology of hip fracture: worldwide geographic variation. *Indian Journal of Orthopaedics, 45*(1), 15–22.
Dyer, S. M., Crotty, M., Fairhall, N., et al. (2016). A critical review of the long-term disability outcomes following hip fracture. *BMC Geriatrics, 16*, 158.
Garrison, I., Domingue, G., & Honeycutt, M. W. (2021). Subtrochanteric femur fractures: current review of management. *EFORT Open Reviews, 6*(2), 145–151.
Kazley, J. M., Banerjee, S., Abousayed, M. M., & Rosenbaum, A. J. (2018). Classifications in brief: Garden classification of femoral neck fractures. *Clinical Orthopaedics and Related Research, 476*(2), 441–445.
Li, J., Tang, S., Zhang, H., et al. (2019). Clustering of morphological fracture lines for identifying intertrochanteric fracture classification with Hausdorff distance-based K-means approach. *Injury, 50*(4), 939–949.
McDonough, C. M., Harris-Hayes, M., Kristensen, M. T., et al. (2021). Physical therapy management of older adults with hip fracture. *Journal of Orthopaedic & Sports Physical Therapy, 51*(2), CPG1–CPG81.
Medical Advisory Secretariat. (2008). Prevention of falls and fall-related injuries in community-dwelling seniors: an evidence-based analysis. *Ontario Health Technology Assessment Series, 8*(2), 1–78.
Sanders, T. G., & Zlatkin, M. B. (2008). Avulsion injuries of the pelvis. *Seminars in Musculoskeletal Radiology, 12*(1), 42–53.
Schnell, S., Friedman, S. M., Mendelson, D. A., Bingham, K. W., & Kates, S. L. (2010). The 1-year mortality of patients treated in a hip fracture program for elders. *Geriatric Orthopaedic Surgery & Rehabilitation, 1*(1), 6–14.
Tinetti, M. E., & Kumar, C. (2010). The patient who falls: "It's always a trade-off." *JAMA, 303*(3), 258–266.
Yu, X., Wang, H., Duan, X., Liu, M., & Xiang, Z. (2018). Intramedullary versus extramedullary internal fixation for unstable intertrochanteric fracture, a meta-analysis. *Acta Orthopaedica et Traumatologica Turcica, 52*(4), 299–307.

CHAPTER 67 QUESTIONS

1. **Your patient is an 80 year old whose daughter is worried about her mother fracturing her hip from a fall. Which of these is NOT a best recommendation for your patient?**
   a. Aquatic exercise
   b. Adequate vitamin D intake
   c. Removing household hazards (ie, throw rugs)
   d. Treating impaired vision

2. **Which of these assessment tools are NOT valid for documenting hip function following surgery for hip fracture?**
   a. Timed Up and Go test
   b. New Mobility Score
   c. Hip extensor manual muscle test
   d. Cumulated Ambulation Score

3. **True or False: A bone scan is more sensitive than MRI for detecting nondisplaced hip. fracture in the first 24 hours after injury.**

TOTAL HIP ARTHROPLASTY

M. Cacko, MPT, OCS, M. Caid, DO, and J.D. Keener, MD, PT

1. **What are some indications for a total hip arthroplasty (THA)?**

   The most common indication for a THA is osteoarthritis, which consists of joint space narrowing, osteophyte formation, subchondral cysts, and sclerosis. Other conditions that can lead to hip arthritis are hip dysplasia, trauma, Legg Calve Perthes, slipped capital femoral epiphysis, rheumatoid arthritis, and avascular necrosis.

2. **What are the pros and cons of the different types of arthroplasty surfaces: metal-on-metal, ceramic-on-ceramic, and metal-on-polyethylene?**

   METAL-ON-METAL

   - Pros—metal-on-metal provides a strong material that resists bending, torsion forces, and fatigue, which allows it to carry a sufficient load. Metal-on-metal has an initial rapid wear period for the first 1 to 2 years, but after this it has a lower and steadier wear. Metal has a 20 to 100 times lower wear rate than conventional polyethylene. Wear rates have been found to be 25 to 35 μm per year for the first 3 years and then 5 μm per year thereafter, or 0.6 mm^3 of metallic wear debris per year, which is an order of magnitude less than that of metal-on-polyethylene.
   - Cons—metal-on-metal does produce metallic debris, which can be cytotoxic, altering the phagocytic activity of macrophages and leading to cell death. Metallosis and its effect on accelerating macrophage response can damage the shell or femoral neck. There are elevated ion levels in the blood and urine, effects of which are unknown. Hypersensitivity responses in the immune system are found in 2 out of 10,000 replacements. There are also possible links to cancer because cobalt and chromium have been found to cause cancer in animals, but more research must be done. The coefficient of friction is approximately two to three times greater than that of polyethylene. Metal-on-metal replacements have a higher cost, are heavier, and are stiffer. Periprosthetic soft tissue reactions can also occur, such as pseudotumor, metallosis, and cyst formation.

   CERAMIC-ON-CERAMIC

   - Pros—ceramic-on-ceramic is resistant to chemical and mechanical dissolution. Ceramic is hard, strong, and resistant to oxidation and has high wettability. It has a low coefficient of friction and a scratch-resistant surface. Wear rates are 5 to 10 μm per year.
   - Cons—ceramic-on-ceramic is brittle, and there is risk of fracture to the femoral head and acetabular component. Chipping can also occur with impingement to the hip. There are a limited number of femoral head and neck lengths and sizes that are ceramic. There is accelerated wear with higher degrees of abduction of the acetabular component. Ceramics are also high in cost and have increased rates of acetabular component loosening.

   METAL-ON-POLYETHYLENE

   - Pros—metal-on-polyethylene has low wear rates, costs less, and provides absence of oxidation. There is better adaptability and a forgiving nature of the bearing surface. There is low friction, long-term stability, and low water absorption. Cross-linked polyethylene has been found to have better wear rates than standard polyethylene.
   - Cons—metal-on-polyethylene has a tendency to scuff the surface, wearing it away. Other cons with polyethylene are aging, creep, breakage, and abrasion. Polyethylene has a wear rate of 0.1 mm per year.

3. **Is highly cross-linked polyethylene superior to conventional polyethylene?**

   In two different studies, it was found that cross-linked polyethylene had decreased wear rates compared with conventional polyethylene. One study showed cross-linked had one-tenth the wear rate compared with conventional after 5 years. The other study demonstrated cross-linked had a 95% reduced wear rate compared with conventional polyethylene after 5 years.

4. **What are the different types of surgical approaches used for hip arthroplasty, and how do they affect rehabilitation?**

   The most common surgical approaches performed today are direct anterior, anterolateral, direct lateral, and posterior.

   - The direct anterior approach uses the interval between the tensor fascia lata and the rectus femoris. This approach has the benefit of not requiring any muscles to be detached and then repaired. This approach has become popular due to faster early recovery, decreased pain scores, and very low dislocation rate.
   - The anterolateral approach is performed by developing an interval between the tensor fascia lata and gluteus medius with either partial reflection of the medius or takedown of the greater trochanter to expose the

underlying hip joint. After the components are placed, the gluteus medius is repaired or the greater trochanter is reattached.

- The posterior approach involves splitting of the gluteus maximus with takedown of the deep hip external rotators and conjoint tendon to expose the posterior aspect of the hip joint. After the components are placed, the posterior capsule and conjoint tendon are repaired.

The anterolateral approach has been shown to have a lower rate of postoperative hip dislocation, as the posterior hip soft tissues are not violated. However, with this approach, time is needed to allow for the gluteus medius repair or greater trochanter osteotomy to heal, often restricting active hip abduction. Failure of this repair can lead to a Trendelenburg gait. The posterior approach preserves the integrity of the gluteus medius and greater trochanter and allows wide exposure of the hip and proximal femur often needed for revision surgery. Dementia, mental retardation, Parkinson's disease, stroke, or seizure disorders are relative contraindications to the posterior approach because of the greater potential for postoperative hip dislocation. Implications for rehabilitation include avoidance of active hip abduction exercises following anterolateral and direct lateral approaches for at least 6 weeks and more stringent adherence to total hip precautions following posterior hip approaches because of the potential for hip dislocation. With the direct anterior approach, medial to the tensor fascia latae (TFL), there is little need for any typical total hip precautions given the extremely low dislocation rate.

5. **Is direct anterior THA superior to THA done from the posterior approach?**
No clear advantage has been consistently proven; the most consistent factor that correlates to a successful outcome after THA is when a high-volume joint reconstruction surgeon does the procedure, regardless of which approach is used. However, direct anterior THAs trends to have reduced pain, faster recovery, decreased dislocation rate, and decreased hospital stay.

6. **What are the advantages and disadvantages of a direct anterior total hip arthroplasty?**
Advantages are that this approach is muscle sparing and does not require a muscle repair at the end of the procedure. Anterior hips have decreased pain and a faster post op recovery. There is also a decreased risk of dislocation with an anterior approach.
Disadvantages are that the anterior approach has been associated with delayed wound healing with higher BMI patients with an abdominal pannus, this can be associated with superficial cellulitis as well. A low percentage of patients can experience thigh numbness and tingling with the anterior approach. This is usually temporary but can be permanent. This is due to the lateral femoral cutaneous nerve being stretched or injured.

7. **Which total hip arthroplasty surgical approach is most likely to cause a limp due to abductor weakness?**
The anterolateral approach is also known as the Watson-Jones approach. This approach has been associated with a Trendelenburg gait and abductor weakness. One reason for this is that it requires the anterior one-third of the abductors to be detached during the procedure. When the abductors do not heal after being repaired or they become injured during the post op period a limp can develop. Another cause is that the superior gluteal nerve is in close proximity during this approach and can be injured.

8. **Which type of THA provides better results, cemented or cementless?**
A long-term study was performed on 171 patients with simultaneous B THA with a cemented stem in one hip, and a cementless in the other with a cementless acetabular component on all hips at a minimum of 25-year follow-up. Survival rate of the acetabular components was 79% for cemented stem group and 78% for the cementless stem group. Survival rate of the femoral components was 96% for cemented stem group and 95% for the cementless stem group. Harris scores were a mean 91 points for cemented stem group and a mean of 93 points for the cementless stem group.

9. **What types of patients are candidates for minimally invasive THA? What are the outcomes with this procedure?**
Patients who qualify for a minimally invasive total hip replacement have a lower average body mass index, are thinner and healthier, and have fewer medical comorbidities. Patients are typically between 40 and 75 years of age and usually do not have larger, muscular frames. Minimally invasive hip replacements reduce blood loss, transfusion requirements, postoperative pain, and hospital stays. Dislocation rates have been found to be between 2% and 10%, and 35% of those patients do not have reoccurrence. Three times more patients ambulate on day 1 and 50% more patients meet all discharge criteria by day 3 with minimally invasive THA. The average time for patients to discontinue the use of crutches was 6 days, 9 days to walk independently without an assistive device, 10 days to resume activities of daily living, and 16 days average time to walk a half mile. Patients were able to return to walking with no limp, secondary to insufficiency of the gluteus medius. Average return to driving was 6 days, compared with between 4 and 12 weeks for THA patients.

10. Is there an advantage to a minimally invasive THA versus conventional THA?

Minimally invasive has an advantage of decreased pain initially after surgery, earlier discharge to home, and less use of an assisted device. Evaluations at 6 weeks and 3 months post operation revealed no differences between the groups. There is no difference with regard to hip function and complication rates between the two groups.

11. What are the outcomes following THA?

Survivorship analysis in multiple studies has shown acetabular and femoral components lasting 15 to 20 years with acceptable rates of survivorship ranging from 85% to 95%. Pain relief and improved function correlate well with survivorship of components for most patients, with good to excellent results in 85% to 95% of patients at 15 to 20 years. Postoperative limp has been associated with takedown of the greater trochanter and hip abductor muscles. Thigh pain has been associated with uncemented femoral stems. It has been found that the strength of the muscles surrounding the operated hip joint was 84% to 89% of the strength of the uninvolved side in men and 79% to 81% of the strength of the uninvolved hip in women. It was also found that significant residual muscle weakness persisted in the operated hip for up to 2 years following surgery. This persistent weakness could contribute to higher rates of component loosening. Physical therapy early in THA does restore range of motion, but significant impairments in postural stability remain 1 year after surgery. It is recommended that muscle-strengthening exercises be continued for at least 1 year after THA.

12. What complications are associated with THA?

There are several serious but relatively infrequent complications, including loosening/osteolysis, dislocation, periprosthetic fractures, sciatic nerve injury, heterotopic ossification, and infection. Dislocation following THA is a multifactorial problem with reported rates of occurrence ranging from 1% to 10%. The majority of dislocations occurs within the first month following surgery. The prevalence of dislocation has been related to posterior surgical approaches, smaller prosthetic femoral head size, surgical technique, revision surgery, and patient compliance. Many dislocations can be treated conservatively with bracing and activity modification, particularly in the early postoperative period. Often, recurrent dislocation requires revision surgery. In a Mayo Clinic study of 19,680 hips, it was found that the incidence of dislocation was 1.8% at 1 year and 7% at 5 years, and increased 1% every subsequent 5-year period. The incidence of dislocation also increased after revision surgery to between 9% and 21%. Of the patients who had a dislocation, 16% to 59% had recurrent dislocations. Nerve injuries occur approximately in 1% of primary total hip replacements and 6% of revisions. The rate of nerve injury is higher in females than males. Functional recovery occurs in approximately 80% of patients. Nerve injuries can increase with approximately 1.5 cm of limb lengthening, and if the limb is lengthened 4 cm, significant nerve injury will be seen in 28% of patients. The femoral nerve and the peroneal branch of the sciatic nerve are more likely to recover than the tibial branch or the entire sciatic nerve. Most patients who recover do so within 7 months, but recovery can continue for 2 to 3 years. Those approached from a direct anterior approach may experience thigh numbness or groin pain.

13. You notice that a patient you are treating following THA has developed increased calf swelling and localized tenderness. What should you do?

An increase in calf swelling, calf pain with dorsiflexion of the ankle, calf tenderness, and/or erythema are all potential signs of deep vein thrombosis (DVT) and should prompt the therapist to contact the physician as soon as possible. These findings warrant the immediate attention of the physician so that appropriate studies may be obtained. The development of DVT following THA is very common despite the use of various types of DVT prophylactic measures (aspirin, warfarin, heparin derivatives, and sequential compression devices). Even with preventive therapy, rates of postoperative DVT following THA range from 10% to 20%. In spite of the high incidence of DVT, the rate of progression to fatal pulmonary embolism in unprotected patients is only 0.34%.

14. What are total hip precautions? Are they necessary?

Instructions given to patients to help minimize the risk of postoperative hip dislocation are termed total hip precautions. The majority of hips that dislocate have a tendency to do so posteriorly. This usually occurs in positions of extreme hip flexion or hip flexion in combination with adduction and/or internal rotation. These hips tend to be stable in positions of extension, abduction, and external rotation. Most patients are instructed not to flex the hip greater than 90 degrees or adduct the leg across midline, especially during the first 6 weeks following surgery, during which time the soft tissues are healing. Patients are instructed not to sleep on the affected hip and to keep pillows between their knees to prevent adduction of the hip. In a systemic review of 6900 patients from 7 studies, with 3517 treated with and 3383 treated without precautions, there was no significant difference in dislocation rates between the two groups. There was a 2.2% rate in the restricted group as compared to 2.0% in the unrestricted group.

Anterior approach THA precautions are to not extend the hip past neutral, ER the hip, and to not cross legs. These patients are recommended to sleep on their surgical side when side lying and to not take large steps laterally with surgical side. Many surgeons don't feel it is necessary to have precautions following anterior hip replacement, so always consult the surgeon.

In a study performed with 2386 patients with 2612 hips replaced with an anterior THA approach, only four dislocations occurred (0.15%). Dislocations occurred between 3 to 12 days postoperatively. Patients were not given any functional restrictions, such as elevated seats, abduction pillows, or driving limits. It was found that a no-restriction protocol did not increase the risk of early dislocation following THA with the anterior approach.

15. **What is the postoperative weight-bearing status of a THA patient?**
Patients with cemented joint replacements can bear weight as tolerated, unless the operative procedure involved a soft tissue repair or internal fixation of bone. Patients with cementless components are also weight bear as tolerated but full ingrowth of the implant takes 2 to 3 months. Elderly osteoporotic patients, specifically women, are at risk for periprosthetic fracture with cementless components.

16. **What are typical hip range of motion goals following total hip arthroplasty (THA)?**
Range of motion following THA usually advances rapidly. By the time of hospital discharge, patients should be able to extend to neutral and easily flex the hip to 90 degrees. Most patients will be able to achieve 110 to 120 degrees of hip flexion and will have the needed 160 degrees of combined hip flexion, abduction, and external rotation motion necessary to put on socks and shoes by 6 weeks after surgery.

17. **What are typical hip flexion range of motion with various activities?**
Hip flexion ranges of motion varies depending on activity. Please keep these ranges of motion in mind when educating patients following THA. Walking requires between 9.9 and 49.3 degrees of flexion. Ambulating upstairs will require between 19.6 and 67.8 degrees of hip flexion. Ambulating downstairs will require 26.2 to 52.4 degrees of hip flexion. Squatting has an average of 120 degrees of flexion. Sit to stand transfers average 103 degrees of flexion range of motion. Getting on/off the toilet has an average maximum of 112.6 degrees of hip flexion. Tying shoes requires 126.1 degrees flexion.

18. **How much force is placed across the hip during routine activities of daily living?**
The force vectors created by contraction of the surrounding hip musculature are the primary determinant of hip joint reactive forces. The double-leg stance has been shown to create hip joint reactive forces of one time the body weight compared with two to three times the body weight for a single-leg stance. Walking produces hip joint reactive forces of two to four times the body weight depending on the pace of gait. Stair-climbing produces forces of three to four times the body weight on the hip joint, in addition to significant torsional forces at the proximal femur. Simply elevating the pelvis to position a bedpan can produce hip joint reactive forces of five to six times body weight as a result of the required hip muscle contractions.

19. **What is the typical recovery and rehabilitation for total hip arthroplasty?**
Initial healing phase following total hip arthroplasty between 0 and 6 weeks consist of controlling pain, swelling, and protecting the healing tissue. During this time follow any surgical precautions provided by the surgeon depending on which surgical approach performed. Patients may be ordered home physical therapy for the initial 2 weeks after surgery. Patient will be weight bearing as tolerated with assistive device initially and progressed from the assistive device as able. Passive range of motion and active assistive range of motion within restrictions muscle activation with heel slides, quad sets, quad sets, isometrics in hook lying, straight leg raises, long arc quadriceps, short arc quadriceps, and progression to close kinetic chain exercises. After 6 weeks, the goal will focus on restoring range of motion soft tissue mobilization and stretching, avoiding aggressive end range stretching. Progress strength, balance, and gait with close kinetic chain exercises progressed to mini squats, and 3-way hip exercises in standing with resistance, and balance on unstable surfaces. During this time there will be focus to improve balance and pain-free range of motion and increase strength to a 4/5 by 12 weeks. After 12 weeks, the goal is to build up strength, range of motion, balance, and gait. Higher intensity training and return-to-sport exercises should be consulted with the surgeon.

20. **When do patients following THA see the greatest results?**
Patients can expect to see the most rapid gain in the first 12 to 15 weeks postoperatively in self-reported and physical performance. Slower recovery occurred in weeks 15 to 20. Patients seem to plateau at 30 to 40 weeks.

21. **When can patients expect to return to sporting activity following total hip arthroplasty?**
Research has shown approximately 40% of patients return to sporting activity between 2 and 3 months after surgery. Approximately 77% of patients return to sporting activity by 6 months after surgery. Approximately 94% of patients are able to return to sporting activity between 6 and 12 months after surgery. Activities that the vast majority of surgeons recommended without limitations or training were walking, swimming, hiking, and level biking. Surgeon recommendations seemed to vary more for sports such as ballroom dancing, cross-country biking, bowling, dancing, e-scooters, fitness/weights, golf, horseback riding, jogging, Pilates, cross-country skiing, table tennis, and yoga. Sports including basketball, boxing, soccer, gymnastics, handball, hockey, squash, climbing, volleyball, tennis, and skiing on slopes were typically not recommended or only with adequate training.

22. **Do high-impact sports affect survivorship after THA?**
    Yes, there is an increase in risk of mechanical failure for patients after THA. Survivorship at 15 years after THA was about 80% for patients participating in high-impact sports, compared with 93.5% for those who did not.

23. **Does exercise before THA improve outcomes?**
    Subjects who exercised before total hip replacement demonstrated progress that was 3 months ahead of that seen in the control group during early rehabilitation. The exercise group had two 1-hour supervised exercise sessions and also performed home exercises two times a week. The exercise group demonstrated greater stride length and gait velocity at 3 weeks after surgery. At 24 weeks postoperatively, in a 6-minute time test the exercise group was able to walk 549.7 meters, as opposed to 485.1 meters for the control group. Gait velocity was also faster in the exercise group at 24 weeks after surgery—1.57 meters per second, compared with 1.36 meters per second in the control group. A gait velocity of 1.22 meters per second is the guideline used by city engineers who set traffic signal crossing times. Patients that participated in preoperative exercises and education had decreased length of hospital stay, less postoperative pain, and improved postoperative function as compared to control group.

Bibliography

Amstutz, H. C., Le Duff, M. J., & Beaulé, P. E. (2005). Prevention and treatment of dislocation after total hip replacement using large diameter balls. *Clinical Orthopaedics and Related Research*, *429*, 108–116.

Barrack, R. L., Burak, C., & Skinner, H. B. (2004). Concerns about ceramics in THA. *Clinical Orthopaedics and Related Research*, *429*, 73–79.

Berger, R. A., Jacobs, J. J., Meneghini, R. M., Della Valle, C., Paprosky, W., & Rosenberg, A. G. (2004). Rapid rehabilitation and recovery with minimally invasive total hip arthroplasty. *Clinical Orthopaedics and Related Research*, *429*, 239–247.

Brand, R. A., & Crowninshield, R. D. (1980). The effect of cane use on hip contact force. *Clinical Orthopaedics*, *147*, 181–184.

Crompton, J., Osagie-Clouard, L., & Patel, A. (2020). Do hip precautions after posterior approach total hip arthroplasty affect dislocation rates? A systemic review of 7 studies with 6,900 patients. *Acta Orthopaedica*, *91*(6), 687–692.

Digas, G., Kärrholm, J., Thanner, J., & Herberts, P. (2007). 5-year experience of highly cross-linked polyethylene in cemented and uncemented sockets: Two randomized studies using radiostereometric analysis. *Acta Orthopaedica*, *78*, 746–754.

Dorr, L. D., Maheshwari, A. V., Long, W. T., Wan, Z., & Sirianni, L. E. (2007). Early pain relief and function after posterior minimally invasive and conventional total hip arthroplasty: A prospective, randomized, blinded study. *Journal of Bone and Joint Surgery (American)*, *89*, 1153–1160.

Harris, W. H. (2004). Highly cross-linked, electron-beam-irradiated, melted polyethylene: Some pros. *Clinical Orthopaedics and Related Research*, *429*, 63–67.

Higgins, B. T., Barlow, D. R., Heagerty, N. E., & Lin, T. J. (2014). Anterior vs. posterior approach for total hip arthroplasty, a systematic review and meta-analysis. *Journal of Arthroplasty*, *30*(3), 419–434.

Jackson-Trudelle, E., Emerson, R., & Smith, S. (2002). Outcomes of total hip arthroplasty: A study of patients one year postsurgery. *Journal of Orthopaedic and Sports Physical Therapy*, *32*, 260–267.

Kennedy, D. M., Stratford, P. W., Robarts, S., & Gollish, J. D. (2011). Using outcome measure results to facilitate clinical decisions the first year after total hip arthroplasty. *Journal of Orthopaedic and Sports Physical Therapy*, *41*(4), 232–239.

Knahr, K., Pospischill, M., Köttig, P., Schneider, W., & Plenk, H., Jr. (2007). Retrieval analysis of highly cross-linked polyethylene ace tabular liners 4 and 5 years after implantation. *Journal of Bone and Joint Surgery (British)*, *89*(8), 1036–1041.

Li, N., & Chen, L. (2012). Comparison of complications in single-incision minimally invasive THA and conventional THA. *Orthopedics*, *35*, e1552–e1558.

Magan, A. A., Radhakrishnan, G. T., Kayani, B., et al. (2021). Time for return to sport following total hip arthroplasty: a meta-analysis. *Hip International*, *33*(2), 221–230.

Magee, D. J. (1997). *Orthopedic physical assessment* (3rd ed.). Philadelphia: WB Saunders.

Malahias, M.-A., Loucas, R., Loucas, M., Denti, M., Sculco, P. K., & Greenberg, A. (2021). Preoperative opioid use is associated with higher revision rates in total joint arthroplasty: A systematic review. *Journal of Arthroplasty*, *36*(11), 1089–1093.

Morshed, S., Bozic, K. J., Ries, M. D., Malchau, H., & Colford, J. M., Jr. (2007). Comparison of cemented and uncemented fixation in total hip replacement: A meta-analysis. *Acta Orthopaedica Scandinavica*, *78*, 315–326.

Moyer, R. (2017). The value of preoperative exercise and education for patients undergoing total hip and knee arthroplasty. A systematic review and meta-analysis. *JBJS Reviews*, *5*(12), e2.

Olliver, M., Frey, S., Parratte, S., Flecher, X., & Argenson, J. -N. (2012). Does impact sport activity influence total hip arthroplasty durability? *Clinical Orthopaedics and Related Research*, *470*, 3060–3066.

Pelligrini, V. D., Clement, D., Lush-Ehmann, C., Keller, G. S., & Mc Collister Evarts, C. (1996). Natural history of hip thromboembolic disease after total hip arthroplasty. *Clinical Orthopaedics*, *333*, 27–40.

Pritchett, J. W. (2004). Nerve injury and limb lengthening after hip replacement: Treatment by shortening. *Clinical Orthopaedics and Related Research*, *418*, 168–171.

Restrepo, C., Mortazavi, S. M. J., Brothers, J., Parvizi, J., & Rothman, R. H. (2011). Hip dislocation: Are hip precautions necessary in anterior approaches? *Clinical Orthopaedics and Related Research*, *469*, 417–422.

Sah, A. P. (2022). How much hip motion is used in real-life activities? Assessment of hip flexion by a wearable sensor and implications after total hip arthroplasty. *Journal of Arthroplasty*, *37*(8S), S871–S875.

Silva, M., Heisel, C., & Schmalzreid, T. P. (2005). Metal-on-metal total hip replacement. *Clinical Orthopaedics and Related Research*, *430*, 53–61.

Tian, P., Li, Z. -J., Xu, G. -J., Sun, X. -L., & Ma, X. -L. (2017). Partial versus early full weight bearing after uncemented total hip arthroplasty: a meta-analysis. *Journal of Orthopaedic Surgery and Research*, *12*(1), 31.

Toossi, N., Adeli, B., Timperley, A. J., Haddad, F. S., Maltenfort, M., & Parvizi, J. (2013). Acetabular components in total hip arthroplasty: Is there evidence that cementless fixation is better? *Journal of Bone and Joint Surgery (American)*, *95*, 168–174.

Vu-Han, T., Hardt, S., Ascherl, R., Gwinner, C., & Perka, C. (2021). Recommendations for return to sports after total hip arthroplasty are becoming less restrictive as implants improve. *Archives of Orthopaedic and Trauma Surgery*, *141*(3), 497–507.

Wang, A. W., Gilbey, H. J., & Ackland, T. R. (2002). Perioperative exercise programs improve early return of ambulatory function after total hip arthroplasty: A randomized, controlled trial. *American Journal of Physical Medicine and Rehabilitation*, *81*, 801–806.
Warrick, D. (1995). Death and thromboembolic disease after total hip replacement: A series of 1162 cases with no routine chemical prophylaxis. *Journal of Bone and Joint Surgery*, *77*(1), 6–10.
Young-Hoo, K., Park, J.-W., Kim, J.-S., & Kim, I.-W. (2016). Twenty-five- to twenty-seven-year results of a cemented vs cementless stem in the same patients younger than 50 years of age. *Journal of Arthroplasty*, *31*(3), 662–667.

CHAPTER 68 QUESTIONS

1. **If you have a patient following posterior approach THA, which of these activities require greater hip flexion ROM than 90 degrees?**
   a. Squatting
   b. Tying shoes
   c. Transfer from toilet
   d. All of the above

2. **The majority of hip dislocations occurs during what time frame?**
   a. 1 to 4 weeks
   b. 5 to 8 weeks
   c. 9 to 12 weeks
   d. After 13 weeks

3. **How much combined range of motion of hip flexion, abduction, and external rotation is required to put on socks and shoes following THA?**
   a. 160
   b. 120
   c. 90
   d. 180

4. **What time frame do over 90% of all patients following THA able to return to sport?**
   a. 2 to 4 months
   b. 4 to 6 months
   c. 6 to 9 months
   d. 6 to 12 months

5. **Which is not an advantage of the direct anterior approach for THA?**
   a. No need for muscle or tendon repair
   b. Lower infection rate
   c. Lower dislocation rate
   d. Lower rate of significant limp

6. **What type of joint replacement has been correlated with the highest amount of cytotoxic debris?**
   a. Ceramic on ceramic
   b. Metal on metal
   c. Metal on polyethylene
   d. Ceramic on polyethylene

FUNCTIONAL ANATOMY OF THE KNEE

D.J. Denton, PT, DPT, EdD, CIDN, CVT, D.E. Jacks, PhD, and T.A. 'TAB' Blackburn, Jr., MED, PT (Life)

1. **What is a plica?**
   The plica is composed of excess tissue identified in some literature as arising from mesenchyme (or embryonic connective tissue) during the development of the knee in the first 4 months of fetal life. The mesenchyme forms the membranes that eventually divide the various compartments of the knee. The membranes that failed to be reabsorbed eventually become inward folds of the synovial lining. The infrapatellar plica originates from the intercondylar notch and enters the inferior aspect of Hoffa's fat pad.

2. **What are the symptoms of an irritated plica?**
   Clinically, the medial patellar plica is associated with carrying clinical significance as a potential cause of anteromedial knee pain, particularly in adolescents. Blunt trauma, a sudden increase in athletic activity, or any form of transient synovitis are associated with plica inflammation. Overuse causing plica inflammation in some cases leads to hypertrophic fibrosis, with the proliferation of nerves and blood vessels. This progression results in an enlarged medial plica that is less elastic and can either become impinged between the medial femoral condyle and the medial facet of the patella during knee flexion or create a shearing force over the medial femoral condyle. The progression has been referenced to be a cause for medial compartment degeneration, or knee osteoarthritis, as the articular cartilage is sloughed off by the medial plica. Clinically, inflammation or irritation of the plica is referred to as plica syndrome, medial shelf syndrome, shelf syndrome, plica synovialis, mediopatellaris syndrome, or synovial plica syndrome.

3. **Describe the patella-trochlear groove contact as the knee moves from full extension to full flexion.**
   Upon full knee extension in standing, the quadriceps muscle is relaxed and the patella is resting on the suprapatellar fat pad. The patella migrates inferiorly as the knee flexes.
   - At 20 to 30 degrees of knee flexion, the patella moves inferiorly, lying in the shallow part of the intercondylar groove, explaining why lateral patella dislocations occur near this range. The patella contacts the femur with its inferior pole.
   - At 60 to 90 degrees knee flexion the patella occupies the intercondylar groove. There is maximum contact between the patella and the intercondylar groove (one third of the posterior surface area of the patella).
   - At 135 degrees of knee flexion (near full knee flexion), the patella contacts the femur with its superior pole and rests below the intercondylar groove.

4. **Patella baja may result from adhesions caused by disruption of what bursa?**
   Patella baja is a term referencing a distally positioned patella concerning the femoral trochlea, which has been reported to result from the shortening of patellar tendon fibers, as well as traumatic and postoperative scarring. This condition can be seen as a genetic birth abnormality or acquired patella baja has been reported to occur as a postoperative complication due to anterior cruciate ligament reconstruction, injury, or weakness to the extensor apparatus, or as a consequence of major knee surgery. In these cases, surgical intervention is recommended because failure to treat patella baja has been reported to result in a limited range of motion (ROM) in extension, persistent anterior knee pain, and accelerated progression of patellofemoral osteoarthritis.
   Soft-tissue procedures including patellar tendon elongation or reconstruction, as well as the proximalization of the tibial tubercle, can be options for treatment.

5. **What portion of the capsular ligament holds the menisci to the tibia?**
   The capsular ligament of the knee is often called the coronary ligament. Anatomically the fibers of the capsule run proximal to distal. The capsule originates on the femur and courses first to the outer edge of the meniscus and then to its distal attachment on the tibia. The two distinct ligaments proximal and distal to the menisci are called the meniscofemoral ligament and the meniscotibial ligament, respectively. The meniscotibial portion of the capsule secures the menisci to the tibial plateau. Injury to the meniscofemoral portion leads to a less stable meniscal tear. If the capsule tears completely, swelling may leave the knee joint completely, giving the appearance of a milder knee injury.

6. **Discuss the role of the posterior oblique ligament.**
   Biomechanics and cadaveric studies have demonstrated that the posterior oblique ligament (POL) can be considered the predominant ligamentous structure on the posterior medial corner of the knee joint. It is located at

the posterior third of the medial collateral ligament, attached proximally to the adductor tubercle of the femur and distally to the tibia and posterior aspect of the joint capsule. The main role of the POL is to control anteromedial rotatory instability (AMRI) and to provide static resistance to the valgus loads when the knee is fully extended. Moreover, the POL plays a small role in preventing posterior translation of the tibia on the femur as a result of the posterior cruciate ligament's (PCL) strength. During a side-step cut, the POL contributes to keeping the pivot leg from opening in valgus, along with semimembranosus muscle activation. Additionally, the POL helps prevent excessive external tibial rotation and internal femoral rotation.

7. What important function does the arcuate complex provide?

Most surgeons view the posterolateral region of the knee as a functional tendoligamentous unit, which is termed the *arcuate ligament complex*. This complex encompasses the lateral collateral ligament; biceps femoris tendon; popliteus muscle and tendon; popliteal meniscal and popliteal fibular ligaments; oblique popliteal, arcuate, and fabellofibular ligaments; and lateral gastrocnemius muscle.

The arcuate ligament is a Y-shaped thickening of the posterior lateral knee capsule. The arcuate complex helps to control internal rotation of the femur on the fixed tibia during closed kinetic chain function (or external rotation of the tibia on the femur during open kinetic chain function). Patients that have injured the arcuate complex will experience instability (feeling that the knee is hyperextending) at heel strike.

8. Does the anatomical positioning of the anterior cruciate ligament dictate its function?

The major functions of the ACL are to 1) stop recurvatum of the knee to control internal rotation of the tibia on the femur during open kinetic chain or nonweight-bearing function (external rotation of the femur on the fixed tibia during closed kinetic chain or weight-bearing function) and 2) stop anterior translation of the tibia on the femur during open kinetic chain or nonweight-bearing function (posterior translation of the femur on the tibia during closed kinetic chain or weight-bearing function). This action stops the pivot-shift phenomenon. Therefore, the position of the ACL in extension of the knee elevates it against the intercondylar notch, acting like a "yard arm" to provide strength to the ligament and prevent recurvatum. Internal rotation of the tibia on the femur causes the ACL to tighten. The two main bundles of the ACL are the anterior medial and posterior lateral bundles. The posterior lateral bundle becomes tauter in extension, and the anterior medial bundle becomes more taut in flexion. This arrangement allows the ACL to control the pivot-shift through the complete knee flexion-extension range of motion. Innovative surgical techniques have been developed to reconstruct individual ACL bundles to improve control of combined internal tibial torque and valgus torque; however, evidence regarding the implications of these techniques on improved patient function is currently lacking.

9. What is the function of the posterior cruciate ligament?

The major function of the PCL is to stop posterior translation of the tibia on the femur during open kinetic chain or nonweight-bearing function or anterior translation of the femur on the fixed tibia during closed kinetic chain or weight-bearing function. Its femoral and tibial attachments in the central knee joint enable it to be an ideal passive decelerator of the femur. The PCL is composed of three bundles, which allow some portion of the ligament to be taut throughout the range of motion. When the knee is in full extension, the posterior medial bundle of the PCL is most taut. Even when all of the other ligaments have been resected, the knee maintains some stability to varus and valgus forces when the posterior medial PCL bundle is intact. As the knee moves into flexion, the anterior lateral bundle becomes more taut. When the femur moves into external rotation during closed kinetic chain or weight-bearing function, or when the tibia moves into internal rotation during open kinetic chain function, the PCL becomes tauter.

10. What is the function of the iliotibial band? How does it contribute to the integrity of the knee?

The iliotibial band (ITB) or tract is a lateral thickening of the fascia lata in the thigh. Proximally it splits into superficial and deep layers, enclosing tensor fasciae latae and anchoring this muscle to the iliac crest. It also receives most of the tendon of the gluteus maximus as it is globally a part of the overall fascia surrounding the entire thigh. The ITB is generally viewed as a band of dense fibrous connective tissue that passes over the lateral femoral epicondyle and attaches to Gerdy's tubercle on the anterolateral aspect of the tibia. ITB friction syndrome is an overuse injury well recognized as a common cause of lateral knee pain that results from repetitive friction between the ITB and the lateral femoral epicondyle, as the fibrous band "rolls over or clicks" over the epicondyle during knee movements.

11. How does the ITB affect the pivot-shift test of the knee?

The pivot-shift test assesses the integrity of the ACL and anterolateral stability to the knee. As the knee flexes during the pivot-shift test, the ITB shifts posteriorly. The ACL and the middle one third of the lateral capsular ligament normally prevent the tibia and femur from shifting. However, in their absence, the pull of the ITB allows the shift to occur, with the tibia moving posteriorly and the femur anteriorly shifting the subluxed tibia back into a normal position.

12. **Describe the anatomic reasons for patellar instability.**
The makeup of the patellofemoral joint is the undersurface of the patella and the cartilaginous anterior surface of the distal femur, comprising the trochlear groove. The proper biomechanics of the patellofemoral joint requires an intact and anatomic trochlear groove and inline congruent forces acting on the patella so that it can glide across the trochlear groove smoothly. Any disruption in this mechanism will produce dislocation of the patella out of the trochlear groove.

The bony structures of the patellofemoral joint provide stability to the patella, and any defect in the bony surface will result in instability. The normal trochlear groove has a large depth and steepness that provides inherent stability to the patellofemoral joint. Trochlear dysplasia and flattening of this groove will cause patellar instability. The major facets (total of seven facets) are medial and lateral, which are further divided into thirds. A seventh facet is on the most medial edge of the patella and is called the odd facet. Any osteochondral fracture or defect will lead to pain and instability and requires fixation.

The quadriceps tendon, patella, and patellar tendon combined make up the extensor mechanism of the knee. Disruption of the extensor mechanism along its length will result in significant patellar instability and maltracking. With regards to stability, the medial patellofemoral ligament (MPFL), patellomeniscal ligament, patellotibial ligament, and retinaculum of the knee capsule all play roles in preventing lateral patella motion and keeping the patella congruent in the trochlear groove. The strongest of these is the MPFL, which originates from the adductor tubercle to insert onto the superior medial border of the patella. Once the patella begins to enter the trochlea at 20 to 30 degrees of flexion, the bony anatomy begins to be the major stabilizer as the patella sits in the trochlear groove. A patella that does not engage in the groove until higher than normal knee flexion (condition patella alta) predisposes the patella to dislocation.

13. **Describe the anatomy of articular cartilage.**
Hyaline articular cartilage is an aneural, avascular, and lymphatic structure. Sixty-five to eighty percent of the weight of articular cartilage is formed by water, with 80% being in the superficial zone and 65% in the deep zones. Water permits load-dependent deformation of the cartilage. It provides nutrition and medium for lubrication, creating a low-friction gliding surface. Ten to 20% of the wet weight of the articular cartilage is formed by collagen. Type II collagen forms the principal component (90%–95%) of the macrofibrillar framework and provides tensile strength to the articular cartilage. Proteoglycans form 10% to 20% wet weight and provide a compressive strength to the articular cartilage. Chondrocytes are highly specialized cells, forming only 1% to 5% of volume, are sparsely spread within the matrix. Chondrocytes organize the collagen, proteoglycans, and noncollagenous proteins into a unique and highly specialized tissue suitable for carrying out the functions stated above.

14. **Describe the arterial blood vessels of the knee.**
The popliteal artery begins at the adductor hiatus as a continuation of the femoral artery. The course of the popliteal artery runs across the popliteal fossa ending at popliteus dividing into anterior and posterior tibial arteries. The five genicular (superior lateral, superior medial, middle, inferior lateral, and inferior medial) supply the capsule and ligaments of the knee. The arteries form genicular anastomosis surrounding the joint providing collateral arterial profusion through full knee flexion even in the event of popliteal artery kinking.

15. **Do the cruciate ligaments cross?**
From their tibial attachment sites at the anterior (ACL) and posterior (PCL) intercondylar areas, the cruciate ligaments cross before they attach to the lateral and medial femoral condyles, respectively. The cruciate ligaments also twist upon themselves during knee flexion and extension.

16. **Describe the alignment of the femur and tibia during weight bearing.**
The knee is most stable in the extended position. In full extension the collateral and cruciate ligaments are taut, and tendons of large muscles provide secondary support. Full extension of the knee medially rotates the femur optimally aligning the condyles of the femur with the tibial plateau. The menisci add depth to the surface of the tibia and aid in the dissipation of force. The increased articulation unloads muscles of the leg and thigh while maintaining moderate stability of the joint. The normal knee joint alignment compared with the mechanical axis is in 2° to 3° of varus. If this alignment is altered by degenerative changes, fracture, or genetic conditions, excessive stress is placed on either the medial or the lateral tibiofemoral joint compartment. Tibial varum or femoral valgus (angle greater than 170–175 degrees) leads to increased medial compartment stress, whereas femoral varum or tibial valgus (angle less than 170–175 degrees) leads to increased lateral compartment stress.

17. **Are there differences between male and female knee joint anatomy and biomechanics?**
No particular anatomic or biomechanical knee joint characteristic is unique to either gender. However, females tend to have a wider pelvis, greater femoral anteversion, more frequent evidence of a coxa varus–genu valgus hip and knee joint alignment with lateral tibial torsion, a greater Q-angle (18 degrees vs 13 degrees), more elastic capsuloligamentous tissues, a narrower femoral notch, and smaller diameter cruciate ligaments.

18. **What is the normal amount of tibial torsion and how does the physical therapist measure it clinically?**
    Tibial torsion can be measured by having the patient sit with their knees flexed to 90 degrees over the edge of an examining table. The therapist then places the thumb of one hand over the prominence of one malleolus and the index finger of the same hand over the prominence of the other malleolus. Looking directly down over the end of the distal thigh, the therapist visualizes the axes of the knee and of the ankle. These lines are not normally parallel but instead form a 12- to 18-degree angle because of lateral tibial rotation. Tibial torsion greater than 30 degrees is referred to as abnormal external tibial torsion. Tibial torsion less than zero degrees is considered abnormal and referred to as internal tibial torsion.

19. **What is the function of the popliteus musculotendinous complex?**
    The popliteus musculotendinous complex functions as a static and dynamic restraint to external rotation especially on knee flexion and as a smaller stabilizer regarding internal rotation anterior translation and varus force. It has been denoted as the "5th ligament of the knee."

Bibliography

Cherian, J. J., Kapadia, B. H., Banerjee, S., Jauregui, J. J., Issa, K., & Mont, M. A. (2014). Mechanical, anatomical, and kinematic axis in TKA: Concepts and practical applications. *Current Reviews in Musculoskeletal Medicine*, *7*(2), 89–95.

Csintalan, R. P., Schulz, M. M., Woo, J., McMahon, P. J., & Lee, T. Q. (2002). Gender differences in patellofemoral joint biomechanics. *Clinical Orthopaedics and Related Research*, *402*, 260–269.

Fairclough, J., Hayashi, K., Toumi, H., et al. (2006). The functional anatomy of the iliotibial band during flexion and extension of the knee: Implications for understanding iliotibial band syndrome. *Journal of Anatomy*, *208*(3), 309–316.

Feger, J., & Marghany, B. (2021). Popliteus tendon. Reference article, Radiopaedia.org. (accessed on 27 Dec 2021). https://doi.org/10.53347/rID-89179

Fox, A. J., Bedi, A., & Rodeo, S. A. (2012). The basic science of human knee menisci: structure, composition, and function. *Sports Health*, *4*(4), 340–351.

Kim, Y. M., Joo, Y. B., Lee, W. Y., Park, I. Y., & Park, Y. C. (2020). Patella-patellar tendon angle decreases in patients with infrapatellar fat pad syndrome and medial patellar plica syndrome. *Knee Surgery, Sports Traumatology, Arthroscopy*, *28*(8), 2609–2618.

Jibri, Z., Jamieson, P., Rakhra, K. S., Sampaio, M. L., & Dervin, G. (2019). Patellar maltracking: An update on the diagnosis and treatment strategies. *Insights into Imaging*, *10*(1), 65.

Logterman, S. L., Wydra, F. B., & Frank, R. M. (2018). Posterior cruciate ligament: Anatomy and biomechanics. *Current Reviews in Musculoskeletal Medicine*, *11*(3), 510–514.

Schindler, O. (2014). "The Sneaky Plica" revisited: Morphology, pathophysiology and treatment of synovial plicae of the knee. *Knee Surgery, Sports Traumatology, Arthroscopy*, *22*(2), 247–262.

Stuberg, W., Temme, J., Kaplan, P., Clarke, A., & Fuchs, R. (1991). Measurement of tibial torsion and thigh-foot angle using goniometry and computed tomography. *Clinical Orthopaedics and Related Research*, *272*, 208–212.

Suero, E. M., Njoku, I. U., Voigt, M. R., Lin, J., Koenig, D., & Pearle, A. D. (2013). The role of the iliotibial band during the pivot shift test. *Knee Surgery, Sports Traumatology, Arthroscopy*, *21*(9), 2096–2100.

Wolfe, S., Varacallo, M., Thomas, J.D., et al. Patellar instability. [Updated 2021 Jul 20]. In: StatPearls [Internet]. Treasure Island (FL): StatPearls Publishing. Available from: https://www.ncbi.nlm.nih.gov/books/NBK482427/

CHAPTER 69 QUESTIONS

1. **The most common symptom associated with an irritated plica is ___________.**
   a. Lateral retinacular laxity
   b. Mechanical joint locking
   c. Medial patellofemoral joint tenderness
   d. Instability of the knee in full extension

2. **The arcuate complex of the knee does not include the ________________.**
   a. Lateral collateral ligament
   b. Extension from the popliteus tendon
   c. Posterior third of the lateral knee joint capsule
   d. Posterior oblique ligament

3. **The posterolateral bundle of the ACL primarily serves to limit ___________.**
   a. Tibial internal rotation during extension
   b. Anterior tibial translation during extension
   c. Tibial external rotation during flexion
   d. Posterior tibial translation during flexion

PATELLOFEMORAL DISORDERS

T.R. Malone, EdD, MS, BS and A.L. Pfeifle, EdD, PT

CHAPTER 70

1. **What is the Q-angle?**
   The Q-angle is measured by extending a line through the center of the patella to the anterior superior iliac spine and another line from the tibial tubercle through the center of the patella. The intersection of these two lines is the Q-angle; the normal value for this angle is 13 to 18 degrees. Men tend to have Q-angles closer to 13 degrees, and women usually have Q-angles at the high end of this range. Because the Q-angle is a measure of bony alignment, it can be altered only through bony realignment surgical procedures. Despite the common opinion among clinicians that excessive Q-angle is a contributing factor to patellofemoral (PF) pain, it has not been shown to be a predictive factor in the outcome of patients with PF pain undergoing rehabilitation. Always remember when they have L pain and an abnormal Q-angle, they have an R side with an approximately equally abnormal Q-angle and are not symptomatic.

2. **What is the tubercle-sulcus angle?**
   A measurement similar to the Q-angle, the tubercle-sulcus angle is reported to be a more accurate assessment of the quadriceps vector. It is measured with the patient sitting and the knee at 90 degrees of flexion. The tubercle-sulcus angle is formed by a line drawn from the tibial tubercle to the center of the patella, which normally should be perpendicular to the transepicondylar axis.

3. **What may cause an increase in the Q-angle?**
   Excessive femoral anteversion, external tibial torsion, genu valgum, and subtalar hyperpronation can contribute to an increase in the Q-angle. When these conditions are found together, a patient is often said to have malicious or "miserable" malalignment syndrome. However, it should be noted that all of these static measures of angles (in isolation or in aggregate) are not strongly predictive of patellofemoral dysfunction—be careful to not overly rely on static measures. The last few years, many additional static measures have been developed using points on the patella (A-Angle—goiniometric assessment) and via imaging (Tibial Tubercle distance to Trochlear Groove, Trochlear depth/width, etc.). Importantly, morphology and kinematics do not often correlate with pain.

4. **What anatomic structures encourage lateral tracking of the patella?**
   Bony factors, such as a dysplastic patella, patella alta, or a shallow intercondylar groove, can contribute to lateral tracking of the patella. Soft tissue structures, such as a tight lateral retinaculum or a tight iliotibial band (which has a fibrous band that extends to the lateral patella), can encourage lateral tracking of the patella.

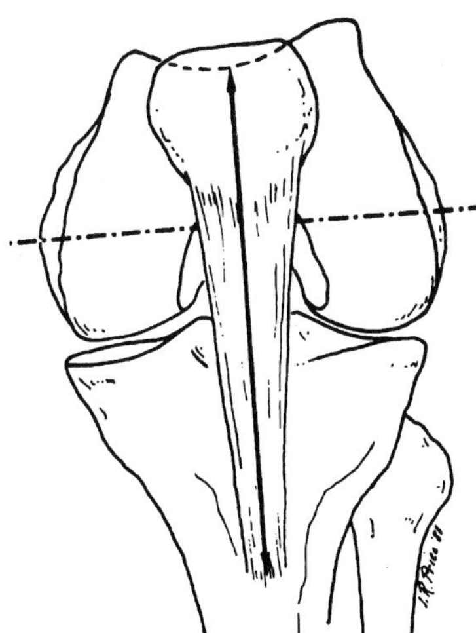

A normal tubercle-sulcus angle at 90 degrees of knee flexion. A line from the tibial tubercle to the center of the patella should be perpendicular to the transepicondylar axis. From Kolowich PA, et al. (1990). Lateral release of the patella: Indications and contraindications, *Am J Sports Med.* 18, 359–365.

5. **Define patella alta.**
Patella alta refers to a cephalad position of the patella. Usually it is diagnosed by radiography and by determining the ratio between the length of the patellar tendon and the vertical length of the patella (Insall-Salvati ratio). The length of the patellar tendon is determined by measuring the distance between the inferior pole of the patella and the most cephalad part of the tibial tubercle. The normal ratio is 1:1. If the ratio is >1:3, the patient has patella alta. Patients with patella alta are more susceptible to patellar instability because the patella is less able to seat itself in the intercondylar groove.

6. **What is the function of the vastus medialis oblique (VMO) muscle?**
In their classic cadaver study of quadriceps function, Lieb and Perry1968 reported that the primary function of the VMO is to counter the pull of the vastus lateralis and thus prevent lateral subluxation of the patella. They concluded that the ability of the VMO to contract and maintain patellar alignment throughout the full range of active knee extension enhanced the ability of the vastus lateralis to produce knee extension. Furthermore, when acting without the other quadriceps muscles, the VMO produced no knee extension. Importantly, we cannot isolate the VMO but rather we strengthen the quadriceps as a whole—all the muscles of the group. It is true that there is high EMG in extension—but it is true of all portions—not just the VMO.

7. **How is chondromalacia classified?**
The four types of chondromalacia are based on arthroscopic appearance:
- Type I—patellar surface intact; softening, swelling, "blister" formation
- Type II—cracks and fissuring in surface but no large cavities
- Type III—fibrillation; bone may be exposed; "crab-meat" appearance
- Type IV—crater formation; underlying bone involvement

8. **How is PF pain classified?**
Merchant classified patients according to five different etiologic factors: 1) trauma, 2) PF dysplasia, 3) idiopathic chondromalacia patellae, 4) osteochondritis dissecans, and 5) synovial plicae. These categories were subdivided into 38 subcategories. Others have classified patients with PF pain according to radiologic findings. A simple classification scheme that helps to determine treatment was proposed by Holmes and Clancy 1998. The three major categories are PF instability, PF pain with malalignment, and PF pain without malalignment. In addition, Wilk et al. proposed a classification system that focuses on the underlying anatomic cause and presenting symptoms. The four major "rehabilitation" categories associated with this system require the clinician to recognize instability, tension, friction, and compression disorders and the specific protocols for their appropriate treatment.

9. **Describe treatment based on the classification scheme of Holmes and Clancy 1998.**
Patellofemoral instability includes patients with patellar subluxation or dislocation—either recurrent or a single episode. First-time or infrequent subluxations and dislocations are treated with rehabilitation. Patients who continue to have problems after exhaustive therapy often require surgery.

PF pain without malalignment includes a number of diagnoses, such as osteochondritis dissecans of the patella or femoral trochlea, fat pad syndrome, patellar tendinitis, bipartite patella, prepatellar bursitis, PF osteoarthritis, apophysitis, plica syndrome, and trauma (eg, quadriceps or patellar tendon rupture, patella fracture, contusion). Most patients are treated conservatively with physical therapy, including hip and quadriceps strengthening, lower extremity stretching, and treatment of potential contributing factors.

PF pain with malalignment includes patients with increased Q-angles, tight lateral retinaculum, grossly inadequate medial stabilizers, patella alta or baja, and dysplastic femoral trochlea. Such patients often are treated with surgery again only after an appropriate trial of rehabilitation.

10. Describe the classification scheme of Wilk et al. 1998.

CATEGORY	AFFECTED ANATOMIC AREA	PRESENTING SYMPTOMS	EXAMINATION	TREATMENT
Instability (hypermobile patella)	Ligamentous structures (passive) or insufficient musculature (active)	Patellar instability (subluxation/ dislocation)	Integrity of static patellar restraints	Avoid terminal knee extension
			Medial and lateral patellar glides	Suggest exercise from 90 to 30 degrees
				Use external support braces (taping, late buttress brace, pain-free ROM)
				Open- and closed-chain exercise
Tension (overload of muscle, tendon, or tendon-bone junction)	Muscle, tendon, or tendon-bone junction	Pain with eccentric actions, particularly maximal efforts	Palpation of inferior patellar pole, patellar ligament, and insertion of patellar ligament onto tibial tuberosity	Open- and closed-chain eccentric exercise emphasized
	Commonly related conditions jumper's knee, patellar tendonitis, and Osgood-Schlatter disease			Plyometrics
				Stretch tight opposing muscles
				Physical agents and electromodalities
Friction (soft tissue rubbing)	Friction points under sliding tissues	Pain with repetitive loaded flexion-extension	Observation of activity that replicates pain	Avoid repeated flexion and extension exercises
	Commonly involved structures: ITB, plica, fat pad		Palpation of structures associated with common friction syndromes	Exercise in pain-free ROM; exercise above and below painful ROM

Continued

CATEGORY	AFFECTED ANATOMIC AREA	PRESENTING SYMPTOMS	EXAMINATION	TREATMENT
Compression (articular and periarticular compression)	Articular surfaces	Osteoarthritis, pain with function under load	Compression testing of PF joint via special clinical tests of functional movements that apply compressive loads to PF joint	Key is to increase quadriceps function to assist in absorbing weight-bearing loads
			Radiographic and other imaging studies helpful	Exercise in pain-free ROM in unloaded environment (pool)

ITB, Iliotibial band; ROM, range of motion.

11. **How can the system of Wilk et al. 1998 be applied to common anterior knee pain disorders?**

GENERAL NAME/DISORDER	TREATMENT CATEGORY
Lateral patellar compression syndrome	Compression
Global patellar pressure syndrome	Compression
Patellar instability	Instability
Patellar trauma (depends on structure)	Compression or friction
Osteochondritis dissecans	Compression
Articular defect	Compression or friction
Suprapatellar plica	Friction
Fat pad irritation	Friction or compression
Medial retinacular pain	Friction
Medial patellofemoral ligament	Friction or instability
Iliotibial band syndrome	Friction
Bursitis	Friction or compression
Muscle strain	Tension
Tendinosis/tendinitis	Tension
Osgood-Schlatter disease (apophysitis)	Tension

12. **What is lateral pressure syndrome?**
Lateral pressure syndrome, which can result in PF pain, is caused by a tight lateral retinaculum that pulls and tilts the patella laterally, increasing pressure on its lateral facet. Treatment includes stretching of the lateral retinaculum, such as medial glides/tilts, and often includes proximal hip musculature through the iliotibial tract to thus "stretch" the distal iliotibial band. McConnell 1986 advocates quadriceps strengthening exercises with a medial glide of the patella with patellar taping. If rehabilitation is not successful, a lateral retinacular release often is performed.

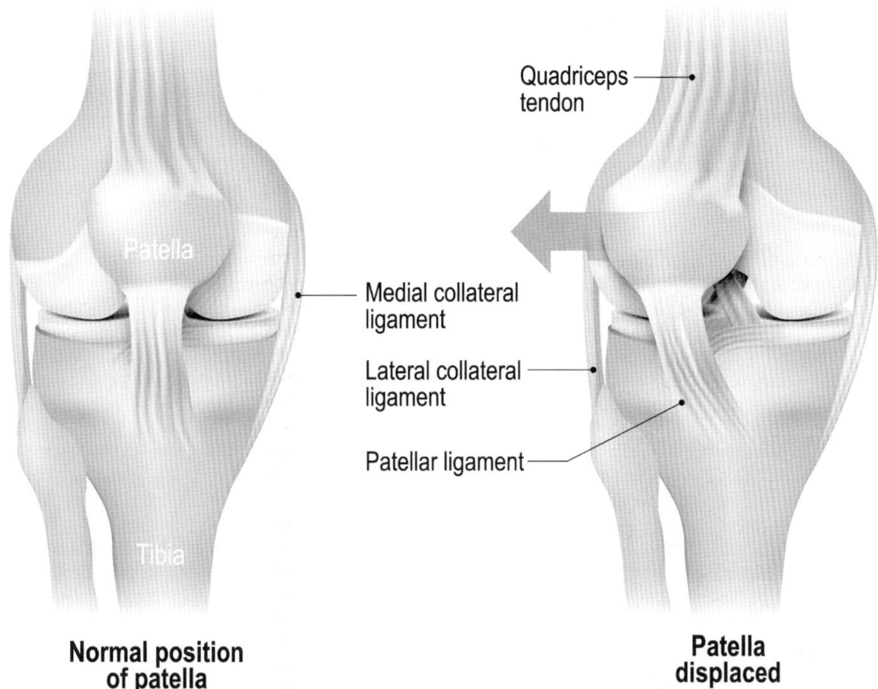

A tight lateral retinaculum can result in a lateral pull increasing pressures resulting in stretching of the medial soft tissues. (From www.istockphoto.com/ttsz.)

13. **Define bipartite patella.**
    Bipartite patellas still have an intact ossification center, most commonly at the superolateral pole. They are present in about 2% of adults and usually are asymptomatic. An anteroposterior radiograph of the bipartite patella may be mistaken for a fracture by the inexperienced eye. Extremely active people may irritate or disrupt this epiphyseal plate, causing PF pain. This area also can become painful after direct trauma to the patella. A bone scan may assist the clinician in diagnosing symptomatic disruption of the bipartite patella. If it remains symptomatic, surgical excision may be performed.

14. **What is Sinding-Larsen-Johansson disease?**
    Sinding-Larsen-Johansson disease is apophysitis of the distal pole of the patella. Physical therapy intervention would consist of relative rest, temporary heel lift, light stretching of the gastroc/soleus, hamstrings and quadriceps muscle groups, and gentle strengthening that is pain free in nature progressing to functional activities. This can be contrasted with apophysitis at the inferior insertion of the patellar ligament to the tibia resulting in Osgood-Schlatter disease, which again typically responds to a comprehensive physical therapy intervention.

15. **Can a leg length discrepancy contribute to PF pain?**
    Few authors describe the precise relationship between PF pain and leg length. However, the common compensations that can result from leg length discrepancy theoretically may contribute to PF pain. Functional shortening of the longer lower extremity may involve excessive subtalar pronation, genu valgus, forefoot abduction, and/or walking with a partially flexed knee. All of these common situations can distort PF mechanics.

16. **Because articular cartilage is aneural, what tissues around the PF joint cause PF pain?**
Normally, healthy articular cartilage absorbs stress across the PF joint. However, when the cartilage is not healthy, stresses are transferred to the subchondral bone, which is highly innervated. Subchondral bone is often thought to be the source of pain arising from the PF joint. Other structures around the PF joint also can cause peripatellar pain, including the infrapatellar fat pad, medial plica, bursa, and distal iliotibial band.

17. **Define Hoffa's disease.**
Hoffa's disease (fat pad syndrome) manifests as pain and swelling of the infrapatellar fat pad, usually from direct trauma to the anterior knee. Tenderness often is present at the anteromedial and anterolateral joint lines and on either side of the patellar tendon. A large fat pad also may become entrapped between the anterior articular surfaces of the knee with forced knee extension.

18. **How is Hoffa's disease treated?**
Treatment normally begins with protection of the anterior knee, particularly during activities where repetitive contusion may occur. Local physical agents such as ice or ultrasound also may be used. Quadriceps strengthening should be performed to prevent weakness or atrophy resulting from disuse. At times, isometrics may be effective in pain-free positions early in the rehabilitation.

19. **Describe the mechanism of pain stemming from the medial plica.**
The medial plica is a crescent-shaped, rudimentary synovial fold extending from the quadriceps tendon to around the medial femoral condyle and inserting into the fat pad. The medial plica can be injured with a direct blow to the knee or through overuse activities such as repetitive squatting, running, cycling (especially with the use of toe clips), or jumping. Inflammation and edema can lead to stiffening and contracture of the plica. Contracted tissue running repetitively over the medial femoral condyle can cause pain and even erosion of the articular surface of the medial femoral condyle.

20. **How is plica syndrome diagnosed?**
Patients with plica syndrome have similar complaints as those with PF joint pain. Pain is aggravated by running, squatting, jumping, and prolonged sitting with the knee flexed. The most frequent clinical sign is tenderness located one finger's breadth medial to the patella. The fold is often palpable, especially when the knee is flexed and the plica is stretched across the medial femoral condyle. Techniques designed to assess the presence of plica syndrome include the stutter test, Hughston's plica test, and the mediopatellar plica test, but their sensitivity and specificity have not been documented via studies with large numbers. However, MRI is reported to have a sensitivity and specificity of up to 95% and 72%, respectively.

21. **Define housemaid's knee.**
Housemaid's knee is the layman's term for prepatellar bursitis. This injury occurs when the prepatellar bursa is subjected to blunt trauma or repetitive microtrauma over the anterior knee, often found in individuals who work on their knees (carpenters or gardeners). Swelling in the prepatellar bursa occurs almost immediately and varies from slight to severe. Treatment consists of protecting the area from further trauma, applying ice, administering antiinflammatory medications, and performing exercises to maintain range of motion and strength.

22. **Describe the mechanism for patellar dislocation.**
The typical mechanism is external rotation of the tibia combined with valgus stress to the knee. Frequently this is actually the result of internal rotation of the femur over the "fixed" tibia with the tibia thus becoming externally rotated and valgus associated with knee positioning. This is often related to strong quadriceps activation. Patellar dislocation also may result from blunt trauma that pushes the patella laterally.

23. **What population is more susceptible to patellar dislocations?**
Patellar dislocations occur slightly more frequently in women than in men. Patellar dislocations typically affect the adolescent population, with the frequency of their occurrence decreasing with age. Patients with patellar dislocation often experience recurrent episodes, especially adolescent patients.

24. **What is the rate of repeat dislocation?**
Reports in the literature on the rate of repeat dislocation vary. Repeat dislocation rates among first-time dislocations treated with immobilization are 20% to 43%. The rate depends to a significant degree on the presence of congenital predisposing factors such as PF dysplasia.

25. **Can hip weakness contribute to PF pain?**
From initial contact to midstance, the hip rotates internally. The external rotators must control this motion eccentrically. If the external rotators are weak, they may not decelerate internal rotation effectively. The result is excessive hip internal rotation, which functionally increases the Q-angle and encourages additional contact

pressures between the lateral patellar facet and the lateral portion of the trochlear groove. Powers has proposed as an analogy for this movement the alteration of a train track under the train.

Hip extension weakness also can contribute to PF pain. During a weight-bearing activity such as climbing stairs, the hip and knee extensors work together to elevate the body. People with weak hip extensors may recruit the knee extensors to a greater degree, thus creating greater PF joint reaction force. By itself this reaction force may not cause a problem; in association with malalignment, however, it may contribute to PF pain.

Several researchers have increasingly examined hip weakness as either a result or a cause of patellofemoral pain syndromes. Proximal strengthening is now often a significant part of PFP rehabilitation. Numerous authors have now documented that utilizing a regional interdependence approach and strengthening the hip abductor, hip extensors, and hip external rotators results in improved function and a reduction of pain in patients suffering from PFP thus documenting clinical success through use of proximally based approaches to PF pain management. It is unknown if PFP causes hip weakness or if proximal hip weakness contributes to or causes PFP. Interestingly, one recent publication outlined that hip weakness may be the result of PFP rather than being related as the cause, so we must be careful in broad statements related to proximal musculature. The Clinical Practice Guidelines for Patellofemoral Pain (2019) strongly indicates that the best approach to management is multidimensional and exercise being paramount to successful outcomes.

26. What criteria are used to assess patellar instability?

1. Static approach—if the examiner can glide the patella laterally >50% of the total patellar width over the edge of the lateral femoral condyle, the patella is said to be unstable.
2. Dynamic technique—examiner observes patellar tracking as the patient moves from approximately 30 degrees of flexion to complete extension. If the patella makes an abrupt lateral movement at terminal extension, it may be considered unstable. This finding also is called a "J" sign because the patella follows the path of an inverted "J." Recognize there is significant subjectivity in this assessment.

27. Are radiologic studies useful?

Routine radiologic studies can show the depth of the intercondylar groove, level of congruence of the PF joint, presence of patella alta or baja, and patellar tilt. When instability is the focus, these tests are helpful as significant structural abnormality may limit the success of conservative measures. Although helpful, there is significant "greyness" in the analyses and applications of these measures and probably are most valuable when very significant differences are identified.

28. What views are best to examine the PF joint?

The Merchant view provides an excellent view of the PF joint. The radiograph is shot with the patient in supine position with the legs over the edge of the examination table and the knees in approximately 45 degrees of flexion. The x-ray beam is aligned parallel to the femoral condyles. From this view, the clinician can see the shape of the articular surface of the patella and femoral condyles, PF joint space, medial and lateral facets, and degree of medial or lateral tilt of the patella.

29. Define the congruence angle.

The congruence angle is measured from a Merchant's view and provides information about patellar position. A normal congruence angle is $\pm$ 6 degrees (see figure). Studies have shown the normal congruence angle to be -6 degrees in men and -10 degrees in women. CT scans delineate this better than radiographs, and higher values tend to be associated with patellar subluxation.

30. Is MRI a useful tool to assess patients with PF pain?

With arthroscopy as the gold standard, McCauley et al. 2001 found that MRI had a sensitivity of 86%, specificity of 74%, and accuracy of 81%. The accuracy of MRI in identifying patients with chondromalacia patellae is excellent (accuracy of 89%) for identifying stage III or IV chondromalacia and poor for identifying stage I or II chondromalacia patellae.

31. Does strengthening of the quadriceps help patients with PF pain?

Almost all rehabilitation programs for patients with PF pain include some type of quadriceps strengthening exercises. Natri et al. 1998 examined 19 factors to determine the best predictors of positive outcome, with quadriceps strength being the single best predictor of outcome. According to Natri et al., the smaller the difference in quadriceps strength between the affected and the unaffected extremity, the better the resultant outcome. Bennett and Stauber reported that a few weeks of concentric/eccentric quadriceps strength training within a pain-free range of motion obliterated an eccentric strength deficit and provided pain relief in patients with PF pain. Thomee compared 12-week isometric and eccentric quadriceps training programs in the rehabilitation of patients with PF pain and found significant increases in vertical jump height, knee extension torque, and activity level and decreases in pain for both groups. Recent reviews of the literature examining evidence for rehabilitation efficacy in these patients demonstrate very good evidence for the positive effects of pain-free strengthening but somewhat limited support for ancillary interventions.

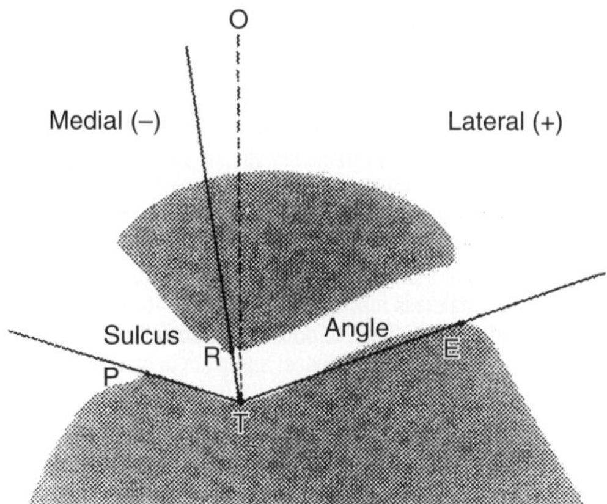

The congruence angle is formed by line TO and TR. A normal value is ±6 degrees. (From Merchant AC. (1988). Classification of patellofemoral disorders. *Arthroscopy*, 4:235–240.)

32. **Do all patients need to perform aggressive quadriceps strengthening exercises?**
The answer can be found by examining the classification schemes for PF pain. Patients should be treated specifically, depending on the particular problem. In patients with patellar instability, aggressive quadriceps strengthening in the safe parts of the range of motion is a key component of rehabilitation. Patients with global patellar pressure syndrome may have a primary flexibility problem. Although quadriceps strengthening exercises are included in this rehabilitation program, stretching and mobility exercises are the main emphasis.

33. **Does electromyographic (EMG) biofeedback strength training help patients with PF pain?**
Few studies support the use of biofeedback training in the rehabilitation of patients with PF pain. Early research suggested a statistically significant increase in recruitment of the VMO compared with the vastus lateralis after 3 weeks of biofeedback training. The increase of 6%, however, is unlikely to be clinically meaningful. Ingersoll and Knight 1991 found that terminal knee extension exercises without EMG biofeedback resulted in a more lateral patellar position than performing the same exercises with VMO EMG biofeedback. The preponderance of the literature supports EMG biofeedback as an adjunct rather than as a primary focus.

34. **What are the advantages of nonweight-bearing exercises for patients with PF pain?**
Traditional nonweight-bearing strengthening exercises, such as seated knee extension, offer many advantages to patients with PF pain. Of primary importance, the knee joint and the quadriceps work independently during nonweight-bearing exercises. The only muscle group that can perform knee extension in the nonweight-bearing position is the quadriceps. Other muscle groups cannot substitute for weak or pain-inhibited quadriceps. Thus a maximal strengthening stimulus is provided for the quadriceps. In addition, ROM can be carefully controlled. Strengthening in a limited range can be easily achieved with most equipment. Finally, the amount of resistance also can be easily controlled with nonweight-bearing quadriceps strengthening.

35. **What are the disadvantages of nonweight-bearing exercises?**
Nonweight-bearing strengthening is often described as nonfunctional. The quadriceps muscles do not work in isolation during normal activities. Strengthening in the nonweight-bearing position does not train the lower extremity muscle groups to work together in synchrony or sequenced recruitment. In addition, in an exercise such as seated knee extension, the quadriceps are working maximally at end-range extension—the position at which the PF joint is most unstable. If the patient has PF instability and/or quadriceps imbalance that directs the patella laterally, the patella may easily track abnormally in complete extension. Thus selective use of open chain/nonweight-bearing exercise and control of the appropriate range of motion used appear vital.

36. **What are the advantages of weight-bearing exercises for patients with PF pain?**
The primary advantage is that the weight-bearing position is the position of function for the knee joint. An exercise such as the lateral step-up allows the quadriceps to train in synchrony with other muscle groups to

complete the activity. Although the research supporting this concept is limited, the law of specificity of training suggests this type of training should lead to the greatest improvement in functional performance. In addition, quadriceps activity is minimal as the knee approaches terminal extension. Therefore minimal quadriceps activity in the least stable position of the PF joint does not encourage lateral tracking of the patella. This advantage is especially important if the patient has patellar hypermobility or muscle imbalance that encourages lateral tracking.

37. **What is the main disadvantage of weight-bearing exercises?**
In the weight-bearing position, other muscle groups, specifically the hip extensors and soleus muscle, can contribute to knee extension force. Therefore patients with weakness or pain inhibition of the quadriceps may rely on other muscles to perform the knee extension. The result is insufficient stimulus for the quadriceps and minimal strength gains.

38. **Are open-chain or closed-chain exercises better for a patient with PF pain?**
Clinicians should focus on interventions that enable pain-free actions and target the underlying "cause" with an appropriate protocol (instability, tension, friction, compression). Integration of both open and closed activities appears optimal whenever possible. A recent review of the current evidence emphasizes the utility of an integrated approach that fits the specific presentation of the patient.

39. **Can the VMO be strengthened in isolation?**
This question is highly controversial. Some studies support the concept of preferential recruitment of the VMO. The VMO is more active than the vastus lateralis during hip adduction. Laprade et al. 1998 reported that the VMO is more active than the vastus lateralis with tibial internal rotation. It remains questionable whether the differences are clinically significant. Many studies do not support the concept of selective recruitment of the VMO over the vastus lateralis. Most clinicians have come to accept that there is very limited opportunity for signficant selectivity—we strengthen the quadriceps.

40. **Is it better to perform quadriceps strengthening in a specific part of the knee's range of motion?**
The answer may depend on the patient's specific problem. If lateral tracking or patellar instability is a concern, the patient should avoid strengthening in the last 40 degrees, where the patella is not well seated in the intercondylar groove. If lateral tracking or patellar instability is not a problem, strengthening in the range of 0 to 90 degrees is generally safe. At the other end of the spectrum, extreme amounts of knee flexion (>90 degrees) result in higher PF joint reaction forces and should be avoided when compressive loading is a concern.

41. **Tightness of which muscles can contribute to PF pain?**
Tightness of several musculotendinous groups has been implicated as a contributing factor to PF pain, including the gastrocnemius-soleus group, hamstrings, and iliotibial band. Inflexible plantar flexors may not allow full ankle dorsiflexion, which may result in a compensatory increase in subtalar pronation. This increase may encourage lateral tracking of the patella. Hamstring inflexibility is thought to cause an increase in quadriceps contraction to overcome the passive resistance of the tight hamstrings. The result is an increase in PF joint reaction force and quadriceps fatigue, as well as a decrease in dynamic patellar stabilization. Finally, the distal iliotibial band has fibers that attach to the lateral retinaculum. Tightness of the distal iliotibial band may encourage lateral tracking of the patella. The distal portion of the iliotibial band can be stretched by performing medial glides of the patella with the hip adducted. Patellar taping also provides a prolonged passive stretch to the retinacular tissues but the actual impact may be neurologic, enabling enhanced muscle activation.

42. **Should physical modalities be a component of the rehabilitation program?**
Ice can be an effective modality to decrease pain and inflammation in patients with patellofemoral pain syndrome. Electrical stimulation may aid in quadriceps muscle reeducation in patients with inhibition of the quadriceps resulting from pain or effusion. Very limited data exist on the efficacy of dry needling in these patients. The randomized trials have not reported an added value and thus use as a primary treatment cannot be recommended—consistent with the recent CPG on patellar pain.

43. **Is patellar taping (McConnell taping) an effective intervention for patients with PF pain syndrome?**
Patellar taping is thought to improve "functional" patellar alignment and decrease pain to allow the patient to perform rehabilitation exercises more effectively. Many studies report a decrease in pain or an increase in knee extension moment with patellar taping. Whether the taping actually alters patellar position or alters neuromuscular responses of the lower limb (facilitation, inhibition, and proprioception) is still unknown. Taping has the advantage over bracing because it can be customized to fit the patient's specific patellar alignment problem. However, the reliability of patellar orientation assessment has been poor. The majority of tape use is probably associated with

attempting to provide a medial pull (taping lateral to medial) on the "patella." Past reviews have suggested that patellar taping is effective at reducing patellofemoral pain; however, most recent reviews indicate that the efficacy as a primary intervention is limited. Taping is probably best thought of as an adjunct to facilitate strengthening.

44. Is kinesio taping an effective intervention for patients with PF pain syndrome?
At this time there is very limited/weak evidence to support the use of kinesio taping for patients with PF pain syndrome. It has a very limited role per recent literature.

45. Is bracing beneficial for the patient with PF pain?
Early reports suggested decreased PF pain in 93% of patients who used an elastic sleeve brace with a patella cutout and lateral pad. Shellock et al. 1994 used MRI to demonstrate centralization of the patella with a patellar realignment brace during active movement. Bracing generally is thought to "more likely" be beneficial in patients with patellar instability than in patients with patellar compression syndromes.

46. How is a patellar tendon strap supposed to alleviate PF pain?
One study reported success in 16 of 17 patients who used an infrapatellar strap. The proposed mechanism for the success of the strap was that it displaced the patella upward and slightly anteriorly. In addition, it was proposed that compression of the patellar tendon altered PF mechanics. Theoretically, elevation of the patella may slightly diminish PF joint reaction force, and compression of the patellar tendon may reduce excessive lateral movement of the tibial tubercle during tibial external rotation. Another publication indicates that patellar tendon straps significantly reduce the measured strain at the site of a "jumper's knee lesion" within a patellar tendon. Thus there are well-supported data indicating this device may be a valuable adjunct.

47. What is the relationship between foot mechanics and PF pain?
Multiple studies have demonstrated a relationship between foot posture and PF pain. Powers et al. 1995 found that patients with PF pain had an increase in rearfoot varus compared with controls without PF pain. Klingman et al. 1997 used radiographic analysis to show that orthotic posting of the subtalar joint in patients with excessive foot pronation results in less lateral displacement of the patella. These data indicate relationships but not necessarily "cause and effects." Further research is required for definitive implications.

48. Are foot orthotics beneficial for patients with PF pain?
Many clinicians treating patients with PF pain provide anecdotal support for using orthotics. The clinician must treat the patient according to the classification of PF pain. If abnormal foot mechanics are suspected as an etiologic factor, orthotics may play a role in treatment. Eng et al. 1993, Lack et al. 2014, and Mills et al. 2012 showed that patients treated with soft orthotics and exercise had better outcomes than patients treated with an exercise program alone. The use of orthotics appears useful at least in some subsets of PFP patients.

49. When are surgical procedures indicated including distal realignment?
Three disorders may require distal realignment procedures: PF instability, PF arthritis, or infrapatellar contracture syndrome. Criteria for considering realignment for each of these categories are outlined next.

PF INSTABILITY

- Three-quadrant medial patellar glide
- Tubercle sulcus angle >0 degrees
- Patella alta combined with generalized ligamentous laxity and flat trochlear groove

PF ARTHRITIS

- Significant PF chondromalacia or arthritis combined with PF instability indicates the need for anterior and medialization of the tibial tubercle.

INFRAPATELLAR CONTRACTURE SYNDROME

- If after lateral release and debridement of the fat pad and infrapatellar tissues there is no change in patellar height, a proximal advancement of the tibial tubercle is indicated.

A fourth procedure, medial patellofemoral ligament reconstruction is utilized when recurrent dislocations occur. This procedure may include a soft tissue autograft or allograft, enabling a true reconstruction of the primary medial stabilizer. Recent literature indicates a very successful result with this reconstruction.

50. What are the long-term results of nonsurgical management of PF disorders?
Patients generally respond well to nonsurgical intervention. The long-term success rate is 75% to 85%. Multiple outcome studies support the importance of strengthening as the primary activity demonstrating efficacy. The recent Patellofemoral Pain Clinical Practice Guideline emphasizes exercise therapy as the most critical element in successful management. Thus it is appropriate to institute an individualized rehabilitation program before surgical intervention. If the rehabilitation program fails to provide adequate symptom relief and functional return, then surgery may be a viable option.

BIBLIOGRAPHY

Aksu, N., Atansay, V., Karalok, I., et al. (2021). Relationships of patellofemoral angles and tibiofemoral rotational angles with jumper's knee in professional dancers: an MRI analysis. *The Orthopaedic Journal of Sports Medicine, 9*(3), 2325967120985229.

Aliberti, G. M., Kraeutler, M. J., Miskimin, C., et al. (2021). Autograft versus allograft for medial patellofemoral ligament reconstruction: A systematic review. *Orthopaedic Journal of Sports Medicine, 9*(10), 23259671211046639.

Arshi, A., Cohen, J. R., Wang, J. C., et al. (2016). Operative management of patellar instability in the United States: An evaluation of national practice patterns, surgical trends, and complications. *Orthopaedic Journal of Sports Medicine, 4*(8), 2325967116662873.

Barton, C., Balachander, V., Lack, S., et al. (2014). Patellar taping for patellofemoral pain: a systematic review and meta-analysis to evaluate clinical outcomes and biomechanical mechanisms. *British Journal of Sports Medicine, 48*, 417–424.

Bennet, J. G., & Stauber, W. T. (1986). Evaluation and treatment of anterior knee pain using eccentric exercise. *Medicine and Science in Sports and Exercise, 18*, 26–30.

Bolgla, L., & Malone, T. (2005). Exercise prescription and patellofemoral pain: Evidence for rehabilitation. *Journal of Sport Rehabilitation, 14*, 72–88.

Callaghan, M. J., & Selfe, J. (2012). Patellar taping for patellofemoral pain syndrome in adults. *Cochrane Database of Systematic Reviews, 18*(4), CD006717.

Clijsen, R., Fuchs, J., & Taeymans, J. (2014). Effectiveness of exercise therapy in treatment of patients with patellofemoral pain syndrome: A systematic review and meta-analysis. *Physical Therapy, 94*(12), 1697–1708.

Diveta, J. A., & Volgelbach, W. D. (1992). The clinical efficacy of the a-angle in measuring patellar alignment. *Journal of Orthopaedic and Sports Physical Therapy, 16*(3), 136–139.

Dutton, R. A. 1, Khadavi, M. J., & Fredericson, M. (2014). Update on rehabilitation of patellofemoral pain. *Current Sports Medicine Reports, 13*(3), 172–178.

Eng, J. J., & Pierrynowski, M. R. (1993). Evaluation of soft orthotics in the treatment of patellofemoral syndrome. *Physical Therapy, 73*, 62–70.

Ernst, G. P., Kawaguchi, J., & Saliba, E. (1999). Effect of patellar taping on knee kinetics of patients with patellofemoral pain syndrome. *Journal of Orthopaedic and Sports Physical Therapy, 20*, 661–667.

Espi-Lopez, G. V., Serra-Ano, P., Vicent-Ferrando, J., et al. (2017). Effectiveness of inclusion of dry needling in a multimodal therapy program for patellofemoral pain: a randomized parallel-group trial. *Journal of Orthopaedic & Sports Physical Therapy, 47*, 392–401.

Fick, C. N., Grant, C., & Sheehan, F. T. (2020). Patellofemoral pain in adolescents: understanding patellofemoral morhololgy and its relationship to maltracking. *American Journal of Sports Medicine, 48*(2), 341–350.

Fulkerson, J. P. (1997). *Disorders of the patellofemoral joint* (3rd ed.). Baltimore: Williams & Wilkins.

Holmes, S. W., & Clancy, W. G. (1998). Clinical classification of patellofemoral pain and dysfunction. *Journal of Orthopaedic and Sports Physical Therapy, 28*, 299–306.

Hughston, J. C., Walsh, W. M., & Puddu, G. (1984). *Patellar subluxation and dislocation.* Philadelphia: WB Saunders.

Ingersoll, C., & Knight, K. (1991). Patellar location changes following EMG biofeedback or progressive resistance exercises. *Medicine and Science in Sports and Exercise, 23*, 1122–1127.

Jee, W. H., Choe, B. Y., Kim, J. M., Song, H. H., & Choi, K. H. (1998). The plica syndrome: Diagnostic value of MRI with arthroscopic correlation. *Journal of Computer Assisted Tomography, 22*, 814–818.

Kannus, N. A., & Jarvinen, M. (1998). What factors predict the long-term outcome in chronic patellofemoral pain syndrome? A 7-yr prospective follow-up study. *Medicine and Science in Sports and Exercise, 30*, 1572–1577.

Klingman, R. E., Liaos, S. M., & Hardin, K. M. (1997). The effect of subtalar joint posting on patellar glide position in subjects with excessive rearfoot pronation. *Physical Therapy, 25*, 185–191.

Lack, S., Barton, C., Woledge, R., Laupheimer, M., & Morrissey, D. (2014). The immediate effects of foot orthoses on hip and knee kinematics and muscle activity during a functional step-up task in individuals with patellofemoral pain. *Clinical Biomechanics, 29*, 1056–1062.

Laprade, J., Elsie, C., & Brouwer, B. (1998). Comparison of five isometric exercises in the recruitment of the vastus medialis oblique in persons with and without patellofemoral pain syndrome. *Journal of Orthopaedic and Sports Physical Therapy, 27*, 197–204.

Lavagnino, M., Arnoczky, S. P., Dodds, J., & Elvin, N. (2014). Infrapatellar straps decrease patellar tendon strain at the site of the jumper's knee lesion: A computational analysis based on radiographic measurements. *Sports Health, 3*(3), 296–302.

Lieb, F. J., & Perry, J. (1968). Quadriceps function: An anatomical and mechanical study using amputated limbs. *Journal of Bone and Joint Surgery, 50*(8), 1535–1548.

McCauley, T. R., Recht, M. P., & Disler, D. G. (2001). Clinical imaging of the articular cartilage in the knee. *Seminars in Musculoskeletal Radiology, 4*, 293–304.

McConnell, J. (1986). The management of chondromalacia patellae: A long term solution. *Australian Journal of Physiotherapy, 32*, 215–223.

Merchant, A. C. (1988). Classification of patellofemoral disorders. *Arthroscopy, 4*, 235–240.

Mills, K., Blanch, P., Dev, P., Martin, M., & Vicenzino, B. (2012). A randomised control trial of short term efficacy of in-shoe foot orthoses compared with a wait and see policy for anterior knee pain and the role of foot mobility. *British Journal of Sports Medicine, 46*(4), 247–252.

Nascimento, L. R., Teixeira-Salmela, L. F., Souza, R. B., & Resende, R. A. (2018). Hip and knee strengthening is more effective than knee strengthening alone for reducing pain and improving activity in individuals with patellofemoral pain: a systematic review with meta-analysis. *Journal of Orthopaedic & Sports Physical Therapy, 48*(1), 19–31.

Natri, A., Kannus, P., & Järvinen, M. (1998). Which factors predict the long-term outcome in chronic patellofemoral pain syndrome? A 7-yr prospective follow-up study. *Medicine and Science in Sports and Exercise, 30*(11), 1572–1577.

Neal, B. S., Lack, S. D., Lankhorst, N. E., Raye, A., Morrissey, D., & van Middelkoop, M. (2019). Risk factors for patellofemoral pain: a systematic review and meta-analysis. *British Journal of Sports Medicine, 53*(5), 270–281.

Peters, J. S. J., & Tyson, N. L. (2013). Proximal exercises are effective in treating patellofemoral pain syndrome: A systematic review. *International Journal of Sports Physical Therapy, 8*(5), 689–700.

Pietrosimone, B., Thomas, A. C., Saliba, S. A., & Ingersoll, C. D. (2014). Association between quadriceps strength and self-reported physical activity in people with knee arthritis. *International Journal of Sports Physical Therapy, 9*(3), 320–328.

Powers, C. M. (2000). Patellar kinematics part I and II. *Physical Therapy, 80*, 956–976.

Powers, C. M., Bolgla, L. A., Callaghan, M. J., Collins, N., & Sheehan, F. T. (2012). Patellofemoral pain: Proximal, distal, and local factors 2nd international research retreat. *Journal of Orthopaedic and Sports Physical Therapy, 42*(6), A1–A20.
Powers, C. M., Ho, K., Chen, Y., Souza, R. B., & Farrokhi, S. (2014). Patellofemoral joint stress during weight-bearing and non-weight-bearing quadriceps exercises. *Journal of Orthopaedic and Sports Physical Therapy, 44*(5), 320–327.
Powers, C. M., Maffucci, R., & Hampton, S. (1995). Rearfoot postures in patients with patellofemoral pain. *Journal of Orthopaedic and Sports Physical Therapy, 22*, 155–160.
Rathleff, M. S., Rathleff, C. R., Crossley, K. M., & Barton, C. J. (2014). Is hip strength a risk factor for patellofemoral pain? A systematic review and meta-analysis. *British Journal of Sports Medicine, 48*, 1088.
Rixe, J. A., Glick, J. E., Brady, J., & Olympia, R. P. (2013). A review of the management of patellofemoral pain syndrome. *The Physician and Sportsmedicine, 41*(3), 19–28.
Saltychev, M., Dutton, R. A., Laimi, K., Beaupré, G. S., Virolainen, P., & Fredericson, M. (2018). Effectiveness of conservative treatment for patellofemoral pain syndrome: A systematic review and meta-analysis. *Journal of Rehabilitation Medicine, 50*(5), 393–401.
Shellock, F. G., Brinkmann, G., Skaf, A., Heller, M., & Resnick, D. (1994). Effect of a patellar realignment brace on patellofemoral relationships: Evaluation with kinematic MR imaging. *Journal of Magnetic Resonance Imaging, 4*, 590–594.
Thomee, R. (1997). A comprehensive treatment approach for patellofemoral pain syndrome in young women. *Physical Therapy, 77*, 1690–1703.
Tomisch, D. A., Nitz, A. J., Threlkeld, A. J., & Shapiro, R. (1996). Patellofemoral alignment: Reliability. *Journal of Orthopaedic and Sports Physical Therapy, 23*, 200–208.
Wilk, K. E., Davies, G. J., Mangine, R. E., & Malone, T. R. (1998). Patellofemoral disorders: A classification system and clinical guidelines for nonoperative rehabilitation. *Journal of Orthopaedic and Sports Physical Therapy, 28*, 307–322.
Willy, R. W., Hoglund, L. T., Barton, C. J., et al. (2019). Patellofemoral pain: clinical practice guidelines linked to international classification of functioning, disability, and health from the Academy of Orthopaedic Physical Therapy of the American Physical therapy Association. *Journal of Orthopaedic and Sports Physical Therapy, 49*(9), CPG 1–CPG 95.
Witvrouw, E., Callaghan, M. J., Stefanik, J. J., et al. (2014). Patellofemoral pain: consensus statement from the 3rd international patellofemoral pain research retreat held in Vancouver, September 2013. *British Journal of Sports Medicine, 48*, 411–414. Followed by Crossley KM, Stefanik JJ, Selfe J, et al 2016 4th Retreat & Powers CM, Witvrouw E, Davis IS, et al. 4th Retreat 2017.

CHAPTER 70 QUESTIONS

1. **During the examination of a female patient with anterior knee pain, you note a relatively flat area medially superior to the patella when she extends against resistance. She exhibits a similar presentation on her less involved side. Her patellae are also somewhat laterally biased as she gets to full extension. The referral was for VMO insufficiency. Which of the rehabilitation strategies is likely the best approach regarding this patient?**

   a. A VMO focus done in full extension to isolate the specific fibers
   b. An integrated proximal and quadriceps program of strengthening
   c. Hip flexor, adductor, and external rotator strengthening with no quadriceps required
   d. VMO isolated strengthening and hip internal rotation strengthening

2. **A 13-year-old male presents with continuing pain of 4 weeks duration associated with the initiation of middle school soccer on dry hard pitch. He describes the pain as worst during practice but also is noted during stair decent. He also plays on a travel team that practices 1 night per week and often plays one or two games on Saturday. Before examining, what do you suspect?**
   a. Medial plica syndrome
   b. IT Band friction syndrome
   c. Apophysitis (Osgood–Schlatter)
   d. Medial meniscal pathology

3. **A cyclist reports to your clinic with a 2 week history of "pain in the front of my knee" that is getting worse. Their typical workout includes hills and sprints but approximately 20 miles daily. Being a great PT, you determine the only workout change was addition of toe clips as it was recommended by a friend to enhance performance. As you begin examination, you are suspecting___________.**
   a. Medial plica syndrome
   b. IT Band friction syndrome
   c. Jumper's knee syndrome
   d. Medial meniscus pathology

MENISCAL INJURIES

P.B. Lonnemann, PT, DPT, OCS, FAAOMPT and D.A. Boyce, PT, EdD, OCS, ECS

CHAPTER 71

1. **How common are meniscal injuries in the United States?**
   The prevalence of meniscal tears is 61 per 100,000. The overall male-to-female incidence is 2.5:1. Peak incidence of meniscal injury in males is between 31 to 40 years of age; for females it is younger, at 11 to 20 years. Currently 850,000 meniscal surgeries are performed each year.

2. **Describe the Anatomy of the meniscus.**
   The menisci are wedges of fibrocartilage located on the articular surface of the tibia. The outer portion of the meniscus is thick and convex, whereas the inner portion is thin and concave. The menisci are composed of cells and an extracellular matrix of collagen, proteoglycans, glycoproteins, and elastin. The collagen content is 90% type I collagen, with the remaining 10% consisting of collagen types II, III, V, and VI. The collagen fibers are oriented circumferentially, which helps to transmit compressive loads. Cell types are fibroblastic in the outer third, chondrocytic in the inner third, and fibrochondrocytic in the middle third. The menisci are attached to the tibia at their anterior and posterior horns. The medial meniscus is more C-shaped, whereas the lateral meniscus is more O-shaped.

3. **What structures attach to the medial meniscus?**
   - Joint capsule
   - Deep medial collateral ligament (MCL)
   - Coronary ligament of patella
   - Transverse "intermeniscal" ligament from anterior horn of medial meniscus to anterior horn of lateral meniscus
   - Meniscopatellar fibers from lateral border
   - Semimembranosus tendon

4. **Is the meniscus avascular?**
   No. The outer third of the meniscus is supplied by the branches of the geniculate arteries. The anterior and posterior horns are vascular, but the posterolateral corner of the lateral meniscus has no blood supply. The outermost third is called the red-red zone, the middle third is the red-white zone, and the inner third is the white-white zone. Healing is greatest at the outermost third and decreases with inward progression because of diminished blood supply.

5. **List the functions of the meniscus.**
   - Helps to transmit loads across the tibiofemoral joint by increasing the contact surface area
   - Viscoelastic properties add to shock-absorbing capacity
   - Serves as secondary restraint to tibiofemoral motion by improving joint fit
   - Helps with roll and glide of tibiofemoral arthrokinematics
   - May assist in nutrition and lubrication of the joint

6. **How important are the menisci in transmitting loads across the knee joint?**
   The medial and lateral menisci are responsible for carrying 50% to 60% of the compressive load across the knee. At 90 degrees of knee flexion, the percentage of the load borne by the menisci increases to 85%.

7. **Do the menisci move with knee joint motion?**
   Yes. The lateral meniscus is more mobile because of its slacker coronary ligament. It does not attach to the lateral collateral ligament (LCL), whereas the medial meniscus attaches to the deep portion of the MCL. The lateral meniscus translates approximately 11 mm versus 5 mm for the medial meniscus. The menisci move posteriorly with knee flexion and anteriorly with extension. External rotation of the tibia is accompanied by anterior translation of the lateral meniscus and posterior translation of the medial meniscus.

8. **What is a discoid meniscus?**
   It is a congenital deformity found most often during adolescence. The abnormal meniscus is the shape of a round disc. It is more commonly found in the lateral than medial meniscus. The abnormality affects the contact stresses and mobility of the menisci. Due to its abnormal shape, the discoid meniscus may cause symptoms of pain, effusion, or snapping. Partial meniscectomy may be required to create a more normal cartilage. If the discoid meniscus is not symptomatic it should not be surgically treated.

9. **What is a meniscal cyst? Where is it likely to occur?**
Meniscal cysts are ganglion-like formations secondary to central degeneration of the meniscus. They may occur on either meniscus but are more common on the lateral meniscus at the midportion or posterior one-third. The patient may be asymptomatic or complain of a dull ache on the side of the cyst (medial versus lateral). Localized extraarticular swelling may be present and is proportional to the patient's activity level. Meniscal cysts are treated surgically via partial meniscectomy or cystectomy.

10. **What is the most common mechanism of meniscal injury?**
The patient describes a turning or twisting maneuver of the leg in weight bearing. Most acute meniscal injuries are associated with ligamentous injury. Additionally, the meniscus may become injured when rising from a squatting position because of excessive compression of the posterior horn in association with an anterior translation of the menisci.

11. **Which meniscus is more commonly injured?**
Tears of the medial meniscus are more common than tears of the lateral meniscus. Reasons for increased injury rates of the medial meniscus are its elongated "c" shape, attachment to the medial collateral ligament, and joint capsule.

12. **What are the signs and symptoms of a meniscal tear?**
The patient complains of symptoms such as catching or locking of the knee joint, pain with twisting of the knee, and tenderness along the joint line (77%–86%). In addition, swelling may be present (50% usually 24 hours after injury), especially with activity. Some patients complain of a "giving-way" sensation secondary to instability. A locked knee that will not fully extend usually indicates a large bucket-handle tear.

13. **Describe the most common meniscal tears.**
Meniscal tears are classified as longitudinal, vertical (transverse), or horizontal. Bucket-handle tears are classified as longitudinal tears that eventually separate and may cause locking of the joint. The parrot-beak tear is a pedunculated tag tear located on the posterior horn.

14. **How accurate is magnetic resonance imaging (MRI) in detecting a meniscal tear?**
MRI has a fair accuracy rate for detecting medial (88%) and lateral (88%) meniscal tears. According to Gelb et al., (1996) MRI has a sensitivity of 82% and a specificity of 87% for an isolated meniscal lesion.

15. **Describe the McMurray test.**
The McMurray test is the classic manipulative test for meniscal tears. The patient lies supine with the knee in full flexion. The tibia is rotated internally, and a varus stress is applied while the knee is extended (lateral meniscus). The procedure is repeated with the knee externally while a valgus stress is applied to the knee while it is extended (medial meniscus). A positive test is a reproduction of symptoms and/or an audible or palpable "thud" or "click." Due to the McMurray test's relatively low sensitivity and specificity, it is of limited clinical value when used in isolation.

16. **What is the sensitivity and specificity of commonly used special tests utilized to detect meniscal pathology?**

Sensitivities and Specificities of Common Meniscal Tear Tests

CLINICAL TEST/SIGN	SENSITIVITY	SPECIFICITY
McMurray test	70%	71%
Joint-line tenderness	85%	30%
Apley test	60%	70%
Thessaly test	53%	64%
Steinman sign	83%	66%

In general, the sensitivity and specificity of the above tests used during clinical examination to detect meniscal pathology are varied and often low. Clustering these tests is recommended to increase the accuracy of detecting meniscal pathology.

17. **What is the Meniscal Pathology Composite Score?**
According to Lowery et al., (2006) a higher composite score of the following tests correlated with the presence or absence of meniscal pathology.

1. Patient report of a history of "catching" or "locking"
2. Pain with forced hyperextension
3. Pain with maximum flexion
4. Pain or an audible click with McMurray's maneuver
5. Joint line tenderness to palpation

When all five of the tests were positive there was a positive predictive value of 92.3%. With three or more positive tests the positive predictive value was 75%. If the patient had Degenerative Joint Disease the values were higher, and lower in the presence of an ACL tear.

18. **What is the typical management strategy for a meniscal tear?**
Management falls into four main categories:
- Nonoperative—degenerative tears in older patients without mechanical symptoms
- Meniscectomy (partial)—symptomatic tears that are unable to be repaired and can preserve meniscal function
- Meniscal repair—most suitable in younger patients with peripheral red-red zone tears
- Meniscal transplant—most suitable in younger patients who have undergone meniscectomy and still have pain or articular cartilage damage in the meniscectomized knee compartment

19. **How effective is nonoperative treatment for meniscal tears?**
Nonoperative treatment has good outcomes in older patients with degenerative tears without mechanical symptoms. Several studies have shown that a structured physical therapy program consisting of strengthening, flexibility, proprioception, and cycling results in the same favorable outcomes (6-month and 5-year follow-up) compared with those individuals undergoing meniscectomy alone or meniscectomy and physical therapy. Additionally, elderly patients with known osteoarthritis of the knee who underwent arthroscopic lavage or debridement were no better than a placebo surgery group (thus surgery may not be warranted in this population). However, it should be noted that approximately 30% of individuals with degenerative meniscal tears who undergo nonoperative treatment initially may require meniscectomy to achieve adequate pain relief. No current evidence exists related to the effectiveness of a conservative treatment approach for acute meniscal tears in younger populations.

20. **What is the most common surgical management of meniscal injury?**
Arthroscopic examination followed by partial meniscectomy is the most typical surgical management of meniscal injury. Short-term results suggest 90% satisfaction. Long-term satisfaction has shown that 50% of patients become symptomatic again at 5 years, and they have either modified or given up their sporting activities. Additionally, radiographic degenerative changes rose from 40% to nearly 90% over that same 5-year period.

21. **When is a partial meniscectomy indicated?**
Partial meniscectomy is indicated for younger or middle-aged patients with symptomatic tears (joint-line catching and pain, effusion, locking, and/or giving way that interferes with daily function) and in those with tears outside of the red-red zone that are not amendable to meniscal repair. Total meniscectomy is no longer considered a treatment option because of the significant increase in contact pressure that results in accelerated articular cartilage damage and pain.

22. **What are the predictors of a poor outcome following partial arthroscopic meniscectomy?**
- Low preoperative activity level
- >40 years old
- Higher than normal body mass index (BMI)
- Varus or valgus knee deformity
- Preexisting articular cartilage damage
- ACL insufficiency
- Radial tears
- Lateral meniscus tear

23. **What is the usual course of rehabilitation following partial meniscectomy?**
Rehabilitation consists of pain and swelling control, short-term use of crutches to insure proper ambulation, self-limiting exercises to regain full range of motion and strength, with progression to functional exercises. Return to full function occurs after a 2- to 6-week time frame.

24. **When is a meniscal repair indicated?**
Indications for repair are peripheral nondegenerative longitudinal tears <3 cm. Short tears of 1 to 2 cm have better success rates, and young patients seem to have the best outcomes.

25. **What are the common forms of meniscal repair, and is one better than the other?**
Meniscal repair is preferable to partial meniscectomy for salvaging the meniscus and preserving the tibiofemoral joint. There are four basic surgical approaches: 1) open (rarely used in contemporary practice), 2) inside-out suture techniques, 3) outside-in suture techniques, and 4) all-inside techniques. A systematic review examining different repair techniques found no differences in clinical failure rates of inside-out or all-inside techniques. It should be noted that more nerve complications have been noted with all inside-out techniques.

26. **What is the clinical success rate following meniscal repair?**
When looking at 10-year follow-ups, approximately 75% to 80% of patients undergoing meniscal repair were considered to be a clinical success. Clinical success was defined as low or absent pain and minimal radiographic changes in the tibiofemoral joint. Improved outcomes are seen in the repaired traumatic versus chronic tears (73% vs 42%) and when acute tears are repaired within 3 months of injury versus those repaired after 3 months (91% vs 58%).

27. **What are contraindications for meniscal repair?**
- Meniscus tears located in the inner-third region
- Chronic degenerative tears
- Longitudinal tears <10 mm in length
- Incomplete radial tears that do not extend into the outer third
- Patients older than 60 years of age
- Patients unwilling to follow postoperative rehabilitation
- BMI >35

28. **Does bleeding stimulate the reparative process of a torn meniscus?**
Yes. It has been shown that bleeding can stimulate the reparative process within a healing meniscus. It has been shown that patients with meniscal repairs performed in conjunction with ACL reconstruction have up to a 93% healing rate compared with 50% healing rates in meniscal repairs alone. Other interventions used to stimulate healing of the meniscus include an exogenous fibrin clot, which is placed at the site of meniscal injury to form a wound hematoma and trephination (shaving of the meniscus to promote bleeding) at the meniscus. Both of these techniques facilitate healing because of the release of local clotting and growth factors.

29. **Can stem cells be used to treat a meniscal tear?**
According to Dai et al., (2021) several animal studies and a few small human studies, with small population sizes, have shown meniscus regeneration and decrease in pain following injection of human mesenchymal stem cells in individuals following partial meniscectomy. Further studies are needed to assess the long-term viability of this treatment.

30. **What are the typical rehabilitation guidelines following meniscal repair?**
No consensus exists on a universal rehabilitation protocol. However, general guidelines/milestones are offered herein. Please note time frames may be slightly longer in complex repairs.
- Long leg brace with lockouts—4 to 6 weeks
- Early protected gradual weight bearing (full weight bearing at approximately 5–6 weeks)
- Full ROM—4 to 6 weeks (90 degrees by 2 weeks, 120 degrees by 4 weeks)
- Mini squats—by 3 to 4 weeks
- Hamstring curls (0–90 degrees)—by 5 to 6 weeks
- Leg press (0–70 degrees)—by 5 to 8 weeks
- Stationary cycling—at 7 to 8 weeks
- Running—4 months
- Return to sport—5 months

31. **Do surgically repaired menisci appear normal on MRI after 10 years?**
A 13-year follow-up study of asymptomatic patients who underwent a previous surgical repair of the meniscus demonstrated abnormal MRI signals even though the meniscus had a stable union. These abnormalities at the site of repair represent edematous scar tissue, not the failure to heal.

32. **What is meniscal repair using a bioabsorbable screw or arrow?**
This is a relatively new technique that uses an all-inside device. All-inside devices for meniscal repair are attractive because they do not require additional incision or arthroscopic knot tying. An arrow or screw is inserted across the torn meniscus to bring the torn edges together and stabilize the tear. Some of the more recent devices have been designed to allow tensioning of the construct after insertion. This approach is less time consuming and has similar pullout strength to that of sutures used in a standard meniscal repair.

33. What are the outcomes of meniscal repair using a bioabsorbable screw or arrow?

Failure rates of all inside techniques are similar and tend to increase after 2 years with failure rates reaching 25% or greater after 5 years regardless of the fixation type. Surgical complications and infections are minimal. A recent study demonstrated a 28% failure rate with postoperative complications, such as chondral scoring, fixator breakage, and postoperative joint-line irritation.

34. If a meniscal repair fails, can it be repaired a second time?

Yes; a case series of 14 patients who underwent a second repair had a success rate of approximately 72% after a 7-year follow-up.

35. What is a meniscal transplant?

For patients >19 to 50 years of age with severe irreparable meniscal injuries and symptoms, cadaveric meniscal implant is a potential option. Still considered controversial, meniscal transplantation in the hands of a trained surgeon may be considered before a total joint replacement. Three types of allografts are utilized: fresh, frozen, and synthetic. Fresh allografts are less favorable due to the required immunosuppression associated with it, and the risk of disease transmission. Although frozen allografts do not show evidence of hyaline cartilage protection, they are favored over fresh allografts. According to Vaquero et al., (2016) synthetic allografts have been approved for use in clinical trials in the United States, but further studies are required to assess their benefit over human tissue allografts. Best results are obtained in those individuals who have a stable knee, no signs of advanced tibiofemoral arthritis, absence of varus and valgus deformities, and a BMI <35. A common surgical technique used in meniscal transplantation consists of drilling holes at the anterior and posterior horn attachments of the meniscus and inserting bone plugs that are attached to the cadaveric meniscal transplant and fixating them in place. Additional stabilization is afforded via soft tissue anchoring to the capsule/surrounding soft tissues or modified bone plug or keyhole techniques.

36. What are the typical rehabilitation guidelines following meniscal transplantation?

No consensus exists on a universal rehabilitation protocol. However, general guidelines/milestones are offered herein.

- Long leg brace with lockouts—4 to 6 weeks
- Early protected gradual weight bearing (full weight bearing at approximately 5 to 6 weeks)
- Full ROM—by 5 to 6 weeks (90 degrees by 2 weeks, 120 degrees by 4 weeks)
- Mini squats—by 5 to 6 weeks
- Hamstring curls (0–90 degrees)/leg press (0–70 degrees)—by 9 to 12 weeks
- Stationary cycling—at 7 to 8 weeks
- Running/sport—7 to 12 months

37. What are the outcomes associated with meniscal transplantation?

Success rates (success being defined as a lack of persistent pain and mechanical integrity of the transplant) following meniscal transplantation vary from 12% to 100% (mean 60%). Long-term studies have shown transplantation survival rates of the lateral (74%–76%), medial (50%–70%), and combined transplants (67%).

38. What are the main focus areas of future research and management of meniscal injuries?

Currently, the most valuable type of orthobiologic treatment for meniscal injury is platelet-rich plasma. Other emerging medical technologies are the use of 3D printing of meniscal transplants and bioengineered artificial transplants.

Bibliography

Anderson, A. B., Gaston, J., LeClere, L. E., & Dickens, J. F. (2021). Meniscal salvage: Where we are today. *Journal of the American Academy of Orthopaedic Surgeons, 29*(14), 596–603.

Arnoczky, S. P., & Warren, R. F. (1982). Microvasculature of the human meniscus. *American Journal of Sports Medicine, 10*, 90–95.

Cavanaugh, J. T. (1991). Rehabilitation following meniscal surgery. In R. P. Engle (Ed.), *Knee ligament rehabilitation*. New York, NY: Churchill Livingstone.

Clark, C. R., & Ogden, J. A. (1983). Development of the menisci of the human knee joint. *Journal of Bone and Joint Surgery, 65*(4), 538–547.

Dai, T.-Y, Pan, Z.-Y, & Yin, F. (2021). In vivo studies of mesenchymal stem cells in the treatment of meniscus injury. *Orthopaedic Surgery, 13*, 2185–2195.

DePhillipo, N. N., LaPrade, R. F., Zaffagnini, S., et al. (2021). The future of meniscus science: international expert consensus. *Journal of Experimental Orthopaedics, 8*, 24.

Fairbank, T. J. (1948). Knee joint changes after meniscectomy. *Journal of Bone and Joint. Surgery, 30B*(4), 664–670.

Fox, A. J., Bedi, A., & Rodeo, S. A. (2012). The basic science of human knee menisci: structure, composition, and function. *Sports Health, 4*(4), 340–351.

Gelb, H. J., Glasgow, S. S., Sapega, A. A., & Torg, J. S. (1996). Magnetic resonance imaging of knee disorders. *American Journal of Sports Medicine, 24*, 99–103.

Goossens, P., Keijsers, E., van Geenen, R. J. C., et al. (2015). Validity of the Thessaly test in evaluating meniscal tears compared with arthroscopy: A diagnostic accuracy study. *Journal of Orthopaedic and Sports Physical Therapy, 45*(1), 18–24.
Gray, J. C. (1999). Neural and vascular anatomy of the menisci of the human knee. *Journal of Orthopaedic and Sports Physical Therapy, 29*, 23–30.
Kelly, M. A., Flock, T. J., Kimmel, J. A., et al. (1991). Imaging of the knee: Clarification of its role. *Arthroscopy, 7*, 78–82.
Lee, S. R., Kim, J. G., & Nam, S. W. (2012). The tips an pitfalls of meniscus allograft transplantation. *Knee Surgery & Related Research, 24*(3), 137–145.
Lowery, D. J., Farley, T. D., Wing, D. W., Sterett, W. I., & Steadman, J. R. (2006). A clinical composite score accurately detects meniscal pathology. *Arthroscopy, 22*(11), 1174–1179.
Majewski, M., Susanne, H., & Klaus, S. (2006). Epidemiology of athletic knee injuries: A 10-year study. *The Knee, 13*(3), 184–188.
Mordecai, S. C., Al-Hadithy, N., Ware, H. E., & Gupte, C. M. (2014). Treatment of meniscal tears: An evidence based approach. *World Journal of Orthopaedics, 5*(3), 233–241.
Nepple, J. J., Dunn, W. R., & Wright, R. W. (2012). Meniscal repair outcomes at greater than five years: a systematic literature review and meta-analysis. *Journal of Bone and Joint. Surgery (American), 94*(24), 2222–2227.
Noyes, F. R., Heckman, T. P., & Barber-Westin, S. D. (2012). Meniscus repair and transplantation: A comprehensive update. *Journal of Orthopaedic and Sports Physical Therapy, 42*(3), 274–290.
Vangsness, C. T., Farr, J., 2nd, Boyd, J., Dellaero, D. T., Mills, C. R., & LeRoux-Williams, M. (2014). Adult human mesenchymal stem cells delivered via intra-articular injection to the knee following partial medial meniscectomy: A randomized double-blinded controlled study. *Journal of Bone and Joint Surgery (American), 96*(2), 90–98.
Vaquero, J., & Forriol, F. (2016). Meniscus tear surgery and meniscus replacement. *Muscles, Ligaments and Tendons Journal, 6*(1), 71–89.
Voloshin, I., Schmitz, M. A., Adams, M. J., & DeHaven, K. E. (2003). Results of repeat meniscal repair. *American Journal of Sports Medicine, 31*, 874–880.
Walker, P. S., & Erkman, P. J. (1975). The role of the menisci in force transmission across the knee. *Clinical Orthopaedics, 109*, 184.

CHAPTER 71 QUESTIONS

1. **Your 26-year-old patient had a meniscal transplantation. He is asking when he can return to running. You tell him that running will most likely begin in:**
   a. 5 to 6 weeks
   b. 10 to 12 weeks
   c. 4 months
   d. 7 months

2. **Your patient is a 58-year-old athletic female with mild OA who is considering a partial meniscectomy for her right lateral meniscus tear. Your advice to her is:**
   a. Meniscectomy is the best option.
   b. Meniscal repair is the best option.
   c. Avoiding surgery is the best option.
   d. Total knee arthroplasty is the best option.

3. **Your patient injured their knee. They report intermittent catching. You note that they are tender over the medial joint line, have pain with passive overpressure into extension, and full flexion. They have a positive McMurray's test. What additional special tests would you do to be more than 90% confident that they have a meniscus tear?**
   a. No additional special tests are needed.
   b. Steinman's
   c. Apley's
   d. Thessaly's

CHAPTER 72

LIGAMENTOUS INJURIES OF THE KNEE

T.J. Manal, PT, DPT, OCS, SCS, FAPTA and W.G. Seymour, PT, DPT, OCS, FAAOMPT

1. **What constitutes a knee ligamentous injury during objective examination and how does biological healing impact recovery prognosis?**
The amount of movement present during ligamentous stress testing is estimated in millimeters and graded accordingly: grade 1+ indicates 3 mm to 5 mm, grade 2+ indicates 5 mm to 10 mm, and grade 3+ indicates >10 mm (absolute values; not different compared to contralateral side).

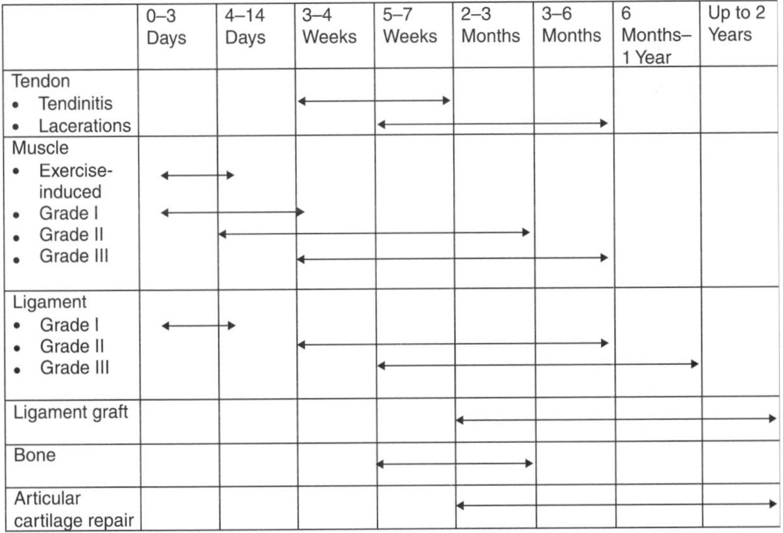

Healing Rates of Tissues

	0–3 Days	4–14 Days	3–4 Weeks	5–7 Weeks	2–3 Months	3–6 Months	6 Months–1 Year	Up to 2 Years
Tendon								
• Tendinitis			←	→				
• Lacerations				←	—	→		
Muscle								
• Exercise-induced	←	→						
• Grade I	←	→						
• Grade II		←	—	—	→			
• Grade III			←	—	—	→		
Ligament								
• Grade I	←	→						
• Grade II			←	—	—	→		
• Grade III				←	—	—	→	
Ligament graft					←	—	—	→
Bone				←	→			
Articular cartilage repair					←	—	—	→

As evaluators, the objective is to resolve impairments as quickly as possible to improve patient's function. The speed of recovery is dependent on pathology and biological healing principles (**Healing Time Rates of Tissues Figure**) and, when applicable, any surgical procedure performed. Adequate biological healing must occur before exposure to forces beyond the tolerance of healing tissue or surgical fixation is allowed. Healing is affected by age and concomitant illness or injury. The pathology and surgical procedure, as well as the soft tissue, bony anatomy, and articular cartilage healing potential, must all be considered when designing a rehabilitation program. Communication between the referring physician and the physical therapist is essential for the exchange of information critical to the rehabilitation process including any information gleaned during the surgical procedures such as tissue quality, healing potential, and fixation strength.

2. **The patient has an MRI-diagnosed cruciate ligament tear. How accurate is magnetic resonance imaging (MRI) in detecting ACL and Posterior Cruciate Ligament (PCL) tears?**
In two meta-analyses, MRI sensitivity for suspected acute ACL sprain/tears ranged from 98% to 87% within the literature, with specificity ranging from 100% and 93%. Within the same meta-analyses, MRI sensitivity and specificity for suspected acute PCL injury were 100%; however MRI sensitivity for chronic PCL tears was shown to be with less sensitive (62.5%).

3. **What patient-reported information is valuable in the care of knee patients? How can this data inform the therapist of patients' needs, progress, or recovery?**
Body region (knee) or pathology/injury-specific specific questionnaires have been specifically developed to ensure that a patient's complaints and level of functional limitations are understood and recovery is meeting key milestones during the duration of care. If the clinician notices a lack of progress in the questionnaire (determined by psychometric properties such as minimally clinical important difference [MCID] or minimal detectable change [MDC]) not predicted by the patient's initial prognosis, a reevaluation or consultation may be necessary. The questionnaire of choice should be as specific to the patient as possible (in terms of condition) and have sufficient psychometric properties of reliability, validity, and responsiveness.
(Table 72-1) (Questionnaires Table) The table contains questionnaires commonly seen in the literature for those after ligamentous injury or postoperative ligamentous reconstruction/repair.
The Patient-Specific Functional Scale (PSFS) allows the person to self-nominate the top three limiting activities. This questionnaire can be used in populations who need to be very specific describing a sport or work action or more generic to daily activities in less active populations.
These patients' reported questionnaires can establish baseline severity when performed during the evaluation and when repeated during appropriate intervals during the episode of care provide insight into the patient's functional change over time.

Table 72-1 Questionnaires Table

INDICES	INDICATION	SCORING	MDC/MCID	COMMENTS
Knee Injury and Osteoarthritis Outcome Score (KOOS)	ACLR, meniscectomy, tibial osteotomy, posttraumatic OA, TKA	**Scale 0–4:** None (0) Mild (1) Moderate (2) Severe (3) Extreme (4) Score can either be reported as a collective or broken into four categories. **Categories** Pain: 0–36 pts Other symptoms: 0–28 pts ADLs: 0–68 pts QOL: 0–16 pts	MDC *ACLR: Salavati et al.* Pain: 6.1 pts Other symptoms: 8.5 pts ADLs: 8.0 pts QOL: 7.2 pts	Valid, reliable, and responsive for pain, stiffness, and physical function in OA
International Knee Documentation Committee (IKDC) questionnaire	Knee ligament injury	Grading found at: http://test.sportsmed.org/Research/IKDC_Forms/	MCID: 11.5 pts	Not sensitive for sports-related function. May overestimate the disability of an injury
Lysholm Knee Score	Ligament and meniscal injuries	Eight items: 0–100 pts Pain (25 points) Instability (25 points) Locking (15 points) Swelling (10 points) Limp (5 points) Stair climbing (10 points) Squatting (5 points) Need for support (5 points)	MDC: 10 pts	Evidence for usefulness inconclusive
Cincinnati Knee Rating System	Nonspecific knee conditions	Scale of 0–10 described on form. Subscales: Pain 0–10 Swelling 0–10 Partial giving way 0–10 Full giving way 0–10	MDC Pain: 2.45 pts Swelling: 2.86 pts Partial giving way: 2.82 pts Full giving way: 2.30 pts	Responsive for changes in pain, swelling, giving way, symptoms, sports function, and overall rating

Table 72-1 Questionnaires Table

INDICES	INDICATION	SCORING	MDC/MCID	COMMENTS
Knee Outcome Survey (KOS)	Nonspecific knee conditions	6 symptom questions 5 = "I Do Not Have the Symptom" 0 = "The Symptom Prevents Me From All Daily Activities" 8 functional questions 5 = "Not Difficult" 0 = "I am Unable to Do the Activity" Total = ___ pts/70 = ___ %	MDC: 8.87 pts MCID: 7.1%	Responsive for functional limits for a variety of impairments
Global Rating of Change	Patients with clinical conditions	11-pt scale: –5, 0, +5 15-pt scale: –7, 0, +7 (– very much/great deal worse) 0 (no change) (+ very much/great deal better)	MDC: 0.45 points on 11-point scale MCID: 2 points on 11-point scale	High test-retest reliability
Patient-Specific Functional Scale	Orthopedic conditions	3 Self Chosen Activities Grade EACH: 0–10; 0 = unable to perform at all 10 = performs at prior level	MDC 2 for average score 3 for single activity score	Useful in multiple populations as patients self-identify most difficult tasks

4. **Patient presents with an acutely inflamed and large knee. Which objective test will determine the presence of this impairment and how does the information inform diagnosis and prognosis?**

   Although many use the terms joint effusion and swelling interchangeably, when defined more strictly they can explain different conditions. Effusion describes increased fluid in the tibiofemoral joint (ie, intracapsular), while swelling is reflecting inflammation and fluid outside of the capsule (ie, extracapsular). Because of this definition, any test for effusion would typically lead the clinician to consider if there has been some form of irritation or trauma to structures within the joint or to the capsule itself. Extracapsular swelling leads the clinician to examine other structures outside of the capsule.

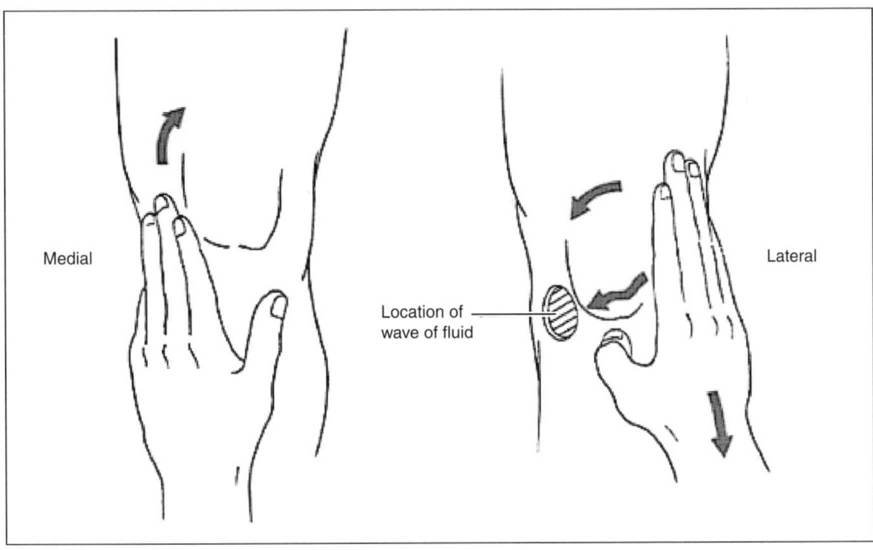

Table 72-2 Sweep Test Results

GRADE	SWEEP TEST RESULT
0	Initial medial sweep does not move any form of fluid, even with multiple attempts.
Trace	Initial medial sweep milks fluid from medial sulcus; lateral sweep moves fluid back but not enough fluid to fill the sulcus.
1+	Initial medial sweep milks fluid from medial sulcus; lateral sweep moves fluid back and fills the entire medial sulcus.
2+	Initial medial sweep milks fluid from medial sulcus; fluid moves back spontaneously. Does not require lateral sweep.
3+	Initial medial sweep cannot move fluid out of medial sulcus; fluid stays even after consistent medial sweeps.

For effusion, Sturgill et al. demonstrated substantial interrater agreement (kappa 0.75) when using a "sweep test" by *"pushing up"* the medial aspect of the knee from a distal to proximal direction with the examiner's hand to attempt to move the swelling from the knee joint area (see Sweep Test Figure). The examiner then sweeps the hand from the mid lateral thigh back down toward the knee joint on the lateral side while watching for a *filling* response on the medial side of the patella. (Table 72-2) (Sweep Test Results) The table demonstrates grading of the test. Additional video reference can be found at: https://www.jospt.org/doi/suppl/10.2519/jospt.2009.3143.

Swelling of the extracapsular areas surrounding the knee can be assessed using girth measurements (at the levels of the superior/mid/inferior patella) or recording general visual observations (eg, loss of patellar dimples or noting an enlarged superior patellar pouch). While girth measurements have shown to be reliable both within individuals with ACL injuries,160,161 the same cannot be said after total knee arthroplasty.

If whole lower extremity swelling is noted, clinicians should consider cellulitis, phlebitis, or deep vein thrombosis (DVT) as a differential diagnosis and consider if the presentation requires a referral or is a contraindication to continue with examination and treatment.

5. **How can the patient's complaint of changing local knee joint or knee joint region pain and soreness guide decision-making related to treatment progressions and dosage?**

The International Association for the Study of Pain (IASP) defines pain as "An unpleasant sensory and emotional experience associated with, or resembling that associated with, actual or potential tissue damage." This definition leaves room for both inflammatory (characterized as redness, swelling, and warmth) or mechanical influences as well as nonphysical factors such as a person's mental state, previous life influences, anxiety, depression, and distress. These factors are important to consider as, at times, pain may be the most significant factor that inhibits the progression or tolerance to exercise.

Pain at most/worst and at best are questions that most clinicians ask their patients on a treatment-by-treatment basis, and evidence supports the validity of these questions while also showing they are responsive to change. The verbal rating scale (VRS) and the numerical rating scale (NRS) describe pain with numbers from 0 = no pain to 10 = worst possible pain. In particular, the VRS has been shown to have an MCID of 10 mm on a 100 mm scale for postsurgical patients, meaning if the patient reports a change of 10 mm or more, the clinician can conclude that a clinically important difference has occurred.

The response of the knee to clinical interventions can provide feedback to guide clinical decisions. Knee Soreness rules have been previously proposed as a rationale for progression of exercise (Table 72-3) (Knee Soreness Rules). These rules are based on soreness of the knee joint, not of the muscles surrounding the knee (eg, quadriceps) and can improve decision-making when coupled with expected responses to increases in activity and exercise dosage or the addition of new activities.

For example, a patient 4 weeks post-anterior cruciate ligament reconstruction (ACLR) complains of knee soreness (not muscular) the day after a physical therapy treatment session. This patient should take 1 day off and not advance their home program to a higher level. If, however, a patient in physical therapy begins to have knee soreness during their warm-up on an exercise bike and the soreness goes away, the patient would stay with the same treatment program that day. If soreness did not improve with an appropriate warm-up, the program should be reduced to a level below their last treatment level.

The use of the soreness rules allows the therapist to correlate the irritability of the knee joint to the components of the treatment and respond accordingly. These rules are also used to assist therapists in allowing patients to progress their home program while following the rules in order to reflect the therapist's advice even in their absence.

Table 72-3 Knee Soreness rules

CRITERION (KNEE JOINT SORENESS, *NOT* MUSCLE SORENESS)	ACTION
Soreness during warm-up that continues	2 days off, drop down 1 step
Soreness during warm-up that goes away	Stay at step that led to soreness
Soreness during warm-up that goes away but redevelops during session	2 days off, drop down 1 step
Soreness the day after lifting (not muscle soreness)	1 day off, do not advance program to the next step
No soreness	Advance as instructed by healthcare provider

6. **How strongly should clinicians suggest functional bracing for their patients for injury prevention or protection after ligamentous injury or surgical reconstruction or repair?**

Functional bracing attempts to provide external support, after intrinsic stability is impacted by collateral or cruciate ligamentous compromise. While these braces can sometimes be distributed prophylactically in an athletic setting, there is no conclusive evidence that suggests functional knee bracing prevents ACL injuries. They are more often utilized during the nonsurgical or postsurgical rehabilitative process. Surgeons may require functional brace usage during different stages of the postoperative rehabilitation; sometimes braces are prescribed acutely with activities of daily living (ADLs) when quadriceps strength is diminished but are more commonly used to help with transitions of return-to-running and return-to-sport. Under low-loading conditions, the use of functional braces has proven to be effective in decreasing the strain on the ACL, supporting consideration of its use until sufficient quadriceps activation and strength are demonstrated. However, the use remains controversial and is generally linked to surgeon preference. Multiple authors have shown no difference in tibial translation or excursion between those who are or are not braced after ACLR; however, some of the same authors still suggest bracing in the first 4 to 5 months after surgery.

The decision to be braced may now more than ever be a collaborative decision between the care team and patient. While Colville et al. reported that 90% of individuals that wear braces believe that the brace is beneficial in reducing the frequency and severity of giving-way episodes, DeCoster et al. reported that 36% of the physicians surveyed had recently decreased their brace prescription practice.

While Colville reported that the patients who brace feel more protected from giving-way episodes while using their prescribed brace, it is unclear if there is relationship between quadriceps strength and the decision to brace. In patients with quadriceps strength less than 80% of their uninvolved side, Cook et al. found improved functional performance with the use of a brace. Risberg et al. also found those who discharged their braces sooner (3 months after ACL surgery) had improved functional measures at 6 months and strength scores at 1 to 2 years compared to those who continued wearing their brace at 1 to 2 years after surgery.

The usefulness of bracing for PCL injury is also unclear. Typically, braces are not prescribed following PCL reconstruction, but when they are used, they are generally discontinued by the fourth postoperative week. Early use of bracing for grade 2 and 3 MCL injuries has also been suggested to provide stabilization to the knee while the ligament heals. Typically braces are locked to avoid knee extension <30° or flexion >90°, thereby diminishing stress on the MCL outside of those ranges. Because the typical soft tissue healing timeframes are 4 to 6 weeks, this is the bracing timeframe when bracing is used after an acute MCL injury.

SCREENING/DIFFERENTIAL DIAGNOSIS QUESTIONS

7. **When should a patient be screened for the risk of deep vein thrombosis as a component of a knee evaluation?**

Wells and colleagues (2006) formed a clinical prediction rule (CPR) for examining appropriateness for referral for DVT investigation (Table 72-4) (Wells and Colleagues DVT CPR). In a primary care setting, confirmed DVT was 26% in patients classified as "low risk" (<2 pts), and 63% in patients classified as "high risk" (≥2 pts) (Table 72-5) (Primary Care DVT CPR).

Clinicians need to be considering these decision-making tools for any patient that has diminished activity levels or immobilization after injury or when completing postoperative rehabilitation. Any patient scored as moderate-to-high risk warrants consultation with the referring physician at a minimum, with communication on steps and decision-making for D-dimer and diagnostic ultrasound to rule out a potential DVT.

Table 72-4 Wells and Colleagues DVT CPR

CLINICAL VARIABLES	POINTS
Active cancer or cancer treated within 6 months	+1
Paralysis, paresis, or recent orthopedic casting of lower extremity	+1
Recently bedridden (>3 days) or major surgery within 12 weeks	+1
Localized tenderness in deep venous system	+1
Swelling of entire leg	+1
Calf swelling 3 cm greater than other leg (measured 10 cm below the tibial tuberosity)	+1
Pitting edema greater in the symptomatic leg	+1
Collateral nonvaricose superficial veins	+1
Previously documented DVT	+1
Alternative diagnosis more likely than DVT: Baker's cyst, cellulitis, musculoskeletal injury, superficial venous thrombosis, postthrombotic syndrome, external venous compression, varicose veins, chronic venous insufficiency, hematoma, heart failure, chronic liver or kidney disease, lymphedema	–2

Score (Points)	Risk Stratification	D-dimer (Blood Test)	Ultrasound (US)
0	Low risk (DVT prevalence ~5%)	Use mod or high sensitivity D-dimer Neg—rule out DVT Pos—proceed to US	Neg- rule out DVT Pos- consider anticoagulation treatment
1–2	Moderate risk (DVT prevalence ~17%	Use high sensitivity D-dimer only Neg—rule out DVT Pos—proceed to US	Neg- rule out DVT Pos- consider anticoagulation treatment
≥3	High risk (DVT prevalence 17%–53%) All get D-dimer and US	High sensitivity D-dimer only ALL proceed to US	Neg D-dimer plus and neg US = rule out Neg D-dimer and positive US consider anticoagulants Pos D-dimer and pos US- use anticoagulants Post D-dimer and neg US- retest in 1 week

Table 72-5 Primary Care Setting DVT CPR

CLINICAL VARIABLES	POINTS
Personal history of DVT	+1
Immobilization in the previous month	+1
Estrogen contraceptive	+2
Active malignancy	+3
Swelling of the calf	+1
Presence of an alternative diagnosis more likely than DVT	–3

8. **Patient's prescription at the time of evaluation says "knee pain"; however, they subjectively report no mechanism of injury. The initial paperwork is unremarkable for an injury event and during an objective examination there is no limitation in knee range of motion, no palpable pain, no pain with resisted knee extension, and no limitations in tibiofemoral or patellofemoral joint mobility. What else should be considered?**

The clinician considers red flag screening that may result in consultation with another health care provider. Questions that could be revisited in this case could include but are not limited to rapid and unexplained weight gain or loss, fever, night pain unrelated to movement, acute and insidious pain, and unexplained joint aching and malaise.

In the absence of a clear injury mechanism or symptom onset, clinicians should be mindful of potential for referred or systemic causes of pain. Examples of these include rheumatoid arthritis, OA, or systemic illness such as lupus or Lyme disease. In 90% of Lyme disease cases, a systemic illness resulting from a deer tick bite causing pain and swelling or migratory polyarthritis, knee pain is a major complaint. Questions that could be revised include exposure to tick areas, any unexplained rashes, and any short flu-like symptoms. At times, referring a patient to rule out Lyme disease is a step in differential diagnosis that adds value to the evaluation.

The clinician should also consider revisiting the subjective and asking questions regarding pain in additional regions and any correlation with their chief complain of knee pain. As far as the objective examination, screening of the neurological system (lower quarter screen) lumbar, sacroiliac, and hip regions should also be considered as potential sources of pain referred to the knee. Referred pain from another adjacent areas is likely when there is unexplained pain and the presence of a negative knee examination.

9. **A 10-year-old boy presents with insidious onset of medial knee pain that has worsened over the past few months until participation in recreation and school sports was impacted. On objective examination, knee range of motion is full and pain-free. Ligamentous testing of medial and lateral collateral ligaments (valgus and varus gapping at 0° and 30°), anterior cruciate ligament (Lachman's), and posterior cruciate ligament (quad activating test) reveals no difference bilaterally and no laxity. Provocative pain testing with palpation (medial joint line, medial plica, pes anserine) and resisted knee extension for patellofemoral pain are negative. What else should be considered?**

In the case of a young person with persistent knee pain and a negative knee examination, the clinician must consider an underlying hip disorder. In this case, slipped capital femoral epiphysis (SCAFE) and Legg-Calve-Perthes disease are potential differential diagnoses. SCAFE, which involves slippage of the femoral head at the growth plate, typically occurs in prepubescent males (8–18 years old) who are either overweight or slender and tall. In the case of an endocrine disorder (diagnosed or undiagnosed) the age can be slightly older. Legg-Calve-Perthes typically occurs in children between 5 and 12 years old and involved avascular necrosis of the femoral head.

The clinician should consider hip clinical tests that either attempt to reproduce symptoms (flexion, abduction, and external rotation ([FABER]) or examine for loss of hip internal rotation (IR) and excessive hip external rotation (ER). This should be completed bilaterally as SCAFE is present bilaterally in as many as 50% of the cases. If this hip examination provokes knee pain, and is significantly limited in hip IR with or without excessive hip ER, the patient needs to be referred for imaging and if positive for surgical consultation.

10. **A patient has sustained a trauma (eg, fall from a ladder) as a cause of injury. Is a referral for radiographs indicated?**

Ottawa knee rules provide guidance for determining referrals for radiographs when blunt trauma or a fall is the mechanism of injury. They have been validated in person >12 years of age and provide 100% sensitivity for ruling-out fractures. The rules have not been validated on injuries older than 7 days; they are for acute injuries. The evaluation includes collecting and identifying the required key indicators (Table 72-6) (Ottawa Knee Rules). If one or more of the key indicators is present, referral for radiographs is indicated. When applied appropriately, these rules actually help to reduce unnecessary radiographs by 78% without missing any needed referrals.

Table 72-6 Ottawa Knee Rules

OTTAWA KNEE RULES (INDICATED FOR BLUNT TRAUMA OR FALL)
1. Age greater than 55 years
2. Isolated tenderness of the patella
3. Tenderness of the fibular head
4. Inability to flex the knee to 90°
5. Inability to weight bear (4 steps) both immediately and in the emergency room/at time of examination

LIGAMENT SPECIFIC QUESTIONS

COLLATERAL LIGAMENTS (LCL, MCL)

11. On evaluation the patient has an isolated collateral ligament injury, what is the anticipated plan of care for this patient?

Injuries to the collaterals without other concomitant injury are usually managed nonoperatively. There is mixed evidence on the results of nonoperative management of isolated lateral collateral ligament (LCL) sprains; however, the evidence is very clear that nonoperative management is recommended for isolated MCL sprains. Paramount to early (~4–6 weeks depending on degree of sprain) nonoperative management is the avoidance of excessive tibiofemoral rotation (MCL: avoid external rotation and extreme IR; LCL: avoid internal rotation) during progressive resistance activities. As with most ligamentous conservative management, normalizing quadriceps strength and facilitating dynamic stabilization is key.

In more rare cases where surgical intervention is deemed necessary, protection of the collateral repair site is important. Early use of an immobilizer is essential to prevent frontal plane stresses. The knee is braced or immobilized in 30° of flexion during weight-bearing activities for 2 to 6 weeks depending on the extent of the repair.

After collateral ligament repair, early ROM is encouraged. Normalizing quadriceps strength is a fundamental part of the rehabilitation process. The evidence for the rehabilitation principles for collateral injury and postsurgical management is theoretical, although based on biological healing principles. The same rehabilitation guidelines are used for MCL repair as for a grade III MCL sprain managed nonoperatively.

MCL

12. Testing for medial knee instability in a 10-year-old boy after a valgus injury demonstrates a pathologic opening of the medial compartment using a valgus stress test. What should be the primary diagnosis?

In a prepubescent individual, primary diagnostic thought should be an epiphyseal plate injury rather than an MCL sprain, as would be suspected in an adult. The reasoning is twofold: 1) the MCL is much stronger than the physes in a younger person, making it more prone to failure in a valgus stress injury mechanism, and 2) an epiphyseal injury is a much more serious injury in a young person than an MCL injury. An epiphyseal injury may require more aggressive medical treatment than an MCL sprain, and therefore immediate referral to an orthopedist is required. Physicians will likely complete radiographs upon referral, and additional CT or MRI may be required if surgical intervention is deemed to be necessary. While CT comes with the complication of radiation exposure to the child, it would allow the physician to determine intraarticular alignment and identify small fracture fragments that could complicate surgical intervention. While MRI can be complicated earlier on because of local swelling, it can be useful to evaluate vascular compromise, periosteal disruption, and surrounding soft-tissue injury.

13. The patient had a knee injury; in describing what happened, which positions place the greatest strain on the MCL leaving it susceptible to injury?

The primary role of the MCL is to restrain valgus stress as well as lateral and medial tibial rotation. While the MCL provides 57% of the resistance to valgus forces at 5° of flexion, it is relied upon even more so at 25° of flexion (78% of the resistance to valgus forces). For this reason, it is important that the valgus stress test be completed at full knee extension as well as 25° to 30° of flexion. Functionally, the MCL endures similar stresses when the patient is either hyperextended or in slight flexion (30°), and external contact or a cut/pivot motion moves the knee into a valgus position.

14. The patient has an ACL injury with a concomitant MCL injury; how would the rehabilitation program be impacted?

The rich blood supply to the MCL provides an opportunity for this ligament to heal following injury and rarely requires surgical intervention. In the case of nonoperative ACL and MCL management, the MCL nonoperative protocol would take precedence to allow for soft tissue healing. Restrictions in sagittal plane motion may be as high as 4 to 6 weeks given the grade of MCL sprain (I-III), and the patient may be asked to complete weight-bearing activities in mid-range internal rotation (placing the MCL on slack) to avoid overstressing the healing ligament. A brace may be applied that limits full extension (30° knee flexion) in order to allow the ligament to heal in a shortened position rather than full extension where it is under tension. In the event the ACL requires reconstruction, surgeons may consider a staged rehabilitation. They will follow the guidelines noted to allow for the MCL to heal and then proceed to an ACL reconstruction after the 4 to 6 week time period. In a staged procedure, recovering MCL sprains would not require modifications in the postoperative ACLR rehabilitation time period. While avoiding early full extension during exercise may be desirable for isolated MCL recovery, concurrent ACLR and MCL repairs will likely not limit full extension ROM secondary to detrimental long-term functional impact. Clinicians may, however, alter sagittal plane motion during exercise with use of IR during weight-bearing exercises is encouraged.

LCL/PLC

15. Describe the signs and symptoms of an LCL injury

The most common signs and symptoms of LCL injury are pain, stiffness, swelling, and tenderness along the lateral joint line of the knee. Walking pain typically is worse on heel strike than other parts of the gait cycle. Patients will present with a (+) varus stress test at both 0° and 30°. Patients typically complain of instability, especially in pivoting activity or change of direction, resulting in the knee "giving way." More severe tears can also cause numbness in the foot along with dorsiflexion and eversion weakness, which can occur if the peroneal nerve is stretched at time of injury or compressed by local edema or tissue post injury.

16. How can the posterior lateral corner be evaluated to determine if it was compromised in a knee injury?

The LCL is the common passive structure that blends the posterior and lateral capsule. The most posterior aspect of the lateral tibiofemoral compartment is a thickened reinforcement made up of both passive and active structures: the arcuate complex (two branches: lateral, posterior); biceps femoris and popliteus tendons. Along with the LCL, the posterolateral corner (PLC) also includes the popliteofibular ligament (PFL) and popliteus tendon.

The PLC provides support to limit excessive hyperextension, varus angulation, and tibial external rotation.

Integrity of the PLC is examined with the patient using the prone external rotation test (dial test). The clinician grasps the patient's distal leg (in prone), flexes the knee, and externally rotates the tibia. External rotation that exceeds 10° greater than the uninvolved side is a positive test. The test should be performed at both 30° and 90° of knee flexion. Increased external rotation at 30° but not at 90° indicates an isolated injury of the PLC. Increased external rotation at both angles suggests a concomitant lesion of the PCL.

Primary PCL reconstruction is unlikely to be sufficient when concomitant PLC injury is present. Rarely do they occur in isolation, but when they do, both can be reconstructed in isolation with successful outcomes. It is important to remember the cruciate ligaments also provide secondary support to frontal plan stresses. Clinicians must then remember to complete this test when any cruciate compromise is suspected as the patient may not be appropriate for long-term nonoperative management when both a cruciate ligament and a PLC injury are present. Nonoperative management of a combined PCL/PLC injury places the patient at more risk for degenerative changes in comparison to an isolated PCL injury.

An undiagnosed PLC injury unmanaged during the cruciate reconstruction can also compromise the successful rehabilitation due to the additional instability contributed by the unchecked laxity. If a prone dial test is positive, even preoperatively in the case of cruciate ligament injury, a referral back to the surgeon with suspicion and recommendation for evaluation for PLC injury is a priority.

POL

17. Where is the posterior oblique ligament (POL) located, what does it resist and why is it important to examine when either collateral or cruciate ligamentous compromise is present?

The POL is a strong reinforcement for the posteromedial tibiofemoral capsule that blends with the semimembranosus tendon. The POL provides resistance to valgus forces near full extension as well as provides stability as the knee moves into flexion given its attachment to the hamstring. Increased excursion during the valgus stress test with external rotation, which is indicative of posteromedial corner compromise, combined with other positive cruciate or collateral findings may indicate that the patient is not a candidate for nonoperative management. This would mean that the patient has compromise to multiple structures that potentially resist valgus stresses and anterior tibial translation. At a minimum the patient should be referred for further surgical consultation and second opinion.

PCL

18. The patient reports hitting their knee on the dashboard during a motor vehicle accident. What differential diagnosis should be considered?

Common tests for PCL rupture include the posterior drawer, posterior sag, and quadriceps activating tests. While all tests have fairly high sensitivity (Sn) and specificity (Sp) scores for evaluating PCL compromise, the quadriceps activating has slightly better psychometric properties (Sn 97.6%, Sp 100%). The test is performed with the patient in supine, with the hip at 45° of flexion and knee at 90° of flexion. In this position, the profile of the knee is examined, and a *sag* of the proximal tibia can be seen. Then the patient is asked to contract the quadriceps, and a positive sign is seen when the proximal tibia moves anteriorly to reduce the sag.

Besides compromise to the PCL, direct tibial posterior translation, such as a dashboard injury, often also results in injuries to secondary restraints such as the PLC. PLC compromise is best tested with the prone dial test explained earlier. Clinicians must then remember to complete this test when patient's cruciate compromise is indicated as the patient may not be appropriate for long-term conservative management. Attempt to treat without surgical intervention and concomitant PCL/PLC injury places the patient at more risk for degenerative changes in comparison to an isolated PCL injury.

19. **The patient has a PCL sprain (Gr I–III); should they be referred for surgical management or proceed with nonsurgical rehabilitation?**

    Full functional recovery with nonoperative management occurs at a higher rate for those who sustain a grade I–II PCL injury when compared to the same approach for management of a complete ACL tear. Chandrasekaran et al. have demonstrated that athletes can return to similar levels of activity and sports while pursuing nonoperative management of PCL injuries. In addition, multiple prospective studies found no association between functional outcomes and posterior laxity.

    Grade I and II tears have a rapid recovery, and the goal is to return-to-sport (RTS) within 2 to 4 weeks after injury. Shelbourne et al. (1999) completed a prospective, 10-year follow-up study of patients with grade I and II PCL tears receiving nonoperative management. A high number of the patients included in the study demonstrated high quadriceps strength symmetry (>90% symmetry compared to contralateral limb), maintained full knee ROM, were able to maintain an active lifestyle, and had a low prevalence of moderate knee OA. While Gr III PCL sprains recover slower (requiring immobilization in full extension for 2–4 weeks to limit hamstring activation that could increase stress in the posterior direction), studies have also shown these individuals can continue with a nonoperative plan of care and return to similar levels of activity. These same studies indicate that there is no association between degree of posterior laxity and long-term functional outcomes.

    The focus of acute management is related to early strengthening and effusion control with knee range of motion. Those with greater quadriceps recovery had greater levels of self-reported knee function. After quadriceps recovery, rehabilitation shifts to balance, coordination, and proprioception during weight-bearing exercises. The coactivation of muscles around the joint loaded during weight bearing helps to reduce the typical shear forces seen with open chain knee flexion and extension. In the case of Grade 3 tears early immobilization in full extension may be used for 2 to 4 weeks to control posterior subluxation during the early healing time. While quadriceps recovery is emphasized, knee flexion past 70° and resisted isolated hamstring exercises are also avoided early in rehabilitation to reduce posterior shear. Those who attempt nonoperative management for PCL sprain usually are able to RTS at about 3 months. If the patient continues to have persistent pain or persistent subjective instability makes the patient unable to continue with RTS, surgical consultation may be considered.

ACL

20. **A patient's imaging notes ACL tear with "kiss lesion"; what is the clinical implication?**

    "Kissing lesion" describes a specific type of bone contusion presentation that typically occurs from contact between the femur and tibia during a hyperextension and valgus type mechanism. This combination of forces likely causes the tibial plateau to strike the anterior aspect of the femoral condyle resulting in this specific type of lesion to occur. They are associated with a higher suspicion of simultaneous ACL compromise and any form of osteochondral finding (not just "kissing lesions") on MRI is more often associated with meniscal involvement. Bone marrow edema, bone bruise, and bone contusion are called a kissing lesion when there are matching components on both joint surfaces. Sixty-five percent of bone contusions are found in knees with ACL injury but they can occur on their own as a result of injury. The rarer kissing lesion (involving both sides of the knee joint) is only 6.5% of bone contusions. The prevalence of a bone bruise has been correlated to more severe joint damage that could impact the joint degenerative process. In a review of long-term outcomes after ACL injury and ACLR, those who present with chondral findings at the time of initial injury were more likely to report higher pain ratings at 2 years; however, function was similar between both groups. Since the injury is multifactorial it is difficult to identify the single source of the less favorable outcomes over time.

21. **The patient is a skeletally immature athlete with an ACL injury; how are they managed differently?**

    In most cases, physicians will decide surgical appropriateness based on closure status of the patient's epiphyseal growth plate. Timelines between initial injury and surgery can be as little as 6 months or as long as a few years. During this waiting period, clinicians may consider similar guidelines as nonsurgical ACL management in skeletally mature adults; the largest goal during this time is minimizing further concomitant injury (eg, tearing a meniscus not injured at the time of the original ACL tear or injury to a collateral ligament).

    A group of surgeons recently published a cluster of four clinical signs that would indicate the need for potential earlier surgical intervention: (1) skeletal age >14 years old, (2) partial tear >1/2 thickness of the original ACL, (3) tear of the posterolateral bundle, and pivot shift grade B/II or greater. If the surgeon determines that ACLR is indicated, modern operative techniques that avoid epiphyseal plate damage may be utilized (ie, Kocher technique, Anderson technique, Ganley technique, Cordasco-Green technique). Rehabilitation following ACLR in the skeletally immature athlete follows a similar timeline for that of an adult.

22. Your patient is deciding on conservative management versus surgical reconstruction after sustaining an ACL injury. What are the potential long-term consequences related to the decision?

A substantial amount of literature has shown patients who sustained an ACL injury are at risk later in life for development of knee osteoarthritis. While there is no definite answer that implies causation, current evidence has found higher association between altered gait mechanics and progressive onset of knee osteoarthritis after ACL injury. This progressive OA onset is not diminished by surgical reconstruction (ACLR) and therefore the patient likelihood of developing knee OA is not impacted by their decision of conservative versus surgical intervention.

23. The patient is considering an ACL reconstruction and has been to two different surgeons. One is offering a single bundle procedure and the other is suggesting a double-bundle procedure. The patient is interested in the evidence between the two and how that may impact their rehabilitation.

Surgeons who touted the double bundle ACLR felt the procedure should reproduce the biomechanical properties of the original ACL. Given that the procedure is more technically demanding and time consuming, the surgeon's experience with the procedure should be considered when a patient is selecting this option. While double bundle reconstructions provide better knee stability based on knee joint arthrometer and pivot shift testing, more objective measures, subjective patient outcomes, and functional test scores were not impacted by single or double bundle ACL reconstruction.

The retear rates after double bundle are similar to single bundle patellar tendon grafts (double bundle 10%, patellar tendon grafts 4%). The debate on the best way to reconstruct the ACL is likely to continue, monitoring cost, mechanical factors (postoperative laxity), and risk associated with long-term OA development and progression. There is currently no evidence to suggest any modifications in rehabilitation between single and double bundle procedures.

24. The patient has an ACL rupture but is not sure they want to undergo a surgical reconstruction. Is there information that can be collected after ACL injury to see who is appropriate to consider nonoperative management?

A screening process developed by Eastlack et al. can help identify those who may be able to return to short-term high levels of activity with nonoperative management (deemed "potential copers," meaning they may be able to cope with ACL deficiency). Clinicians need to consider that these patients must meet specific criteria before this nonoperative rehabilitation is initiated. The screening protocol is presented in (Table 72-7) (Potential Coper Screening After Confirmed ACL Compromise).

When these patients are first seen, acute impairments are notable, and it may be multiple weeks after the time of initial evaluation before the person can achieve these milestones and is then appropriate for screening to be evaluated as a "potential coper." The screen is typically administered within 2 months of the injury although some patients can reach these milestones much sooner (within days from injury). With this criteria-based screen, no patient in 20 years has extended their injury during the testing.

After screening occurs, a specialized 10-session, neuromuscular re-training program deemed "perturbation training" (Table 72-8) (Perturbation Training) was devised to assist with the potential coper's return-to-sport goals. This program consists of applying destabilizing forces to the patient's involved limb while the patient stands on tilt boards or roller boards.

At the completion of the training program, the patient is screened to see if they are appropriate for return-to-activity/sport at that time (Table 72-9) (Return-to-Activity/Sport Criteria). If not, they should continue with an impairment-based, individualized program until this status is achieved.

If or when patients complete these criteria, patients must resume full participation in their sport for a full year to be considered *true copers*.

25. How successful are patients in attempting short-term return to sport after ACL injury with nonoperative management?

Hurd et al. reported on a 10-year, prospective trial where individuals were screened for "potential coper" status developed by Eastlack et al. after ACL injury. Those that were deemed as rehabilitation candidates at the time of screening [(1) No more than one episode of giving way; (2) $\geq$80% involved/uninvolved leg during timed hop test, (3) >80% KOS ADLs scale, (4) $\geq$60% for the global rating] moved forward to 10 sessions of strengthening and neuromuscular training. After these training sessions, patients were screened for return-to-sport status and were allowed to return to high-level sporting activities. Seventy-two percent (63/88) of the potential copers who pursued nonoperative care successfully returned to high-level sports activities. None sustained additional chondral or meniscal injuries. Of note, over 10 years based on all prescreening criteria and screening criteria, approximately 10% of subjects in the study returned to full sport participation. This included those who chose not to try and opted for surgery along with those unable to pass the set criteria. These rates of return to sport are comparable to after ACLR, where studies vary in return rates from 63% to 83%. Of note, over 10 years based on

Table 72-7 Potential Coper Screening After Confirmed ACL Compromise

POTENTIAL COPER SCREENING AFTER CONFIRMED ACL COMPROMISE*			
Patient must meet the following criteria to be considered for screening: • MRI confirmation of an isolated tear of the ACL (ie, no repairable meniscal injury and or concomitant ligamentous damage) • Minimal knee effusion (Zero-Trace) • Ability to hop on injured leg without pain • Full knee range of motion • ≥70% involved/uninvolved quadriceps strength ratio			
Test	**Description**	**Rehabilitation Candidate**	**Non-Candidate**
Timed Hop Test	Part of Noyes et al. four single-limb hop tests: single, cross-over, triple, and timed hop	≥80% (involved/ uninvolved leg)	Failure of **any one** of the criteria for a rehabilitation candidate; consider surgical intervention or mitigation of activity
Knee Outcome Survey (KOS)	A patient questionnaire self-rating performance of the knee during ADLs	≥80%	
Global Rating Survey (GRS)	The patient's self-assessment of knee function during ADLs on a scale from 0 to 100, with 100 being equal to preinjury functional level	≥60%	
Episodes of Giving Way	Record the number of giving-way episodes after the one at the time of injury	≤1	

Reprinted with permission of the University of Delaware Physical Therapy Clinic—modified from *Eastlack M, Axe M, Snyder-Mackler L. Laxity, instability, and functional outcome after ACL injury: copers versus noncopers. *Med Sci Sports Exerc*, 1999;31(2):210–215.

Table 72-8 Perturbation Training

PERTURBATION TRAINING			
	EARLY (EST. SESSIONS: 1–3)	**MIDDLE (EST. SESSIONS: 4–7)**	**LATE (EST. SESSIONS: 8–10)**
A/P and M/L roller board	Position: Patient on board (bilateral stance 1st treatment, progress to unilateral) with eyes straight ahead. Application: Inform patient of direction and timing of roller board movement with straight planes of movement and slow, low magnitude, application of force. Observe: Cue patient to avoid massive cocontraction at knees. Do no overstress beyond limit of stability. Do not induce fall.	Position: Unilateral stance (avoid forefoot abduction/ adduction). Application: Unexpected forces with rapid increasing magnitude of force application, alternate planes of movement (start A/P, then M/L, progress to ER/IR), and short delay between subsequent force applications. Add rotational and diagonal movement. Distraction: May begin to add distraction (ball toss, stick work). Observe: Observe difficulty with recovery but do not allow falls.	Position: Unilateral stance. Application: Increase magnitude of force application with random direction and little to no delay between applications. Distraction: Increase speed and magnitude of distraction (consider sport specific positions). Observe: Look for dissociation of hip, knee, and ankle.

Table 72-8 Perturbation Training

PERTURBATION TRAINING	EARLY (EST. SESSIONS: 1–3)	MIDDLE (EST. SESSIONS: 4–7)	LATE (EST. SESSIONS: 8–10)
A/P and M/L tilt board	Position: Begin bilateral stance, progress to unilateral with eyes straight ahead. Application: Inform patient of direction and timing of tilting with less force medial than lateral and overall slow. Low magnitude application of force. Observe: Cue patient to maintain balance and recover quickly from the disturbance. Cue patient to avoid massive co-contraction at the knee.	Position: Unilateral stance (avoid forefoot abduction/adduction). Application: Unexpected forces with rapid, increasing magnitude of force application. Hold the board to the floor in one direction and unexpectedly release. Distraction: May begin to add distraction (ball toss, stick work). Observe: Look for rapid return to a stable base after perturbation, looking for dissociation of hip, knee, and ankle.	Position: Begin to place foot at a diagonal. Application: Increase magnitude of force application with random direction movements and little to no delay between applications. Distraction: Increase speed and magnitude of direction (consider sport-specific positions). Observe: Look for minimal sway from stable stance at rest following any perturbation.
Roller board and stationary platform set-up: The involved leg is placed on either the roller board or stationary platform and after three sets of 1 minute, the legs switch positions and the treatment is repeated. Instructions: "*Meet my force; don't beat my force. When I push the roller board, resist the exact movement in speed and magnitude. The board should remain in the same place. Do not overpower me and move the roller board away and do not let me overpower you.*"	Position: One foot on roller board, the other foot on the platform with eyes straight ahead, equal weight bearing on both lower extremities. Application: Inform patient of direction and timing of movement performing slow, low magnitude application of force. Perform all directions A/P, M/L, IR/ER, diagonals. Observe: Cue patient to maintain equal weight bearing bilaterally (watch for unweighting of involved limb as level of difficulty increases). Do not overpower the patient. The board should not move more than 1 or 2 inches.	Position: One foot on roller board, the other foot on the platform with eyes straight ahead, equal weight bearing on both lower extremities. Application: Do not inform the patient of the direction and consider combining directions (eg, anterior/lateral). Distraction: Begin distraction with ball tosses during the activity. Observe: Equal weight bearing on both lower extremities, be sure patient does not just stiffen leg to stop board from moving but responds to directions introduced by the therapist.	Position: One foot on roller board, the other on the platform with eyes straight ahead, equal weight bearing on both lower extremities. Application: Increase magnitude of force application with random direction movements and little to no delay between applications. Distraction: Increase speed and magnitude of distraction. Consider sport-specific stance—forward split, backward split. Observe: Cue patient to maintain equal weight bearing bilaterally (watch for unweighting of the involved limb as difficulty level increases). Cue patient to react as you remove force (avoid rebound board movement).
Concurrent Treatment Within-Session	Above treatment coupled with a patient-specific and progressive agility program as well as an impairment based lower extremity strengthening program.		

Reprinted with permission of the University of Delaware Physical Therapy Clinic.

Table 72-9 Return-to-Activity/Sport Criteria

RETURN-TO-ACTIVITY/SPORT CRITERIA*		
ACTIVITY OR SCORE	**DESCRIPTION**	**REQUIREMENT**
Single-Limb Hop Tests	Noyes et al. four single-limb hop tests: single, cross-over, triple, and timed hop tests	>90% for all four single-limb hop tests (involved/uninvolved leg)
Knee Outcome Survey (KOS)	A patient questionnaire self-rating performance of the knee during ADLs	>90%
Global Rating Survey (GRS)	The patient's self-assessment of knee function during ADLs on a scale from 0 to 100, with 100 being equal to preinjury functional level	>90%
Quadriceps Strength Symmetry	Isometric quadriceps strength testing; electrodynamometer, HHD or 1RM (90-0 deg OR 90-45 deg)	>90% (involved/uninvolved leg)

Reprinted with permission of the University of Delaware Physical Therapy clinic modified from *Fitzgerald GK, Axe MJ, Snyder-Mackler L. Proposed practice guidelines for nonoperative anterior cruciate ligament rehabilitation of physically active individuals. *JOSPT.* 2000; 30:194–203.

all prescreening criteria and screening criteria, approximately 10% of subjects in the study returned to full sport participation. This included those who chose not to try and opted for surgery along with those unable to pass the set criteria and those who tried and were unsuccessful. This is not an option for all patients after ACL injury but may be an option for those who meet the criteria.

Rehabilitation Questions

26. The patient has been diagnosed with a lateral collateral ligament injury. Should they be referred for surgical repair?

Most LCL injuries are managed conservatively, focusing on addressing acute impairments and minimizing varus and rotational forces for up to 6 to 8 weeks to allow for healing. In grade III LCL sprains or rarer cases, surgical intervention may be deemed necessary. Similarly, after surgery protection of the collateral repair site is important. In most cases, an immobilizer is used to prevent frontal plane stresses. The knee is braced or immobilized in 30° of flexion during weight bearing to allow the ligament to heal in a shortened position and during activities for 2 to 6 weeks depending on the extent of the repair. After collateral ligament repair, early ROM is encouraged. Normalizing quadriceps strength is a fundamental part of the rehabilitation process. The evidence for the rehabilitation principles for collateral injury and postsurgical management is theoretical, although based on biological healing principles.

If the tear occurs mid tendon, the ends are typically approximated with sutures arthroscopically. In more severe grade 3 injury, where the LCL cannot be repaired, the lateral knee requires reconstruction, which is an open knee procedure and cannot be completed arthroscopically. Tendon autografts are typically harvested from the quadriceps or the hamstrings. The grafts are passed through bone tunnels in the femur and fibula and fixated using screws or posts, or sutures are tied around a post.

Most LCL injuries are managed conservatively; however, research is mixed on the superiority of nonoperative versus operative approaches. With both approaches, collateral repair site protection is important with diminishing valgus and varus forces as well as excessive rotation of the tibiofemoral joint for 6 to 8 weeks of healing. In most postoperative cases, an immobilizer is used to prevent frontal plane stresses. This is normally done with a hinged knee brace, which can be locked in 0° to 30° of flexion during weight bearing to allow the ligament to heal in a shortened position and during activities for 2 to 6 weeks. Outcomes on nonoperative use of similar braces show mixed effectiveness. These principles are considered while implementing both weight-bearing and nonweight-bearing activities.

The focus of rehabilitation, with either approaches to management, should be an impairment-based approach that focuses on normalizing quadriceps strength and facilitating dynamic stabilization. If surgery is deemed necessary the lateral knee may require reconstruction, which is an open knee procedure (nonarthroscopic), and may use a variety of graft choices.

27. The patient had a PCL injury during skiing and had surgical reconstruction. What are the key considerations following PCL reconstruction that influence rehabilitation choices?

While many PCL injuries are caused by motor vehicle accidents (45%), athletic injuries are the next most common cause of injury (40%). Those who have a grade II tear, who are mildly symptomatic or avoid high-demand participation in sport, may be able to pursue nonoperative management. Surgical intervention is indicated for any of the following scenarios: acute tibial translation of >12 mm, concomitant injuries of the meniscus, capsuloligament injuries, or symptomatic chronic PCL injuries.

PCL laxity is known to occur following rehabilitation following reconstruction. The focus of rehabilitation is a slow progression of ROM, especially knee flexion. The graft is typically placed on tension between 70° and 90°of knee flexion; so flexion beyond that range is limited for 2 to 4 weeks as it will directly place stress on the healing graft, which tends to stretch out over time anyway. Range of motion in knee flexion is often performed in prone to minimize the posterior translation that occurs during knee flexion in supine where the tibia is loaded posteriorly by gravity.

Quadriceps recovery is a goal in PCL reconstruction recovery; however, since posterior shear forces are higher, beyond 60° knee flexion, resisted knee extension is limited to 0° to 60° range. The hamstrings provide direct attachments to contribute to posterior translation of the tibia on the femur, stressing the healing PCL, therefore, resisted knee flexion is routinely avoided for 8 weeks after surgery and high resistance loads for as long as 4 months.

28. A patient had a motorcycle accident resulting in a knee dislocation that required concurrent ACL and PCL reconstructions. Which postoperative guidelines take precedence for clinicians to follow?

When a patient has a concurrent ACLR and PCL reconstruction, the PCL rehabilitation guidelines take precedent. In general, this is because graft laxity after PCL reconstruction is typically worse in comparison to ACLR so to protect the structure least likely to recover as well, the protection of the PCL is prioritized. Acutely, active knee flexion past 70° should be initially avoided. Resisted knee flexion exercises should be approached with caution until adequate healing of the PCL (2 to 4 months after PCL reconstruction) because of the excessively high PCL stress that occurs with hamstring contractions. With the importance we commonly place on quadriceps strengthening, it is important to note that PCL shear is still noted during OKC quadriceps strengthening, with the peak value at 85° to 95°. Given this information OKC quad strengthening may be best to complete from 60° to 0° where PCL shear forces are lower.

29. A patient is slow to progress with full knee extension after ligamentous reconstruction/ repair. Are there clinical implications and consequences that require an enhanced focus on this impairment?

A preponderance of evidence demonstrates negative implications on extension range-of-motion (ROM) loss on patient postoperative function. With the status of this evidence, many protocols have early clinical milestones for regaining full active and passive knee extension ROM to avoid risk of arthrofibrosis or a more ACLR-specific issue, like a cyclops lesion. In the absence of motion occurring with movement of the knee through range of motion, scar tissue can grow and impinge on the intercondylar notch (Cyclops lesion) impinging on the graft and limiting range of motion after ACL reconstruction. Early prolonged low load positioning or stretching in full extension is universally recommended after ligamentous surgery until full knee extension is achieved (see Low-Load-Long-Duration Knee Extension Stretch "Bag Hang" Figure). When range of motion is not progressing early in the postoperative period, modified approaches and elongated stretching times and the inclusion of low loads superimposed on the stretching are encouraged. This can be in the form of bag hangs or other stretching protocols.

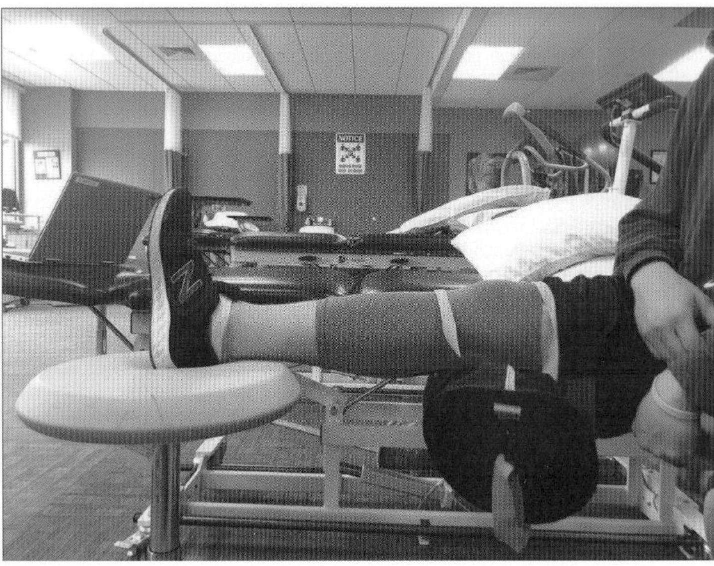

Drop-out casting is the use of an external load created by a removable cast to overcome the resistance to stretch for prolonged periods of the day and can be a useful and aggressive tool for clinicians who are attempting to help patients avoid arthroscopic debridement or a manipulation under anesthesia (see Drop Out Case Figure). The cast provides a low-load, long-duration stretching into extension by using a 3-point fulcrum system and used by the patient as much long as 23 hours a day.

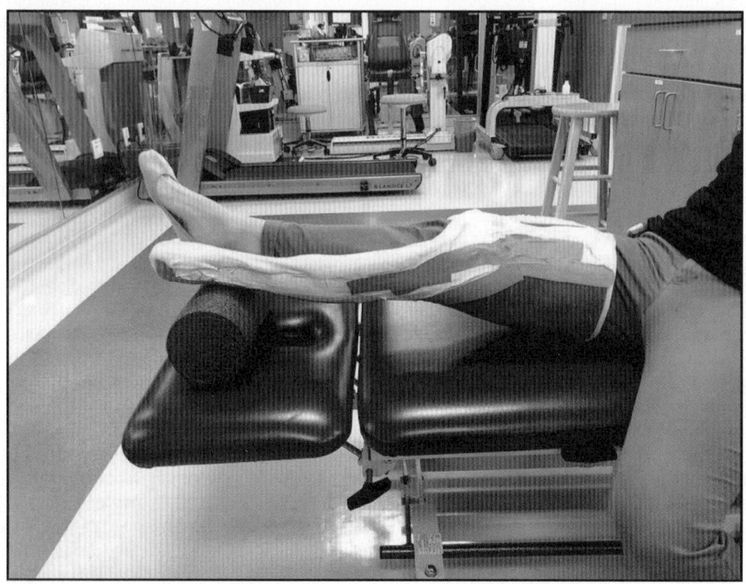

It is crafted through bivalving a long-leg cylindrical cast that may be fabricated in the clinician's or physician's office. To assess the gain made with any intervention for range of motion recovery, the use of pre- and postintervention measurements can be meaningful for assessment of the value of the intervention. For example, if a patient is lacking 10° of knee extension, after patellar mobilizations the range can again be measured. If knee extension gains are achieved, the technique would be continued; however, if gains are not made the value of the mobilizations would be questioned as a necessary component to overcome the current deficit. This can be done with each intervention included in a program aimed at knee extension gains (patellar mobilizations, tibiofemoral mobilizations, overpressure stretching, prolonged low load bag hangs, and so on). A systematic approach evaluating the individual and sequential contributions of each intervention aimed at range gains may provide insight into the order and best components to be included for gains in an individual patient situation. Gains in knee ROM are expected following each intervention, and gains are also expected to be maintained from treatment to treatment if the home program is successful in either maintaining clinical gains or contributing independently to overall gains.

30. The patient appears to have difficulty with quadriceps strength return after ligamentous injury. What accurate and reliable methodologies can be used to measure and track over time to determine if key milestones are met before patients can return to activities such as running (RTR) or return to sport (RTS)?

The significance of resolving quadriceps strength and activation impairments for those rehabilitating after knee injury or surgery cannot be overstated. The literature supporting superior clinical outcomes, assisting with RTR and RTS by striving for symmetrical quadriceps strength, is substantial. It becomes equally as important for clinicians to have reliable and systematic methods to measure and track progressions in quadriceps strength over time. Manual resistance muscle testing (break or make testing) cannot discern small or even large deficits in quadriceps muscle strength; therefore, it should not be considered as an option for postoperative patients or those with complaints of pain or instability. Instead, the use of a mechanical device is recommended for quantifying these deficits.

Small hand-held dynamometers (HHDs) can be both accurate and reliable, with standardized positions with adequate stabilization. Larger electromechanical dynamometers can also be utilized in measuring isokinetic, isotonic, or isometric quadriceps strength. These methods provide reproducibility and standardization that results in highly accurate measurements of volitional strength and symmetry (involved/uninvolved). The downfall to these forms of dynamometers is the cost and access in many clinical settings.

To address measurement access concerns, Sinacore et al. compared reliability of quadriceps strength symmetry index (involved/uninvolved) on an electromechanical dynamometer, HHD, a 1-repetition maximum (RM) test on a knee extension machine, and 1RM test on a leg press machine. In particular, the authors wanted to investigate if there would be differences in hallmark clinical decisions of RTR and RTS based on the symmetry findings of each method compared to electromechanical dynamometry as the gold standard. HHD and 1RM testing on a knee extension machine both resulted in an 8% to 10% overestimation of quadriceps strength symmetry (involved/uninvolved side) when compared to an electrodynamometer. It is important to note that 1RM testing on a leg press machine resulted in a substantially larger overestimation of quadriceps strength (23%–27%) and therefore may be less clinically useful when attempting to make decisions about RTR or RTS. A 1RM knee extension machine and HHD testing are usable alternatives for quadriceps strength measures when an electromechanical dynamometer is not available with consideration that the results include an overestimation that should be recognized and included in the final analysis.

31. Would my patient benefit from neuromuscular electrical stimulation (NMES) after knee ligamentous injury (without or without surgery)? How is this modality best incorporated into a program?

Clinicians should consider augmenting a quadriceps strengthening program with NMES for any patient presenting with weakness, including those after ligamentous injury. This is particularly true for those who demonstrate quadriceps strength deficits of ≥15% to 20% (involved compared to uninvolved). Faster quadriceps strength gains were noted when NMES augmented a strength program for those after ACLR. The use of NMES is typically discontinued when the quadriceps force output of the involved leg is ≥80% of the uninvolved quadriceps force (eg, side to side comparison).

Quadriceps NMES is typically performed while on an electrodynamometer or knee extension machine, and after a maximum voluntary isometric contraction (MVIC) or 1-repetition max (1-RM) is completed. Sinacore et al. described forms of 1-RM testing that can be utilized for this purpose. Testing before performance is important for establishing the dosage of NMES. During the electrical stimulation procedure, 10 contractions of 10 seconds each are elicited on a resting muscle and the intensity (milliamps) is increased until the electrically generated contraction creates at least 50% of the previously tested MVIC or 1-RM. For example, if a patient's 1-RM on a knee extension machine is 100 lbs on the day of treatment, NMES alone should be able to initiate movement at 50 lbs or greater on the machine for proper dosage. After this is accomplished, the clinician can simply complete the full intervention isometrically by raising the resistance to anything >50%, which will limit any knee extension motion during the NMES treatment.

Depending on the injury or procedure, the angle of the knee may be altered. Electrodes are normally placed over the VMO and 3 to 4 inches distal to the anterior superior iliac spine on the rectus femoris Russian-type stimulation parameters have been used with a burst-modulated current with a pulse duration of 400 microseconds, 75 pulses per second, and a 2-second ramp time. Inclusive of ramp time, a 12 second on time and a rest period of 50 seconds are used to allow recovery between contractions and to optimize strength gains.

Typically, the literature describes the electrical stimulation being performed isometrically (no movement of the knee during the procedure) at angles between 90° and 30° of knee range. Completing quadriceps NMES in full extension has also been described. When performed, the dosage is determined by subjective patient max tolerance after a full, sustained, tetanic contraction resulted in a superior patellar glide. Since maximal volitional contracts are difficult to perform and measure in this position, the intensity is set to maximal tolerable. Fitzgerald et al. (2003) noted inferior clinical outcomes when compared to groups where force output was used to determine NMES dosage in positions of greater knee flexion; however, if those positions are not tolerated by the patient due to pain or range limitations, those receiving electrical stimulation still outperformed those receiving volitional exercise alone. Therefore, electrical stimulation in full extension without recording force output is better than nothing; however, creatively measuring force and dosing the electrical stimulation compared to a force output remains the goal.

Precautions for NMES use include uncontrolled hyper/hypotension, excessive adipose tissue, pregnancy (location dependent), severe osteoporosis, and impaired sensation. Contraindications for its use for patients with knee conditions include a history of demand-type pacemaker implantation, known history of peripheral vascular disease, known neoplasm or infection in the area, skin integrity limitations, and the patient's inability to provide clear feedback on response to intensity or dosage.

32. The patient requires intense quadriceps strengthening following ACL reconstruction. Should the rehabilitation program only include closed kinetic chain exercises (CKC) to protect the healing graft while enhancing muscle recovery?

Until recently, many clinicians speculated that forms of open kinetic chain (OKC) quadriceps strengthening had negative consequences on surgically reconstructed ACL grafts, which could result in graft loosening. More recent work has compared ACL graft strain during OKC strengthening to typical postsurgical activities. It was discovered that normal walking exerted three times greater ACL strain compared to OKC quadriceps exercise. Peak strain noted in these studies was up to 10% to 13% between heel contact and midstance of the gait cycle. Other systematic reviews and meta-analyses also concluded there was no significant difference in anterior tibial laxity when programs incorporated OKC strengthening after ACL reconstruction.

Beynnon et al. (1997) found similar levels of ACL peak strain levels (3%–5%) at 10° knee flexion for both OKC and CKC exercises. Given the data, the avoidance of OKC strengthening exercises for most cases after ACL has no clinical basis. There is also evidence to show clinicians who choose to avoid OKC quadriceps strengthening after ACL reconstruction may be delaying patient recovery. Snyder-Mackler et al. (1995) demonstrated that weight-bearing exercises were not sufficient to restore quadriceps strength after ACLR. Because the graft is the weakest at 12 weeks postoperatively, full recovery of the quadriceps musculature must be reached by this time point so dynamic stability can help protect the graft. While weight-bearing exercise may be beneficial by addressing proprioception and incorporating multijoint movement patterns, nonweight-bearing exercises (OKC) isolate quadriceps function during knee extension. A comprehensive rehabilitation program should include a combination of weight-bearing and nonweight-bearing exercises and is likely to improve both strength and coordinated movement.

33. The patient has weak quadriceps after knee ligamentous injury. Should rehabilitation prioritize eccentric quadriceps strengthening exercises and are eccentric exercises superior to concentric?

Previous literature has suggested that eccentric muscle training can be more effective at addressing muscular hypertrophy and strength testing than concentric or isometric exercise. A more recent systematic review of the topic indicated no differences when compared to other forms of muscular loading programs. Programs focused on a combination of both concentric heavy slow resistance straining and eccentric loading demonstrated superior patient satisfaction, strength, and function compared to an isolated eccentric program.

At the same time, when chosen with clinical reasoning, eccentric strengthening can be a helpful adjunct in rehabilitation after ligamentous injury. Clinicians may find eccentrics beneficial if pain and activation deficits result in the patient's diminished ability to complete an exercise with a normal concentric contraction. Such impairments in quadriceps activation and patellofemoral pain are common after ligamentous injury or surgical intervention. For example, if a patient after ACLR cannot complete a long arc quad on a knee extension machine unilaterally, focusing on the lowering or eccentric contraction may be completed in the short term until the patient can activate the concentric leg raise on their own.

The patellar tendon is also commonly involved after ACLR, with the growing use of bone-patellar tendon-bone grafts (BPTB) in younger individuals. Longer-lasting patellar tendinopathy can impact the ability to strengthen the quadriceps. In these scenarios, clinical presentations of patellar tendinopathy may be present as a result of compensations or substitutions with ADLs or gait over time. It has been suggested that the use of a decline board, with a unilateral squat, can be a helpful exercise in recovery from this condition.

While the addition of decline squats may be valuable in patellar tendon recovery, the superiority of an eccentric program has not been established in this population. Instead, based off the work of Silbernagel et al., a pain monitoring model is advocated for addressing pain patellar tendinopathy. This includes the use of a visual-analogue-scale (VAS) to ensure pain does not surpass 5/10 during exercise and using a combination of slow-heavy-concentric and eccentric resistance training.

In Table 72-10 (Eccentric Loading Patellar Tendon Programs) below are program examples of studies for patellar tendon rehabilitation where eccentric programs were utilized, and sufficient parameters were reported to allow clinicians to recreate loading programs.

34. When should clinicians think to incorporate blood flow restriction (BFR) therapy into treatment after ligamentous injury or surgery?

Many clinicians have recently adopted BFR therapy into their clinical practice to promote hypertrophy and reach therapeutic levels of exercise with submaximal resistance. To complete lower extremity BFR, some form of tourniquet is placed around the proximal thigh and a percentage of vascular occlusion (percentage based on recommendations) is superimposed on the patient while completing exercises. While the exact mechanism for hypertrophy is unknown, it is thought to be a combination of both mechanical and metabolic stresses on the system.

To date, BFR shows no superior outcomes or additive value in hypertrophy or function when compared to a traditional high-load (high resistance, low repetition) training program. However, evidence for BFR programs is substantial for hypertrophy and improved function when compared to a low-load training program. Most clinicians normally would not support low-load programs for strengthening as they are subtherapeutic for the desired effect; however, some patients are unable to tolerate high-load programs (eg, patellofemoral pain, sarcopenia in the elderly population). In these cases, the addition of BFR may allow them to strengthen when they would otherwise be unable to achieve therapeutic responses due to underdosing.

Table 72-11 (Lower Extremity Blood Flow Restriction [BFR] Guidelines) provides guidelines on parameters for lower extremity BFR use. It should be noted that due to occluding vascular supply to the lower extremity, therapists should consult with referring physicians/surgeons if the patient presents with a history of cardiovascular issues or they present post surgery.

Table 72-10 Eccentric Loading Patellar Tendon Programs

PROGRAMS	TYPE OF EXERCISE	SETS, REPETITIONS	FREQUENCY	PROGRESSION	PAIN
Alfredson	Eccentric	3,15	Two times daily	Load	Enough load to achieve up to moderate pain
Stanish & Curwin	Eccentric-concentric power	3,10–20	Daily	Speed then load	Enough load to be painful in the third set
Sibernagel	Eccentric-concentric, eccentric, faster eccentric-concentric, balance exercise, plyometric	Various	Daily	Volume, type of exercise	Acceptable if within defined parameters*
Heavy Slow Resistance	Eccentric-concentric	4,15–16	Three times per week	15–16 repetitions of maximum	Acceptable if pain was not worse after

*Moderate (<5 of 10 on a visual analog scale, 10 = worst pain imaginable); subsided by the following day.
Reprinted with Permission of the University of Delaware Physical Therapy Clinic.

(1) *Alfredson, Håkan. "Chronic midportion Achilles tendinopathy: an update on research and treatment."* Clinics in sports medicine 22.4, *2003;727–741.*

(2) *Stanish, William D., Sandra Curwin, and M. Rubinovich. "Tendinitis: the analysis and treatment for running."* Clinics in sports medicine 4.4 *1985; 593–609.*

(3) *Silbernagel KG, Thomeé R, Eriksson BI, Karlsson J. Continued sports activity, using a pain-monitoring model, during rehabilitation in patients with Achilles tendinopathy: a randomized controlled study.* Am J Sports Med. *2007;35(6):897–906.* http://doi.org/10.1177/0363546506298279.

Table 72-11 Lower Extremity Blood Flow Restriction (BFR) Guidelines

Exercise % 1-Repetition Maximum	15%–30%
Repetitions per sets	30-15-15-15
Rest between sets	30 sec
% arterial occlusion	60%–80% *(80% preferred)*

*No suggested use of a tourniquet without known % occlusion
Based on Fujita et al., Madarama et al., and Wilson et al.

(1) *Fujita T, Brechue W, Kurita K, Sato Y, Abe T: Increased muscle volume and strength following six days of low-intensity resistance training with restricted muscle blood flow.* Int J KAATSU Train Res, *2008; 4:1–8.*

(2) *Madarame H, Kurano M, Takano H, et al. Effects of low-intensity resistance exercise with blood flow restriction on coagulation system in healthy subjects.* Clin Physiol Funct Imaging, *2010; 30(3):210–213.*

(3) *Wilson JM, Lowery RP, Joy JM, Loenneke JP, Naimo MA: Practical blood flow restriction training increases acute determinants of hypertrophy without increasing indices of muscle damage.* J Strength Cond Res, *2013; 27(11):3068–3075.*

35. The patient had a bone-patellar-tendon bone ACL reconstruction and complains of pain during strengthening and quadriceps loading. How can a patient's pain be managed without reducing their training loads to subtherapeutic levels?

Anterior knee pain is a common patient complaint about patients after ACLR, particularly in those where the BPTB autografts were utilized. Before attempting symptom modulation strategies, it is important for clinicians to consider if they have truly met clinical milestones earlier in the rehabilitative process (resolving ROM, effusion, patellar mobility, quadriceps strength deficits), as foregoing these recommendations may increase a patient's likelihood for setbacks in later strengthening phases.

Patellar taping is successful in decreasing complaints of pain in patients with PFP. Recently published CPGs gave patellofemoral taping a grade of B for enhancing short-term (4 weeks) outcomes and assisting with decreasing pain so a person can return to an exercise program.

While the exact mechanism for improvement is unknown, taping is thought to relieve knee pain by unloading irritated tissues or altering patellar stresses. Clinicians may use a *comparable sign* (eg, lateral step-down test, squatting, pain during the specific strengthening/loading exercise), which is performed pre and post taping. The purpose of this assessment is to confirm that the taping is having a positive impact on the pain complaint. Even the best clinicians may require multiple attempts to find the most effective, and patient-specific, taping application. Application and reapplication of tape to relieve symptoms, not alter patellar position, is the clinical goal. When patients are unable to tolerate higher-load training (in this case secondary to pain, BFR is another intervention that should be considered (please see above for BFR considerations and evidence-based parameters).

36. **How can functional testing be used to compare a patient's performance to the normative population or cluster their performance for determining readiness for return to activity?**
For some time, clinical literature has attempted to discern and validate a particular battery of tests that either decreases or eliminates risk of reinjury when returning to a high level of activity (sport). While there is no gold standard battery of testing for all forms of athletes, the most commonly used functional tests to help with this clinical decision-making are a series of 1-legged hops described by Noyes et al. (1991). The test requires a 6-inch wide, 6-meter long line and a stopwatch. Before completion of each test, the patient performs two practice trials on each side to allow for warm up and learning of the activities. The patient performs two trials of each of the following four hop tests: single hop for distance, triple hop for distance, crossover triple hop for distance, and a timed 6-meter hop (see Hop Tests Figure).

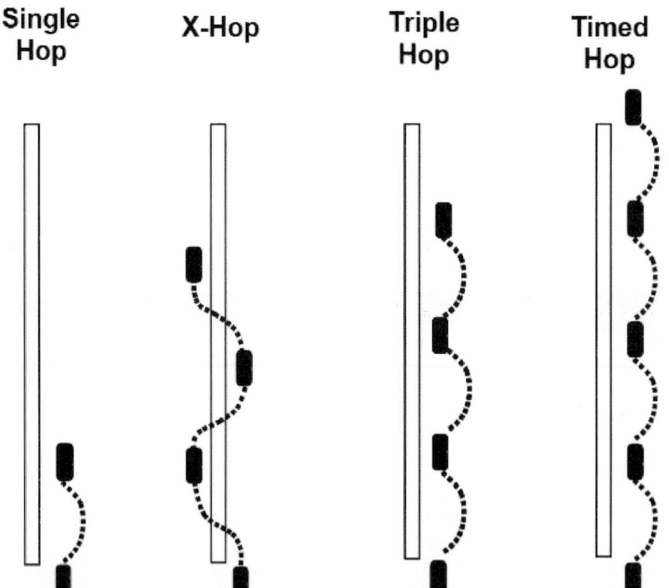

The two trials are averaged for each side and either the raw distance or time can be used or, when appropriate, a comparison between the involved and uninvolved side can be calculated to demonstrate how the involved leg performed as a percentage of the "uninvolved."

Patient likelihood of reinjury when returning to a level 1 sport (>50 hours per year, sports that require jumping, hard pivoting, and cutting, eg, soccer, football, basketball) after ALCR is reduced by 84% if symmetry (involved/uninvolved) of these four hop tests are combined in a battery of measures for RTS criteria: (1) ≥90% symmetry on all four single limb hop tests, (2) ≥90% quadriceps strength, (3) ≥90% KOS-ADLs score, (4) ≥90% global rating scale.

While symmetry is normally considered for this decision-making, clinicians may also find utility in having normative values for younger athletes. The normative values of high school and collegiate basketball and soccer players are provided below (Table 72-12) (Hop Test Normative Values for Collegiate and Highschool Athletes).

A continued deficit in lower extremity hop performance would trigger adjustments to the rehabilitation program; however, symmetry recovery alone is not the only criteria for return to activity. It is important to consider that

Table 72-12 Hop Test Normative Values for Collegiate and High School Athletes

	MALE COLLEGE	FEMALE COLLEGE	MALE HIGH SCHOOL	FEMALE HIGH SCHOOL
Single Hop Test	1.92 m +/- 20 cm	1.49 m +/- 17 cm	1.81 m +/- 20 cm	1.29 m +/- 18 cm
	6 ft 4 in +/- 8 in	4 ft 11 in +/- 7 in	5 ft 11 in +/- 8 in	4 ft 3 in +/- 7 in

Adapted from the International Journal of Sports Physical Therapy. Myers BA, Jenkins WL, Killian C, Rundquist P. Normative data for hope tests in high school and collegiate basketball and soccer players. Int J Sports Phys Ther. 2014;9(5):596-603. c 2014, IJSPT.

return to activity decision-making is multifactorial, and clinicians likely need to consider biological healing, strength assessments, and even self-efficacy along with these functional measures. Grindem et al. demonstrated that reinjury rate after ACLR is reduced by 51% for each month RTS is delayed until 9 months post surgery. So, while these criteria are a starting point of discussion between the patient and care team, strictly delaying RTS until 9 months or longer after ACLR should be a priority in addition to passing formal objective RTSC.

37. The athletic patient is nearing the end of rehabilitation after ACL reconstruction and preparing to return to sport. What could be included in the rehabilitation to decrease the risk of reinjury or secondary injury?

The rate of ipsilateral ACL graft rupture or contralateral knee ligamentous injury continues to be high in those with a previous reconstructed ACL injury who return to level 1 athletics. Webster et al. (2014) found younger female cohorts (<20 years) were more susceptible to ACL injury after initial ACL reconstruction (29% more likely). Given these data, it is essential to educate athletes on RTS risks, particularly for sports requiring cutting and pivoting. While fewer studies have specifically looked at an RTS programs ability to decrease reinjury risk, a recent cohort (ACL-SPORT) provided 10 additional training sessions of: (1) progressive strengthening, (2) sport-specific agilities, and (3) plyometrics before discharge from ACL rehabilitation. Those with the additional specific training had diminished ACL retear rates compared to more traditional postoperative rehabilitative cohorts (23% vs 32%–33%). Clinicians should consider these categories of activities and attempt to be as sport specific as possible when providing an RTS program for patients who have met milestones and are preparing to return to sport after ACL reconstruction.

JOSPT has recently published clinical practice guidelines that provide evidence-based knee injury prevention programs across different populations derived recommended court and field prevention programs (https://www.jospt.org/doi/suppl/10.2519/jospt.2018.0303). A recent meta-analysis of eight meta-analyses found a combined ACL injury reduction rate of 50% when some form of an ACL injury prevention training program was completed. Even more impactful, the same study indicated a combined 67% reduction in noncontact ACL injuries in female athletes when a prevention program was included in the process.

Evidence suggests successful prevention programs:

(1) incorporate multiplanar components
(2) include both unilateral and bilateral activities due to the increased incidence of ACL injuries in single limb stance positions
(3) incorporate unanticipated or reaction type movements to simulate game scenarios due to higher incidence of ACL injuries in game compared to practice
(4) emphasize correct foot positioning and muscle coordination during cutting and dynamic movements
(5) consider the implications of playing surface, fatigue, and prophylactic bracing.

As we continue to see a high rate of second ACL injuries after RTS, clinicians are also in search of programs that help with secondary injury prevention. In a recent study, secondary ACL injury rates were compared in different cohorts. Those who received 10 additional training sessions of progressive strengthening, sport-specific agilities, and plyometrics (ACL-SPORT cohort) had diminished ACL retear rates compared to more traditional postoperative rehabilitative cohorts (23% vs 32%–33%).

38. The patient has a second ACL injury after returning from a primary ACL reconstruction. Is this atypical and how should rehabilitation be altered?

Despite all the advancements in surgical intervention and rehabilitation, second ACL injury rates continue to be high among those who attempt to return to preinjury, high-level sports function (4× increased likelihood of reinjury when returning to level 1 sport after ACLR). Young athletes that RTS after ACLR are four times as likely to sustain a second ipsilateral ACL rupture and five times as likely to sustain a contralateral ACL rupture. Clinicians should be particularly aware that younger females (aged 6–19) have a significantly high rate of second ACL injury, up to 32%. Consideration should be given on slowing down the rate of RTS in these populations and drawing out the later rehabilitative process focused on strength and neuromuscular control.

In the event a second ACL injury occurs, the ACLR revision rehab guidelines are modified and prolonged after surgery. Weight-bearing status is slowed by prolonging crutch and brace use (~2 weeks or longer) to protect the already compromised graft fixation and allow biological healing to occur as most revisions have poorer surgical fixation than the original and therefore the graft requires protection and longer healing. CKC and weighted loading exercises in a less controlled environment should be deferred until 4 weeks after surgery. Running, hop testing, and agility drills are delayed by 4 weeks or longer. Return to sport is also significantly delayed and may be up to 1 year or beyond.

39. **What patient data can be collected to better predict recovery and success in return to sport?**
Studies to assist with return-to-sport decision-making use criterion-based clearance to determine readiness for returning to activity. It is important to remember that return-to-sport criteria (RTSC) used in many of these studies require greater than 90% on all four single limb hop tests (Noyes) and for quadriceps strength (see strength measurement question), KOS-ADLs score, global rating scale, and IKDC 2000 score. The Knee Outcome Survey (KOS) has a sport and activities of daily living subscale. The global rating scale is a scale of 0 to 100 where 100 = the preinjury level of performance and the patient self-rates their current functional level concerning preinjury levels. While those that return to level 1 sports (>50 hours per year, sports that require jumping, hard pivoting, and cutting, eg, soccer, football, basketball) after ACLR are four times more likely to reinjure over 2 years, passing these RTSC before participating in sports reduces this risk by 84%.

40. **A patient is 9 months after ACLR and working on returning back to sport but is cautious and hesitant during sport-specific movements. How can you quantify the potential psychological impact of this challenge?**
The psychological aspects of rehabilitation are an emerging topic of within the medical community, and the ACL-Return to Sport after Injury (ACL-RSI) scale was designed for specifically this clinical challenge. This clinical tool was developed to measure an athlete's psychological readiness to return to sport after ACL and ACLR. It asks questions about the athlete's opinion on their readiness to play sport without concern for their knee at their previous level and asks about their nervousness and fear of reinjury with sport participation.
The tool demonstrates good internal consistency and reliability; however, there currently is no clear cutoff for abnormal fear of activity or a cut score for return-to-play clinical decision-making. Recently, Webster and Feller (2018) did show that at 6 months ACL-RSI score possessed "fair-to-good" predictive ability to both determine: (1) If someone would return to their preinjury level of competition at 12 months (62 pts: Sn 57%, Sp 81%); (2) if someone would fail RTS criteria at 12 months (42 pts: Sn 57% Sp 78%). Therefore, the best use of the ACL-RSI is to provide an objective measure of the patient's current feeling toward return to sport and allow clinicians to use the information to drive discussions or even graded exposure opportunities to reduce the athlete's concerns and demonstrate progressive success in return-to-sport activities.

41. **The patient is athletic and has had many friends who have had ACL injuries. They are interested in an evaluation and recommendations to prevent an ACL injury. What components are in evidence-based ACL injury prevention programs?**
Given the high rate of initial injury or subsequent reinjury within certain athletic patient populations, literature has been published over the last 5 to 10 years in attempts to formulate a program to minimize the risk ligamentous injury in active populations. A recent evaluation of meta-analyses, which included eight meta-analyses, found an ACL injury prevention training program could have an overall 50% reduction in ACL injury across all sports and both sexes and a 67% reduction in noncontact ACL injury in female athletes.
Sugimoto and colleagues concluded that ACL prevention programs should be structured with the following specific recommendations: (1) incorporate multiplanar components, (2) include both unilateral and bilateral activities due to the increased incidence of ACL injuries in single limb stance positions, (3) incorporate unanticipated or reaction type movements to simulate game scenarios due to higher incidence of ACL injuries in game compared to practice, (4) emphasize correct foot positioning and muscle coordination during cutting and dynamic movements, and (5) consider the implications of playing surface, fatigue, and prophylactic bracing.

CHAPTER 72 QUESTIONS

1. **Your patient was in a motor vehicle accident and hit their knee on the dashboard during the impact. You note bruising at the proximal tibia on evaluation. You suspect a PCL injury and confirm it with a quadriceps activating test. ACL is ruled out with a Lachman test. Which condition should be evaluated to rule it out as a secondary injury that can complicate the nonoperative management of this condition? Which test will provide you the information?**
a. Posterior lateral corner (PLC) injury is suspected, perform a pivot shift test
b. Posterior lateral corner (PLC) injury is suspected, perform a prone dial test
c. Lateral collateral ligament injury is suspected, perform a valgus stress test
d. Medial collateral ligament injury is suspected, perform a varus stress test

2. **The test is positive, and the patient is returned to the surgeon with this information for further evaluation. The patient returns after surgical management. Early after surgical reconstruction, range of motion of knee flexion is limited to which angle?**
   a. Knee flexion beyond 15° is limited early after surgical reconstruction
   b. Knee flexion beyond 30° is limited early after surgical reconstruction
   c. Knee flexion beyond 50° is limited early after surgical reconstruction
   d. Knee flexion beyond 70° is limited early after surgical reconstruction

3. **Your patient has come to rehabilitation after a double bundle anterior cruciate ligament reconstruction surgery. What changes to your rehabilitation program are necessary?**
   a. There is no evidence to suggest any modification in rehabilitation is needed.
   b. Limit resisted knee flexion (hamstring) exercise early in the postoperative time period.
   c. Keep patient on crutches for 3 months postoperatively.
   d. Limit weightbearing on the reconstructed limb for 4 to 6 months postoperatively.

4. **The rehabilitation program is progressing; however, the patient is unable to tolerate a high resistance strengthening program. In order to supplement the low load resistance program you are planning to incorporate blood flow restriction. The parameters you are considering….**
   a. Arterial occlusion of 40% and resistance of 20% 1-repetition maximum
   b. Arterial occlusion of 60% and resistance of 10% 1-repetition maximum
   c. Arterial occlusion of 70% and resistance of 25% 1-repetition maximum
   d. Arterial occlusion of 90% and resistance of 30% 1-repetition maximum

5. **Your 40-year-old patient fell onto the ground this morning from the side of a boat trailered in a boat yard onto their leg. They complain of knee pain. You are determining if the person should be referred for radiographs. They have no isolated tenderness of the patella, no tenderness of the fibular head, and have knee flexion of 115°. Which of the following would necessitate a referral for radiographs?**
   a. Knee effusion
   b. Inability to weight bear and walk four steps
   c. Pain in the back of the knee
   d. Inability to perform a strong quadriceps muscle contraction

6. **The radiographs were negative, and the ligaments were evaluated without any significant clinical findings. The knee recovers quickly and as you are prepared to return the patient to their jogging program they get "knee soreness that begins with the warm up that continues as they try to do their program." Using this information for your decision-making for their running program, you will advise the patient…**
   a. Advance the program by 10% tomorrow
   b. Take 1 day off and repeat this step of the program do not progress to the next step
   c. Take 2 days off, drop down one step in the program
   d. Stay at this step, repeat this program tomorrow, and do not progress to the next step

Bibliography

Adams, D., Logerstedt, D., Hunter-Giordano, A., Axe, M. J., & Snyder-Mackler, L. (2012). Current concepts for anterior cruciate ligament reconstruction: a criterion-based rehabilitation progression. *Journal of Orthopaedic & Sports Physical Therapy, 42*(7), 601–614.

Albright, J. P., Powell, J. W., Smith, W., et al. (1994). Medial collateral ligament knee sprains in college football. Effectiveness of preventative braces. *American Journal of Sports Medicine, 22*(1), 12–18.

Arundale, A. J. H., Bizzini, M., Giordano, A., et al. (2018). Exercise-based knee and anterior cruciate ligament injury prevention. *Journal of Orthopaedic & Sports Physical Therapy, 48*(9), A1–A25.

Arroll, B., Robb, G., & Sutich, E. (2003). The diagnosis and management of soft tissue knee injuries: internal derangements. New Zealand Guidelines Group. https://www.moh.govt.nz/notebook/nbbooks.nsf/0/CF4EAA928B2FFEFECC257ECD0077A665/$file/Diagnosis%20and%20management%20of%20soft%20tissue%20knee%20injuries.pdf.

Axe, M., & Snyder-Mackler, L. (2005). Operative and postoperative management of the knee In M. A. Wilmarth (Ed.), *ISC 15.3, Postoperative Management of Orthopaedic Surgeries.* Orthopedic Section, APTA.

Axe, M. J., Snyder-Mackler, L., Konin, J. G., & Strube, M. J. (1996). Development of a distance-based interval throwing program for Little League-aged athletes. *American Journal of Sports Medicine, 24*(5), 594–602.

Bach, J. M., Hull, M. L., & Patterson, H. A. (1997). Direct measurement of strain in the posterolateral bundle of the anterior cruciate ligament. *Journal of Biomechanics, 30*(3), 281–283.

Baker, C. L., Norwood, L. A., & Hughston, J. C. (1984). Acute combined posterior cruciate and posterolateral instability of the knee. *American Journal of Sports Medicine, 12*(3), 204–208.

Banos, J. E., Bosch, F., Canellas, M., Bassols, A., Ortega, F., & Bigorra, J. (1989). Acceptability of visual analogue scales in the clinical setting: a comparison with verbal rating scales in postoperative pain. *Methods and Findings in Experimental & Clinical Pharmacology, 11*(2), 123–127.

Barber-Westin, S. D., Noyes, F. R., & McCloskey, J. W. (1999). Rigorous statistical reliability, validity, and responsiveness testing of the Cincinnati knee rating system in 350 subjects with uninjured, injured, or anterior cruciate ligament-reconstructed knees. *American Journal of Sports Medicine, 27*(4), 402–416.

Beynnon, B. D., Fleming, B. C., Johnson, R. J., Nichols, C. E., Renstrom, P. A., & Pope, M. H. (1995). Anterior cruciate ligament strain behavior during rehabilitation exercises in vivo. *American Journal of Sports Medicine, 23*(1), 24–34.

Beynnon, B. D., Johnson, R. J., Fleming, B. C., Stankewich, C. J., Renstrom, P. A., & Nichols, C. E. (1997). The strain behavior of the anterior cruciate ligament during squatting and active flexion-extension. A comparison of an open and a closed kinetic chain exercise. *American Journal of Sports Medicine, 25*(6), 823–829.

Branch, T., Hunter, R., & Reynolds, P. (1988). Controlling anterior tibial displacement under static load: a comparison of two braces. *Orthopedics, 11*(9), 1249–1252.

Briggs, K., Kocher, M., Rokey, W., & Steadman, J. (2006). Reliability, validity and responsiveness of the Lysholm Knee score and Tegner activity scale for patients with meniscal injury of the knee. *Journal of Bone and Joint Surgery (American), 88*(4), 698–705.

Campos, J. C., Chung, C. B., Lektrakul, N., et al. (2001). Pathogenesis of the Segond fracture: anatomic and MR imaging evidence of an iliotibial tract or anterior oblique band avulsion. *Radiology, 219*(2), 381–386.

Capin, J. J., Khandha, A., Zarzycki, R., et al. (2018). Gait mechanics and tibiofemoral loading in men of the ACL-SPORTS randomized control trial. *Journal of Orthopaedic Research, 36*(9), 2364–2372.

Centner, C., Wiegel, P., Gollhofer, A., & Konig, D. (2019). Effects of blood flow restriction training on muscular strength and hypertrophy in older individuals: a systematic review and meta-analysis. *Sports Medicine, 49*(1), 95–108.

Chandrasekaran, S., Ma, D., Scarvell, J. M., Woods, K. R., & Smith, P. N. (2012). A review of the anatomical, biomechanical and kinematic findings of posterior cruciate ligament injury with respect to non-operative management. *Knee, 19*(6), 738–745.

Chatman, A. B., Hyams, S. P., Neel, J. M., et al. (1997). The patient-specific functional scale: Measurement properties in patients with knee dysfunction. *Physical Therapy, 77*(8), 820–829.

Clancy, W., Melster, K., & Raythorne, C. (1995). Posteriorlateral corner and collateral ligament reconstruction In D. Jackson D (Ed.), *Reconstructive Knee Surgery* (pp. 87–102). Raven Press.

Colliander, E. B., & Tesch, P. A. (1990). Effects of eccentric and concentric muscle actions in resistance training. *Acta Physiologica Scandinavica, 140*(1), 31–39.

Colliander, E. B., & Tesch, P. A. (1991). Responses to eccentric and concentric resistance training in females and males. *Acta Physiologica Scandinavica, 141*(2), 149–156.

Collins, N. J., Misra, D., Felson, D. T., Crossley, K. M., & Roos, E. M. (2011). Measures of knee function: International Knee Documentation Committee (IKDC) Subjective Knee Evaluation Form, Knee Injury and Osteoarthritis Outcome Score (KOOS), Knee Injury and Osteoarthritis Outcome Score Physical Function Short Form (KOOS-PS), Knee Ou. *Arthritis Care and Research (Hoboken), 63*(Suppl 11), S208–228.

Colville, M. R., Lee, C. L., & Ciullo, J. V. (1986). The Lenox Hill brace. An evaluation of effectiveness in treating knee instability. *American Journal of Sports Medicine, 14*(4), 257–261.

Cook, F. F., Tibone, J. E., & Redfern, F. C. (1989). A dynamic analysis of a functional brace for anterior cruciate ligament insufficiency. *American Journal of Sports Medicine, 17*(4), 519–524.

Costa, L. O. P., Maher, C. G., Latimer, J., et al. (2008). Clinimetric testing of three self-report outcome measures for low back pain patients in Brazil: which one is the best? *Spine (Phila Pa 1976), 33*(22), 2459–2463.

Covey, C. D., & Sapega, A. A. (1993). Injuries of the posterior cruciate ligament. *Journal of Bone and Joint Surgery (American), 75*(9), 1376–1386.

Crawford, C., Nyland, J., Landes, S., et al. (2007). Anatomic double-bundle ACL reconstruction: A literature review. *Knee Surgery, Sports Traumatology, Arthroscopy, 15*(8), 946–964.

Decoster, L., Vailas, J., & Swartz, W. (1995). Functional ACL bracing. A survey of current opinion and practice. *American Journal of Orthopaedics, 24*(11), 838–843.

Delincé, P., & Ghafil, D. (2012). Anterior cruciate ligament tears: conservative or surgical treatment? A critical review of the literature. *Knee Surgery, Sports Traumatology, Arthroscopy, 20*(1), 48–61.

Delluc, A., Le Pape, F., Le Bras, A., et al. (2012). Validation d'un score de prédiction clinique de la thrombose veineuse profonde des membres inférieurs spécifique à la médecine générale [Validation of a clinical prediction rule for the diagnosis of deep vein thrombosis of the lower limbs in primary care]. *Revue de Médecine Interne, 33*(5), 244–249.

DePhillipo, N. N., Cinque, M. E., Godin, J. A., Moatshe, G., Chahla, J., & LaPrade, R. F. (2018). Posterior tibial translation measurements on magnetic resonance imaging improve diagnostic sensitivity for chronic posterior cruciate ligament injuries and graft tears. *American Journal of Sports Medicine, 46*(2), 341–347.

Divi, S. N., & Bielski, R. J. (2016). Legg-Calve-Perthes disease. *Pediatric Annals, 45*(4), e144–e149.

Eastlack, M., Axe, M., & Snyder-Mackler, L. (1999). Laxity, instability, and functional outcome after ACL injury: copers versus noncopers. *Medicine & Science in Sports & Exercise, 31*(2), 210–215.

Edson, C. J. (2001). Postoperative rehabilitation of the multiligament-reconstructed knee. *Sports Medicine and Arthroscopy Review, 9*(3), 247–254.

Ekhtiari, S., Horner, N. S., de Sa, D., et al. (2017). Arthrofibrosis after ACL reconstruction is best treated in a step-wise approach with early recognition and intervention: a systematic review. *Knee Surgery, Sports Traumatology, Arthroscopy, 25*(12), 3929–3937.

Emparanza, J. I., & Aginaga, J. R. (2001). Validation of the Ottawa knee rules. *Annals of Emergency Medicine, 38*(4), 364–368.

Englander, Z. A., Garrett, W. E., Spritzer, C. E., & DeFrate, L. E. (2020). In vivo attachment site to attachment site length and strain of the ACL and its bundles during the full gait cycle measured by MRI and high-speed biplanar radiography. *Journal of Biomechanics, 98*, 109443.

Fanelli, G. C., Giannotti, B. F., & Edson, C. J. (1996). Arthroscopically assisted combined posterior cruciate ligament/posterior lateral complex reconstruction. *Arthroscopy, 12*(5), 521–530.

Fees, M., Decker, T., Snyder-Mackler, L., & Axe, M. J. (1998). Upper extremity weight-training modifications for the injured athlete. A clinical perspective. *American Journal of Sports Medicine, 26*(5), 732–742.

Ferraz, R. B., Gualano, B., Rodrigues, R., et al. (2018). Benefits of resistance training with blood flow restriction in knee osteoarthritis. *Medicine & Science in Sports & Exercise, 50*(5), 897–905.

Filardo, G., Andriolo, L., di Laura Frattura, G., Napoli, F., Zaffagnini, S., & Candrian, C. (2019). Bone bruise in anterior cruciate ligament rupture entails a more severe joint damage affecting joint degenerative progression. *Knee Surgery, Sports Traumatology, Arthroscopy, 27*(1), 44–59.

Fischer, D., Stewart, A. L., Bloch, D. A., Lorig, K., Laurent, D., & Holman, H. (1999). Capturing the patient's view of change as a clinical outcome measure. *JAMA, 282*(12), 1157–1162.

Fitzgerald, G. K., Axe, M. J., & Snyder-Mackler, L. (2000a). The efficacy of perturbation training in nonoperative anterior cruciate ligament rehabilitation programs for physically active individuals. *Physical Therapy, 80*(2), 128–151.

Fitzgerald, G. K., Axe, M. J., & Snyder-Mackler, L. (2000b). Proposed practice guidelines for nonoperative anterior cruciate ligament rehabilitation of physically active individuals. *Journal of Orthopaedic & Sports Physical Therapy, 30*, 194–203.

Fitzgerald, G. K., Piva, S. R., & Irrgang, J. J. (2003). A modified neuromuscular electrical stimulation protocol for quadriceps strength training following anterior cruciate ligament reconstruction. *Journal of Orthopaedic & Sports Physical Therapy, 33*(9), 492–501.

Fitzgibbons, R. E., & Shelbourne, K. D. (1995). "Aggressive" nontreatment of lateral meniscal tears seen during anterior cruciate ligament reconstruction. *American Journal of Sports Medicine, 23*(2), 156–159.

Frank, C. B., Hart, D. A., & Shrive, N. G. (1999). Molecular biology and biomechanics of normal and healing ligaments—a review. *Osteoarthritis Cartilage, 7*(1), 130–140.

Gagne, P., Simon, L., Le Pape, F., Bressollette, L., Mottier, D., Le Gal, G., & pour le groupe Géné-GETBO, (2009). Réalisation d'un score clinique de prédiction de thrombose veineuse profonde des membres inférieurs spécifique à la médecine générale [Clinical prediction rule for diagnosing deep vein thrombosis in primary care]. *La Presse Médicale, 38*(4), 525–533.

Gagnier, J. J., Shen, Y., & Huang, H. (2018). Psychometric properties of patient-reported outcome measures for use in patients with anterior cruciate ligament injuries: A systematic review. *JBJS Reviews, 6*(4), e5.

Garrick, J., & Requa, R. (1988). Prophylactic knee bracing. *American Journal of Sports Medicine, 16*(Suppl 1), S118–123.

Giles, L., Webster, K. E., Mcclelland, J., & Cook, J. L. (2017). Quadriceps strengthening with and without blood flow restriction in the treatment of patellofemoral pain: a double-blind randomized trial. *British Journal of Sports Medicine, 51*(23), 1688–1694.

Gottsegen, C. J., Eyer, B. A., White, E. A., et al. (2008). Avulsion fractures of the knee: imaging findings and clinical significance. *Radiographics, 28*(6), 1755–1770.

Graf, B. K., Ott, J. W., Lange, R. H., & Keene, J. S. (1994). Risk factors for restricted motion after anterior cruciate reconstruction. *Orthopedics, 17*(10), 909–912.

Grawe, B., Schroeder, A. J., Kakazu, R., & Messer, M. S. (2018). Lateral collateral ligament injury about the knee: anatomy, evaluation, and management. *Journal of the American Academy of Orthopaedic Surgeons, 26*(6), 127.

Griffith, C. J., LaPrade, R. F., Johansen, S., Armitage, B., Wijdicks, C., & Engebretsen, L. (2009). Medial knee injury: Part 1, static function of the individual components of the main medial knee structures. *American Journal of Sports Medicine, 37*(9), 1762–1770.

Grindem, H., Snyder-Mackler, L., Moksnes, H., Engebretsen, L., & Risberg, M. A. (2016). Simple decision rules can reduce reinjury risk by 84% after ACL reconstruction: the Delaware-Oslo ACL cohort study. *British Journal of Sports Medicine, 50*(13), 804–808.

Grood, E. S., Noyes, F. R., Butler, D. L., & Suntay, W. J. (1981). Ligamentous and capsular restraints preventing straight medial and lateral laxity in intact human cadaver knees. *Journal of Bone and Joint Surgery (American), 63*(8), 1257–1269.

Grood, E. S., Stowers, S. F., & Noyes, F. R. (1988). Limits of movement in the human knee. Effect of sectioning the posterior cruciate ligament and posterolateral structures. *Journal of Bone and Joint Surgery (American), 70*(1), 88–97.

Harner, C. D., & Hoher, J. (1998). Evaluation and treatment of posterior cruciate ligament injuries. *American Journal of Sports Medicine, 26*(3), 471–482.

Harner, C. D., Xerogeanes, J. W., Livesay, G. A., et al. (1995). The human posterior cruciate ligament complex: an interdisciplinary study. *American Journal of Sports Medicine, 23*(6), 736–745.

Harner, C. D., Vogrin, T. M., Hoher, J., Ma, B. C., & Woo, S. L. Y. (2000). Biomechanical analysis of a posterior cruciate ligament reconstruction: Deficiency of the posterolateral structures as a cause of graft failure. *American Journal of Sports Medicine, 28*(1), 32–39.

Hauger, A. V., Reiman, M. P., Bjordal, J. M., Sheets, C., Ledbetter, L., & Goode, A. P. (2018). Neuromuscular electrical stimulation is effective in strengthening the quadriceps muscle after anterior cruciate ligament surgery. *Knee Surgery, Sports Traumatology, Arthroscopy, 26*(2), 399–410.

Hefti, E., Muller, W., Jakob, R. P., & Staubli, H. U. (1993). Evaluation of knee ligament injuries with the IKDC form. *Knee Surgery, Sports Traumatology, Arthroscopy, 1*(3-4), 226–234.

Henning, C. E., Lynch, M. A., & Glick, K. R., Jr. (1985). An in vivo strain gage study of elongation of the anterior cruciate ligament. *American Journal of Sports Medicine, 13*(1), 22–26.

Higbie, E. J., Cureton, K. J., Warren, G. L., & Prior, B. M. (1996). Effects of concentric and eccentric training on muscle strength, cross-sectional area, and neural activation. *Journal of Applied Physiology, 81*(5), 2173–2181.

Hinman, R. S., Bennell, K. L., Crossley, K. M., & McConnell, J. (2003). Immediate effects of adhesive tape on pain and disability in individuals with knee osteoarthritis. *Rheumatology (Oxford), 42*(7), 865–869.

Hughston, J. C. (1993). *Knee ligaments: Injury and repair.* Mosby.

Hughes, L., Paton, B., Rosenblatt, B., Gissane, C., & Patterson, S. D. (2017). Blood flow restriction training in clinical musculoskeletal rehabilitation: A systematic review and meta-analysis. *British Journal of Sports Medicine, 51*(13), 1003–1011.

Hurd, W. J., Axe, M. J., & Snyder-Mackler, L. (2008). A 10-year prospective trial of a patient management algorithm and screening examination for highly active individuals with anterior cruciate ligament injury: Part 1, outcomes. *The American Journal of Sports Medicine, 36*(1), 40–47.

Iannitto, J., Loyd, B., Johnson, R., et al. (2017). Assessment of commonly used measures of lower extremity swelling following total knee arthroplasty. *FASEB Journal, 31*, 903–904.

Indelicato, P. A. (1983). Non-operative treatment of complete tears of the medial collateral ligament of the knee. *Journal of Bone and Joint Surgery (American), 65*(3), 323–329.

International Association for the Study off Pain. IASP Terminology. Part III: Pain terms, a current list with definitions and notes on usage. Accessed June 2, 2021. https://www.iasp-pain.org/Education/Content.aspx?ItemNumber=1698

Irrgang, J. J., Snyder-Mackler, L., Wainner, R. S., Fu, F. H., & Harner, C. D. (1998). Development of a patient-reported measure of function of the knee. *Journal of Bone and Joint Surgery (American), 80*(8), 1132–1145.

Irrgang, J. J., Anderson, A. F., Boland, A. L., et al. (2002). Development and validation of the International Knee Documentation Committee Subjective Knee Form. *American Journal of Sports Medicine, 29*(5), 600–613.

Irrgang, J. J., Anderson, A. F., Boland, A. L., et al. (2006). Responsiveness of the International Knee Documentation Committee Subjective Knee Form. *American Journal of Sports Medicine, 34*(10), 1567–1573.

Jakobsen, B. W., Lund, B., Christiansen, S. E., & Lind, M. C. (2010a). Anatomic reconstruction of the posterolateral corner of the knee: a case series with isolated reconstructions in 27 patients. *Arthroscopy, 26*(7), 918–925.

Jakobsen, T. L., Christensen, M., Christensen, S. S., Olsen, M., & Bandholm, T. (2010b). Reliability of knee joint range of motion and circumference measurements after total knee arthroplasty: Does tester experience matter? *Physiotherapy Research International, 15*(3), 126–134.

James, E. W., LaPrade, C. M., & LaPrade, R. F. (2015). Anatomy and biomechanics of the lateral side of the knee and surgical implications. *Sports Medicine and Arthroscopy Review, 23*(1), 2–9.

Janousek, A. T., Jones, D. G., Clatworthy, M., Higgins, L. D., & Fu, F. H. (1999). Posterior cruciate ligament injuries of the knee joint. *Sports Medicine, 28*(6), 429–441.

Johnson, J. L., Capin, J. J., Arundale, A. J. H., Zarzycki, R., Smith, A. H., & Snyder-Mackler, L. (2020). A secondary injury prevention program may decrease contralateral anterior cruciate ligament injuries in female athletes: 2-year injury rates in the ACL-SPORTS randomized controlled trial. *Journal of Orthopaedic & Sports Physical Therapy, 50*(9), 523–530. https://doi.org/10.2519/jospt.2020.9407.

Kaeding, C. C., Pedroza, A. D., Reinke, E. K., Huston, L. J., & Spindler, K. P. (2015). Risk factors and predictors of subsequent ACL injury in either knee after ACL reconstruction: Prospective analysis of 2488 primary ACL reconstructions from the MOON cohort. *American Journal of Sports Medicine, 43*(7), 1583–1590.

Kamper, S. J., & Mackay, G. (2009). Global rating of change scales. *Australian Journal of Physiotherapy, 55*(4), 289.

Kannus, P. (1989). Nonoperative treatment of Grade II and III sprains of the lateral ligament compartment of the knee. *American Journal of Sports Medicine, 17*(1), 83–88.

Kennedy, M. I., Bernhardson, A., Moatshe, G., Bukely, P. S., Engebretsen, L., & LaPrade, R. F. (2019). Fibular collateral ligament/posterolateral corner injury: when to repair, reconstruct, or both. *Clinics in Sports Medicine, 38*(2), 261–274.

Kim, K. M., Croy, T., Hertel, J., & Saliba, S. (2010). Effects of neuromuscular electrical stimulation after anterior cruciate ligament reconstruction on quadriceps strength, function, and patient oriented outcomes: A systematic review. *Journal of Orthopaedic & Sports Physical Therapy, 40*(7), 383–391.

Kondo, E., Yasuda, K., Azuma, H., Tanabe, Y., & Yagi, T. (2008). Prospective clinical comparisons of anatomic double-bundle versus single-bundle anterior cruciate ligament reconstruction procedures in 328 consecutive patients. *American Journal of Sports Medicine, 36*(9), 1675–1687.

Kues, J. M., Rothstein, J. M., Lamb, R. L., & Minor, S. D. (1992). Obtaining reliable measurements of knee extensor torque produced during maximal voluntary contractions: An experimental investigation. *Physical Therapy, 72*(7), 492–501. discussion 501–504.

Levangie, P., & Norkin, C. (2019). *Joint structure and function: A comprehensive analysis* (6th ed.). FA Davis Co.

Loder, R. (1998). Slipped capital femoral epiphysis. *American Family Physician, 57*(9), 21–42.

Logerstedt, D., & Sennett, B. J. (2007). Case series utilizing drop-out casting for the treatment of knee joint extension motion loss following anterior cruciate ligament reconstruction. *Journal of Orthopaedic & Sports Physical Therapy, 37*(7), 404–411.

Lohmander, L. S., Ostenberg, A., Englund, M., & Roos, H. (2004). High prevalence of knee osteoarthritis, pain, and functional limitations in female soccer players twelve years after anterior cruciate ligament injury. *Arthritis & Rheumatology, 50*(10), 3145–3152.

Lohmander, L. S., Englund, P. M., Dahl, L. L., & Roos, E. M. (2007). The long-term consequence of anterior cruciate ligament and meniscus injuries: osteoarthritis. *American Journal of Sports Medicine, 35*(10), 1756–1769.

Lunden, J. B., Bzdusek, P. J., Monson, J. K., Malcomson, K. W., & LaPrade, R. F. (2010). Current concepts in the recognition and treatment of posterolateral corner injuries of the knee. *Journal of Orthopaedic & Sports Physical Therapy, 40*(8), 502–516.

Lynch, A. D., Chmielewski, T., Bailey, L., et al. (2017). Current concepts and controversies in rehabilitation after surgery for multiple ligament knee injury. *Current Reviews in Musculoskeletal Medicine, 10*(3), 328–345.

Malliaras, P., Barton, C. J., Reeves, N. D., & Langberg, H. (2013). Achilles and patellar tendinopathy loading programs: a systematic review comparing clinical outcomes and identifying potential mechanisms for effectiveness. *Sports Medicine, 43*(4), 267–286.

Marx, R. G., Jones, E. C., Allen, A. A., et al. (2001). Reliability, validity, and responsiveness of four knee outcome scales for athletic patients. *Journal of Bone and Joint Surgery (American), 83*(10), 1459–1469.

Mayr, H. O., Stueken, P., Munch, E. O., et al. (2014). Brace or no-brace after ACL graft? Four-year results of a prospective clinical trial. *Knee Surgery, Sports Traumatology, Arthroscopy, 22*(5), 1156–1162.

McCullough, K. A., Phelps, K. D., Spindler, K. P., et al. (2012). Return to high school- and college-level football after anterior cruciate ligament reconstruction: A Multicenter Orthopaedic Outcomes Network (MOON) cohort study. *American Journal of Sports Medicine, 40*(11), 2523–2529.

McKinnis, L. (1997). *Fundamentals of Orthopedic Radiology*. FA Davis Co. https://radiopaedia.org/articles/segond-fracture?lang=us.

Meier, W., Mizner, R. L., Marcus, R. L., Dibble, L. E., Peters, C., & Lastayo, P. C. (2008). Total knee arthroplasty: muscle impairments, functional limitations, and recommended rehabilitation approaches. *Journal of Orthopaedic & Sports Physical Therapy, 38*(5), 246–256.

Meleiro, S. A., Mendes, V. T., Kaleka, C. C., Cury, R. P., & Brazilian Society of Orthopedics and Traumatology, (2015). Treatment of isolated lesions of the posterior cruciate ligament. *Revista da Associacao Medica Brasileira (1992), 61*(2), 102–107.

Meszler, D., Manal, T., & Snyder-Mackler, L. (1998a). Disorders of the tibiofemoral joint: evaluation, diagnosis, and intervention. *Orthopaedic Physical Therapy Clinics of North America, 7*, 347–366.

Meszler, D., Manal, T. J., & Snyder-Mackler, L. (1998b). Rehabilitation after revision anterior cruciate ligament reconstruction: Practice guidelines and procedure-modified, criterion-based progression. *Operative Techniques in Sports Medicine, 6*(2), 111–116.

Myers, B. A., Jenkins, W. L., Killian, C., & Rundquist, P. (2014). Normative data for hop tests in high school and collegiate basketball and soccer players. *International Journal of Sports Physical Therapy, 9*(5), 596–603.

Miller, M. D., Bergfeld, J. A., Flowler, P. J., Harner, C. D., & Noyes, F. R. (1999). The posterior cruciate ligament injured knee: principles of evaluation and treatment. *Instructional Course Lectures, 48*, 199–207.

Mohtadi, N. G., & Chan, D. S. (2019). A randomized clinical trial comparing patellar tendon, hamstring tendon, and double-bundle ACL reconstructions: patient-reported and clinical outcomes at 5-year follow-up. *Journal of Bone and Joint Surgery (American), 101*(11), 949–960.

Myles, P. S., Myles, D. B., Galagher, W., et al. (2017). Measuring acute postoperative pain using the visual analog scale: The minimal clinically important difference and patient acceptable symptom state. *British Journal of Anaesthesia, 118*(3), 424–429.

Nakayama, H., Kambara, S., Iseki, T., Kanto, R., Kurosaka, K., & Yoshiya, S. (2017). Double-bundle anterior cruciate ligament reconstruction with and without remnant preservation—comparison of early postoperative outcomes and complications. *Knee, 24*(5), 1039–1046.

Nguyen, J. C., Markhardt, B. K., Merrow, A. C., & Dwek, J. R. (2017). Imaging of pediatric growth plate disturbances. *Radiographics, 37*(6), 1791–1812.

Noyes, F. R., & Barber-Westin, S. D. (1995). The treatment of acute combined ruptures of the anterior cruciate and medial ligaments of the knee. *American Journal of Sports Medicine, 23*(4), 380–389.

Noyes, F. R., McGinniss, G. H., & Mooar, L. A. (1984). Functional disability in the anterior cruciate insufficient knee syndrome review of knee rating systems and projected risk factors in determining treatment. *Sports Medicine, 1*(4), 278–302.

Noyes, F. R., Barber, S. D., & Mangine, R. E. (1991). Abnormal lower limb symmetry determined by function hop tests after anterior cruciate ligament rupture. *American Journal of Sports Medicine, 19*(5), 513–518.

Pache, S., Aman, Z. S., Kennedy, M., et al. (2018). Posterior cruciate ligament: Current concepts review. *Archives of Bone and Joint Surgery, 6*(1), 8–18.

Palmitier, R. A., An, K. N., Scott, S. G., & Chao, E. Y. (1991). Kinetic chain exercise in knee rehabilitation. *Sports Medicine, 11*(6), 402–413.

Papalia, R., Torre, G., Vasta, S., et al. (2015). Bone bruises in anterior cruciate ligament injured knee and long-term outcomes. A review of the evidence. *Open Access Journal of Sports Medicine, 6*, 37–48.

Paulos, L. E., France, E. P., Rosenberg, T. D., Jayaraman, G., Abbott, P. J., & Jaen, J. (1987). The biomechanics of lateral knee bracing. Part I: Response of the valgus restraints to loading. *American Journal of Sports Medicine, 15*(5), 419–429.

Perriman, A., Leahy, E., & Semciw, A. I. (2018). The effect of open-versus closed-kinetic-chain exercises on anterior tibial laxity, strength, and function following anterior cruciate ligament reconstruction: A systematic review and meta-analysis. *Journal of Orthopaedic & Sports Physical Therapy, 48*(7), 552–566.

Phelan, N., Rowland, P., Galvin, R., & O'Byrne, J. M. (2016). A systematic review and meta-analysis of the diagnostic accuracy of MRI for suspected ACL and meniscal tears of the knee. *Knee Surgery, Sports Traumatology, Arthroscopy, 24*(5), 1525–1539.

Phillips, N., Benjamin, M., Everett, T., & Van Deursen, R. W. M. (2000). Outcome and progression measures in rehabilitation following anterior cruciate ligament injury. *Physical Therapy in Sport, 1*(4), 106–118.

Pierce, C. M., O'Brien, L., Griffin, L. W., & Laprade, R. F. (2013). Posterior cruciate ligament tears: functional and postoperative rehabilitation. *Knee Surgery, Sports Traumatology, Arthroscopy, 21*(5), 1071–1084.

Raj, M. A., Mabrouk, A., & Varacallo, M. (2021). Posterior cruciate ligament knee injuries: *StatPearls [Internet]*. Treasure Island (FL): StatPearls Publishing. Available from https://www.ncbi.nlm.nih.gov/books/NBK430726/.

Rehabilitation Practice Guidelines: MCL Gr 1-3 & Rehabilitation after ACL Reconstruction: Practice Guidelines: University of Delaware Physical Therapy Clinic. (2021). Rehab Guidelines & Protocols. Accessed 2021. https://sites.udel.edu/ptclinic/professionals/guidelines/.

Risberg, M. A., Holm, I., Steen, H., Eriksson, J., & Ekeland, A. (1999). The effect of knee bracing after anterior cruciate ligament reconstruction: A prospective, randomized study with two years' follow-up. *American Journal of Sports Medicine, 27*(1), 76–83.

Roberts, C. C., Towers, J. D., Spangehl, M. J., et al. (2007). Advanced MR imaging of the cruciate ligaments. *Radiologic Clinics of North America, 45*(6), 1003–1016. vi–vii.

Roos, E. M., & Toksvig-Larsen, S. (2003). Knee injury and Osteoarthritis Outcome Score (KOOS)—validation and comparison to the WOMAC in total knee replacement. *Health and Quality of Life Outcomes, 1*, 17.

Rosenthal, M. D., Rainey, C. E., Tognoni, A., & Worms, R. (2012). Evaluation and management of posterior cruciate ligament injuries. *Physical Therapy in Sport, 13*(4), 196–208.

Rubinstein, R. A., Shelbourne, K. D., McCarroll, J. R., Vanmeter, C. D., & Rettig, A. C. (1994). The accuracy of the clinical examination in the setting of posterior cruciate ligament injuries. *American Journal of Sports Medicine, 22*(4), 550–557.

Sahrmann, S. A. (1988). Diagnosis by the physical therapist—A prerequisite for treatment. A special communication. *Physical Therapy, 68*(11), 1703–1706.

Salavati, M., Akhbari, B., Mohammadi, F., Mazaheri, M., & Khorrami, M. (2011). Knee injury and Osteoarthritis Outcome Score (KOOS); reliability and validity in competitive athletes after anterior cruciate ligament reconstruction. *Osteoarthritis and Cartilage, 19*(4), 406–410.

Sanders, T. G., Medynski, M. A., Feller, J. F., & Lawhorn, K. W. (2000). Bone contusion patterns of the knee at MR imaging: footprint of the mechanism of injury. *Radiographics, 20(Spec No)*, S135–151.

Scarvelis, D., & Wells, P. S. (2006). Diagnosis and treatment of deep-vein thrombosis. *Canadian Medical Association Journal, 175*(9), 1087–1092.

Schechinger, S. J., Levy, B. A., Dajani, K. A., Shah, J. P., Herrera, D. A., & Marx, R. G. (2009). Achilles tendon allograft reconstruction of the fibular collateral ligament and posterolateral corner. *Arthroscopy, 25*(3), 232–242.

Schierl, M., Petermann, J., Trus, P., Baumgartel, F., & Gotzen, L. (1994). Anterior cruciate and medial collateral ligament injury. ACL reconstruction and functional treatment of the MCL. *Knee Surgery, Sport Traumatology, Arthroscopy, 2*(4), 203–206.

Schmitt, J., & Abbott, J. H. (2015). Global ratings of change do not accurately reflect functional change over time in clinical practice. *Journal of Orthopaedic & Sports Physical Therapy, 45*(2), 106–111. D1–3.

Seaberg, D. C., & Jackson, R. (1994). Clinical decision rule for knee radiographs. *American Journal of Emergency Medicine, 12*(5), 541–543.

Shantanu, K., Singh, S., Srivastava, S., & Saroj, A. K. (2021). The validation of clinical examination and MRI as a diagnostic tool for cruciate ligaments and meniscus injuries of the knee against diagnostic arthroscopy. *Cureus, 13*(6), e15727.

Shelbourne, K. D., & Johnson, G. E. (1994). Outpatient surgical management of arthrofibrosis after anterior cruciate ligament surgery. *American Journal of Sports Medicine, 22*(2), 192–197.

Shelbourne, K. D., & Patel, D. V. (1999). Treatment of limited motion after anterior cruciate ligament reconstruction. *Knee Surgery, Sport Traumatology, Arthroscopy, 7*(2), 85–92.

Shelbourne, K. D., Davis, T. J., & Patel, D. V. (1999). The natural history of acute, isolated, nonoperatively treated posterior cruciate ligament injuries. A prospective study. *American Journal of Sports Medicine, 27*(3), 276–283.

Shelbourne, K. D., Gray, T., & Haro, M. (2009). Incidence of subsequent injury to either knee within 5 years after anterior cruciate ligament reconstruction with patellar tendon autograft. *American Journal of Sports Medicine, 37*(2), 246–251. https://doi.org/10.1177/0363546508325665.

Shelbourne, K. D., Clark, M., & Gray, T. (2013). Minimum 10-year follow up of patients after an acute, isolated posterior cruciate ligament injury treated nonoperatively. *American Journal of Sports Medicine, 41*(7), 1526–1533.

Shen, W., Jordan, S., & Fu, F. (2007). Review article: anatomic double bundle anterior cruciate ligament reconstruction. *Journal of Orthopaedic Surgery (Hong Kong), 15*(2), 216–221.

Silbernagel, K. G., Thomee, R., Eriksson, B. I., & Karlsson, J. (2007). Continued sports activity, using a pain-monitoring model, during rehabilitation in patients with achilles tendinopathy: A randomized controlled study. *American Journal of Sports Medicine, 35*(6), 897–906.

Sinacore, J. A., Evans, A. M., Lynch, B. N., Joreitz, R. E., Irrgang, J. J., & Lynch, A. D. (2017). Diagnostic accuracy of handheld dynamometry and 1-repetition maximum tests for identifying meaningful quadriceps strength asymmetries. *Journal of Orthopaedic & Sports Physical Therapy, 47*(2), 97–107.

Sitler, M., Ryan, J., Hopkinson, W., et al. (1990). The efficacy of a prophylactic knee brace to reduce knee injuries in football. A prospective, randomized study at West Point. *American Journal of Sports Medicine, 18*(3), 310–315.

Slichter, M. E., Wolterbeek, N., Auw Yang, K. G., Zijl, J. A. C., & Piscaer, T. M. (2018). Rater agreement reliability of the dial test in the ACL-deficient knee. *Journal of Experimental Orthopaedics, 5*(1), 18.

Snyder-Mackler, L., Ladin, Z., Schepsis, A., & Young, J. (1991). Electrical stimulation of the thigh muscles after reconstruction of the anterior cruciate ligament. Effects of electrically elicited contraction of the quadriceps femoris and hamstring muscles on gait and on strength of the thigh muscles. *Journal of Bone and Joint Surgery, 72*(7), 1025–1036.

Snyder-Mackler, L., Delitto, A., Stralka, S. W., & Bailey, S. L. (1994). Use of electrical stimulation to enhance recovery of quadriceps femoris muscle force production in patients following anterior cruciate ligament reconstruction. *Physical Therapy, 74*(10), 901–907.

Snyder-Mackler, L., Delitto, A., Bailey, S., & Stralka, S. (1995). Strength of the quadriceps femoris muscle and functional recovery after reconstruction of the anterior cruciate ligament. A prospective, randomized clinical trial of electrical stimulation. *Journal of Bone and Joint Surgery, 77*(8), 1166–1173.

Sood, G., & O'Donnell, J. (2001). Clinical controversies in Lyme Disease. *Hospital Physician, 37*(6), 62–74.

Stiell, I. G., Greenberg, G. H., Wells, G. A., et al. (1996). Prospective validation of a decision rule for the use of radiography in acute knee injuries. *JAMA, 275*(8), 611–615.

Stiell, I. G., Wells, G. A., Hoag, R. H., et al. (1997). Implementation of the Ottawa Knee Rule for the use of radiography in acute knee injuries. *JAMA, 278*(23), 2075–2079.

Stratford, P. (1995). Assessing disability and change on individual patients: a report of a patient specific measure. *Physiotherapy Canada, 47*(4), 258–263.

Sturgill, L. P., Snyder-Mackler, L., Manal, T. J., & Axe, M. J. (2009). Interrater reliability of a clinical scale to assess knee joint effusion. *Journal of Orthopaedic & Sports Physical Therapy, 39*(12), 845–849.

Sugimoto, D., Myer, G. D., Barber Foss, K. D., & Hewett, T. E. (2015). Specific exercise effects of preventive neuromuscular training intervention on anterior cruciate ligament injury risk reduction in young females: Meta-analysis and subgroup analysis. *British Journal of Sports Medicine, 49*(5), 282–289.

Tardy, N., Thaunat, M., Sonnery-Cottet, B., Murphy, C., Chambat, P., & Fayard, J. -M. (2016). Extension deficit after ACL reconstruction: is open posterior release a safe and efficient procedure? *Knee, 23*(3), 465–471.

Taylor, K. A., Cutcliffe, H. C., Queen, R. M., et al. (2013). In vivo measurement of ACL length and relative strain during walking. *Journal of Biomechanics, 46*(3), 478–483.

Tegner, Y., & Lysholm, J. (1985). Rating systems in the evaluation of knee ligament injuries. *Clinical Orthopaedics and Related Research, 198*, 43–49.

Terzidis, I. P., Christodoulou, A. G., Ploumis, A. L., Metsovitis, S. R., Koimtzis, M., & Givissis, P. (2004). The appearance of kissing contusion in the acutely injured knee in the athletes. *British Journal of Sports Medicine, 38*(5), 592–596.

Tippett, S. R. (1994). Referred knee pain in a young athlete: a case study. *Journal of Orthopaedic & Sports Physical Therapy, 19*(2), 117–120.

Torg, J., Barton, T., Pavlov, H., & Stine, R. (1989). Natural history of the posterior cruciate ligament-deficient knee. *Clinical Orthopaedics and Related Research, 246*, 208–216.

University of Delaware Physical Therapy Clinic. (2021). Rehab Guidelines & Protocols. https://sites.udel.edu/ptclinic/professionals/guidelines/

Van Cant, J., Dawe-Coz, A., Aoun, E., & Esculier, J. F. (2020). Quadriceps strengthening with blood flow restriction for the rehabilitation of patients with knee conditions: A systematic review with meta-analysis. *Journal of Back and Musculoskeletal Rehabilitation, 33*(4), 529–544.

Vegso, J. J., Genuario, S. E., & Torg, J. S. (1985). Maintenance of hamstring strength following knee surgery. *Medicine & Science in Sports Exercise, 17*(3), 376–379.

Visnes, H., & Bahr, R. (2007). The evolution of eccentric training as treatment for patellar tendinopathy (jumper's knee): a critical review of exercise programmes. *British Journal of Sports Medicine, 41*(4), 217–223.

Wadsworth, C. T., Krishnan, R., Sear, M., Harrold, J., & Nielsen, D. H. (1987). Intrarater reliability of manual muscle testing and hand-held dynametric muscle testing. *Physical Therapy, 67*(9), 1342–1347.

Webster, K. E., & Feller, J. A. (2016). Exploring the high reinjury rate in younger patients undergoing anterior cruciate ligament reconstruction. *American Journal of Sports Medicine, 44*(11), 2827–2832.

Webster, K. E., & Feller, J. A. (2018). Development and validation of a short version of the anterior cruciate ligament return to sport after injury (ACL-RSI) scale. *Orthopaedic Journal of Sports Medicine, 6*(4) 2325967118763763.

Webster, K. E., & Hewett, T. E. (2018). Meta-analysis of meta-analyses of anterior cruciate ligament injury reduction training programs. *Journal of Orthopaedic Research, 36*(10), 2696–2708.

Webster, K. E., Feller, J. A., & Lambros, C. (2008). Development and preliminary validation of a scale to measure the psychological impact of returning to sport following anterior cruciate ligament reconstruction surgery. *Physical Therapy in Sport, 9*(1), 9–15.

Webster, K. E., Feller, J. A., Leigh, W. B., & Richmond, A. K. (2014). Younger patients are at increased risk for graft rupture and contralateral injury after anterior cruciate ligament reconstruction. *American Journal of Sports Medicine*, *42*(3), 641–647.

Webster, K. E., Feller, J. A., Kimp, A. J., & Whitehead, T. S. (2018). Revision anterior cruciate ligament reconstruction outcomes in younger patients: medial meniscal pathology and high rates of return to sport are associated with third ACL injuries. *American Journal of Sports Medicine*, *46*(5), 1137–1142.

Wells, P. S., Hirsh, J., Anderson, D. R., et al. (1995). Accuracy of clinical assessment of deep-vein thrombosis. *The Lancet*, *345*, 1326–1330.

Wells, P. S., Owen, C., Doucette, S., Fergusson, D., & Tran, H. (2006). Does this patient have deep vein thrombosis? *JAMA*, *295*(2), 199–207.

Wellsandt, E., Gardinier, E. S., Manal, K., Axe, M. J., Buchanan, T. S., & Snyder-Mackler, L. (2016). Decreased knee joint loading associated with early knee osteoarthritis after anterior cruciate ligament injury. *American Journal of Sports Medicine*, *44*(1), 143–151.

Wilk, K. E. (1994). Rehabilitation of isolated and combined posterior cruciate ligament injuries. *Clinics in Sports Medicine*, *13*(3), 649–677.

Wilk, K. E., Andrews, J. R., Clancy, W. G., & Conner, J. A. (1996). Non-operative and postoperative rehabilitation of the collateral ligaments of the knee. *Operative Techniques in Sports Medicine*, *4*(3), 192–201.

Willy, R. W., Hoglund, L. T., Barton, C. J., et al. (2019). Patellofemoral pain. *Journal of Orthopaedic & Sports Physical Therapy*, *49*(9), CPG1–CPG95.

Wilson, T., Carter, N., & Thomas, G. (2003). A multicenter, single-masked study of syndrome in individuals with patellofemoral pain medial, neutral, and lateral patellar taping. *Journal of Orthopaedic & Sports Physical Therapy*, *33*(8), 437–443. discussion 444–448.

Wind, W. M., Jr, Bergfeld, J. A., & Parker, R. D. (2004). Evaluation and treatment of posterior cruciate ligament injuries: Revisited. *American Journal of Sports Medicine*, *32*(7), 1765–1775.

World Health Organization. (2001). International Classification of Functioning, Disability and Health. https://apps.who.int/iris/bitstream/handle/10665/42407/9241545429.pdf

Wylie, J. D., Marchand, L. S., & Burks, R. T. (2017). Etiologic factors that lead to failure after primary anterior cruciate ligament surgery. *Clinics in Sports Medicine*, *36*(1), 155–172.

Xie, X., Liu, X., Chen, Z., Yu, Y., Peng, S., & Li, Q. (2015). A meta-analysis of bone-patellar tendon-bone autograft versus four-strand hamstring tendon autograft for anterior cruciate ligament reconstruction. *Knee*, *22*(2), 100–110.

Yack, H. J., Collins, C. E., & Whieldon, T. J. (1993). Comparison of closed and open kinetic chain exercise in the anterior cruciate ligament-deficient knee. *American Journal of Sports Medicine*, *21*(1), 49–54.

Yaras, R. J., O'Neill, N., & Yaish, A. M. (2021). Lateral collateral ligament knee injuries: *StatPearls [Internet]*. Treasure Island (FL): StatPearls Publishing.

CHAPTER 73

TOTAL KNEE ARTHROPLASTY

M. Cacko, MPT, OCS, M. Caid, DO, and J.D. Keener, MD, PT

1. **What are the indications for total knee arthroplasty?**
   Pain, limited function, limited range of motion (ROM) or deformity in the setting of osteoarthritis, inflammatory arthritis, posttraumatic arthritis, or avascular necrosis that has failed conservative management.

2. **What is the most common approach for total knee arthroplasty?**
   The medial parapatellar approach is the most common and allows for extensile exposure of the knee. After a midline skin incision is made, incision is then made along the medial aspect of the quadriceps tendon and medial patellar border leaving a cuff of tendon to be repaired. This incision is carried down along the medial aspect of the patellar tendon and along the proximal medial tibia. Medial and lateral releases are performed and the infrapatellar fat pat retracted or excised. The patella can then be inverted and the knee flexed to allow exposure of the knee joint. Variants including a subvastus approach leave the vastus medialis intact and a potentially improved extensor mechanism. Variations such as a lateral parapatellar approach and VY-plasty can be used in certain circumstances or revision cases. Minimally invasive techniques utilize similar exposure with special instrumentation to allow accurate placement of components.

3. **Is the patella typically resurfaced at the time of total knee arthroplasty (TKA)? What are the outcome differences?**
   Most surgeons advocate resurfacing the patella, especially in the presence of patellar chondromalacia, rheumatoid arthritis, and obesity. The decision of whether or not to resurface the patella has been investigated in several randomized trials. Some studies have shown no difference in subjective performance (ascending or descending stairs) or the incidence of anterior knee pain between resurfaced and nonresurfaced groups with short-term follow-up. Some studies have shown decreased pain and improved extensor mechanism strength in nonresurfaced compared with resurfaced groups. However, several authors have documented persistent anterior knee pain requiring repeat operation for patellar resurfacing following knee arthroplasty. Patella thickness less than 12 mm has been associated with fracture; this is a catastrophic complication. In this situation surgeons may decide not to resurface the patella to avoid fracture.

4. **What is the difference between a posterior cruciate-substituting (PS) and a posterior cruciate-retaining (CR) knee replacement? How do they affect rehabilitation?**
   PS systems require removal of both cruciate ligaments at the time of surgery. Knee stability is obtained through a design that allows the tibial intercondylar eminence to articulate within the femoral intercondylar box during knee flexion, thus preventing posterior translation of the tibia in relation to the femur. CR designs spare the posterior cruciate ligament, allowing the ligament to retain its functional purpose. Clinical trials have demonstrated excellent results with both design types. Posterior cruciate-retaining devices have the theoretical advantage of maintaining the proprioceptive function of the ligament. Additionally, posterior femoral rollback facilitated by the posterior cruciate ligament during knee flexion potentially allows greater knee flexion range of motion and improves the mechanical advantage of the quadriceps mechanism. One study has shown improved knee kinematics while ascending stairs in patients with posterior cruciate-retaining knee replacements versus those with substituting designs. Proponents of posterior cruciate substituting designs cite greater ease of surgery, greater ability to correct deformities, and, most importantly, potentially decreased polyethylene wear rates as advantages of these designs. Rehabilitation protocols are generally identical for both design types. Because of the rare reports of posterior knee dislocation in cruciate-substituted knees, some studies advocate avoidance of resistant hamstring strengthening in positions of extreme knee flexion.

5. **What is a rotating platform total knee arthroplasty?**
   A mobile-bearing rotating platform total knee replacement consists of a dual-surface articulation between a polyethylene insert and a metallic femoral tibial tray. The tibial tray has a conical cavity that articulates with the central cone of the one-piece polyethylene insert. This design increases articulation conformity, decreases polyethylene wear, and minimizes the shear stress at the tibial tray-bone cement interface. Rotating platforms provide unlimited axial rotation but with limited anterior, posterior, medial, and lateral translation of the femoral polyethylene insert. This was designed to approximate the kinematics of a natural knee. Dislocation rates were found to range between 0.5% and 4.65% and usually occurred in the early stage of total knee replacement, between 6 days and 2 years, although late dislocation has also been known to occur. Dislocation rates are higher in those patients with a preoperative valgus deformity and greater age at surgery. Average range of motion has

been determined to be between 107 and 115 degrees of knee flexion. Survival rates have varied from 89.5% at 12 years, to 92.1% at 15 years, to 97.7% at 20 years. There has been no superiority found from a mobile-bearing rotating platform total knee replacement compared with a fixed total knee arthroplasty.

6. **Are robotic-assisted TKAs superior to manual TKAs?**
   There is no consensus data to indicate superiority of robotic TKAs versus manual TKAs. Most research shows equivocal patient outcomes. Robotic TKAs have been shown to have more precise bone resections but this has not corresponded to superior patient reported outcomes.

7. **Which type of total knee arthroplasty provides better results cemented or cementless?**
   Cement has been considered the gold standard over the years, but cementless has significantly improved recently with improved implant design and better biological function. There is no statistical difference between the two with long-term survivorship up to 16 years. Cement is preferred for older patients, osteoporosis, less active individuals, and those with bone growth not sufficient enough to hold the implant. Cementless is recommended for morbidly obese, obese, and younger/active patient. Cementless total knee arthroplasty may cause more postoperative pain secondary to biological fixation that equalizer within a year.

8. **What are the risks and benefits of simultaneous TKA versus staged TKA?**
   Patients receiving simultaneous TKA have a higher risk for cardiac complications, pulmonary complications, and mortality. Males have a higher complication rate than females. Other risk factors included advanced age (>65), presence of coronary artery disease, pulmonary hypertension, and congestive heart failure when considering simultaneous TKA. Simultaneous TKA did demonstrate a decreased risk for infection, respiratory complications, and decreased time with rehabilitation. There were no significant differences in revision, superficial infection, arthrofibrosis, cardiac complications, neurological complications, and urinary complications between procedures.

9. **What are the outcomes of total knee arthroplasty?**
   Outcomes following total knee arthroplasty are excellent in appropriately selected patients. Most clinical studies following total knee arthroplasty report survival rates between 80% and 95% for the tibial and femoral components at 10 to 15 years' follow-up. Approximately 10% of patients will have pain local to the patellofemoral joint. Up to 94% survival rates of tibial and femoral components at 18 to 20 years have been reported following cemented posterior stabilized total knee arthroplasty, with overall survival rates of 90% when patellar revisions were included. Lower rates of success have been demonstrated in certain well-defined patient populations.
   It is found that the greatest amount of improvement is seen within the first 3 to 6 months after surgery, with more gradual improvements occurring up to 2 years after surgery. Walking speeds for patients with total knee arthroplasties were found to be 13% and 18% slower at normal and fast speeds, compared with subjects without knee pathology. Stair climbing was compromised by 43% to 51% with patients following total knee replacement compared with other subjects. Men with total knee arthroplasty were 37% to 39% weaker and women were 28% to 29% weaker in their knee extensors compared with healthy individuals.

10. **How long do total knee arthroplasties last?**
    Mont in 2014 found a cemented survivorship at 10 years of 95.3% and cementless survivorship of 95.6%. Twenty-year survivor rate for cemented was 71% and 76% for cementless. Sartaw found survivorship at 15 years for posteriorly stabilized total knee arthroplasty was 98% and 100% survivorship for cruciate-retaining total knee arthroplasty. Young Hoo Kim in 2021 found patients with mobile bearing knees had 94.5% survivorship at 27 years and fixed bearing survivorship was at 93.1%. Christian Liu in 2022 found 95% to 97% survivorship after total knee arthroplasty at 20 years.

11. **What complications are associated with total knee arthroplasty?**
    There are many complications that are relatively uncommon, including peroneal nerve palsy (0.5%), vascular injury (0.03%–0.2%), infection (1%–5%), periprosthetic fracture, extensor mechanism dysfunction, wound healing complications, and arthrofibrosis. Peroneal nerve palsy is a serious complication that can lead to permanent dorsiflexion weakness also called "foot drop." The prevalence of peroneal nerve palsy after total knee arthroplasty has been reported to be around 0.5%. The development of nerve palsy has been associated with several risk factors, including preoperative valgus knee alignment, preoperative knee flexion contracture, and epidural anesthesia for postoperative pain control. In many instances, nerve function will return if diagnosed early and treated accordingly. The extensor mechanism is the most common source of continued postoperative knee pain and can be related to patella fracture, patellar tracking problems, parapatellar soft tissue impingement, and failure of patellar components. Arthrofibrosis relates to scar tissue formation in and around the knee, resulting in restriction of range of motion. This is treated with manipulation, aggressive physical therapy, and arthroscopic release of scar tissue. Infection is a dreaded complication following total knee arthroplasty, with reported rates of 1% to 5% depending on the patient population. Risk factors include revision surgery, delays in wound healing, skin ulcers, rheumatoid arthritis, and, in some studies, urinary tract infections and diabetes mellitus.

Early infections can sometimes be treated with debridement and antibiotics, with later infections often requiring removal of components.

12. **You notice that a patient you are treating following knee arthroplasty has developed increased calf swelling and localized tenderness. What should you do?**
An increase in calf swelling, calf pain with dorsiflexion of the ankle, calf tenderness, and/or erythema are all potential signs of deep vein thrombosis (DVT) and should prompt the therapist to contact the physician as soon as possible. DVT following total knee arthroplasty is very common, despite the use of various types of DVT prophylaxis (aspirin, warfarin, heparin derivatives, and sequential compression devices). Rates of postoperative asymptomatic DVT, without preventive therapy, range from 10% to 80% of patients following total knee arthroplasty. DVT after total joint arthroplasty with preventive therapy ranges from .05% to 1.5%. The incidence of asymptomatic and symptomatic pulmonary embolism is from .4 to 23% in patient receiving prophylaxis. The risk of fatal pulmonary embolism in unprotected patients is as low as 0.19% in some studies. The reliability of physical examination findings for the detection of a DVT is notoriously inaccurate.

13. **What are the common knee range of motion goals following total knee arthroplasty?**
Most patients who are able to achieve 75 degrees of knee flexion at the time of discharge will have at least 90 degrees of knee flexion at 1 year after surgery. The amount of knee flexion needed to perform various activities of daily living has been shown to range from 50 degrees while walking, to 80 to 90 degrees for stair-climbing, to 100 to 110 degrees for activities such as rising from a chair or tying a shoe. Most orthopedists consider 105 to 110 degrees the best long-term goal for knee flexion that will optimize patient function.
If the patient does not reach an acceptable range of motion the surgeon can elect to perform a manipulation under anesthesia (MUA). During an MUA, the surgeon manually flexes the knee to break up scar tissue and increase range of motion for the patient after they have been sedated.

14. **What are indications for manipulation under anesthesia for a total knee arthroplasty? What are expected gains?**
After a total knee arthroplasty the knee can become stiff. Increased scar tissue leads to what is known as arthrofibrosis and it limits range of motion of the knee. Unacceptable flexion of the knee is typically less than 90 degrees. MUA is when IV sedation is used and the surgeon manually flexes the knee to break up scar tissue and increase motion. A MUA should be done at or before 12 weeks post op. On average, knee flexion gains were found to be 22 to 35 degrees, and extension was 4 degrees. Knee range of motion after manipulation is similar to preoperative range of motion levels.

15. **What characteristics are commonly found in patients with knee flexion contractures following TKA? Are there surgical procedures to help prevent this?**
Patients with flexion contractures following TKA typically have preoperative contractures, are more likely to be female, and have a BMI of $\geq$30 kg/m^2. Flexion contractures greater than 5 degrees are correlated with poorer outcomes. Surgical techniques used to address preoperative flexion contractures include bone resection, posterior capsule release, ligamentous release, and removal of posterior osteophytes.

16. **Will the use of a continuous passive motion (CPM) machine after a total knee arthroplasty increase range of motion of the knee?**
Research has shown some early increases in range of motion with the use of CPM but no overall increase in motion after 8 weeks. CPM and non-CPM patients had no statistically significant difference in knee motion at 8 weeks post op. High-quality physical therapy that starts as soon as possible has been shown to be the most effective way to maximize ROM after a total knee arthroplasty.

17. **Does following an exercise program before total knee replacement surgery improve outcome?**
Studies have found that there was a significant statistical difference identified in knee flexion, timed-up-and-go, Knee Injury and Osteoarthritis Outcome Score (knee-associated life quality and functions in sports and recreation), as well as decreased length of hospital stay for the group that performed a preoperative exercise program. There was no significant statistical difference identified in pain scores, 6-min walk, knee extension, the Knee Injury and Osteoarthritis Outcome Score (pain, symptoms, and function of daily living), and Western Ontario and McMaster Universities Osteoarthritis Index score (WOMAC) after TKA between the two groups.

18. **What is the weight-bearing status of most patients following total knee arthroplasty?**
Most total knee arthroplasty components are placed using cement fixation. Cement fixation is stable immediately, allowing most patients to bear weight as tolerated on the involved lower extremity. Uncemented components are also weight bear as tolerated. Due to the increased force used to implant these components they have a higher rate of periprosthetic fracture.

19. **What is a typical rehabilitation program following total knee arthroplasty?**
The first 2 weeks of care following total knee arthroplasty focuses on controlling pain and protecting healing tissue and activating muscles of the knee. Patients often have home physical therapy at this time but can proceed to outpatient physical therapy if they are progressing well. The goal is to improve knee extension to 20 degrees and knee flexion up to 90 degrees with active range of motion/passive range of motion exercises. Exercises in this phase consist of quad sets, heel slides, glute sets, etc. Patients will typically use an assistive device. Outpatient physical therapy typically starts after 2 weeks with progression of range of motion, strength, and gait. Between weeks 2 and 6, range of motion should increase to 100 to 110 degrees. Exercise will continue to focus on hip/knee strengthening in close kinetic chain, bike, proprioception, and functional exercises. Progression from cane depends on patient's limp with gait. Weeks 6 to 12 focus on improving/progressing strength and increasing range of motion to 115 to 120 degrees. Exercise then progresses to more functional and single-leg activity as tolerated for balance and proprioception. Patients will start to decrease use of assistive devices by weeks 4 to 8. After 12 weeks, the patient may continue to make progress in strength and function. Return to sports should be consulted with the surgeon.

20. **Can a patient kneel after total knee arthroplasty?**
Recent studies show that after 1 year 36.8% of patients were able to kneel after TKA. After 3 years 47.6% of patients were able to kneel. Ability to kneel improves as pain and numbness decreases, which is greatest in the first year after surgery. Range of motion was a mean of 114 degrees in patients who could kneel comfortably and 110 degrees for subjects who could not kneel comfortably. The odds of kneeling were greater for patients undergoing an anterolateral incision compared with an anteromedial incision, a transverse incision compared with a longitudinal incision, and a shorter incision compared with a longer incision. The odds of kneeling were worse for a mobile prosthesis compared with a fixed platform design. Most patients avoid kneeling secondary to pain, numbness, fear of harming prosthesis, and third-party advice in order to protect the prosthesis.

21. **What are preoperative predictors for return to work following TKA and unicompartmental knee arthroplasty (UKA)?**
Return to work was noted at a mean of 7.7 weeks after TKA and 5.9 weeks following UKA. Most patients return to work within 12 weeks after surgery. Factors that promoted return to work were rehab, desire, necessity, self-employed, availability of light duty, and higher income. Factors impeding return to work were pain, fatigue, medical restrictions, standing job, and physical demands of job.

22. **When is it safe for a patient to return to driving after total knee arthroplasty?**
Classic teachings and literature have suggested 6 to 8 weeks postop before driving, with majority of patients driving by 12 weeks. Factors associated with return to driving are confidence, gender, comfort, and laterality. Break reaction time returned to baseline levels at 4 weeks and 88% of patients return to drive by 6 weeks. Brake pedal force baseline was reached after 6 weeks. Normal break time returned by 4 weeks for right total knee arthroplasty and as early as 2 weeks for left total knee arthroplasty. Break reaction time was met at 2 weeks for most patients and by all by 4 weeks.

23. **When can patients with total knee arthroplasty and unilateral knee arthroplasty return to sporting activity?**
Patients with both TKA and UKA may return to sporting activity. UKA patients are more likely to return to sport as compared to TKA. There is no difference between which sports are recommended to return to between the two groups. Return for low-impact sports such as walking, biking, swimming, and golf were 12 weeks for UKA and 13 weeks for TKA. Return to moderate-impact sports such as doubles tennis and downhill skiing were recommended with previous experience of the sport. High-impact sports return was recommended to be discussed with the surgeon. The biggest predictor of return to sports was patient's previous experience participating in the sport.

24. **Does preoperative opioid use affect recovery in total joint replacement?**
Studies have shown that preoperative opioid use (within 30 days of operation) has been associated with higher overall revision rates for aseptic loosening, periprosthetic fractures, dislocation, and infection. Preoperative opioid consumption was also significantly associated with chronic postoperative use following total hip and total knee arthroplasty.

25. **What are the indications for UKA?**
The indications have expanded due to improved survivorship. However, the classic indications are:
- Greater than 60 years old
- Arthritis limited to one compartment of the knee
- Patient who is not overweight or a heavy-demand laborer
- Knee ROM >90 degrees with less than a 5-degree flexion contracture
- Angular deformity <10 degrees
- A functional ACL

26. What are the outcomes of UKA?

UKA may be converted to TKA with somewhat less difficulty than a proximal tibial osteotomy. Augmentation with metal wedges is required in approximately 20% of the cases, and pain relief and function are similar to those for primary TKA. UKA are less invasive, preserve the bone stock, are more cost-effective, and have faster recovery times. Survivorship at 10 years after surgery for patients <55 years old has been reported to be 87.5% to 96%, and for patients ≥60 years old survivorship rates are 94% to 98%. Average range of motion is 114 to 125 degrees after UKA. Patients have shown a loss of torque of approximately 30% in extension and flexion at 60 to 180 degrees/sec of isokinetic testing compared with individuals without knee pathology. Patients with UKAs showed no significant difference with regard to proprioceptive testing compared with normal controls. UKA also preserve normal knee kinematics, which are significantly changed in total knee replacements. A common cause of failure that would lead to revision is progression of arthritis at the patellofemoral joint and the contralateral compartment. Progression of arthritis to the lateral compartment can result from slight overcorrection into valgus, and better results are found when the knee is slightly undercorrected. It has been found that neutral to slight valgus is the optimal alignment for unicompartmental knee arthroplasty for anterior medial osteoarthritis. Overcorrection can shift the mechanical axis to the unreplaced compartment.

27. What are the indications for proximal tibial osteotomy?

- Less than 60 years old
- Arthritis limited to one compartment of the knee
- Patient who is not overweight or a heavy-demand laborer
- Knee ROM >90 degrees
- Varus angle deformity of 10 to 15 degrees
- Flexion contracture <15 degrees
- Enough strength to successfully use walker or crutches

28. What are the outcomes of proximal tibial osteotomy?

Typically there is approximately a 73% survivorship at 10 to 14 years, thus significantly delaying TKA for the appropriately chosen patient. Good to excellent results are slightly lower after conversion to TKA (63%) versus primary TKA (88%).

Bibliography

Andriacchi, T. P., Galante, J. O., & Fermier, R. W. (1982). The influence of total knee replacement design on walking and stair climbing. *Journal of Bone and Joint Surgery, 64*(9), 1328–1336.

Ayers, D. L., Dennis, D. A., Johanson, N. A., & Pellegrini, V. D., Jr. (1997). Common complications of total knee arthroplasty. *Journal of Bone and Joint Surgery, 79*(2), 278–311.

Barrack, R. L., Wolfe, M. W., Waldman, D. A., Milicic, M., Bertot, A. J., & Myers, L. (1997). Resurfacing the patella in total knee arthroplasty: a prospective randomized double-blind study. *Journal of Bone and Joint Surgery, 79*(8), 1121–1131.

Cates, H. E., & Schmidt, J. M. (2009). Closed manipulation after total knee arthroplasty: outcomes and affecting variables. *Orthopedics, 32*, 398.

Collier, M. B., McAuley, J. P., Szuszczewicz, E. S., & Engh, G. A. (2004). Proprioceptive deficits are comparable before unicondylar and total knee arthroplasties, but greater in the more symptomatic knee of the patient. *Clinical Orthopaedics and Related Research, 423*, 138–143.

Collins, R. A., Walmsley, P. J., Amin, A. K., Brenkel, I. J., & Clayton, R. A. E. (2012). Does obesity influence clinical outcome at nine years following total knee replacement? *Journal of Bone and Joint. Surgery (British), 94*(10), 1351–1355.

Dugdale, E. M., Siljander, M. P., & Trousdale, R. T. (2021). Factors associated with early return to driving following total joint arthroplasty. *Journal of Arthroplasty, 36*(10), 3392–3400.

Fuchs, S., Frisse, D., Laass, H., Thorwesten, L., & Tibesku, C. O. (2004). Muscle strength in patients with unicompartmental arthroplasty. *American Journal of Physical Medicine and Rehabilitation, 83*, 650–654.

Goudie, S. T., Deakin, A. H., Ahmad, A., Maheshwari, R., & Picard, F. (2011). Flexion contracture following primary total knee arthroplasty: risk factors and outcomes. *Orthopedics, 34*, e855–e859.

Huang, C. H., Ma, H. -M., Leen, Y. -M., & Ho, F. -Y. (2003). Long-term results of low contact stress mobile-bearing total knee replacements. *Clinical Orthopaedics and Related Research, 416*, 265–270.

Jones, C. A., Voaklander, D. C., & Suarez-Alma, M. E. (2003). Determinants of function after total knee arthroplasty. *Physical Therapy, 83*, 696–706.

Keating, E. M., Ritter, M. A., Harty, L. D., et al. (2007). Manipulation after total knee arthroplasty. *Journal of Bone and Joint Surgery (American), 89*, 282–286.

Khaw, F. M., Moran, C. G., Pinder, I. M., & Smith, S. R. (1993). The incidence of fatal pulmonary embolism after knee replacement with no prophylactic anticoagulation. *Journal of Bone and Joint Surgery, 75*(6), 940–942.

Kim, Y. -H., Park, J. -W., & Kim, J.-S. (2012). Computer-navigated versus conventional total knee arthroplasty: a prospective randomized trial. *Journal of Bone and Joint Surgery (American), 94*, 2017–2024.

Lester, D., Barber, C., Sowers, C. B., et al. (2021). Return to sport post-knee arthroplasty: an umbrella review for consensus guidelines. *Bone & Joint Open, 3*(3), 245–251.

Liu, C., Varady, N., Antonelli, B., Thornhill, T., & Chen, A. F. (2022). Similar 20 year survivorship for single and bilateral total knee arthroplasty. *Knee, 35*, 16–24.

Liu, L., Liu, H., Zhang, H., Song, J., & Zhang, L. (2019). Bilateral total knee arthroplasty: simultaneous or staged? A systematic review and meta-analysis. *Medicine (Baltimore), 98*(22), e15931.

McGonagle, L., Convery-Chan, L., DeCrus, P., Haebich, S., Fick, D. P., & Khan, R. J. K. (2019). Factors influencing return to work after hip and knee arthroplasty. *Journal of Orthopaedics and Traumatology, 20*(1), 9.

Meehan, J. P., Danielsen, B., Tancredi, D. J., Kim, S., Jamali, A. A., & White, R. H. (2011). A population-based comparison of the incidence of adverse outcomes after simultaneous-bilateral and staged-bilateral total knee arthroplasty. *Journal of Bone and Joint Surgery (American), 93*, 2203–2213.

Memtsoudis, S. G., Ma, Y., Chiu, Y. -L., Poultsides, L., Della Valle, A. G., & Mazumdar, M. (2011). Bilateral total knee arthroplasty: Risk factors for major morbidity and mortality. *Anesthesia and Analgesia, 113*, 784–790.

Miller, A. J., Stimac, J. D., Smith, L. S., Feher, A. W., Yakkanti, M. R., & Malkani, A. L. (2018). Results of cemented versus cementless primary total knee arthroplasty using the same implant design. *Journal of Arthroplasty, 33*(4), 1089–1093.

Mont, M. A., Pivec, R., Issa, K., Kapadia, B. H., Maheshwari, A., & Harwin, S. F. (2014). Long-term implant survivorship of cementless total knee arthroplasty: a systematic review of the literature in meta-analysis. *Journal of Knee Surgery, 27*(5), 369–376.

Nadeem, S., Mundi, R., & Chaudhry, H. (2021). Surgery-related predictors of kneeling ability following total knee arthroplasty: a systematic review and meta-analysis. *Knee Surgery & Related Research, 33*(1), 36.

Naudie, D., Guerin, J., Parker, D. A., Bourne, R. B., & Rorabeck, C. H. (2004). Medial unicompartmental knee arthroplasty with the Miller-Galante prosthesis. *Journal of Bone and Joint Surgery, 86*(9), 1931–1935.

Palmer, S. H., Servant, C. T., Maguire, J., Parish, E. N., & Cross, M. J. (2002). Ability to kneel after total knee replacement. *Journal of Bone and Joint Surgery, 84*(2), 220–222.

Prasad, A. K., Tan, J. H. S., Bedair, H. S., Dawson-Bowling, S., & Hanna, S. A. (2020). Cemented vs. cementless fixation in primary total knee arthroplasty: a systematic review and meta-analysis. *EFORT Open Reviews, 5*(11), 793–798.

Polkowski, G. G., II, Ruh, E. L., Barrack, T. N., Nunley, R. M., & Barrack, R. L. (2013). Is pain and dissatisfaction after TKA related to early-grade preoperative osteoarthritis? *Clinical Orthopaedics and Related Research, 471*, 162–168.

Sartawi, M., Zurakowski, D., & Rosenberg, A. (2018). Implant survivorship and complication rates after total knee arthroplasty with a third-generation cemented system: 15-year follow-up. *American Journal of Orthopedics (Belle Mead NJ), 47*(3).

Sorrells, R. B., Voorhorst, P. E., Murphy, J. A., Bauschka, M. P., & Greenwald, A. S. (2004). Uncemented rotating-platform total knee replacement: a five to twelve-year follow-up study. *Journal of Bone and Joint Surgery, 86*(10), 2156–2162.

Su, E. P. (2012). Fixed flexion deformity and total knee arthroplasty. *Journal of Bone and Joint Surgery, 94*(11 Suppl A), 112–115.

Su, W., Zhou, Y., Qiu, H., & Wu, H. (2022). The effects of preoperative rehabilitation on pain and functional outcome after total knee arthroplasty: a meta-analysis of randomized controlled trials. *Journal of Orthopaedic Surgery and Research, 17*(1), 175.

Thompson, N. W., Wilson, D. S., Cran, G. W., Beverland, D. E., & Stiehl, J. B. (2004). Dislocation of the dislocating platform after low contact stress total knee arthroplasty. *Clinical Orthopaedics and Related Research, 425*, 207–211.

Tibbo, M. E., Limberg, A. K., Salib, C. G., et al. (2019). Acquired idiopathic stiffness after total knee arthroplasty. *Journal of Bone and Joint Surgery (American), 101*(14), 1320–1330.

Walsh, M., Woodhouse, L. J., Thomas, S. G., & Finch, E. (1998). Physical impairments and functional limitations: a comparison of individuals 1 year after total knee arthroplasty with control subjects. *Physical Therapy, 78*, 248–258.

Wülker, N., Lambermont, J. P., Sacchetti, L., Lazaró, J. G., & Nardi, J. (2010). A prospective randomized study of minimally invasive total knee arthroplasty compared with conventional surgery. *Journal of Bone and Joint Surgery (American), 92*, 1584–1590.

CHAPTER 73 QUESTIONS

1. **How much knee flexion (degrees) is needed to ambulate stairs following TKA?**
   a. 60 to 70
   b. 70 to 80
   c. 80 to 90
   d. 90 to 100

2. **What type of incision improves odd with kneeling?**
   a. Anterolateral
   b. Anteromedial
   c. Longitudinal
   d. Longer

3. **When is the latest a manipulation under anesthesia should occur after TKA?**
   a. 8 weeks
   b. 10 weeks
   c. 12 weeks
   d. 16 weeks

4. **When do patients typically return to low-impact sports following TKA?**
   a. 12 weeks
   b. 13 weeks
   c. 15 weeks
   d. 16 weeks

5. **Which is an indication for UKA?**
   a. Age less than 50
   b. Overweight
   c. Angular deformity >15 degrees
   d. Functioning ACL

6. **What is a contraindication for proximal tibia osteotomy?**
   a. Flexion contracture >15 degrees
   b. Unicompartmental arthritis
   c. Age less than 60
   d. Varus deformity of 10 to 15 degrees

7. **How much knee range of motion is needed to get up from a chair?**
   a. 80 degrees
   b. 90 degrees
   c. 100 degrees
   d. 120 degrees

KNEE FRACTURES AND DISLOCATIONS

R.C. Hall, DPT, ATC and J. Placzek, MD, PT

PATELLAR FRACTURES

1. **List, in order of frequency of occurrence, the five types of patellar fractures.**
   - Transverse
   - Comminuted or stellate
   - Vertical
   - Osteochondral
   - Polar (apical or basal)

2. **List the two major mechanisms of injury that result in patellar fractures.**
   - Direct trauma (blow or fall) to the patella with significant articular cartilage damage
   - Indirect force (jumping) resulting in a displaced or transverse fracture

3. **When is nonsurgical treatment indicated for a patellar fracture?**
   - Minimal displacement (<2–3 mm)
   - Intact extensor mechanism
   - Minimal articular step-off (1–2 mm)

4. **Describe the course of conservative treatment for patellar fractures.**
   - Aspiration of hematoma and full extension in a long-leg cylinder cast or brace for 3 to 6 weeks
   - Quadriceps set and straight-leg raises with return to weight bearing as tolerated
   - Gradual progression of active knee flexion and strengthening after cast removal
   - Progression of closed-chain exercises (eg, biking) at 6 weeks, with a goal of return to full range of motion (ROM) and strength at 12 weeks

5. **What are the common sequelae of patellar fractures?**
   The typical sequelae of patellar fractures is the following: patellofemoral arthritis, instability, decreased knee ROM, quadriceps weakness, and difficulty with stairs, downhill walking, and kneeling.

6. **How is a bipartite patellar differentiated from a fracture?**
   On radiographs a bipartite patellar shows well-rounded, smooth margins, and usually has one fragment in the superolateral position. Bipartite patellas occur in 0.05% to 2% of the population and are bilateral in 43% of the cases.

7. **Describe the outcomes for nonoperative treatment of nondisplaced patellar fractures.**
   Most patients have full ROM and return to normal quadriceps strength without patellofemoral problems. Complications, such as nonunion or patellofemoral problems, occur in <2% of cases. Patient satisfaction has been reported as high as 95% or greater.

8. **What are the outcomes for open reduction and internal fixation (ORIF) of patellar fractures?**
   Good to excellent results (return to full function within 6–9 months) are reported in 70% to 80% of all cases. Fair to poor results are reported in 20% to 30% of cases, and loss of the extensor mechanism is reported in 20% to 49% of cases. In one study, late displacement occurred in 7.4% of cases. Refracture has been reported in 5%. Prolonged immobilization (>8 weeks) increases the likelihood of poor results. Hyperalgesia can continue long term in a significant number of patients.

9. **By what mechanism does the tension-banding technique stabilize patellar fractures?**
   The wires are placed in such a fashion that with knee flexion (increased quadriceps tension) the tension in the wires increases to intensify compression of the fragments and facilitate fracture healing.

10. **How does rehabilitation differ between patients with nondisplaced fractures and patients with severely comminuted fractures?**
    Nondisplaced fractures are treated with knee immobilization in full extension, early weight bearing as tolerated, and isometric quadriceps exercises with a gradual increase in active assisted ROM at 4 to 6 weeks. Severely

comminuted fractures with ORIF are treated like nondisplaced fractures but require partial weight bearing for the first 6 weeks and a gradual increase in active assisted ROM at 3 to 6 weeks (with demonstration of stable fixation). All other patients with ORIF may begin active assisted ROM at 1 to 2 weeks.

11. **What are the outcomes for patellectomy?**
Good to excellent outcomes have been reported in 22% to 85% of cases and fair to poor outcomes in 14% to 60%. Loss of quadriceps strength has been reported averaging 50% decrease in peak torque. ROM is similar to those who undergo ORIF. As a result, rehabilitation and return to function may be prolonged up to 6 to 8 months or longer.

12. **At what age does a quadriceps tendon rupture typically occur? How do patients present?**
Eighty percent of quadriceps tendon ruptures occur in patients older than 40 years. The mechanism of injury is forced knee flexion with maximal quadriceps contraction. Presentation includes intense pain, inability to walk, swelling, palpable defect, and hemarthrosis. Patients usually seek immediate medical attention.

13. **How is a quadriceps tendon rupture treated? What is the expected outcome?**
Repair is often primary anastomosis, with the knee immobilized in full extension for a minimum of 6 weeks, followed by 6 months of rehabilitation for full recovery. Acute repairs usually result in good recovery of ROM and strength sufficient for activities of daily living. A 20% decrease in quadriceps strength was reported in 50% of patients in one case series. Late repairs are at risk for significant extension deficit. Potential complications include infection, heterotopic ossification, and failure of the repair.

14. **At what age does a patellar tendon rupture typically occur? How do patients present?**
Patellar tendon ruptures most commonly occur in people younger than 40 years of age with a history of patellar tendonitis or steroid injections. Other pathogenesis includes long-standing tendinopathy, mucoid degeneration, and tendolipomatosis. Tendon ruptures are associated with high-energy trauma. Presentation is similar to that of a quadriceps tendon rupture, with a palpable defect and superiorly displaced patellar.

15. **What is the incidence of repeat patellar tendon rupture following surgical repair?**
The rerupture rate of patellar tendon rupture repairs is reported at less than 10%.

16. **How are patellar tendon ruptures repaired? What is the expected outcome?**
Ligament is sutured to bone, and the knee is immobilized in full extension for 6 to 8 weeks with <50% weight bearing. Earlier repairs have better outcomes than late repairs. Complications include decreased knee flexion and patellar baja.

DISTAL FEMORAL FRACTURES

17. **What is the typical direction of displacement for a supracondylar distal femoral fracture? Why?**
The distal fragment is flexed by the gastrocnemius, causing posterior displacement and angulation. The pull of the quadriceps and hamstrings causes the femur to shorten.

18. **How are closed supracondylar fractures treated after reduction?**
A cast brace is used for 6 to 8 weeks. If displaced and not reducible, supracondylar fractures may require ORIF. Skeletal traction is used less often.

19. **What are the primary goals of operative treatment of distal femoral fractures?**
- Anatomic reduction of joint surfaces
- Rigid fixation
- Restoration of limb length
- Early knee motion

20. **What injuries are commonly associated with distal femoral fractures?**
- Ipsilateral hip fracture or dislocation
- Peroneal nerve injury
- Vascular injury
- Damage to the quadriceps apparatus

21. **Describe the age distribution of distal femoral fractures.**
The age distribution is bimodal: 1) young males have a higher incidence of high-energy trauma and intraarticular damage, and 2) elderly women have a higher incidence of low-energy trauma with fractures secondary to osteopenia.

22. **What are the indications and contraindications for operative and nonoperative treatment of distal femoral fractures?**
- Operative indications—absolute: displaced intraarticular fractures, open fractures, neurovascular injury, ipsilateral lower extremity fractures, and pathologic fractures; relative: isolated extraarticular fractures and severe osteoporosis
- Operative contraindications—preexisting infection, marked obesity, comorbid conditions, poor bone quality, and systemic infections
- Nonoperative indications—nondisplaced or incomplete fractures, impacted stable fractures in elderly osteopenic patients, significant underlying medical disease (cardiac, pulmonary, neurologic), advanced osteoporosis, selected gunshot wounds, and nonambulatory patients

23. **Why is fat embolism such a concern with femoral fractures?**
The pathogenesis of fat embolism is a subject of conjecture and controversy. Most investigators agree that the bone marrow is the source of the fat. Fat embolism is associated more often with intramedullary instrumentation of the femur than with fracture. Fat embolism typically occurs in high-energy tibial or femoral fractures among patients between the ages of 20 and 40. Embolism is also common among elderly patients (60–80 years old) with low-energy hip fractures.

24. **What are the outcomes for low-profile minimally invasive plating for distal femoral fractures?**
ROM averages 1 to 109 degrees, 93% heal without bone grafting, nearly all maintain fixation, malreduction occurs in approximately 6%, and infection occurs in 3% of patients.

25. **How do distal femoral fractures present in children? What is the incidence of distal femoral fractures in children? What are the common mechanisms of injury?**
Presenting symptoms for distal femoral fractures in children include inability to bear weight, maintaining the knee in flexion, gross deformity, and occasionally neurovascular compromise. Salter-Harris type II fractures are the most common category of distal femoral fractures in children (54%), with physeal fractures accounting for 1% to 6% of all physeal injuries in children.

Mechanisms of injury include indirect varus or valgus stress, breech birth, and minimal trauma in conditions that weaken the growth plate (osteomyelitis, leukemia, myelodysplasia).

26. **Describe the nonoperative treatment of nondisplaced and displaced distal femoral fractures in children.**
- Nondisplaced fractures are treated with a long-leg cast or hip spica cast for 4 to 6 weeks.
- Displaced Salter-Harris type I and II fractures are treated with closed reduction with traction and gentle manipulation, followed by immobilization with or without percutaneous pinning. The position of immobilization depends on the direction of the displacement.
- Displaced Salter-Harris type III and IV fractures are treated with open anatomic reduction.

27. **What are the indications for ORIF of distal femoral fractures in children?**
Irreducible Salter-Harris type II fractures, unstable reductions, and Salter-Harris type III and IV fractures are all candidates for ORIF.

28. **What complications are associated with distal femoral fractures in children?**
- Acute—peroneal nerve palsy (3%) from traction or attempts at reduction, recurrent displacement, and popliteal artery injuries (<2%) associated with hyperextension injuries.
- Late—angulation deformity (19%–24%), leg length discrepancy (24%–30%), knee stiffness (16%), avascular necrosis (rare), and nonunion (rare). Up to 50% of injuries may have growth arrest. Growth plate arrest is 4x higher in displaced fractures compared to nondisplaced fractures.

PROXIMAL TIBIAL FRACTURES

29. **What are the general types of proximal tibial fractures?**
- Extraarticular—tibial spine, tibial tubercle, and subcondylar
- Articular—condylar, bicondylar, and comminuted
- Intraarticular—epiphyseal

30. **What kinds of condylar fractures are often seen in the elderly?**
Insufficiency fractures of the medial tibial condyle are often found in the elderly. Varus deformity on examination usually indicates a depression or split-depression fracture (more common).

31. **What injuries are associated with condylar fractures?**
Meniscal injuries occur in up to 50% of all condylar fractures and ligamentous injuries in 30%. Peroneal nerve neurapraxia and popliteal artery injury are also associated injuries.

32. **Which tibial condyle is fractured more frequently? Why?**
The lateral condyle is fractured 70% to 80% more often because of weaker trabeculation, valgus orientation of the knee, and valgus-directed external forces.

33. **Describe conservative treatment of nondisplaced condylar fractures.**
    - Early passive exercise to maintain mobility and strength without weight bearing; weight bearing delayed until the fracture heals (6–12 weeks)
    - Nonweight-bearing cast immobilization (long-leg foot-groin cast, 5 degrees of flexion) for 3 to 6 weeks, followed by 2 to 4 weeks of nonweight-bearing rehabilitation, with progressive weight bearing from 9 to 16 weeks
    - Traction with passive exercise for 6 weeks, followed by nonweight bearing at about 12 weeks; return to full weight bearing when tissue healing is evident
    - Cast bracing with initial nonweight bearing and progressive weight bearing for up to 12 weeks; full weight bearing when tissue healing is evident

34. **Describe the outcomes of low-profile minimally invasive plating for proximal tibia fractures.**
Approximately 91% heal without major complication, some malalignment occurs in 10%, need for hardware removal occurs in 5%, and infection is seen in 4%. Mean final ROM is approximately 1 to 122 degrees, with full weight bearing allowed an average of 12.6 weeks postoperatively.

35. **Traumatic avulsions of the tibial tubercle are seen most often in what age group? Describe the mechanism and rate of injury for proximal tibial physeal fractures in children.**
Traumatic avulsions of the tibial tubercle are most often seen in young patients. Injury results from a strong quadriceps contraction with a slight degree of knee flexion. The sustained or sudden force disrupts either the tibial apophysis or the proximal tibial epiphysis. Preexisting apophysitis may be a predisposing factor. Proximal tibial physeal fractures account for 3% of all physeal injuries. Hyperextension forces the metaphysis posteriorly. Salter-Harris type II fractures are most common (35%).

36. **How are proximal tibial physeal fractures in children treated?**
    - Type I and II are treated with closed reduction followed by immobilization.
    - Type III and IV are treated with closed reduction, percutaneous pinning, and immobilization with an above-the-knee cast in 10 to 20 degrees of flexion for 6 to 8 weeks.

37. **What complications are associated with proximal tibial physeal fractures?**
Vascular compromise occurs in 5% to 7% of cases, angular deformity in 28% of cases, and leg length discrepancy in 19% of cases.

38. **Describe the weight-bearing progression for the various fractures about the knee.**

Weight-Bearing Status of Knee Fractures

	SURGICAL FIXATION			NONOPERATIVE TREATMENT		
Fracture	NWB	PWB	FWB (weeks)	NWB (weeks)	PWB	FWB
Patella	—	Immediate	6	—	Immediate	As tolerated
Distal femur	—	Immediate	12	—	2–3 weeks	8 weeks
Proximal tibia	2–4 weeks	9 weeks	16*	4–6† 12–16‡	—	Dependent on healing

NWB, nonweight bearing; PWB, partial weight bearing; FWB, full weight bearing.
*Based on signs of healing.
†Minimally displaced fractures.
‡After traction.

KNEE DISLOCATIONS

39. **What is the frequency of vascular and nerve injury following knee dislocation?**
One large retrospective study of 267 patients who had knee dislocations in the United States reported associated knee vascular injury at 3.3%. Other studies show vascular injuries in up to 18% of patients and nerve injury in up to 38%.

40. **How does disruption of a popliteal artery after knee dislocation present? Describe the emergent treatment.**
Disruption of a popliteal artery presents with absent or decreased distal pulses and signs of ischemia. The artery must be repaired within 8 hours of injury to avoid limb amputation. If timing allows, a vascular surgeon may elect to perform an arteriogram to rule out an intimal tear. In clinically ischemic legs, however, the surgeon may proceed directly to open exploration and repair.

41. **Should repair of ligament tears be acute or delayed in knee dislocations?**
This issue is somewhat controversial. Some authors advocate acute repair of arterial structures with delayed repair of ligamentous structures to allow better healing of vascular repairs. Others advocate acute repair of both vascular and ligamentous structures with limited early motion, depending on the extent of the vascular repair. The literature slightly favors acute ligamentous repair, because early motion results in fewer postoperative complications.

42. **Does the use of a hinged external fixator provide for better outcomes in knee dislocations?**
Although the use of a hinged external fixator does significantly reduce ligament reconstruction failure in knee dislocations, overall it does not appear to enhance the chances of return to full function in patients with such devastating injuries.

PATELLAR DISLOCATIONS AND SUBLUXATIONS

43. **What are the anatomic characteristics of typical patients with patellar dislocations?**

Genu valgum	Shallow patellar groove
Shallow lateral femoral condyle	Deformed patellar
Elongated patellar tendon	Pes planus
Deficient vastus medialis	Increased Q-angle
Lateral insertion of patellar tendon	Ligamentous laxity

44. **What type of fracture is frequently associated with acute patellar dislocations?**
Osteochondral fractures of the medial facet of the patellar have been reported in up to 66% of all patellar dislocations. Osteochondral fractures of the lateral femoral condyle are also common.

45. **What are the two main mechanisms of patellar dislocation and subluxation?**
- Direct trauma or blow to the patellar with the knee in slight flexion
- Powerful quadriceps contraction combined with slight flexion and external rotation of the tibia on the femur

46. **Describe the typical conservative course of treatment for a first-time patellar dislocation.**
The course of treatment for first-time patellar dislocation is as follows: in the absence of osteochondral fracture, 6 weeks of brace immobilization in full extension; progressive weight bearing as tolerated; early quadriceps isometrics, with straight leg raising (SLR) as pain allows; passive pain-free ROM progressing to full active ROM and aggressive closed-chain strengthening at 6 weeks.

47. **What factors contribute to recurrent instability after acute patellar dislocation?**
Anatomic factors include trochlear dysplasia, patellar alta, injury to the medial patellofemoral ligament, connective tissue disorders, overall limb alignment, and poor muscle tone. Additionally, first-time dislocations have lower recurrence rates, and individuals experiencing two or more dislocations have a 50% higher risk of reinjury.

48. **What are the indications for surgery with a patellar dislocation?**
- First-time dislocation with significant osteochondral fracture
- First-time dislocation with inadequate or unstable reduction

- Recurrent dislocation not responding to nonoperative treatment
- Disruption of the medial patellofemoral ligament on magnetic resonance imaging

49. What are the indications and contraindications for lateral retinacular release?
- Indications—intractable patellofemoral pain with lateral tilt, lateral compression syndrome, persistent subluxations, patellar dislocations
- Contraindications—patellofemoral pain without lateral tilt, advanced patellofemoral arthrosis, lateral hypermobile patellar, normal tracking patellar, patellar subluxation, and dislocation with significant extensor mechanism malalignment

50. How effective is reconstruction of the medial patellofemoral ligament (MPFL) for the treatment of instability?
MPFL reconstruction is somewhat technically demanding, with complication rates being reported around 26%. Complications include fracture, graft failure, loss of ROM, persistent anterior knee pain, as well as persistent instability. Proper patient selection has been reported to enhance success. Patients with severe trochlea dysplasia, femoral anteversion, and obesity lend to poor outcomes. Factors for success include accurate graft placement and tensioning to avoid overloading the medial patellar facet or increasing the chance of a medial patellar subluxation.

51. What is the typical progression of rehabilitation following a lateral retinacular release?

WEEKS 1–2	WEEKS 3–5	6 WEEKS
Weight bear as tolerated	Full weight bearing	Sport-specific activities
Early AROM 1–115 degrees	Full AROM	Functional/isometric eval
Multiangle isometrics	Closed-chain exercises	Brace for activity
Patella mobilization	Aerobic reconditioning	Agility drills
Control pain/swelling	Isometric strength eval	

52. When is a tibial tubercle osteotomy indicated, and what kind of outcomes can be expected?

Patients who have instability such as an increased tibial tubercle to trochlea groove distance of 20 mm or greater, patellar alta, or damage to distal lateral articular cartilage may benefit from this procedure. Long-term follow-up has reported that 70% to 80% of patients get good to excellent results. Recurrent instability can occur in 1% to 4% of patients.

53. What is the average recurrence rate after lateral retinacular release for recurrent patellar dislocation?
Published studies show a recurrence rate of as much as 5%, with a range of 14 to 48 months of follow-up.

54. What degree of tubercle-sulcus angle (Q-angle at 90 degrees) indicates potential patellar instability?
A tubercle-sulcus angle <10 degrees indicates potential patellar instability.

55. What radiographic view is used to assess patellar malalignment?
The Mercer-Merchant patellar view at 45-degree knee flexion angle is used to assess patellar malalignment.

56. What are the outcomes of medial retinacular repair with lateral retinacular release for acute patellar dislocation?
Good to excellent results have been reported in 81% to 91% of cases, with <2% redislocation rates. Some comparative studies show little difference in redislocation rates of those repaired to those treated without surgery although surgical repairs tend to function at a higher level.

BIBLIOGRAPHY

Aglietti, P., & Buzzi, R. (1993a). Fractures of the femoral condyles. In J. N. Insall (Ed.), *Surgery of the knee* (pp. 983–1034). New York: Churchill Livingstone.

Aglietti, P., & Buzzi, R. (1993b). Fractures of the tibial plateau. In J. N. Insall (Ed.), *Surgery of the knee* (pp. 1035–1084). New York: Churchill Livingstone.

Basener, C. J., Mehlman, C. T., & DiPasquale, T. G. (2009). Growth disturbance after distal femoral growth plate fractures in children: a meta-analysis. *Journal of Orthopaedic Trauma, 23*(9), 663–667.

Brotzman, S. B., & Wilk, K. E. (Eds.). (2003). *Clinical orthopaedic rehabilitation* (2nd ed., pp. 346–350). Philadelphia: Mosby.

Carpenter, J., Kasman, R., & Mathews, L. (1993). Fractures of the patellar. *Journal of Bone and Joint Surgery, 75*(10), 1550–1561.

Cole, P. A., Zlowodzki, M., & Kregor, P. J. (2004). Treatment of proximal tibia fractures using the less invasive stabilization system: Surgical experience and early clinical results in 77 fractures. *Journal of Orthopaedic Trauma, 2004*, 528–535.

Deng, X., Zhu, L., Hu, H., et al. (2021). Comparison of total patellectomy and osteosynthesis with tension band wiring in patients with highly comminuted patella fractures: A 10-20-year follow-up study. *Journal of Orthopaedic Surgery and Research, 16*(1), 497.

Fithian, D. C., Paxton, E. W., Stone, M. L., et al. (2004). Epidemiology and natural history of acute patellar dislocation. *American Journal of Sports Medicine, 32*(5), 1114–1121.

Helfet, D., & Novak, K. (1991). The management of fractures of the tibial plateau. *International Journal of Orthopaedic Trauma, 1*, 148.

Hing, C. B., Smith, T. O., Donell, S., & Song, F. (2011). Surgical versus non-surgical interventions for treating patellar dislocation. *Cochrane Database of Systematic Reviews*, (11), CD008106.

Hsu, K., Wang, K. C., Ho, W. P., & Hsu, R. W. (1994). Traumatic patellar tendon ruptures: A follow-up study of primary repair and a neutralization wire. *Journal of Trauma, 36*, 658–660.

Kahan, J. B., Schneble, C. A., Li, D., et al. (2021). Increased neurovascular morbidity is seen in documented knee dislocation versus multiligamentous knee injury. *Journal of Bone and Joint Surgery (American), 103*(10), 921–930.

Koh, J. L., & Stewart, C. (2014). Patellar instability. *Clinics in Sport Medicine, 33*(3), 461–476.

Larsen, P, Vedel, J, Vistrup, S, & Elsoe, R (2017). Long-lasting hyperalgesia is common in patients following patella fractures. *Pain Medicine*, 19, 429–437.

Magee, D. L. (1997). Knee: *Orthopedic physical assessment* (pp. 506–571). Philadelphia: WB Saunders.

Mangine, R. E., Eifert-Mangine, M., Burch, D., Becker, B. L., & Farag, L. (1998). Postoperative management of the patellofemoral patient. *Journal of Orthopaedic and Sports Physical Therapy, 28*, 323–335.

Markmiller, M., Konrad, G., & Sudkamp, N. (2004). Femur-LISS and distal femoral nail for fixation of distal femoral fractures: Are there differences in outcome and complications? *Clinical Orthopaedics and Related Research, 426*, 252–257.

Medina, O., Arom, G. A., Yeranosian, M. G., Petrigliano, F. A., & McAllister, D. R. (2014). Vascular and nerve injury after knee dislocation: A systemic review. *Clinical Orthopaedics and Related Research, 472*(9), 2621–2629.

Natsuhara, K. M., Yeranosin, M. G., Cohen, J. R., Wang, J. C., McAllister, D. R., & Petrigliano, F. A. (2014). What is the frequency of vascular injury after knee dislocation? *Clinical Orthopaedics and Related Research, 472*(9), 2615–2620.

Reid, D. C. (1992). Bursitis and knee extensor mechanism pain syndromes: *Sports injury assessment and rehabilitation* (pp. 399–401). New York: Churchill Livingstone.

Reilly, J. P. (1994). Tibial plateau fractures. In W. N. Scott (Ed.), *The knee* (pp. 1369–1392). St. Louis: Mosby.

Rockwood, C. A. (Ed.), (1996). *Rockwood and Green's fractures in adults* Vol. 2, (4th ed., pp. 1919–2178). Philadelphia: Lippincott-Raven.

Scheinberg, R. R., & Bucholz, R. W. (1994). Fractures of the patellar. In W. N. Scott (Ed.), *The knee* (pp. 1393–1403). St. Louis: Mosby.

Sillanpaa, P. J., Peltola, E., Mattila, V. M., et al. (2009). Femoral avulsion of the medial patellofemoral ligament after primary traumatic patellar dislocation predicts subsequent instability in men: A mean 7-year nonoperative follow-up study. *American Journal of Sports Medicine, 37*(8), 1513–1521.

Simon, R. R., & Koenigsknecth, S. J. (1987). *Emergency orthopedics: The extremities* (2nd ed. pp. 234–387). Norwalk, CT: Appleton & Lange.

Stanitski, C. L., & Paletta, G. A., Jr. (1998). Articular cartilage injury with acute patellar dislocation in adolescents: Arthroscopic and radiographic correlation. *American Journal of Sports Medicine, 26*, 52–55.

Stannard, J. P., Nuelle, C. W., McGwin, G., & Volgas, D. A. (2014). Hinged external fixation in the treatment of knee dislocations: A prospective randomized study. *Journal of Bone and Joint Surgery (American), 96*(3), 184–191.

CHAPTER 74 QUESTIONS

1. **A 45-year-old man presents as nonambulatory stating that he slipped and hyperflexed his knee while jumping off his tractor. Examination reveals a large swollen knee, inability to actively extend it, and a palpable defect superior to the patellar. Which injury is most likely?**
   a. Patella tendon rupture
   b. Bipartite patellar
   c. Quadriceps tendon rupture
   d. Tibial tubercle avulsion

2. **Which type of weight-bearing status best describes treatment for a nonoperative minimally displaced proximal tibial fracture?**
   a. Immediate partial weight bearing for 2 weeks
   b. 4 to 6 weeks nonweight bearing progressing to full weight bearing depending on healing
   c. Immediate partial weight bearing for 12 weeks
   d. Full weight bearing as soon as tolerated

3. **Which of the following is true with regard to patellar dislocations?**
   a. Patellar dislocations usually occur with the knee in full extension.
   b. First-time patellar dislocations require 6 weeks of nonweight bearing.
   c. Medial patellofemoral ligament reconstruction has excellent outcomes.
   d. A shallow lateral femoral condyle is a predisposing factor to dislocation.

4. **What is the growth arrest rate of the distal femoral epiphysis after fracture?**
    a. 0% to 10%
    b. 10% to 20%
    c. 20% to 50%
    d. 60% to 80%

5. **Bipartite patella occurs in what percent of the general population?**
    a. 2%
    b. 10%
    c. 25%
    d. 50%

6. **Peak extension torque after patellectomy is approximately**
    a. 10%
    b. 30%
    c. 50%
    d. 80%

NERVE ENTRAPMENTS OF THE LOWER EXTREMITY

J.S. Halle, PT, PhD, ECS (Emeritus) and D.G. Greathouse, PT, PhD, ECS, FAPTA

1. **What nerve entrapments are found in the lower extremity?**
   - Lateral cutaneous nerve of the thigh mononeuropathy (meralgia paresthetica)—lateral cutaneous nerve of the thigh (lateral femoral cutaneous nerve) is compressed medial to the anterior superior iliac spine as it passes under the inguinal ligament
   - Femoral nerve entrapment—femoral nerve is a mixed nerve that can be entrapped in the anterior abdominal wall as it passes under the inguinal ligament or in the femoral triangle
   - Obturator nerve entrapment—obturator nerve, although not usually compromised, is a mixed nerve that can become entrapped in the obturator foramen and as it passes around the obturator externus muscle
   - Saphenous nerve entrapment—saphenous nerve is a cutaneous nerve that can become entrapped in the distal thigh as it passes through the adductor canal; it is the distal extension of the femoral nerve
   - Piriformis syndrome—sciatic nerve can become entrapped as it passes through the piriformis muscle
   - Common fibular (peroneal) neuropathy—both the superficial and the deep fibular nerve branches can become compressed as they pass around the fibular head
   - Fibular neuropathy (superficial branch)—superficial fibular nerve can be compressed as it passes through the deep fascia of the anterolateral leg to become subcutaneous
   - Fibular neuropathy (deep branch)—compression can affect the deep fibular nerve in the anterior compartment
   - Ski boot syndrome (anterior tarsal tunnel syndrome)—deep fibular (peroneal) nerve can become entrapped at the ankle, most commonly as a result of tight-fitting shoes
   - Tarsal tunnel syndrome—medial and/or lateral plantar nerve can be compressed at the ankle
   - Sural nerve compression—purely cutaneous sural nerve can be compressed as it passes through the deep investing fascia of the leg or by an extrinsic source such as tight boots

2. **How does lateral cutaneous nerve of the thigh mononeuropathy (meralgia paresthetica) present clinically? Describe its pathogenesis.**
   Presenting symptoms typically include altered or absent sensation over the lateral aspect of the mid thigh. Other sensory symptoms may include burning pain, dull ache, itching, and tingling over the cutaneous nerve field supplied by the lateral cutaneous nerve of the thigh (lateral femoral cutaneous nerve). The nerve is purely cutaneous and becomes superficial to supply the skin of the lateral thigh about 10 cm distal to the inguinal ligament. No loss in voluntary motor function should occur with isolated involvement of this nerve, apart from possible guarding secondary to pain with hip extension, which may increase symptoms. Visceral motor function can be impacted by the compression neuropathy.

3. **Describe the cause and prognosis of lateral cutaneous nerve of the thigh mononeuropathy (meralgia paresthetica).**
   The cause may be tight clothing (tight underwear or tight jeans), pendulous abdomen, or rapid increase in weight. A variant in the normal path of exit from the pelvis also may increase the likelihood of entrapment. With the recent changes in the anterior approach to hip arthroplasty, there have been a number of studies reporting damage to the lateral cutaneous nerve of the thigh. The damage occurs either from direct injury to the nerve or as a result of traction of the nerve during the surgical procedure. Although rare, injury to the contralateral lateral cutaneous nerve of the thigh during total hip arthroplasty has been reported, due to the obesity of the patient and the surgical positioning. The prognosis is good in the vast majority of patients when the predisposing cause has been identified and removed, and the majority of paresthesias associated with surgery also resolve within a year. The peak incidence occurs during middle age, when progressive weight gains are also frequently observed. The incidence is equivalent on both right and left sides; symptoms may occur intermittently over a period of years, either unilaterally or bilaterally. Other forms of treatment include injection of an anesthetic agent with or without a corticosteroid in the area of suspected involvement.

4. **What causes femoral nerve entrapment?**
   The femoral nerve can become compressed anywhere along its course by such diverse factors as tumors, psoas abscesses, lymph node enlargement, hematoma, or penetrating trauma. The nerve also can be compressed at the inguinal ligament or stretched when it is subjected to excessive hip abduction and external rotation (eg, during

vaginal deliveries). With the move to the muscle-sparing approach provided by anterior hip arthroplasty, there have been a number of studies reporting damage to the femoral nerve. The observed damage may be due to the femoral nerve block used to deliver anesthesia, traction of the nerve during the surgical procedure, or direct injury to the nerve. The femoral nerve can also be damaged by tourniquet-related injury following knee surgery. Weakness in knee extension and possibly hip flexion, because of the involvement of the rectus femoris, may be noted. Sensation may be affected on the medial aspect of the knee and the anterior aspect of the thigh, which are supplied by the saphenous branch of the femoral nerve and the anterior cutaneous nerve of the thigh, respectively.

5. **What is the prognosis of a femoral nerve injury?**
The prognosis of a femoral nerve neuropathy depends on the location (intrapelvic or extrapelvic, ie, distal to the inguinal ligament) and severity of the lesion. Electrophysiological studies of the femoral nerve may show increased femoral nerve motor latency, reduced amplitude of the compound muscle action potential, and evidence of denervation in the femoral nerve innervated muscles. In general, two thirds of patients with a femoral nerve injury show functional improvement in 2 years. The estimated axon loss based on compound muscle action potential amplitude and EMG testing is a good measure of prognosis.

6. **How does an obturator nerve entrapment present?**
Obturator nerve entrapments are rare. When they occur, they usually are associated with acute trauma attributable to an event such as childbirth, pelvic trauma, or surgery. The adductor muscles supplied by the obturator nerve may be weakened, and sensation may or may not be decreased in the middle portion of the medial thigh. Problems noted by the patient include pain in the region of the inguinal ligament, instability of the lower extremity during gait, and atrophy of the adductor muscles.

7. **What clinical manifestations are associated with entrapment of the saphenous nerve?**
Before passing through the adductor hiatus, the saphenous nerve pierces the tough connective tissue layer between the sartorius and gracilis muscles to supply the skin of the anteromedial knee, medial leg, and medial side of the foot as distally as the metatarsal phalangeal joint. In some cases, the nerve also may pass through the sartorius muscle. The possible site of entrapment at this location is the point where the nerve passes through the thick connective tissue of the investing fascia and undergoes a sharp angulation. It is also possible to have a second site of entrapment as the infrapatellar branch of the saphenous nerve passes through the sartorius tendon. In this case symptoms are restricted to the infrapatellar region.
The most common complaint is knee pain, which may or may not be associated with sensory changes in the distribution of the saphenous nerve. Vigorous palpation at the point where the nerve pierces the adductor canal may reproduce the patient's symptoms. Treatments range from injection of an anesthetic with or without corticosteroid to surgical decompression.

8. **List four sites of potential fibular (peroneal) nerve entrapment.**
   - In the popliteal space behind the knee
   - At the fibular head
   - In the anterior compartment of the leg (as the deep fibular nerve)
   - In the lateral compartment of the leg (as the superficial fibular nerve)

The common fibular nerve is the most commonly injured nerve in the lower extremity. Patients may present with clinical findings of weakness of the ankle dorsiflexors and toe extensors (eg, footdrop), which may also be a consequence of a lumbar (L5) radiculopathy. The clinical and electrophysiologic evidence distinguishing between a common fibular nerve (peroneal nerve) mononeuropathy and an L5 radiculopathy is weakness and denervation in one or more of the proximal muscles of the lower extremity that have L5 innervation in the case of a radiculopathy (eg, tensor fascia lata, gluteus medius, semitendinosus, and short head of the biceps femoris). In addition, since the tibialis posterior muscle (L4-L5, tibial nerve) is a primary L5 innervated muscle, EMG testing of the tibialis posterior muscle would also assist in identifying an L5 nerve root radiculopathy from a common fibular nerve mononeuropathy. A number of studies have shown that this nerve is susceptible to dysfunction from other causes, such as prolonged ice pack application, cysts, ankle sprains, cancer and the associated weight loss that accompanies it, and direct trauma. Some treatments, such as a short leg walking cast that distributes inappropriate pressure to the common fibular nerve just distal to the knee, can also result in a common fibular neuropathy.

9. **Describe the clinical presentation of compression of the superficial sensory fibular nerve.**
Approximately at the junction between the middle and distal third of the leg, the cutaneous continuation of the superficial sensory fibular nerve passes through the deep fascia to become subcutaneous. At this site, the fascia may be tough or restrictive, creating a potential point of entrapment. The terminal extensions of the superficial fibular nerve are the medial and lateral cutaneous branches, which supply the distal two thirds of the anterolateral leg and the dorsum of the foot, apart from the web space between the great and second toes. Symptoms are present along the distribution supplied by the nerve—over the distal leg and

dorsum of the foot. Common injuries, such as an inversion sprain of the ankle, may stress this nerve at the point where it passes through the fascial opening.

10. **Describe the clinical presentation of a deep fibular nerve injury.**
Once the nerve has left the region of the fibular head and entered the anterior compartment, it is relatively protected and rarely entrapped, apart from problems associated with the anterior compartment. Again, distinguishing between a deep fibular nerve mononeuropathy and an L5 radiculopathy is paramount for both the clinical and the electrophysiological examinations. Anatomically, a compartment is created with the tibia medially, the fibula laterally, the interosseous membrane posteriorly, and a tough fascial layer anteriorly. Insults that involve this compartment can affect deep fibular nerve or anterior tibial artery function or muscle tissue directly. The muscle weakness pattern includes weakness of ankle dorsiflexion (tibialis anterior) and toe extensors (extensor digitorum longus, extensor halluces longus, and extensor digitorum brevis/halluces; and could result to a complete "foot drop" with severe muscle weakness. Examples range from anterior tibialis strain (shin splints: a mild form of anterior compartment syndrome) to muscle inflammation secondary to prolonged exercise, direct trauma to the leg, snake bites, or arterial bleeding. Significant increases in pressure are treated with fasciotomy—an incision of the anterior fascia of the leg.

11. **Describe the tarsal tunnel.**
The tarsal tunnel can be anatomically described as an anterior tarsal tunnel (ATT) and a posterior tarsal tunnel (PTT). The more common and traditional use of the term tarsal tunnel syndrome relates to the nerve and vascular structures that may be compromised in the PTT. The ATT is located anterior to the talotibial and talonavicular joints where the deep fibular (deep peroneal) nerve and dorsalis pedis artery pass beneath the inferior extensor retinaculum of the ankle. The PTT or tibiotalocalcaneal tunnel is posterior to the medial malleolus of the tibia. The tibial nerve usually branches into its four divisions—medial plantar, lateral plantar, medial calcaneal, and inferior calcaneal nerves—within the confines of the PTT. In the PTT, the posterior tibial artery usually branches into the medial plantar, lateral plantar, and medial calcaneal arteries.

12. **What is anterior tarsal tunnel syndrome?**
Anterior tarsal tunnel syndrome (ATTS), also known as ski boot syndrome, is caused by compression of the deep fibular nerve (DFN) as it passes deep to the inferior extensor retinaculum. ATTS is also seen in runners and soccer players who wear tight-fitting shoes, compressing the nerve in the region of the anterior ankle. After the deep fibular nerve passes through the ATT, it will provide motor function to the extensor digitorum brevis (EDB) and extensor hallucis brevis (EHB) and sensation to the web space between the great and second toes. The most common presentation involves only the sensory component; numbness and tingling are identified in the web space between the great and second toes. However, both motor and sensory fibers may be involved, in which case weakness may be identified in the EDB and EHB. Electrophysiologic testing, including sensory and motor nerve conduction studies of the DFN and needle EMG studies of the EDB and EHB, can be used to identify involvement of the distal aspect of the deep fibular nerve. Clinically, this nerve is sometimes compromised after repeated ankle sprains.

13. **What is PTT syndrome?**
The PTT is the region where the muscular, vascular, and nerve structures of the posterior compartment of the leg continue into the foot, passing between the medial malleolus and calcaneus in a tunnel created by the flexor retinaculum. In 90% of individuals, the tibial nerve splits into the medial plantar, lateral plantar, medial calcaneal, and inferior calcaneal nerves while still within the PTT. The medial calcaneal branch of the tibial nerve may bifurcate in this region, but its origin is highly variable and may occur proximal to, within, or distal to the PTT. Thus entrapment of the nervous structures in this region may affect the medial plantar nerve, lateral plantar nerve, medial calcaneal branch, or inferior calcaneal branch, or any combination of these nerves. Symptoms involving the plantar nerves include pain, burning, and paresthesias, often in the distribution of one or both plantar nerves. Recent studies have demonstrated effective techniques that facilitate the electrophysiologic examination of this region, including the medial plantar nerve, lateral plantar nerve, and the medial calcaneal nerve. The focus of these procedures has been to improve the consistency of the measurements and electrophysiologic signals.

14. **Is tarsal tunnel syndrome a common problem? What branch of the plantar nerve is preferentially involved?**
The diagnosis of posterior tarsal tunnel syndrome (PTTS) is not particularly easy because there are no hallmarks of the disorder. Athul et al. (2005) looked at the usefulness of EMG and NCS in the evaluation of PTTS and determined that sensory NCS may be useful in the identification of PTTS. However, EMG and motor nerve conduction studies are of limited benefit.

An area of potential controversy is the actual extent of the PTT. Some clinicians refer only to the region under the flexor retinaculum as the PTT. Others refer to the entire region from the flexor retinaculum proximally to the metatarsophalangeal joint distally as the PTT. Both methods of describing the PTT are accepted although electrophysiologic testing of these structures may specifically demonstrate involvement of the individual plantar or calcaneal nerves. Sensory nerve conduction is the most sensitive electrodiagnostic examination for possible compromise of the medial plantar nerve, lateral plantar nerve, or calcaneal nerve in the region of the ankle or foot.

The medial plantar nerve may be involved more frequently than the lateral plantar nerve, although the overall incidence of plantar neuropathies is relatively low. Sensory NCS may be useful in the identification of PTTS, while EMG and motor nerve conduction studies are typically of limited benefit. Incidence rates for PTTS using EMG/NCS studies are approximately 0.5% with one large study reporting only 51 confirmed cases following 8727 electromyographic examinations (0.58%). Because repetitive pronation or foot hypermobility may stress the medial plantar nerve in activities such as jogging or jumping, the constellation of symptoms associated with medial plantar neuropathy has been called "jogger's foot." Determination of the extent of nerve involvement is an electrodiagnostic challenge that requires detailed examination and meticulous technique.

15. What causes entrapment of the sural nerve?

In general, passage through the fascia of the leg is not a common site of entrapment; thus sural nerve compressions are relatively rare. When an entrapment occurs, it usually is associated with factors such as a ganglion cyst, tight combat boots, or stretch injury. An important clinical point is that the sural nerve is often evaluated when generalized polyneuropathy is suspected. A decrease in nerve conduction velocity in this nerve as well as other major nerves of the leg (eg, tibial and deep fibular) suggests polyneuropathy.

16. Are there regions of the lower extremity that have a tendency to generate electrophysiologic false positives?

Yes. Recent research identified that 21% of patients have abnormal needle electromyographic (EMG) results that suggested denervation, when examining the abductor hallucis intrinsic muscle of the foot. These abnormal electrophysiologic findings additionally appeared to increase with age, being most noticeable in individuals over the age of 60. A second muscle examined, the fibularis (peroneus) tertius, also demonstrated positive findings in normal subjects over the age of 60 but at a much lower rate of 9%. The reasons for these findings and the anecdotal reports of spontaneous abnormal EMG in the foot are unclear, but the findings may be associated with the fact that we ambulate on some of the intrinsic muscles of the foot or that these muscles and their vascular and nerve supplies are restricted by structures such as shoes.

Other studies have demonstrated a much more conservative prevalence of only 2% when examining foot intrinsics in normal subjects. Regardless of the cause, false positives are possible and relatively common with EMG of the small muscles of the foot.

17. What neurologic conditions should be considered in patients with bilateral lower limb numbness, tingling, and pain?

- Spinal stenosis
- Spinal cord tumor
- Radiculopathy
- Mononeuropathy multiplex
- Peripheral neuropathy

18. What are the various causes of lower limb peripheral neuropathy?

- Metabolic and endocrine disorders: diabetes, metabolic liver, and thyroid disease
- Small vessel disease: caused by diabetes and vasculitis
- Autoimmune diseases: Sjögren's, lupus, and rheumatoid arthritis; acute conditions like Guillain-Barré; chronic conditions like chronic inflammatory demyelinating polyneuropathy (CIDP)
- Kidney disease
- Cancer: can trigger global immune responses; radiation treatment can also lead to neuropathic conditions
- Infections (viruses/bacteria): HIV, Lyme disease, diphtheria, leprosy, or West Nile virus
- Medication toxicity: chemotherapy (30%–40% of all patients receiving chemotherapy develop neuropathy); medications used to fight infections, heart and blood pressure abnormalities, and anticonvulsants
- Environmental toxins: lead, mercury, arsenic, and insecticides
- Heavy alcohol consumption
- Inherited peripheral neuropathies: Charcot-Marie-Tooth, Dejerine-Sottas, and Friedreich's ataxia

19. How does a sciatic nerve injury present?

The most common presentation of a sciatic nerve injury is footdrop. It can often be confused with L5 radiculopathy and fibular nerve injury. In severe sciatic nerve injuries, patients will also exhibit (in addition to weak ankle dorsiflexion) weak ankle plantar flexion and knee flexion, decreased ankle jerk reflex, and sensory loss of the lateral leg and dorsal and plantar aspects of the foot.

20. **What are the most common causes of sciatic nerve injury?**
The most common causes of sciatic nerve injury are hip trauma and surgery. Sciatic nerve injury can occur up to 3% of the time following total hip replacement. The next most common injuries are external compression and penetrating injuries (ie, gunshot, knife, injections). Least common are tumors in adults; however, in the pediatric population a tumor is the most common cause of sciatic neuropathy.

21. **What are common nerve conduction and electromyography findings in patients with sciatic nerve injury?**
NCS findings:
Derivatives of the sciatic nerve such as the sural and superficial fibular sensory nerves will have reduced amplitudes or, in severe injuries, absent responses. Because sciatic nerve injuries most often involve the fibular portion versus the tibial portion of the sciatic nerve, the fibular motor nerve amplitude will be significantly reduced, and the tibial nerve and tibial H-reflex will demonstrate normal or near normal values. Fibular F-waves will be abnormal.
EMG findings:
Sampling of the lumbar paraspinals (lumbar dorsal rami), gluteus maximus (inferior gluteal nerve), tensor fascia latae (superior gluteal nerve), and quadriceps (femoral nerve) will test normal because they are not innervated by the sciatic nerve. Muscles showing denervation will primarily be fibular innervated muscles (94%–100% of patients), such as the biceps femoris short head and pretibial and lateral lower leg compartment muscles. Tibial innervated muscles (medial hamstring muscles, posterior and medial leg compartment muscles) can and will be involved in severe sciatic nerve injuries (74%–84% of patients).

22. **What is the prognosis for patients who have sustained a sciatic nerve injury?**
The prognosis is dependent on the severity of the injury (not location). However, most individuals have a good outcome 3 years following injury, whereas 30% of individuals sustaining sciatic nerve injury have near normal function 1 year post injury. The best outcomes occur in those patients with a common fibular nerve conduction response that is obtainable from the extensor digitorum brevis muscle and the absence of paralysis of the pretibial and/or posterior compartment muscles.

23. **Differentiating a lower extremity focal neuropathy from a polyneuropathy.**
Generalized peripheral polyneuropathy (GPPN) involves multiple nerves in multiple extremities (BUE and BLE). The pathophysiology of GPPN may be primary demyelination, primary axon degeneration, or a combination of both demyelination and axon degeneration. Polyneuropathies are classified as general medical conditions (diabetes and renal disease), autoimmune (Guillain-Barre syndrome), metabolic and toxic (alcohol abuse), hereditary or inherited (Charcot-Marie-Tooth disease), and idiopathic. GPPN may also be classified using electrophysiologic terminology as demyelinating or axon degeneration and involving motor or sensory fibers. Since the pathophysiology of GPPN is based on diseases, the patients with GPPN present with symptoms that are diffuse, symmetrical, typically involve all four extremities, and typically affect BLE before BUE. On physical examination of patients with GPPN, the "triad of polyneuropathy" may be seen and includes: (1) sensory changes in a stocking or glove distribution; (2) distal weakness; and (3) hypo-reflexia (depressed or absent muscle stretch reflexes). During the evaluation and treatment of patients with GPPN, the physical therapist must be aware of the "triad of polyneuropathy" and the effects that GPPN may have on the interventions and prognosis of these patients.

24. **Describe why neuromuscular ultrasound (NMUS) is an emerging adjunctive technique to complement electrodiagnosis for select lower extremity entrapments.**
Ultrasound is a modality that was first used medically in the 1940s and it is a procedure that uses sound waves to produce an image. Resolution and increased clarity of direct imaging of nerves improved to where the first reported clinical evaluation of a nerve was referenced in 1991. Since that case approximately three decades ago, ultrasound (referred to as neuromuscular ultrasound [NMUS] or high-resolution nerve ultrasound [HRUS], has increased in use in some electrophysiologic laboratories as a complement to the standard electrophysiologic study due to machine availability, reduced cost of the procedure, ease of use, and the fact that the procedure is noninvasive and is not painful. There are several clear advantages for the addition of NMUS to the evaluation of a patient with a potential entrapment; since the modality allows direct visualization of the nerve in question, it permits improved nerve conduction studies by identifying variable nerve anatomy for structures such as the lateral cutaneous nerve of the thigh, and while electrodiagnostics may not be applicable in the first few weeks following a traumatic injury, NMUS visualization can be used immediately to facilitate optimal patient care. This advantage of being able to directly visualize lower extremity entrapments can provide structural confirmation of neuromas, peripheral nerve entrapments, Baker's cysts, intra and extraneural cysts, artery aneurysms, deep vein thrombosis, and other patient problems. One study has shown that with the NMUS added to the clinical and electrophysiological evaluation, the diagnosis and treatment provided was modified in 42.3% of the cases, and it had a confirmatory role in 40% of the cases. Thus, when the two procedures were combined, there was improved accuracy of the diagnosis and potentially improved therapeutics.

25. What does NMUS add to electrodiagnostics (EDX) and in what types of lower extremity entrapment conditions is this modality potentially warranted?

Simply stated, the clinical and electrophysiological evaluations assess function, with nerve parameters assessed including the speed of conduction (eg, latency and nerve conduction velocity), signal size (amplitude), shape, and duration. While these parameters assess how the peripheral nerve is working (functioning), no direct information is provided about the structure of the nerve under investigation. Neuromuscular ultrasound (NMUS), on the other hand, complements EDX by providing direct visualization of the underlying nerve anatomy. Nerve enlargement is the most important diagnostic marker associated with peripheral nerve dysfunction, and entrapment neuropathies are the most common indication for NMUS to assist with localization of the problem. Thus, assessment of the cross-sectional area (CSA) along suspected regions of the nerve under investigation is essential. Cross-sectional area enlargement is typically a feature of demyelinating conditions more than in axonal dysfunctions. An abridged list of nerves where ultrasound has been an adjunctive technique in the lower extremity include the femoral nerve, sciatic nerve, fibular (peroneal) nerve, lateral femoral cutaneous nerve, sural nerve, saphenous nerve, tibial nerve, medial and lateral plantar nerves. Nerve enlargement is also evident in other conditions like Charcot-Marie-Tooth (CMT) disease, chronic inflammatory demyelinating polyneuropathy (CIDP), and diabetic polyneuropathy. Ultrasound is most useful on more superficially located nerves, with limitations in nerves under significant tissue masses such as the lumbar plexus, lumbar roots, and small nerves located deep within an extremity.

Bibliography

Akyuz, G., Us, O., Türan, B., Kayhan, O., Canbulat, N., & Yilmar, I. T. (2000). Anterior tarsal tunnel syndrome. *Electromyography and Clinical Neurophysiology, 40*, 123–128.

Amato, A. A. (2002). Approach to peripheral neuropathy (Chapter 21). In D. Dumitru, A. Amato, & M. Zwarts (Eds.). *Electrodiagnostic medicine* (2nd ed.). Philadelphia, PA: Hanley & Belfus.

American Association of Electrodiagnostic Medicine. (1993). Practice parameters for electrodiagnostic studies in carpal tunnel syndrome—summary statement. *Muscle and Nerve, 16*, 1390–1391.

Atul, P., Gaines, K., Malamut, R., Park, T. A., Del Toro, D. R., Holland, N., American Association of Neuromuscular and Electrodiagnostic Medicine, (2005). Usefulness of electrodiagnostic techniques in the evaluation of suspected tarsal tunnel syndrome. An evidence based review. *Muscle and Nerve, 32*(2), 236–240.

Bereend, K. R., Kavolus, J. J., Morris, M. J., & Lombardi, A. V., Jr. (2013). Primary and revision anterior supine total hip arthroplasty: An analysis of complications and reoperations. *Instructional Course Lectures, 62*, 251–263.

Bhargava, T., Goytia, R. N., Jones, L. C., & Hungerford, M. W. (2010). Lateral femoral cutaneous nerve impairment after direct anterior approach for total hip arthroplasty. *Orthopedics, 13*(7), 472.

Boon, A., & Harper, C. (2003). Needle EMG of abductor hallucis and peroneus tertius in normal subjects. *Muscle and Nerve, 27*, 752–756.

Brull, R., McCartney, C. J., Chan, V. W., & El-Beheiry, H. (2007). Neurological complications after regional anesthesia: Contemporary estimates of risk. *Anesthesia and Analgesia, 104*(4), 965–974.

Burakqazi, A. Z., Kelly, J. J., & Richardson, P. (2012). The electrodiagnostic sensitivity of proximal lower extremity muscles in the diagnosis of L5 radiculopathy. *Muscle and Nerve, 45*(6), 891–893.

Casciere, B. (2014). Normative data for trans-tarsal conduction velocity of the medial and lateral plantar nerves recorded from the flexor hallucis brevis and first dorsal interosseous. Provo, UT: Rocky Mountain University of Health Professions. Unpublished dissertation.

Carroll, A. S., & Simon, N. G. (2020). Current and future applications of ultrasound imaging in peripheral nerve disorders. *World Journal of Radiology, 12*(6), 101–129.

Dalley, A. F., & Agur, A.M.R. (2023). Moore's clinically oriented anatomy (9th ed.). Philadelphia PA: Wolters Kluwer.

Dillingham, T. (2002). Electrodiagnostic approach to patients with suspected radiculopathy. *Physical Medicine and Rehabilitation Clinics of North America, 13*, 567–588.

Distad, B. J., & Weiss, M. D. (2013). Clinical and electrodiagnostic features of sciatic neuropathies. *Physical Medicine and Rehabilitation Clinics of North America, 24*, 107–120.

Dumitru, D. (2002). Peripheral nervous system's reaction to injury (Chapter 4). In D. Dumitru, A. Amato, & M. Zwarts (Eds.), *Electrodiagnostic medicine* (2nd ed.). Philadelphia, PA: Hanley & Belfus.

Dumitru, D., Diaz, C., & King, J. (2001). Prevalence of denervation in paraspinal and foot intrinsic musculature. *American Journal of Physical Medicine and Rehabilitation, 80*, 482–490.

Dumitru, D., & Zwarts, M. (2002). Focal peripheral neuropathies (Chapter 24). In D. Dumitru, A. Amato, & M. Zwarts (Eds.), *Electrodiagnostic medicine* (2nd ed.). Philadelphia, PA: Hanley & Belfus.

Fritz, J., & Wainner, R. (2001). Examining diagnostic tests: An evidence-based perspective. *Physical Therapy, 81*, 1546–1564.

Galloway, K. M., & Greathouse, D. G. (2006). Tibial nerve motor conduction with recording from the first dorsal interosseous: A comparison with standard tibial studies. *Neurology, Neurophysiology, and Neuroscience, 10*, 2.

Girolami, M., Galletti, S., Montanari, G., et al. (2013). Common peroneal nerve palsy due to hematoma at the fibular neck. *Journal of Knee Surgery, 26*(Suppl 1), S132–S135.

Gonzalez, N. L., & Hobson-Webb, L. D. (2019). Neuromuscular ultrasound in clinical practice: A review. *Clinical Neurophysiology Practice, 4*, 148–163.

Goulding, K., Beaule, P. E., Kim, P. R., & Fazeka, A. (2010). Incidence of lateral femoral cutaneous nerve neuropraxia after anterior approach hip arthroplasty. *Clinical Orthopaedics and Related Research, 468*(9), 2397–2404.

Greathouse, D. G., Ernst, G., Halle, J. S., & Shaffer, S. W. (2020). Electrophysiological testing (nerve conduction and electromyographic studies). In W. Boissonnault (Ed.), *Primary care for the physical therapist (Examination and triage)* (3rd ed.). Philadelphai, PA: Elsevier Sanders.

Halle, J., & Greathouse, D. (2021). Principles of electrophysiologic evaluation and testing (Chapter 8). In W. E. Prentice, W. S. Quillen, & F. Underwood (Eds.), *Therapeutic modalities in rehabilitation* (6th ed.). New York, NY: McGraw Hill.

Hallert, O., Li, Y., Brismar, H., & Lindgren, U. (2012). The direct anterior approach: Initial experience of a minimally invasive technique for total hip arthroplasty. *Journal of Orthopaedic Surgery and Research, 7*, 17.

Hannaford, A., Vucic, S., Kiernan, M. C., et al. (2021). Review article "spotlight on ultrasonography in the diagnosis of peripheral nerve disease: The evidence to date". *International Journal of General Medicine, 14*, 4597–4604.
Jablecki, C., Andary, M., & So, Y. (1993). Literature review of the usefulness of nerve conduction studies and electromyography for the evaluation of patients with carpal tunnel syndrome. *Muscle and Nerve, 16*, 1392–1414.
Kimura, J. (2013). *Electrodiagnosis in diseases of nerve and muscle* (4th ed.). New York, NY: Oxford University Press.
Kramer, M., Grimm, A., Winter, L. D., et al. (2019). Nerve ultrasound as helpful tool in polyneuropathiews. *Diagnostics, 11*, 211.
Kuntzer, T. (1994). Carpal tunnel syndrome in 100 patients: Sensitivity, specificity on multi-neurophysiological procedures and estimation of axonal loss of motor, sensory and sympathetic median nerve fibers. *Journal of Neurological Sciences, 20*, 221–229.
Mingo-Robinet, J., Castaneda-Cabrero, C., Alvarez, V., Leon Alonso-Cortes, J. M., & Monge-Casares, E. (2013). Tourniquet-related iatrogenic femoral nerve palsy after knee surgery: Case report and review of the literature. *Case Reports in Orthopedics, 2013*, 368290.
Mitsiokapa, E. A., Mavrogenis, A. F., Antonopoulos, D., Tzanos, G., & Papagelopoulos, P. J. (2012). Common peroneal nerve palsy after grade I inversion ankle sprain. *Journal of Surgical Orthopaedic Advances, 21*(4), 261–265.
Moore, A. E., & Stringer, M. D. (2011). Iatrogenic femoral nerve injury: A systematic review. *Surgical and Radiologic Anatomy, 33*(8), 649–658.
Mulligan, E. P., & McCain, K. (2012). Common fibular (peroneal) neuropathy as the result of a ganglion cyst. *Journal of Orthopaedic and Sports Physical Therapy, 42*(12), 1051.
Netter, F. (2014). *Atlas of human anatomy* (6th ed.). Philadelphia, PA: Elsevier.
Oh, S. J. (2003a). Uncommon nerve conduction studies: Techniques and normal values (Chapter 11). In S. Oh (Ed.), *Clinical electromyography: Nerve conduction studies* (3rd ed.). Philadelphia, PA: Lippincott Williams & Wilkins.
Oh, S. J. (2003b). Nerve conduction in focal neuropathies. In S. Oh (Ed.), *Clinical electromyography: Nerve conduction studies* (3rd ed.). Philadelphia, PA: Lippincott Williams & Wilkins.
Padua, L., Liotta, G., Di Pasquale, A., et al. (2012). Contribution of ultrasound in the assessment of nerve diseases. *European Journal of Neurology, 19*(1), 47–54.
Portney, L., & Watkins, S. (2009). Validity of measurements (Chapter 6). In L. Portney & M. Watkins (Eds.), *Foundations of clinical research: Applications to practice* (3rd ed.). Saddle River, NJ: Pearson & Prentice Hall.
Simmons, C., Jr., Izant, T. H., Rothman, R. H., Booth, R. E., Jr., & Balderston, R. A. (1991). Femoral neuropathy following total hip arthroplasty. Anatomic study, case reports and literature review. *Journal of Arthroplasty, 6*(Suppl), S57–S66.
Simon, N. G., & Kieman, M. C. (2012). Common peroneal neuropathy and cancer. *Internal Medicine Journal, 42*(7), 837–840.
Steinitz, E., Singh, S., & Saeed, M. (1999). Diagnostic tests help clarify tarsal tunnel mystery. *Biomechanics, 10*, 43.
Suk, J. I., Walker, F. O., & Cartwright, M. S. (2013). Ultrasound of peripheral nerves. *Current Neurology and Neuroscience Reports, 13*(2), 328.
Swenson, C., Sward, L., & Karlsson, J. (1996). Cryotherapy in sports medicine. *Scandinavian Journal of Medicine and Science in Sports, 6*(4), 193–200.
Weier, C. A., Jones, L. C., & Hungerford, M. W. (2010). Meralgia paresthetica of the contralateral leg after total hip arthroplasty. *Orthopedics, 33*(4).
Yi, C., Aqudelo, J. F., Dayton, M. R., & Morgan, S. J. (2013). Early complications of anterior supine intermuscular total hip arthroplasty. *Orthopedics, 36*(3), e276–e281.

CHAPTER 75 QUESTIONS

1. **In a patient with footdrop (ie, weakness of ankle dorsiflexors and toe extensors), the clinical and electrophysiologic evidence distinguishing between a common fibular nerve (peroneal nerve) mononeuropathy and an L5 radiculopathy is:**
   a. Weakness and denervation in the tibialis anterior, EDL, and EHL
   b. Weakness and denervation in the EDB and EHB
   c. Weakness and denervation in the tensor fascia lata and tibialis anterior
   d. Loss of sensation over the dorsum of the foot

2. **A patient presents with numbness and tingling on the dorsal aspect of his foot between the first and second toe and 2/5 MMT of the extensor digitorum brevis muscle. No other weakness or loss of sensation is noted in the involved lower limb. What is the MOST likely lower limb nerve entrapment?**
   a. L5 radiculopathy
   b. Fibular nerve injury at the fibular head
   c. Deep fibular nerve injury at the ankle
   d. Tarsal tunnel syndrome

3. **Following a routine arthroscopic knee surgery, a patient reports loss of sensation along the medial aspect of the lower limb. There is no motor weakness of the involved lower limb and reflexes are intact. What is the most likely nerve injury?**
   a. Femoral nerve
   b. Lateral cutaneous nerve of the thigh
   c. Obturator nerve
   d. Saphenous nerve

4. **Ultrasound coupled with electrophysiological evaluation provides increased clinical insight in all of the following areas except:**
   a. Underlying anatomy can be visualized.
   b. Nerve function can be directly assessed.
   c. Cross-sectional area of a nerve along its course can be determined.
   d. Extraneural structures associated with the potential entrapment can be documented.

FUNCTIONAL ANATOMY OF THE FOOT AND ANKLE

T.A. Brosky, Jr., PT, DHSc, SCS

1. **What are the main cooperative functions provided by the foot/ankle complex?**
   Together, the foot/ankle complex provides the following general functions:
   Provides a base of support for upright posture
   Serves as a torque converter controlling rotation of leg during stance phase of gait
   Provides the flexibility required to adapt to uneven terrain
   Serves as an important functional shock absorber during weight bearing
   Provides a rigid lever for push-off

2. **What are the major anatomic divisions of the bones of the foot?**
   The rear foot (tarsus) consists of the talus and calcaneus. The midfoot (lesser tarsus) consists of the navicular (or scaphoid), cuboid, and three cuneiforms (medial, intermediate, and lateral). Distal to the midfoot are the metatarsals and phalanges. The foot also may be divided into medial and lateral columns. The medial column is composed of the talus, navicular, three cuneiforms, and metatarsals 1 to 3, along with their respective phalanges. The lateral column consists of the calcaneus, cuboid, and metatarsals 4 to 5 along with their respective phalanges.

3. **What are the four muscular layers, from superficial to deep, from the plantar aspect of the foot?**
   FIRST LAYER (3 MUSCLES)
   - Abductor hallucis
   - Flexor digitorum brevis
   - Abductor digiti minimi

   SECOND LAYER (2 MUSCLES)
   - Quadratus plantae
   - Lumbricals

   Note anatomic location: the tendons of the flexor hallucis longus and the flexor digitorum longus, which are considered extrinsic foot muscles located in the leg, pass through this layer.
   THIRD LAYER (3 MUSCLES)
   - Flexor hallucis brevis
   - Adductor hallucis
   - Flexor digiti minimi brevis

   FOURTH LAYER (2 MUSCLES)
   - Plantar interossei (3 muscles; PAD = Plantar ADduct)
   - Dorsal interossei (4 muscles; DAB = Dorsal ABduct)

   Note anatomic location: the tendons of the peroneus longus and tibialis posterior, which are considered extrinsic foot muscles located in the leg, pass through this layer.

4. **What is the axis of movement and range of motion (ROM) of the foot and ankle?**

	TALOCRURAL	SUBTALAR	MIDTARSAL	TARSOMETA-TARSAL
ROM	PF: 0–50 degrees	IN: 0–35 degrees	IN: 0–20 degrees	PF: 0–15 degrees
	DF: 0–20 degrees	EV: 0–15 degrees	EV: 0–10 degrees	DF: 0–3 degrees
Axis	80 degrees from vertical reference (10 degrees, up from horizontal), 84 degrees from longitudinal reference of foot	40–45 degrees superior from horizontal reference, 15–18 degrees medially from longitudinal reference (sagittal plane)	15 degrees superior from horizontal reference, 9 degrees to midline for IN/EV	Similar to subtalar joint

PF, Plantar flexion; DF, dorsiflexion; IN, inversion; EV, eversion; ROM, range of motion.

5. **What are the resting and close-packed positions of the talocrural joint, the subtalar joint, and the first metatarsophalangeal (MTP) joint?**

	RESTING	CLOSE
Talocrural joint	10 degrees plantar flexion	Maximum dorsiflexion
	neutral inversion/eversion	
Subtalar joint	Midway between extremes of motion	Full supination
First MTP joint	10 degrees dorsiflexion	Maximal dorsiflexion

6. **How much talocrural ROM is typically required for normal gait?**
Although compensations may occur in the lower limb, pelvis, or lumbar spine to accommodate for a restricted talocrural joint, approximately 6 to 10 degrees of dorsiflexion and 20 to 30 degrees of plantar flexion are required for normal gait.

7. **How much subtalar ROM is required for normal gait?**
Although compensations may occur in the lower limb, pelvis, or lumbar spine to accommodate for a restricted subtalar joint, a total of 4 to 6 degrees of inversion/eversion is generally required for normal gait.

8. **What is the correct terminology to use when referring to or describing foot and ankle motion?**
It is correct to use the suffix "-us" or "-ed" when describing or referring to a static position (eg, supinatus or pronated) and "-ion" and "-ing" when describing or referring to motion or a movement (eg, supination or pronating).

9. **How is pronation and supination concerning the rear foot defined?**
Pronation and supination are the triplane motions in the subtalar joint, the so-called universal joint of the lower extremity. In weight bearing, pronation occurs at initial contact through the loading response during gait. Internal rotation of the lower leg produces talar adduction and plantar flexion relative to the calcaneus, and the calcaneus everts and abducts. This process typically occurs during the first 25% of the stance phase of gait, as the foot adapts to the ground.

Supination during gait occurs from the start of the midstance phase of gait (foot flat) through terminal stance. This process occurs as the lower leg starts to rotate externally, leading to talar abduction (dorsiflexion relative to the calcaneus), and the calcaneus inverts and adducts. In the nonweight-bearing or swing phase, the talus is relatively fixed in the ankle mortise, and supination/pronation occurs through the subtalar joint by movement of the calcaneus and foot around the subtalar joint axis of motion. In supination, the calcaneus and foot move through a combination of inversion, adduction, and plantar flexion in relation to the fixed talus. In pronation, the calcaneus moves through eversion, abduction, and dorsiflexion relative to the fixed talus.

10. **What is the windlass mechanism of the foot?**
The windlass mechanism of the foot refers to the seemingly simple maneuver of dorsiflexion of the toes of the foot, most specifically related to passive hallux extension that elevates the medial longitudinal arch through hindfoot supination when the calcaneus inverts. The plantar fascia and intrinsic foot musculature are supinators around the subtalar joint axis of motion. Hence, dorsiflexion of the digits produces supination, which creates the medial longitudinal arch of the foot through midtarsal joint motion.

11. **What are the common arches of the normal foot?**
There are four primary arches of the normal foot supported by myoligamentous structures. The two longitudinal arches are the medial longitudinal arch (MLA) and the lateral longitudinal arch (LLA). The calcaneus is common to both longitudinal arches. The MLA is formed by the medial columnar structures of the calcaneus, talus, navicular, three cuneiforms, and metatarsals 1, 2, and 3. The MLA is primarily involved in weight bearing. The LLA is formed by the calcaneus, cuboid, and metatarsals 4 and 5. There are two transverse arches: the proximal transverse arch, formed by the bony structures of the navicular, three cuneiforms, and cuboid, and the distal transverse arch, formed by the heads of the five metatarsals.

12. **What are the main noncontractile or passive supports of the longitudinal arches?**
The noncontractile passive supports of the longitudinal arches are the: (1) plantar aponeurosis, (2) long plantar ligament, (3) short plantar ligament, and (4) plantar calcaneonavicular ligament, also commonly known as the "spring" ligament.

13. **What are the main dynamic support structures of the longitudinal arches of the foot?**
The dynamic support structures of the foot include the intrinsic muscles (four layers) and the muscles and tendons of the fibularis longus, posterior tibialis, flexor hallucis longus, and flexor digitorum.

14. **What is pes planus?**
Pes planus (flatfoot) describes a foot that exhibits no longitudinal arch and an ankle that is everted (valgus). It can be classified as rigid or flexible. A rigid flatfoot is often associated with a tarsal coalition or a vertical talus, and a flexible flatfoot is considered a normal variant. Pes planus is normal in children up to 6 to 7 years of age. A rigid flatfoot is always flat but a flexible flatfoot appears normal when nonweight bearing but becomes flat when standing. If a flexible flatfoot is asymptomatic, no treatment is warranted, but if it is symptomatic, then arch supports are often incorporated. If the deformity is rigid, then the underlying cause (eg, tarsal coalition, vertical talus) must be addressed.

15. **What is pes cavus?**
Pes cavus refers to a high arch foot. This can be a benign condition that merely describes a foot type exhibiting an abnormally high arch or can be related to muscle imbalances in the immature foot, although it is important to rule out the possibility of underlying neuromuscular disease (such as Charcot-Marie-Tooth disease). The presentation is typically an 8- to 10-year-old child who complains of ankle pain, habitually toe-walks, and exhibits tight Achilles tendon and limited ankle dorsiflexion. A clinical workup may be needed that includes radiographs, EMG/NCS, and MRI of the spine to rule out occult neuromuscular disease. Treatment may include bracing/ankle-foot orthoses (AFOs) or osteotomies and tendon transfers in more severe cases.

16. **What is the ideal position for ankle fusion (eg, arthrodesis)?**
The ideal position for ankle arthrodesis is neutral dorsiflexion (or slight plantar flexion if heeled shoes are preferred, eg, by women), slight valgus (0–5 degrees), and external rotation of approximately 5 to 10 degrees.

17. **What percentage of weight does the fibula bear?**
The fibula supports approximately 12% to 17% of the axial load.

18. **What is Fick's angle?**
Normally when an individual stands, the posture of the foot assumes a slight toe-out position, and this angle, approximately 12 to 18 degrees in the adult (5 degrees in children), is sometimes referred to as Fick's angle.

19. **What is the function of the deltoid ligament?**
The deltoid or medial collateral ligament of the rear foot consists of a superficial and a deep ligament complex. The superficial deltoid ligament consists of the ligament attachment to the distal tibia (medial malleolus) with insertions onto the navicular, sustentaculum tali, and talus. The majority of these ligament fibers are vertically oriented and therefore prevent or limit excessive rear-foot eversion in the frontal plane. The deep deltoid ligament consists of relatively transversely oriented fibers deep to the superficial band from the medial malleolus anteriorly and posteriorly along the medial body of the talus. Thus it resists excessive transverse plane rotation (abduction) of the talus. The deltoid ligament may be sprained under excessive loading of the ankle and rear foot in eversion

or may avulse a portion of the medial malleolus as part of an ankle fracture (four components: tibionavicular, tibiocalcaneal, anterior tibiotalar, and posterior tibiotalar).

20. **What are the lateral collateral ligaments of the ankle and rear foot?**
The lateral collateral complex of rear-foot and ankle ligaments consists of the anterior and posterior talofibular ligaments and the calcaneofibular ligament. The anterior talofibular ligament and calcaneofibular ligaments are most commonly sprained in inversion ankle injuries. The horizontally oriented anterior talofibular ligament and the more vertically oriented calcaneofibular ligaments provide reciprocal stability to the rear foot. In a plantar-flexed position of the ankle, the anterior talofibular ligament (flat, fan-shaped capsular ligament) is the primary stabilizer to rear-foot inversion. In a dorsiflexed position, the cordlike calcaneofibular ligament is the stabilizer to rear-foot inversion.

21. **What is the Lisfranc ligament?**
The Lisfranc ligament is the plantar tarsometatarsal ligament, spanning the medial cuneiform to the base of the second metatarsal. In fractures and dislocations of the Lisfranc joint, this ligament commonly avulses a fragment of bone from the plantar medial base of the second metatarsal.

22. **What is the spring ligament?**
The spring ligament is another name for the calcaneonavicular ligament, which extends from the plantar aspect of the sustentaculum tali (on the calcaneus) to the navicular. It provides support to the plantar head of the talus and talonavicular joint and is a primary static stabilizer, reinforcing the medial longitudinal arch.

23. **What is the bifurcate ligament?**
The bifurcate ligament is Y-shaped and originates from the anterior floor of the sinus tarsi and anterior process of the calcaneus. It extends and divides distally into two distinct bands that attach to the cuboid laterally and navicular medially. This ligament provides important stability to the rear foot.

24. **What are the Chopart and Lisfranc joints?**
The Chopart joint is the midtarsal joint, which consists of the talonavicular and calcaneocuboid joints. The Lisfranc joint is the tarsometatarsal joint, which consists of the three cuneiforms and metatarsals 4 and 5.

25. **What is a Lisfranc joint sprain?**
The Lisfranc joint sprain, also referred to as a midfoot sprain, is often missed as it sometimes accompanies an inversion/plantarflexion ankle injury also involving a hyperflexion or torsion (twisting) of the midfoot. The injury is located at the articulation of the first and second metatarsal with the medial (or first) cuneiform and may involve a small fracture. This area should be closely evaluated with all ankle injuries and often requires a longer healing time and occasionally immobilization and/or surgical fixation.

26. **How does the weight-bearing surface of the ankle change after syndesmotic injury of the ankle?**
Mortise widening, resulting in a 1-mm lateral shift of the talus, decreases the weight bearing surface of the talus by 40%, a 3-mm shift by >60%, and a 5-mm shift by approximately 80%. Increased contact pressures may lead to early degenerative joint disease.

27. **Why is the anterior talus subject to impingement?**
The anterior portion of the talus is 2.5 mm wider than the posterior talus. With dorsiflexion, the space available in the anterior mortise is decreased. This space can be further compromised by osteophytes, scar tissue, or overly compressed open reduction and internal fixation (ORIF) to the syndesmosis after ankle fracture. The compression/distraction of the ankle joint (talocrural joint) that occurs with normal walking may be important for normal lubrication of the joint.

28. **What is the sinus tarsi?**
The sinus tarsi is a funnel-shaped opening in the rear foot between the talus and calcaneus. It is widest anterolaterally and narrows as it passes posteromedially between the talus and calcaneus, separating the anterior and middle facets of the subtalar joint from the posterior facet. The narrow posteromedial section of this space often is called the tarsal canal. Through this area pass the interosseous talocalcaneal ligament and the major blood supply to the body of the talus (the anastomosis between the artery of the tarsal canal and the artery of the tarsal sinus).

29. **What are the contents of the tarsal tunnel?**
From superficial to deep and anterior to posterior, the contents of the tarsal tunnel can be remembered by the mnemonic "Tom, Dick, And Very Nervous Harry":
Tom = posterior Tibial tendon
Dick = flexor Digitorum longus
And Very Nervous = posterior tibial Artery, Vein, and Nerve
Harry = flexor Hallucis longus

30. **How would one describe the structure of the tarsal tunnel?**
The tarsal tunnel is bounded by the distal tibia (medial malleolus) anteriorly and the Achilles tendon posteriorly; it is roofed by the flexor retinaculum (laciniate ligament). The flexor retinaculum divides into fibrous (septae) bands that separate the contents of the tarsal tunnel into individual compartments.

31. **What are the five nerves that cross into and supply the motor and sensory fibers to the foot?**
    1. Sural nerve—sensory (posterolaterally)
    2. Superficial peroneal nerve—motor and sensory (anterolaterally)
    3. Deep peroneal nerve—motor and sensory (anteriorly, traveling with the dorsalis pedis artery)
    4. Saphenous nerve—sensory (anteromedially, as the long continuation of the femoral nerve distally)
    5. Posterior tibial nerve—motor and sensory (posteromedially, dividing to supply the foot distally as the medial and lateral plantar nerves)

32. **What is porta pedis?**
The porta pedis is the anatomic opening into the plantar aspect of the foot beneath the belly of the abductor hallucis muscle. Through this opening pass the medial and lateral plantar nerves and arteries/veins distally from the tarsal tunnel into the foot. The porta pedis is a potential site for compression of the plantar nerves and may also be a cause of heel pain.

33. **What structure is referred to as "freshman's nerve"?**
The plantaris muscle tendon, which often appears like a nerve to new dissectors of the human cadaver, is referred to as "freshman's nerve." However, its location, flat, firm appearance, and consistency reveal that it is a tendon. It travels deep to the gastrocnemius and superficially to the soleus to lie medially to the Achilles tendon, where it attaches onto the medial aspect of the posterior calcaneal tuberosity.

34. **What is meant by an accessory bone of the foot?**
An accessory bone is a small ossicle or extra bone that separates from the normal bone (most commonly caused by fracture or a secondary ossification center). Accessory bones are more frequently found in the foot than anywhere else in the body. The most common are the os trigonum (from the posterior talus), the os tibiale externum (from the navicular tuberosity), the bipartite medial cuneiform (superior/inferior), the os vesalianum pedis (tuberosity of the base of the fifth metatarsal), the os sustentaculum (sustentaculum tali), and the os supranaviculare (dorsum of talonavicular joint).

35. **What is an exostosis and where are they most commonly located in the foot?**
An exostosis is an abnormal or bony growth (osteophyte or "spur") that results in response to excessive pressure, overuse, or localized trauma. In some cases the cause may be unknown or related to family history, then referred to as hereditary multiple exostosis(es). Common locations in the foot include the dorsal aspect of the tarsometatarsal joint, head of the fifth metatarsal, dorsum of the first metatarsophalangeal joint, the posterior lateral calcaneus (ie, "pump bump" or Haglund's deformity), dorsal aspect of the navicular, and the anteromedial aspect of the calcaneus at the insertion of the plantar fascia. These exostoses can also often be the result of wearing improper footwear (too large or too small) and can be treated with shoe modifications or pressure relief pads.

36. **How would one describe the function of the sesamoids?**
The sesamoids are located beneath the head of the first metatarsal. The two functions of the sesamoids are (1) to transfer loads through the soft tissues to the metatarsal head and (2) to increase the lever arm of the flexor hallucis brevis to aid in push-off.

37. **What is the master knot of Henry?**
The master knot of Henry is a fibrous band on the plantar aspect of the foot adjoining the flexor digitorum longus and flexor hallucis longus tendons in the second layer of the intrinsic foot muscles.

38. What is the effect of an increasing hallux valgus on plantar flexion force at push-off?
A hallux valgus angle of 40 degrees decreases push-off strength of the great toe by 78%. Adding a 30-degree pronation deformity decreases the plantar flexion strength to 5% of normal.

39. What is Toygar's triangle?
On the lateral radiograph of the foot and ankle, Toygar's triangle is the hypodense radiographic triangle bordered by the more radiodense Achilles tendon posteriorly, the superior border of the calcaneus at its base, and the posterior border of the mid to distal tibia. When the triangle is not apparent on the lateral radiograph, the usual cause is accumulation of fluid along the tarsal tunnel, which may suggest inflammation from ankle, subtalar joint, or retrocalcaneal bursitis. The triangle may be obliterated by hematoma or swelling around an Achilles tendon rupture.

40. What are the normal forces (relative to body weight) acting on the ankle joint during functional activities, such as walking, running, and jumping?
Compressive forces during normal walking are 1 to 1.2 times body weight, running 2 times body weight, and jumping (from a height of about 24 inches) 4 to 5 times body weight.

41. How many muscles attach to the talus?
None. One of the unique features of the talus is articular cartilage covers approximately 60% of its surface and there are no musculotendinous attachments to it.

42. What is metatarsus adductus?
This refers to one of the most common pediatric foot disorders and describes the position of the forefoot in varus and adduction. It is often associated with intrauterine position and clinically presents with a "kidney-bean" appearance, depicting the nature of the deformity and an in-toeing gait. Most will resolve with normal development, minor shoe modifications, or serial casting. Rarely is surgical intervention (eg, midfoot osteotomy) required.

43. What is the function of the interossei and lumbrical muscles?
The dorsal interossei (DAB, four muscles) are abductors of the toes, while the plantar interossei (PAD, three muscles) perform adduction of the toes. The combined primary actions of the lumbricals and interossei are plantar flexion of the metatarsophalangeal joints and extension at the proximal interphalangeal and distal interphalangeal joints. These intrinsic muscles provide stability, support, and integrity to the arches of the foot.

44. Describe the functional anatomy of the anterior talofibular ligament.
Bone is less dense at the fibular attachment, but the enthesis fibrocartilage is more prominent. Fibrocartilage is present at the site where the ligament wraps around the lateral talar articular margin in the plantar-flexed and inverted foot, likely as a result of compression in this region. Avulsion fractures are less common at the talar end because the bone in this area is denser and stress is dissipated away from the talar enthesis by the fibrocartilaginous character of the ligament near the talus.

45. What is the relationship between metatarsal length and midfoot arthrosis?
Patients with midfoot arthrosis have a significantly higher ratio of second metatarsal to first metatarsal length compared with controls. Studies have shown the functional length of the second metatarsal was 18.6% greater than the first metatarsal in the arthrosis group, compared with 4.1% for the control group.

46. List the anatomical compartments of the leg and the key structures located within each.
There are four anatomical compartments in the leg that are enclosed by osteo-fascial tissue and bordered in part by an interosseus membrane and the tibia and fibula. The four compartments include the anterior, lateral, deep posterior, and superficial posterior.
Anterior Compartment:
Muscular: tibialis anterior, extensor hallucis longus, extensor digitorum longus, and peroneus tertius
Neurovascular: deep fibular nerve and anterior tibial artery and vein
Lateral Compartment:
Muscular: fibularis longus and fibularis brevis
Neurovascular: superficial fibular nerve
Deep Posterior Compartment:
Muscular: tibialis posterior, flexor hallucis longus, flexor digitorum longus and popliteus
Neurovascular: tibial nerve, posterior tibial artery and vein
Superficial Posterior Compartment:
Muscular: gastrocnemius, plantaris, soleus
Neurovascular: sural nerve

47. Describe compartment syndrome and the common signs and symptoms.

Compartment syndrome can be exertional (gradual onset with exercise/activity) or from acute trauma and occurs when compartmental pressures become elevated resulting in insufficient oxygenated blood supply to muscles and nerves. About three quarters of the time, acute compartment syndrome is caused by acute trauma such as a leg fracture or trauma to the soft tissue. Chronic or exertional compartment syndrome may be caused by regular, vigorous exercise.

Common signs and symptoms of exertional compartment syndrome include the "6 P's": pain, pallor (pale skin color), paresthesia (numbness), pulselessness, paralysis (muscular weakness), and poikilothermia (local tissue temperature change). Differential diagnosis of exertional compartment syndrome of the leg includes "shin splints" or medial tibial stress syndrome and stress fracture.

48. What mechanisms are involved that result in injury to the syndesmosis or a "high ankle" sprain?

While several mechanisms of syndesmosis injury have been reported, the two most common are external rotation of the planted foot with accompanied internal rotation of the leg and hyper-dorsiflexion of the ankle. When the foot is forced into external rotation and the leg is internally rotated with ankle dorsiflexed, calcaneal eversion at the subtalar joint may force the talus against the distal fibula, creating a widening stress at the tibiofibular mortise. The structures injured often involve the anterior inferior and posterior inferior tibiofibular ligaments along with the inferior interosseus ligament and the inferior transverse tibiofibular ligament. In some cases, injury to the proximal fibula can occur including the presence of a Maisonneuve fracture. Evaluation of severe ankle injuries warrants close evaluation of the distal syndesmotic complex and entire fibula as these injuries often require modifications in rehabilitation and a prolonged recovery.

49. What is a Maisonneuve injury?

A Maisonneuve is characterized by fractures of the proximal fibula and rupture of the anterior inferior tibiofibular ligament along with the deltoid ligament. The mechanism of injury involves a pronation-external rotation. This is considered an unstable injury and requires surgical intervention.

Bibliography

Brosky, T., Nyland, J., Nitz, A., & Caborn, D. N. (1995). The ankle ligaments: consideration of syndesmotic injury and implications for rehabilitation. *Journal of Orthopaedic & Sports Physical Therapy, 21*(4), 197–205.

Davitt, J. S., Kadel, N., Sangeorzan, B. J., Hansen, S. T., Jr., Holt, S. K., & Donaldson-Fletcher, E. (2005). An association between functional second metacarpal length and midfoot arthrosis. *Journal of Bone and Joint Surgery (American), 87*, 795–800.

Epomedicine. (2020). 6 Ps and 3 As of Compartment Syndrome [Internet]. https://epomedicine.com/medical-students/compartment-syndrome-mnemonic/.

He, J. Q., Ma, X. L., Xin, J. Y., et al. (2020). Pathoanatomy and injury mechanism of typical Maisonneuve fracture. *Orthopaedic Surgery, 12*(6), 1644–1651.

Kapandji, I. A. (1987). *The physiology of the joints* (Vol. 2). New York. NY: Churchill Livingstone.

Kumai, T., Takakura, Y., Rufai, A., Milz, S., & Benjamin, M. (2002). The functional anatomy of the human anterior talofibular ligament in relation to ankle sprains. *Journal of Anatomy, 200*, 457–465.

Magee, D. J. (Ed.), (2014). *Orthopedic physical assessment* (6th ed.). Philadelphia PA: Elsevier Science.

Mizel, M. S., Miller, R. A., & Scioli, M. W. (Eds.), (1998). *Orthopaedic knowledge update—foot and ankle II.* Rosemont. IL: American Academy of Orthopedic Surgeons.

Neumann, D. A. (2017). *Kinesiology of the musculoskeletal system: foundations for rehabilitation* (3rd ed.). St. Louis, MO: Elsevier Inc. ISBN.

Nordin, M., & Frankel, V. H. (Eds.). (1989). *Basic biomechanics of the musculoskeletal system.* Philadelphia. PA: Lea & Febiger.

Rajasekaran, S., & Hall, M. M. (2016). Nonoperative management of chronic exertional compartment syndrome: a systematic review. *Current Sports Medicine Reports, 15*(3), 191–198.

Rockwood, C. A. Greenwood, D.P., Bucholz, R.W., & Heckman, J.D. (Eds.). (1996). *Fractures in adults.* Philadelphia. PA: Lippincott-Raven.

Thompson, J. C. (2002). *Netter's concise atlas of orthopaedic anatomy.* Teterboro, NJ: Icon Learning Systems.

Snowden, J., Becker, J. A., Brosky, J. A., & Hazle, C. (2014). Chronic leg pain in a division ii field hockey player: a case report. *International Journal of Sports Physical Therapy, 9*(1), 125–134.

CHAPTER 76 QUESTIONS

1. **A construction worker slipped and turned his ankle while stepping off a ladder. They reported "feeling and hearing a pop" on the side (lateral) of their ankle. Swelling increased gradually over the next few hours and while the ankle was very painful, they were able to walk with a significant limp. Examination the next day reveals tenderness over the soft tissues in the sinus tarsi and some visible ecchymosis (bruising). An anterior drawer test and talar tilt is determined to be negative (no laxity). Based on mechanism and history what is the likely diagnosis?**
   a. Deltoid ligament sprain
   b. Distal fibular fracture
   c. Compartment syndrome
   d. Anterior talofibular ligament sprain

2. **A distance runner notes some pain in the anterior and lateral aspect of the leg that seems to be consistently getting worse over the past several weeks. The runner notes she has been increasing her hill running recently. The pain is described as nonspecific but is associated with tightness and cramping that gets worse after about 10 to 15 minutes of running but reportedly improves after a few hours of rest. What should be considered in the differential diagnosis as the possible condition?**
   a. Medial tibial stress syndrome ("shin splints")
   b. Stress fracture
   c. Exertional compartment syndrome
   d. All of the above

3. **Which of the following ankle ligaments of the lateral complex is most likely to be injured with an inversion mechanism with the foot in a plantar-flexed position?**
   a. Anterior talofibular ligament
   b. Posterior talofibular ligament
   c. Calcaneofibular ligament
   d. Anterior inferior tibiofibular ligament

4. **Which of the following ligaments supports both the medial longitudinal arch and the plantar aspect of the talonavicular joint?**
   a. Long plantar ligament
   b. Short plantar ligament
   c. Bifurcate ligament
   d. Calcaneonavicular ligament

5. **A rigid flatfoot is often an indication of which of the following underlying pathologies?**
   a. Tarsal coalition
   b. Lisfranc sprain
   c. Charcot-Marie-Tooth
   d. Os trigonum

COMMON ORTHOPAEDIC FOOT AND ANKLE DYSFUNCTIONS

S. Mais, BS, BA, MS, DPT

CHAPTER 77

1. **What is the difference between Achilles tendonitis, tendinosis, and tendinopathy?**

Tendinopathy is a general term that describes tendon degeneration characterized by a combination of pain, swelling, and impaired performance. Tendinosis is described as a localized intrinsic degeneration of unknown etiology, characterized by localized swollen tendon nodes. Several studies have shown that tendon biopsies taken at surgery lack inflammatory cells. While true tendonitis is rare, it can exist due to acute overuse activities or related to a specific disease process, such as rheumatic diseases. The signs of tendonitis are pain on palpation, swelling, warmth, and pain on active contraction of the muscle-tendon complex. Passive stretching may also induce pain. The clinical practice guidelines of the American Physical Therapy Association (APTA) in 2018 have established that tendonitis or tendinosis is misleading and should be replaced with "tendinopathy," unless histologic evidence has proven otherwise.

In Achilles tendinopathy the patient may report mild pain and stiffness with his or her desired level of activity, and it may progress to limiting activity considerably. There may be an appearance of thickening of the tendon, but this is not swelling related to the inflammation. MRI findings may show signal changes inside the tendon.

2. **What is the pathophysiology causing Achilles tendinopathy?**

In 2009 Cook and Purdam proposed a continuum model for staging tendinopathy based on the changes and distribution of disorganization within the tendon. However, classifying tendinopathy based on structure in what is primarily a pain condition has been challenged. Cook and Purdam in 2016 revisited the model to explain the relationship between structure, pain, and function. Their model describes structural changes in the tendon from a ***reactive tendon*** to ***tendon disrepair***, which can progress to a ***degenerative tendon***. A *reactive tendon* is a patient who has acute overload and the tendon responds by increasing the cells and matrix. This patient will need unloading and settling down. They are usually younger and athletic with no history of a swollen tendon.

If the tendon continues to be overloaded the tendon can go into a phase of *disrepair* that is characterized by collagen disorganization and the phenomenon of neovascularization—the attempt of the tendon to heal by bringing blood vessels to the damaged areas. It is speculated that nerve fibers, which accompany these new blood vessels, are the source of long-term pain experienced in these patients. If the tendon is not allowed to heal then the progression of the continuum will lead to an irreversible cell death or *degeneration* of the tendon. Their updated model includes the new phase of *reactive on degenerative* tendon that illustrates that not all of the tendons will be in the same phase of the continuum. Rehab can still target the unaffected part of the tendon that can respond favorably to load, so all is not lost. These patients with a degenerative pathology will often be older with a history of tendon pain and they will do better with starting with a loading program. It is clinically most important to look at symptoms and irritability when assessing and planning a rehabilitation program. This refers to clinical cases where the structurally normal portion of the tendon may drift in and out of a reactive response.

3. **What is the difference between midsubstance tendinopathy and insertional tendinopathy, and what are the treatment implications?**

Midsubstance tendinopathy occurs 4 to 6 cm proximal to the achilles insertion. Distal tendinopathy or insertional tendinopathy is located where the tendon inserts into the calcaneous, and often calcification is found in the tendon. Treatment for insertional tendinopathy has included modification of shoe wear, heel lifts, orthosis, antiinflammatory medication, rest, night splints, and trial of iontophoresis and ice. Frequently, rigid heel lifts of ½ inch either in shoes or attached to the outer sole and clinically have been observed to reduce symptoms.

It is suggested that stretching the achilles with gastroc and soleus stretches should be **AVOIDED**. A recent randomized controlled study confirmed that the addition of eccentric training for patients with insertional pain did not lead to further improvements. Haglund's "triad," which occurs at the site of the calcaneous and includes Haglund's deformity (pump bump) retrocalcaneal bursitis with insertional tendonitis should be considered and unloading that area with a modification of the heel counter and activity reduction is indicated.

4. **What is the best way to diagnose midportion Achilles tendinopathy?**

Pain and stiffness are gold standard subjective reports. Tenderness to palpation of the midportion of the Achilles tendon are the gold standard objective signs.

A patient will often have pain and weakness with the heel rise test, and for higher level or less irritable patients, a single leg hop test like in jumping rope would be indicated. The goal with recovery would be 10 single leg hops without pain. The VISA-A questionnaire is a valid and reliable tool to evaluate the clinical severity of Achilles tendinopathy.

5. **What other findings should be assessed with Achilles tendon pain?**

Dorsiflexion range of motion, subtalar joint range of motion, plantar flexion strength and endurance, static arch height, and forefoot alignment should also be assessed.

There may be an appearance of thickening of the tendon, but this is not swelling related to the inflammation. Most patients will report a failure of NSAIDs to provide relief. While the literature agrees that clinical signs and symptoms are adequate to diagnose tendinopathy, MRI findings may show signal changes inside the tendon. In addition, high-resolution ultrasound is more commonly used and identifies this pathology more clearly. The tendon may have hyperechoic areas, indicating disorganization of the collagen fibers. While imaging may be helpful in some cases, there is a limitation with imaging, because if you image someone without pain degeneration is frequently present.

6. **What are the risk factors for developing Achilles tendinopathy and what are factors affecting recovery?**

Achilles tendinopathy is an injury that frequently occurs in athletes performing sport activities that include running or jumping, but has also been demonstrated in physically inactive individuals.

Intrinsic risk factors associated with Achilles tendinopathy include abnormal ankle dorsiflexion range of motion, abnormal subtalar joint range of motion, decreased ankle plantar flexion strength, increased foot pronation, and abnormal tendon structure. Obesity, hypertension, hyperlipidemia, and diabetes are intrinsic factors associated with Achilles tendinopathy. Clinicians also should consider training errors, environmental factors, and faulty equipment as extrinsic risk factors associated with Achilles tendinopathy.

There are many adverse factors affecting the recovery of the tendon. These include predisposing factors of genetic and reduced physiological blood supply in specific areas. There are also both extrinsic (heavy sport activities, environmental conditions, training errors in athletes) and intrinsic (age, osteoarticular pathologies, and systemic factors affecting microcirculation or collagen metabolism. This explains why subjects respond differently to overloading, and the threshold for repair may vary largely from one subject to another.

7. **What is the best program for midsubstance Achilles tendinopathy?**

While much of the earlier research focused on eccentric training based on the work of Alfredson et al., current studies are strongly showing successful outcomes with heavier loading with either eccentric or both eccentric and concentric protocols. The key is that there is heavy tension and it is increased over a long period of time. Given the low metabolic rate of tendons, the optimal conditions for good healing are adequate recovery time; absence of excessive overloading; and good metabolism and blood supply. When these conditions are not met, the healing mechanisms fail.

In developing the exercise program, you want to load the tendon based on their activity. For example, for the running athlete we want to include repetitive fatiguing exercises. For the jumping athlete, we want to include plyometrics.

To supplement strengthening, manual therapy to increase ankle and subtalar range of motion (ROM) is indicated. Taping techniques either to offload the tendon or to limit ankle ROM and/or taping the arch have all been clinically beneficial. It is also the responsibility of the physical therapist to assess the function of the entire lower extremity to identify whether there are other impairment findings in the lower extremity (hip/knee weakness; flexibility issues) that may have contributed to the cause of the tendon dysfunction.

8. **What is a sample exercise protocol for effective Achilles tendon loading?**

Silbernagel and Crossley (2015) have consistently affirmed the effectiveness of a heavy-loading protocol with patients who could perform 10 heel rise but have pain.

The exercises consist mainly of 2-legged, 1-legged, eccentric, and fast-rebounding heel raises. The intensity is increased successively by increasing the range of motion (starting standing on the floor and then performing the exercise standing on stairs), increasing the number of repetitions (starting at three sets of maximum amount tolerated, up to 15 repetitions maximum per set), and increasing the load (with use of either a backpack or weight machine and by increasing the speed of loading).

Phase 1: Weeks 1 to 2

Patient status: Pain and difficulty with all activities, difficulty performing ten 1-legged heel raises.

Goal: Start to exercise, gain understanding of their injury and of pain-monitoring model.

Treatment program: Perform exercises every day,

Pain-monitoring model information and advice on exercise activity,

Circulation exercises (moving foot up/down), 2-legged toe raises standing on the floor (3 sets × 10–15 repetitions/set), 1-legged toe raises standing on the floor (3 × 10), Sitting toe raises (3 × 10), Eccentric toe raises standing on the floor (3 × 10)

Phase 2: Weeks 2 to 5

Patient status: Pain with exercise, morning stiffness, pain when performing toe raises,

Goal: Start strengthening.

Treatment program: Perform exercises every day, 2-legged toe raises standing on edge of stair (3 × 15), 1-legged toe raises standing on edge of stair (3 × 15), Sitting toe raises (3 × 15), Eccentric toe raises standing on edge of stair (3 × 15), Quick-rebounding toe raises (3 × 20)

Phase 3: Weeks 3 to 12 (longer if needed)

Patient status: Handled the phase 2 exercise program, no pain distally in tendon insertion, possibly decreased or increased morning stiffness.

Goal: Heavier strength training, increase or start running and/or jumping activity.

Treatment program: Perform exercises every day and with heavier load 2 to 3 times/week, 1-legged toe raises standing on edge of stair with added weight (3 × 15), Sitting toe raises (3 × 15), Eccentric toe raises standing on edge of stair with added weight (3 × 15), Quick-rebounding toe raises (3 × 20), Plyometric training

Phase 4: Week 12 to 6 months (longer if needed)

Patient status: Minimal symptoms, morning stiffness not every day, can participate in sports without difficulty.

Goal: Maintenance exercise, no symptoms.

Treatment program: Perform exercises 2 to 3 times/week, 1-legged toe raises standing on edge of stair with added weight (3 × 15), Eccentric toe raises standing on edge of stair with added weight (3 × 15), Quick-rebounding toe raises (3 × 20)

For heavy load activity researchers recommend 3× a week with rest days in between to allow building up their tolerance. The program could be adjusted every 3 weeks accordingly. The patient must understand that tendons "heal" very slowly, and this process will take time.

9. What is the advantage of eccentric training and what is a typical eccentric protocol for Achilles tendinopathy?

Eccentric training appears to be more effective at increasing muscle mass than concentric training. The superiority of eccentric training to produce adaptations in strength and muscle mass is possibly mediated by the higher forces developed during this type of exercise. So, a patient may not be able to perform a heel rise without significant pain, but they could perform a heel lowering exercise successfully.

It is also theorized that the eccentric exercise helps to stop blood flow when the ankle joint is in dorsi flexion, which may act with a mechanism similar to sclerosing therapy, that is, through reducing neoangiogenesis. Maffulli and colleagues, however, claim that tendons respond to mechanical forces by adapting both their metabolism and by altering gene expression, so that eccentric training could work both metabolically and mechanically (Maffulli and Longo 2008).

The typical heel drop exercise is done with the patient standing on a block or a step. The patient is instructed to go up as high as he or she can on both feet and then come down slowly on the affected side, only to drop the heel below the step.

This original protocol developed by Dr. Alfredson et al. (1998) recommends the completion of three sets of 15, twice a day for 12 weeks, with the leg both flexed and extended (a total of 180 daily heel drops). Pain is actually expected with the exercise and should be expected after exercise. Progression of the exercise should be when the exercise is pain free and increased repetitions or a load can be added. Recently, Stevens and Tan (2014) reported that a "6-week, as tolerated" program of eccentric exercise was as effective and less uncomfortable than the Alfredson protocol for midportion Achilles tendinopathy. Patients are asked to perform as many heel drops as they could tolerate. This program may be appropriate for patients who have trouble executing the full Alfredson protocol.

10. How do you know if you have pushed the patient too hard or not hard enough?

Make sure that the 24-hour behavior of the tendon is not be worse, ideally not greater than 3/10. If the tendon is not irritable the next day, then increase the load.

Load that is slow and heavy will be good, but for the athlete or runner you also will need quick load on the tendon, like plyometrics with jumping and even skipping or stair running. Make sure to quantify load and only change one thing at a time.

Initially, for the very irritable patient, isometrics will be beneficial. It can take up to a year for recovery, and there is much variability, so it is necessary to educate the patients appropriately.

11. Is it necessary for Achilles tendon patients who are athletes to rest from their sport initially before starting the heavy loading protocol?

The research shows it is not necessary for athletes to rest from their sport or activity. Silbernagel and colleagues in 2007 compared similar groups, one who rested from their sports for 6 weeks and then started high-load training and the other group who did not rest from their activity. This randomized study could not demonstrate any negative effects from allowing the patients to continue Achilles tendon–loading activity (such as running and jumping) when using the pain-monitoring system.

The underlying effects of exercise are not fully known, but mechanical loading on tendons appears to be important in both the healing process and in improving strength of the tendons. In several studies, Malliaras et al. (2013) have shown that exercise activity on tendons in healthy individuals produces an acute increase in the tendon collagen synthesis and they have also shown convincingly that immobilization causes negative effects on tendons. It is wise to tell the patient that if they have gone a year without symptoms then they are fully recovered.

12. What is an acceptable pain level during rehabilitation?

Pain is very common during mechanical loading exercises of the tendon and research has shown you need to load the tendon or it won't heal and that it is typically painful. The pain monitoring model introduced by Silbernagel

(2007) has shown to be effective in many studies. The **acceptable pain level during rehabilitation** has shown a level of 4–5 during exercises and 3–4 during activity or sport. This is based on the visual analog scale (VAS), where 0 is no pain and 10 is the worst pain imaginable. However, it is most important for the patient to document how much pain or discomfort they have 24 hours later and to monitor exercises based on this response.

13. **What about adjunct treatment for tendinopathy?**
According to Hay et al. (1999) and Rompe et al. (2008), nonsteroidal antiinflammatory drugs and steroids may be beneficial for pain and function in the early phases of disease but are usually ineffective later. Boesen et al. (2017) used a randomized controlled trial that showed that treatment with either a combination of steroid, saline, and local anesthetic or PRP in combination with eccentric training in chronic AT was more effective in reducing pain, improving activity level, and reducing tendon thickness and intratendinous vascularity than eccentric training alone. They also conclude that the combination high volume injection may be more effective in improving outcomes of chronic AT than PRP in the short term. In advanced cases with an average length of pain for 33 months, treatment using sclerosing injections into the tendon targeting the area with neovascularization of the Achilles tendon led to significantly reduced pain during tendon-loading activity. Clinical improvement corresponded with elimination of the color doppler appearance of neovascularization (destroyed new vessels and nerves).

14. **Is Achilles tendinopathy a precursor to rupture?**
While it can occur, the most common scenario is that patients do NOT have achilles tendinopathy prior to rupture. It appears that people who have had ruptures have not commonly had achilles tendon pain.

15. **What is the differential diagnosis for those with heel and posterior lower leg pain who don't have Achilles tendinopathy?**
- Acute Achilles tendon rupture
- Partial tear of the Achilles tendon
- Retrocalcaneal bursitis
- Haglund's deformity—a protuberance of bone originating on the calcaneus at the tendocalcaneal junction that can cause friction between the Achilles tendon and the shoe
- Posterior ankle impingement by osseous abnormalities including os trigonum syndrome
- Irritation or neuroma of the sural nerve
- Accessory soleus muscle
- Achilles tendon ossification
- Systemic inflammatory disease
- Insertional Achilles tendinopathy
- S1 radiculopathy

16. **What are the common rupture sites of the Achilles tendon complex?**
The most common site is a complete midsubstance rupture of the Achilles tendon. This area is 2 to 6 cm proximal to the insertion site and is most susceptible to injury because it is hypovascular. The second most common site is the proximal musculotendinous interface, followed by the rare avulsion of the tendon from the bone. An incomplete rupture of the Achilles tendon also can evolve from chronic tendinosis in the midsubstance area.

17. **Describe the typical patient with Achilles tendon rupture.**
The typical patient is male between 30 and 50 years of age who engages in a physical activity or sport. Predisposing factors include advanced age, weekend athletes, history of tendonitis or tendinosis, and loss of flexibility in the Achilles tendon.

18. **How is an Achilles tendon rupture diagnosed?**
According to the American Academy of Orthopedic Surgeons, the following tests are recommended to arrive at the diagnosis of Achilles tendon rupture:
- Thompson's test—The patient is positioned prone with the foot hanging off the table. The examiner squeezes the widest girth of the calf and observes for plantar flexion to occur. If no plantar flexion occurs, the test is positive for rupture.
- Decreased plantar flexion strength—The patient will most likely be unable to perform a heel rise while standing.
- Presence of palpable gap, defect, or lack of contour of the achilles tendon.
- Increased passive ankle dorsiflexion.

The evidence surrounding the use of MRI, ultrasound, and radiographs in the diagnosis of achilles tendon rupture is inconclusive.

19. **Is operative treatment necessary for acute Achilles tendon ruptures?**
Although surgical repair is more common, it is not necessary. Controversy continues with regard to the optimal treatment for acute Achilles tendon ruptures (ATR). In a meta-analysis of randomized controlled trials, Khan et al.

(2005) reported that surgical treatment decreases the risk for re-rupture more than nonsurgical treatment (re-rupture rate: 3.5% vs 12.6%, respectively). However, the majority of the patients treated for ATRs never sustain a re-rupture, and it appears to be the surgeon's preference combined with the surgical risk for infections that directs the choice for surgery or nonoperative management.

Surgery can be classified into operative (open or minimally invasive/percutaneous) and nonoperative. Postoperative support can be divided into cast immobilization and functional bracing. Weight-bearing status also varies, depending on the surgeon.

Primary repair seems to be the "gold standard" of care; however, surgically repaired tendons rarely recover functionality similar to the previous state. Most patients with an Achilles tendon rupture seldom achieve full function 2 years after surgery; moreover, results after the first year are quite variable. Poor results have been attributed to overstretching the tendon or alterations in the cellular organization within the tendon that occur at the time of injury and during early healing stages. In the future, tissue engineering, such as human growth hormones, may lead to improved management of these injuries.

20. What is a recommended nonoperative and operative rehabilitation protocol after achilles tendon rupture?

There is no clear consensus regarding the optimal rehabilitation protocol for this injury. Traditionally, patients have been placed in a cast with the ankle in plantar flexion for the first 6 to 8 weeks nonweight bearing. However, more recent literature advocates for accelerated early range of motion exercises and weight-bearing protocol for both operative and nonoperative management. Additionally, outcomes appear very similar for these two groups.

- 0–2 weeks: NWB in plantar-flexion-posterior splint
- 2–4 weeks: CAM boot with 2-inch heel lift, PWB with crutches, and active ROM (plantar and dorsiflexion) to neutral
- 4–6 weeks: WBAT in CAM boot; continue active ROM to neutral
- 6–8 weeks: remove heel lift; dorsiflexion stretching, hydrotherapy, and graduated resistance exercises
- 8–12 weeks: wean off boot, continue active ROM, strength, proprioception, and prn crutches
- 12 weeks: sport-specific training

This accelerated protocol focuses on early movement of the ankle between neutral and plantar flexion and while in a brace for 6 weeks. Prospective studies and randomized controlled trials have shown that, compared with cast immobilization, the use of early postoperative ROM and weight bearing actually showed significant improvement in health-related quality of life in the early postoperative period, posed no additional risks, and demonstrated a trend toward a reduction in lost work days and an earlier return to sports.

21. What is the goal for functional outcome after Achilles tendon rupture with appropriate rehabilitation?

A systematic review of the literature performed by the American Academy of Orthopedic Surgeons (AAOS) in 2009 found that patients who participate in sports are able to return to jogging as early as 3 to 4 months, with the majority returning at 6 to 8 months. However, it must be noted that studies confirm continued calf weakness in both operative and nonoperative management. Khan et al. (2004) identified that the strength deficit of the calf musculature after an ATR was approximately 10% to 30% on the injured side compared with the uninjured side, and the deficit appears to be difficult to overcome. Gait abnormalities have also been found 24 months after injuries in patients with surgically treated ATRs. This could indicate that regardless of treatment, therapists and patients should understand the long-term sequelae of ATR and the susceptibility of compensations and future injuries in other areas of the kinetic chain.

22. What are the most important considerations with rehabilitation of the Achilles tendon rupture?

The goal is to prevent overlengthening of the Achilles tendon. Protection of the ankle is very important, and heel lifts can be used to reduce stress on the repair while the patient progresses in weight-bearing status. Early overstretching of the tendon with calf stretches can be detrimental to the length-tension relationship and have permanent consequences on recovery. Stretching of the Achilles tendon during the first 4 months after repair is not recommended.

23. Describe symptoms for tarsal tunnel syndrome.

Pain in the area of the tarsal tunnel or into the foot is the most commonly reported symptom. Some patients also may complain of paresthesia in the foot.

24. What factors may contribute to tarsal tunnel syndrome?

Mechanical factors (such as foot pronation) may cause compression of the tibial nerve and its branches in this location. Trauma to the lower leg—from fracture, sprain, or other soft tissue injury—may also lead to increased swelling. The abnormal swelling of the lower leg may cause compression on the nerve in this closed space. In addition, more proximal pathology may be associated with tarsal tunnel syndrome. A thorough review of systems is essential in identification of tarsal tunnel syndrome. Rheumatic disease may also cause swelling around the nerve or a peripheral neuropathy can present with similar symptoms; both should be ruled out. For example, patients with other nerve lesions, such as a lumbar spine pathology, may also have concomitant symptoms in the area of the tarsal tunnel. In closer proximity to the tarsal tunnel is the soleus hiatus, where the tibial nerve can be compressed because it is surrounded by a fibromuscular tunnel.

25. What is posterior tibialis tendon dysfunction (PTTD)?

PTTD is a progressive degeneration of the posterior tibial tendon and is the most common cause of painful and debilitating acquired flatfoot deformity in adults. The dysfunction is often progressive and may result in collapse of the plantar arch associated with tendon rupture. Many practitioners have currently labeled this sequela as adult-acquired flatfoot disorders (AAF) because not only is the posterior tendon involved, but many of the structures of the foot are affected. Before rupture, the tendon undergoes attenuation and degeneration, resulting in frequent episodes of debilitating pain.

26. What are the different stages of PTTD?

Johnson and Strom (1989) originally described the progressive clinical stages of posterior tibial tendon dysfunction. In stage I the patient has mild swelling and medial ankle pain but no deformity. There is mild weakness and the length of the tendon is normal; however, degeneration is present. A patient may be able to perform a single heel rise, but this movement is painful. Stage II is progressive flattening of the arch, with an abducted midfoot. In this stage the tendon is ruptured or functionally incompetent. The foot is still flexible and correctable, but the patient is unable to perform a single heel rise because the tendon is functionally incompetent. In stage III all of the signs of stage II occur; however, the hindfoot deformity becomes fixed. Myerson (1989) added stage IV for those patients who progressed to valgus tilt of the talus in the ankle mortise, leading to lateral tibiotalar degeneration.

Stages I and II are most amenable to conservative treatment, while III and IV often require surgery.

27. What causes PTTD?

Patients with excessive pronation are likely predisposed to the condition because pronation changes the alignment of the foot and, over time, can lead to adult-acquired flatfoot deformity. When the foot is excessively pronated, the balance between the tibialis posterior tendon and the fibularis longus is lost. The pronated foot then changes the alignment of the gastroc/soleus tendon relative to the axis of rotation, and then, instead of being an invertor of the foot, the Achilles tendon is lateral to the axis and pulls the foot into further eversion. Overload of the posterior tibial tendon then occurs, causing the other supporting structures of the foot, such as the spring ligament, and plantar aponeurosis to take over and the deformity progresses. Another predisposition is a critical area of hypovascularity in the tendon posterior and distal to the medial malleolus. In addition, medical factors linked with PTTD include hypertension, obesity, diabetes, steroid exposure, and inflammatory arthritides.

28. What should be considered when evaluating PTTD?

- Observation—arch height and foot posture including the "too many toes sign" (as seen from behind, the toes are seen laterally indicating abduction of the forefoot).
- Location of symptoms—medial ankle pain and swelling behind the medial malleolus is the hallmark. However, in very later stages, patients may have pain laterally because of impingement of the fibula or lateral talar process by the anterior process of the calcaneus.
- Palpation—tenderness in the same area as well as more proximally in the muscle and possible pain in other arch-supporting structures of the foot, such as the plantar fascia, because of overload of these tissues.
- Ability to perform a pain-free heel rise—the calcaneus should be in an inverted position with full range of motion. This should be compared to the uninvolved side first. Common compensations of knee flexion or pushing with the upper extremities should be observed. Repeated heel rise for endurance should also be tested.
- Manual muscle test of the tibialis posterior in plantarflexion with inversion.
- ROM and mobility of the ankle, subtalar, and first MTP as well as lower extremity strength and endurance, especially the gluteal muscles.

29. What is the best evidence-based treatment for PTTD?

Initially, immobilization and rest of the tendon are necessary to prevent excessive pronation and to decrease demand on the posterior tibialis. Techniques include taping to support the arch, custom-made foot orthotics, a custom-made ankle-foot orthosis, or even complete immobilization with a cast or walking boot. The Richie Brace®, an AFO with a custom-contoured footplate, is a lightweight, low-profile design that is suited to control the abnormal pronation forces and is recommended for support and comfort. Calf stretching with both the knee straight and flexed should be implemented. After immobilization, progressive strengthening in the pain-free range of the posterior tibialis as well as strengthening of the foot intrinsics is beneficial. For patients with stage I and II PTTD, strengthening both eccentrically and concentrically has proven to be effective without harmful effects.

Kulig and colleagues (2004) have clearly demonstrated that the best exercise to selectively and effectively train the tibialis posterior is resisted foot adduction with the foot in contact with the floor, in a windshield-wiper type of motion. The use of an arch support or orthoses during this exercise will recruit the tibialis posterior more effectively. In addition, studies have confirmed that women with PTTD have impaired ability to perform single-leg stance and diminished hip strength and endurance bilaterally, so strengthening weak proximal muscles would be indicated.

30. **What causes peroneal tendon subluxation?**
Both the longus and brevis tendons are at risk for subluxation or dislocation from the fibular retromalleolar sulcus. The most frequent cause is a skiing injury, but subluxation has been reported in several other sports (eg, soccer, football, basketball, tennis, and gymnastics). The most commonly described mechanism is sudden, forceful passive dorsiflexion of the everted foot with sudden, strong reflex contraction of the peroneal muscles. The injury also has been described with forced inversion, which also causes sudden contraction of the peroneals.

31. **How is peroneal tendon subluxation diagnosed?**
An acute subluxating peroneal tendon frequently is misdiagnosed as an ankle sprain. The patient usually describes a traumatic injury with lateral swelling and ecchymosis, which often are associated with popping or snapping sounds. Often patients with a subacute condition also have sprained the lateral collateral ligaments. Most patients complain of pain behind the fibula and above the joint line, which differentiates it from the pain of a lateral ankle sprain. The patient's presenting symptoms usually include swelling and tenderness posterior to the lateral malleolus. Provocative tests should be done but may not be helpful in the acute setting. Dislocation of the peroneal tendon is evident during a stress test of inversion. Testing is done by resisting eversion with a dorsiflexed ankle.

32. **Summarize the differential diagnosis for plantar heel pain.**
Plantar heel pain is one of the most common musculoskeletal disorders of the foot and ankle.
- Inflammation or microtrauma of the plantar fascia
- Entrapment neuropathy of the tibial nerve or branches
- Fat pad atrophy
- Heel spur
- Stress fracture
- Tarsal tunnel syndrome
- Systemic problems (Reiter syndrome, rheumatoid arthritis, and gout; more common bilaterally)
- Radiculopathy of S1

33. **What is plantar fasciitis?**
Although the term "fasciitis" denotes inflammation, like Achilles tendon problems, cells associated with inflammation are typically not present. Plantar fasciitis is one of the most common foot-related disorders seen in the outpatient setting. The most common location of pain is at the origin of the plantar fascia at the medial plantar tubercle of the calcaneus. Pain at the midportion of the plantar fascia can occur but is less common.

34. **Besides the plantar fascia, what other structures can be involved with this syndrome?**
Pain may arise from one or more of the following structures: subcalcaneal bursa, fat pad, tendinous insertion of the intrinsic muscles, long plantar ligament, medial calcaneal branch of the tibial nerve, or nerve to abductor digiti minimi. True plantar fasciitis is characterized by progressive pain with weight bearing as well as pain with the first few steps upon rising from a sitting position.

35. **What are the risk factors associated with plantar fasciitis?**
According to the APTA guidelines, the multifactorial risks include limited ankle dorsiflexion and a high body mass index in nonathletic populations. Running and work-related weight-bearing activities that occur under conditions of poor shock absorption are also risk factors. However, clinically many patients are not overweight and there appear to be other structural alignment issues in the foot and up the chain that could contribute to excessive stress on the plantar fascia.

36. **What tests and measures are useful in the diagnosis of plantar fasciitis?**
According to the updated 2014 guidelines published by the orthopaedic section of the APTA, the following test and measures are recommended to diagnose plantar fasciitis:
- Palpation of proximal plantar fascia insertion
- Active and passive talocrural dorsiflexion
- Tarsal tunnel test
- Windlass mechanism
- Longitudinal arch angle
- Foot posture index

37. What is the best evidence-based treatment for plantar heel pain?

According to the APTA Clinical Practice Guidelines for Heel Pain, the following clinical practices are recommended based on the strength of the evidence:

- Manual therapy—talocrural joint posterior glides, subtalar joint lateral glide, anterior and posterior glides of the tarsometatarsal joint distraction manipulation; Level A evidence
- Night splints—use of a night splint for 1 to 3 months; Level A evidence
- Foot orthosis—orthosis with medial longitudinal arch and heel cushion; Level A evidence
- Taping—antipronation taping of the foot and kinesio taping of the gastroc/soleus and plantar fascia; Level A evidence
- Stretching—plantar fascia specific stretching and gastroc/soleus stretching; Level A evidence

Modalities such as ultrasound, phonophoresis, low-level laser, and iontophoresis have limited evidence to support their use; Level C evidence.

38. What is the best way to tape for plantar fasciitis?

Like foot orthoses, it is thought that supportive tape reduces the symptoms of plantar heel pain by reducing strain in the plantar fascia during loading. Low-Dye taping has shown to be effective for the short-term treatment of the common symptom of "first-step" pain in patients with plantar heel pain and has shown to decrease the pain to allow increased weight bearing. It can be used as an inexpensive short-term treatment for plantar heel pain while patients wait for foot orthoses. In our clinical experience the Johnson and Johnson Zonas™ is the best tape for the modified Low Dye. Step 1: Four strips of 1½ in tape are placed horizontally along the plantar aspect of the foot under the arch from the metatarsal heads to the proximal calcaneus. Step 2: Three strips of 1 in tape are anchored, one on top of each other, from the lateral heel and wrapped obliquely across the plantar foot brand ending under the plantar aspect of the base of the fifth metatarsal. Step 3: Step 1 is repeated. Step 4: Two 1½ inch anchors, approximately 3 inches in length, are placed on the lateral and medial aspects of the foot to secure all of the tape.

39. What nerves are involved with plantar heel pain?

There is a clear distinction between entrapment of the medial calcaneal nerve and the first branch of the lateral plantar nerve (ie, the nerve to the abductor digiti quini brevis). The medial calcaneal nerve innervates the skin under the heel and may innervate the subcalcaneal bursa. In most cases, this nerve plays no role in plantar heel pain. More likely, the heel pain is from irritation of the first branch of the lateral plantar nerve (known as Baxter's nerve) or the inferior calcaneal nerve. It innervates the plantar fascia at its origin on the calcaneus, and it also innervates the periosteum of the calcaneus. It often becomes entrapped during chronic plantar fasciitis. With this pathology, patients will deny first-step pain but, on the contrary, they will complain of symptoms worsening with prolonged activity. They may complain of laterally radiating pain or paresthesia and may be unable to abduct the fifth digit. Traditional treatment for plantar heel pain, as described, would be helpful as well as neural mobilization.

40. How can adverse neurodynamics cause plantar heel pain, and why do patients feel better with neural mobilization?

Chronic irritation may cause reduced microcirculation, decreased axonal transport, and altered mechanics, resulting in a painful cycle. In addition, the nerve is a continuum with multiple sites of potential compression that may result in a double-crush phenomenon, exacerbating the pain. It is hypothesized that sliding between the neural tissue and interface tissue can decrease adhesions and promote healing. Neural tissue can shorten and lengthen and has considerable remodeling capabilities. Restoring normal neural mobility appears to be important in abolishing symptoms.

41. Describe the common cause and usual management of heel pain in children.

Calcaneal apophysitis of the os calcis (Sever's disease) is related to activity. The child usually complains of pain with running or jumping as well as tenderness over the insertion of the Achilles tendon. The patient should be referred to a physician. Radiographs are useful for diagnosis when pain has been prolonged and recalcitrant. Treatment should include decreased activity guided by the child's symptoms, foot taping, or, in severe cases, immobilization with a brace. A heel lift or improved shoe wear also helps reduce the traction pull on the tendinous apophyseal attachment. The key is to restore heel cord flexibility.

42. What are some clinically useful outcome measures that can be used for patients with heel pain or plantar fasciitis?

- Foot and Ankle Measure (FAAM)
- Foot Health Status Questionnaire (FHSQ)
- Foot Function Index (FFI)

43. **What is the incidence and impact of an ankle sprain?**
Over 2 million ankle sprains are treated yearly in emergency departments in the United States and the United Kingdom. Ankle sprain is associated with significant socioeconomic cost in addition to the acute debilitating symptoms (which include pain, swelling, and impaired function).

Findings from the recent systematic review by Dohtery (2014) indicate that the three most common clinical classifications of ankle sprain are lateral ankle sprain followed by syndesmotic (high) ankle sprain and finally deltoid (medial) ligament sprain. Both computer simulation and cadaveric models have shown that plantarflexion and inversion increase strain on the lateral ligaments of the ankle, and the higher risk of sustaining a lateral ligament sprain can be attributed to relative lower load to failure rate of the lateral ligamentous complex when compared with the medial and syndesmotic ligament groups. There is also reduced arthrokinematic restriction of the talus within the ankle mortise in the plantar-flexed and inverted position.

The long-term prognosis of acute ankle sprain is poor, with a high proportion of patients (up to 70%) reporting persistent residual symptoms and injury recurrence.

44. **What other structures should be considered following ankle inversion sprain?**
- Subtalar joint ligament injury
- Osteochondral fracture of the talus
- Distal fibula fracture
- Avulsion fracture of the fifth metatarsal
- Jones fracture (metaphyseal-diaphyseal junction of the fifth metatarsal)
- Peroneal tendon injury
- High ankle sprain of the anteroinferior tibial fibular ligament
- Peroneal or sural nerve irritation
- Cuboid subluxation
- Achilles tendon injury
- Medial ligament injury
- Lisfranc fracture/dislocation

45. **What are the risk factors for acute lateral ankle sprain?**
Recommendation based on moderate evidence from the APTA Clinical Practice Guidelines, patients who are at risk for a lateral ankle sprain include the following:

(1) have a history of a previous ankle sprain, (2) do not use an external support, (3) do not properly warm up with static stretching and dynamic movement before activity, (4) do not have normal ankle dorsiflexion range of motion, and (5) do not participate in a balance/proprioceptive prevention program when there is a history of a previous injury.

46. **How do we diagnose and grade an acute lateral ankle sprain?**
Grade 1: no loss of function, no ligamentous laxity (ie, negative anterior drawer and talar tilt tests), little or no hemorrhaging, no point tenderness, decreased total ankle motion of 5 degrees or less, and swelling of 0.5 cm or less.

Grade 2: some loss of function, positive anterior drawer test (anterior talofibular ligament involvement), negative talar tilt test (no calcaneofibular ligament involvement), hemorrhaging, point tenderness, decreased total ankle motion greater than 5 degrees but less than 10 degrees, and swelling greater than 0.5 cm but less than 2.0 cm.

Grade 3: near total loss of function, positive anterior drawer and talar tilt tests, hemorrhaging, extreme point tenderness, decreased total ankle motion greater than 10 degrees, swelling greater than 2.0 cm. Grade III injuries have been further divided according to stress radiograph results, with anterior drawer movement of 3 mm or less being IIIA and greater than 3 mm of movement being IIIB. Grade 3 would be a complete rupture with significant instability that would involve other ligamentous structures in addition to the ATF.

47. **How do we know if the person sustained a simple ATFL sprain in isolation?**
Simple ATFL sprains encompass 65% of all sprains and the recovery should be straightforward. The patient should be improving with dorsiflexion and functional activities within 2 weeks. If the patient is not hitting these milestones, you should consider the possibility of other damaged structures with the most common being osteochondral defect, subtalar sprain, or syndesmosis involvement.

48. **When are radiographs warranted for ankle and foot injuries?**
The Ottawa ankle and foot rules are 100% sensitive and 40% specific in the identification of ankle and foot fractures.

Radiography of the ankle is indicated if any of the following is present on physical examination:
- Bone tenderness of the distal 6 cm of the posterior medial malleolus
- Bone tenderness of the distal 6 cm of the posterior lateral malleolus
- Inability to bear weight

Radiography of the foot is indicated if any of the following is present on physical examination:

- Tenderness at the base of the fifth metatarsal
- Tenderness over the navicular
- Inability to bear weight

49. **What impairments should we assess and treat following an ankle sprain?**
When evaluating a patient with an acute or subacute lateral ankle sprain over an episode of care, assessment of impairment of body function should include objective and reproducible measures of ankle swelling, ankle range of motion, talar translation and inversion, and single-leg balance.

Specifically, recent studies have shown the value of assessing and working on ankle plantarflexion range of motion after ankle sprain, which is often overlooked.

Postural control should be assessed with the Y balance or the Star Excursion tests at baseline and balance can be assessed accordingly. Strength assessment is also very important both in inversion and eversion strength. Inversion strength is also often overlooked because that's a position where the sprained ankle occurs but is important to assess and treat. Weakness after an acute sprain has also been identified in the gluteal muscles

A systematic review noted balance is not only impaired on the injured extremity but may also be impaired on the uninjured extremity after an acute lateral ankle sprain.

50. **What is the best evidence-based treatment for ankle sprains?**
In a recent systematic review with meta-analysis Doherty et al. in 2017 summarized that there is strong evidence for nonsteroidal antiinflammatory drugs and early mobilization and moderate evidence supporting exercise and manual therapy techniques for pain, swelling, and function. Exercise therapy and bracing are supported in the prevention of CAI.

51. **What outcome measures should clinicians incorporate after ankle sprain?**
Validated functional outcome measures, such as the Foot and Ankle Ability Measure and the Lower Extremity Functional Scale, should be a standard clinical examination. These should be utilized before and after interventions intended to alleviate the impairments of body function and structure, activity limitations, and participation restrictions associated with ankle sprain and instability. The Cumberland Ankle Instability Tool (The CAIT) is a 9-item scale measuring the severity of functional ankle instability. The total score ranges from 0 to 30. Items focus on the degree of difficulty in performing different physical activities per ankle.

52. **What are the guidelines for return to activities and sports after ankle sprains, and what is the best evidence to prevent recurrent sprains?**
It is important that they have full dorsiflexion. The Hop for distance, height and/or star excursion tests that match their sport of running, jumping, or cutting should be utilized.

Cumberland ankle instability tool is very helpful, and you want the scores above 26 or 27.

Although each patient should be treated individually, suggested criteria for return to sports after an ankle sprain include:

- Full range of active and passive motion at the ankle
- No limp with walking
- Strength equal to 90% of the uninvolved side
- Single-leg hop, high jump test, and 30-yard zig-zag test at least 90% of the uninvolved side
- Ability to reach maximal running and cutting speeds

Coordination/balance training and bracing have been proven to help reduce the severity of future ankle sprains. It is also necessary to strengthen all muscles of the lower extremity. For example, if the hip abductors are weak, one may compensate with lateral trunk flexion, which causes the center of mass to deviate laterally, potentially creating an inversion force to the ankle and hindfoot.

53. **What is chronic ankle instability (CAI)?**
Chronic ankle instability (CAI) is the encompassing term used to describe the chronic symptoms that may develop following an acute ankle sprain, with injury recurrence at the hallmark of the chronic condition. The residual symptoms of CAI are "giving way" and feelings of ankle joint instability and should be present for a minimum of 1 year after initial sprain.

It has been demonstrated that CAI negatively alters central mechanisms of motor control, leading to an increased risk of falls, and has been confirmed that CAI is a leading cause of posttraumatic ankle joint osteoarthritis. The incidence of residual symptoms following acute ankle sprain is variable but has been reported with rates of between 40% and 50%.

54. **What impairments may cause chronic pain after an ankle sprain?**
    - Tension neuropathy of the superficial peroneal nerve—Inversion sprains may stretch the superficial peroneal nerve and lead to chronic pain localized to the dorsum of the foot. Compression is found most often at the site

where the nerve exits the deep fascia of the anterior compartment of the leg. Pain most often is localized to the anterolateral ankle and radiates to the anterior foot. It can be reproduced by plantar flexion and reduced by dorsiflexion. Careful physical examination and local nerve blocks are most helpful in correct diagnosis.

- Anterior or lateral soft tissue impingement—Hypertrophied synovial tissue or scarring of the ATFL can become entrapped in the joint during dorsiflexion. Entrapment is most severe in the anterolateral gutter of the ankle. A less common cause of pain is talar impingement by the anteroinferior tibiofibular ligament. Bassett and Spear (1993) hypothesized that after severe sprain, the ATFL has increased laxity, which causes the talar dome to protrude more anteriorly. During dorsiflexion, the distal fascicle of the anteroinferior tibiofibular ligament may cause impingement on the talus. Management requires removal of the fascicle.
- Cuboid subluxation—This fairly common, but often unrecognizable, condition has been reported in the literature. Most commonly the cuboid is subluxated in the plantar direction and requires dorsal manipulation. The peroneals are often weak as a result of the displaced bone.

55. What is a syndesmotic ankle sprain?

Injury of the anterior and posterior inferior tibiofibular ligaments and damage to the interosseous membrane are known as a high ankle sprain. The common mechanism is external rotation of the tibia on a planted foot. High ankle sprains are common in football and baseball. They must be differentiated from routine lateral ankle sprains. Patients have tenderness and swelling over the anterior distal leg and may have swelling and ecchymosis on both sides of the ankle. External rotation of the foot while the leg is stabilized creates pain at the syndesmosis. The squeeze test is pain elicited distally over the syndesmosis with compression of the tibia and fibula at midcalf level.

It may be critical to rule out concurrent fracture of the fibula. Patients with a syndesmotic sprain should be referred to an orthopaedic surgeon. Complete diastasis of the syndesmosis should be evaluated by radiograph, and instability may require surgery. The syndesmotic sprain typically produces longer disability than the more routine ankle sprain.

56. What is a midfoot (Lisfranc) injury and what is the mechanism of injury?

Lisfranc injury occurs when there is disruption of the soft tissues and/or bones about the tarsometatarsal joint complex. Lisfranc (midfoot) injuries result if bones in the midfoot are broken or ligaments that support the midfoot are sprained or ruptured. The severity of the injury can vary from a simple injury that affects only a single joint to a complex injury that disrupts multiple different joints and includes multiple fractures.

These injuries can happen with a simple twist and fall or in sport when someone stumbles over the top of the athlete's foot and the athlete is turning at the same time. More severe mechanisms and injury can occur with severe bending stress, which can occur in equestrian or in sail-boarding accidents when the foot is fixed in a stirrup. Injury can also result from direct trauma, such as a fall from a height. These high-energy injuries can result in multiple fractures and dislocations of the joints.

A Lisfranc injury is often mistaken for a simple sprain, especially if the injury is a result of a straightforward twist and fall. However, injury to the Lisfranc joint is not a simple and can be commonly missed and in severe injury may take many months to heal and require surgery to treat.

57. How does one diagnose a tarsometatarsal (Lisfranc) injury?

Examine the midfoot for swelling or bruising, especially the plantar aspect. Observe the ability to fully load the forefoot, especially during the terminal stance phase of gait, and heel raise is often painful. Pain is often reproduced with dorsal palpation along the first and second tarsometatarsal (Lisfranc) joints, squeezing of the midfoot, and passive motion of the forefoot with a stabilized rearfoot. Often nonweight-bearing films are normal, and these findings do not rule out tarsometatarsal joint injury. Weight-bearing films and/or MRI are needed to identify a diastasis at the junction of the base of the second metatarsal and the medial and middle cuneiforms and Lisfranc ligament tear. The more Lisfranc-involved injuries, if left untreated, may result in secondary degenerative joint changes and persistent disability. Surgical intervention is often necessary with more severe disruption of the ligaments and bone fracture.

58. What does conservative management for Lisfranc involve?

If there are no fractures or dislocations in the joint and the ligaments are not completely torn, nonsurgical treatment may be all that is necessary for healing. Conservative management includes rigid taping to support the first and second tarsometatarsal joints.

A nonsurgical treatment plan includes wearing a nonweight-bearing cast or boot for 6 weeks and then progressing to weight-bearing in a removable cast boot or an orthotic. For athletes, physical therapy should aim to address typical return to sport of at least 4 months, even if the diagnosis is a minor sprain.

59. What are shin splints?

"Shin splints" is not a specific diagnosis. The evidence is clear that shin splint pain has many different causes from tibial stress fractures to compartment syndrome. It is preferable to describe shin splint pain by location and etiology, for example, lower medial tibial pain, resulting from periostitis or upper lateral tibial pain caused by elevated compartment pressure.

60. **What is the most common cause of tibial overuse syndromes?**
Tibial overuse injuries are a recognized complication of chronic, intensive, weight-bearing exercise or training, commonly practiced by athletic and military populations. The most common tibial overuse injuries are anterior stress syndrome and posterior medial stress syndrome.

61 **Why is anterior tibial stress syndrome (shin splints) often associated with runners?**
Reber et al. (1993) using fine-wire EMG, identified that during running, the tibialis anterior muscle increased in activity and fired above the fatigue threshold for 85% of the time. This may account for the high number of fatigue-related injuries to the tibialis anterior muscle seen in runners.

62. **What is the cause of posterior medial tibial stress syndrome?**
Beck and Osternig (1994) identified that the soleus, the flexor digitorum longus, and the deep crural fascia were found to attach most frequently at the site where symptoms of medial tibial stress syndrome occur. These data contradict the contention that the tibialis posterior contributes more to this particular condition. Also, research has specifically shown overactive FHL with medial stress syndrome; therefore it is recommended to strengthen the intrinsic foot muscles.

63. **What is the best treatment for shin splints?**
Generally, the most effective treatment is considered to be rest, often for prolonged periods. In a recent review of the literature, Thacker et al. (2002) found limited evidence for the use of shock-absorbent insoles, foam heel pads, heel cord stretching, and alternative footwear as well as graduated running programs among the military. They did identify the most encouraging evidence for effective prevention of shin splints was the use of shock-absorbing insoles.

64. **What is the importance of intrinsic foot strengthening and how do you identify weakness?**
New research has shown that strengthening the intrinsic muscles of the foot acts to stiffen the foot and propel the foot forward, and aids with quick change of direction of the body, and helps with improving balance in the general population, especially the elderly. Many studies have also identified the following diagnoses that are related to intrinsic foot muscle weakness and the need for intrinsic foot strengthening.

1. Plantar fascia pain
2. Metatarsal stress fracture
3. Ankle sprain
4. Medial tibial stress syndrome
5. Balance issues, especially in the elderly

One method to identify weak foot intrinsics is the overactivity of the long toe extensors or flexors. A heel raise test is a good method for testing for overactive long FHL and weak toe intrinsics. Have the patient perform a single heel raise and look for big toe clawing, especially with multiple reps. Another method to observe the muscle imbalance of the dorsal aspect of the foot is to observe the movement task of sit to stand. If the patient has an overactivity of the long toe extensors, you will see extension of the log toes and clawing. The best treatment in these cases is with movement reeducation of the functional tasks of heel raise and/or sit to stand with having the patient cue in to keeping the toes flat and grounded against the ground.

Recommendation for specific strengthening is to place a theraband around the big toe in a sitting position and have the patient attempt to isolate big toe flexion at the MTP joint with avoiding PIP flexion or movement of the other toes. If the patient can manage 10 reps with red progress to blue theraband and then also progress to the same motion with the pinky toe followed by individual MTP flexion of each toe.

Therapeutic exercise of the plantar intrinsic foot muscles has been traditionally described as occurring during toe flexion exercises such as towel curls and marble pick-ups. While these exercises certainly do activate some of the plantar intrinsic muscles, they also involve substantial activation of the flexor hallucis longus and flexor digitorum longus muscles that will lead to muscle imbalance. Recently, the "short foot exercise" has been described as a means to isolate contraction of the plantar intrinsic muscles. The foot is "shortened" by using the intrinsic muscles to pull the first metatarsophalangeal joint towards the calcaneus as the medial longitudinal arch is elevated. As the arch raises during this exercise, it is also referred to as "foot doming" and has shown to be helpful in the above diagnoses.

65. **Define sinus tarsi syndrome.**
The sinus tarsi is an oval space laterally between the talus and the calcaneus and continuous with the tarsal tunnel. The sinus tarsi and tarsal canal are filled with fatty tissue, subtalar ligaments, an artery, a bursa, and nerve endings. Tenderness in the tarsal sinus indicates disruption or dysfunction of the subtalar complex. Chronic ankle

sprains have been cited as a common cause of sinus tarsi syndrome. Arthroscopic reports indicate scarring and synovial inflammation in the lateral talocalcaneal recess.

66. **Define tarsal coalition.**
In this structural abnormality, a fibrous or osseous bar abnormally spans two of the tarsal bones, most commonly the talocalcaneal or calcaneonavicular joint. It is most often recognized in the early teenage years. Ankle sprains, slight trauma, or growth-plate ossification are common factors that provoke pain and lead to the discovery of this condition via radiograph. Typically the pain is unrelenting. Common findings are loss of rear-foot motion and concomitant rigid pes planus. A talocalcaneal coalition is difficult to identify on radiographs; magnetic resonance imaging or computed tomography may be required. Treatment focuses initially on rest and then on treatment to increase flexibility and decrease stiffness. Surgery may be necessary to resect the bar; extreme cases may require fusion.

67. **Describe the normal mobility of the first ray. How is it assessed clinically?**
The first metatarsal should lie in the same plane as the lesser metatarsals. Normal mobility is assessed with stabilization of the lateral four toes while the examiner's other hand applies dorsal or plantar force on the first metatarsal. Motion in plantar and dorsal directions should be equal, and during dorsal testing, the inferior aspect of the first metatarsal should reach the plane of the lesser metatarsals.

68. **What are hallux rigidus and hallux limitus, and what is the best treatment?**
Hallux limitus is restriction in metatarsophalangeal (MTP) extension. Normal walking requires 65 degrees of extension during terminal stance. Hallux rigidus is further loss of motion, characterized by the development of osteoarthritis, as evidenced by spurring or loss of joint space. Common problems associated with these two disorders include trauma to the forefoot, congenital variations in the head of the first metatarsal, and a dorsiflexed first ray.

Conservative treatment for both should focus on strengthening of the flexor hallucis longus, and taping the great toe (at the MTP joint) into flexion can limit painful dorsiflexion. Mobilization of the proximal phalange in a plantar direction to increase extension is indicated in hallux limitus. However, in hallux rigidus the arthritic joint needs to be protected. In most cases, mobilizing the joint will not reduce symptoms and may cause irritation.

In more chronic cases, treatment is focused on decreasing the force to the MTP by using a stiff-soled shoe, external metatarsal bar, or orthotic modifications such as a metatarsal bar and full-contact orthoses.

69. **What is the consequence of a hypomobile first ray?**
Patients with a hypomobile first ray present with callus formation under the first metatarsal and hallux, suggesting shear and compressive forces. The problems result from inability of the first ray to dorsiflex with weight acceptance, which causes increased plantar pressure under the first ray. Patients report pain with walking, primarily at the end of stance, and with passive extension as well as decreased range of motion in dorsiflexion of the first MTP joint.

70. **Describe bunions and hallux abducto valgus (HAV) deformity and discuss risk factors.**
A bunion refers to just the bony prominence or exostosis on the medial aspect of the first MTP. A bursa can form over the enlarged joint, which can then become inflamed and painful.

HAV deformity consists of abduction or medial deviation of the first metatarsal and adduction or lateral deviation of the hallux (phalanges), which then can lead to the bunion. HAV deformity is one of the most common and disabling pathologies of the foot.

The cause of HAV is multifactorial but commonly includes genetics and improper shoe wear. It is interesting that the incidence of HAV is approximately 2% in cultures that do not wear shoes and 44% in women and 22% in men who wear shoes. Abnormal biomechanics with excessive pronation and first ray hypermobility contribute to altered forces that can stretch the MTP joint ligaments and weaken the intrinsic muscles of the foot. In addition, the altered positioning shifts the forces at the MTP joint, changes the moment arms angles, and thus leads to excessive pronation and abnormal alignment of the MTP joint out of the sagittal plane.

There are many other conditions associated with developing HAV from arthritic causes like RA, OA, neuromuscular conditions such as MS and CVA, and genetic causes such as Down syndrome. Therefore, any disorder that can affect the balance of the toe flexors and extensors can lead to HAV.

71. **Should you treat asymptomatic HAV?**
No, treatment is not warranted.

72. **What interventions are helpful in those with painful HAV?**
The goal of nonoperative treatment is to stop or even reverse the progression of degeneration at the first MTP and the compensatory overload on the second toe and resultant second toe deformities.

- To treat the pain and immediate symptoms
- Night splint to align the MTP joint and balance the pull of ligaments

- Wider shoe to decrease pressure on irritated bunion
- Padding the bunion to reduce direct pressure
- Taping arch or taping MTP sesamoids or combination for stabilization
- To treat the progression of the problem
- Foot exercises to balance muscle strength and improve proximal hip stability and first ray stability
- Seated calf raises with focus on first MTP joint extension
- Foot fists to work on foot intrinsics
- Lunge progression with foot in neutral arch and plantarflexed first ray
- Gait training with focus on shifting weight under the first MTP joint at preswing
- Achilles and soleus stretching if short or stiff
- A custom-made, full-contact orthosis to decrease abnormal pronation. An extension under the first MTP joint may be helpful
- Manual therapy
- Plantar glides of first metatarsal head with goal of increasing first MTP motion
- Sesamoid glides: proximal and distal
- Talocrural glides or mobilization with movement with goal of improving normal ankle ROM

73. What is the typical surgery for a bunion or HAV?

It is very important to differentiate surgery for a bunion verses surgery for HAV.

Surgery to remove the bony prominence and/or inflamed bursa at the base of the MTP joint is called a bunionectomy. On the other hand, many different surgical techniques exist for HAV. The most common is an osteotomy to realign the bones of the foot that are causing the deformity. Repair of tendons and ligaments, which are imbalanced, is often combined with an osteotomy. Other corrections may be removal of bone from the end of the first metatarsal, reshaping the MTP joint (resection arthroplasty), fusion of the MTP joint, fusion of the first cuneiform and first metatarsal (Lapidus procedure) or implant of an artificial joint. It is important to communicate with the surgeon to understand the precise surgery performed on your patient.

74. What should be considered with rehabilitation after HAV?

The recovery from HAV surgery can be painful and often more involved than the patient expected. The foot is initially protected for the first 3 to 4 weeks in a stiff walking shoe or boot.

Active and passive ROM of the first MTP is started early on to avoid irreversible stiffness. In the early stages, patient education regarding swelling and pain management should be implemented.

Patients are often fearful to bear weight medially under the first metatarsal, so gait training is key. The goal is to restore balance, strength, and normal biomechanics to the foot and the entire lower kinetic chain. Schuh et al. (2009) recently confirmed by plantar pressure analysis that postoperative physical therapy and gait training lead to improved function and weight bearing of the first ray after hallux valgus surgery.

75. Describe the windlass mechanism. How can abnormal mechanics lead to pathology?

From midstance to terminal stance in gait, full body weight is transferred to the metatarsal heads. As a result, the MTPs extend and activate the windlass mechanics, tightening the tissues on the plantar aspect of the foot and elevating the arch.

Dorsal movement of the navicular results in plantar flexion of the first ray. Plantar flexion of the first ray allows the phalanges to glide, resulting in dorsiflexion of the first MTPs. If plantar flexion of the first ray is not achieved, dorsiflexion cannot occur at the MTPs, and the windlass mechanism is lost. This leads, in turn, to loss of the structural stability of the foot. If the foot remains excessively pronated for any number of reasons, the windlass loses its effect. The loss of the windlass mechanism may result in the following clinical pathologies:

- Joint laxity of the metatarsals
- Metatarsalgia
- Formation of hallux valgus

76. Describe hammer toes and mallet toes. How are they treated?

A hammer toe is MTP extension with proximal interphalangeal (PIP) flexion, which may be a flexible or fixed deformity. Pain often results from a callus on the dorsum of the PIP and under the metatarsal head. Hammering of the second toe is often accompanied by a hallux valgus deformity. A mallet toe is a toe deformity that results in flexion of the distal interphalangeal (DIP). Treatment for hammer and mallet toes includes stretching of the dorsal extrinsics in a position of ankle plantar flexion and MTP extension, strengthening of the intrinsics, padding over the dip or pip, and toe tip, and wearing a deeper shoe.

77. Define claw toes. How are they treated?

Claw toe is also an extension deformity of the MTP joint with concomitant flexing or “clawing” of the toe at both the proximal and distal interphalangeal joints. The claw toe results from muscle imbalance in which the active extrinsics are stronger than the deep intrinsics (lumbricals; interosseus) and may indicate a neurologic disorder. It is commonly seen with high arches (cavus foot). Stretching, as with the hammer toe, is often successful with flexible deformities, and shoes should avoid unnecessary pressure.

78. What is sesamoiditis?

Active people may develop a problem in the two small bones (sesamoids) that lie in the tendon of the flexor hallucis brevis muscle under the first MTP joint. The medial digital plantar nerve also runs in close proximity to the medial sesamoid and can be irritated. Patients with an inflamed sesamoid find it quite painful to ambulate. They have palpable pain at the first MTP joint, pain on extension of the great toe, and often swelling at the head of the first metatarsal. The differential diagnosis should include fracture of the sesamoid and bipartite medial sesamoid.

79. What is metatarsalgia?

Metatarsalgia refers to an acute or chronic pain syndrome involving most commonly the second and third metatarsal heads. Pain also prevents extension at the MTP joint and is provoked by gait. The various causes include overuse, anatomic misalignment, foot deformity, and degenerative changes. Other nonmechanical causes include RA, gout, or other arthropathies. A cavus foot, which places more weight on the distal end, is commonly seen with this disorder.

Metatarsalgia of the first MTP joint often results from a traumatic episode or degenerative arthritis. Patients should be screened for a hallux valgus rigidus as well as sesamoiditis.

80. In general, what is the best conservative treatment for forefoot disorders?

- Change pressure under the tender area with a metatarsal pad proximal to the pain or cut-out under orthoses.
- Change ill-fitting shoes and educate on improper shoe wear, such as avoiding high heels and shoes that are too flexible.
- Improve MTP flexion and IP extension by strengthening intrinsics with manual and weight-bearing exercises.
- Maintain correct arch position by strengthening in an arched or short-foot position.
- Taping to unload fat pad or claw-hammer toe correction.
- Taping for arch support with the modified low-dye technique.
- Joint mobilization: first MTP joint, sesamoid glides, and subtalar and ankle mobilization joints and calf stretching to allow for normal progression over foot during gait.

81. Where is the most common site of a neuroma? Describe the symptoms of a neuroma.

Neuromas are found most commonly in the third web space between the third and fourth metatarsals. Neuromas at the first and fourth web spaces are rare. Patients complain of deep burning pain and may have paresthesia extending into the toe. The main symptom is pain in the plantar aspect of the foot, which is increased by walking and relieved by rest. The neuroma is secondary to irritation of the intermetatarsal plantar digital nerve as it travels under the metatarsal ligament. Pain often is elicited with MTP extension, which tightens the ligament and compresses the nerve.

82. How is a neuroma diagnosed?

Palpation in the interspace as opposed to over the joint should provoke the patient's pain. Mulder's sign is where the clinician squeezes the forefoot while palpating the involved interspace with the thumb and index finger of the other hand. A positive test is reproduction of pain and a possible audible click.

83. What is the suggested treatment for neuromas?

Physical therapy intervention includes shoe modification (specifically a wider toe box), metatarsal pads, and orthosis. Foot orthotic therapy can be very effective and, compared with metatarsal pads, can reduce plantar pressures across the forefoot and restore loading of the first metatarsal.

Joint mobilization to increase intertarsal motion is often necessary as well as deep soft tissue mobilization. Neurodynamics should be assessed and treated because the nerve may be compressed more proximally as well as locally. Steroid injection is often helpful to decrease inflammation, and, in chronic, unrelenting cases, referral for surgical neurectomy may be necessary.

84. How is the level of protective sensation tested?

The Semmes-Weinstein microfilament test is a simple, inexpensive, and effective method for assessing sensory neuropathy in patients at risk for developing foot ulcers. Patients unable to feel the nylon filament with a 10-gram bending force are diagnosed with loss of protective sensation. They benefit from protective footwear and a foot care education program.

85. What about foot pain in the elderly?

Foot problems, particularly foot pain, hallux valgus, and lesser toe deformity, are associated with falls in older people. Higher odds of recurrent falls are observed in older adults with foot pain, especially severe foot pain, as well as in individuals with planus foot posture, indicating that both foot pain and foot posture may play a role in increasing the risk of falls among older adults. Foot problems are associated with frailty level and decreased motor performance in older adults. There are age-related lower extremity muscle strength and power changes, specifically hallux and ankle muscle strength, which are found to contribute to decreases in balance/gait.

Recommendation is to strengthen large LE muscles as well as foot and ankle muscles, assess shoe wear, and work on balance.

Bibliography

Abate, M., Silbernagel, K. G., Siljeholm, C., et al. (2009). Pathogenesis of tendinopathies: Inflammation or degeneration?*Arthritis Research & Therapy*, *11*(3), 235.

Alfredson, H., & Ohberg, L. (2005). Sclerosing injections to areas of neo-vascularisation reduce pain in chronic Achilles tendinopathy: A double-blind randomised controlled trial. *Knee Surgery, Sports Traumatology, Arthroscopy*, *13*(4), 338–344.

Alfredson, H., Pietilä, T., Jonsson, P., & Lorentzon, R. (1998). Heavy-load eccentric calf muscle training for the treatment of chronic Achilles tendinosis. *American Journal of Sports Medicine*, *26*, 360–366.

Barfod, K. W., Bencke, J., Lauridsen, H. B., Ban, I., Ebskov, L., & Troelsen, A. (2014). Nonoperative dynamic treatment of acute achilles tendon rupture: The influence of early weight-bearing on clinical outcome: A blinded, randomized controlled trial. *Journal of Bone and Joint Surgery (American)*, *96*(18), 1497–1503.

Bassett, F. H. D., & Speer, F. P. (1993). Longitudinal rupture of the peroneal tendons. *American Journal of Sports Medicine*, *21*, 354–357.

Beck, B. R., & Osternig, L. R. (1994). Medial tibial stress syndrome. The location of muscles in the leg in relation to symptoms. *Journal of Bone and Joint Surgery*, *76*(7), 1057–1061.

Boesen, A. P., Hansen, R., Boesen, M. I., Malliaras, P., & Langberg, H. (2017). Effect of high-volume injection, platelet-rich plasma, and sham treatment in chronic midportion Achilles tendinopathy: A randomized double-blinded prospective study. *The American Journal of Sports Medicine*, *45*(9), 2034–2043.

Bonnin, M., Tavernier, T., & Bouysset, M. (1997). Split lesions of the peroneus brevis tendon in chronic ankle laxity. *American Journal of Sports Medicine*, *25*, 699–703.

Brumann, M., Baumbach, S. F., Mutschler, W., & Polzer, H. (2014). Accelerated rehabilitation following Achilles tendon repair after acute rupture—Development of an evidence-based treatment protocol. *Injury*, *45*(11), 1782–1790.

Carcia, C. R., Martin, R. L., Houck, J., & Wukich, D. K. (2010). Orthopaedic section of the American Physical Therapy Association: Achilles pain, stiffness, and muscle power deficits: Achilles tendinitis. *Journal of Orthopaedic and Sports Physical Therapy*, *40*(9), A1–A26.

Cetti, R., Christensen, S. E., Ejsted, R., Jensen, N. M., & Jorgensen, U. (1993). Operative versus nonoperative treatment of Achilles tendon rupture: A prospective randomized study and review of the literature. *American Journal of Sports Medicine*, *21*, 791–799.

Chandler, T. J. (1998). Iontophoresis of 0.4% dexamethasone for plantar fasciitis. *Clinical Journal of Sport Medicine*, *8*, 68.

Cheung, R. T. H., Sze, L. K. Y., Mok, N. W., & Ng, G. Y. F. (2016). Intrinsic foot muscle volume in experienced runners with and without chronic plantar fasciitis. *Journal of Science and Medicine in Sport/Sports Medicine Australia*, *19*(9), 713–715.

Cleland, J. A., Abbott, J. H., Kidd, M. O., et al. (2009). Manual physical therapy and exercise versus electrophysical agents and exercise in the management of plantar heel pain: A multicenter randomized clinical trial. *Journal of Orthopaedic and Sports Physical Therapy*, *39*(8), 573–585.

Cook, J. L., Rio, E., Purdam, C. R., & Docking, S. I. (2016). Revisiting the continuum model of tendon pathology: What is its merit in clinical practice and research? *British Journal of Sports Medicine*, *50*(19), 1187–1191.

Cornwall, M. W., & McPoil, T. G. (1999). Plantar fasciitis: Etiology and treatment. *Journal of Orthopaedic and Sports Physical Therapy*, *29*, 756–760.

Davenport, T. E., Kulig, K., Matharu, Y., & Blanco, C. E. (2005). The EdUReP model for nonsurgical management of tendinopathy. *Physical Therapy*, *85*(10), 1093–1103.

DiGiovanni, B. F., Nawoczenski, D. A., Lintal, M. E., et al. (2003). Tissue-specific plantar fascia-stretching exercise enhances outcomes in patients with chronic heel pain. A prospective, randomized study. *Journal of Bone and Joint Surgery*, *85*(7), 1270–1277.

Doherty, C., Delahunt, E., Caulfield, B., Hertel, J., Ryan, J., & Bleakley, C. (2014). The incidence and prevalence of ankle sprain injury: A systematic review and meta-analysis of prospective epidemiological studies. *Sports Medicine*, *44*(1), 123–140.

Doherty, C., Bleakley, C., Delahunt, E., & Holden, S. (2017). Treatment and prevention of acute and recurrent ankle sprain: An overview of systematic reviews with meta-analysis. *British Journal of Sports Medicine*, *51*(2), 113–125.

Don, R., Ranavolo, A., Cacchio, A., et al. (2007). Relationship between recovery of calf-muscle biomechanical properties and gait pattern following surgery for achilles tendon rupture. *Clinical Biomechanics*, *22*(2), 211–220.

Fallat, L., Grimm, D. J., & Saracco, J. A. (1998). Sprained ankle syndrome: Prevalence and analysis of 639 acute injuries. *Journal of Foot and Ankle Surgery*, *37*, 280–285.

Gebauer, M., Beil, F. T., Beckmann, J., et al. (2007). Mechanical evaluation of different techniques for Achilles tendon repair. *Archives of Orthopaedic and Traumatic Surgery*, *127*, 795–799.

Geideman, W. M., & Johnson, J. E. (2000). Posterior tibial tendon dysfunction. *Physical Therapy*, *30*, 68–77.

Gerber, J. P., Williams, G. N., Scoville, C. R., Arciero, R. A., & Taylor, D. C. (1998). Persistent disability associated with ankle sprains: A prospective examination of an athletic population. *Foot and Ankle International*, *19*, 653–660.

Greenberg, E. T., & Queller, H. R. (2016). Tarsometatarsal (Lisfranc) joint injury in an athlete with persistent foot pain. *Journal of Orthopaedic and Sports Physical Therapy*, *46*(6), 494.

Habets, B., van Cingel, R. E. H., Backx, F. J. G., van Elten, H. J., Zuithoff, P., & Huisstede, B. M. A. (2021). No difference in clinical effects when comparing Alfredson eccentric and Silbernagel combined concentric-eccentric loading in Achilles tendinopathy: A randomized controlled trial. *Orthopaedic Journal of Sports Medicine*, *9*(10), 23259671211031254.

Hay, E. M., Paterson, S. M., Lewis, M., Hosie, G., & Croft, P. (1999). Pragmatic randomised controlled trial of local corticosteroid injection and naproxen for treatment of lateral epicondylitis of elbow in primary care. *BMJ*, *319*(7215), 964–968.

Huffer, D., Hing, W., Newton, R., & Clair, M. (2017). Strength training for plantar fasciitis and the intrinsic foot musculature: A systematic review. *Physical Therapy in Sport*, *24*, 44–52.

Järvinen, T. A. H., Kannus, P., Maffulli, N., & Khan, K. M. (2005). Achilles tendon disorders: Etiology and epidemiology. *Foot and Ankle Clinics*, *10*(2), 255–266.

Johnson, K. A., & Strom, D. E. (1989). Tibialis posterior tendon dysfunction. *Clinical Orthopaedics*, *239*, 196–206.

Johnston, E. C., & Howell, S. J. (1999). Tendon neuropathy of the superficial peroneal nerve: Associated conditions and results of release. *Foot and Ankle International*, *20*, 576–582.

Kedia, M., Williams, M., Jain, L., et al. (2014). The effects of conventional physical therapy and eccentric strengthening for insertional achilles tendinopathy. *International Journal of Sports Physical Therapy*, *9*(4), 488–497.

Khan, R. J. K., Fick, D., Keogh, A., Crawford, J., Brammar, T., & Parker, M. (2005). Treatment of acute achilles tendon ruptures. A meta-analysis of randomized, controlled trials. *Journal of Bone and Joint Surgery (American)*, *87*(10), 2202–2210.

Kulig, K., Burnfield, J. M., Requejo, S. M., Sperry, M., & Terk, M. (2004). Selective activation of tibialis posterior: Evaluation by magnetic resonance imaging. *Medicine & Science in Sports & Exercise*, *36*, 862–867.

Kulig, K., Burnfield, J. M., Reischl, S., Requejo, S. M., Blanco, C. E., & Thordarson, D. B. (2005). Effect of foot orthoses on tibialis posterior activation in persons with pes planus. *Medicine and Science in Sports and Exercise*, *37*(1), 24–29.

Kulig, K., Reischl, S. F., Pomrantz, A. B., et al. (2009). Nonsurgical management of posterior tibial tendon dysfunction with orthoses and resistive exercise: A randomized controlled trial. *Physical Therapy*, *89*(1), 26–37.

Kulig, K., Popovich, J. M., Jr., Noceti-Dewit, L. M., Reischl, S. F., & Kim, D. (2011). Women with posterior tibial tendon dysfunction have diminished ankle and hip muscle performance. *Journal of Orthopaedic and Sports Physical Therapy*, *41*(9), 687–694.

Kulig, K., Lee, S. P., Reischl, S. F., & Noceti-DeWit, L. (2014). Effect of tibialis posterior tendon dysfunction on unipedal standing balance test. *Foot and Ankle International*, *36*(1), 83–89.

Lentell, G., Baas, B., Lopez, D., McGuire, L., Sarrels, M., & Snyder, P. (1995). The contributions of proprioceptive deficits, muscle function, and anatomic laxity to functional instability of the ankle. *Journal of Orthopaedic and Sports Physical Therapy*, *21*, 206–215.

Maffulli, N., & Longo, U. G. (2008). How do eccentric exercises work in tendinopathy? [Review of *How do eccentric exercises work in tendinopathy?*]. *Rheumatology*, *47*(10), 1444–1445.

Malliaras, P., Barton, C. J., Reeves, N. D., & Langberg, H. (2013). Achilles and patellar tendinopathy loading programmes: A systematic review comparing clinical outcomes and identifying potential mechanisms for effectiveness. *Sports Medicine*, *43*(4), 267–286.

Mandelbaum, B. R., Myerson, M. S., & Forster, R. (1995). Achilles tendon ruptures: A new method repair, early range of motion, and functional rehabilitation. *American Journal of Sports Medicine*, *23*, 392–395.

Maquirriain, J. (2011). Achilles tendon rupture: Avoiding tendon lengthening during surgical repair and rehabilitation. *Yale Journal of Biology and Medicine*, *84*(3), 289–300.

Martin, R. L., Davenport, T. E., Paulseth, S., Wukich, D. K., Godges, J. J., & Orthopaedic Section American Physical Therapy Association., (2013). Ankle stability and movement coordination impairments: ankle ligament sprains. *Journal of Orthopaedic and Sports Physical Therapy*, *43*(9), A1–A40.

Martin, R. L., Davenport, T. E., Reischl, S. F., et al. (2014). Heel pain—plantar fasciitis: Revision 2014. *Journal of Orthopaedic and Sports Physical Therapy*, *44*(11), A1–A33.

McKeon, P. O., Hertel, J., Bramble, D., & Davis, I. (2015). The foot core system: A new paradigm for understanding intrinsic foot muscle function. *British Journal of Sports Medicine*, *49*(5), 290.

McPoil, T. G., Martin, R. L., Cornwall, M. W., Wukich, D. K., Irrgang, J. J., & Godges, J. J. (2008). Heel pain—plantar fasciitis: Clinical practice guidelines linked to the international classification of function, disability, and health from the orthopaedic section of the American Physical Therapy Association. *Journal of Orthopaedic and Sports Physical Therapy*, *38*(10), 648.

Metz, R., van der Heijden, G. J., Verleisdonk, E. J., Tamminga, R., & van der Werken, C. (2009). Recovery of calf muscle strength following acute Achilles tendon rupture treatment: A comparison between minimally invasive surgery and conservative treatment. *Foot & Ankle Specialist*, *2*(5), 219–226.

Mulligan, E. P., & Cook, P. G. (2013). Effect of plantar intrinsic muscle training on medial longitudinal arch morphology and dynamic function. *Manual Therapy*, *18*(5), 425–430.

Myerson, M. G., Solomon, G., & Shereff, M. (1989). Posterior tibial tendon dysfunction: Its association with seronegative inflammatory disease. *Foot & Ankle*, *9*, 219–225.

Ohberg, L. R., Lorentzon, R., & Alfredson, H. (2004). Eccentric training in patients with chronic Achilles tendinosis: Normalized tendon structure and decreased thickness at follow up. *British Journal of Sports Medicine*, *38*, 8–11. discussion 11.

Okamura, K., Kanai, S., Hasegawa, M., Otsuka, A., & Oki, S. (2018). The effect of additional activation of the plantar intrinsic foot muscles on foot dynamics during gait. *The Foot*, *34*, 1–5.

Pfeffer, G. P., Bacchetti, P., Deland, J., et al. (1999). Comparison of custom and prefabricated orthoses in the initial treatment of proximal plantar fasciitis. *Foot and Ankle International*, *20*, 214–221.

Pugia, M. L., Middel, C. J., Seward, S. W., et al. (2001). Comparison of acute swelling and function in subjects with lateral ankle injury. *Journal of Orthopaedic and Sports Physical Therapy*, *31*, 384–388.

Radford, J. A., Landorf, K. B., Buchbinder, R., & Cook, C. (2006). Effectiveness of low-Dye taping for the short-term treatment of plantar heel pain: A randomised trial. *BMC Musculoskeletal Disorders*, *7*, 64.

Reber, L., Perry, J., & Pink, M. (1993). Muscular control of the ankle in running. *American Journal of Sports Medicine*, *21*, 805–810. Discussion 810.

Richie, D. H., Jr. (2007). Biomechanics and clinical analysis of the adult acquired flatfoot. *Clinics in Podiatric Medicine and Surgery*, *24*(4), 617–644.

Riddle, D. L., Pulisic, M., Pidcoe, P., & Johnson, R. E. (2003). Risk factors for Plantar fasciitis: A matched case-control study. *Journal of Bone and Joint Surgery (American)*, *85*(5), 872–877.

Robinson, J. M., Cook, J. L., Purdam, C., et al. (2001). The VISA-A questionnaire: A valid and reliable index of the clinical severity of Achilles tendinopathy. *British Journal of Sports Medicine*, *35*(5), 335–341.

Rompe, J. D., Furia, J. P., & Maffulli, N. (2008). Mid-portion Achilles tendinopathy – current options for treatment. *Disability and Rehabilitation*, *30*(20-22), 1666–1676.

Safran, M. R., Benedetti, R. S., Bartolozzi, A. R., 3rd, & Mandelbaum, B. R. (1999). Lateral ankle sprains: A comprehensive review. Part 1: Etiology, pathoanatomy, histopathogenesis, and diagnosis. *Medicine & Science in Sports & Exercise*, *31*, S429–S437.

Safran, M. R., O'Malley, D., Jr., & Fu, F. H. (1999). Peroneal tendon subluxation in athletes: New exam technique, case reports, and review. *Medicine & Science in Sports & Exercise*, *31*(7 Suppl), S487–S492.

Schuh, R., Hofstaetter, S. G., Adams, S. B., Jr., et al. (2009). Rehabilitation after hallux valgus surgery: Importance of physical therapy to restore weight bearing of the first ray during the stance phase. *Physical Therapy*, *89*(9), 934–945.

Silbernagel, K., & Crossley, K. M. (2015). A proposed return-to-sport program for patients with midportion achilles tendinopathy: Rationale and implementation. *The Journal of Orthopaedic and Sports Physical Therapy, 45*(11), 876–886.
Silbernagel, K. G., Thomeé, R., Eriksson, B. I., & Karlsson, J. (2007). Continued sports activity, using a pain-monitoring model, during rehabilitation in patients with Achilles tendinopathy: A randomized controlled study. *The American Journal of Sports Medicine, 35*(6), 897–906.
Soroceanu, A., Sidhwa, F., Aarabi, S., Kaufman, A., & Glazebrook, M. (2012). Surgical versus nonsurgical treatment of acute Achilles tendon rupture: A meta-analysis of randomized trials. *Journal of Bone and Joint Surgery (American), 94*(23), 2136–2143.
Stevens, M., & Tan, C. W. (2014). Effectiveness of the Alfredson protocol compared with a lower repetition-volume protocol for midportion Achilles tendinopathy: A randomized controlled trial. *Journal of Orthopaedic & Sports Physical Therapy, 44*, 59–67.
Suchak, A. A., Bostick, G. P., Beaupre, L. A., et al. (2008). The influence of early weight- bearing compared with non-weightbearing after surgical repair of the Achilles tendon. *Journal of Bone and Joint Surgery (American), 90*(9), 1876–1883.
Thacker, S. B., Gichrest, J., Stroup, D. F., & Kimsey, C. D. (2002). The prevention of shin splints in sports: A systematic review of literature. *Medicine & Science in Sports & Exercise, 34*, 32–40.
Wadsworth, D. J. S., & Eadie, N. T. (2005). Conservative management of subtle Lisfranc joint injury: A case report. *Journal of Orthopaedic and Sports Physical Therapy, 35*(3), 154–164.
Willits, K., Amendola, A., Bryant, D., et al. (2010). Operative versus nonoperative treatment of acute Achilles tendon ruptures: A multicenter randomized trial using accelerated functional rehabilitation. *Journal of Bone and Joint Surgery (American), 92*(17), 2767–2775.

CHAPTER 77 QUESTIONS

1. **A 45-year-old male runner patient presents with an insidious onset of pain distal to the medial malleolus and into the arch and slightly into the foot that worsens 75% into a 5-mile run. Which is the most likely diagnosis?**
   a. Deltoid ligament sprain
   b. Plantar fasciitis
   c. Posterior tibial tendinosis
   d. Pain from accessory navicular

2. **A physical therapist evaluates a 22-year-old college basketball player who presents with midportion Achilles tendinopathy. What treatment is most appropriate for this athlete?**
   a. Remove from sport, rest, and start strength training when pain is absent.
   b. Remove from sport, rest, and start calf and Achilles stretching.
   c. Remove from sport, rest, and start eccentric strength training allowing 4/10 pain during exercise.
   d. Allow return to sport limiting pain over 3/10 and perform heavy load eccentric and concentric exercise allowing pain to 4/10 with monitoring 24-hour pain now going above 3/10.

3. **A therapist evaluates a 55-year-old male who is s/p 4–6 weeks s/p Achilles tendon repair. Which is the most appropriate intervention?**
   a. Calf and Achilles stretching and high-volume eccentric exercise
   b. Calf and Achilles stretching and high-volume concentric and eccentric exercise
   c. Avoid Achilles stretching, progressive weight bearing with a heel lift for walking
   d. Progressive strengthening, Achilles stretching and heel lift for walking

4. **A physical therapist evaluates a 40-year-old female with complaints of heel pain for the past 6 months. Her pain is worse in the morning when first getting out of bed and later in the day after her job as an RN. Which intervention would be** *most effectivemost effective* **according to the APTA Guidelines for heel pain?**
   a. Iontophoresis
   b. Intrinsic foot exercises
   c. Laser therapy
   d. Foot orthotics

5. **A physical therapist is assisting with a health prescreen for high school athletes. All of the following are risk factors for acute lateral ankle sprain EXCEPT:**
   a. Has a history of a previous ankle sprain
   b. Does not use an external support
   c. Does not have normal ankle dorsiflexion range of motion
   d. Does not have enough inversion range of motion

6. **A physical therapist is evaluating a 55-year-old patient with stage II PTTD? Which of the following is the most appropriate exercise for this patient?**
   a. Open chain plantar flexion and inversion with a theraband
   b. An open chain resisted foot adduction, a windshield-wiper type of motion

c. Resisted foot adduction with the foot also pressing down into the floor, in a windshield-wiper type of motion with high-volume strengthening
d. Eccentric heel lowering
e. Exercise should not be performed in this stage

7. **A physical therapist evaluates a 50-year-old woman with a new onset of heel pain and a diagnosis of plantar fasciitis. Which of the following is most likely contributing to her pain?**
   a. Excessive pronated foot posture
   b. Excessive supinated foot posture
   c. BMI of 26 kg/m^2
   d. Lack of ankle plantar flexion compared to the uninvolved foot
   e. Lack of ankle dorsiflexion compared to the uninvolved foot

8. **A 66-year-old woman presents with pain on the plantar aspect of the forefoot, which is increased by walking and relieved by rest. Her symptoms increase when the forefoot is squeezed and causes some tingling. What is the best treatment for this patient with a neuroma?**
   a. Dorsiflexion stretching
   b. Plantarflexion strengthening
   c. Intrinsic strengthening
   d. Increasing the toe box of the shoe and using a metatarsal pad

CHAPTER 78

FRACTURES AND DISLOCATIONS OF THE FOOT AND ANKLE

R.T. Hockenbury, MD

1. **How are ankle fractures classified?**
   Ankle fractures are described by the number of malleoli involved:
   - Single malleolar fracture is a lateral malleolar, medial malleolar, or posterior malleolar fracture (posterior aspect of the distal tibial articular surface).
   - Bimalleolar fracture is a fracture of two of the malleoli.
   - Trimalleolar fracture is a fracture of the lateral malleolus, medial malleolus, and posterior malleolus.

   There are two major classification systems for ankle fractures: the Weber/AO classification and the Lauge-Hansen classification (more complex). Fractures are classified in order to dictate treatment, simplify communication between medical personnel treating the fracture, and predict outcome.

   The Weber/AO classification is the simplest method to classify ankle fractures:
   - Weber A—below the level of the tibiotalar joint
   - Weber B—at or near the level of the tibiotalar joint; 50% have disruption of the syndesmosis
   - Weber C—above the level of the tibiotalar joint; >50% have disruption of the syndesmosis

   The four Lauge-Hansen classes are (the first term in parentheses refers to the foot position during injury and the second term describes the external force applied to the ankle):
   - Supination-Adduction (SA, 10% to 20%)
   - Supination-External Rotation (SER, 40% to 75%)
   - Pronation-Abduction (PA, 5% to 20%)
   - Pronation-External Rotation (PER, 5% to 20%)

2. **Describe the anatomy of the ankle syndesmosis and how it affects ankle stability**
   The distal fibula articulates with the lateral distal tibia at the syndesmosis. The anterior-inferior tibiofibular ligament (AITFL), interosseous ligament (IOL), interosseous membrane, posterior-inferior tibiofibular ligament (PITFL), and inferior transverse ligament provide stability at the syndesmosis. If an external rotation and/or abduction ankle injury occurs, the syndesmotic ligaments can be disrupted and the ankle joint mortise becomes widened and unstable. The ankle depends on exact articular surface contact between the tibia and talus. A 1 mm lateral talar shift results in 40% decrease in tibiotalar contact and results in abnormal joint mechanics, leading to early posttraumatic tibiotalar joint arthritis. It is crucial to diagnose and restore syndesmotic stability during treatment of ankle fractures.

3. **Describe the radiographic views and alignment guides used in assessing syndesmotic stability.**
   ANTEROPOSTERIOR VIEW
   - Measured 1 cm proximal to the ankle joint, the tibiofibular overlap should be >6 mm.
   - Measured 1 cm proximal to the ankle joint, the tibiofibular clear space should be <6 mm.
     - Medial tibiofibular clear space should be <5 mm and should be symmetrical to the superior tibiotalar space
     - If the above measurements are undiagnostic and a high index of suspicion exists, external rotation stress views are taken. See below. Abnormalities of the above measurements indicate instability of the ankle syndesmosis that typically requires surgical stabilization.

   LATERAL VIEW
   - Assess joint line congruity. Assess for talus, calcaneus, and posterior tibial fracture.

   MORTISE VIEW
   - Tibiofibular line should be continuous
   - Talocrural angle—normally 8 to 15 degrees or within 2 to 3 degrees of opposite side
   - Medial clear space—normally equal to the superior clear space (should be <5 mm)
   - Tibiofibular overlap should be >1 mm

   SPECIALIZED STRESS VIEWS
   - External rotation stress test is performed by stabilizing the distal tibia and externally rotating the foot while taking a mortise radiograph. Widening of the medial tibiotalar clear space greater than 5 mm indicates a tear of the deep deltoid ligament. This finding in conjunction with a distal fibular fracture is called a bimalleolar equivalent fracture.

4. **What are the indications for surgical treatment of an ankle fracture?**
   - Intraarticular displacement of the distal tibial surface of 2 mm or more requires surgical intervention.
   - Syndesmotic injury causing widening of the ankle mortise is an indication for surgery.
   - Any injury that causes two breaks in the ankle joint "ring" requires surgery. The ankle is a hinge joint in which the malleoli are connected to the talus through the lateral and medial collateral ligaments. Bimalleolar fractures are inherently unstable and require surgical stabilization. A fibular fracture combined with a deltoid ligament tear is a bimalleolar equivalent fracture and also requires surgery.
   - Any fracture that allows the talus to shift laterally or medially in the mortise is treated surgically.
   - Ankle fractures that involve only one malleolar fracture and do not disturb the stability of the ankle mortise are treated nonoperatively; the patient wears a short-leg walking cast or fracture boot for 6 weeks.

5. **Describe other fracture patterns around the ankle**
   - Maisonneuve—pronation-external rotation fracture with fracture of the proximal fibula
   - Curbstone—isolated posterior malleolus fracture
   - Le Fort-Wagstaffe—anterior fibular avulsion, supination-external rotation injury
   - Tillaux-Chaput—anterior tibial avulsion
   - Pronation-dorsiflexion fracture—fracture of anterior articular surface
   - Nutcracker fracture—avulsion fracture of the navicular with comminuted compression fracture of the cuboid
   - Pilon—high-energy compression fracture through tibial plafond
   - Snowboarder's fracture—lateral talar process fracture

6. **What is a pilon ankle fracture and how is it treated?**
   A pilon fracture is an intraarticular fracture of the distal tibia produced by dorsiflexion and/or axial loading forces. The term pilon refers to the talus as the pestle driving into the mortar-like ankle mortise, producing a fracture of the weight-bearing surface of the tibia.
   The Ruedi-Allgower classification describes pilon fractures as follows:
   - Type I—nondisplaced
   - Type II—displaced
   - Type III—displaced with joint surface comminution and impaction

   The recommended treatment of displaced fractures is surgery. Most patients are initially treated with a two-stage protocol of immediate external fixation to restore length and achieve temporary reduction, which allows for soft tissue healing. Second stage of treatment entails ORIF with plates and screws.

7. **What complications can occur following pilon fractures?**
   The most frequent complication following pilon fracture treatment is posttraumatic arthritis (50% to 70%). Other complications include wound healing problems, dehiscence, nonunion, malunion, and pin tract infections. In type III fractures, the goal is often to achieve soft tissue healing and sufficient bony healing of the metaphyseal bone to allow fusion or ankle replacement at a later date.

8. **How does the presence of diabetes affect ankle fracture outcomes?**
   It is estimated that one-third of the U.S. population born after 2000 will develop diabetes. The presence of diabetic neuropathy or vasculopathy complicates soft tissue and bony healing following an ankle fracture. Diabetics have higher complication rates including infection rates, nonunions, delayed unions, delayed wound healing, and amputations. Postoperative emphasis on blood sugar control is important to optimize wound healing. Neuropathic patients may benefit from superconstructs using multiple syndesmotic screws, rigid locked plating, intramedullary nails, or external fixation in conjunction with internal fixation. A longer period of postoperative immobilization and nonweight bearing is needed with diabetic patients compared to nondiabetic patients following internal fixation to insure bony healing. Due to the presence of diabetic neuropathy, these patients have decreased postoperative pain and may ambulate against medical advice leading to internal fixation failure and redisplacement of the fracture. The presence of morbid obesity in many diabetics may also preclude their ability to remain nonweight bearing on the injured extremity.

9. **What common fractures are frequently misdiagnosed as ankle sprains?**
   - Talar osteochondral fracture (a divot fracture involving bone and cartilage usually from the anterolateral or posteromedial talar dome)
   - Lateral talar process fracture
   - Anterior calcaneal process fracture
   - Posterior talar process fracture
   - "Flake fracture" of the posterior distal fibular rim, indicating a tear of the superior peroneal retinaculum and peroneal tendon dislocation
   - Navicular fracture
   - Lateral or medial malleolar fracture

10. How are talar fractures classified?

Talar fractures account for 3% to 6% of all foot fractures. Fractures of the talus are characterized by location. The different types of fractures are talar neck fractures (50%); talar body fractures (25%); fractures of the lateral talar process, fractures of the posterior talar process, osteochondral fractures of the talar dome, and talar neck fractures (combined make up the remaining 25%). Any of these fractures may be misdiagnosed as an ankle sprain. Talar neck fractures are usually caused by a hyperdorsifexion of the ankle.

Hawkins and Canale (1970) have classified talar neck fractures as four types:

- Type I—nondisplaced vertical fracture of talar neck
- Type II—displaced talar neck fracture with subluxation or dislocation of the subtalar joint
- Type III—displaced talar neck fracture with dislocation of both subtalar and ankle joints
- Type IV—type III fracture with talonavicular subluxation or dislocation

11. How are talar fractures treated?

It is essential to diagnose talar fracture displacement to plan treatment. A radiographic view called a Canale view provides optimal visualization of the talar neck. The radiograph is taken with the foot in maximal plantar flexion and pronated at 15 degrees; the x-ray tube is directed 15 degrees cephalad to the vertical. CT scans are usually obtained following closed reduction of fractures and dislocations.

Treatment of displaced fractures is usually surgical because of problems with late displacement and prolonged immobilization. Anatomic reduction and stable internal fixation of displaced fractures are crucial to prevent malalignment and subsequent subtalar joint or ankle joint arthritis. Due to the tenuous blood supply of the talus, the risk of avascular necrosis is high and correlates with the initial displacement of the fracture fragments. The risk of avascular necrosis (AVN) increases with Hawkins type (type I = 0% to 13%, type II = 20% to 50%, type III = 20% to 100%). Approximately 50% to 100% of patients suffer late subtalar arthritis.

Type I fractures of the talar neck are treated with immobilization for 3 months. Type II to IV fractures are treated with closed reduction. If an acceptable reduction is achieved, nonweight-bearing cast immobilization is used for 3 months. In the case of displaced fractures, ORIF is indicated.

12. What is Hawkins sign?

Hawkins sign is the appearance of talar dome subchondral lucency on the ankle AP view at 6 to 8 weeks following talar fracture. This indicates that the talar body is vascular and excludes the diagnosis of osteonecrosis, also known as avascular necrosis. If the talar body appears more dense and sclerotic than the surrounding bone, then osteonecrosis is present. In cases of talar body osteonecrosis, 44% will spontaneously revascularize without collapse. Treatment of symptomatic AVN is difficult. Options include core decompression, bone grafting, osteochondral allograft, vascularized bone grafting, fusion, talectomy, and tibiocalcaneal fusion or total talar implant.

13. Describe the pathophysiology of calcaneal fractures

Calcaneal fractures occur during falls or during high-energy motor vehicle accidents. Seventy-five percent of calcaneal fractures are intraarticular, causing damage to the subtalar joint articular cartilage. A primary fracture line courses anterolateral to posteromedial through the calcaneus and the lateral portion of the posterior calcaneal facet drives downward into the calcaneal body causing subtalar joint incongruity and shortening of the calcaneal height. A secondary fracture line that exits just posterior to the posterior facet produces a joint depression fracture. A secondary fracture line that exits through the posterior tuberosity produces a tongue type fracture. Other secondary fractures also occur causing calcaneal widening, calcaneocuboid joint displacement, and peroneal tendon impingement. The calcaneal tuberosity typically rotates into varus. If a calcaneus fracture is left unreduced, the patient develops subtalar joint arthritis, peroneal tendon impingement, anterior ankle impingement, widening of the heel, and heel varus.

14. How are calcaneal fractures classified?

Calcaneal fractures are classified according to whether they are open or closed, extraarticular or intraarticular, and whether they are displaced or undisplaced. Standard AP, lateral, oblique, and calcaneal axial views are taken. The Böhler angle is the angle formed by a line drawn between the superior-most aspect of the anterior process of the calcaneus and the posterior facet and a line drawn along the superior border of the tuberosity to the posterior facet on a lateral radiograph. Typically, a normal Böhler angle ranges from 20 to 40 degrees. This angle decreases when the posterior facet is driven down into the calcaneal body. The angle of Gissane is the angle drawn between the two cortical columns that are inferior to the lateral process of the talus on a lateral radiograph, which correlates with the sinus tarsi. A normal angle of Gissane ranges from 95 to 110 degrees.

The Essex-Lopresti classification divides fractures into joint depression and tongue types. CT scans are required for classification and surgical planning.

Any displaced calcaneal fracture should be evaluated with a CT scan to determine the degree of posterior facet displacement and comminution. The Sanders' classification uses CT scanning in the coronal plane to describe the number of posterior facet fragments and their location. Sanders (1992) classifies an extraarticular fracture as a type I. A posterior calcaneal facet fracture with two pieces is a type II; a fracture with three pieces is a type III; and a fracture with four pieces is a type IV. Using this system, Sanders has reported results of ORIF of displaced intraarticular fractures by fracture type: 73% of type II fractures had a good or excellent result, 70% of type III fractures had a good or excellent result, and only 9% of type IV fractures had a good or excellent result.

15. **What injuries are commonly associated with calcaneal fractures?**
The calcaneus is the most fractured tarsal bone. Approximately 75% of calcaneal fractures are intraarticular. Approximately 10% of patients have associated fractures of the spine, 25% have extremity injuries, 10% are bilateral, and 5% are open.

16. **How are calcaneal fractures treated?**
   - Nondisplaced fracture—6 weeks of splinting, elevation, nonweight bearing, and early motion typically yield acceptable results.
   - Displaced fractures—Treatment is controversial. Surgery is performed 10 to 21 days post injury to allow for edema resolution and healing of fracture blisters. Displaced fractures of the posterior calcaneal tuberosity may cause tenting of the posterior heel skin and require immediate ORIF to avoid skin breakdown and infection. Operative treatment of displaced intraarticular fractures through an extensile L-shaped incision yields excellent exposure but carries a higher risk of complications than nonoperative treatment. These complications include wound infection, sural nerve injury, malunion, nonunion, osteomyelitis, and amputation. A large prospective study comparing surgical and nonsurgical treatment of displaced intraarticular calcaneal fractures showed no overall difference between patients in the two treatment groups at 2- to 8-year follow-up. However, among patients who did not have a workers' compensation claim, surgical treatment led to better satisfaction scores than nonsurgical treatment. It is known that patients with posterior facet displacement, articular incongruity, and increasing levels of comminution have poor outcomes. Most surgeons agree that patients with displaced intraarticular calcaneal fractures do not have good outcomes with nonoperative management. Calcaneal reductions through smaller incisions and percutaneous techniques have been developed to avoid wound complications while allowing for fracture reduction to prevent posttraumatic subtalar joint arthritis. Contraindications for calcaneal open reduction internal fixation include poor vascular supply, poorly controlled diabetes, tobacco abuse, drug abuse, venous stasis, neuropathy, unhealed fracture blisters, and elderly or inactive patients.
   - Open calcaneal fractures—Immediate operative debridement, intravenous antibiotics, temporary fracture stabilization, and temporary wound coverage are the initial course of treatment. No internal fixation or limited percutaneous fixation are used in grade III open fractures because of the significant risk of wound dehiscence, infection, chronic osteomyelitis, and amputation. Grade I and II open fractures with medial wounds can be treated with staged ORIF after initial wound management. Open calcaneal fractures have a much higher complication rate than closed calcaneal fractures. A recent study of 115 surgically treated open fractures found superficial wound infection in 9.6%, deep infection in 12.2%, and culture-positive osteomyelitis in 5.2%. Six patients (5.2%) required amputation.

17. **What are expected outcomes after calcaneal fractures?**
Sanders type II and III fractures have shown good to excellent results in 70% to 85% of patients. This compares favorably to 40% to 60% acceptable results following nonoperative management.

18. **What is the pathophysiology of stress fractures of the foot?**
A stress or fatigue fracture is a break that develops in bone after cyclical, submaximal loading. In states of increased physical activity, bone is resorbed faster than it is replaced, which results in physical weakening of the bone and the development of microfractures. With continued physical stress these microfractures coalesce to form a complete stress fracture. Middle-aged and older adult patients with osteoporosis, diagnosed with a T score of lower than −2.5 on dual photon spectrometry (DXA scan), are also at risk for stress fractures. Amenorrheic athletes are predisposed to stress fractures; amenorrhea is present in up to 20% of vigorously exercising women and may be as high as 50% in elite runners and dancers.

19. **What are common locations for stress fractures of the foot?**
Common locations for foot stress fractures are the metatarsals, calcaneus, and navicular. Distal tibial stress fractures and lateral malleolar fractures are less common. Symptoms of stress fracture are localized pain and swelling with weight bearing of insidious onset. A thin sclerotic line may be seen in a stress fracture of metaphyseal bone. Although initial radiographs may be negative, a technetium bone scan is positive as early as 48 to 72 hours after onset of symptoms. MRI is now more commonly used to diagnose stress fractures in symptomatic patients with normal radiographs. MRI shows bone edema, periosteal reaction, and cortical breaks in the area of stress fracture.

20. **How are stress fractures treated?**
Most stress fractures of the foot will heal with a 4- to 8-week period of weight-bearing immobilization in a walking boot or orthopedic shoe. The exceptions are navicular stress fractures and stress fractures of the proximal fifth metatarsal. Navicular stress fractures can be difficult to diagnose as most initial radiographs are normal. These patients will have a nickel-sized area of tenderness (the N spot) over the dorsal central navicular. Single-leg hopping is a useful provocative test. MRI may be required to make the diagnosis. Navicular stress fractures are treated in a nonweight-bearing short leg cast for 6 to 8 weeks. Recalcitrant fractures may require screw fixation.

21. **What fractures of the foot are at risk for avascular necrosis and why?**
In the foot the bones at risk for AVN are the talus and the navicular. The talus is 60% to 70% articular cartilage and has no tendinous attachments. Most of the talar body blood supply enters the undersurface of the talar neck and flows posteriorly. The talus is at particular risk for osteonecrosis with displaced fractures of the talar neck and dislocations of the talar body. The weakened bone of the osteonecrotic segment of the talar dome may then collapse, causing pain and arthritis in the ankle and subtalar joints. In some instances, talar osteonecrotic segments will heal spontaneously over a course of 2 to 3 years in a process known as "creeping substitution," in which the dead bone is resorbed and replaced by live bone. The large articular surface area of the navicular also limits blood supply to the dorsal and plantar aspects. Blood perfusion is diminished to the central third of the navicular. AVN with late partial collapse of the navicular is common in comminuted navicular fractures.

22. **What is a Lisfranc joint injury?**
The Lisfranc joint, or tarsometatarsal joint, consists of the articulations between the five metatarsals, three cuneiforms, and cuboid. Stability is enhanced by the archlike configuration of the joint in the coronal plane and by the dorsal and plantar tarsometatarsal and intermetatarsal ligaments. The recessed second metatarsal base is connected to the medial cuneiform by the important Lisfranc ligament. Most Lisfranc injuries occur by forceful external rotation and pronation of the foot. A fall onto a maximally plantar-flexed foot can cause dorsal displacement of the metatarsals. Direct crushing injuries are less frequent causes of Lisfranc injury. Injury to the Lisfranc ligament results in an increased space between the second metatarsal base and medial cuneiform. Injury to other tarsometatarsal ligaments will cause subluxation of metatarsal bases relative to their respective cuneiforms and cuboid. Additionally, injury to the intercuneiform ligaments can result in instability of these joints as well.

23. **Why are Lisfranc injuries sometimes hard to diagnose?**
The clinician should have a high index of suspicion for a patient who has sustained a foot injury and now has pain, midfoot swelling, and limited ability to bear weight. This patient often has normal nonweight-bearing radiographs. The most important imaging studies to order are bilateral standing foot x-rays. Any increased space between the second metatarsal base and medial cuneiform compared to the normal side is diagnostic of a Lisfranc injury. Plain radiographs may show a fleck sign, which is an avulsed piece of bone between the medial cuneiform and second metatarsal, which is an indication of Lisfranc joint injury. MRI may show Lisfranc ligament injury and has been correlated with Lisfranc joint instability. Stress examination under anesthesia can also be used if studies are inconclusive and Lisfranc instability is suspected.

24. **What are the classification patterns and treatment for Lisfranc injuries?**
Lisfranc injuries are classified into three injury patterns:
- Homolateral—All metatarsals are displaced in the same direction.
- Divergent—Metatarsals are displaced in both sagittal and coronal planes in differing directions.
- Isolated—One or more metatarsals are separated from the remaining Lisfranc complex.

An anatomic reduction is required for the best result. Surgery entails ORIF with fixation across joints using screws and/or bridge plating. This hardware is typically removed at a later date. Despite anatomic reduction some patients will develop arthritis necessitating fusion. Some studies have shown better results with immediate reduction and fusion of the first through third tarsometatarsal joints.

25. **What is a Jones fracture and how is it treated?**
The fifth metatarsal metaphyseal-diaphyseal region is a watershed area of blood supply, which makes this fracture location notorious for delayed union and nonunion. The anatomic location of the fracture determines treatment. A type I fracture involves the tuberosity and extends into the metatarsocuboid joint. A type II fracture (true Jones fracture) extends into the fourth to fifth metatarsal joint. A type III fracture involves the proximal fifth metatarsal shaft and is distal to the fourth to fifth metatarsal joint. Type III fractures may also occur as a stress fracture in athletes. The more the distal the fracture, the greater the risk of nonunion. Type I fractures can be successfully managed in a fracture boot or postoperative shoe for 6 to 8 weeks or until healing occurs.
Type II and III fractures should be managed with a period of nonweight-bearing cast immobilization or immediate intramedullary screw fixation. Recent studies suggest that screw fixation is the preferred treatment for the acute

type II or III fracture in the athlete. Intramedullary screw fixation is also recommended for treatment of delayed union or nonunion of these fractures.

26. **What is Charcot neuroarthropathy and how is it classified?**
A Charcot or neuropathic arthropathy is a process of chronic, noninfective, painless joint destruction. Charcot first described this condition associated with tabes dorsalis in 1868. Approximately 0.1% to 0.5% of diabetic patients will develop a neuroarthropathic joint. Three theories explain the development of a Charcot joint. The neurotraumatic theory states that decreased protective sensation and cumulative mechanical trauma lead to fracture and joint destruction. The neurovascular theory states that a neurally initiated vascular reflex leads to increased resorption by osteoclasts. The inflammatory cytokine theory postulates that elevated levels of alpha tumor necrosis factor and interleukin 1 stimulate osteoclasts to increase bone resorption. Studies have shown increased osteoclastic activity without a concomitant increase in osteoblastic bone formation in the feet of diabetic patients.

The presenting symptoms of a Charcot foot include the spontaneous onset of a warm, swollen foot associated with no pain or vague pain. The midfoot is most commonly involved, followed by the hindfoot and ankle. The midfoot will lose its arch over time as the hindfoot assumes an equinus position and the forefoot dorsiflexes and abducts, producing a rocker-bottom foot deformity. The patient is then predisposed to plantar ulceration over the plantar bony prominence. The Charcot ankle may develop a significant varus or valgus deformity with eventual corresponding pressure ulceration over the prominent malleolus.

Early radiographs may show osteopenia with intact joints. Later radiographs will show fractures, joint subluxation or dislocation, bone destruction, and fragmentation. Eichenholtz described the following clinical and radiographic stages of Charcot joints:

- Stage 0—neuropathic patient with a history of sprain or fracture
- Stage 1—inflammatory stage with edema, hyperemia, erythema, and bone fragmentation on x-ray
- Stage 2—reparative stage with less swelling and erythema; radiographs show new bone formation at site of fracture and dislocation
- Stage 3—consolidation phase with resolution of swelling; radiographs show bony healing of fractures and dislocations

Brodsky (2006) has classified the Charcot foot based on anatomic location. Type 1 involves the tarsometatarsal and naviculocuneiform joints. Type 2 involves the subtalar and/or Chopart joint. Type 3A involves the ankle joint.
Type 3B involves a fracture of the calcaneal tuberosity.

27. **How is Charcot neuroarthropathy diagnosed and treated?**
The key to treatment of the Charcot foot is making the diagnosis. A clinician should have a high index of suspicion for the neuropathic patient with a warm, swollen foot. The acute Charcot foot is warm, erythematous, and swollen, mimicking a diabetic foot infection. Radiographs, bone scans, and MRI scans show findings indistinguishable from osteomyelitis. Charcot patients will typically be afebrile, have a normal white blood cell count, normal C-reactive protein, and normal erythrocyte sedimentation rate. The swelling and erythema in a Charcot foot will usually resolve with bed rest and elevation. A combination three-phase Technetium bone scan and Indium-labeled WBC scan has been shown to have a high sensitivity and specificity rates for differentiating Charcot from infection. A bone biopsy is the definitive test to differentiate Charcot from bone infection in those patients with open wounds and Charcot. The mainstay treatment of Eichenholtz Stage 1 Charcot is a total contact cast. This type of cast incorporates felt padding over the malleoli and tibial crest, unloads plantar prominences with a plastizote insert, and encloses the toes. The cast is changed every 2 to 4 weeks for 2 to 4 months until radiographic healing progresses to Eichenholtz Stage 2. Weight bearing is allowed in the cast. A Charcot restraint orthopedic walker (CROW) boot is an alternative to total contact casting. In Stage III, the patient may progress to walking in an extra depth shoes with custom diabetic inserts. Surgical treatment is reserved for patients with recalcitrant ulceration, unbraceable deformities, acute fractures and dislocations, and infections. Surgery ranges form the simple removal of a bony prominence through plantar exostectomy to extensive midfoot or hindfoot fusion with internal or external fixation.

28. **How are osteochondral talar dome fractures classified?**
Osteochondral talar dome fractures or talar osteochondritis dessicans lesions are believed to be caused by trauma, although idiopathic avascular necrosis may also be a factor. Location in the talar dome is either posteromedial or anterolateral. Most anterolateral lesions are traumatic. Medial lesions may be posttraumatic or idiopathic. The classic Brendt and Harty classification is based on plain radiographic appearance and is most commonly used to classify these lesions:

- Type I—compression of subchondral bone
- Type II—incomplete fracture
- Type III—complete, nondisplaced fracture
- Type IV—completely detached, displaced fragment

These lesions are best evaluated by CT scan or MRI. More recent CT classifications include subchondral cystic lesions in the talar dome.

29. **How are osteochondral talar dome fractures treated?**
Initial treatment is immobilization of nondisplaced acute lesions (types I to III); type IV fractures require surgery. If patients remain symptomatic after a period of immobilization, arthroscopy is indicated. Ankle arthroscopy allows inspection and treatment of the lesion with removal of loose cartilage or bone and drilling of the subchondral bone to stimulate growth of fibrocartilage. In cystic lesions with intact articular cartilage, drilling and bone grafting can be achieved through the talar body. For lesions larger than 10 mm diameter, drilling is inadequate to restore cartilage coverage of the lesion, and osteochondral grafting taken from the ipsilateral femoral condyle or from osteochondral allografts is indicated. Use of juvenile particulate cartilage allograft, adult particulate cartilage allograft, and autologous chondrocyte implantation have also been proposed as treatment options.

30. **What is compartment syndrome of the foot and how is it diagnosed?**
When a foot is subjected to significant blunt trauma, crush injuries, or high-energy fracture, swelling occurs that leads to increased compartment pressure. Pressures greater than 30 to 40 mm Hg for longer than 8 hours result in permanent muscle injury, loss of sensation, and muscle contractures.

The foot has five muscle compartments—medial, central, lateral, interosseous, and calcaneal. Classic signs of compartment syndrome are swelling, pain out of proportion to injury, pain on passive stretch of toes, and paresthesias or sensory loss. Loss of pulse or poor capillary refill is not a sign of compartment syndrome, but of vascular compromise. Definitive diagnosis is made by measurement of compartment pressures using a handheld pressure monitor. Surgical compartment release is accomplished surgically through two longitudinal dorsal forefoot incisions and one medial midfoot incision. Wounds are left open for later secondary closure or skin grafting.

BIBLIOGRAPHY

Adelaar, R. S. (1989). The treatment of complex fractures of the talus. *Orthopedic Clinics of North America, 20*(4), 691–707.

Agren, P. H., Wretenberg, P., & Sayed-Noor, A. S. (2013). Operative versus nonoperative treatment of displaced intraarticular calcaneal fractures. A prospective, randomized, controlled multicenter trial. *Journal of Bone and Joint Surgery (American), 95*(15), 1351–1357.

Al-Shaikh, R. A., Chou, L. B., Mann, J. A., Dreeben, S. M., & Prieskorn, D. (2002). Autologous osteochondral grafting for talar cartilage defects. *Foot & Ankle International, 239*, 381–389.

Arendt, E. A., & Griffiths, H. J. (1997). The use of MR imaging in the assessment and clinical management of stress reactions of bone in high performance athletes. *Clinics in Sports Medicine, 16*(2), 291–306.

Arntz, C. T., Veith, R. G., & Hansen, S. T. (1988). Fractures and fracture dislocations of the tarsometatarsal joint. *Journal of Bone and Joint Surgery, 70*(2), 174.

Böhler, L. (1931). Diagnosis, pathology, and treatment of fractures of the os calcis. *Journal of Bone and Joint. Surgery (American), 13*(1), 75–89.

Boraiah, S., Kemp, T. J., Erwteman, A., Lucas, P. A., & Asprinio, D. E. (2010). Outcome following open reduction and internal fixation of open pilon fractures. *Journal of Bone and Joint Surgery (American), 92*(2), 346–352.

Brodsky, J.W. (2006). The diabetic foot. In M. J. Coughlin, R. A. Mann, & C. L. Saltzman (Eds.). *Surgery of the foot and ankle* (ed 8, p. 1341). St. Louis, MO: Mosby.

Buckley, R., Tough, S., McCormack, R., et al. (2002). Operative compared with nonoperative treatment of displaced intra-articular calcaneal fractures: a prospective, randomized, controlled multicenter trial. *Journal of Bone and Joint Surgery (American), 84*(10), 1733–1744.

Charcot., J. -M. (1868). Sur quelques arthropathies qui paraissant depende d'une lesion du cerveau de la moelle epininiere. *Archives de Physiologie Normale et Pathologique, 1*, 161–178.

Chauhary, S. B., Liporace, F. A., Gandhi, A., Donley, B. G., Pinzur, M. S., & Lin, S. S. (2008). Complications of ankle fracture in patients with diabetes. *Journal of the American Academy of Orthopaedic Surgeons, 16*, 159–170.

Csizy, M., Buckley, R., Tough, S., et al. (2003). Displaced intra-articular calcaneal fractures: Variables predicting late subtalar fusion. *Journal of Orthopaedic Trauma, 17*(2), 106–112.

Den Hartog, B. D. (2009). Fracture of the proximal fifth metatarsal. *Journal of the American Academy of Orthopaedic Surgeons, 17*(7), 458–464.

DiGiovanni, C. W. (2004). Fractures of the navicular. *Foot and Ankle Clinics of North America, 9*, 25–63.

Eisele, S. A., & Sammarco, G. J. (1993). Fatigue fractures of the foot and ankle in the athlete. *Journal of Bone and Joint Surgery, 75*(2), 290–298.

Etter, C., & Ganz, R. (1991). Long term results of tibial plafond fractures treated with open reduction and internal fixation. *Archives of Orthopaedic and Trauma Surgery, 110*, 277–283.

Frawley, P. A., Hart, J. A., & Young, D. A. (1995). Treatment outcome of major fractures of the talus. *Foot & Ankle International, 16*(6), 339–345.

French, B., & Tornetta, P., 3rd (2000). Hybrid external fixation of tibial pilon fractures. *Foot and Ankle Clinics, 5*, 853–871.

Giannini, S., & Vannini, E. (2004). Operative treatment of osteochondral lesions of the talar dome. *Foot and Ankle International, 25*, 168–175.

Gough, A., Abraha, H., Li, F., et al. (1997). Measurement of markers of osteoclast and osteoblast activity in patients with acute and chronic diabetic Charcot neuroarthropathy. *Diabetic Medicine, 14*, 527–531.

Hawkins, L. G. (1970). Fractures of the neck of the talus. *Journal of Bone and Joint Surgery, 52*(5), 991–1002.

Heier, K. A., Infante, A. F., Walling, A. K., et al. (2003). Open fractures of the calcaneus: soft-tissue injury determines outcome. *Journal of Bone and Joint Surgery (American), 85*, 2276–2282.

Khan, K. M., Brukner, P. D., Kearney, C., Fuller, P. J., Bradshaw, C. J., & Kiss, Z. S. (1994). Tarsal navicular stress fracture in Athletes. *Sports Medicine, 17*(1), 65–76.
Lauge-Hansen, N. (1950). Fractures of the ankle: 2. Combined experimental-surgical and experimental-roentgenolgic investigations. *Archives of Surgery, 60,* 957–985.
Lauge-Hansen, N. (1953). Fractures of the ankle: 5. Pronation dorsiflexion fractures. *Archives of Surgery, 67,* 813–820.
Lee, K.B., Byun, J.W., Lee, T.H. (2014). Osteonecrosis of the Talus. In L.B. Chou (Ed.). *Orthopaedic Knowledge Update: Foot and Ankle 5.* Rosemont, IL: American Academy of Orthopaedic Surgeons, pp 283–293.
Lindvall, E., Haidukewych, G., DiPasquale, T., Herscovici, D., Jr., & Sanders, R. (2004). Open reduction and stable internal fixation of isolated, displaced talar neck and body fractures. *Journal of Bone and Joint Surgery (American), 86*(10), 2229–2234.
Ly, T. V., & Coetzee, J. C. (2006). Treatment of primarily ligamentous Lisfranc joint injuries: primary arthrodesis compared with open reduction and internal fixation. A prospective, randomized study. *Journal of Bone and Joint Surgery (American), 88*(3), 514–520.
Manoli, A., II. (1990). Compartment syndromes of the foot: current concepts. *Foot & Ankle, 10,* 340–344.
Myerson, M. S., Fisher, R. T., Burgess, A. R., & Kenzora, J. E. (1986). Fracture dislocations of the tarsometatarsal joints: end results correlated with pathology and treatment. *Foot & Ankle, 6,* 225.
Quill, G. E., Jr. (1995). Fractures of the fifth metatarsal. *Orthopedic Clinics of North America, 26,* 353–361.
Raikin, S. M., Elias, I., Dheer, S., Besser, M. P., Morrison, W. B., & Zoga, A. C. (2009). Prediction of midfoot instability in the subtle Lisfranc injury: comparison of magnetic resonance imaging with intraoperative findings. *Journal of Bone and Joint Surgery (American), 91*(4), 892–899.
Ramsey, P. L., & Hamilton, W. (1976). Changes in tibiotalar area of contact caused by lateral talar shift. *Journal of Bone and Joint Surgery (American), 58*(3), 356–357.
Ruedi, T. P., & Allgower, M. (1969). Fractures of the lower end of the tibia into the ankle joint. *Injury, 1,* 92–99.
Rutledge, E. W., Templeman, D. C., & Souza, L. J. (1999). Evaluation and treatment of Lisfranc fracture-dislocation. *Foot and Ankle Clinics, 4,* 603–615.
Sanders, R. (1992). Intra-articular fractures of the calcaneus: present state of the art. *Journal of Orthopaedic Trauma, 6,* 252–265.
Sandlin, M. I., Charlton, T. P., Taghavi, C. E., & Giza, E. Management of osteochondral lesions of the talus. 1027 AAOS Instructional Course Lectures, Vol. 66, Chap. 23: 293–299.
Sangeorzan, B. J., Benirschke, S. K., Mosca, V., Mayo, K. A., & Hansen, S. T., Jr. (1989). Displaced intra-articular fractures of the tarsal navicular. *Journal of Bone and Joint Surgery (American), 71*(10), 1504–1510.
Stephen, D. (2000). Ankle and foot injuries. In J. F. Kellam, T. J. Fischer, P. Tornetta III, M. J. Bosse, & M. B. Harris (Eds.), *Orthopedic Knowledge update: Trauma* (2, pp. 210). Rosemont, Il: American Academy of Orthopaedic Surgeons.
Torg, J. S., Balduini, F. C., Zelko, R. R., Pavlov, H., Peff, T. C., & Das, M. (1984). Fractures of the base of the fifth metatarsal distal to the tuberosity: classification and guideline for non-surgical management. *Journal of Bone and Joint Surgery (American), 66,* 209–214.
Tornetta, P., & Silver, S. (1999). Calcaneal fractures. *Foot and Ankle Clinics, 4,* 571–585.
Vallier, H. A., Reichard, S. G., Alysse, J. B., & Moore, T. A. (2014). A new look at the Hawkins classification for talar neck fractures: which features of injury and treatment are predictive of osteonecrosis? *Journal of Bone and Joint Surgery (American), 96*(3), 192–197.
van der Ven, A., Chapman, C. B., & Bowker, J. H. (2009). Charcot neuroarthropathy of the foot and ankle. *Journal of the American Academy of Orthopaedic Surgeons, 17,* 562–571.
Wiersema, B., Brokaw, D., Weber, T., et al. (2011). Complications associated with open calcaneus fractures. *Foot & Ankle International, 32*(11), 1052–1057.
Wukich, D. K., & Kline, A. J. (2008). The management of ankle fractures in patients with diabetes. *Journal of Bone and Joint Surgery (American), 90*(7), 1570–1578.
Zhang, T., Su, Y., Chen, W., Zhang, Q., Wu, Z., & Zhang, Y. (2014). Displaced intra-articular calcaneal fracture treated in a minimally invasive fashion. Longitudinal approach versus sinus tarsi approach. *Journal of Bone and Joint Surgery (American), 96*(4), 302–309.

CHAPTER 78 QUESTIONS

1. **Why do ankle fractures in poorly controlled diabetic patients have poorer outcomes than nondiabetic patients?**
   a. Wound healing in diabetic patients is compromised.
   b. Diabetics with neuropathy are more likely to be noncompliant and walk on their injured extremity against medical advice.
   c. Infection rates are higher in diabetic patients.
   d. All of the above

2. **Which of the following bones in the foot and ankle are not prone to nonunion?**
   a. Lateral malleolus
   b. Talus
   c. Navicular
   d. Fifth metatarsal base

3. **A diabetic patient with numb feet presents to the ER with a minimally painful, warm, swollen, red foot. Foot radiographs show severely displaced fracture dislocations of the Lisfranc joint. The skin is intact. The patient is afebrile and has a normal leukocyte count. When the patient is placed at bed rest with the foot elevated, the swelling and erythema both improve. The most likely diagnosis is:**
   a. Osteomyelitis of the midfoot
   b. A destructive neoplasm of the midfoot

c. Gangrene of the foot
d. Charcot arthropathy, or neuropathic arthropathy, of the midfoot

4. **A pole vaulter complains of the insidious onset of atraumatic anterior ankle pain and dorsal midfoot pain. He has not responded to rest or physical therapy. He cannot comfortably hop on his painful extremity. Foot radiographs are normal. He has pain over the N spot. Which of the following statements are false?**
   a. An MRI is the imaging modality of choice to diagnose his problem.
   b. His injured bone is at risk for nonunion.
   c. He may require nonweight-bearing short leg cast immobilization.
   d. He may require screw fixation of the injured bone.
   e. Weight bearing as tolerated in a fracture boot is appropriate treatment.

5. **A football lineman sustains a twisting injury during practice. He has pain and swelling over his midfoot. He has difficulty bearing weight on his injured foot. Initial nonweight-bearing radiographs are normal. He has pain over the second metatarsal base. What is the most important thing to do next?**
   a. Start immediate range of motion and strengthening exercises in physical therapy.
   b. Obtain bilateral standing foot radiographs.
   c. Return the patient to practice on a limited schedule.
   d. Start dry needling of the midfoot.
   e. Refer the patient for immediate surgery.

FOOT BIOMECHANICS, ORTHOSES, AND SHOE DESIGN

J.A. Bailey, PT, DPT, OCS, CSCS, CPed

1. **Define the subtalar neutral position. Why is it important?**
   The subtalar neutral position is the position in which the head of the talus is aligned with the navicular. Radiographically, it is defined as the position where the joint lines of the talonavicular joint and the calcaneocuboid joint are continuous. The subtalar joint neutral position is used by clinicians to evaluate the amount of pronation and supination on either side of neutral position. This position is used to assess the foot for structural deformities. Subtalar neutral position also is used during weight-bearing assessment to evaluate foot structure and to determine how far from neutral the patient is functioning. It is considered to be best practice for a foot to be maintained in the subtalar joint neutral position while casting for most types of foot orthoses.

2. **How is subtalar neutral position determined?**
   Other than radiographic analysis, there are two common clinical methods: (1) Divide the total amount of heel eversion (pronation) and inversion (supination) into thirds. The position is found by positioning the rearfoot in a position that is one third from maximal pronation or two thirds from maximal supination. (2) Palpate "congruency" at the talonavicular joint. This procedure is based on creating the talonavicular alignment described above. The head of the talus is palpated on its medial and lateral aspects. Then the foot is moved between a pronated and a supinated position until the examiner feels talonavicular alignment or "congruency." It has been purported that the talonavicular and subtalar joints are at maximal congruency at the same times during passive range of motion assessment (Elveru et al., 1988).

3. **How reliable and valid are these methods?**
   Concerns have been raised about the validity of the first method noted above (Smith-Orrichio & Harris, 1990). The validity has been questioned secondary to variability of the subtalar joint's axis of inclination. For the second method, the interrater reliability is poor to moderate. Intrarater reliability is much higher and may allow each clinician to develop a repeatable method for his or her own use. The reliability of the second method appears to be positively related to examiner experience.

4. **What is the primary goal of a foot orthosis?**
   The common goal of most orthotics would be to improve the overall function of the foot/feet. Functionally, foot orthoses are often utilized to facilitate and normalize the speed and magnitude of motion about the subtalar joint and midtarsal joints during gait (Michaund, 1993). They are used, in this format, to facilitate more normal amounts of pronation during the initial part of stance and supination during the latter part of stance. A recent meta-analysis demonstrated that there is notable evidence that indicates that specifically molded orthotics can be utilized to decrease loading rates and vertical impact forces.

5. **Does the subtalar joint function around neutral position?**
   This well-accepted principle of foot function has been questioned as a result of continued research in human locomotion. Two independent research groups found that the subtalar joint demonstrates the predicted pronation/supination pattern but usually functions in a pronated position. Pierrynowski and Smith, 1996 found that the subtalar joint usually was pronated during stance. During stance the "normal" foot is pronated (position) but is supinating (motion) for a longer period of time during the gait cycle. McPoil and Cornwall, 1994 demonstrated that the subtalar joint did not reach a supinated position before heel rise and that it had a tendency to function around the relaxed standing position. These findings may indicate that the total arc of motion and the speed of such motion may be of greater importance than the position. Despite this evidence, the principle of assessing the cause of abnormal motion and reducing the amount and speed of motion has not changed.

6. **Do orthotics control motion?**
   Many studies demonstrate no effect, whereas others document significant reduction in subtalar joint motion. Possible reasons for contradictory findings are errors in methodology, measurement of shoe motion instead of bone motion, measurement of skin over bone versus actual bone or joint motion, differences in the composition and type of orthoses, lack of specific orthotic prescription, and the patient's need for foot orthoses based on foot structure. The last factor is extremely important. If a patient has no need for foot orthoses and is functioning optimally, it is unreasonable to anticipate notable improvement. Several studies have demonstrated that the effects of medially posted foot orthoses on reducing motion were "small" and "subject specific." Orthotic

specificity requirements render randomized clinical trials difficult to manage, at best. It has been demonstrated that anti-pronation devices fabricated with both rearfoot and forefoot varus posting have the greatest positive effects.

7. **How do foot orthoses control motion?**
Motion at the subtalar joint occurs in all three cardinal planes but primarily in the frontal and transverse planes. The amount of motion expected in these planes can vary depending on the subtalar joint's axis of inclination, which ranges from 20 degrees to as much as 70 degrees. Since pronation and supination are motions occurring in all three cardinal planes simultaneously, controlling motions in either the frontal or transverse planes will reduce the total amount of motion. For this reason, a medial (varus) motion, which reduces the amount of eversion in the frontal plane, also reduces the motions in the other planes.

8. **When can a foot orthosis be utilized to "increase" motion?**
When a patient has a rigid forefoot valgus or similar dysfunction, pronation of the subtalar joint may be blocked when the medial side of the forefoot contacts the ground. A foot orthosis that includes a forefoot valgus post allows proper lateral-to-medial loading of the forefoot, minimizing the supinatory moment of the forefoot valgus. This allows the subtalar joint to pronate in a more normal fashion.

9. **Why do orthotics function better in the clinical setting than a research setting?**
Elimination of symptoms requires a reduction of the stress on the symptomatic tissue. Stress may result from the amount, speed, or timing of subtalar and/or midtarsal joint(s) motion. Alteration in any of these variables may reduce the stress below the symptomatic threshold or to a level that allows healing. The studies that demonstrate the greatest effect of orthoses are performed with patients instead of subjects. If foot orthoses are designed for a specific patient, considering the function of the entire lower extremity as well as foot structure, the chance for resolution of symptoms is maximized.

10. **Does exercise prescription provide an added benefit to foot orthoses application?**
Exercise involving the proximal joints of the lower extremity, as well as trunk, have been employed to treat symptoms caused by excessive tissue stress. Clinical judgments regarding the magnitude of dysfunction must be made to determine whether to use exercises alone, foot orthoses only, or both in providing the most efficacious care to patients. Consider the thought that a foot that excessively pronates will develop a morphologically shortened Achilles tendon and a shortened Achilles tendon will produce an increase in speed and/or magnitude of overpronation. Thus, it is critical to ensure that a patient has adequate available dorsiflexion prior to the application of foot orthotics. Often, static stretching or dynamic stretching should be employed to achieve maximal clinical results.

11. **Are there any clinical tests that, if positive, suggest that a patient requires foot orthoses?**
The rotary stability (or pronation/supination test) is a test that can be used to determine if orthotic intervention is needed. The patient stands and is asked to rotate the trunk in the transverse plane as far as possible. This trunk rotation should cause a reaction at the Subtalar joint (STJ). When the trunk is rotated to the right, the right STJ should supinate and the left STJ should pronate. If the foot does not react, it most likely indicates that the feet are impacting lower extremity function, and an orthotic may be required. The use of foot orthoses is not precluded if the feet do react. There are other functional tests such as a heel rise test, maximum pronation test, or the foot function index that may indicate further biomechanical assessment is indicated but they do not necessarily predict the need for orthotic intervention.

12. **What is the significance of heel eversion in a relaxed standing position?**
Eversion of the calcaneus well past a vertical position indicates that the rearfoot is compensating for another structure because the calcaneus is resting in a less-than-optimal position for its own stability. Reasons include eversion to bring a forefoot varus deformity to the ground, compensation for a severely tight calf group by pronating to unlock the MTJ, functional shortening of a long leg, and transverse plane problems in the spine, pelvis, and hip that cause the leg to rotate internally.

13. **Why do some patients stand with most of the weight on the outside of the feet?**
The patient may be in a supinated position to compensate for a rigid forefoot valgus, partially compensated rearfoot varus, or uncompensated rearfoot varus. The subtalar joint may also be volitionally held supinated to avoid pain (eg, heel pain syndrome). However, the foot may not actually be supinated because a foot with cavus architecture looks similar. To distinguish between supinated position of the subtalar joint and architecture, place the subtalar joint in a neutral position and assess the compensation from neutral to relaxed position.

14. **To allow for the use of a wider variety of shoes, does it make more sense to fabricate smaller orthoses?**
It is generally accepted that the larger depth, width, and length of an orthotic will produce more control. Conversely, a shallow, narrow, and short device will allow for lesser levels of motion control. Although less bulky devices are convenient, they often produce less effect.

15. **In what situation does the heel evert very little while the STJ pronates excessively?**
In patients with a more vertical inclination of the subtalar joint axis, the frontal plane component (eversion) decreases and the transverse plane (abduction) component of pronation increases. Because clinicians usually assess and measure only the frontal plane component, the amount of subtalar joint pronation is often underestimated. In addition, feet with a compensated rearfoot varus deformity typically pronate excessively to reach the supporting surface. Although notable pronation has occurred, this is similarly underestimated as the foot appears very normal in weight bearing. In many cases, these types of feet require more rearfoot varus posting than indicated by minimal heel eversion. A deep heel on the orthotic shell also may enhance control of the predominantly transverse plane motion.

16. **Why does a rearfoot with a varus position fail to pronate at the STJ during weight bearing?**
Ligamentous structures, osseous structures, or pathology such as arthrofibrosis may restrict the STJ motion (Tiberio, 1988). A rigid forefoot valgus may prevent use of available pronation. In addition, a patient with pain or limited hip internal rotation may voluntarily prevent pronation. Given that pronation is a necessary and expected motion, loss of adequate pronation can be dysfunctional and lend to poor shock attenuation.

17. **With restricted calcaneal motion caused by limited STJ pronation, would there ever be a case for posting the heel medially?**
Using a medial (varus) wedge when there is insufficient pronation would seem to be contraindicated. However, the patient may develop symptoms at end range or may avoid end range by voluntarily limiting pronation. In these cases, a medial wedge that prevents the STJ from reaching end range but does not limit the beneficial pronation can be very effective at eliminating symptoms. There is some evidence that utilizing a softer compound, total contact shell is also beneficial in these cases.

18. **Can a foot that pronates excessively still lack enough pronation?**
When a foot has a large forefoot and/or rearfoot varus deformity, all the motion available may be used just to get the foot to the ground. During locomotion this would be seen as excessive pronation. With the foot on the ground, any attempt to pronate further, for example, in order to jump, would be blocked. For the function of jumping, this abnormally pronated foot does not have enough available motion to allow for additional pronation. This is detrimental as the foot is functioning at end range during high demand activities.

19. **Can a foot that relaxes close to STJ neutral be abnormal and require orthotic intervention?**
A foot that has a rearfoot varus and a rigid forefoot valgus has a tendency to relax in STJ neutral position during weight bearing. The rearfoot varus wants the STJ to pronate, but the forefoot valgus does not allow pronation. Orthotic posting is required in the rearfoot and forefoot for normal functioning during gait. Specifically, an orthosis with a rearoot varus post and a forefoot valgus post is indicated. The forefoot valgus post allows more normal pronation, but the rearfoot varus post prevents excessive pronation.

20. **What is the difference between forefoot varus and forefoot supinatus?**
Traditionally, forefoot varus is described as a single-plane (inversion) bony deformity, whereas forefoot supinatus is described as a triplanar soft tissue contracture. Assessment of joint mobility and symmetry of motion may distinguish between the two conditions. The orthotic treatment differs because the soft tissue supinatus may resolve, but the varus will not (Tiberio, 1988).

21. **Are posting strategies different in children?**
Most children pronate more than adults (Astrom & Arvidson, 1995). As the calcaneus and talus endure developmental derotations, the pronation decreases. In designing orthoses for children with rearfoot and forefoot varus deformities, it is likely better to post the rearfoot more aggressively and to use smaller forefoot posts in the hope that the forefoot varus will decrease. Except for special circumstances, the concept of treating the cause of the pronation does not change. It is important to note that the smaller mass of a child produces much lower ground reaction forces than an adult. For this reason, many children can be treated with a modifiable over-the-counter device versus a custom-made orthotic.

22. **What is the role of the arch of the orthotic shell?**
The arch of the shell plays an important role in capturing the inclination angle of the calcaneus, to control the amount of mobility at the talonavicular articulation, and to capture the architecture of the foot to optimize the

effects of corrective posts. There is some evidence that suggests an orthotic shell that is total contact in nature controls the speed of foot motion more effectively (Janisse, 1988). In most patients, the decrease in arch height is not the cause of pronation but rather a result of STJ and midtarsal joint pronation. If the shell is used as the primary corrective component, it may need to be fabricated from a more flexible material to be tolerated by the patient.

23. **What is an extended forefoot post and when is it indicated?**
In most orthoses, the shell ends behind the metatarsal heads. Therefore, the forefoot posting exerts its influence on the metatarsal shafts. Some orthoses are fabricated with a flexible post that extends under the metatarsal heads, often called a runner's wedge or a foot post to the sulcus. This type of post may be more effective because it exerts its influence directly under the metatarsal heads. This also places correction further under the forefoot, which can prevent pronation late into the stance phases when ground reaction forces are higher. A primary limitation of this orthotic feature is that the orthotic has more bulk and thus is more difficult to fit into certain types of shoes.

24. **How does function improve with a first ray cut-out?**
Propulsion occurs off the medial side of the foot. As much as 60% to 70% of forefoot stresses are through the first ray. As the heel rises from the ground, the first metatarsophalangeal (MTP) joint dorsiflexes (up to 70 degrees). The first metatarsal must plantar flex to allow normal MTP dorsiflexion. If the patient has a rigid plantar-flexed first ray, excessive weight bearing under the first metatarsal head may prevent the typical plantar flexion of the first metatarsal that would occur with great toe extension during terminal stance. The first ray cut-out increases weight bearing under the second metatarsal head and provides room for requisite plantar flexion of the first metatarsal.

25. **What is more important in orthotic fabrication: material selection, posting, or specific contouring of the device?**
Although there is evidence that suggests that both custom molding a device to the contours of a patient's foot and posting are both effective strategies for fabrication, Mündermann et al, suggest a total contact design may be the most effective component. There is some evidence that suggests that more rigid devices do not necessarily provide greater levels of control. Device rigidity is likely a factor of patient tolerance and comfort.

26. **What are the pros and cons for intrinsic posting in an orthotic?**
The greatest benefit of fabricating an intrinsic post is that it can reduce the overall bulk of the orthotic, which in turn may allow the orthotic to be used in a larger variety of shoes. Some limitations include greater levels of skill required during the fabrication process, loss of total contact of the shell, and inability to easily modify the device.

27. **Why is it so important to address ankle mobility when applying orthotics to treatment overpronation?**
Many patients with severe pronation gradually acquire a morphological shortening of the calf muscles producing a loss of dorsiflexion at the talocrural joint. Dorsiflexion at the MTJ (the lateral aspect) compensates for loss of ankle dorsiflexion as the oblique midtarsal joint moves in exactly the same planes as the TC joint. One objective of the orthosis is to stabilize the MTJ. When walking with the orthosis, a patient that lacks sufficient ankle dorsiflexion may attempt to pronate on top of the orthosis, producing the feeling of sliding laterally (transverse plane movement) as well as producing a complaint of an increase in local arch pressure. This compensation may also cause blisters under the shaft of the first metatarsal. These symptoms are common when a foot orthosis has been applied but normal TC mobility has not been restored.

28. **Why should the midtarsal joint be considered when designing an orthosis?**
Motion between the rearfoot and forefoot occurs at the MTJ. The ability of the MTJ to compensate for surface irregularities, foot deformities, and orthotic posts depends on the amount of available motion. The amount of available motion is a function of the position of the STJ and general flexibility characteristics. Midtarsal joint mobility may influence the magnitude of both rearfoot and forefoot posts, depending on the particular posting strategies of individual clinicians.

29. **How many miles can a running shoe sustain?**
Generally, the average running shoe is built for a male to weigh approximately 185 pounds and a female to weigh approximately 150 pounds. Given these averages, midsoles predominately made of EVA will last approximately 400 miles. In recent years, many shoe manufacturers have reduced the amount of EVA in the midsoles and replaced this material with neocomposites that are possibility longer lasting.

30. **How can orthotics relieve symptoms of a Morton's neuroma?**
The first metatarsal is purported to bear 60% to 70% of the weight at toe-off in the gait cycle. With excessive or abnormal pronation at toe-off, the hallux assumes a more dorsiflexed position and the lesser metatarsals bear

more weight than they are designed to sustain. Relative varus of the forefoot causes excessive STJ pronation at toe-off, thus creating a mobile lever at push-off instead of a rigid lever. Thus, the medial longitudinal and transverse arches of the foot are compromised, causing compression, and shearing of the interdigital nerves. The most severely compromised area is the third metatarsal interspace, where the medial and lateral plantar nerves converge. A biomechanical orthosis addresses the faulty mechanics, and a metatarsal pad placed proximal to the involved metatarsal heads elevates the metatarsal shafts, reducing stress to the interdigital nerves. The apex of the metatarsal pad should be placed between the affected metatarsals or slightly more proximal (1–1.5 cm).

31. **What is the function of an external metatarsal or rocker bar?**
The function of the metatarsal bar is to delay and decrease loading of the metatarsal heads during gait as well as to decrease early MTP joint extension as the foot moves from midstance to toe-off. The bar is placed at an apex point proximal to all five metatarsal heads and thus shifts foot pressure proximally. External metatarsal bars significantly change the dynamics of the gait cycle and require increased patient balance; therefore, they should be used only as a secondary treatment option.

32. **List common problems with foot orthotics and their possible causes.**
    - Arch pain or blisters on plantar foot surface—Probably the arch or medial posting is too high and needs to be lowered, or the patient did not follow the break-in procedure of increasing wear by 1 hour per day for a 2-week period. This is also a common symptom when the patient lacks appropriate levels of DF and compensation is occurring through the oblique midtarsal joint.
    - Sensation of rolling to the outside of the foot—This sometimes may be normal because the medial longitudinal arch is not accustomed to weight bearing. This symptom will commonly resolve without intervention within the first few weeks. However, it also may indicate that the medial post is too high, that the orthotic shell is too rigid for the patient's foot type or body weight.
    - Sensation that the heel is coming out of the shoe—Wearing a shoe that has a low throat and heel quarter or using an orthotic that is too thick or slick may cause this sensation.
    - Symptoms persist—Reevaluate biomechanics and determine whether more correction is necessary.
    - Pain or blisters under metatarsal heads—Ensure that all rigid shell materials end slightly proximal to the metatarsal heads.

33. **Are injury rates reduced with minimalist shoes?**
Not necessarily. Running barefooted may potentially reduce running injury. However, running barefooted and wearing a minimalist shoe are not the same. Barefoot running may produce a forefoot strike pattern. Forefoot striking during running has been demonstrated to decrease torques at the knee as well as vertical impact forces. The evidence is inconsistent that minimalist shoes will produce or alter a forefoot strike pattern. Those who are prone to injuries or symptoms in the forefoot or Achilles tendon are not likely to tolerate barefoot running or the use of a minimalist shoe. There is mounting evidence that run training or instruction may be more correlated with positive results than shoe selection.

34. **What effects do wearing high-heeled shoes have on the body?**
In a normal standing position, approximately 50% of the weight is borne by the rearfoot and 50% by the forefoot. A 2-inch heel results in a significant change in normal weight distribution (10% rearfoot and 90% forefoot). With a flat-soled shoe, the angle between the body's weight line and the horizontal is 90 degrees. With a 2-inch heel, the angle is changed to 70 degrees. Thus, the body must compensate by changing joint position and muscle functions of the feet, ankles, hips, and spine to maintain erect position. Furthermore, a 2-inch heel tilts the pelvis forward 20 degrees. High-heeled shoes also force the knees to stay in relative knee flexion throughout the gait cycle. Chronic wearing of high-heeled shoes causes shortening of the Achilles tendon, reduces normal heel-to-toe gait pattern, and necessitates muscle and joint compensations of the lower quadrant.

35. **How should the shoe wear patterns be assessed?**
A normal sole is worn just laterally to the center of the heel, bisecting the sole and running medially toward the ball and great toe of the foot. Check the heel first to see that it is worn slightly lateral off center, indicating that the heel is supinated at heel strike. Next check the counter, making sure that it is firm and positioned perpendicular to the sole and has not migrated medially or laterally. A medially migrated counter or one that leans inward may indicate increased pronation during gait. Check the stability and flexibility of the sole by grasping the shoe from heel and toe; then twist and bend the shoe. The normal shoe should provide stability through the midfoot and shank area but flexibility at the toe break and forefoot. The front quarters should have a slight crease from the first MTP to the fifth MTP. An oblique crease may indicate a shoe that is too long or a condition such as hallux rigidus. The front quarter also should be perpendicular to the sole without medial or lateral migration. A front quarter that has migrated laterally is also an indication of an increased pronation response as the foot excessively abducts in the transverse plane. Finally, check the arch and midsole to make sure that the arch of the foot is not collapsing over the sole.

36. **How do you properly fit a shoe?**
    - Fit a shoe only after you have been active or at the end of the day so that your foot size and shape are typical. This is when the foot is at its largest as well.
    - Allow one half an inch between the longest toe and the end of the toe box to ensure proper toe-off without jamming of the toes into the toe box of the shoe.
    - The widest part of the shoe should coincide with the widest part of the forefoot.
    - The shoe should be snug along the instep; therefore, the dimensions from the heel to the ball of the foot and the shoe instep should be equal.
    - The quarter, vamp, and toe box of the shoe should not gap or fold excessively.
    - The heel counter should be rigid and should fit snugly around the heel of the foot, limiting excessive heel motion and slippage. Allow space for only one finger to slip beside the calcaneus and the heel counter of the shoe.
    - When standing in the shoe, perform a pinch test at the fifth metatarsal head. You should be able to slightly pucker the material, indicating that there is adequate width.
    - Purchase a shoe that was designed for your foot type and that is immediately comfortable. Do not try to "break in" your shoes.

    A normal foot lengthens and widens with age, so assessing shoe fit routinely is critical.

37. **What is the leading cause of diabetic foot ulcers? What are the appropriate recommendations for therapeutic footwear?**

    Most diabetic ulcers result from peripheral neuropathy, which leads to an insensate foot. The insensate foot is unable to recognize increased shear and pressure forces that cause skin breakdown and ulceration. Skin breakdown is most common over the bony prominences of the metatarsal heads, which bear most of the weight during walking. Once the ulcer has healed, therapeutic shoe wear is essential to prevent recurrence. Patients who return to normal footwear have a recurrence rate of 90%, whereas those who use modified shoes and orthosis have a recurrence rate of 15% to 20%. Therapeutic footwear should fulfill the following objectives:
    - Redistribute and relieve high-pressure areas by using an accommodative total contact orthosis.
    - Provide shock absorption by decreasing vertical load forces.
    - Reduce shear by decreasing horizontal movement of the foot in the shoe.
    - Accommodate deformities such as loss of fatty tissue or ligamentous support.
    - Stabilize and support flexible deformities toward a more normal or neutral position while accommodating rigid deformities.
    - Reduce painful joint motion or stress.

38. **What is a last?**

    A last is a three-dimensional positive model or mold from which the upper and lower aspects of the shoe are constructed. There are three basic last types: a straight last, a standard last, and an inwardly curved last. The forefoot and rearfoot are in neutral alignment with a straight last, whereas a curved last is angled medially at the forefoot. In general, the straighter the last, the greater the stability and control the shoe will have; the curved last is more mobile during the gait cycle. The mechanism by which lasts is constructed has changed dramatically over time. Initially, most lasts were made of wood. Presently, nearly all 3D models are printed. Lasts may vary significantly from one brand of shoe to another.

39. **Describe the anatomy and construction of the shoe.**

    The upper portion of the shoe includes the quarter, counter, vamp, throat, toe box, and top lining. The quarter is a horseshoe-shaped material that cradles the heel of the foot. The counter is a rigid piece of material surrounding the heel posteriorly to stabilize motion. Shoes often include an extended medial heel counter to limit midfoot motion in the overpronator. The vamp is the portion of the shoes that covers the dorsum of the foot to the upper ball of the foot. The throat is the line that connects the proximal portion of the vamp and distal portion of the quarter. The two most common styles are Blucher and Balmoral. The Blucher style is designed for a wider forefoot; the front edges of the quarter are placed on top of the vamp and not sewn together, yielding more room at the throat and instep. In the Balmoral style, the quarter panels are sewn together on the back edge of the vamp. The toe box then covers the end of the toes and refers to the depth of the toe region Figure.

    The sole of the shoe includes the outsole, midsole, innersole, and shankpiece. The outsole is the portion of the shoe that contacts the ground. Important outsole properties should include stability, flexibility, durability, and traction. The outsole is made of various materials, depending on the function of the shoe. Outsoles are typically made of leather or a synthetic material. Shankpieces are commonly used in dress and orthopedic shoes to provide rigidity to the midsection of the shoe. The shankpiece helps to reduce the twisting or torsion of the forefoot in relation to the rearfoot as well as provides support for the midfoot region. The shank refers to the portion of the shoe from the heel to the metatarsal heads. In athletic shoes, the midsole replaces the use of the shank. The midsole is made of differing materials, depending on individual needs. For example, the overpronator may benefit from an athletic shoe that uses a dual-density midsole. A dual-density midsole uses a softer durometer material

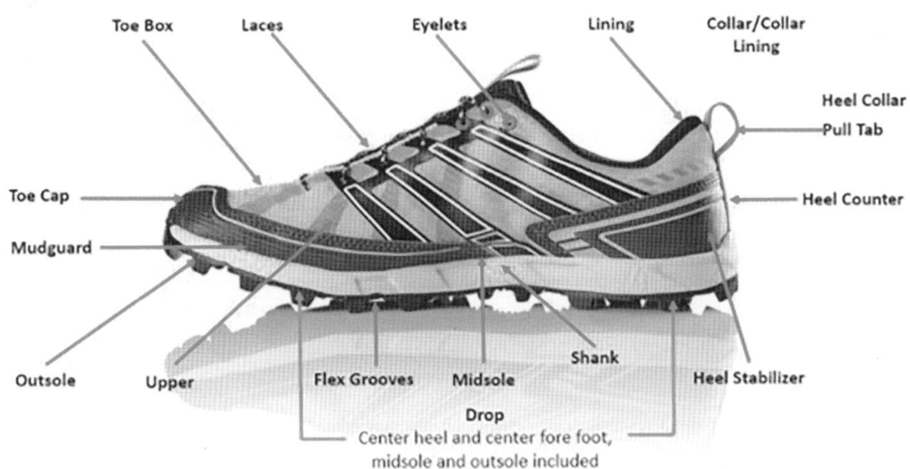

on the lateral side to decrease the lever arm ground reaction forces at heel strike and decrease the rate of pronation. The medial side of the midsole is made of a more dense or firmer durometer material to decrease the magnitude of pronation. The innersole attaches the upper part of the shoe to the soling and acts as a smooth filler for the foot to rest upon.

40. **What is driving the trend toward maximalist shoes as compared to minimalist shoes?**
Minimalist shoes flooded the market from 2010 to 2015. With this time of increase in sales there was also some weak evidence that there would be a correlated reduction in injury. This type of evidence was largely not consistency produced and the Minimalist philosophy slowly faded. From 2016 to 2021, there has been a growing level of affection for maximalist shoes. Maximalist shoes generally have midsole thicknesses greater than 30 mm. Over time, these shoes have become more stable and offer higher levels of shock absorption. There is a small amount of data that even suggest that Maximalist shoes produce higher levels of efficiency while running. The softer feel of the shoe and limited alterations to running strides continue to make them a popular choice among runners.

41. **What is a rocker sole?**
A rocker sole is used to facilitate a heel-to-toe gait pattern while reducing the proportion of internal energy of the foot and ankle for the gait cycle. The toe of the shoe is curved upward to simulate dorsiflexion and allow the metatarsal heads to move through a decreased range of motion at toe-off. Ground reaction forces also are reduced on the ankle because the take-off point is moved posteriorly. In addition, a rocker sole may be used to reduce pressure on specific areas of the foot, such as the heel, midfoot, metatarsals, and toes. Two of the more common types of rocker soles include the forefoot rocker sole and the heel-to-toe rocker sole. A forefoot rocker sole reduces shock at toe-off by placing the apex of the rocker sole just proximal to the metatarsal heads. A forefoot rocker provides stability at midstance but unloads the forefoot at toe-off. A heel-to-toe rocker sole uses a rocker at both the posterior aspect of the heel and just proximal to the metatarsal heads. This type of rocker sole is able to dissipate ground reaction forces at heel strike and increase propulsion at toe-off.

42. **What mechanisms can be used to capture an impression of the patient's foot to fabricate an orthotic?**
There are five basic approaches that one might capture an impression of the patient's foot. These types include suspension slipper casting with plaster, foam crush boxes, digital scanning of the foot, tracings of the foot (manually or with a digital photograph), and wax impressions. Wax impressions are, by far, the least common. The gold standard approach is considered to be negative suspension slipper plaster casting with the foot in a subtalar neutral position. This may be performed in either prone or supine positions with equal results. Foam crush boxes can be utilized effectively, specifically for more rigid foot types. The quality of digital impression, captured by a scanner, is highly variable.

43. **What are the proposed mechanisms by which a foot orthotic has a positive effect on pain and function in patients with patellofemoral knee pain?**
Some of the most common theories on how foot orthotics decrease knee pain and increase function in patients with patellofemoral knee pain include the following: (1) reduction of lower limb internal rotation; (2) reduction in Q-angle; (3) decrease in laterally directed soft tissue tension forces of the vastus lateralis, iliotibial band, and patellar tendon; and (4) reduction in lateral patellofemoral contact forces. There could be an argument made that a reduction in shock absorption requirements at the knee would also be beneficial to the anterior knee pain.

44. **Does the prophylactic use of a foot orthotic reduce the incidence of lower limb stress reactions in younger, active adults?**
It appears the use of a shock-absorbing orthotic can reduce the incidence of lower limb stress reactions, especially in military recruits. The best outcomes are associated with a total contact shell and rearfoot and forefoot posting as indicated. As far as over-the-counter products, comfort seems to be the most important variable. The use of a shock-absorbing orthotic as a preventative measure may be a wise choice for those participating in activities that often cause stress reactions of the lower limbs (e.g., running, walking—especially in boots).

45. **Does the type of prophylactic foot orthosis have any effect on the incidence of lower limb overuse injuries?**
The limited research in this area suggests that there is not a significant difference in overuse injury rates based on the type of orthotic used (soft custom, soft prefabricated, semirigid biomechanical, and semirigid prefabricated). Because there is no significant difference between the various types of orthotics, clinical judgment is likely the key deciding factor. Due to methodological issues within the research, and often-small sample sizes definitive conclusions are unable to be drawn.

46. **Are laterally wedged orthotics helpful to patients with medial knee osteoarthritis?**
Yes, there appears to be strong evidence to suggest that treating symptomatic medial compartment DJD of the knee with laterally wedged insoles can be effective in reducing pain. A laterally wedged orthotic would likely have a greater overall outcome than a lateral heel wedge alone (Marks & Penton, 2004). The magnitude of heel wedge should not exceed the total amount of eversion motion available passively.

47. **Do lacing pattern produce functional changes in running shoes?**
There is moderate evidence to support that lacing patterns can impact how the foot moves within the shoe (Fuller, 1994). The evidence suggests that certain lacing techniques may assist in the reduction in the speed and magnitude of pronation (Hagen & Hennig, 2009) (Figure).

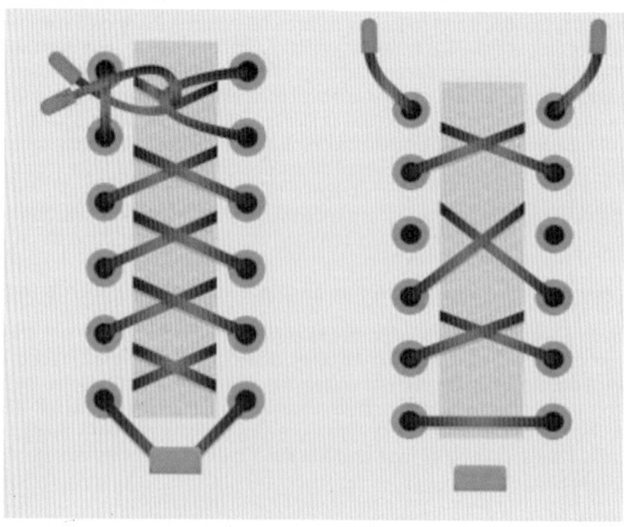

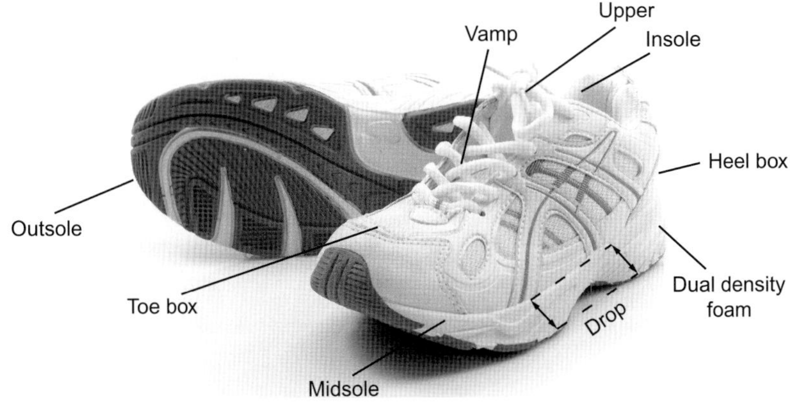

48. What is the main difference between hiking shoes and other shoes utilized for sport or recreation?

Hiking shoes or boots historically have a rock plate within the midsole. This rock plate is typically made of polyurethane or carbon fiber and designed to protect the foot in event that one steps on a sharp rock. This improves the comfort as well as tolerance to hiking on even or difficult terrain. Additionally, the rock plate adds torsional control, which can be a useful choice for unstable feet.

Bibliography

Astrom, M., & Arvidson, T. (1995). Alignment and joint motion in the normal foot. *Journal of Orthopedic and Sports Physical Therapy, 22*(5), 216–222.

Barton, C. J., Bonanno, D., & Menz, H. B. (2009). Development and evaluation of a tool for the assessment of footwear characteristics. *Journal of Foot and Ankle Research, 2*, 10.

Baxter, M. L., Ribeiro, D. C., & Milsavijevic, S. (2012). Do orthotics work as an injury prevention strategy for the military? *Physical Therapy Review, 17*, 241–251.

Bonacci, J., Saunders, P. U., Hicks, A., Rantalainen, T., Vicenzino, B. G. T., & Spratford, W. (2012). Running in a minimalist and lightweight shoe is not the same as running barefoot: A biomechanical study. *British Journal of Sports Medicine, 10*, 1136.

Crawford, F., & Thomson, C. (2005). Interventions for treating plantar heel pain. *Cochrane Database of Systematic Reviews, 3*, CD003674.

D'hondt, N. E., Struijs, P. A., Kerkhoffs, G. M., et al. (2002). Orthotic devices for treating patellofemoral pain syndrome. *Cochrane Database of Systematic Reviews* CD002267.

Ekenman, I., Milgrom, C., Finestone, A., et al. (2002). The role of biomechanical shoe orthoses in tibial stress fracture prevention. *American Journal of Sports Medicine, 30*, 866–870.

Eng, J. J., & Pierrynowski, M. (1993). Evaluation of soft foot orthotics in the treatment of patellofemoral pain syndrome. *Physical Therapy, 73*, 62–68.

Elveru, R. A., Rothstein, J. M., Lamb, R. L., & Riddle, D. L. (1988). Methods for taking subtalar joint measurements: A clinical report. *Physical Therapy, 68*, 678–682.

Finestone, A., Novack, V., Farfel, A., Berg, A., Amir, H., & Milgrom, C. (2004). A prospective study of the effect of foot orthoses composition and fabrication on comfort and the incidence of overuse injuries. *Foot & Ankle International, 25*, 462–466.

Fuller, E. A. (1994). A review of biomechanics of shoes. *Clinics in Podiatric Medicine and Surgery, 11*, 241–258.

Gross, M. T. (1995). Lower quarter screening for skeletal malalignment: Suggestions for orthotics and shoe wear. *Journal of Orthopaedic & Sports Physical Therapy, 21*, 389–405.

Gross, M. T., & Foxworth, J. L. (2003). The role of foot orthoses as an intervention for patellofemoral pain. *Journal of Orthopaedic & Sports Physical Therapy, 33*, 661–670.

Hagen, M., & Hennig, E. M. (2009). Effects of different shoe-lacing patterns on the biomechanics of running shoes. *Journal of Sports Sciences, 27*(3), 267–275.

Hunter, S., Dolan, M. G., & Davis, J. M. (1995). *Foot orthotic in therapy and sport.* Champaign, IL: Human Kinetics.

Janisse, D. (1988). *Introduction to pedorthics.* Columbia, MD: Pedorthic Footwear Association.

Kerrigan, D. C., Franz, J. R., Keenan, G. S., Dicharry, J., Croce, U. D., & Wilder, R. P. (2009). The effect of running shoes on lower extremity joint torques. *PM & R, 12*, 1058–1063.

Luther, L. D., Mizel, M. S., & Pfeffer, G. B. (1994). *Orthopedic knowledge update: Foot and ankle.* Rosemont: American Academy of Orthopedic Surgeons.

Marks, R., & Penton, L. (2004). Are foot orthotics efficacious for treating painful medial compartment knee osteoarthritis? A review of the literature. *International Journal of Clinical Practice, 58*(1), 49–57.

Mills, K., Blanch, P., Chapman, A. R., McPoil, T. G., & Vicenzino, B. (2010). Foot orthoses and gait: A systematic review and meta-analysis of literature pertaining to potential mechanisms. *British Journal of Sports Medicine, 44*, 1035–1046.

Mündermann, A., Wakeling, J.M., Nigg, B.M., Humble, R.N., & Stefanyshyn, D.J. (2006). Foot orthoses affect frequency components of muscle activity in the lower extremity. *Gait Posture*, 23(3), 295–302. In press.

McPoil, T. G., & Cornwall, M. W. (1994). The relationship between subtalar joint neutral position and rearfoot motion during walking. *Foot & Ankle International, 15*, 141–145.
Michaund, T. M. (1993). *Foot orthoses and other forms of conservative foot care.* Baltimore, MD: Williams & Wilkins.
Milgrom, C., Finestone, A., Lubovsky, O., Zin, D., & Lahad, A. (2005). A controlled randomized study of the effect of training with orthoses on the incidence of weight bearing induced back pain among infantry recruits. *Spine, 30*, 272–275.
Nester, C. J., van der Linden, M. L., & Bowker, P. (2003). Effect of foot orthoses on the kinematics and kinetics of normal walking gait. *Gait and Posture, 17*, 180–187.
Northwestern University Medical School, Prosthetic-Orthotic Center, (1998). *Management of foot disorders: Theory and clinical concepts.* Chicago: Northwestern University.
Picciano, A. M., Rowlands, M. S., & Worrell, T. (1993). Reliability of open and closed kinetic chain subtalar joint neutral positions and navicular drop test. *Journal of Orthopaedic & Sports Physical Therapy, 18*, 553–558.
Pierrynowski, M. R., & Smith, S. B. (1996). Rear foot inversion/eversion during gait relative to the subtalar joint neutral position. *Foot & Ankle International, 17*, 406–412.
Smith-Orrichio, K., & Harris, B. A. (1990). Inter-rater reliability of subtalar neutral, calcaneal inversion and eversion. *Journal of Orthopaedic & Sports Physical Therapy, 12*, 10–15.
Stacoff, A., Reinschmidt, C., Nigg, B. M., et al. (2000). Effects of foot orthoses on skeletal motion during running. *Clinical Biomechanics, 15*, 54–64.
Tiberio, D. (1988). Pathomechanics of structural foot deformities. *Physical Therapy, 68*, 1840–1849.

CHAPTER 79 QUESTIONS

1. **Which of the following is true regarding the proper "fitting" of a shoe?**
   a. Allow ⅛ inch between the longest toe and the end of the toe box.
   b. Allow space for two fingers to slip between the calcaneus and the heel counter.
   c. Fit a shoe only after you have been active or at the end of the day.
   d. In standing, pinch the first and the fifth MTP together; there should be no puckering of material.

2. **After 5 days of wearing a new orthotic, a patient reports blisters on the sole of their foot and arch pain. What is the most likely cause?**
   a. Orthotic is too thick.
   b. Orthotic shell is too flexible.
   c. Arch is too low.
   d. Medial posting is too high.

3. **Minimalist shoes:**
   a. Decrease injury of the posterior tibial tendon
   b. Increase stress to the Achilles tendon and metatarsals
   c. Mimic barefoot running exactly
   d. Produce a forefoot strike pattern

ANSWERS TO QUESTIONS

CHAPTER 1: 1. A, 2. B, 3. D

CHAPTER 2: 1. C, 2. C, 3. B, 4. B

CHAPTER 3: 1. C, 2. B, 3. C

CHAPTER 4: 1. C, 2. D, 3. B

CHAPTER 5: 1. A, 2. A, 3. D, 4. C, 5. A, 6. D, 7. B

CHAPTER 6: 1. D, 2. B, 3. D, 4. B, 5. B, 6. A, C and D are True, B is False.

CHAPTER 7: 1. C, 2. C, 3. A, 4. C, 5. D

CHAPTER 8: 1. C, 2. B, 3. C

CHAPTER 9: 1. A, 2. D, 3. B

CHAPTER 10: 1. D, 2. C, 3. B

CHAPTER 11: 1. A, 2. D, 3. C, 4. C

CHAPTER 12: 1. E, 2. C, 3. A

CHAPTER 13: 1. B, 2. D, 3. D, 4. B

CHAPTER 14: 1. C, 2. A, 3. D, 4. A, 5. D

CHAPTER 15: 1. B, 2. B, 3. D, 4. B, 5. A, 6. B

CHAPTER 16: 1. C, 2. D, 3. C, 4. D, 5. True, HA1C provides a 2 to 3 month "history" or snapshot of patients' blood glucose control. This is helpful as various HA1C values correlate with an average blood glucose value over the past 2 to 3 months., 6. B

CHAPTER 17: 1. B, 2. D, 3. B

CHAPTER 18: 1. D, 2. A, 3. B

CHAPTER 19: 1. B, 2. B, 3. C

CHAPTER 21: 1. D, 2. A, 3. C, 4. B, 5. D, 6. B

CHAPTER 22: 1. C, 2. D, 3. A

CHAPTER 23: 1. C, 2. C, 3. A, 4. D, 5. D

CHAPTER 24: 1. D, 2. C, 3. A, 4. C, 5. E, 6. B

CHAPTER 25: 1. B, 2. B, 3. B, 4. A

CHAPTER 26: 1. A, 2. D, 3. B

CHAPTER 27: 1. A, 2. F, 3. A

CHAPTER 28: 1. B, 2. A, 3. D

CHAPTER 29: 1. D, 2. B, 3. A

CHAPTER 30: 1. C, 2. A, 3. B

CHAPTER 31: 1. C, 2. A, 3. D

CHAPTER 32: 1. A, 2. B, 3. C

CHAPTER 33: 1. B, 2. B, 3. C, 4. C

CHAPTER 35: 1. B, 2. D, 3. C

CHAPTER 36: 1. D, 2. B, 3. C, 4. B, 5. D, 6. C

CHAPTER 37: 1. B, 2. C

CHAPTER 38: 1. C, 2. A, 3. A, 4. D, 5. C, 6. D, 7. D

CHAPTER 39: 1. D, 2. C, 3. D, 4. D, 5. D, 6. C

CHAPTER 40: 1. C, 2. A, 3. C, 4. A, 5. D, 6. A

CHAPTER 41: 1. C, 2. C, 3. A

CHAPTER 42: 1. C, 2. B, 3. A

CHAPTER 43: 1. C, 2. D, 3. E, 4. B, 5. B, 6. D

CHAPTER 44: 1. C, 2. B, 3. B

CHAPTER 45: 1. A, 2. D, 3. B, 4. C, 5. D, 6. C

CHAPTER 46: 1. A, 2. A, 3. D

CHAPTER 47: 1. B, 2. C, 3. D, 4. B, 5. C, 6. D

CHAPTER 48: 1. D, 2. A, 3. B

CHAPTER 49: 1. C, 2. C, 3. D, 4. B, 5. C, 6. A, 7. B

CHAPTER 50: 1. B, 2. A, 3. D, 4. B

CHAPTER 51: 1. B, 2. D, 3. B, 4. C, 5. A, 6. D

CHAPTER 52: 1. B, 2. B, 3. D

CHAPTER 53: 1. D, 2. D, 3. D, 4. C, 5. A, 6. D

CHAPTER 54: 1. B, 2. C, 3. D, 4. A

CHAPTER 55: 1. E, 2. C, 3. D, 4. C

CHAPTER 56: 1. A, 2. C, 3. B

CHAPTER 57: 1. C, 2. D, 3. B, 4. C

CHAPTER 58: 1. B, 2. D, 3. A

CHAPTER 59: 1. A, 2. C, 3. A

CHAPTER 60: 1. C, 2. B, 3. D, 4. D, 5. A

CHAPTER 61: 1. B, 2. C, 3. D

CHAPTER 62: 1. C, 2. B, 3. C, 4. E, 5. D, 6. A, B, C and E

CHAPTER 63: 1. A, 2. A, 3. D

CHAPTER 64: 1. D, 2. B, 3. B

CHAPTER 65: 1. C, 2. A, 3. D

CHAPTER 66: 1. B, 2. D, 3. C

CHAPTER 67: 1. A, 2. C, 3. False

CHAPTER 68: 1. D, 2. A, 3. A, 4. D, 5. B, 6. B

CHAPTER 69: 1. C, 2. C, 3. A

CHAPTER 70: 1. B, 2. C, 3. A

CHAPTER 71: 1. D, 2. C, 3. A

CHAPTER 73: 1. C, 2. A, 3. C, 4. B, 5. D, 6. A, 7. C

CHAPTER 74: 1. C, 2. B, 3. D, 4. C, 5. A, 6. C

CHAPTER 75: 1. C, 2. C, 3. D, 4. B

CHAPTER 76: 1. D, 2. D, 3. A, 4. D, 5. A

CHAPTER 77: 1. C, 2. D, 3. C, 4. D, 5. D, 6. C, 7. E, 8. D

CHAPTER 78: 1. D, 2. A, 3. D, 4. E, 5. B

CHAPTER 79: 1. C, 2. D, 3. B

INDEX

Note: Page numbers followed by *f* indicate figures, *t* indicate tables, and *b* indicate boxes.

F

I

Q

R

U